DIASTOLOGY

EDITION 2

DIASTOLOGY

Clinical Approach to Heart Failure with Preserved Ejection Fraction

ALLAN L. KLEIN, MD, FRCP (C), FACC, FAHA, FASE, FESC
Professor of Medicine
Cleveland Clinic Lerner College of Medicine of Case Western University
Director, Center for the Diagnosis and Treatment of Pericardial Diseases
Department of Cardiovascular Medicine
Heart, Vascular, and Thoracic Institute
Past-President of the American Society of Echocardiography
Cleveland Clinic
Cleveland, Ohio

MARIO J. GARCIA, MD
Professor of Medicine and Radiology
Albert Einstein College of Medicine
Chief, Division of Cardiology
Co-Director, Montefiore-Einstein Center for Heart and Vascular Care
Bronx, New York

ELSEVIER

1600 John F. Kennedy Blvd.
Ste 1800
Philadelphia, PA 19103-2899

DIASTOLOGY: CLINICAL APPROACH TO HEART FAILURE WITH PRESERVED EJECTION FRACTION, SECOND EDITION

ISBN: 978-0-323-64067-1

Executive Content Strategist: Robin Carter
Content Development Specialist: Sara Watkins
Publishing Services Manager: Deepthi Unni
Senior Project Manager: Haritha Dharmarajan
Book Designer: Ryan Cook

Printed in The United States of America

Last digit is the print number: 9 8 7 6 5 4 3 2 1

LIST OF CONTRIBUTORS

Øyvind Senstad Andersen, MD
Cardiology
Oslo University Hospital
Cardiologic Department and Institute of Surgical Research
Oslo, Norway

Bonita A. Anderson, DMU (Cardiac), MAppSc (Med Ultrasound), ACS, FASE, FASA
Clinical Fellow
Faculty of Health
School of Clinical Sciences
Queensland University of Technology
Advanced Cardiac Scientist
Cardiac Sciences Unit
The Prince Charles Hospital
Brisbane, Queensland, Australia

Christopher P. Appleton, MD, FACC, FASE
Professor of Medicine
Mayo Clinic School of Medicine
Department of Cardiovascular Diseases
Mayo Clinic Arizona
Phoenix, Arizona

Craig R. Asher, MD, FACC, FASE
Department of Cardiology
Medical Director Hypertrophic Cardiomyopathy Clinic
Cleveland Clinic Florida
Weston, Florida

Gerard P. Aurigemma, MD
Division of Cardiovascular Medicine
Department of Medicine
University of Massachusetts Medical School
Worcester, Massachusetts

Catalin F. Baicu, PhD
Research Associate Professor of Medicine
Division of Cardiology
Department of Medicine
Medical University of South Carolina
Charleston, South Carolina

Ruxandra Beyer, MD, PhD
Department of Cardiology
Heart Institute
University of Cluj-Napoca
Cluj-Napoca, Romania

Pavan Bhat, MD, FACC
Staff Physician
Section of Heart Failure and Transplantation Medicine
Department of Cardiovascular Medicine
Heart, Vascular, and Thoracic Institute
Cleveland Clinic
Cleveland, Ohio

Christopher Michael Bianco, DO
Assistant Professor of Medicine
West Virginia University School of Medicine
Department of Cardiology
Heart and Vascular Institute
Morgantown, West Virginia

Barry A. Borlaug, MD
Professor of Medicine
Director of Circulatory Failure Research
Department of Cardiovascular Medicine, Mayo Clinic
Rochester, Minnesota

Amy D. Bradshaw, PhD
Professor
Medicine Division of Cardiology
Division of Cardiology
Medical University of South Carolina
Charleston, South Carolina

Darryl J. Burstow, MBBS, FRACP, FCSANZ, FASE
Associate Professor
Department of Medicine, University of Queensland
Eminent Cardiologist
Department of Cardiology
The Prince Charles Hospital
Brisbane, Queensland, Australia

Shemy Carasso, MD, FESC, FASE
Clinical Associate Professor of Medicine
The Azrieli Faculty of Medicine in the Galilee, Zefat, Israel
Head, Non-invasive Cardiac Imaging Unit
Cardiovascular Division
B Padeh Medical Center, Poriya, Israel

Manuel D. Cerqueira, MD, FACC, MASNC
Professor of Medicine and Radiology
Cleveland Clinic Lerner College of Medicine of Case Western Reserve University
Chairman of Nuclear Medicine Depart
Imaging Institute
Staff Cardiologist
Department of Cardiovascular Medicine
Heart, Vascular, and Thoracic Institute
Cleveland Clinic
Cleveland, Ohio

Michael Chetrit, MD
Assistant Professor of Medicine, McGill University
Cardiologist, McGill University Health Centre
Co-Director, McGill Amyloidosis Project
Monteral, Quebec, Canada

Patrick Collier, MD, PhD, FASE, FESC, FACC
Associate Professor of Medicine
Cleveland Clinic Lerner College of Medicine of Case Western Reserve University
Co-Director Cardio-oncology Center
Associate Director Echo Lab
Department of Cardiovascular Medicine
Heart, Vascular, and Thoracic Institute
Cleveland Clinic
Cleveland, Ohio

Kristine Y. DeLeon-Pennell, PhD
Assistant Professor
Division of Cardiology
Department of Medicine
Medical University of South Carolina
Charleston, South Carolina

Hisham Dokainish, MD, FRCPC, FACC, FASE
Director, Cardiology and Echocardiography Laboratory
Circulate Cardiac and Vascular Centre
Burlington, Ontario, Canada

Frank A. Flachskampf, MD, FESC, FACC
Senior Cardiology Consultant
Department of Medical Sciences
Uppsala University and Uppsala University Clinic
Uppsala, Sweden

Mark K. Friedberg, MD
Professor of Pediatrics
Labatt Family Heart Centre
Department of Pediatrics, The Hospital for Sick Children and University of Toronto
Toronto, Ontario, Canada

Andrea C. Furlani, MD
Diagnostic Radiology Resident
Department of Radiology
Montefiore Medical Center
Albert Einstein College of Medicine
Bronx, New York

Mario J. Garcia, MD
Professor of Medicine and Radiology
Albert Einstein College of Medicine
Chief, Division of Cardiology
Co-Director, Montefiore-Einstein Center for Heart and Vascular Care
Bronx, New York

Eiran Z. Gorodeski, MD, MPH, FACC, FHFSA
Associate Professor of Medicine
Case Western Reserve University School of Medicine
Department of Medicine
Harrington Heart and Vascular Institute
University Hospitals Cleveland Medical Center
Cleveland, Ohio

Stephen H. Gregory, MD
Assistant Professor of Anesthesiology
Washington University in St. Louis
Department of Anesthesiology
St. Louis, Missouri

Richard A. Grimm, DO, FACC, FASE
Charles and Loraine Moore Endowed Chair in Cardiovascular Imaging
Chief Medical Information Officer
Director, Echocardiography Laboratory
Department of Cardiovascular Medicine
Heart, Vascular, and Thoracic Institute
Cleveland Clinic
Cleveland, Ohio

Jong-Won Ha, MD, PhD, FESC
General Director
Severance Hospital
Professor of Medicine
Department of Cardiology
Yonsei University College of Medicine
Seoul, Korea

Manhal Habib, MD, PhD
Cardiology Department
Peter Munk Cardiac Center
Toronto General Hospital
Toronto, Ontario, Canada

Serge C. Harb, MD, FACC
Assistant Professor of Medicine
Cleveland Clinic Lerner College of Medicine of Case Western Reserve University
Staff, Section of Cardiovascular Imaging
Department of Cardiovascular Medicine
Heart, Vascular, and Thoracic Institute
Cleveland Clinic
Cleveland, Ohio

Cesar J. Herrera, MD, FACC, CEDIMAT
Director, Clinical Associate Professor of Medicine (Adjunct)
Department of Cardiology
CEDIMAT Cardiovascular Center
Albert Einstein College of Medicine-Montefiore Center for Heart and Vascular Care
Santo Domingo, Dominican Republic
Albert Einstein College of Medicine
Montefiore Center for Heart and Vascular Care
Bronx, New York

Brian D. Hoit, MD
Professor of Medicine and Physiology and Biophysics
Case Western Reserve University
Department of Medicine
Division of Cardiology
University Hospitals Cleveland Medical Center
Harrington Heart and Vascular Center
Cleveland, Ohio

Massimo Imazio, MD, FESC
Professor of Cardiology
Referral Senior Consultant for Myopericardial Diseases and Cardiovascular Multimodality Imaging
University Cardiology, Cardiovascular and Thoracic Department
AOU Citta'della Salute e della Scienza di Torino
Torino, Italy

Katsuji Inoue, MD, PhD
Associate Professor
Department of Cardiology, Pulmonology, Hypertension, and Nephrology
Ehime University Graduate School of Medicine
Toon, Japan

Wael A. Jaber, MD, FACC, FESC, FASE
Professor of Medicine
Cleveland Clinic Lerner College of Medicine of Case Western Reserve University
Director, Nuclear Cardiology and Imaging CoreLab
Department of Cardiovascular Medicine
Heart, Vascular, and Thoracic Institute
Cleveland Clinic
Cleveland, Ohio

Garvan C. Kane, MD, PhD, FAHA, FASE
Professor of Medicine
Mayo Clinic College of Medicine
Director, Echocardiography Laboratory & Chair, Division of Cardiovascular Ultrasound
Department of Cardiovascular Medicine
Mayo Clinic
Rochester, Minnesota

Allan L. Klein, MD, FRCP (C), FACC, FAHA, FASE, FESC
Professor of Medicine
Cleveland Clinic Lerner College of Medicine of Case Western University
Director, Center for the Diagnosis and Treatment of Pericardial Diseases
Department of Cardiovascular Medicine
Heart, Vascular, and Thoracic Institute
Past-President of the American Society of Echocardiography
Cleveland Clinic
Cleveland, Ohio

Lara C. Kovell, MD
Assistant Professor of Medicine
Division of Cardiovascular Medicine
Department of Medicine
University of Massachusetts Medical School
Worcester, Massachusetts

Deborah H. Kwon, MD, FACC, FSCMR, FASE
Associate Professor of Medicine
Cleveland Clinic Lerner College of Medicine of Case Western Reserve University
Director of Cardiac MRI
Co-Director, Center for the Diagnosis & Treatment of Pericardial Diseases
Department of Cardiovascular, Medicine and Radiology
Heart, Vascular, and Thoracic Institute
Cleveland Clinic
Cleveland, Ohio

Cameron T. Lambert, MD
Fellow
Cardiac Electrophysiology and Pacing
Department of Cardiovascular Medicine
Heart, Vascular, and Thoracic Institute
Cleveland Clinic
Cleveland, Ohio

Benjamin D. Levine, MD, FACC, FAHA, FACSM
Professor of Medicine and Cardiology
Distinguished Professorship in Exercise Science
The University of Texas Southwestern Medical Center
Director, Institute for Exercise and Environmental Medicine
S. Finley Ewing Jr. Chair for Wellness at Texas Health Presbyterian Dallas
Harry S. Moss Heart Chair for Cardiovascular Research
Dallas, Texas

Martin M. LeWinter, MD
Professor of Medicine and Molecular Physiology and Biophysics Emeritus
Department of Medicine
Larner College of Medicine at the University of Vermont
Attending in Cardiology
University of Vermont Medical Center
Burlington, Vermont

James P. MacNamara, MD
Division of Cardiology
University of Texas Southwestern
Institute of Exercise and Environmental Medicine
Dallas, Texas

Mohammed Makkiya, MD
General Cardiology and Advance Imaging Fellow
Department of Cardiology and Hospital Medicine
Albert Einstein College of Medicine
Bronx, New York

Dimitrios Maragiannis, MD, FESC, FASE, FACC, FAHA
Department of Cardiology
401 General Army Hospital
Athens, Greece

Vojtech Melenovsky, MD, PhD
Associate Professor of Medicine
Department of Cardiology
Institute for Clinical and Experimental Medicine – IKEM
Charles University, Prague, Czech Republic

Donald R. Menick, PhD, FAHA
Professor of Medicine
Director of the Gazes Cardiac Research Institute
Research Health Scientist
Ralph H. Johnson VA Medical Center
Department of Medicine/Division of Cardiology
Medical University of South Carolina
Charleston, South Carolina

William R. Miranda, MD
Assistant Professor of Medicine Department of Cardiovascular Diseases
Mayo Clinic
Rochester, Minnesota

Sandhya Murthy, MD
Assistant Professor of Medicine
Montefiore Medical Center
Albert Einstein College of Medicine
Department of Medicine
The Center for Heart and Vascular Care
Director, Pulmonary Hypertension Center
Bronx, New York

Sherif F. Nagueh, MD, FACC, FASE, FAHA
Professor of Medicine
Weill Cornell Medical College
Medical Director Echocardiography Laboratory
Houston Methodist DeBakey Heart and Vascular Center
Houston, Texas

Satoshi Nakatani, MD, PhD, FACC, FESC, FASE (hon)
Professor Emeritus, Osaka University
Director of Saiseikai Senri Hospital
Saiseikai Senri Hospital
Suita, Osaka, Japan

Lakshmi Nambiar, MD
Fellow
Weill Cornell Medicine
Department of Cardiology
New York-Presbyterian Hospital/Weill Cornell Medical Center
New York City,
New York

Kazuaki Negishi, MD, PhD
Professor of Medicine
Head of Discipline of Medicine
Nepean Clinical School
Cardiologist
Department of Medicine and Health
University of Sydney
New South Wales, Australia

Masaru Obokata, MD, PhD
Department of Cardiovascular Medicine
Mayo Clinic
Rochester, Minnesota

Jae K. Oh, MD, FACC, FAHA, FESC, FASE
Samsung Professor of Cardiovascular Diseases
Director, Echo Core Lab
Director, Pericardial Diseases Clinic
President, Asian Pacific Association of Echocardiography
Department of Cardiovascular Medicine
Mayo Clinic
Rochester, Minnesota

Ileana Piña, MD, MPH, FAHA, FACC, FHFSA
Professor of Medicine
Senior Staff Fellow, Medical Officer
Department of Medicine
Wayne State University
Detroit, Michigan

Zoran B. Popović, MD, PhD
Associate Professor of Medicine
Cleveland Clinic Lerner College of Medicine of Case Western Reserve University
Staff Department of Cardiovascular Medicine
Heart, Vascular, and Thoracic Institute
Cleveland Clinic
Cleveland, Ohio

Miguel A. Quinones, MD, MACC, FASE
Winters Family Distinguished Centennial Chair In Cardiovascular Education
Professor of Medicine
Weil Cornell Medicine
Department of Cardiology
Houston Methodist Hospital
Houston, Texas

Harry Rakowski, MD, FACC, FASE, ED
Professor of Medicine
Department of Medicine
University of Toronto
Douglas Wigle Research Chair in Hypertrophic Cardiomyopathy
Development Director, Peter Munk Cardiac Imaging Centre
Division of Cardiology
Department of Medicine
Toronto General Hospital, University Health Network
Toronto, Ontario, Canada

Yogesh NV Reddy, MBBS, MSc
Assistant Professor of Medicine
Department of Cardiovascular Diseases
Mayo Clinic
Rochester, Minnesota

Leonardo Rodriguez, MD
Program Director Advanced Imaging Fellowship
Associated Director, Transesophageal Echocardiography Laboratory
Department of Cardiovascular Medicine
Heart, Vascular, and Thoracic Institute
Cleveland Clinic
Cleveland, Ohio

Satyam Sarma, MD
Assistant Professor of Medicine
Department of Internal Medicine, Division of Cardiology
University of Texas Southwestern Medical
Dallas, Texas

Aldo L. Schenone, MD
Chief Non-invasive Cardiovascular Imaging Fellow
Non-invasive Cardiovascular Imaging Department
Brigham and Women's Hospital/Harvard Medical School
Boston, Massachusetts

Partho Sengupta, MD
Professor of Medicine
J.W. Ruby Memorial Hospital
Chief, Division of Cardiology
Director, Cardiovascular Imaging
J.W. Ruby Memorial Hospital
WVU Heart and Vascular Institute
Morgantown, West Virginia

Otto A. Smiseth, MD, PhD, FESC, FACC, FASE
Professor of Medicine
Division Head
Division of Cardiovascular and Pulmonary Diseases
Oslo University Hospital
Oslo, Norway

Randall C. Starling, MD, MPH, FACC, FAHA, FESC, FHFSA
Professor of Medicine
Cleveland Clinic Lerner College of Medicine of Case Western Reserve University
Department of Cardiovascular Medicine
Heart, Vascular, and Thoracic Institute
Cleveland Clinic
Cleveland, Ohio

Marie Stugaard, MD, PhD, FESC
Doctor of Medicine
Department of Health Sciences
Osaka University Graduate School of Medicine
Suita, Osaka, Japan

Madhav Swaminathan, MD, MMCi, FASE, FAHA
Professor
Vice chair, Faculty Development
Department of Anesthesiology
Duke University
Durham, North Carolina

Edlira Tam, DO, MS
Division of Cardiology
Montefiore-Einstein Heart Center
Bronx, New York

W.H. Wilson Tang, MD FACC, FAHA, FHFSA
Professor of Medicine
Cleveland Clinic Lerner College of Medicine of Case Western Reserve University
Research Director
Section of Heart Failure and Cardiac Transplantation Medicine
Department of Cardiovascular Medicine
Heart, Vascular, and Thoracic Institute
Cleveland Clinic
Cleveland, Ohio

Harsh V. Thakkar, MBBS
Clinical Lecturer
School of Medicine
University of Tasmania
Department of Cardiology
The Royal Hobart Hospital
Hobart CBD, Tasmania, Australia

James D. Thomas, MD, FACC, FASE
Professor of Medicine
Feinberg School of Medicine
Northwestern University
Director, Center for Heart Valve Disease and Co-director
Center for Artificial Intelligence in Cardiovascular Disease
Division of Cardiology in the Bluhm Cardiovascular Institute
Northwestern Medicine
Chicago, Illinois

Lynne Williams, MBBCh, FRCP, PhD
Consultant Cardiologist
Department of Cardiology
Royal Papworth Hospital NHS Foundation Trust
Cambridge, United Kingdom

Dmitry M. Yaranov, MD
Advanced Heart Failure Failure and Transplant Cardiologist
Advanced Heart Failure, Heart Transplant, Mechanical Circulatory Support
Baptist Memorial Hospital
Memphis, Tennessee

Laura Young, MD
Clinical Instructor of Medicine
Cleveland Clinic Lerner College of Medicine of Case Western Reserve University
Interventional Cardiology Fellow
Department of Cardiovascular Medicine
Heart, Vascular, and Thoracic Institute
Cleveland Clinic
Cleveland, Ohio

Michael R. Zile, MD
Charles Ezra Daniel Professor of Medicine
Distinguished University Professor
Medical University of South Carolina
Chief, Division of Cardiology
RHJ Department of Veterans Affairs Medical Center
Charleston, South Carolina

FOREWORD

Diastolic dysfunction and its clinical cousin, heart failure with preserved ejection fraction (HFpEF), are among the most baffling of topics in clinical cardiology. Is it primarily a cardiac condition? Related to comorbidities? A manifestation of poor peripheral muscular oxygen extraction? Maybe a bit of each. And so many cardiac parameters to consider: E wave, A wave, tissue Doppler, LA size, torsion, RV pressure, diastolic strain rate, just to name a few! How to put them together in a unified way is nearly impossible. It is rare to find a resource that addresses all the myriad manifestations of diastolic function: basic principles from cellular physiology to the physics of intracardiac blood flow, multimodality assessment and diagnosis, as well as standard and evolving therapies for this challenging syndrome. In 2008, Drs. Allan Klein and Mario Garcia brought forth their landmark book *Diastology,* which for the first time brought all aspects of diastolic function, especially the diagnostic aspects, under one cover. It's hard to believe it's been 12 years since that initial publication, but the science of diastology has progressed rapidly in that time. Building on the great achievement of the first edition of *Diastology,* Allan and Mario now bring us their second edition, completely updated with the latest basic and clinical information. In addition to updating all the chapters from the first edition, they bring out four new chapters. These include the diastolic function stress test, the perioperative assessment of diastolic function, and the important entity of pulmonary hypertension in HFpEF. An important new chapter addresses the ASE/EACVI Diastolic Guidelines (of which there have been two since the first edition), examining the strengths and limitations of these important formulations.

On a personal note, I congratulate dear friends Allan and Mario on this great achievement. I have known Allan for over 30 years and well recall planning the first conference on diastolic function in 1992, where we coined for the first time (I think) the word *diastology*. Soon thereafter, Mario joined us at the Cleveland Clinic, and together the three of us and our colleagues produced some of the landmark research and education in diastolic function. With this book, Allan and Mario continue their masterful scholarship into the science of diastolic function. It is thus with great enthusiasm that I commend the second edition of *Diastology* to you.

James D. Thomas, MD, FASE, FACC, FESC
Professor of Medicine
Feinberg School of Medicine
Northwestern University
Director, Center for Heart Valve Disease and
Co-director, Center for Artificial Intelligence in Cardiovascular Disease
Division of Cardiology in the Bluhm Cardiovascular Institute
Northwestern Medicine
Chicago, Illinois

FOREWORD

I am pleased to say a few words about the 2nd Edition of *Diastology* edited by Allan Klein and Mario Garcia. I have known both editors for more than 20 years and have followed their careers with great pride. The first edition of this book in 2008 was a magnificent achievement. Diastolic heart failure at that time had evolved substantially to a point where we were beginning to better understand how to define it and manage its various phenotypes. New and improved imaging techniques, including magnetic resonance imaging and use of echo to image strain rate were quickly evolving. The book very much captured our attention regarding the diagnosis and management of this very important clinical syndrome as it emerged from a somewhat obscure clinical entity in the 1970s to a major diagnostic entity with multiple etiologies by 2008.

Now it is 2020, and the clinical syndrome of diastolic heart failure is one of the more common diagnoses in cardiology. Heart failure with preserved ejection fraction (HFpEF) is now similar in prevalence to heart failure with reduced ejection fraction (HFrEF) in terms of hospitalization for heart failure in the United States. Hospitalization for HFrEF has steadily declined between 2002 and 2013, while increases in heart failure hospitalizations are now being driven by more cases of HFpEF. Of course, other conditions such as amyloidosis, hypertrophic cardiomyopathy, left ventricular hypertrophy due to long-standing hypertension, chronic renal disease, coronary disease as well as primary restrictive, infiltrative and storage cardiomyopathies are also now well recognized as etiologies of diastolic dysfunction leading to the development of heart failure. Valvular heart disease and pericardial disorders are still with us and may also lead to diastolic dysfunction and heart failure.

Each of these entities are discussed in great detail by expert contributing authors in the new edition of *Diastology*. Clinical and laboratory diagnoses are also featured in great detail and treatment options are carefully discussed. Each of the contributing authors brings substantial experience to bear in describing the subtleties of diastolic dysfunction. The book is richly endowed with many tables and figures.

This very comprehensive book is the best we have in the field of Diastology. Doctors Klein, Garcia and their contributing authors are to be congratulated for their magnificent contribution. It will be most useful for clinicians, but others will find it to be the definitive text in this complex but important field of cardiac relaxation and filling. Trainees, internists, cardiologists and sonographers will benefit from this wholly updated and outstanding text.

Gary S. Francis, M.D.
Professor of Medicine
University of Minnesota
Minneapolis, Minnesota

PREFACE

A 56-year-old obese woman with exertional dyspnea was referred for evaluation of suspected heart failure with preserved LV ejection fraction. She had a past medical history of Crohn disease, hypothyroidism, and asthma. She had been medically treated for hypertension for several years. Over the last several years, she was hospitalized several times with pneumonia and exacerbations of asthma. Between these admissions, she was experiencing shortness of breath on moderate activity, which was attributed to the combination of moderate asthma and obesity. She was referred to echocardiography to determine if cardiac dysfunction contributed to her dyspnea.

Echocardiography revealed normal systolic function, with LV EF of 54%. She had moderate LV hypertrophy with septal wall thickness of 1.3 cm. Peak mitral early diastolic velocity (E) was 73 cm/sec, mitral early diastolic velocity/atrial velocity ratio (E/A) was 0.9 with an E deceleration time (DT) of 222 msec. Septal mitral annulus velocity (e′) was 7 and lateral e′ 8 cm/sec. Previously using the ASE/EACVI 2009 guidelines, this patient would not have met diagnostic criteria for elevated LV filling pressure, since mitral E/A was 0.9. However, in the 2016 ASE/EACVI guidelines by following Algorithm B in the setting of myocardial pathology (LVH), she is in the intermediate diastolic function group where three additional criteria—E/e′ (10), left atrial (LA) volume (35 mL/m^2), and peak tricuspid regurgitation (TR) velocity (2.9 cm/sec)—need to be considered to assess for grade 2 diastolic dysfunction and elevated filling pressures (see Chapter 19).

Since the first edition of *Diastology,* published over a decade ago, there have been significant advances in our general understanding of the pathophysiologic mechanisms, epidemiology, and diagnostic approaches to the syndrome of diastolic heart failure, now reclassified as "heart failure with preserved ejection fraction (HFpEF)." Like in the previous edition, this textbook comprehensively discusses the basic molecular and hemodynamic assessment principles, epidemiology, clinical presentation, diagnostic approaches, and treatment of the different cardiovascular diseases that lead to HFpEF. The content of this book is targeted to a broad audience encompassing noninvasive and invasive cardiologists, physiology scientists, cardiology fellows, and cardiac sonographers.

Why is the study of diastology relevant? The answer is that a complete understanding of the pathophysiology of diastolic function and a complete characterization through diagnostic imaging are fundamental to the management of all patients with congestive heart failure syndromes, independent of etiology.

HISTORICAL PERSPECTIVE

As early as the Renaissance, Leonardo da Vinci described how the lower cardiac chambers of the heart filled with blood by drawing it from the upper chambers. In the 1940s, Carl J. Wiggers proposed the term *inherent elasticity* to describe the passive properties of the heart. In the 1970s, cardiac physiologists assessed the properties of active ventricular relaxation and passive filling using invasive quantification of intracavity pressure and volume. During the following decade, clinicians recognized that diastolic heart failure was an important cause of congestive heart failure, and Doppler echocardiography emerged as an important noninvasive method to assess the diastolic filling properties of the heart. The term *diastology* was coined in the early 1990s; imaging modalities, such as Doppler echocardiography and cardiac magnetic resonance imaging (MRI), advanced our understanding of diastolic function. Over the past decade, newer methods such as myocardial strain imaging, contrast cardiac MRI, and nuclear scintigraphy have been able to enhance our ability to establish the diagnosis of HFpEF and diagnose infiltrative disorders at earlier stages of the disease. Recent results from large-scale clinical trials have now identified targeted treatment for many HFpEF patients, leading to improved outcomes.

ABOUT THE AUTHORS

In the late 1980s, Allan Klein started his interest in this field as a Canadian Heart Foundation fellow at the Mayo Clinic studying Doppler assessment of LV filling during acute myocardial infarction and after reperfusion. His first impression was that the quick bedside echocardiographic evaluation, including the mitral E/A ratio and deceleration time, was a simple but powerful measure of LV diastolic filling, relaxation, and prognosis. Also, he was struck by how the grades of diastolic filling related to the clinical exam, including the extra heart sounds (S_3 and S_4). As a student of the field, he also learned that the study of diastolic function was more complex than the simple analysis of the mitral E/A ratio. During his training, Dr. Klein was very fortunate to have excellent mentors, including Liv Hatle, Jamil Tajik, and James Seward.

Dr. Mario Garcia developed his interest in the field while at the Cleveland Clinic in the early days of tissue Doppler echocardiography, color M mode Doppler, and strain rate imaging. His clinical observations and hemodynamic validation of early annular velocities (e′) and the slope of the flow propagation (Vp) as well as the relationship of mitral early filling/annular e-wave (E/e′) and mitral early filling/flow propagation slope (E/Vp) as measures of LV filling pressure were important for the advancement of the field. Their work as well as that of the other leaders who have contributed to the new edition of *Diastology* makes this textbook an essential read for all cardiovascular specialists.

CONTENTS OF THE BOOK

In this second edition, *Diastology* is organized into five main sections: basic determinants, noninvasive and invasive diagnosis, specific cardiac disease, emerging topics, and treatment. It includes a comprehensive analysis of the major areas of knowledge in the field from the molecular, genetic, and cellular mechanisms to clinical presentation and treatment of HFpEF. The book discusses traditional and newer diagnostic methods, including 2-D and 3-D Doppler echocardiography, LV and LA strain imaging, and nuclear and cardiac MRI techniques. The strengths and weaknesses of the ASE/EACVI 2016 guidelines on diastolic function are analyzed in depth. A review of the prototypical diseases that show diastolic dysfunction, including hypertension, coronary artery disease, hypertrophic cardiomyopathy, restrictive cardiomyopathies, diabetes mellitus, and pericardial disease provide an important clinical perspective. Newer topics, including the effect of pacing, aging, pulmonary hypertension, and perioperative assessment, are also included. General treatment, analyzing the results of clinical trials such as I-PRESERVE, TOPCAT, and PARAGON, and future therapies are reviewed. Of note, the book includes 50 interactive cases and 150 review questions.

Finally, it is important to recognize that the field of HFpEF is a fast-moving target. We have made a concerted effort to keep the content current and to avoid overlap between chapters.

We surely hope that you enjoy our latest version of the book.

ACKNOWLEDGMENTS

We would like to especially thank our parents Jean and Sam Klein as well as Marilyn, Jared, Lauren, and Jordan Klein, Anna Kezerashvili and Melinda, and Olivia Garcia for their inspiration and encouragement and unwavering support of our careers. We especially would like to express our thanks to Marie Phillips, who helped and guided us in the journey of putting this book together. Finally, we would like to express our gratitude to the editors of Elsevier including Robin Carter, Sara Watkins and Haritha Dharmarajan for their guidance in making the second edition of this book.

CONTENTS

Part IV: Emerging Topics in HFpEF

Part V: Treatment of HFpEF

Part VI: Cases of Diastolic Heart Failure

VIDEO TABLE OF CONTENTS

1

Molecular, Gene, and Cellular Mechanism

Amy D. Bradshaw, Kristine Y. DeLeon-Pennell, and Donald R. Menick

OUTLINE

Although heart failure (HF) has been traditionally affiliated with reduced contractile function and dilation of the left ventricle (LV) resulting in reduced ejection fraction (HFrEF), nearly half of HF patients have an ejection fraction that is normal. These patients present with abnormal LV relaxation, diastolic distensibility, or diastolic stiffness.[1] The number of patients hospitalized and the mortality risk for patients with heart failure with preserved ejection fraction (HFpEF) is equivalent to patients with HFrEF (~50% die within 3 years).[2–4] Importantly, whereas HFrEF patients treated with angiotensin-converting enzyme (ACE) inhibitors, angiotensin receptor blockers (ARBs), and mineralocorticoid receptor antagonist have improved clinical outcomes,[5] no such benefit has been seen in patients with HFpEF.[6,7] Therefore determining the signaling pathways and molecular mechanisms that trigger the decline into diastolic HF is one of the major challenges facing cardiovascular medicine. The identification of these pathways will hopefully lead to new therapies for this dramatically growing health problem.

Multiple risk factors are associated with HFpEF, including age (>65), hypertension, renal disease, and diabetes mellitus, and HFpEF presents more often in women than in men. But the significance of each risk factor, in terms of molecular mechanisms, remains uncertain in part because access to live human heart tissue at various times during disease progression is limited, and animal models do not fully recapitulate the integrative complexity of human disease. To point, the majority of animal models in use focus on a single defect such as pressure overload (PO), hypertension, obesity, diabetes, renal insufficiency, or age. For technical reasons and efforts to limit confounding variables, rarely are multiple defects combined in animal models. Nonetheless, this chapter will focus on the leading contributors that have been identified in the research setting, including myocyte stiffness, reactive oxygen species (ROS), age, mitochondrial dysfunction, myocardial interstitial fibrosis, and inflammation.

MYOCYTE STIFFNESS

Myocardial stiffness is a hallmark of diastolic heart disease and an important contributor to HFpEF. The contributors of myocardial stiffness and impaired diastolic filling are naturally divided into those specific to the myocyte itself and those factors affecting the extracellular matrix (ECM). We will first discuss myocyte-specific factors identified as determinants of myocyte stiffness, which include calcium dysregulation, mitochondrial energetics, posttranslational modification of titin and other sarcomeric proteins, and infiltration of amyloids.

Calcium Dysregulation

Calcium (Ca^{2+}) plays a central role in the excitation-contraction and repolarization-relaxation of the myocardium.[8] Hence factors that regulate Ca^{2+} flux in myocytes are poised to be critical regulators of diastolic function. Depolarization of the sarcolemma results in Ca^{2+} influx into the cytosol via the voltage-gated L-type channels. This inward Ca^{2+} current (I_{Ca}) promotes the release of Ca^{2+} from the sarcoplasmic reticulum (SR) by Ca^{2+}–induced Ca^{2+}–release via the ryanodine receptor 2 (RYR). The I_{Ca} and SR Ca^{2+} release raise intracellular free Ca^{2+} allowing Ca^{2+} to bind to the myofilament protein troponin C (TnC). When cytosolic Ca^{2+} is low, the troponin-tropomyosin complex inhibits the formation of the actinomyosin complex. When Ca^{2+} binds to TnC, it releases the inhibition and allows cross-bridge cycling and

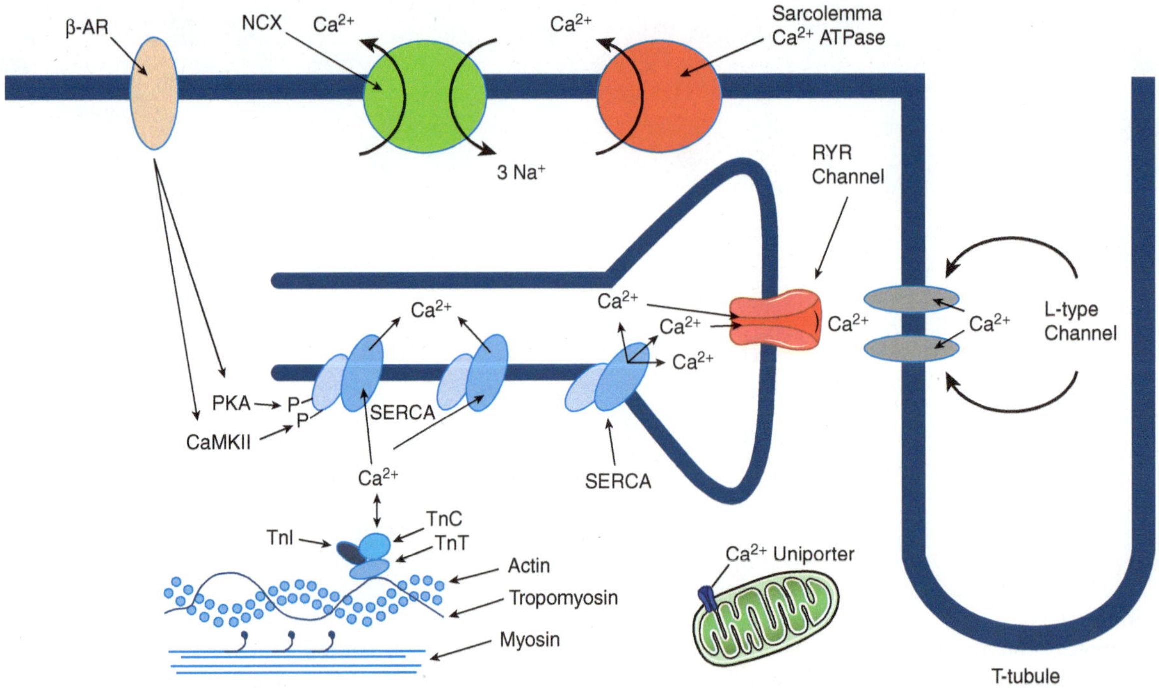

Fig. 1.1 Diagram of cardiomyocyte Ca^{2+} flux during excitation-contraction coupling. Ca^{2+} enters via L-type Ca channels, which triggers Ca^{2+}-induced Ca^{2+} release from the sarcoplasmic reticulum (SR). The increase in cytosolic Ca^{2+} results in Ca^{2+} binding to troponin C *(TnC)* initiating myofilament activation. For relaxation, cytosolic Ca^{2+} is transported into the SR via SR Ca^{2+}-ATPase *(SERCA)* and into the extracellular space via sarcolemmal Na/Ca exchanger. *β-AR,* β-Adrenergic; *NCX,* Na/Ca exchanger; *PKA,* protein kinase A; *RYR,* ryanodine receptor; *TnT,* troponin T; *TnI,* troponin I.

contraction of the sarcomeres. In cardiac relaxation, cytosolic free Ca^{2+} must decline to result in Ca^{2+} dissociation from TnC. Ca^{2+} is transported from the cytosol by four pathways: (1) SR Ca^{2+}-ATPase (SERCA), (2) sarcolemmal Na/Ca exchanger (NCX), (3) sarcolemmal Ca^{2+}-ATPase, and (4) mitochondrial Ca^{2+} uniporter (Fig. 1.1). For Ca^{2+} homeostasis at each heart beat, the amount of Ca^{2+} pumped back into the SR by SERCA must equal the amount released through the RYR2 channel, and levels of Ca^{2+} extruded from the cell must equal the amount that entered via the L-type channel.

During relaxation Ca^{2+} is pumped back into the SR lumen by SERCA, which is regulated by phospholamban (PLN). When PLN is dephosphorylated it binds to SERCA and inhibits its Ca^{2+} affinity. Phosphorylation of PLN relieves SERCA inhibition and enhances Ca^{2+} sequestration in the SR increasing the rate of relaxation. PLN is phosphorylated by cyclic adenosine monophosphate (cAMP) activated–protein kinase A (PKA) and Ca-CaM–dependent protein kinase (CaMK) as a result of β-adrenergic stimulation. The major substrates for the cAMP-PKA axis include PLN, L-type Ca channels, RYR, troponin I (TnI), and myosin-binding protein C (cMyBP-C). The relaxant effect of PKA is mediated mainly by phosphorylation of PLN and TnI. PLN phosphorylation (at Ser-16) speeds up SR Ca^{2+} sequestration, while phosphorylation of TnI speeds up dissociation of Ca^{2+} from the myofilaments. CaMKII phosphorylation of PLN (at Thr-17) also increases SR Ca^{2+}-ATPase activity. Both PKA and CaMKII are likely to be coactivated during normal sympathetic stimulation (β adrenergic), creating synergy between these important regulatory signaling pathways (see Fig. 1.1). SERCA expression and function is decreased in most HF models. Several studies have also shown reduced SERCA/PLN ratio with age. In addition, there are data that point to reduced phosphorylation state of PLN in HF.[9] This would result in reduced Ca^{2+} sensitivity of SERCA and lower SR Ca^{2+} uptake at physiologic cytoplasmic Ca^{2+} levels $[Ca]_I$. The reduction of SERCA activity is consistent with the characteristic slowed relaxation and $[Ca]_I$ seen in diastolic HF. In animal models when SERCA expression is increased or PLN expression is decreased, myocardial relaxation and $[Ca]_I$ decline are accelerated resulting in improved diastolic function.[9] Consequently, factors that might target SERCA and other mediators of Ca^{2+} flux are an active area of research for therapeutic opportunities.

Posttranslational Modification of Myofibrillar Proteins

The sarcomeric protein titin is the largest known protein with a length greater than 1 um. It spans half the sarcomere connecting the Z-line to the M-line. It functions as a very large molecular spring contributing to force transmission at the Z-line and resting tension in the I-band region.[10] Titin limits the range of sarcomere motion and is a major molecular contributor to myocyte passive stiffness. Titin activity can be modulated both by isoform expression and by phosphorylation. The differences in titin isoforms are correlated with the differences in the mechanical properties of cardiac, skeletal, and smooth muscle and differences of cardiac passive tension across species.[11] Importantly, phosphorylation of titin by PKA, PKG, and PKC-α modulates its stiffness.[12–15] Consequently, the activity of these kinases in myocytes has a direct influence on diastolic parameters. For example, PKA activated by β-adrenergic stimulation can phosphorylate titin as well as thick and thin filaments of the sarcomere.[16] Nitric oxide (NO) and natriuretic peptides initiate signaling pathways activating PKG, which phosphorylates some of the same titin residues in the N2B spring element as PKA. Phosphorylation of the N2B element by either PKA or PKG results in a reduction in passive tension. α-Adrenergic stimulation activates PKC-α in cardiomyocytes, which is known to phosphorylate titin in the proline-valine-glutamate-lysine (PVEK) sequence increasing titin-based passive tension (Fig. 1.2). Therefore phosphorylation of the N2B

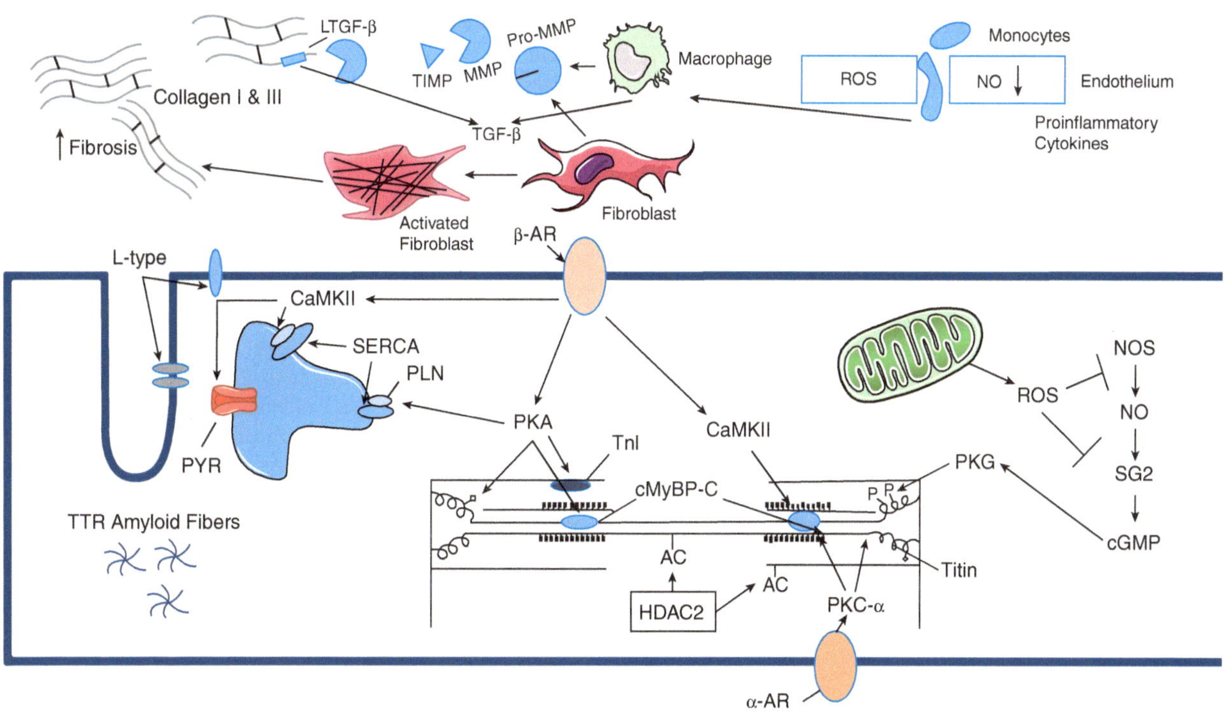

Fig. 1.2 Diagram of pathways contributing to diastolic dysfunction. *Intersitial response:* Cardiac connective tissue, composed primarily of collagen types I and III, is maintained by resident cardiac fibroblasts. In response to pressure overload (PO), the recruitment of monocytes through activated endothelium occurs, triggered by increases in cytokine expression, and results in increases in macrophage populations as well as activation of resident fibroblasts. These cell types express extracellular matrix (ECM) components, matricellular proteins, and matrix metalloproteinases *(MMPs)*, which drive remodeling of the myocardium. Sequestered factors in the ECM such as latent TGF-β *(LTGF-β)*, are released through the action of MMPs to further propagate remodeling events. Tissue inhibitors of MMPs *(TIMPs)*, also act to modulate myocardial remodeling by limiting MMP activity on both sequestered cytokines and structural ECM components. Macrophages also contribute fibrotic deposition of collagen in the PO myocardium through matricellular protein and MMP production. *Myocyte response:* Increased levels of nitric oxide *(NO)* promote myocyte relaxation through activation of protein kinase G *(PKG)* and phosphorylation of titin. Increased production of reactive oxygen species *(ROS)* can foster diastolic dysfunction by reducing the bioavailability of NO. PKA activated by β-adrenergic *(β-AR)* stimulation can phosphorylate titin decreasing passive tension. α-Adrenergic stimulation activates PKC-α in cardiomyocytes, which is known to phosphorylate titin, increasing titin-based passive tension. β-AR stimulated activation of CaMKII and protein kinase *(PKA)*, also results in the phosphorylation of phospholamban *(PLN)*, the ryanodine receptor *(RYR)*, and L-type calcium channels, which increases diastolic cytosolic Ca^{2+} content consistent with the characteristic slowed relaxation seen in diastolic HF. *α-AR*, α-Adrenergic; *cGMP*, cyclic guanosine monophosphate; *cMyBP-C*, myosin-binding protein C; *HDAC2*, histone deacetylase 2; *NOS*, nitric oxide synthase; *SERCA*, SR Ca^{2+}-ATPase SG2, soluble guanylate cyclase; *TGF-β*, transforming growth factor-β; *TnI*, troponin I.

element in titin by PKA or PKG decreases passive tension, whereas phosphorylation of titin's PEVK element by PKC-α increases passive tension.[11] The increased oxidative pressure or ROS in diastolic dysfunction has been proposed to deplete NO reserve, lowering PKG activity and leading to hypophosphorylation of the N2B element and titin stiffing in HFpEF.[14,17] Increased ROS can also result in the oxidation of cysteine residues in the N2B element resulting in disulfide bond formation and increased passive tension in mouse models.[18,19]

In addition to titin, posttranslational modification of thick and thin filaments of myofibrils can affect cardiomyocyte relaxation. As mentioned, TnI and cMyBP-C are targets for phosphorylation by β-adrenergic stimulation. Phosphorylation of cardiac TnI at serine 23/24 by PKA reduces TnC-TnI interaction strength while reducing calcium sensitivity. The weakened C-I interaction may slow thin filament activation and result in faster relaxation kinetics thus increasing early phase relaxation with β-adrenergic stimulation.[20] The cardiac cMyBP-C is a thick filament accessory protein that when unphosphorylated represses both cross-bridge attachment and detachment. It is phosphorylated by multiple kinases, including PKA, PKC, PKD, CaMKII, glycogen synthase kinase 3β, and ribosomal S6 kinase. Phosphorylation of cMyBP-C results in increased rates of cross-bridge cycling.[21] Hypophosphorylation of cMyBP-C is associated with diastolic dysfunction in human patients.[22] A recent study examined phosphorylation-deficient and phosphomimetic mutants of PKA-targeted cMyBP-C sites. They found that PKA phosphorylation of cMyBP-C threonine 35 results in accelerated cross-bridge detachment of myosin and actin, thereby enhancing relaxation.[23]

Other Posttranslational Modifications

Advanced aging is associated with increased posttranslational modifications and has been associated with a systemic proinflammatory state (inflamm-aging) and development of HFpEF. Inflammation of the coronary microvascular endothelial cells leads to increased production of ROS. Oxidative stress can promote diastolic dysfunction by reducing the bioavailability of NO. Cardiac relaxation is regulated by NO. ROS can affect NO-related signaling at multiple sites. NO is generated by NO synthase (NOS), which requires tetrahydrobiopterin as a cofactor for the reaction. Hypertension and activation of the renin-angiotensin system lead to a depletion of tetrahydrobiopterin. The loss of tetrahydrobiopterin leads to NOS uncoupling, the production of superoxide instead of NO, and diastolic dysfunction.[24] Some of the mechanisms of how NO modulates myofilament contractility have been recently revealed. Depletion of tetrahydrobiopterin in hypertension can repress NO synthesis and is associated with S-glutathionylation of MyBP-C, which reduces cross-bridge cycling. S-glutathionylation is an oxidative posttranslation modification of cysteines. Tetrahydrobiopterin supplementation lowers S-glutathionylation of MyBP-C, reduces the changes in actin-myosin cross-bridge cycling, and improves diastolic dysfunction.[25] Further, excessive ROS leads to oxidation of guanylate cyclase and affects its responsiveness to NO to synthesize cyclic guanosine monophosphate (cGMP).[26] Lower cGMP level decreases PKG activity in cardiomyocytes leading to hypophosphorylation of titin resulting in increased cardiac stiffness.

Many cardiac myofibrillar proteins are posttranslationally modified by acetylation in the healthy heart.[27–29] Unfortunately, we know very little about the changes in acetylation with cardiac pathologies. One recent study demonstrated that histone deacetylase (HDAC) inhibitors were efficacious in two murine models of diastolic dysfunction. In addition, the investigators showed that HDAC2 copurified with myofibrils. Although the target(s) were not identified, the study showed that ex vivo deacetylation of isolated myofibrils with recombinant HDAC2 significantly increased the rate of myofibril relaxation, whereas acetylation with recombinant p300 decreased myofibril relaxation duration.[30] Hence HDAC inhibitors might be a promising avenue for future research into potential HFpEF therapies.

Transthyretin Amyloidosis

Cardiac amyloid deposition has also been linked with HFpEF. Over 30 different proteins have been shown to form amyloid fibrils and five (immunoglobulin light chain, immunoglobulin heavy chain, transthyretin, serum amyloid A, and apolipoprotein AI) have been found to infiltrate the heart.[31] Autopsy from patients who were diagnosed with HFpEF revealed that transthyretin amyloidosis was present in 32% of those greater than 75 years of age.[32] Another study using nuclear scintigraphy to detect amyloids has indicated that 13% of hospitalized patients with HFpEF have transthyretin amyloidosis.[33] Interestingly, some HF patients have amyloidosis caused by a mutation in transthyretin. Over 80 transthyretin mutations, with autosomal dominant inheritance, have been associated with tissue amyloid deposition, some within the heart.[34] Nearly 25% of African Americans with cardiac transthyretin amyloidosis were heterozygous for a transthyretin V122I mutation.[34] Although this condition is rare, interstitial deposition of wild-type and mutant transthyretin is an underrecognized trigger of HF in the elderly.[35]

Mitochondrial Dysfunction and Age

As evidenced in the preceding sections, there are many factors that contribute to cellular changes observed in HFpEF. However, the fact that aging is a critical and overarching factor in the development of HFpEF is clearly noted.[36] LV diastolic stiffness increases and LV diastolic filling rate decreases with age.[37,38] Kaushik et al. showed that age-related increases in vinculin, a cytoskeletal protein, was linked to cortical stiffening and contractility.[39] Vinculin is found localized to integrin-mediated cell–ECM and cadherin-mediated cell–cell adhesions. Vinculin acts as one of several proteins involved in anchoring F-actin to the membrane. Senescent rats have twofold the ECM content in the myocardium compared to younger rats.[40] The senescent myocardium has increased levels of ROS, which can activate transforming growth factor-β (TGF-β), inducing conversion of cardiac fibroblast to myofibroblasts, an activated fibroblast phenotype.[41] The aging heart has lower responsiveness to β-adrenergic stimulation. There is lowered PKA and CaMKII phosphorylation of PLN and RYR receptor. Together this results in a lowering of the Ca^{2+} uptake and relaxation rate.[42]

The mitochondrial deoxyribonucleic acid (DNA) in aging hearts in both man and mice have up to 16-fold more point mutations and deletions than those of younger animals. Myocardial energetics have been examined as a potential mechanism for reduced systolic reserve in HFpEF with increased age. Patients with HFpEF have been shown to have a reduced phosphocreatine/adenosine triphosphate (ATP) ratio when compared to controls.[43] Several studies suggest that abnormal skeletal muscle performance is a contributor to exertional intolerance rather than just limited cardiac reserve.[44] One study found that HFpEF patients had reduced type I oxidative muscle fibers, type I/II fiber ratio, and a reduced capillary to fiber ratio in skeletal muscle compared with controls.[45]

Comorbid diseases, including hypertension and renal failure, are much more common in the elderly. There is increased inflammation with increasing age. Although the cellular mechanisms are not yet clearly defined, myocardial aging is interconnected to molecular events that influence both myocyte contractility and changes in the collagenous ECM (see upcoming discussion) that appear to provide a favorable milieu for the development of HFpEF, particularly when in combination with other comorbitidies such as hypertension and diabetes.

MYOCARDIAL COLLAGEN

Cardiac Fibrillar Collagen

Fibrillar collagens play a vital role in homeostatic function and pathologic dysfunction in the heart. Collagen types I, III, and V are the most highly represented myocardial fibrillar collagens.[46] These three types of collagens form composite fibrils that then form the collagen fibers of the heart. Three categories of collagen fibers in and around myocytes have been described based on their morphologic characteristics: coils, struts, and weaves.[47] Presumably each category of collagen fiber has a unique role in providing structural support to myocytes. A perimysial fibrillar collagen weave composed of smaller collagen fibers surrounds each myocyte, whereas the larger collagen fibers present as struts and coils to connect adjacent myocytes and blood vessels. Myocytes are organized in aligned bundles within the myocardium. The bundles are further organized into sheets that slide by one another during each heartbeat to generate the torsional motion to expel blood from the ventricles. Collagen fibers likely also participate in the organization of higher order structures such as bundles and sheets, although these types of structures are more difficult to identify in traditional two-dimensional tissue sections. Recent advances in generating and imaging decellularized hearts have afforded opportunities to visualize cardiac collagenous ECM in three dimensions where these structures can be better appreciated. As imaging technologies advance, the ability to visualize collagen structures in living human hearts in three dimensions will provide critical information for diagnosing and evaluating myocardial fibrosis in patients.

Age-related changes in the cardiac ECM have been observed both in man and in animal models.[48] In mice, levels of fibrillar collagen were found to be low in neonatal hearts where abundant levels of fibronectin were detected.[49] In adult hearts, fibronectin was significantly decreased, whereas fibrillar collagen levels increased to become the dominant fibrillar ECM component. Interestingly, in aged hearts, levels of fibrillar collagen further increased in comparison to adult ages, and increases were also noted in levels of fibronectin. Increases in fibrillar collagen in aged hearts were associated with increases in tissue stiffness even in the absence of hypertension or PO suggesting a tendency for the development of myocardial fibrosis with age alone.[50] Accordingly, age-dependent changes in ECM, coupled with those in myocytes, appear to set the stage for increases in myocardial stiffness that is further exacerbated by comorbid conditions.

Collagen Deposition in HFpEF

In patients diagnosed with HFpEF, increases in fibrillar collagen content are significant. In the study by Zile et al., collagen volume fraction was assessed in patient biopsies recovered from three groups: referent control, hypertensive heart disease only, and hypertensive heart disease with HF.[51] Collagen content and myocardial stiffness were significantly increased only in biopsies from patients with hypertensive heart disease with HF. Furthermore, collagen-dependent stiffness was measured and shown to make a significant contribution to overall muscle stiffness when the sarcomeric component was removed.[51] These results are consistent with increases in collagenous ECM observed in the myocardium of HFpEF patients making a critical contribution to diastolic stiffness.

Similarly, animal models of PO that recapitulate many aspects of human fibrotic disease also support a key role for fibrillar collagen in diastolic stiffness. Resident cardiac fibroblasts are the primary cardiac cell type that produces fibrillar collagen both in homeostasis and in hearts subjected to PO.[52] Activated fibroblasts, often referred to as myofibroblasts, express elevated levels of contractile cytoskeletal elements and ECM components. Although activated fibroblasts are strongly implicated in cardiac remodeling following infarction, the role of activated fibroblasts in PO is less clear.[53] Nonetheless, resident cardiac fibroblasts are the primary producers of fibrillar collagen and, with the assistance of inflammatory cells, are a critical mediator of collagen degradation (see Fig. 1.2).

Although imperfect, animal models provide a platform for evaluating cause-and-effect mechanisms of cardiac collagen deposition. Accumulation of ECM derives from (1) increases in transcription, translation, and secretion of ECM proteins; (2) procollagen processing and deposition to insoluble ECM in the extracellular space; and (3) degradation of ECM by myocardial matrix metalloproteinases (MMPs). Evidence that each of these mechanisms might contribute to increases in collagen content in response to PO has been shown in animal models.

Transcriptional Regulation of Collagen I

Transcriptional control of messenger ribonucleic acid (mRNA) encoding procollagen I is one mechanism by which levels of secreted procollagen can increase. Measurements of mRNA encoding the subunits of collagen I have been shown to significantly increase as soon as 3 days following the induction of PO.[54] The increased levels of mRNA encoding fibrillar collagen subunits coincide with significant increases in MMP expression indicative of extensive ECM remodeling that accompanies hypertrophic growth of the myocardium.[55] The expansion of individual myocytes by addition of sarcomeres requires renewed synthesis of basal lamina surrounding each myocyte as well as ECM in and around blood vessels. Likely the interstitial connective tissue also undergoes remodeling in response to hypertrophic growth. Interestingly, the increase in mRNA encoding fibrillar collagens at day 3 does not immediately result in an increase in collagen deposition in the extracellular space.[54] Significant increases in levels of collagen protein incorporated into collagen fibers is not detected until 1 week after induction of PO. Hence, transcriptional control of fibrillar collagen genes is not the sole mechanism that controls levels of myocardial collagen.

Postsynthetic Procollagen Processing and Deposition

Studies from Laurent et al. suggested that deposition of collagen protein into an insoluble ECM is a critical step in controlling the amount of collagen deposited following PO.[56] In the heart, ~50% of newly synthesized collagen is degraded prior to incorporation into the ECM.[56] Upon induction of PO, the amount of procollagen degraded decreases accompanied by increases in insoluble collagen deposition. These studies suggest that the efficiency of procollagen processing increases in response to PO and results in increases in collagen content. Procollagen maturation in the extracellular space requires cleavage of both the N-terminal and C-terminal propeptides from the procollagen monomer.[57] In addition, modification of amino acids by enzymes that facilitate collagen crosslinking, such as lysyl oxidase, occurs during procollagen processing.[58] Other proteins secreted into the extracellular space influence assembly of collagen into insoluble fibrils and include matricellular proteins such as SPARC and periostin as well as other collagen family members and proteoglycans.[59] Proteins involved in procollagen processing and assembly are essential factors influencing myocardial collagen content in homeostasis and in response to fibrotic stimuli. For example, the absence of SPARC expression results in reduced amounts of insoluble myocardial collagen deposited in response to PO.[60] Likewise, a decrease in insoluble collagen in SPARC-null hearts correlated with a reduction in myocardial stiffness in comparison to wild-type hearts. Hence, like in humans, increases in collagen content in mice is also associated with increases in myocardial stiffness.

ECM Degradation

Matrix Metalloproteinases

Once collagen has been incorporated into an insoluble ECM, the only known biologic mechanism for reducing collagen content is through enzymatic degradation. MMPs are zinc-dependent endopeptidases primarily responsible for ECM degradation. Of note, HFpEF patients have been found to have elevated levels of circulating MMP-1, MMP-2, MMP-8, and MMP-9.[61–64] In addition to ECM degradation, MMPs also perform proteolytic cleavage of inflammatory mediators, matricellular proteins, and other MMPs within the myocardium.[65,66] Hence increases in MMP activity are associated with active remodeling of the myocardial ECM that does not necessarily lead directly to reductions in ECM. For example, MMP-dependent cleavage of latent TGF- β, a potent profibrotic cytokine sequestered in the ECM, can lead to increases in ECM production.

Of the 25 MMPs described to date, MMP-2 and MMP-9 are the most widely studied (see Refs. 55 and 66). Interestingly, circulating MMP-2 has been shown to be elevated to a higher extent in patients with severe diastolic dysfunction as well as those with diastolic HF.[62] Increased MMP-2 activity has also been shown to induce cardiomyocyte hypertrophy and degrade contractile and structural proteins (i.e., TnI, myosin light chain 1, α-actinin, and titin) resulting in decreased cardiac function.[67,68] Hence a prominent function of this MMP in cardiac remodeling beyond ECM degradation alone is suggested. In a murine model of LV PO, genetic deletion of MMP-2 actually reduced the degree of myocardial fibrillar collagen accumulation and improved indices of diastolic function.[69]

Neutrophils and monocyte-derived macrophages are a major source of MMP-[94]. In aged mice, MMP-9 deletion was found to attenuate the age-related decline in diastolic function through a reduction in TGF-β signaling. Reductions in the profibrotic matricellular proteins, periostin and CCN2 (connective tissue growth factor [CTGF]), were detected in the absence of MMP-9.[70] MMP-9 is thought to regulate inflammation through its proteolytic activity on both ECM components and cytokine substrates. For example, in a mouse model of myocardial infarction (MI) MMP-9 mediated the post-MI degradation of CD36 leading to a decrease in macrophage phagocytosis of apoptotic neutrophils.[71] Although a number of MMP-9 substrates have been identified, including collagens (type I, IV, V, VII, X, and XIV), fibronectin, elastin, interleukin (IL)-8, Cxcl4, and IL-1β, the mechanisms whereby MMP-9 modulates LV remodeling and diastolic dysfunction have not been completely elucidated.[72–75]

Other MMPs implicated in diastolic dysfunction include MMP-1, which has the highest affinity for fibrillar collagens and preferentially degrades collagens type I and III. Increased MMP-1 activity results in excessive collagen deposition and diastolic dysfunction.[76] In addition, MMP-8, a collagenase primarily secreted by neutrophils, negatively correlates with development of HFpEF.[64,77] Similarly, MMP-12 inhibition exacerbates cardiac dysfunction by prolonging neutrophil-mediated inflammation highlighting the importance of MMPs in regulation of inflammation and the subsequent development of cardiac dysfunction.[78] Taken together, MMPs are critical mediators of myocardial ECM content and might represent a viable target for therapeutic intervention in future applications.

Tissue Inhibitors of Metalloproteinases

MMP activity is dependent not only on the concentration of active enzymes but also on the levels of a family of naturally occurring tissue inhibitors of metalloproteinases (TIMPs).[79] After chronic stimulation of proinflammatory cytokines, TIMP levels increase leading to decreased MMP/TIMP ratio and increases in fibrillar collagen deposition.[80] For example, the interaction between MMP-1 and TIMP-1 is of critical relevance in the maintenance of the integrity of the cardiac collagen network. TIMP-1 colocalizes with MMP-1 in healthy myocardium and is expressed by cardiac fibroblasts and myocytes.[81–84] Circulating levels of TIMP-1 closely associate with markers of systemic inflammation, diastolic dysfunction, and HF severity.[62,85] In hypertensive subjects with HFpEF, TIMP-1 moderately predicts the presence of HF.[86] Using a single MMP to TIMP ratio, however, can be somewhat misleading as there are multiple MMPs and TIMPs present in diseased myocardium.

In addition to TIMP-1, TIMP-2 levels correlate with deposition of cardiac ECM.[87] In response to angiotensin II infusion, TIMP-2 deleted mice showed enhanced hypertrophy, reduced collagen crosslinking, and suppressed collagen deposition resulting in impaired active relaxation.[88] TIMP-3 has cardioprotective functions, as TIMP-3 deletion leads to spontaneous dilated cardiomyopathy,[89] whereas TIMP-4 levels increase with hypertrophy and decrease with the onset of HF in spontaneously hypertensive rats.[90]

Inflammatory Mediators in HFpEF

A significant role for inflammatory mediators in the heart following MI has been well established in a number of studies where inflammation has been shown to be a major component contributing to healing and scar formation.[91–95] Initiation of the inflammatory response following MI is necessary for adequate wound healing, yet too much or too little inflammation can result in increased dilation and poor cardiac function highlighting the importance of a balanced immune response to injury.[96] Relatively less is known about the role of inflammatory mediators in HFpEF although this actively expanding area of research will certainly lead to new discoveries that are likely to influence treatment strategies.

As mentioned, aging is a risk factor for HFpEF and has been linked to increased systemic inflammation termed inflamm-aging. Inflamm-aging is defined as elevated levels of proinflammatory markers in the blood and other tissues often detected in older individuals. It is hypothesized that this increase in inflammation is the common biologic factor responsible for the decline and the onset of cardiovascular diseases, frailty, multimorbidity, and decline of physical and cognitive function in the elderly. Possible mechanisms potentially underlying inflamm-aging include genomic instability, cell senescence, mitochondria dysfunction, NLRP3 inflammasome activation, and primary dysregulation of immune cells.

Obesity is another risk factor for HFpEF that has been linked to an increase in baseline systemic inflammation.[97] More than 80% of patients with HFpEF are overweight or obese. Visceral fat produces proinflammatory and chemotactic compounds and is infiltrated by inflammatory cells such as macrophages and lymphocytes.[98] Older, obese HFpEF patients that underwent a 20-week caloric restriction diet had significantly improved peak oxygen consumption and quality of life scores. This improvement was found to correlate with reduced body fat mass, increased percent lean body mass, higher thigh muscle/intermuscular fat ratio, and lower biomarkers of inflammation supporting the hypothesis that systemic inflammation due to obesity contributes to exercise intolerance in HFpEF.[99] As mentioned, inflammatory cells produce MMPs, which have a significant impact on cardiac remodeling. Studies that support a function for inflammatory cell types in contributing to fibrotic deposition of cardiac collagen are emerging, particularly for neutrophil and macrophage populations.

Neutrophils

In response to ischemia, neutrophils are the first cells to respond to the site of injury.[100,101] Similarly, neutrophils might also be an important early contributor to PO-induced hypertrophy. In a murine model of PO, the recruitment of neutrophils was characterized as an early event as increases in neutrophil numbers noted at day 1, decreased by day 3.[102] Early infiltration of neutrophils was also associated with detection of neutrophil extracellular traps (NETs) in the heart. The release of chromatin by neutrophils in the form of NETs is thought to be an antimicrobial defense mechanism. However, NETs are also thought to lead to further recruitment of platelets and other types of inflammatory cells. In the study by Martinod et al., transgenic mice that were unable to form NETs demonstrated significant reductions in myocardial collagen content in comparison to wild-type mice after 4 weeks of PO.[102] Whether neutrophil activity and NET deposition might also contribute to human disease is yet to be established.

Macrophages

Similar to neutrophils, increasing evidence that macrophages might also influence fibrotic deposition of collagen after PO is emerging. In a murine model of PO induced by transverse aortic constriction (TAC), cardiac macrophage populations were increased at day 6.[103] McDonald et al. also reported increases in macrophage populations at 1 week after TAC.[54] Importantly, the time course of collagen accumulation paralleled that of macrophage expansion in the PO myocardium.[54] Macrophage expression of the matricellular protein SPARC, a key regulator of myocardial fibrosis, was also found suggesting that macrophage expression of SPARC might increase procollagen processing and enhance collagen deposition in PO hearts.

Evidence that macrophages might also contribute to fibrosis in humans was supported by an increase in macrophages in biopsies from patients diagnosed with HFpEF.[104] Tissue samples from referent controls and from those with hypertension in the absence of HFpEF did not demonstrate significant increases in myocardial macrophages. Hulsmans et al. went on to show, in another murine model of diastolic dysfunction, an association with macrophage recruitment and cardiac fibrosis. In mice with macrophage-specific deletion of IL-10, an improvement in diastolic function was found.[104] Hence a growing body of evidence suggests that macrophages are a critical inflammatory cell population influencing the development of myocardial fibrosis and diastolic dysfunction.

FUTURE DIRECTIONS

Cellular mechanisms that influence diastolic function are multivariant in nature. A decrease in cardiomyocyte number, cardiomyocyte hypertrophy, increased collagen deposition, and functional changes at the cellular level can all contribute to LV stiffness and abnormal diastolic function. Determining what factors trigger the decline into HF has never been more important. Clearly, factors that render the aged myocardium more susceptible to diastolic dysfunction include changes in myocyte contractility, age-related ECM remodeling, and inflammation. New strategies that arise from basic research into cellular mechanisms of diastolic dysfunction are highly likely to lead to significant advances for the treatment of patients diagnosed with HFpEF in the coming years.

KEY POINTS

- Heart failure with preserved ejection fraction (HFpEF) is characterized by increases in myocardial stiffness contributed by both cellular and molecular mechanisms that arise from alterations in myocytes and in extracellular matrix.
- Myocardial energetics are a potential mechanism for reduced systolic reserve in HFpEF with increased age.
- A reduction of SERCA activity is consistent with the characteristic slowed relaxation and $[Ca]_I$ seen in diastolic HF. In animal models when SERCA expression is increased or PLN expression is decreased, myocardial relaxation and $[Ca]_I$ decline are accelerated resulting in improved diastolic function.
- Phosphorylation of the N2B element of titin by PKA or PKG decreases passive tension, whereas phosphorylation of titin's PEVK element by PKC-α increases passive tension.
- Cardiac transthyretin amyloid deposition is linked with HFpEF.
- Three primary cellular mechanisms contribute to increases in myocardial collagen accumulation:
  1. Increased transcription, translation, and secretion of collagen proteins
  2. Increased procollagen processing in the extracellular space
  3. Decreases in extracellular matrix degradation
- Procollagen processing is influenced by expression of collagen-binding proteins, such as the matricellular protein SPARC, that drives collagen deposition in response to pressure overload.
- ECM degradation is controlled by the balance between matrix metalloproteinases (MMPs) and tissue inhibitor of MMPs (TIMPs).
- Cardiac fibroblasts are the primary cell type producing fibrillar collagen in the heart; however, expression of collagen-binding proteins, MMPs, and TIMPs by resident and infiltrating immune cells can influence levels of myocardial ECM.
- Increases in fibrillar collagen and alterations in ECM assembly, such as differential collagen crosslinking, contribute to fibrotic ECM and myocardial dysfunction in HFpEF.

REVIEW QUESTIONS

1. How does NO regulate cardiac relaxation?
   a. Generation of NO by NO synthase requires a cofactor, tetrahydrobiopterin, which can reduce actin-myosin cross-bridge cycling
   b. Through depletion of tetrahydrobiopterin and oxidation of guanylate cyclase
   c. Through NO synthase uncoupling and production of superoxide
2. What are the important steps for procollagen I production, processing, and deposition (in sequential order)?
   i. Transcription and translation inside the cell
   ii. Cleavage by MMPs
   iii. Incorporation into extracellular matrix enhanced by matricellular proteins
   iv. Cleavage by propeptidases
      a. i, ii, iv
      b. ii, iv, iii, i
      c. i, iv, iii
      d. iv, ii, iii
      e. i, ii, iii, iv
3. What are NETs?
   a. Release of chromatin by neutrophils
   b. Antimicrobial defense mechanism
   c. Neutrophil extracellular traps
   d. All the above

REFERENCES

1. Sharma K, Kass DA. Heart failure with preserved ejection fraction: mechanisms, clinical features, and therapies. *Circ Res.* 2014;115:79–96.
2. Owan TE, Hodge DO, Herges RM, Jacobsen SJ, Roger VL, Redfield MM. Trends in prevalence and outcome of heart failure with preserved ejection fraction. *N Engl J Med.* 2006;355:251–259.
3. Bhatia RS, Tu JV, Lee DS, et al. Outcome of heart failure with preserved ejection fraction in a population-based study. *N Engl J Med.* 2006;355:260–269.
4. Steinberg BA, Zhao X, Heidenreich PA, et al. Trends in patients hospitalized with heart failure and preserved left ventricular ejection fraction: prevalence, therapies, and outcomes. *Circulation.* 2012;126:65–75.
5. McMurray JJ, Packer M, Desai AS, et al. Angiotensin-neprilysin inhibition versus enalapril in heart failure. *N Engl J Med.* 2014;371: 993–1004.
6. Pitt B, Pfeffer MA, Assmann SF, et al. Spironolactone for heart failure with preserved ejection fraction. *N Engl J Med.* 2014;370: 1383–1392.
7. Paulus WJ, Tschope C. A novel paradigm for heart failure with preserved ejection fraction: comorbidities drive myocardial dysfunction and remodeling through coronary microvascular endothelial inflammation. *J Am Coll Cardiol.* 2013;62:263–271.
8. Bers DM. Cardiac sarcoplasmic reticulum calcium leak: basis and roles in cardiac dysfunction. *Ann Rev Physiol.* 2014;76:107–127.

9. Kranias EG, Hajjar RJ. Modulation of cardiac contractility by the phospholamban/SERCA2a regulatome. *Circ Res.* 2012;110:1646–1660.
10. Borbély A, van der Velden J, Papp Z, et al. Cardiomyocyte stiffness in diastolic heart failure. *Circulation.* 2005;111:774–781.
11. Hidalgo C, Granzier H. Tuning the molecular giant titin through phosphorylation: role in health and disease. *Trends Cardiov Med.* 2013;23: 165–171.
12. Krüger M, Kötter S, Grützner A, et al. Protein kinase G modulates human myocardial passive stiffness by phosphorylation of the titin springs. *Circ Res.* 2009;104:87–94.
13. Hidalgo C, Hudson B, Bogomolovas J, et al. PKC phosphorylation of titin's PEVK element: a novel and conserved pathway for modulating myocardial stiffness. *Circ Res.* 2009;105(7): 631–638 + 17 pp.
14. Hamdani N, Bishu KG, von Frieling-Salewsky M, Redfield MM, Linke WA. Deranged myofilament phosphorylation and function in experimental heart failure with preserved ejection fraction. *Cardiov Res.* 2013;97:464–471.
15. Hamdani N, Krysiak J, Kreusser MM, et al. Crucial role for Ca2(+)/calmodulin-dependent protein kinase-II in regulating diastolic stress of normal and failing hearts via titin phosphorylation. *Circ Res.* 2013;112:664–674.
16. Yamasaki R, Wu Y, McNabb M, Greaser M, Labeit S, Granzier H. Protein kinase A phosphorylates titin's cardiac-specific N2B domain and reduces passive tension in rat cardiac myocytes. *Circ Res.* 2002;90:1181–1188.
17. van Heerebeek L, Franssen CP, Hamdani N, Verheugt FW, Somsen GA, Paulus WJ. Molecular and cellular basis for diastolic dysfunction. *Curr Heart Failure Rep.* 2012;9:293–302.
18. Grutzner A, Garcia-Manyes S, Kötter S, Badilla CL, Fernandez JM, Linke WA. Modulation of titin-based stiffness by disulfide bonding in the cardiac titin N2-B unique sequence. *Biophys J.* 2009;97:825–834.
19. Nedrud J, Labeit S, Gotthardt M, Granzier H. Mechanics on myocardium deficient in the N2B region of titin: the cardiac-unique spring element improves efficiency of the cardiac cycle. *Biophys J.* 2011;101:1385–1392.
20. Rao V, Cheng Y, Lindert S, et al. PKA phosphorylation of cardiac troponin I modulates activation and relaxation kinetics of ventricular myofibrils. *Biophys J.* 2014;107:1196–1204.
21. Tong CW, Stelzer JE, Greaser ML, Powers PA, Moss RL. Acceleration of crossbridge kinetics by protein kinase A phosphorylation of cardiac myosin binding protein C modulates cardiac function. *Circ Res.* 2008;103:974–982.
22. Donaldson C, Palmer BM, Zile M, et al. Myosin cross-bridge dynamics in patients with hypertension and concentric left ventricular remodeling. *Circ Heart Failure.* 2012;5:803–811.
23. Rosas PC, Liu Y, Abdalla MI, et al. Phosphorylation of cardiac myocin-binding protein-C is a critical mediator of diastolic function. *Circ Heart Failure.* 2015;8:582–594.
24. Silberman GA, Fan TH, Liu H, et al. Uncoupled cardiac nitric oxide synthase mediates diastolic dysfunction. *Circulation.* 2010;121: 519–528.
25. Jeong EM, Monasky MM, Gu L, et al. Tetrahydrobiopterin improves diastolic dysfunction by reversing changes in myofilament properties. *J Molecul Cell Cardiol.* 2013;56:44–54.
26. Tsai EJ, Liu Y, Koitabashi N, et al. Pressure-overload-induced subcellular relocalization/oxidation of soluble guanylyl cyclase in the heart modulates enzyme stimulation. *Circ Res.* 2012;110:295–303.
27. Choudhary C, Kumar C, Gnad F, et al. Lysine acetylation targets protein complexes and co-regulates major cellular functions. *Science (New York, N.Y.).* 2009;325:834–840.
28. Foster DB, Liu T, Rucker J, et al. The cardiac acetyl-lysine proteome. *PLoS One.* 2013;8:e67513.
29. Lundby A, Lage K, Weinert BT, et al. Proteomic analysis of lysine acetylation sites in rat tissues reveals organ specificity and subcellular patterns. *Cell Rep.* 2012;2:419–431.
30. Jeong MY, Lin YH, Wennersten SA, et al. Histone deacetylase activity governs diastolic dysfunction through a nongenomic mechanism. *Sci Transl Med.* 2018 Feb 7;10(427):eaao0144.
31. Maurer MS, Elliott P, Comenzo R, Semigran M, Rapezzi C. Addressing common questions encountered in the diagnosis and management of cardiac amyloidosis. *Circulation.* 2017;135:1357–1377.
32. Mohammed SF, Mirzoyev SA, Edwards WD, et al. Left ventricular amyloid deposition in patients with heart failure and preserved ejection fraction. *JACC. Heart Failure.* 2014;2:113–122.
33. González-López E, Gallego-Delgado M, Guzzo-Merello G, et al. Wild-type transthyretin amyloidosis as a cause of heart failure with preserved ejection fraction. *Eur Heart J.* 2015;36:2585–2594.
34. Buxbaum J, Jacobson DR, Tagoe C, et al. Transthyretin V122I in African Americans with congestive heart failure. *J Am Coll Cardiol.* 2006;47: 1724–1725.
35. Quarta CC, Buxbaum JN, Shah AM, et al. The amyloidogenic V122I transthyretin variant in elderly black Americans. *N Engl J Med.* 2015;372:21–29.
36. Loffredo FS, Nikolova AP, Pancoast JR, Lee RT. Heart failure with preserved ejection fraction: molecular pathways of the aging myocardium. *Circ Res.* 2014;115:97–107.
37. Redfield MM, Jacobsen SJ, Borlaug BA, Rodeheffer RJ, Kass DA. Age- and gender-related ventricular-vascular stiffening: a community-based study. *Circulation.* 2005;112:2254–2262.
38. Bursi F, Weston SA, Redfield MM, et al. Systolic and diastolic heart failure in the community. *JAMA.* 2006;296:2209–2216.
39. Kaushik G, Spenlehauer A, Sessions AO, et al. Vinculin network-mediated cytoskeletal remodeling regulates contractile function in the aging heart. *Sci Trans. Med.* 2015 Jun 17;7:(292):292ra99.
40. Biernacka A, Frangogiannis NG. Aging and cardiac fibrosis. *Aging Dis.* 2011;2:158–173.
41. Cucoranu I, Clempus R, Dikalova A, et al. NAD(P)H oxidase 4 mediates transforming growth factor-beta1-induced differentiation of cardiac fibroblasts into myofibroblasts. *Circ Res.* 2005;97:900–907.
42. Chu G, Lester JW, Young KB, Luo W, Zhai J, Kranias EG. A single site (Ser16) phosphorylation in phospholamban is sufficient in mediating its maximal cardiac responses to beta-agonists. *J Biol Chem.* 2000;275:38938–38943.
43. Phan TT, Abozguia K, Nallur Shivu G, et al. Heart failure with preserved ejection fraction is characterized by dynamic impairment of active relaxation and contraction of the left ventricle on exercise and associated with myocardial energy deficiency. *J Am Coll Cardiol.* 2009;54:402–409.
44. Bhella PS, Prasad A, Heinicke K, et al. Abnormal haemodynamic response to exercise in heart failure with preserved ejection fraction. *Eur J Heart Failure.* 2011;13: 1296–1304.
45. Kitzman DW, Nicklas B, Kraus WE, et al. Skeletal muscle abnormalities and exercise intolerance in older patients with heart failure and preserved ejection fraction. *Am J Physiol. Heart Circ Physiol.* 2014;306:H1364–H1370.
46. Eghbali M, Weber KT. Collagen and the myocardium: fibrillar structure, biosynthesis and degradation in relation to hypertrophy and its regression. *Molecul Cell Biochem.* 1990;96:1–14.
47. Caulfield JB, Borg TK. The collagen network of the heart. *Lab Invest.* 1979;40:364–372.
48. Gazoti Debessa CR, Mesiano Maifrino LB, Rodrigues de Souza R. Age related changes of the collagen network of the human heart. *Mech Ageing Develop.* 2001;122:1049–1058.
49. Trombetta-Esilva J, Eadie EP, Zhang Y, Norris RA, Borg TK, Bradshaw AD. The effects of age and the expression of SPARC on extracellular matrix production by cardiac fibroblasts in 3-D cultures. *PLoS One.* 2013;8:e79715.
50. Bradshaw AD, Baicu CF, Rentz TJ, Van Laer AO, Bonnema DD, Zile MR. Age-dependent alterations in fibrillar collagen content and myocardial diastolic function: role of SPARC in post-synthetic procollagen processing. *Am J Physiol. Heart Circ Physiol.* 2010;298: H614–H622.
51. Zile MR, Baicu CF, Ikonomidis J, et al. Myocardial stiffness in patients with heart failure and a preserved ejection fraction: contributions of collagen and titin. *Circulation.* 2015;131:1247–1259.
52. Moore-Morris T, Guimarães-Camboa N, Banerjee I, et al. Resident fibroblast lineages mediate pressure overload-induced cardiac fibrosis. *J Clin Invest.* 2014;124:2921–2934.

53. Kanisicak O, Khalil H, Ivey MJ, et al. Genetic lineage tracing defines myofibroblast origin and function in the injured heart. *Nature Comm.* 2016;7:12260.
54. McDonald LT, Zile MR, Zhang Y, et al. Increased macrophage-derived SPARC precedes collagen deposition in myocardial fibrosis. *Am J Physiol. Heart Circ Physiol.* 2018.
55. Lindsey ML. Assigning matrix metalloproteinase roles in ischaemic cardiac remodelling. *Nat Rev. Cardiology.* 2018;15:471–479.
56. Bishop JE, Rhodes S, Laurent GJ, Low RB, Stirewalt WS. Increased collagen synthesis and decreased collagen degradation in right ventricular hypertrophy induced by pressure overload. *Cardiov Res.* 1994;28:1581–1585.
57. Bradshaw AD. The extracellular matrix. *Encycl Cell Biol.* 2016;2:694–703.
58. Eyre DR, Paz MA, Gallop PM. Cross-linking in collagen and elastin. *Ann Rev Biochem.* 1984;53:717–748.
59. Bradshaw AD. The role of SPARC in extracellular matrix assembly. *J Cell Comm Signal.* 2009;3:239–246.
60. Bradshaw AD, Baicu CF, Rentz TJ, et al. Pressure overload-induced alterations in fibrillar collagen content and myocardial diastolic function: role of secreted protein acidic and rich in cysteine (SPARC) in post-synthetic procollagen processing. *Circulation.* 2009;119:269–280.
61. Gonzalez A, López B, Querejeta R, Zubillaga E, Echeverria T, Diez J. Filling pressures and collagen metabolism in hypertensive patients with heart failure and normal ejection fraction. *Hypertension.* 2010;55:1418–1424.
62. Martos R, Baugh J, Ledwidge M, et al. Diastolic heart failure: evidence of increased myocardial collagen turnover linked to diastolic dysfunction. *Circulation.* 2007;115:888–895.
63. Martos R, Baugh J, Ledwidge M, et al. Diagnosis of heart failure with preserved ejection fraction: improved accuracy with the use of markers of collagen turnover. *Eur J Heart Failure.* 2009;11:191–197.
64. Zile MR, Desantis SM, Baicu CF, et al. Plasma biomarkers that reflect determinants of matrix composition identify the presence of left ventricular hypertrophy and diastolic heart failure. *Circ Heart Failure.* 2011;4:246–256.
65. Newby AC. Metalloproteinases promote plaque rupture and myocardial infarction: a persuasive concept waiting for clinical translation. *Matrix Biol: J Int Soc Matrix Biol.* 2015;44–46:157–166.
66. Rohani MG, Parks WC. Matrix remodeling by MMPs during wound repair. *Matrix Biol.* 2015;44–46:113–121.
67. Wang W, Schulze CJ, Suarez-Pinzon WL, Dyck JR, Sawicki G, Schulz R. Intracellular action of matrix metalloproteinase-2 accounts for acute myocardial ischemia and reperfusion injury. *Circulation.* 2002;106:1543–1549.
68. Wang GY, Bergman MR, Nguyen AP, et al. Cardiac transgenic matrix metalloproteinase-2 expression directly induces impaired contractility. *Cardiov Res.* 2006;69:688–696.
69. Matsusaka H, Ide T, Matsushima S, et al. Targeted deletion of matrix metalloproteinase 2 ameliorates myocardial remodeling in mice with chronic pressure overload. *Hypertension.* 2006;47:711–717.
70. Chiao YA, Ramirez TA, Zamilpa R, et al. Matrix metalloproteinase-9 deletion attenuates myocardial fibrosis and diastolic dysfunction in ageing mice. *Cardiov Res.* 2012;96:444–455.
71. DeLeon-Pennell KY, Tian Y, Zhang B, et al. CD36 is a matrix metalloproteinase-9 substrate that stimulates neutrophil apoptosis and removal during cardiac remodeling. *Circ Cardiov Gen.* 2016;9:14–25.
72. de Castro Brás LE, Ramirez TA, DeLeon-Pennell KY, Chiao YA, et al. Texas 3-step decellularization protocol: looking at the cardiac extracellular matrix. *J Proteomics.* 2013;86:43–52.
73. DeLeon KY, Yabluchanskiy A, Winniford MD, Lange RA, Chilton RJ, Lindsey ML. Modifying matrix remodeling to prevent heart failure. In: Li R, Weisel RD, eds. *Cardiac Regeneration and Repair. Volume I: Pathology and Therapies.* Woodhead Cambridge, England; 2013.
74. Lindsey ML, Iyer RP, Zamilpa R, et al. A novel collagen matricryptin reduces left ventricular dilation post-myocardial infarction by promoting scar formation and angiogenesis. *J Am Coll Cardiol.* 2015;66:1364–1374.
75. Zamilpa R, Lopez EF, Chiao YA, et al. Proteomic analysis identifies in vivo candidate matrix metalloproteinase-9 substrates in the left ventricle post-myocardial infarction. *Proteomics.* 2010;10:2214–2223.
76. Reed AL, Tanaka A, Sorescu D, et al. Diastolic dysfunction is associated with cardiac fibrosis in the senescence-accelerated mouse. *Am J Physiol. Heart Circ Physiol.* 2011;301:H824–H831.
77. Erkol A, Pala S, Oduncu V, et al. Relation of plasma matrix metalloproteinase-8 levels late after myocardial infarction with left ventricular volumes and ejection fraction. *Turk Kardiyol Dern Ars.* 2013;41(7):617–624.
78. Iyer RP, Patterson NL, Zouein FA, et al. Early matrix metalloproteinase-12 inhibition worsens post-myocardial infarction cardiac dysfunction by delaying inflammation resolution. *Int J Cardiol.* 2015;185:198–208.
79. Visse R, Nagase H. Matrix metalloproteinases and tissue inhibitors of metalloproteinases: structure, function, and biochemistry. *Circ Res.* 2003;92:827–839.
80. Mann DL. Inflammatory mediators and the failing heart: past, present, and the foreseeable future. *Circ Res.* 2002;91:988–998.
81. Lindsey ML, Goshorn DK, Squires CE, et al. Age-dependent changes in myocardial matrix metalloproteinase/tissue inhibitor of metalloproteinase profiles and fibroblast function. *Cardiov Res.* 2005;66:410–419.
82. Tyagi SC, Kumar SG, Banks J, Fortson W. Co-expression of tissue inhibitor and matrix metalloproteinase in myocardium. *J Mol Cell Cardiol.* 1995;27:2177–2189.
83. Tyagi SC, Kumar S, Glover G. Induction of tissue inhibitor and matrix metalloproteinase by serum in human heart-derived fibroblast and endomyocardial endothelial cells. *J Cell Biochem.* 1995;58:360–371.
84. Romanic AM, Burns-Kurtis CL, Gout B, Berrebi-Bertrand I, Ohlstein EH. Matrix metalloproteinase expression in cardiac myocytes following myocardial infarction in the rabbit. *Life Sci.* 2001;68:799–814.
85. Cavusoglu E, Ruwende C, Chopra V, et al. Tissue inhibitor of metalloproteinase-1 (TIMP-1) is an independent predictor of all-cause mortality, cardiac mortality, and myocardial infarction. *Am Heart J.* 2006;151(1101):e1–e8.
86. Janicki JS, Brower GL. The role of myocardial fibrillar collagen in ventricular remodeling and function. *J Cardiac Failure.* 2002;8:S319–S325.
87. Peterson JT, Li H, Dillon L, Bryant JW. Evolution of matrix metalloprotease and tissue inhibitor expression during heart failure progression in the infarcted rat. *Cardiov Res.* 2000;46:307–315.
88. Fan D, Takawale A, Basu R, et al. Differential role of TIMP2 and TIMP3 in cardiac hypertrophy, fibrosis, and diastolic dysfunction. *Cardiov Res. 2014.* 2014;103:268–280.
89. Eckhouse SR, Purcell BP, McGarvey JR, et al. Local hydrogel release of recombinant TIMP-3 attenuates adverse left ventricular remodeling after experimental myocardial infarction. *Sci Transl Med.* 2014;6:223ra21.
90. Mujumdar VS, Tyagi SC. Temporal regulation of extracellular matrix components in transition from compensatory hypertrophy to decompensatory heart failure. *J Hyperten.* 1999;17:261–270.
91. Lindsey ML, Saucerman JJ, DeLeon-Pennell KY. Knowledge gaps to understanding cardiac macrophage polarization following myocardial infarction. *Biochim Biophys Acta.* 2016;1862:2288–2292.
92. DeLeon-Pennell KY, Meschiari CA, Jung M, Lindsey ML. Matrix metalloproteinases in myocardial infarction and heart failure. *Prog Mol Biol Transl Sci.* 2017;147:75–100.
93. Lindsey ML. Regulating macrophage infiltration to alter wound healing following myocardial infarction. *Cardiov Res.* 2018;114:1571–1572.
94. Mouton AJ, Rivera OJ, Lindsey ML. Myocardial infarction remodeling that progresses to heart failure: a signaling misunderstanding. *Am J Physiol Heart Circ Physiol.* 2018;315:H71–H79.
95. Kain V, Liu F, Kozlovskaya V, et al. Resolution agonist 15-epi-Lipoxin A4 programs early activation of resolving phase in post-myocardial infarction healing. *Sci Rep.* 2017;7:9999.
96. Grzybowski M, Welch RD, Parsons L, et al. The association between white blood cell count and acute myocardial infarction in-hospital mortality: findings from the National Registry of Myocardial Infarction. *Acad Emerg Med.* 2004;11:1049–1060.
97. Pandey A, Patel KV, Vaduganathan M, et al. Physical activity, fitness, and obesity in heart failure with preserved ejection fraction. *JACC Heart Fail.* 2018;6:975–982.

98. Surmi BK, Hasty AH. Macrophage infiltration into adipose tissue: initiation, propagation and remodeling. *Future Lipidol.* 2008;3: 545–556.
99. Kitzman DW, Brubaker P, Morgan T, et al. Effect of caloric restriction or aerobic exercise training on peak oxygen consumption and quality of life in obese older patients with heart failure with preserved ejection fraction: a randomized clinical trial. *JAMA.* 2016;315:36–46.
100. Borregaard N, Cowland JB. Granules of the human neutrophilic polymorphonuclear leukocyte. *Blood.* 1997;89:3503–3521.
101. Faurschou M, Borregaard N. Neutrophil granules and secretory vesicles in inflammation. *Microbes Infect.* 2003;5:1317–1327.
102. Martinod K, Witsch T, Erpenbeck L, et al. Peptidylarginine deiminase 4 promotes age-related organ fibrosis. *J Experiment Med.* 2017;214:439–458.
103. Weisheit C, Zhang Y, Faron A, et al. Ly6C(low) and not Ly6C(high) macrophages accumulate first in the heart in a model of murine pressure-overload. *PLoS One.* 2014;9:e112710.
104. Hulsmans M, Sager HB, Roh JD, et al. Cardiac macrophages promote diastolic dysfunction. *J Experiment Med.* 2018;215:423–440.

2

Pathophysiology of Heart Failure With a Preserved Ejection Fraction: Measurements and Mechanisms Causing Abnormal Diastolic Function

Michael R. Zile and Catalin F. Baicu

OUTLINE

INTRODUCTION

Heart failure (HF) can be defined physiologically as an inability of the heart to provide sufficient forward output to meet the perfusion and oxygenation requirements of the tissues at rest and during exercise while maintaining normal diastolic filling pressures. Patients with chronic HF can be divided into two broad groups: heart failure with reduced ejection fraction (HFrEF) and heart failure with preserved ejection fraction (HFpEF). Classifying patients in these two broad categories should be based on characteristic changes in cardiovascular (CV) structure and function (Table 2.1).[1,2]

Patients with HFrEF are characterized by progressive chamber dilation, eccentric remodeling, and abnormalities in systolic function. Clinical manifestations of left ventricular (LV) systolic dysfunction include decreased cardiac output, increased heart rate, and peripheral vasoconstriction. In addition, patients with HFrEF frequently have symptoms of shortness of breath at rest or with exertion. These symptoms of pulmonary congestion are due, at least in part, to LV diastolic dysfunction and increased diastolic filling pressures. Therefore patients with HFrEF (particularly when they have symptomatic decompensation) do not have an isolated abnormality in systolic function; rather, from the pathophysiologic point of view, they have abnormalities in systolic properties and eccentric remodeling, with associated or secondary abnormalities in diastolic function and increased diastolic filling pressures.

By contrast, patients with HFpEF are characterized by normal LV volume, concentric remodeling, normal LV ejection fraction at rest, but abnormalities in diastolic function.[3–16] These patients have abnormalities in diastolic relaxation, filling, and/or distensibility. Clinical manifestations of LV diastolic dysfunction include shortness of breath at rest or with exertion and peripheral edema. However, abnormalities in regional systolic function at rest (such as midwall shortening, longitudinal/circumferential strain, and strain rate) have also been identified in patients with HFpEF. In addition, blunted augmentation in systolic function during exercise has been demonstrated in HFpEF patients. Therefore patients with HFpEF do not have isolated abnormalities in diastolic properties; rather, from the pathophysiologic point of view, they have abnormalities in diastolic properties, concentric remodeling, and diastolic dysfunction-dependent limitations in the ability to augment systolic function during exercise.

TABLE 2.1 Differences in Structure and Function Differentiate HFrEF Versus HFpEF

	HFrEF	HFpEF
LV end diastolic volume	↑	↔
LV mass	↑	↑
Geometry	Eccentric	Concentric
LV ejection fraction	↓	↔
LV diastolic pressure	↑	↑

HFpEF, Heart failure with preserved ejection fraction; *HFrEF,* heart failure with reduced ejection fraction; *LV,* left ventricular.

TABLE 2.2 Definitions

Diastolic Dysfunction: Abnormal diastolic properties of LV (abnormal relaxation, filling dynamics, distensibility).
- EF may be normal or low.
- Patient may be symptomatic or asymptomatic.

Heart Failure With a Preserved Ejection Fraction: Clinical heart failure, preserved EF, abnormal diastolic function.

Systolic Dysfunction: Abnormal systolic properties of LV (abnormal performance, function, contractility).
- EF is low (and diastolic dysfunction may coexist).
- Patient may be symptomatic or asymptomatic.

Heart Failure With a Reduced Ejection Fraction: Clinical heart failure, reduced EF, abnormal systolic function.

Diastolic dysfunction and *HFpEF* are not synonymous terms. Diastolic dysfunction indicates a functional abnormality of diastolic relaxation, filling, or distensibility of the left ventricle—regardless of whether the EF is normal or abnormal and regardless of whether the patient is asymptomatic or has symptoms and signs of HF. Thus diastolic dysfunction refers to abnormal mechanical (diastolic) properties of the ventricle and is present in virtually all patients with HF. HFpEF denotes a patient with the signs and symptoms of clinical heart failure who has a normal EF, normal LV volume, and LV diastolic dysfunction. Similar distinctions apply to the terms *systolic dysfunction* and *HFrEF* (Table 2.2).

The pathophysiology of HFpEF will be reviewed here, beginning with a discussion of normal diastolic relaxation, filling, and distensibility. Understanding normal diastolic function permits an easier understanding of some of the clinical features of HFpEF. The pathophysiologic mechanisms that cause the development of HFpEF are reflected in changes in LV relaxation and filling; LV and LA structural remodeling and altered geometry; changes in LV, systemic, and pulmonary vascular compliance; skeletal muscle and endothelial function; and proinflammatory and profibrotic signaling (Fig. 2.1).[17,18]

NORMAL DIASTOLIC FUNCTION

Cardiac function is critically dependent upon diastolic physiologic mechanisms to provide adequate LV filling (cardiac input) in parallel with LV ejection (cardiac output) both at rest and during exercise. During diastole, the left ventricle, left atrium, and pulmonary veins form a common chamber, which is continuous with the pulmonary capillary bed. LV diastolic pressure is determined by the volume of blood in the left ventricle during diastole and the diastolic distensibility or compliance of the entire CV system (principally the left ventricle but may also include the left atrium, pulmonary vessels, right ventricle, and systemic arteries). Thus an increase in LV diastolic pressure (whether this occurs at rest or during exercise) will increase pulmonary capillary pressure, which if high enough causes dyspnea, exercise limitation, pulmonary congestion, and edema.

Relaxation of the contracted myocardium begins at the onset of diastole. This is a dynamic process that takes place during isovolumic relaxation (the period between aortic valve closure and mitral valve opening during which LV pressure declines with no change in volume), and then continues during auxotonic relaxation (the period between mitral valve opening and mitral valve closure, during which the left ventricle fills at variable pressure) (Fig. 2.2). The rapid pressure decay and the concomitant untwisting and elastic recoil of the left ventricle produce a suction effect that augments the left atrial (LA)–ventricular pressure gradient, pulling blood into the ventricle thereby promoting diastolic filling (Fig. 2.3). During exercise in normal patients, relaxation rate is increased, and early diastolic pressures decrease, augmenting elastic recoil and diastolic suction and resulting in more rapid filling during a shortened diastolic filling period at increasing heart rates.

During the later phases of diastole, the normal left ventricle is composed of completely relaxed cardiomyocytes and is very compliant and easily distensible, offering minimal resistance to LV filling over a normal volume range. Atrial contraction near the end of diastole contributes 20% to 30% to total LV filling volume and increases diastolic pressures by less than 5 mmHg. As a result, LV filling can normally be accomplished by very low filling pressures in the left atrium and pulmonary veins, preserving a low pulmonary capillary pressure (<12 mmHg) and a high degree of lung distensibility. Loss of normal LV diastolic relaxation and distensibility, due to structural and functional causes, impairs LV pressure decline and filling, resulting in increases in LV diastolic, left atrial, and pulmonary venous pressures, which directly increase the pulmonary capillary pressure.

MEASUREMENTS OF LV RELAXATION AND FILLING

LV relaxation is an active, energy-dependent process that begins with the decay of force-generating capacity, follows the completion of the ejection phase of systole, and continues through isovolumic pressure decline and the rapid filling phase. LV filling is dependent both on active relaxation and on the recoil/suction that results from the release of potential energy stored during systole by contraction. Thus blood is effectively pulled into the left ventricle.[19] In normal hearts, over a range of normal heart rates, relaxation and recoil are adequate to allow LA pressures to remain normal. In addition, catecholamine-induced enhancement of relaxation and recoil during exercise lowers LV pressures in early diastole, thereby increasing the LA-to-LV pressure gradient without increasing LA pressures as well as enhancing filling during exercise. By contrast, in patients with HFpEF, relaxation and recoil are abnormal at rest and are not enhanced during increased HR or exercise. As a result, filling can be maintained only by increased LA pressure; blood must be pushed into the left ventricle.

Relaxation and filling can be assessed using measurements of LV diastolic pressure and LV volume using invasive and/or noninvasive methods to measure:

Rate of isovolumic relaxation: peak $(-)dP/dt$, the time constant of the isovolumic LV pressure decay (τ) and the isovolumic relaxation time (IVRT). When relaxation rate is decreased,
$(-)dP/dt$ and τ are increased (Fig. 2.4).

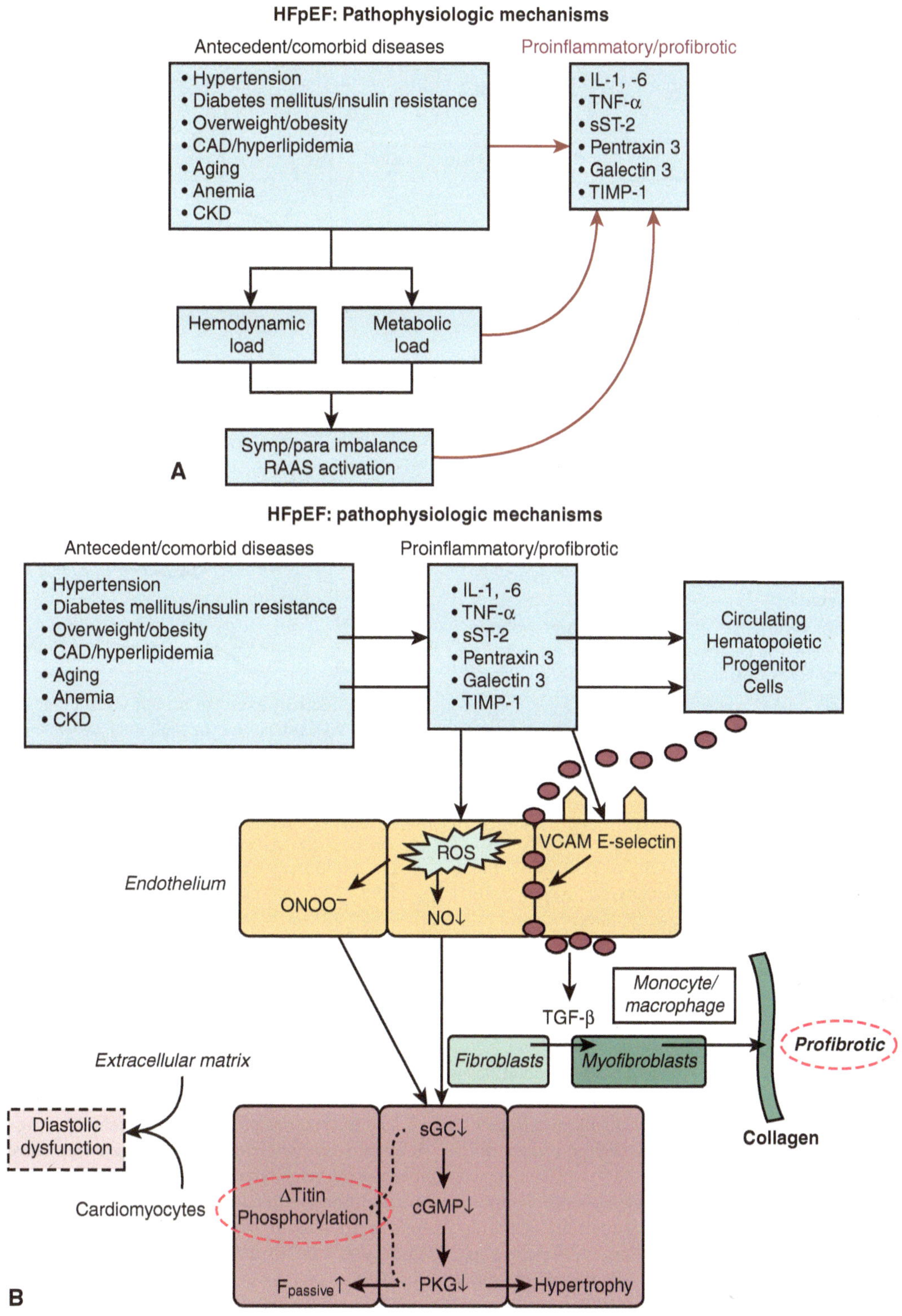

Fig. 2.1 Pathophysiologic mechanisms underlying the development of HFpEF. (A) Antecedent and comorbid diseases create both a hemodynamic and metabolic load that causes sympathetic and renin-angiotensin-aldosterone activation *(RAAS)* and parasympathetic activation. These factors create a proinflammatory and profibrotic milieu as evidenced by changes in typical circulating biomarkers (such as soluble ST-2 and TIMP-1). *CAD,* Coronary artery disease; *CKD,* chronic kidney disease; *TIMP,* tissue inhibitor of metalloproteinase; IL-1, Interleukin-1; IL-6, Interleukin-6; TNF-alpha, Tumor necrosis factor - alpha. (B) Proinflammatory and profibrotic signaling effects recruitment of circulating hematopoietic progenitor cells, alters endothelial function, increases reactive oxygen species *(ROS)*, all of which in turn alters the extracellular matrix (ECM) homeostasis that favors fibrosis and promotes abnormal cardiomyocyte function, including abnormal calcium and energetic regulation, myofilament structure and function, and intracellular signaling. In aggregate, these changes in the ECM and cardiomyocyte result in abnormal diastolic function and promote the development of HFpEF. *VCAM,* Vascular cell adhesion molecule sGC, soluble guanylate cyclase; cGMP, cyclic guanosine monophosphate; PKG, protein kinase G; TGF-beta, transforming growth factor- beta; NO, nitric oxide; ONOO-, peroxynitrite; IL-1, Interleukin-1; IL-6, Interleukin-6; TNF-alpha, Tumor necrosis factor - alpha. (Modified and reproduced with permission from Paulus WJ, Tschöpe C. A novel paradigm for heart failure with preserved ejection fraction: comorbidities drive myocardial dysfunction and remodeling through coronary microvascular endothelial inflammation. *J Am Coll Cardiol.* 2013;62:263–271.)

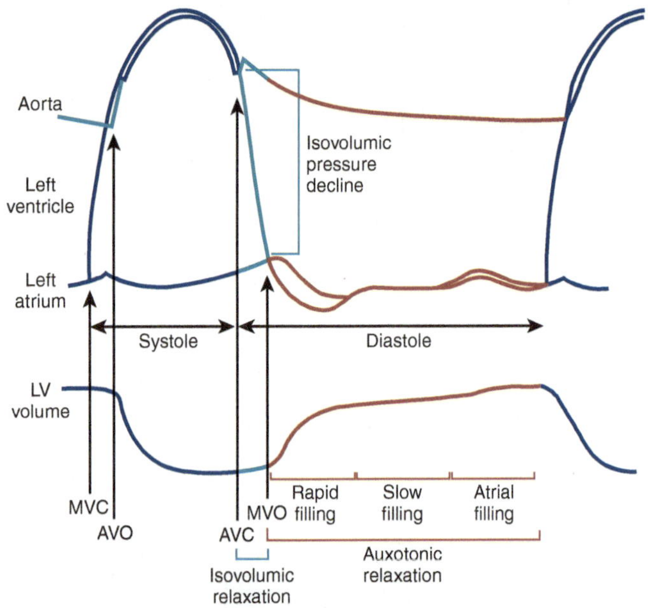

Fig. 2.2 Changes in left ventricular *(LV)* pressure and volume throughout the cardiac cycle. The cardiac cycle is divided into systole, the time period from mitral valve closure *(MVC)* to aortic valve closure *(AVC)*, and diastole. Diastole is further divided into isovolumic relaxation (the time period from AVC to mitral valve opening *[MVO]*, during which LV pressure declines with no change in volume) and auxotonic relaxation (the time period from MVO to MVC during which LV volume increases at variable pressure). *AVO*, Aortic valve opening.

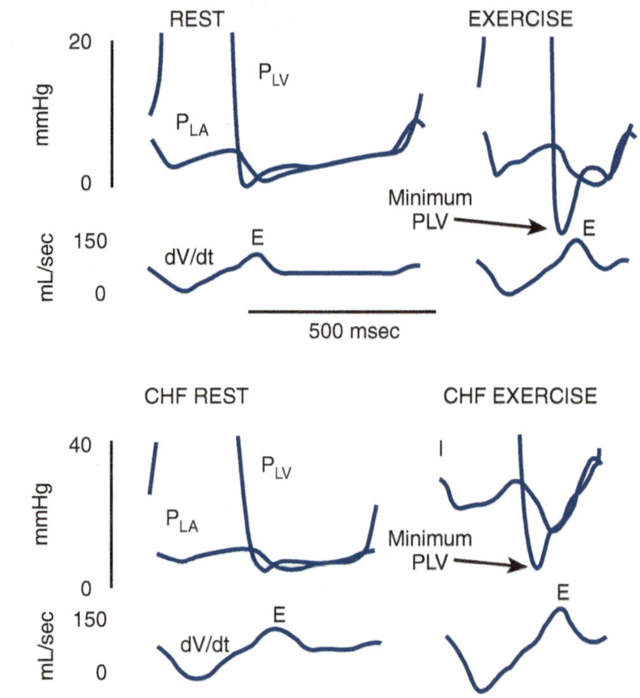

Fig. 2.3 Effects of exercise on left ventricular *(LV)* filling dynamics. Changes in LV pressure *(PLV)*, left atrial pressure *(PLA)*, and the rate of change of PLV (dV/dt) at rest and during exercise. *Top panel:* During exercise in normals, minimal PLV decreases without any change in PLA, leading to an increase in the peak mitral valve gradient and producing a higher peak filling rate (E). *Bottom panel:* In chronic heart failure *(panel B)*, the peak LV filling rate (E) increases during exercise due to an increase in the early transmitral valve pressure gradient. However, the gradient is produced by an increase in left atrial pressure instead of a reduction in PLV as occurs in normals. (Reproduced with permission from Cheng CP, Igarash Y, Little WC. Mechanism of augmented rate of left ventricle filling during exercise. *Circ Res.* 1992;70:9–19.)

Rate and extent of LV filling: filling rate, the time-to-peak filling rate (TPFR), transmitral flow velocity, tissue velocity, strain, and strain rate. When there is prolonged relaxation, early filling rate and extent are decreased, TPFR is prolonged, and the filling rate and extent that result from atrial contraction are increased (Fig. 2.5).

Isovolumic Pressure Decline

The time course of isovolumetric pressure decline has been quantitatively described by the peak rate of pressure fall (dP/dt min) and the time constant τ (tau) of the exponential fall in LV isovolumetric pressure. Each of these requires that LV pressure be measured using a micromanometer-tipped catheter.

dP/dt min measures the rate of pressure decline at a single point in time, is strongly influenced by the LV pressure at the time of aortic valve closure, and therefore like all indices of diastolic function, is afterload-dependent. Patients with HFpEF have a larger dP/dt min, signifying that relaxation rate is decreased.

The time constant τ describes the rate of LV pressure decline throughout isovolumic relaxation. Pressure (P) and time (t) data during the period from end systole (aortic valve closure) to the onset of LV filling (mitral valve opening) are fit to an exponential equation such as the following: LV pressure $= P_0e^{-t/\tau}$, where P_0 is LV pressure at end ejection and τ is the exponential time constant. The larger the value of τ, the longer it takes for the LV pressure to fall, and the more impaired is relaxation. A normal value for τ is less than 40 msec in most age groups, suggesting that relaxation is nearly complete by $3.5 \times \tau$ (<140 msec).

The IVRT also can be estimated by echo techniques as the time between aortic valve closure and mitral valve opening. Although less precise than τ, IVRT is useful in the noninvasive assessment of diastolic properties. However, IVRT depends not only on the rate of LV relaxation but also on the aortic pressure at the time of aortic valve closure and the LA pressure at mitral valve opening. Thus IVRT can be increased by an elevation of aortic pressure or decreased by an increase in LA pressure.

The time course of LV pressure decline during isovolumetric relaxation can also be characterized using noninvasive Doppler measurement of the velocity of a regurgitant jet across the mitral valve. In this method, the modified Bernoulli equation is used to approximate LV pressure during isovolumetric relaxation, allowing calculation of the maximum rate of LV pressure decline and the exponential time constant.

LV Filling

The normal left ventricle has a characteristic pattern of filling and inflow velocities. LV inflow velocity and the rate of LV filling are greatest early (E) in diastole (see Chapters 5, 9 and 17), immediately after mitral valve opening, and are responsible for the normally tall E wave of the transmitral inflow Doppler echocardiogram (echo) (Fig. 2.6). Since most atrial-to-ventricular transfer of blood occurs in early and mid-diastole, the amount of blood transported by atrial contraction is relatively small, the velocity imparted by the atrial contraction (the A wave of the transmitral inflow Doppler echo) is relatively low, and the normal E/A wave ratio is greater than 1 and approaches a value of 2 in younger individuals.

Doppler echo assessment of LV filling has limitations, since diastolic filling parameters are influenced by multiple factors, the most

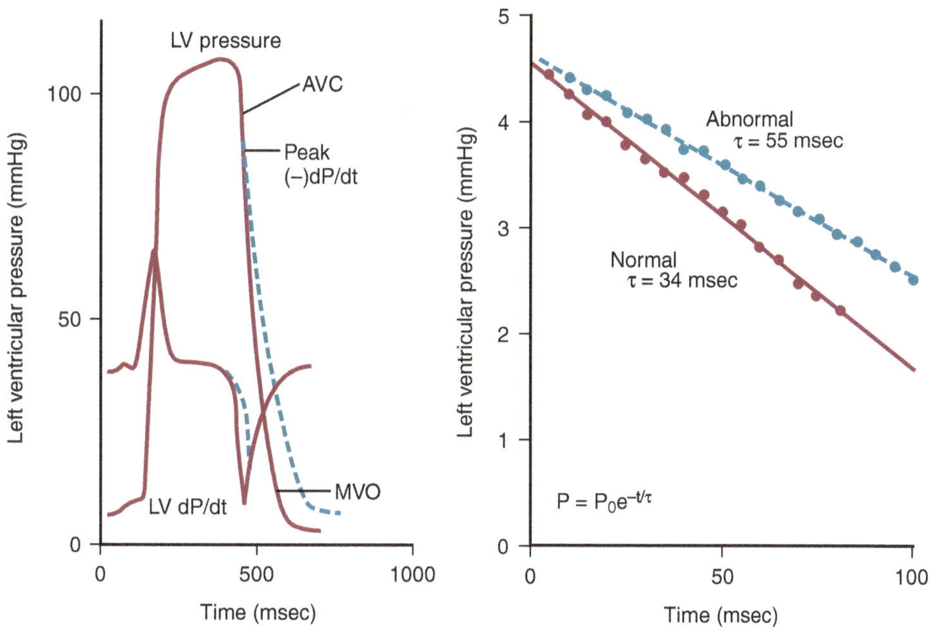

Fig. 2.4 Left ventricular *(LV)* isovolumic relaxation. LV pressure versus time and the rate of change of LV pressure (dP/dt) in a normal subject *(solid line)* versus a patient with heart failure with preserved ejection fraction (HFpEF, *dashed line*) *(left panel)*. Isovolumic relaxation can be quantified by calculating the peak instantaneous rate of LV pressure decline (peak −dP/dt) and the time constant of LV isovolumic pressure decline (τ). When the natural log of LV diastolic pressure is plotted versus time, τ equals the slope of this linear relationship *(right panel)*. Stated in more conceptual terms, τ is the time required for LV pressure to fall by approximately two-thirds of its initial value. When isovolumic relaxation is abnormal, LV pressure decline is slower, (−)dP/dt has a more negative value and the time constant τ is prolonged, and its numerical value is increased *(depicted by the dashed lines in both figure panels)*.

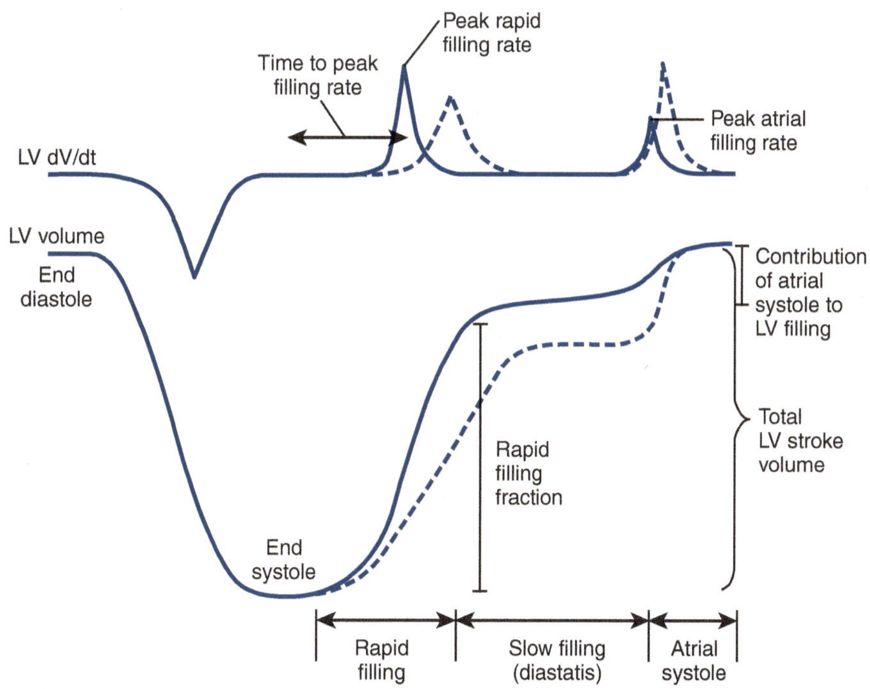

Fig. 2.5 Left ventricular *(LV)* filling dynamics. LV volume versus time and the rate of change of LV volume (dV/dt) in a normal subject *(solid line)* versus a patient with heart failure with preserved ejection fraction (HFpEF, *dashed line*). With the onset of systole, the LV volume decreases and reaches its minimum at the end systole. Diastolic filling has three distinct phases: rapid filling phase during which the LV fills rapidly, dV/dt reaches it maximum, and the peak filling rate occurs; slow filling phase (diastasis), during which there is little change in LV volume; and atrial systole phase during which active atrial contraction fills the left ventricle and allows it to attain its end-diastolic volume. Important diastolic parameters include the peak filling rate, the time-to-peak filling rate, the rapid filling fraction (percent of total stroke volume reached during rapid filling), and the percent contribution of atrial systole to LV filling.

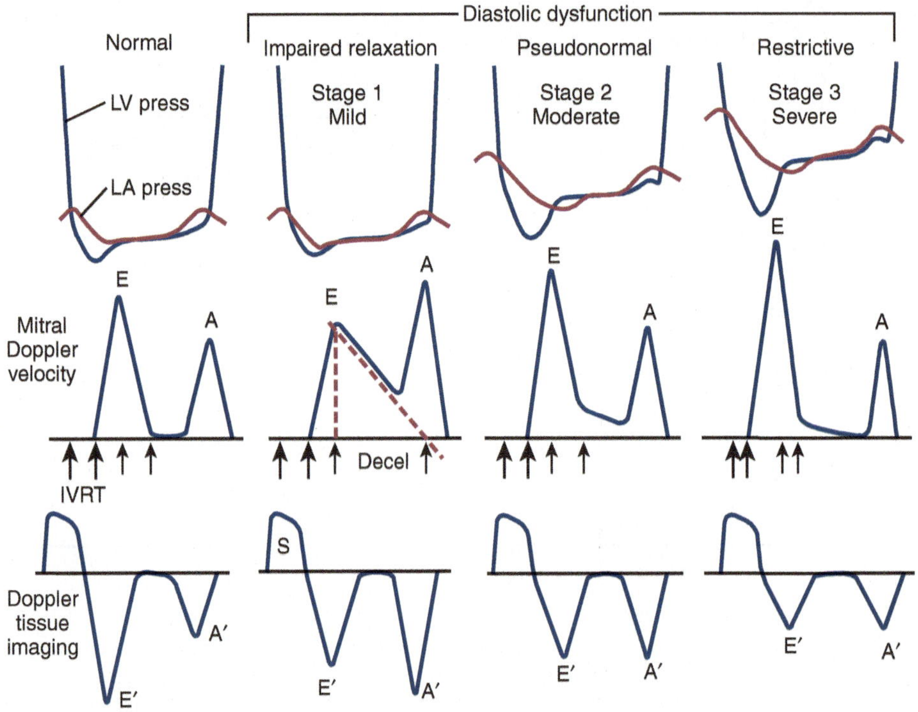

Fig. 2.6 Doppler findings in heart failure with preserved ejection fraction (HFpEF). Schematic representation of left ventricular *(LV)* and left atrial *(LA)* pressures during diastole *(top panel)*, transmittal Doppler LV inflow velocity *(middle panel)*, and Doppler tissue velocity *(bottom panel)* in normals and in different types of diastolic dysfunction. E indicates peak early diastolic flow velocity; A, peak late diastolic flow velocity caused by atrial contraction; E Decel, E wave diastolic deceleration time; S, myocardial velocity during systole; E′, myocardial velocity during early filling; A′, myocardial velocity during filling produced by atrial contraction. This schema divides patients into four filling patterns: (1) normal pattern of relaxation and filling *(column 1 far left)*, (2) impaired relaxation or type I mild diastolic dysfunction, (3) pseudonormal relaxation or type II moderate diastolic dysfunction, and (4) restrictive filling pattern or type III severe diastolic dysfunction. Patients with an impaired filling pattern have a reduced peak early diastolic flow velocity (E), a prolonged E wave diastolic deceleration time of early diastolic filling (E Decel), and an increased peak diastolic flow velocity with atrial contraction (A). Pseudonormal filling pattern is denoted by an increased E wave in the face of a decreased E′. A restrictive filling pattern is denoted by an even larger E wave and even smaller E′, with a shortened isovolumic relaxation time *(IVRT)* and a decreased E Decel time. (Reproduced with permission from Zile MR, Brutsaert DL. New concepts in diastolic dysfunction and heart failure with a preserved ejection fraction: part I: diagnosis, prognosis, and measurements of diastolic function. *Circulation.* 2002;105:1387–1393. Copyright © 2002 Lippincott Williams & Wilkins.)

important of which are loading conditions. The typical, but nonspecific, mitral filling pattern associated with diastolic dysfunction (termed *abnormal relaxation*) is a pattern of increased isovolumic relaxation time and decreased E/A ratio. However, this pattern can be altered or pseudonormalized by changes in LA pressure. When diastolic dysfunction occurs, relaxation is slowed and incomplete, early LV diastolic pressures rise, early diastolic suction falls, and LV filling becomes increasingly dependent on an increase in LA pressure to push blood into the left ventricle during diastole. As LA pressures rise, the value of the E wave increases, and E/A increases to a pseudonormal value. When LA pressures are severely increased, a restrictive pattern may develop in which the isovolumic relaxation time may be decreased and the E/A ratio is further increased. Doppler echo techniques help distinguish these three patterns of abnormal LV filling.

When transmitral Doppler flow patterns are examined in concert with tissue Doppler echo techniques, patterns of normal versus impaired relaxation versus pseudonormal versus restriction can be determined because tissue Doppler provides independent information about LV relaxation properties. Other complementary techniques that are useful to estimate LV filling pressure and the LA–LV diastolic pressure gradient include measuring pulmonary venous flow velocity, tissue Doppler myocardial velocity, strain and strain rate, and color M-mode flow acceleration patterns. In particular, myocardial velocity measures made by tissue Doppler imaging (TDI) appear less sensitive to alteration in LV loading conditions. The TDI peak early diastolic mitral annular velocity (e′) measures the rate of early diastolic myocardial lengthening and, when combined with transmitral Doppler E wave data, can be used to estimate pulmonary capillary wedge pressure (PCWP) = 2 + 1.3 (E/e′) (see Chapter 13).

Recoil and Suction

During systole, potential energy is stored in the elastic elements of the cardiomyocytes and extracellular matrix (ECM).[20] The elastic elements are compressed and twisted during systolic contraction. During relaxation, this potential energy is released as the elastic elements recoil and return to their original length and orientation. Recoil causes LV pressure to fall rapidly during isovolumetric relaxation. Furthermore, for the first 30 to 40 msec after mitral valve opening, the relaxation of LV wall tension normally is rapid enough to cause LV pressure to continue to decline despite an increase in LV volume. This fall in LV pressure produces an early diastolic pressure gradient from the LA that extends to the LV apex. This accelerates blood out of the LA and produces rapid early diastolic flow that quickly propagates to the apex. Because the diastolic intraventricular pressure gradient pulls blood to the apex, it can be considered a measure of LV suction. It is reduced in both experimental models and in patients with ischemia, hypertrophic cardiomyopathy,[19] and HF, including HFpEF.[21–23] The intraventricular pressure gradient can be measured noninvasively from the diastolic spatial-temporal velocity map obtained using apical color M-mode echo (see Chapter 11).

Because the LV apex remains fixed during the cardiac cycle, the mitral annular velocity provides a measure of the long-axis lengthening rate.[24] Under normal conditions, e′ occurs coincidentally with or before the mitral E.[25,26] This is a manifestation of the symmetric expansion of the left ventricle in early diastole as blood moves rapidly to the LV apex in response to a progressive pressure gradient from the left atrium to the LV apex. In addition, the rapid recoil of the mitral annulus and valve into the left atrium early in diastole relocates blood from the left atrium into the left ventricle. Under normal circumstances, both E and e′ respond to changes in the LA-to-LV pressure gradient. For example, both E and e′ normally increase in response to increased volume load and exercise.[26–28]

The extent to which contraction creates potential energy that subsequently is realized during diastole as recoil and is reflected by measures of systolic strain and strain rate measured in the long or circumferential axis. In symptomatic HFpEF, systolic strain and strain rate are commonly abnormal; however, this abnormality in the presence of a normal EF does not alter LV chamber systolic pump performance (at least at rest) but does decrease recoil/suction during diastole. Thus while abnormalities in systolic strain and strain rate occur in systole, their consequent effects are most important during diastole and primarily effect diastolic function in HFpEF patients.

PATHOPHYSIOLOGIC DETERMINANTS OF LV RELAXATION AND FILLING

LV relaxation and filling are under the control of multiple factors that include hemodynamic load (early diastolic load and afterload), myofiber inactivation, and the uniformity of the distribution of load and inactivation in space and time (dyssynchrony, dyssynergy, treppe). Each of these determinants may affect indices of diastolic relaxation, recoil, and filling.

Hemodynamic Load

Both isovolumic pressure decline and early filling are affected by afterload (LV systolic stress). An increase in LV systolic stress results in a delay in and slowed rate of pressure decline and early filling. Increases in systolic load may have different effects, depending on when the load is imposed during systole. Increases in LV pressure late in systole hasten the onset of LV relaxation, but relaxation occurs at a slower rate (increased τ). Increases in LV pressure late in systole occur with aging because of age-related vascular stiffening, which alters the timing of the reflected pressure wave in the vascular tree so that the reflected wave arrives in late systole rather than diastole. In clinical practice, an acute increase in blood pressure either at rest or during exercise will impair ejection, slow pressure decline, prolong time to complete relaxation, and reduce recoil. These changes in relaxation decrease the LA-to-LV gradient, decrease early filling, and result in increased LV diastolic and LA pressure. In addition, the load present at the time of mitral valve opening (LA-to-LV gradient) (i.e., early diastolic load) affects early LV filling.

Heterogeneity

Synchrony (timing of relaxation of the different myocardial segments) and synergy (extent to which myocardial segments relax) will enhance LV relaxation, whereas dyssynchrony or dyssynergy (e.g., caused by infarction, ischemia, asymmetry of hypertrophy, or conduction abnormalities) will impair global LV relaxation. Dyssynchrony, measured using a variety of echo measurements, may be present in patients with HFpEF, particularly those with left bundle branch block (LBBB) or right ventricular (RV) pacing.[29] Whether treatment aimed at resynchronization (i.e., cardiac resynchronization therapy) will affect clinical improvement in patients with HFpEF has not been fully investigated.

Cardiomyocyte Inactivation

Myofiber inactivation refers to the many cellular processes that ultimately influence the process by which the left ventricle, its constitutive cardiomyocytes, and individual sarcomeres return to a normal end-diastolic length with minimum cross-bridge cycling and low force generation. To accomplish this state of complete relaxation requires: (1) calcium resequestration into the sarcoplasmic reticulum, followed by calcium extrusion into the extracellular space; (2) availability of sufficient adenosine triphosphate (ATP); (3) normal myofilament function; and (4) normal elastic properties of the cardiomyocyte and the ECM.

MEASUREMENT OF LV DIASTOLIC STIFFNESS, COMPLIANCE, DISTENSIBILITY, AND PRESSURE

Chamber Stiffness

The passive characteristics of the left ventricle during diastole can be described by the passive diastolic pressure-volume relationship (DPVR).[7,19] Optimally, this relationship should be constructed from points that are obtained after relaxation is complete and at slow filling rates, so that viscous effects are not present. In practice, this can be approximated using points obtained late in diastole, when relaxation is assumed to be complete, by correcting pressure data affected by incomplete relaxation[7] or by using data from variably loaded beats at end diastole. The resultant DPVR is nonlinear and can be approximated by an exponential function. LV stiffness is defined as the ratio of LV diastolic pressure and LV diastolic volume (LV dP/dV) at any given LV diastolic volume. LV compliance is the reciprocal of stiffness (LV dV/dP). Because the DPVR can be approximated as an exponential, stiffness will increase as the left ventricle fills to higher LV diastolic volumes; thus as the left ventricle fills, it becomes stiffer. LV diastolic distensibility is defined as the end-diastolic pressure required to distend the left ventricle to an end-diastolic volume. Patients with HFpEF have reduced distensibility, indicated by a normal or reduced end-diastolic volume and an elevated end-diastolic pressure.[3–9,30] Because the DPVR can be approximated by an exponential function, its position and shape can be described by the constants within an equation such as the following: $P = \alpha \times e\beta V$, where α and β represent the stiffness constants. It should be recognized that β does not indicate stiffness but instead describes how rapidly stiffness increased with increases in volume ($\beta = [dP/dV]/V$). The stiffness constants derived in this fashion can be used to compare passive diastolic properties in different patients or patient groups. The end-diastolic pressure-vs.-volume ratio (instantaneous operative distensibility) also can be used in comparing patients or patient groups. Patients with HFpEF have abnormal DPVRs with elevated β and abnormal distensibility (Fig. 2.7).

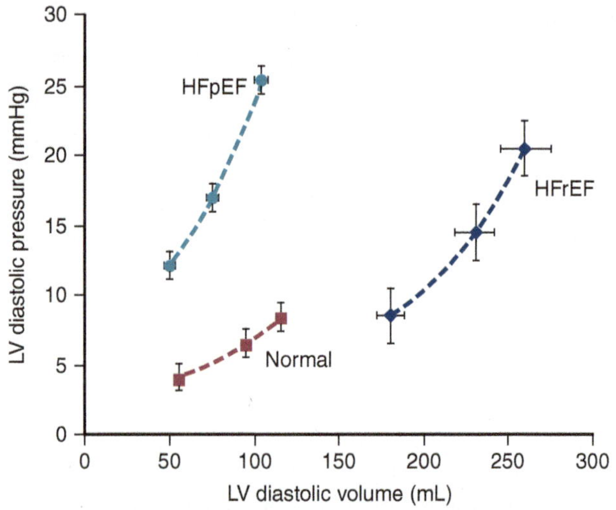

Fig. 2.7 Diastolic pressure versus volume relationships in chronic heart failure patients. Difference in diastolic chamber distensibility in patients with heart failure with preserved ejection fraction (HFpEF) *(red)* versus HF with reduced EF *(HFrEF) (black)* versus age-matched and gender-matched referent controls *(green)*. Compared with that in the controls, the diastolic pressure-volume relationship (DPVR) in patients with HFpEF is shifted upward and to the left, such that for any given left ventricular *(LV)* volume, pressure is higher in HFpEF, indicating decreased distensibility (increased stiffness). By contrast, in patients with HFrEF, the DPVR is shifted to the right, indicating increased distensibility. (Reproduced with permission from Zile MR, Baicu CF, Gaasch WH. Diastolic heart failure—abnormalities in active relaxation and passive stiffness of the left ventricle. *N Engl J Med.* 2004;350:1953–1959; Aurigemma GP, Zile MR, Gaasch WH. Contractile behavior in the left ventricle in diastolic heart failure: with emphasis on regional systolic function. *Circulation* 2006;113:296–304.)

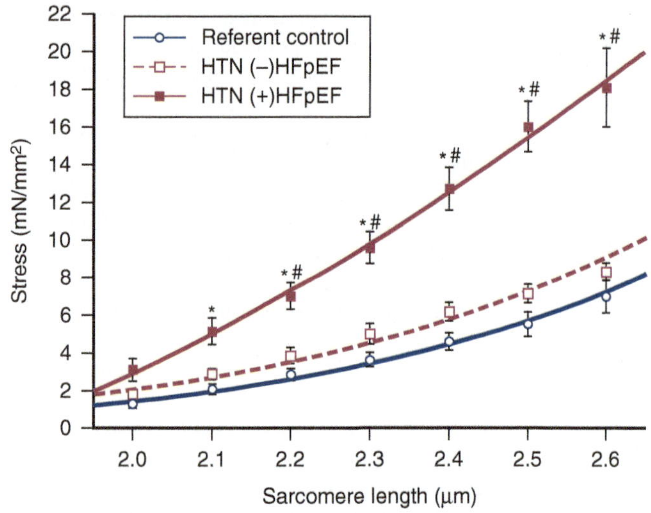

Fig. 2.8 Contributions of changes in collagen and titin to the increased myocardial stiffness in heart failure with preserved ejection fraction *(HFpEF)* patients. Total myocardial stiffness expressed as the relationship between myocardial stress versus cardiomyocyte sarcomere length for referent control patients *(open circle, solid blue line)*, patients with hypertension, but without heart failure and a preserved ejection fraction (HTN(−)HFpEF, *closed circle, dashed red line*), and patients with hypertension and HFpEF (HTN(+)HFpEF, *closed squares, solid red line*). As sarcomere length increases, the slope increases most rapidly in the HTN(+)HFpEF group. Patients with HTN(+)HFpEF had an increase in total myocardial stiffness as indicated by a leftward shift in the stress versus sarcomere length relationship. There were no significant differences between HTN(−)HFpEF versus referent control patients; hypertension in the absence of HFpEF did not alter passive myocardial stiffness. *, # = $p < 0.01$ versus referent control and HTN(−)HFpEF. (Reproduced with permission from Zile MR, Baicu CF, Ikonomidis JS, et al. Myocardial stiffness in patients with heart failure and a preserved ejection fraction: contributions of collagen and titin. *Circulation.* 2015;131(14):1247–1259.)

Myocardial Stiffness

Two of the determinants associated with an upward and leftward shift of the DPRV in patients with HFpEF are (1) the presence of LV and cardiomyocyte concentric remodeling and hypertrophy and (2) changes in the material properties of the myocardial muscle itself (i.e., myocardial stiffness). Myocardial diastolic stiffness can be determined by assessing the myocardial diastolic LV stress-versus-strain relationship. The stress-strain relationship represents the resistance of the myocardium to stretch (increase in length) when subjected to stress (distending force). Calculation of stress requires the use of a geometric model of the LV, and the calculation of strain requires assumption of the unstressed LV volume, which cannot be directly measured in the intact circulation. In addition to these potential theoretical limitations, these calculations require accurate measurements over a wide range of LV pressures, volumes, dimensions, and wall thicknesses. These challenges in determining myocardial stress-strain relationships have limited their clinical application, but they remain important to basic and translational research efforts. Recently, techniques have been developed that allow assessment of myocardial stiffness and determination of the mechanisms that alter myocardial stiffness to be examined using LV myocardial biopsies in patients with clinical heart disease and patients with HFpEF. These translational studies examined the contribution that changes in the cardiac ECM (such as fibrillar collagen and cardiomyocyte cellular structure) and processes (such as calcium homeostasis, energetics, and myofilament and cytoskeletal proteins such as titin and microtubules) make to the abnormalities in myocardial stiffness present in patients with HFpEF (Fig. 2.8).[18]

PATHOPHYSIOLOGIC DETERMINANTS OF DIASTOLIC STIFFNESS

Myocardial Versus Extramyocardial Processes Effecting Diastolic Stiffness

Patients with HF and an increased LV diastolic pressure can be divided into four groups defined by patterns of DPVR (Fig. 2.9).[31] DPVR in patients with HFrEF typically is characterized by the graphed curve D in Fig. 2.9, in which eccentric remodeling results in a shift of the DPVR to the right, representing an increase in distensibility. It should be recognized that although the ventricle is more distensible, the LV end-diastolic volume in these patients typically is very large, and the end-diastolic stiffness in the operating region is high. DPVR in patients with HFpEF may be characterized by curves A to C in Fig. 2.9. Pericardial constraint causes a parallel upward shift in the DPVR. In patients with HFpEF, when relaxation is markedly prolonged and diastole is abbreviated, LV diastolic pressure falls throughout diastole but remains increased. In the most prevalent pattern in HFpEF, the DPVR is shifted upward and to the left, indicating reduced distensibility, where LV pressure is increased at any LV volume.

Cardiomyocyte

The significant abnormalities in LV diastolic function observed at the chamber level are paralleled by the abnormalities in cardiomyocyte

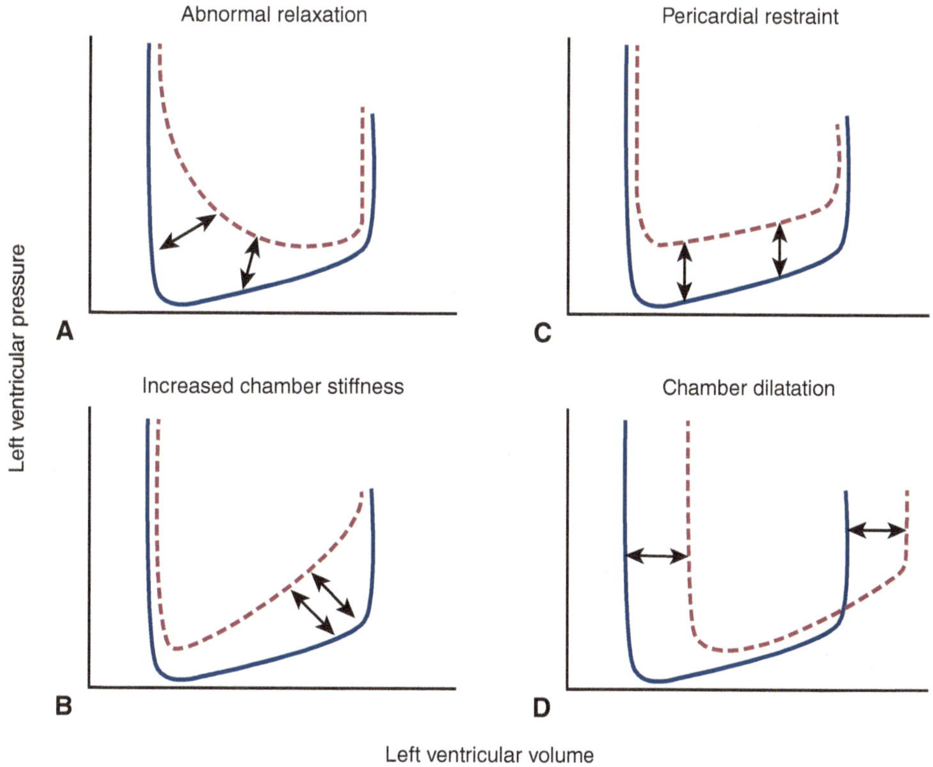

Fig. 2.9 Mechanisms that result in increased left ventricular (LV) diastolic pressure. Among patients with heart failure and an increased LV diastolic pressure, four patterns of a diastolic pressure-volume relationship (DPVR) can be discerned. DPVR in patients with HFpEF may be characterized by graphed curves (A) and (B). In the most prevalent pattern in HFpEF, represented by curve (B), the DPVR is shifted upward and to the left, indicating reduced distensibility, where LV pressure is increased at any LV volume. In patients with HFpEF, when relaxation is markedly prolonged and diastole is abbreviated, as shown in curve (A), LV diastolic pressure falls throughout diastole but remains increased. In curve (C), pericardial constraint causes a parallel upward shift in the DPVR. DPVR in patients with HFrEF typically is characterized by curve (D), in which eccentric remodeling results in a shift of the DPVR to the right, representing an increase in distensibility. It should be recognized that although the ventricle is more distensible, the end-diastolic volume in these patients typically is very large and the end-diastolic stiffness in the operating region is high. (Reproduced with permission from Carroll JD, Lang RM, Neumann AL, et al. The differential effects of positive inotropic and vasodilator therapy on diastolic properties in patients with congestive cardiomyopathy. *Circulation.* 1986;74:815–825.)

diastolic function observed at the cellular level. Cardiomyocyte diastolic function was directly addressed in two studies in which patients with HFpEF underwent endomyocardial biopsy, and single cardiomyocytes were isolated to assess cellular diastolic performance.[32] The cardiomyocytes had an increased resting tension in the absence of calcium that was almost twice as high as control cardiomyocytes. These in vitro cell data corresponded to an in vivo increase in LV end-diastolic pressure in these patients with HFpEF. These data indicate that cardiomyocytes from patients with HFpEF have increased cardiomyocyte stiffness and decreased distensibility compared with normal cardiomyocytes. Therefore these clinical studies, along with studies using animal models of HFpEF, showed that there are clear parallels in the abnormalities in diastolic function between the LV chamber and individual cardiac muscle cells, which constitute the myocardium.

Changes in myofilament proteins, extramyofilament proteins, and proteins that govern calcium homeostasis and myocardial energetics can contribute to the development of diastolic dysfunction and increased diastolic stiffness. These factors are discussed in more detail in other chapters. One particularly important myofilament protein that has been examined in clinical studies in HFpEF patients and may prove to be an important therapeutic target is the giant myocardial protein titin that spans the Z-lines and serves as a molecular spring that resists distension, thereby contributing to LV stiffness. A number of factors, including titin isoform switches (to a less compliant N2B isoform) and titin phosphorylation state, affect diastolic stiffness. Such alterations in titin phosphorylation are present in HFpEF contributing to increased LV diastolic stiffness.[33,34] These changes in titin phosphorylation are not present in patients with antecedent disease processes such as hypertensive heart disease alone but develop only after patients make the transition to HFpEF.[18] Interaction of titin with other signaling molecules and with ion channels also may contribute to diastolic stiffness. The role of alterations in titin and the interactions of titin with the ECM in patients with HFpEF constitute an important area of investigation. In addition to titin, other cardiomyocyte structural proteins and changes in their phosphorylation state may affect diastolic stiffness. These include changes in myosin-binding proteins, microtubules, and others.

Extracellular Matrix

The ECM consists of fibrillar proteins, including collagen type I and type III, elastin, and proteoglycans; basement membrane proteins such as collagen type IV, laminin, and fibronectin; and a large number of bioactive peptides and proteins such as matrix metalloproteinases (MMPs), tissue inhibitors of metalloproteinases (TIMPs), and signaling

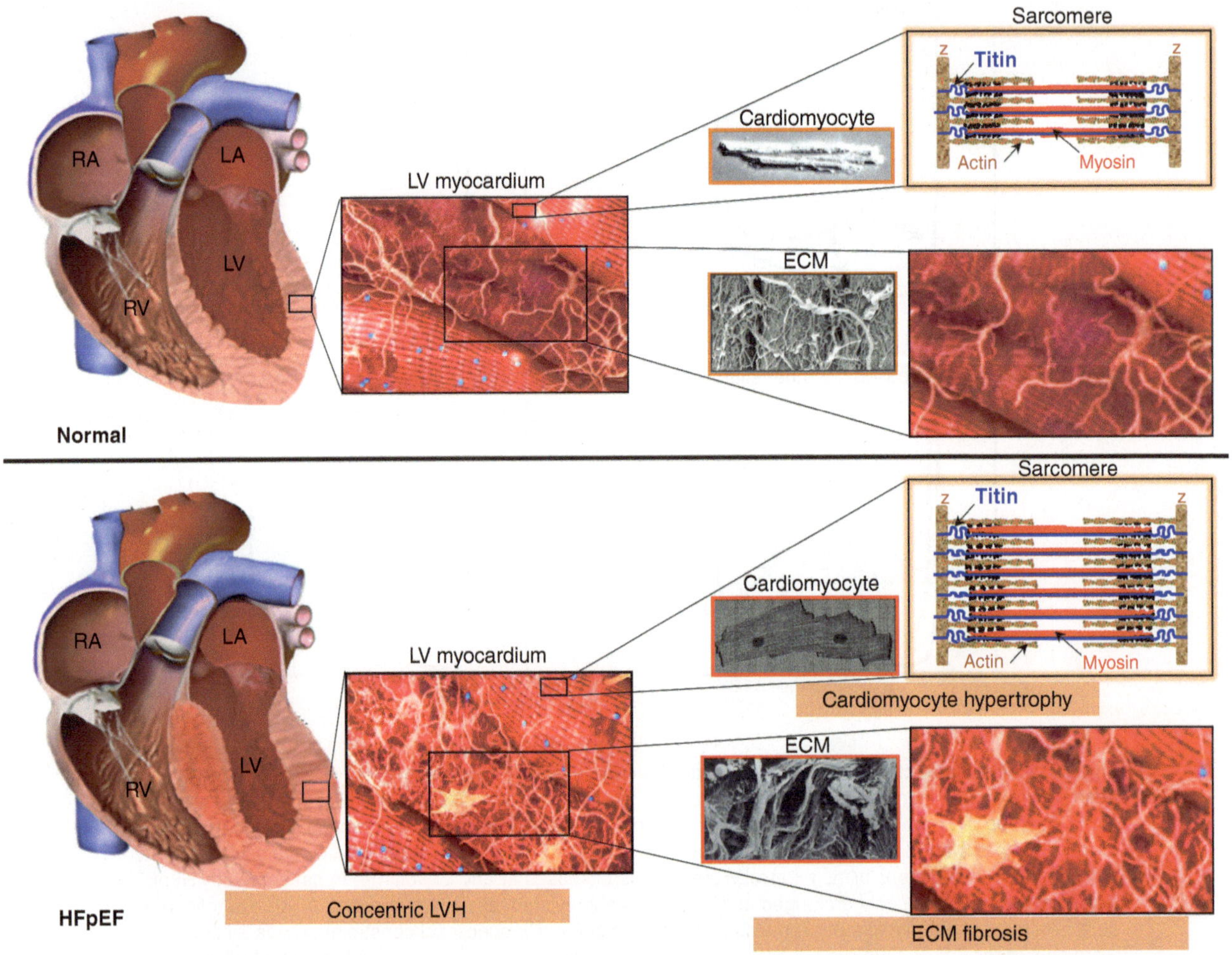

Fig. 2.10 Ventricular, cellular, extracellular matrix *(ECM)*, and molecular structural changes in patients with heart failure with preserved ejection fraction (HFpEF). Compared with age-matched and gender-matched normal controls *(upper panel)*, HFpEF patients *(lower panel)* are characterized frequently by concentric hypertrophy or remodeling at the left ventricular *(LV)* and cardiomyocyte level. The left ventricle is increased in wall thickness with no change in volume; cardiomyocytes have increased diameter but no change in length. These structural cellular changes are accompanied by alterations in titin phosphorylation. In addition, there are structural changes in the ECM, including increased fibrillar collagen content, thickness, and number. These ECM structural changes are associated with alterations in fibroblast function that lead to interstitial fibrosis. *LA*, Left atrium; *LVH*, LV hypertrophy; *RA*, right atrium; *RV*, right ventricle. (Modified and reproduced with permission from Aurigemma GP, Zile MR, Gaasch WH. Contractile behavior in the left ventricle in diastolic heart failure: with emphasis on regional systolic function. *Circulation*. 2006;113:296–304; Zile MR, Baicu CF, Ikonomidis JS, et al. Myocardial stiffness in patients with heart failure and a preserved ejection fraction: contributions of collagen and titin. *Circulation*. 2015;131:1247–1259.)

proteins such as transforming growth factor-β (TGF-β) and cytokines. The myocardial collagen network is composed of endomysial fibers surrounding individual myocytes and capillaries; perimysial fibers, which interweave muscle bundles; and epimysial fibers, which form a matrix adjacent to the epicardial and endocardial surfaces. ECM structure is dynamic and regulated by physical, neurohormonal, and inflammatory mediators. These modulate the four steps in collagen homeostasis: collagen synthesis, postsynthetic processing, posttranslational crosslinking, and degradation.[35–38] The ECM fibrillar collagen content is increased in patients with HFpEF (Fig. 2.10; also see Fig. 2.8). These changes in fibrillar collagen are not present in patients with antecedent disease processes such as hypertensive heart disease alone but develop only after patients make the transition to HFpEF (see Fig. 2.10).[18] Experimental studies have shown that acute degradation of collagen fibers by collagenase perfusion or activation of MMPs results in decreased LV stiffness. Animal models have demonstrated that interventions associated with increases or decreases in myocardial fibrosis are associated with increased or decreased LV diastolic stiffness. Thus evidence that the ECM can contribute to diastolic dysfunction by increasing diastolic stiffness or contributing to impairment in relaxation by altering regional loading or uniformity is strong and supports the potential therapeutic strategy of preventing or reducing fibrosis in the therapy of HFpEF.

ABNORMAL DIASTOLIC FUNCTION LIMITS EXERCISE IN HFpEF

Abnormal diastolic dysfunction during exercise represents important mechanisms that result in exercise dyspnea and limitations in exercise tolerance. A normal response to exercise requires a significant (severalfold) increase in cardiac output to meet the enhanced needs of

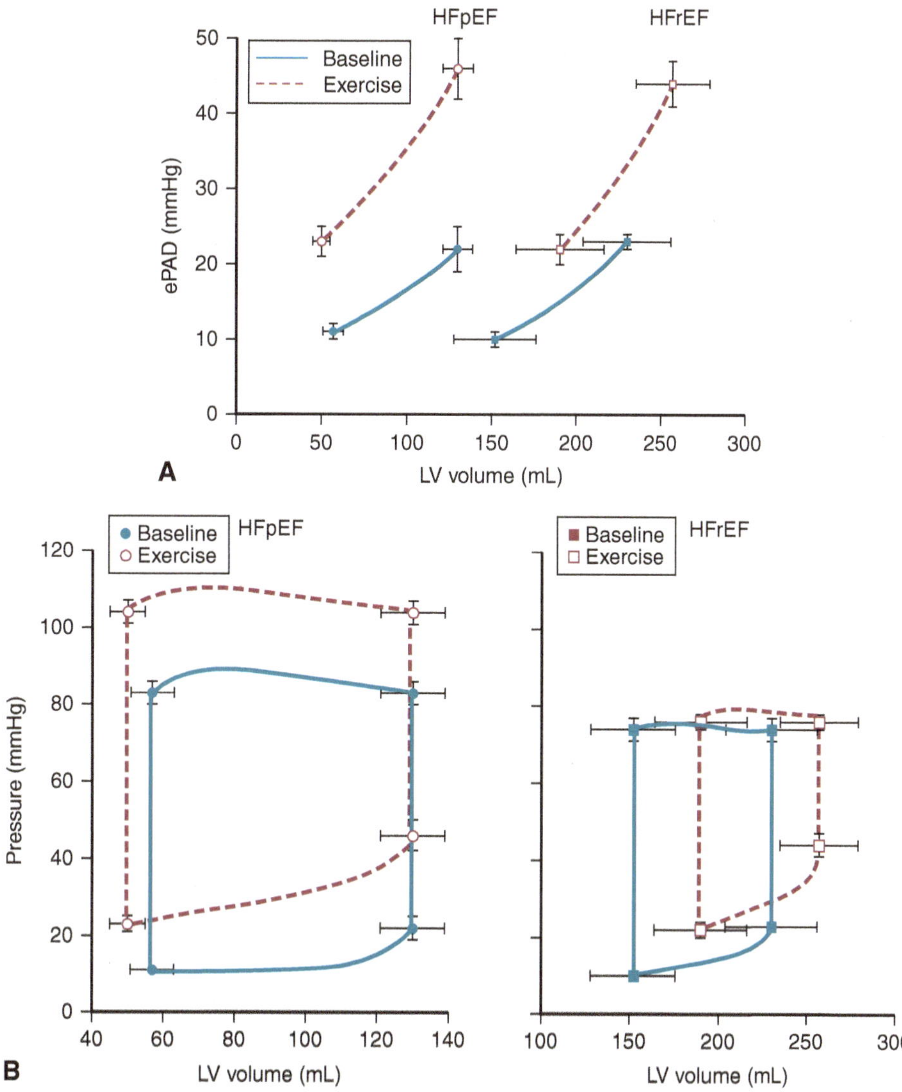

Fig. 2.11 Pressure versus volume response to exercise. (A) Diastolic pressure versus volume data during diastole in patients with heart failure and a preserved ejection fraction (HFpEF; *circles*) versus patients with heart failure and a reduced ejection fraction (HFrEF; *squares*) at baseline *(solid lines)* and during exercise *(dashed lines)*. Estimated pulmonary artery diastolic pressure (ePAD) increased during exercise in all patients with heart failure; and pressure increased without an increase in LV diastolic volume in HFpEF, but with an increase in left ventricular (LV) diastolic volume in HFrEF. Data points = Mean ± SE. Connecting lines between data points were stylized curved lines rather than straight lines. (B) Pressure versus volume throughout the cardiac cycle in patients with heart failure and a preserved ejection fraction (HFpEF; *circles*) versus patients with heart failure and a reduced ejection fraction (HFrEF; *squares*) at baseline *(solid lines)* and during exercise *(dashed lines)*. Data points = Mean ± SE. Connecting lines between data points were stylized curved lines rather than straight lines. *LV,* Left ventricular. (Reproduced with permission from Zile MR, Kjellstrom B, Bennett T, et al. Effects of exercise on left ventricular systolic and diastolic properties in patients with heart failure and a preserved ejection fraction versus heart failure and a reduced ejection fraction. *Circ Heart Fail.* 2013;6:508–516.)

exercising muscle. Multiple factors contribute to this normal response: an increase in heart rate and stroke volume, a reduction in peripheral vascular resistance, an increase in LV relaxation rate, filling rate and diastolic suction, a reduction in early diastolic pressure, and no significant change in LV diastolic pressure. In HFpEF patients, abnormalities in all of these mechanisms, particularly those in diastole, conspire to limit exercise tolerance and cause exercise dyspnea.

HFpEF patients have an increased incidence of chronotropic incompetence, which severely limits their ability to increase heart rate (and cardiac output) during exercise. In addition, the passive diastolic material properties of the left ventricle in HFpEF patients (evidenced by increased LV stiffness) prevents the recruitment of Starling forces by increased LV end-diastolic volume and prevents increased stroke volume (and cardiac output) during exercise (Figs. 2.11 and 2.12).[39,40] Abnormalities in several cellular and myocardial diastolic mechanisms result in significantly increased LV diastolic pressures during exercise in HFpEF patients (Fig. 2.13).[41]

To increase LV diastolic filling rates, there must be a corresponding increase in the transmitral diastolic pressure gradient. In normal patients, this is accomplished by exercise-induced enhancement of diastolic recoil

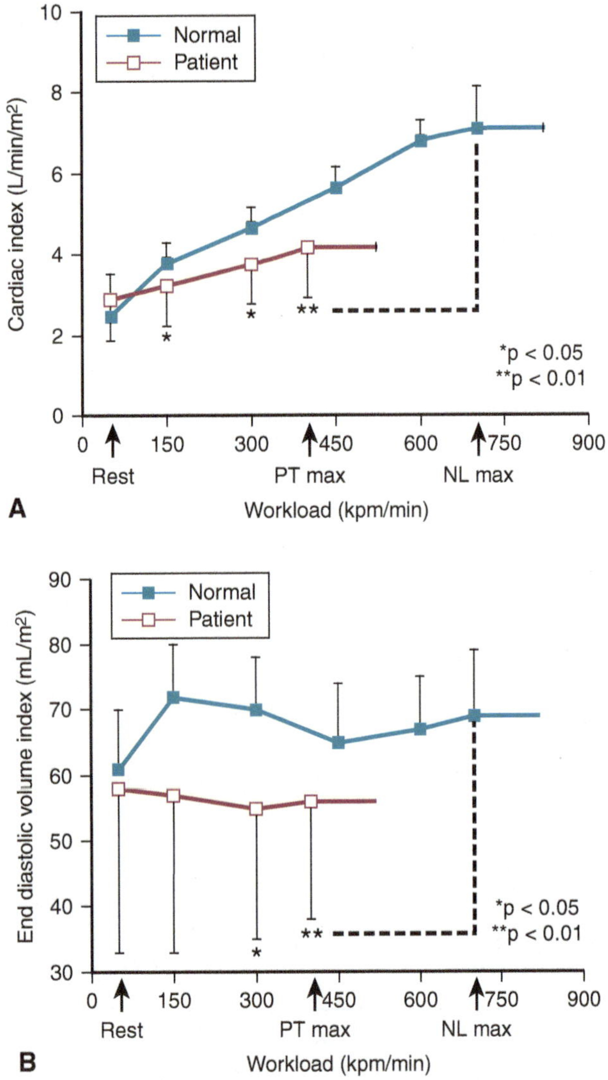

Fig. 2.12 Cardiac index and end-diastolic volume response to exercise. (A) In HFpEF patients, exercise-induced increases in cardiac output are severely limited in part because these patients are not able to recruit Starling forces. (B) HFpEF patients have a decreased ability to recruit Starling forces because increased LV diastolic stiffness only allows negligible increases in end-diastolic volume. (Reproduced with permission from Kitzman DW, Higginbotham MB, Cobb FR, Sheikh KH, Sullivan MJ. Exercise intolerance in patients with heart failure and preserved left ventricular systolic function: failure of the Frank-Starling mechanism. *J Am Coll Cardiol.* 1991;17:1065–1072.)

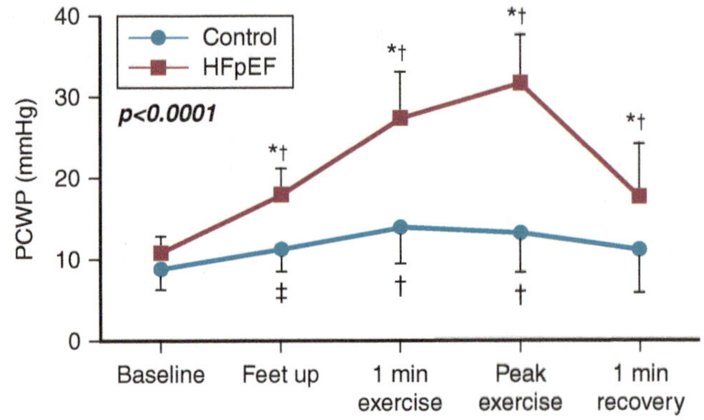

Fig. 2.13 Exercise in HFpEF versus age/gender referent control. Exercise-induced diastolic dysfunction in heart failure with preserved ejection fraction *(HFpEF)* patients using invasive measurement of diastolic function (bicycle ergometry in catheterization lab with right heart catheter in place). Exercise response of pulmonary capillary wedge pressure *(PCWP)* in HFpEF patients *(yellow squares)* versus referent controls *(blue circles)*. (Reproduced with permission from Borlaug BA, Nishimura RA, Sorajja P, et al. Exercise hemodynamics enhance diagnosis of early heart failure with preserved ejection fraction. *Circ Heart Fail.* 2010;3:588–595.)

and relaxation, which results in decreased LV early diastolic pressure creating a relative LV suction effect, which enhances the transmitral pressure gradient without increasing LA pressure. These changes do not happen in HFpEF patients (see Fig. 2.3).[42–45]

During exercise in HFpEF patients, myocardial relaxation is not properly enhanced because there are abnormalities in calcium homeostasis. These include decreased rate of calcium uptake by the sarcoplasmic reticulum (SR), decreased cyclic adenosine monophosphate (cAMP) generated by the β-adrenergic response to exercise, and abnormal phosphorylation of the regulatory SR membrane protein phospholamban, which all lead to the decrease of the rate of calcium uptake by the SR during diastole. These abnormalities in relaxation together with less augmentation in systolic shortening (less of a decrease in end-systolic volume, less of an increase in systolic strain) lead to a reduction in restoring forces, recoil, and suction.

The tachycardia itself (even though it may be blunted in many HFpEF patients) contributes to the rise in LV diastolic pressures and diastolic stiffness. With increased heart rates diastole is shorter, the time for filling reduced, and filling rates must be augmented. This only happens in HFpEF patients at the cost of markedly increased diastolic pressures. In addition, treppe (force-frequency) relationships are abnormal in HFpEF. In normal patients, the relationship between the heart rate (or frequency of contraction) and LV pressure (or systolic force development) and ejection fraction (or shortening) is associated with an increase in stroke volume over a physiologic range of heart rate. In addition, the same mechanism governs the relationship between heart rate and diastolic relaxation rate, where increased heart rate in a normal heart is associated with an increased relaxation rate, which in part allows LV diastolic pressures and PCWP to remain normal during exercise. However, in HFpEF, this treppe relationship is abnormal, with increased heart rates leading to increased diastolic pressures over physiologic heart rate ranges.

In summary, the normal heart during exercise has an elegant balance of physiologic mechanisms to ensure that cardiac input keeps pace with cardiac output, with preservation of a low pulmonary capillary pressure. These mechanisms result in an increase in measured LV distensibility, as manifested by a downward shift of the LV diastolic P-V curve, especially during early diastole.[46,47] The opposite occurs in HFpEF. HFpEF patients are not able to increase LV end-diastolic volume, recruit Frank-Starling forces, increase relaxation rate, or increase filling rate. Consequently, exercise results in a marked increase in diastolic pressure, a limited ability to increase cardiac output, and marked truncation of exercise capacity. These abnormal responses to exercise are made worse by the exaggerated increase in arterial blood pressure that frequently accompanies exercise in most patients with HFpEF.

ABNORMAL DIASTOLIC FUNCTION CAUSES ACUTE DECOMPENSATED HFpEF

Acute decompensated heart failure (ADHF) occurs frequently in HFpEF patients; requires urgent treatment in the hospital, emergency

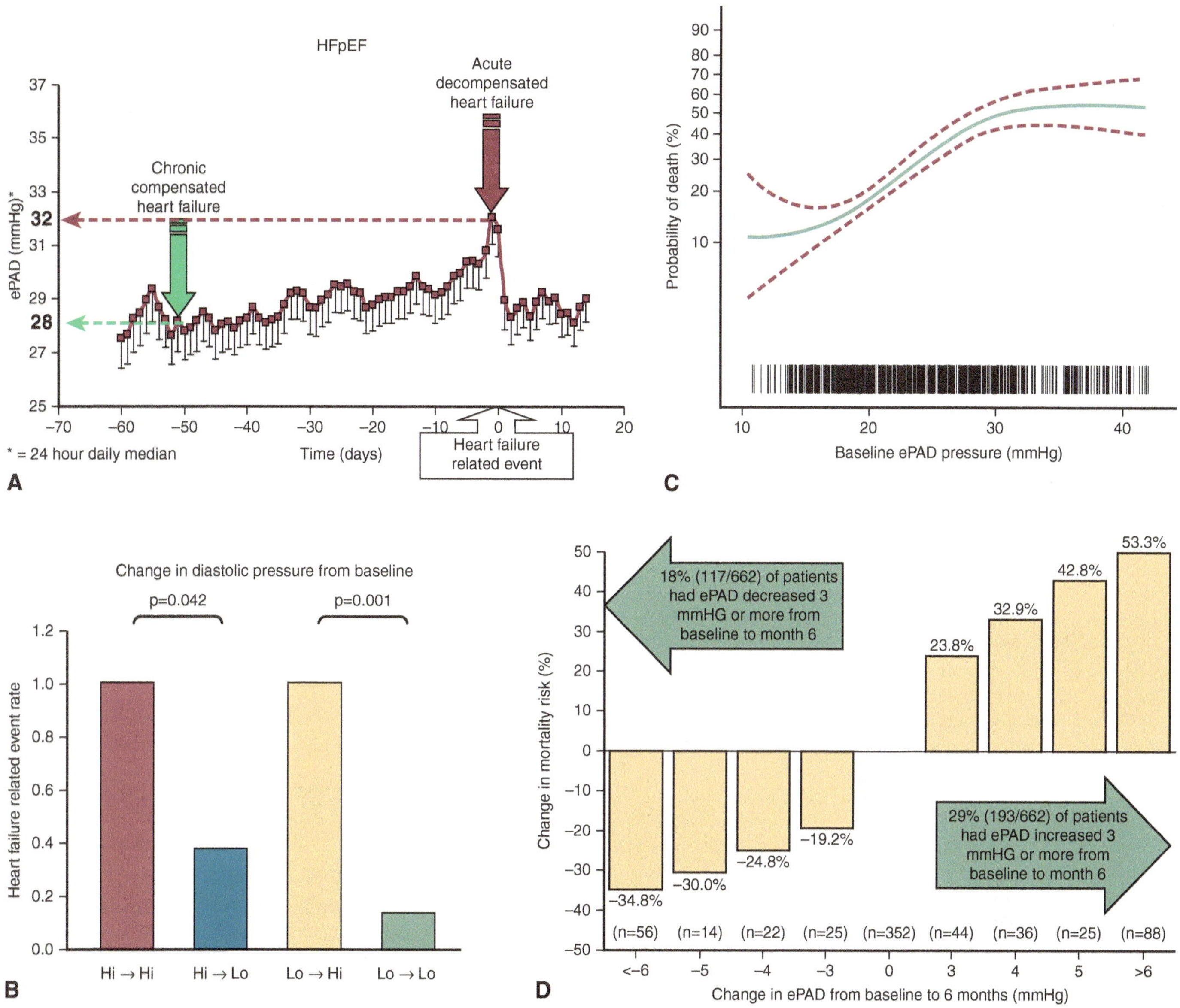

Fig. 2.14 Left ventricular (LV) diastolic pressures in heart failure with preserved ejection fraction *(HFpEF)* patients predict mortal and morbid events. (A) Patients with HFpEF have increased LV diastolic pressure (indexed here as *ePAD,* estimated pulmonary artery diastolic pressure) even when considered in good compensation by their physician and experience further increases in pressure with the development of acute decompensated heart failure (ADHF) necessitating hospital admission. (B) Both baseline LV diastolic filling pressure and changes in filling pressure are sensitive predictors of future ADHF events. (C, D) Both baseline LV diastolic filling pressure and changes in filling pressure are sensitive predictors of all-cause mortality. (A, Reproduced with permission from Zile MR, Bennett TD, St John Sutton M, et al. Transition from chronic compensated to acute decompensated heart failure: pathophysiological insights obtained from continuous monitoring of intracardiac pressures. *Circulation.* 2008;118:1433–41. B, Reproduced with permission from Stevenson LW, Zile M, Bennett TD, et al. Chronic ambulatory intracardiac pressures and future heart failure events. *Circ Heart Fail.* 2010;3:580. C and D, Reproduced with permission from Zile MR, Bennett TD, Hajj SE, et al. Intracardiac pressures measured using an implantable hemodynamic monitor: relationship to mortality in patients with chronic heart failure. *Circ Heart Fail.* 2017;10(1):e003594.)

department, or outpatient office setting; and is associated with increased mortality. A majority of patients hospitalized for ADHF have preexisting heart failure, and recurrent hospitalizations are frequent (50% in 6 months after initial hospitalization); however, some patients with HFpEF may be minimally symptomatic between episodes of ADHF or have significant movement in New York Heart Association (NYHA) class. In 85% or more of HFpEF patients, ADHF is due to volume overload that accompanies increases in LV diastolic filling pressure (Fig. 2.14A).[48] The time course of ADHF is acute only from the point of view of significant changes in symptoms. Changes in diastolic pressures begin from an elevated value, over a time course of 4 to 8 weeks; they occur in small, steady increases in pressure, and only precipitate symptoms over a few days prior to hospitalization (see Fig. 2.14A). Both baseline LV diastolic filling pressure and changes in filling pressure are sensitive predictors of future ADHF events and mortality (see Fig. 2.14B); treatment/prevention of increased diastolic filling pressures have been shown to reduce HF hospitalization and CV mortality (see Fig. 2.14C and D). ADHF in patients with HFpEF can result from increased filling pressure with or without significant changes in body weight, total blood volume, or LV diastolic volume.[49] In contrast, increased LV diastolic pressure and volume can result from increases in total intravascular volume or shifts of intravascular volume due to splanchnic vasoconstriction.

Acute decompensated HFpEF may be caused by both cardiovascular and noncardiovascular factors/mechanisms (or triggers), which act on the already existing structural and functional abnormalities (or substrate) to precipitate the development of ADHF. The substrate in patients with HFpEF consists of structural remodeling of the LV chamber and of the constituent cardiomyocytes and ECM that compose the chamber. These structural changes are associated with significant abnormalities in LV diastolic function, which worsen during ADHF. The mechanisms responsible for these changes include worsening diastolic dysfunction, increased neurohormonal activation, and poorly controlled comorbid disease. These include uncontrolled arterial hypertension, myocardial ischemia, diabetes mellitus, increased salt and water intake, tachyarrhythmias, chronic renal failure, anemia, and coexistent lung disease.[10,50–54] Atrial arrhythmias can result in loss of atrial function and stimulate compensatory increases in diastolic filling pressure to maintain LV filling and maintain cardiac output. Decreased LV diastolic function and abnormal LA function can result in neurohormonal activation, which plays an important role in ADHF by producing increased sodium and water retention, increased venous return, increased splanchnic tone, and arterial vasoconstriction. These comorbidities act upon the substrate to precipitate ADHF. It should be noted, however, that these triggers, in the absence of this substrate, do not result in ADHF or HFpEF. For example, an increase in salt and water intake in the absence of concentric remodeling or diastolic dysfunction does not result in HFpEF. In patients with HFpEF, arterial hypertension can act on preexisting structural and functional abnormalities to cause deterioration in LV diastolic function and precipitate ADHF. Even after normal volume status is restored and neurohormonal activation is suppressed, the inciting comorbid condition may remain and can influence the subsequent clinical course. This ongoing process may contribute to a high rate of non-HF–related rehospitalizations after a HF episode.

Further changes in diastolic function occur when patients develop decompensated HFpEF. Under these circumstances, the rise in pressure causes a significant change in transmitral Doppler flow pattern (as described earlier). There is pseudonormalization of the ratio of ventricular to atrial filling velocities (E/A ratio) and when atrial pressures are extremely increased, to a frankly restrictive pattern. These changes in relaxation and filling are associated with changes in distensibility. During compensated HFpEF, the LV diastolic pressure-volume relationship is shifted upwards, indicating decreased diastolic distensibility. During the development of decompensated HFpEF initially (during the phase of worsening HFpEF), LV volume may increase along a similar abnormal diastolic pressure volume curve. Later, when acute pulmonary edema develops in decompensated HFpEF, there may be a marked upward shift in the diastolic pressure vs. volume relationship, indicating a further decrease in LV distensibility. Once patients with decompensated HFpEF are adequately treated, for example, with diuretics and nitrates, the LV diastolic pressure volume relationship moves back to the compensated HFpEF state. Even after treatment of ADHF yields a status judged by HF specialists as "compensated" HFpEF (NYHA class II–III), abnormal relaxation, filling, and stiffness persist and lead to persistently increased diastolic pressures (see Fig. 2.14).

PREVALENCE OF DIASTOLIC DYSFUNCTION IN HFpEF

The exact prevalence of abnormalities in diastolic function described earlier has been examined in large epidemiologic and randomized clinical trials; these studies, plus small pathophysiologic studies, suggest that abnormalities in diastolic function are present in nearly all or a substantial plurality (≥2/3) of patients with HFpEF. The frequency distribution of diastolic dysfunction grade, increased peak RV systolic pressure, and LA volume varies according to the characteristics of the population studied, that is, the patient's level of hemodynamic compensation and severity of disease. A truly normal diastolic function profile, however, is uncommon in patients with HFpEF. For example, an abnormal diastolic dysfunction grade was found in 60% to 70% of the patients enrolled in the TOP-CAT, I-Preserve, and CHARM studies; LA enlargement was present in 66%; and either diastolic dysfunction of grade II to IV or LA enlargement was found in 85%.[14–16] The metrics that reflect diastolic function serve as critical components of the diagnostic criteria used to make the diagnosis of HFpEF as described in HF guidelines. There are convincing and robust data that indicate the measures of diastolic function described in this chapter have important prognostic value, which complement clinical, biomarker, or other noninvasive measurements. Both baseline metrics that reflect diastolic function and changes from baseline hold prognostic value.

PROGNOSTIC VALUE OF ABNORMAL DIASTOLIC FUNCTION IN HFpEF

Direct Measures of Diastolic Function

Diastolic filling pressures can be continuously and remotely assessed using implantable hemodynamic monitors (IHM) placed in the pulmonary artery or left atrium; these provide direct measures of diastolic function.[48,55–59] Data derived from these IHMs in HFpEF patients (such as those shown in Fig. 2.14) have provided clear evidence that both baseline and change from baseline values of pulmonary artery diastolic and left atrial pressures have important prognostic value for predicting both HF hospitalizations and cardiovascular mortality (see Fig. 2.14).[60–62] In fact, management strategies based on knowledge of these pressures have been developed that aim to decrease elevated baseline pressure and prevent (or modulate) subsequent increases in pressures that occur over time. This pressure-based management strategy has been demonstrated to reduce morbidity and mortality and improve symptom status.[63–66]

Indirect Measures of Diastolic Function

Knowledge of LV diastolic pressure in patients with known or suspected HFpEF is important for establishing diagnosis, predicting prognosis, and directing therapy. However, because direct measures of diastolic pressure are invasive and not suitable for all patients and all situations, noninvasive echo and echo Doppler measurements that reflect diastolic function and diastolic pressure have been developed and clinically applied. The measurements used in the diastolic grading system have prognostic value and can be used to estimate LV diastolic filling pressures and to follow the progression of disease and response to therapy (Fig. 2.15).[14,15] Pseudonormalized and restrictive filling

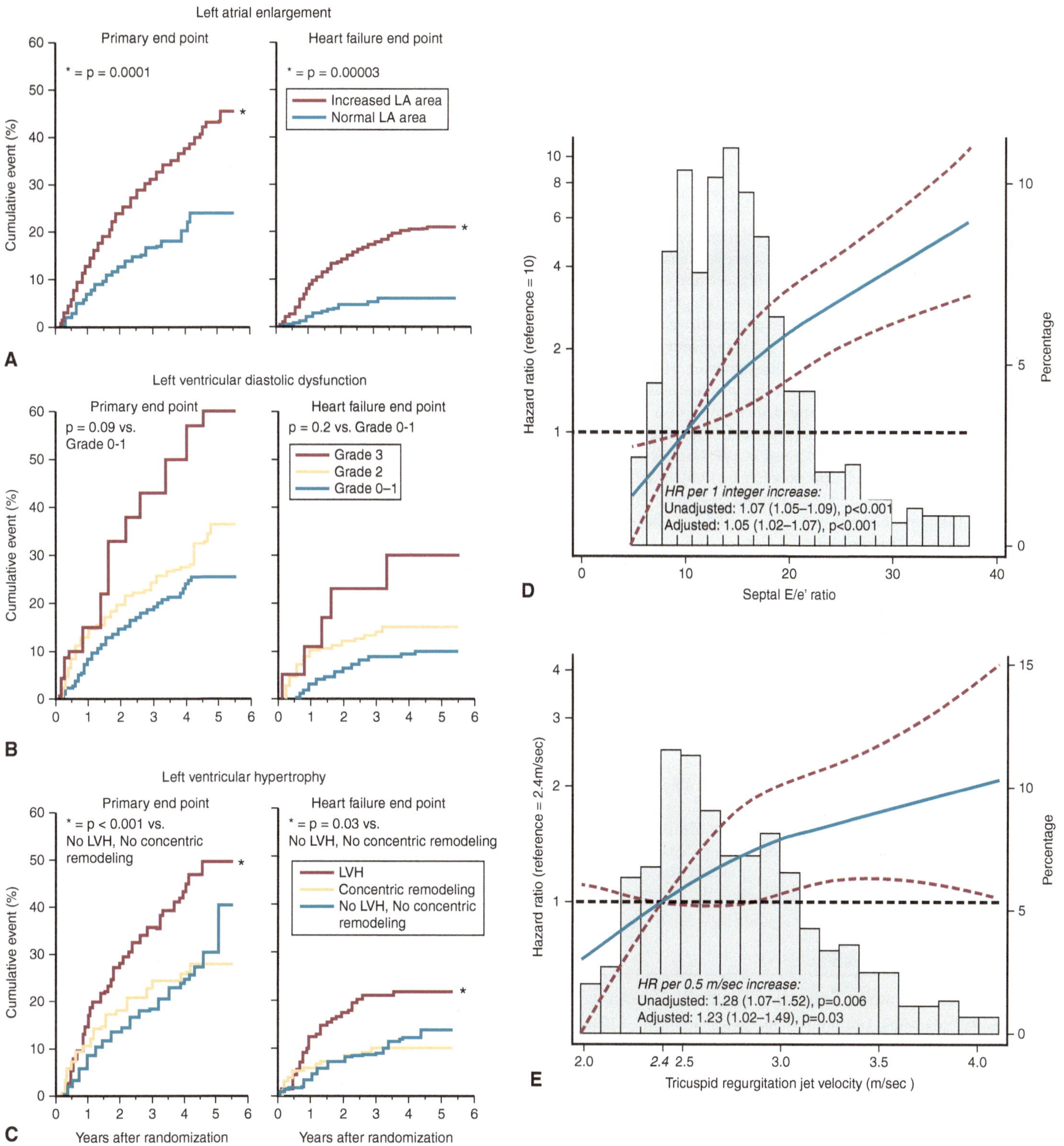

Fig. 2.15 Noninvasive echocardiographic predictors of clinical outcome in HFpEF patients. (A–C) The presence of an increased left atrial *(LA)* area was associated with increased cumulative event rate of the primary study end point (A) in patients with HFpEF. The presence of diastolic dysfunction grade 3 increased the cumulative event rate of the primary study end point (B) in patients with HFpEF. The presence of left ventricular hypertrophy *(LVH)* was associated with an increased cumulative event rate of the primary study end point (C) in patients with HFpEF. (D, E) Restricted cubic spline analysis demonstrating the unadjusted hazard ratio *(HR)* for the primary composite end point of heart failure (HF) hospitalization, aborted cardiac arrest, or cardiovascular death associated with (D) septal E/E′ ratio (n = 502), and (E) peak tricuspid regurgitation jet velocity (n = 450). *P for nonlinearity <0.05. Values presented are a linear approximation. Histograms demonstrate the distribution of each measure in the study population. Multivariable analysis is adjusted for age, sex, race, randomization strata (prior HF hospitalization or biomarker criteria), region of enrollment (Americas vs. Russia or Georgia), randomized treatment assignment, core laboratory left ventricular ejection fraction, history of atrial fibrillation, heart rate, New York Heart Association class, history of stroke, creatinine, and hematocrit. (Reproduced with permission from Zile MR, Gottdiener JS, Hetzel SJ, et al. for the I-PRESERVE Investigators. Prevalence and significance of alterations in cardiac structure and function in patients with heart failure and a preserved ejection fraction. *Circulation.* 2011;124:2491–2501; Shah AM, Claggett B, Sweitzer NK, et al. Cardiac structure and function and prognosis in heart failure with preserved ejection fraction: findings from the echocardiographic study of the Treatment of Preserved Cardiac Function Heart Failure with an Aldosterone Antagonist [TOPCAT] trial. *Circ Heart Fail.* 2014;7:740–751.)

patterns indicate the presence of both diastolic dysfunction and elevated LA pressure. By contrast, the impaired relaxation pattern indicates diastolic dysfunction without a marked elevation in LA pressure. Echo Doppler estimates of peak RV systolic pressure (PRVSP, from the tricuspid regurgitation velocity) and measurements of LA volume both have prognostic value (see Fig. 2.15). Diastolic dysfunction grade and PRVSP estimate instantaneous diastolic pressure. Changes in LA volume reflect longer term changes in LV filling pressures. LA volume is dependent on the product of diastolic pressure and time, so the longer pressures are increased and the higher they are increased, the larger the LA volume. Increased LA volume is highly prevalent in patients with HFpEF and has significant prognostic value (see Fig. 2.15).

All of the foregoing measures are useful in identifying patients with or without elevations of diastolic filling pressure. However, the most commonly used and easily interpretable parameter is the E/e′ ratio. E/e′ has been found to correlate with PCWPs in a wide range of patients studied in multiple laboratories. An E/e′ greater than 15 has been found to clearly indicate elevated PCWP, whereas E/e′ less than 8 is associated with normal LA pressure (see Fig. 2.6). In some situations, however, E/e′ may not provide an accurate assessment of PCWP. The clinical settings in which this application of E/e' may be inaccurate are well described in Chapter 13.

There are other indirect measures of diastolic function that should be considered; these include peripheral biomarkers (discussed here) and sensor technology (discussed later in the chapter).[67–73] Both are critical components of HFpEF diagnostic criteria, have significant prognostic value, and may serve as important targets of management. The best studied peripheral biomarkers in HFpEF are the natriuretic peptides (NPs), both BNP and NT-proBNP. There is a direct correlation between BNP/NT-proBNP and LV end-diastolic wall stress (and its component determinants, including LV diastolic pressure). Both baseline NPs and change from baseline values have significant prognostic value in HFpEF patients and predict both morbidity and mortality (Fig. 2.16).[67] Other biomarkers, such as sST-2, galectin-3, collagen propeptides and teleopeptides, and MMPs and TIMPs, may also reflect at least some of the underlying pathophysiologic changes seen in HFpEF, such as myocardial fibrosis (see Chapter 29). However, their roles in diagnostic criteria and prognosis are yet to be fully defined.

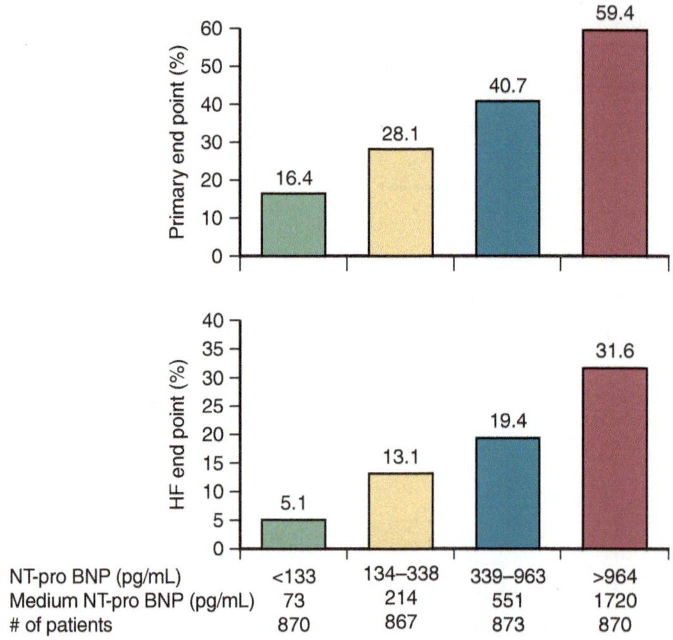

Fig. 2.16 Relationship between NT-proBNP and clinical outcomes in HFpEF patients. Crude event rates for the primary composite outcome *(top panel)* and HF composite outcome *(bottom panel)* by quartile of baseline NT-proBNP. *HF,* Heart failure; *NT-proBNP,* N-terminal pro-brain natriuretic peptide. (Reproduced with permission from Anand IS, Rector TS, Cleland JG, et al. Prognostic value of baseline plasma amino-terminal pro-brain natriuretic peptide and its interactions with irbesartan treatment effects in patients with heart failure and preserved ejection fraction: findings from the I-PRESERVE trial. *Circ HF.* 2011;4:569–577.)

FUTURE DIRECTIONS

Composite Measures Reflecting Diastolic Function

Wearable, cutaneous, and implantable sensor technology have been developed that can provide measurements that reflect baseline and change from baseline values of diastolic function and pressure. Both individual measurements and a composite of multiple measurements have been shown to provide diagnostic and prognostic utility.[72,73] For example, impedance measured in the intravascular and extravascular space has been shown to reflect changes in volume status and has prognostic value in HFpEF, predicting both morbidity and mortality (Fig. 2.17). When impedance is combined in a multisensory analytic array, the resultant composite metric score has acceptable predictive value for HF hospitalizations. The sensor-based metrics that are combined in this composite score include such measurements as heart rate, atrial fibrillation detection and duration, heart rate variability, position, activity, third and fourth heart sounds, impedance, and respiratory rate. In HFpEF patients that make the transition from compensated to decompensated heart failure, the time versus risk score pattern is very similar to the time versus filling pressure pattern, strongly suggesting that the risk score value closely reflects changes in diastolic function and pressure (Fig. 2.18).

Direct Measurements of Diastolic Function as a Target for Management of HFpEF

Increased diastolic filling pressures at rest and/or during exertion are one principle pathophysiologic cause of the symptoms present in HFpEF patients. Therefore lowering these pressures and/or preventing their rise over time should represent important targets for management strategies to improve symptom status and reduce morbidity and mortality in HFpEF. Management using IHM-guided therapy that directly targeted lowering LV diastolic filling pressures has been demonstrated to reduce morbidity and mortality and improve functional status.[64–66] Implantation of interatrial septostomy devices has also reduced exercise-induced diastolic filling pressures and improved symptom status in proof of concept studies; pivotal studies are ongoing.[74,75]

Composite Measurements Reflecting Diastolic Functions as a Target for Management of HFpEF

Several sensor-based technologies provide measurements that change in relation to changes in LV diastolic filling pressures. These include intravascular and extravascular impedance, activity, third heart sound S3, position, respiratory rate, and other measures.[72,73] When used individually (such as impedance) or as a risk composite (HeartLogic, triage HF) to facilitate management of increased diastolic filling pressures, it is expected that this management scheme will improve symptoms and facilitate management strategies that reduce the risk of morbidity and mortality. This is a fertile area for technology development and application to clinical utility.

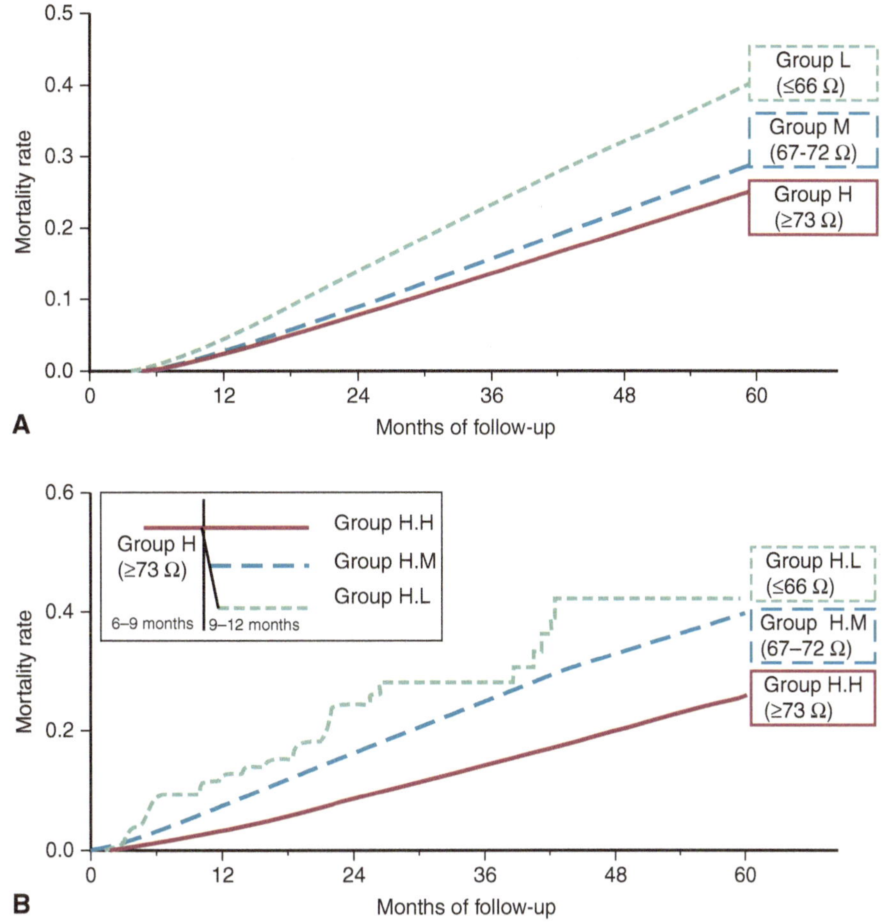

Fig. 2.17 Prognostic value of baseline impedance and change from baseline in predicting mortality. (A) Kaplan-Meier estimate of all-cause mortality in the primary mortality analysis. Patients were divided into tertiles based on average baseline measured impedance from 6 to 9 months after implantation: Group L measured impedance ≤65 ohms; group M, 66 to 72 ohms; and group H, ≥73 ohms. (B) Kaplan-Meier estimate of all-cause mortality in the secondary mortality analysis for patients with changes in baseline measured impedance of ≥73 ohms. Decreased measured impedance resulted in increased mortality (group H.L vs. H.M and H.H). (Reproduced with permission from Zile MR, Sharma V, Johnson JW, et al. Prediction of all-cause mortality based on the direct measurement of intrathoracic impedance. *Circ Heart Fail.* 2016;9 (1):e002543.)

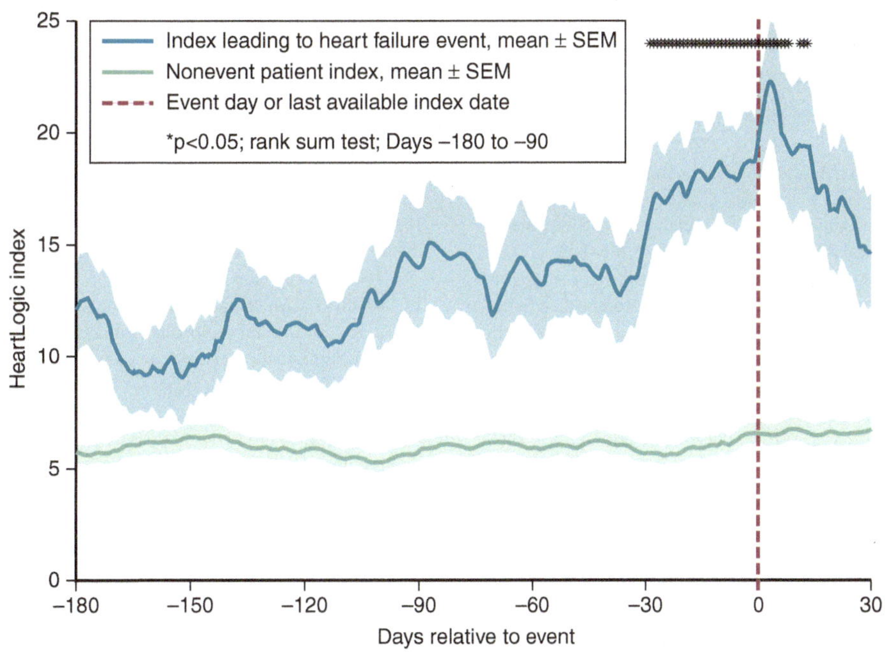

Fig. 2.18 Prognostic value of multisensor-based risk score. Multisensor-based composite risk score (HeartLogic index) in patients with usable heart failure events (HFE, *blue line*) aligned by the date of the HFE *(vertical line)* at day 0; HeartLogic index in patients without HFE *(black line)* aligned by the last available HeartLogic index date for each patient (day 30). Days related to heart failure events (HFEs) with the HeartLogic index are significantly greater ($p < 0.05$, rank sum test) than a 3-month baseline period ending 90 days before the HFE and are indicated by *asterisks*. Data are displayed as mean ± SEM. The *shaded regions* represent the SEM. (Reproduced with permission from Boehmer JP, Hariharan R, Devecchi FG, et al. A multisensor algorithm predicts heart failure events in patients with implanted devices: results from the MultiSENSE study. *JACC-HF* 2017;5:216–225.)

KEY POINTS

- Diastolic dysfunction and HFpEF are not synonymous terms. Diastolic dysfunction indicates a functional abnormality of diastolic relaxation, filling, or distensibility—regardless of the EF or the patient's symptomatic status. HFpEF indicates the presence of clinical HF with a normal EF.
- The relationship between LV diastolic volume and diastolic pressure from mitral valve opening to mitral valve closure defines the stiffness of the LV chamber; patients with HFpEF have a normal or reduced end-diastolic volume and an elevated end-diastolic pressure, indicating an increase in LV diastolic stiffness.
- Management of HFpEF patients using IHM-guided therapy that directly targeted lowering diastolic filling pressures and preventing their rise over time has been demonstrated to reduce morbidity and mortality and improve functional status. Prior to HF hospitalizations, diastolic filling pressures may begin to rise over a period of 4 to 6 weeks. The risks for HF hospitalization are proportional to the area under the pressure versus time relationship.

REVIEW QUESTIONS

1. The echocardiogram of a 75-year-old woman is read as demonstrating normal LV volume, mass, and EF; the transmitral Doppler and tissue Doppler patterns indicate a decreased E and decreased e′. The patient has hypertension, diabetes, and chronic obstructive pulmonary disease (COPD), but has no symptoms of dyspnea on exertion (DOE) or edema, normal lung sounds, no jugular vein distention (JVD) or edema, and normal exercise tolerance for age. Which of the following should be done to manage this patient?
   a. Begin diuretic therapy to treat HFpEF
   b. Carefully manage blood pressure (BP) and hemoglobin A1C (HgbA1C)
   c. Refer to cardiac rehab
   d. Perform diagnostic right heart cath +/- bicycle ergometry
2. A 65-year-old woman underwent surgical aortic valve replacement (AVR) for bicuspid aortic valve stenosis at 10 a.m. She is now in the surgical ICU at 6 pm with a reduced cardiac output and BP that necessitates support with inotropes after successful extubation and PO_2 of 100% on 4 L nasal cannula (NC). A bedside echo shows an end-diastolic volume index (EDVi) of 50 mL/m^2, an EF of 75%, LVH, and a septal wall motion abnormality. Her indwelling right heart catheter shows a PCWP of 18 mmHg. Which of the following should be done to manage this patient?
   a. Discontinue inotropes
   b. Perform cardiac cath to treat STEMI
   c. Increase volume infusion to raise PCWP to 25 mmHg
   d. Start vasodilator therapy
3. A 68-year-old man with HFpEF and recurrent admissions for acute decompensated HF recently had implantation of a CardioMEMS hemodynamic monitor. At the time of implantation, he had well-compensated NYHA class II symptoms with no JVD, rales, or peripheral edema, and his pulmonary artery diastolic pressure (PADP) was 21 mmHg. Over the ensuing 4 weeks, his PADP varies between 22 and 25 mmHg with the last reading =25 mmHg. During the office visit follow-up (at 4 weeks postimplant), he remains NHYA class II symptoms and has no JVD, rales, or peripheral edema. Which of the following should be done to manage this patient?
   a. Perform repeat right heart cath to recalibrate the CardioMEMS
   b. Make no changes in medications
   c. Perform echocardiogram to r/o pericardial effusion
   d. Increase diuretic therapy to reduce PADP

REFERENCES

1. Yancy CW, Jessup M, Bozkurt B, et al. 2017 ACC/AHA/HFSA focused update of the 2013 ACCF/AHA guideline for the management of heart failure: a report of the American College of Cardiology/American Heart Association Task Force on Clinical Practice Guidelines and the Heart Failure Society of America. *J Am Coll Cardiol.* 2017;70:776–803.
2. Ponikowski P, Voors AA, Anker SD, et al. 2016 ESC guidelines for the diagnosis and treatment of acute and chronic heart failure: the task force for the diagnosis and treatment of acute and chronic heart failure of the European Society of Cardiology (ESC). Developed with the special contribution of the Heart Failure Association (HFA) of the ESC. *Eur J Heart Fail.* 2016;18:891–975.
3. Aurigemma GP, Zile MR, Gaasch WH. Contractile behavior of the left ventricle in heart failure with a preserved ejection fraction: with emphasis on regional systolic function. *Circulation.* 2006;113:296–304.
4. Zile MR, Gaasch WH, Carroll JD, et al. Heart failure with a normal ejection fraction. Is measurement of diastolic function necessary to make the diagnosis of heart failure with a preserved ejection fraction? *Circulation.* 2001;104:779–782.
5. Zile MR. Heart failure with preserved ejection fraction: is this diastolic heart failure? *J Am Coll Cardiol.* 2003;41:1519–1522.
6. Aurigemma GP, Gaasch WH. Heart failure with a preserved ejection fraction. *N Engl J Med.* 2004;351:1097–1105.
7. Zile MR, Baicu CF, Gaasch WH. Heart failure with a preserved ejection fraction—abnormalities in active relaxation and passive stiffness of the left ventricle. *N Engl J Med.* 2004;350:1953–1959.
8. Baicu CF, Zile MR, Aurigemma GP, Gaasch WH. Left ventricular systolic performance, function, and contractility in patients with heart failure with a preserved ejection fraction. *Circulation.* 2005;111:2306–2312.
9. Zile MR, Baicu CF, Bonnema DD. Heart failure with a preserved ejection fraction: definitions and terminology. *Progr Cardiov Dis.* 2005;47:307–313.
10. Bhatia RS, Tu JV, Lee DS, et al. Outcome of heart failure with preserved ejection fraction in a population-based study. *N Engl J Med.* 2006;355:260–269.
11. Redfield MM, Jacobsen SJ, Burnett JC Jr, Mahoney DW, Bailey KR, Rodeheffer RJ. Burden of systolic and diastolic ventricular dysfunction in the community: appreciating the scope of the heart failure epidemic. *JAMA.* 2003;289:194–202.
12. Kitzman DW, Little WC, Brubaker PH, et al. Pathophysiological characterization of isolated heart failure with a preserved ejection fraction in comparison to heart failure with a reduced ejection fraction. *JAMA.* 2002;288:2144–2150.
13. Brucks S, Little WC, Chao T, et al. Contribution of left ventricular diastolic dysfunction to heart failure regardless of ejection fraction. *Am J Cardiol.* 2005;95:603–606.
14. Zile MR, Gottdiener JS, Hetzel SJ, et al. Prevalence and significance of alterations in cardiac structure and function in patients with heart failure and a preserved ejection fraction. *Circulation.* 2011;124:2491–2501.
15. Shah AM, Claggett B, Sweitzer NK, et al. Cardiac structure and function and prognosis in heart failure with preserved ejection fraction: findings from the echocardiographic study of the treatment of preserved cardiac function heart failure with an Aldosterone Antagonist (TOPCAT) trial. *Circulation. Heart Failure.* 2014;7:740–751.

16. Solomon SD, Rizkala AR, Lefkowitz MP, et al. Baseline characteristics of patients with heart failure and preserved ejection fraction in the PARAGON-HF trial. *Circulation. Heart Failure.* 2018;11(7):e004962.
17. Paulus WJ, Tschöpe C. A novel paradigm for heart failure with preserved ejection fraction: comorbidities drive myocardial dysfunction and remodeling through coronary microvascular endothelial inflammation. *J Am Coll Cardiol.* 2013;62:263–271.
18. Zile MR, Baicu CF, Ikonomidis JS, et al. Myocardial stiffness in patients with heart failure and a preserved ejection fraction: contributions of collagen and titin. *Circulation.* 2015;131:1247–1259.
19. Rovner A, Smith R, Greenberg NL, et al. Improvement in diastolic intraventricular pressure gradients in patients with HOCM after ethanol septal reduction. *Am J Physiol. Heart Circ Physiol.* 2003;285:H2492–H2499.
20. Little WC. Diastolic dysfunction beyond distensibility: adverse effects of ventricular dilatation. *Circulation.* 2005;112:2888–2890.
21. Yotti R, Bermejo J, Antoranz JC, et al. A noninvasive method for assessing impaired diastolic suction in patients with dilated cardiomyopathy. *Circulation.* 2005;112:2921–2929.
22. Ohara T, Ohte N, Little WC. Pulmonary hypertension in heart failure with preserved left ventricular ejection fraction: diagnosis and management. *Curr Opin Cardiol.* 2012;27:281–287.
23. Stewart KC, Kumar R, Charonko JJ, Ohara T, Vlachos PP, Little WC. Evaluation of LV diastolic function from color M-mode echocardiography. *JACC. Cardiov Imaging.* 2011;4:37–46. 2011.
24. Little WC, Oh JK. Echocardiographic evaluation of diastolic function can be used to guide clinical care. *Circulation.* 2009;120:802–809.
25. Hasegawa H, Little WC, Ohno M, et al. Diastolic mitral annular velocity during the development of heart failure. *J Am Coll Cardiol.* 2003;41:1590–1597.
26. Masutani S, Little WC, Hasegawa H, Cheng HJ, Cheng CP. Restrictive left ventricular filling pattern does not result from increased left atrial pressure alone. *Circulation.* 2008;117:1550–1554.
27. Fukuta H, Little WC. Elevated left ventricular filling pressure after maximal exercise predicts increased plasma B-type natriuretic peptide levels in patients with impaired relaxation pattern of diastolic filling. *J Am Soc Echocardiograph.* 2007;20:832–837.
28. Opdahl A, Remme EW, Helle-Valle T, et al. Determinants of left ventricular early-diastolic lengthening velocity. *Circulation.* 2009;119:2578–2586.
29. Shen L, Jhund PS, Docherty KF, et al. Prior pacemaker implantation and clinical outcomes in patients with heart failure and preserved ejection fraction. *JACC. Heart Failure.* 2019;7:418–427.
30. Westermann D, Kasner M, Steendijk P, et al. Role of left ventricular stiffness in heart failure with normal ejection fraction. *Circulation.* 2008;117:2051–2060.
31. Carroll JD, Lang RM, Neumann AL, Borow KM, Rajfer SI. The differential effects of positive inotropic and vasodilator therapy on diastolic properties in patients with congestive cardiomyopathy. *Circulation.* 1986;74:815–825.
32. Hamdani N, Paulus WJ. Myocardial titin and collagen in cardiac diastolic dysfunction: partners in crime. *Circulation.* 2013;128:5–8. 2013.
33. Borbely A, Falcao-Pires I, van Heerebeek L, et al. Hypophosphorylation of the stiff N2B titin isoform raises cardiomyocyte resting tension in failing human myocardium. *Circ Res.* 2009;104:780–786.
34. Borbely A, van Heerebeek L, Paulus WJ. Transcriptional and posttranslational modifications of titin: implications for diastole. *Circ Res.* 2009;104: 12–14.
35. Bradshaw AD, Baicu CF, Rentz TJ, et al. Pressure-overload induced alterations in fibrillar collagen content and myocardial diastolic function: role of SPARC in post-synthetic procollagen processing. *Circulation.* 2009;119:269–280.
36. Bradshaw AD, Baicu CF, Rentz TJ, Van Laer AO, Bonnema DD, Zile MR. Age-dependent alterations in fibrillar collagen content and myocardial diastolic function: role of SPARC in post-synthetic procollagen processing. *Am J Physiol. Heart Circ Physiol.* 2010;298:H614–H622.
37. Baicu CF, Li J, Zhang Y, et al. Time course of right ventricular pressure-overload induced myocardial fibrosis: relationship to changes in fibroblast dependent post-synthetic procollagen processing. *Am J Physiol. Heart Circ Physiol.* 2012;303:H1128–1134.
38. McDonald LT, Zile MR, Zhang Y, et al. Increased macrophage-derived SPARC precedes collagen deposition in myocardial fibrosis. *Am J Physiol. Heart Circ Physiol.* 2018;315(1): H92–H100.
39. Zile MR, Kjellstrom B, Bennett T, et al. Effects of exercise on left ventricular systolic and diastolic properties in patients with heart failure and a preserved ejection fraction versus heart failure and a reduced ejection fraction. *Circulation. Heart Failure.* 2013;6:508–516.
40. Kitzman DW, Higginbotham MB, Cobb FR, Sheikh KH, Sullivan MJ. Exercise intolerance in patients with heart failure and preserved left ventricular systolic function: failure of the Frank-Starling mechanism. *J Am Coll Cardiol.* 1991;17:1065–1072.
41. Borlaug BA, Nishimura RA, Sorajja P, Lam CS, Redfield MM. Exercise hemodynamics enhance diagnosis of early heart failure with preserved ejection fraction. *Circulation. Heart Failure.* 2010;3:588–595.
42. Cheng CP, Igarash Y, Little WC. Mechanism of augmented rate of left ventricle filling during exercise. *Circ Res.* 1992;70:9–19.
43. Cheng CP, Noda T, Nozawa T, Little WC. Effect of heart failure on the mechanism of exercise induced augmentation of mitral valve flow. *Circ Res.* 1993;72:795–806.
44. Little WC, Cheng CP. Modulation of diastolic dysfunction in the intact heart. In: Lorell BH, Grossman W, eds. *Diastolic Relaxation of the Heart.* 2d ed. Boston: Kluwer Academic Publishers; 1994:167–176.
45. Little WC. Diastolic dysfunction beyond distensibility: adverse effects of ventricular dilatation. *Circulation.* 2005;112:2888–2890.
46. Carroll JD, Hess OM, Hirzel HO, Krayenbuehl HP. Dynamics of LV filling at rest and during exercise. *Circulation.* 1983;68:59–67.
47. Carroll JD, Hess OM, Hirzel HO, Krayenbuehl HP. Exercise-induced ischemia: the influence of altered relaxation on early diastolic pressures. *Circulation.* 1983;67:521–528.
48. Zile MR, Bennett TD, St John Sutton M, et al. Transition from chronic compensated to acute decompensated heart failure: pathophysiological insights obtained from continuous monitoring of intracardiac pressures. *Circulation.* 2008;118:1433–1441.
49. Gandhi SK, Powers JC, Nomeir AM, et al. The pathogenesis of acute pulmonary edema associated with hypertension. *N Engl J Med.* 2001;344:17–22.
50. Owan TE, Hodge DO, Herges RM, Jacobsen SJ, Roger VL, Redfield MM. Trends in prevalence and outcome of heart failure with preserved ejection fraction. *N Engl J Med.* 2006;355:251–259.
51. Yancy CW, Lopatin M, Stevenson LW, De Marco T, Fonarow GC. for the ADHERE Scientific Advisory Committee and Investigators. Clinical presentation, management, and in-hospital outcomes of patients admitted with acute decompensated heart failure with preserved systolic function: a report from the Acute Decompensated Heart Failure National Registry (ADHERE) Database. *J Am Coll Cardiol.* 2006;47:76–84.
52. Shah SJ, Kitzman DW, Borlaug BA, et al. Phenotype-specific treatment of heart failure with preserved ejection fraction: a multiorgan roadmap. Contribution of cardiac and extra-cardiac disease burden to risk of cardiovascular outcomes varies by ejection fraction in heart failure. *Circulation.* 2016;134:73–90.
53. Wolsk E, Claggett B, Køber L, et al. Contribution of cardiac and extra-cardiac disease burden to risk of cardiovascular outcomes varies by ejection fraction in heart failure. *Eur J Heart Failure.* 2018;20:504–510.
54. Mentz RJ, Kelly JP, von Lueder TG, et al. Noncardiac comorbidities in heart failure with reduced versus preserved ejection fraction. *J Am Coll Cardiol.* 2014;64:2281–2293.
55. Stevenson LW, Zile M, Bennett TD, et al. Chronic ambulatory intracardiac pressures and future heart failure events. *Circulation. Heart Failure.* 2010;3:580–587.
56. Zile MR, Adamson PB, Cho YK, et al. Hemodynamic factors associated with acute decompensated heart failure: Part 1—insights into pathophysiology. *J Cardiac Failure.* 2011;17: 282–291.
57. Adamson PB, Zile MR, Cho YK, et al. Hemodynamic factors associated with acute decompensated heart failure: Part 2—use in automated detection. *J Cardiac Failure.* 2011;17:366–373.
58. Ritzema J, Troughton R, Melton I, et al. Physician-directed patient self-management of left atrial pressure in advanced chronic heart failure. *Circulation.* 2010;121:1086–1095.

59. Dickinson MG, Allen LA, Albert NA, et al. Remote monitoring of patients with heart failure: a white paper from the heart failure Society of America Scientific Statements Committee. *J Cardiac Failure.* 2018;24:682–694.
60. Zile MR, Sharma V, Johnson JW, Warman EN, Baicu CF, Bennett TD. Prediction of all-cause mortality based on the direct measurement of intrathoracic impedance. *Circulation. Heart Failure.* 2016;9:e002543.
61. Zile MR, Bennett TD, El Hajj S, et al. Intracardiac pressures measured using an implantable hemodynamic monitor: relationship to mortality in patients with chronic heart failure. *Circulation. Heart Failure.* 2017;10:e003594.
62. Givertz MM, Stevenson LW, Costanzo MR, et al. Pulmonary artery pressure-guided management of patients with heart failure and reduced ejection fraction. *J Am Coll Cardiol.* 2017;70:1875–1886.
63. Bourge RC, Abraham WT, Adamson PB, et al. Randomized controlled trial of an implantable continuous hemodynamic monitor in patients with advanced heart failure: The COMPASS-HF study. *J Am Coll Cardiol.* 2008;51:1073–1079.
64. Abraham WT, Adamson PB, Bourge RC, et al. Wireless pulmonary artery haemodynamic monitoring in chronic heart failure: a randomized controlled trial. *Lancet (London, England).* 2011;377:658–666.
65. Adamson PB, Ginn G, Anker SD, Bourge RC, Abraham WT. Remote haemodynamic-guided care for patients with chronic heart failure: a meta-analysis of completed trials. *Eur J Heart Failure.* 2017;19:426–433.
66. Desai AS, Bhimaraj A, Bharmi R, et al. Ambulatory hemodynamic monitoring reduces heart failure hospitalizations in "real-world" clinical practice. *J Am Coll Cardiol.* 2017;69:2357–2365.
67. Anand IS, Rector TS, Cleland JG, et al. Prognostic value of baseline plasma amino-terminal pro-brain natriuretic peptide and its interactions with irbesartan treatment effects in patients with heart failure and preserved ejection fraction: findings from the I-PRESERVE trial. *Circulation. Heart Failure.* 2011;4:569–577.
68. Zile MR, Jhund PS, Baicu CF, et al. Plasma biomarkers reflecting profibrotic processes in heart failure with a preserved ejection fraction: data from the prospective comparison of ARNI with ARB on management of heart failure with preserved ejection fraction study. *Circulation. Heart Failure.* 2016;9:e002551.
69. Chow SL, Maisel AS, Anand I, et al. Role of biomarkers for the prevention, assessment, and management of heart failure: a scientific statement from the American Heart Association. *Circulation.* 2017;135:e1054–e1091.
70. Ferreira JP, Duarte K, Graves TL, et al. Natriuretic peptides, 6-min walk test, and quality-of-life questionnaires as clinically meaningful endpoints in HF trials. *J Am Coll Cardiol.* 2016;68:2690–2707.
71. Zile MR, Jhund PS, Baicu CF, et al. Plasma biomarkers reflecting profibrotic processes in heart failure with a preserved ejection fraction: data from the prospective comparison of ARNI with ARB on management of heart failure with preserved ejection fraction study. *Circulation. Heart Failure.* 2016;9(ii):e002551.
72. Boehmer JP, Hariharan R, Devecchi FG, et al. A multisensor algorithm predicts heart failure events in patients with implanted devices: results from the MultiSENSE study. *JACC. Heart Failure.* 2017;5:216–225.
73. Virani SA, Sharma V, McCann M, Koehler J, Tsang B, Zieroth S. Prospective evaluation of integrated device diagnostics for heart failure management: results of the TRIAGE-HF study. *ESC Heart Failure.* 2018;5:809–817.
74. Shah SJ, Feldman T, Ricciardi MJ, et al. One-year safety and clinical outcomes of a transcatheter interatrial shunt device for the treatment of heart failure with preserved ejection fraction in the reduce elevated left atrial pressure in patients with heart failure (REDUCE LAP-HF I) trial: a randomized clinical trial. *JAMA Cardiol.* 2018;3:968–977.
75. Kaye DM, Petrie MC, McKenzie S, et al. Impact of an interatrial shunt device on survival and heart failure hospitalization in patients with preserved ejection fraction. *ESC Heart Failure.* 2018;6:62–69.

3

Role of the Pericardium in Diastolic Dysfunction

Massimo Imazio

OUTLINE

INTRODUCTION

Pericardial diseases are often underdiagnosed and confused with other pathologic entities such as chronic liver diseases, heart failure, and restrictive cardiomyopathies especially in the setting of complicated pericarditis with evolution to constrictive pericarditis.[1,2] The main reasons for these misunderstandings are related to both the rarity of the diseases and the lack of specific skills and knowledge of pericardial diseases, which are often considered the "Cinderella of cardiovascular diseases." Nevertheless, the development of first prospective cohort studies,[3–8] randomized controlled trials (RCTs),[9–11] international guidelines,[1,12,13] and especially the development of multimodality imaging of pericardial diseases[1,13] has greatly improved the awareness and knowledge of these conditions. This chapter will further contribute to assess the importance of the pericardium in the study of diastolic function of the heart (Chapter 36).

Case Study

A 34-year-old man, a bricklayer coming from Western Europe, is referred for second opinion because of recurrent episodes of pleuritic chest pain, unexplained peripheral edema, and signs of right heart failure. He is a smoker with a previous chest trauma due to an accident at work 5 years earlier. On physical examination the patient shows elevated jugular venous pressure, a pericardial knock on auscultation, and 2+ peripheral leg edema (Fig. 3.1A and B). On electrocardiogram (ECG), a sinus rhythm is evident with nonspecific ST-T changes (see Fig. 3.1C). Chest x-ray shows pericardial calcifications (see Fig. 3.1D).

ANATOMY AND PHYSIOLOGY OF THE PERICARDIUM

The **pericardium** (from the Greek περί, "around" and κάρδιον, "heart") is a double-walled sac containing the heart and the roots of the great vessels. The pericardium is the external layer of the heart providing protection and support to inner structures. It is composed of an external fibroserosal part (parietal pericardium) and an internal serosal part (visceral pericardium) (Fig. 3.2). The internal serosal layer is also named epicardium, which has direct connection with the myocardium. The parietal pericardium has an inner serosal part that is in continuity with the epicardium and an external fibrous part. Between the visceral and parietal pericardial layers, a virtual pericardial cavity is filled by 20 to 30 mL of plasma ultrafiltrate (pericardial fluid) that acts as a lubricant allowing myocardial contraction without irritation of the surrounding anatomic structures.[14–16] The pericardial fluid is produced by the serosal pericardium, which is conformed by mesothelial cells with microvilla and cilia that further expand the available pericardial surface. The reflection of the visceral pericardium into the parietal pericardium over the great vessels is responsible for the creation of spaces, where pericardial fluid can accumulate and be detected by imaging studies.[17,18] Greater spaces are called **sinuses**, while smaller spaces between adjacent anatomic structures are called **recesses**. The main sinuses include the **transverse sinus**, located between the aorta and pulmonary trunk anteriorly, the atria and veins posteriorly, and the **oblique sinus** located behind the left atrium and between the pulmonary veins and the inferior vena cava. Both sinuses may be accessed for electrophysiology purposes for ablation of cardiac arrhythmias.[17]

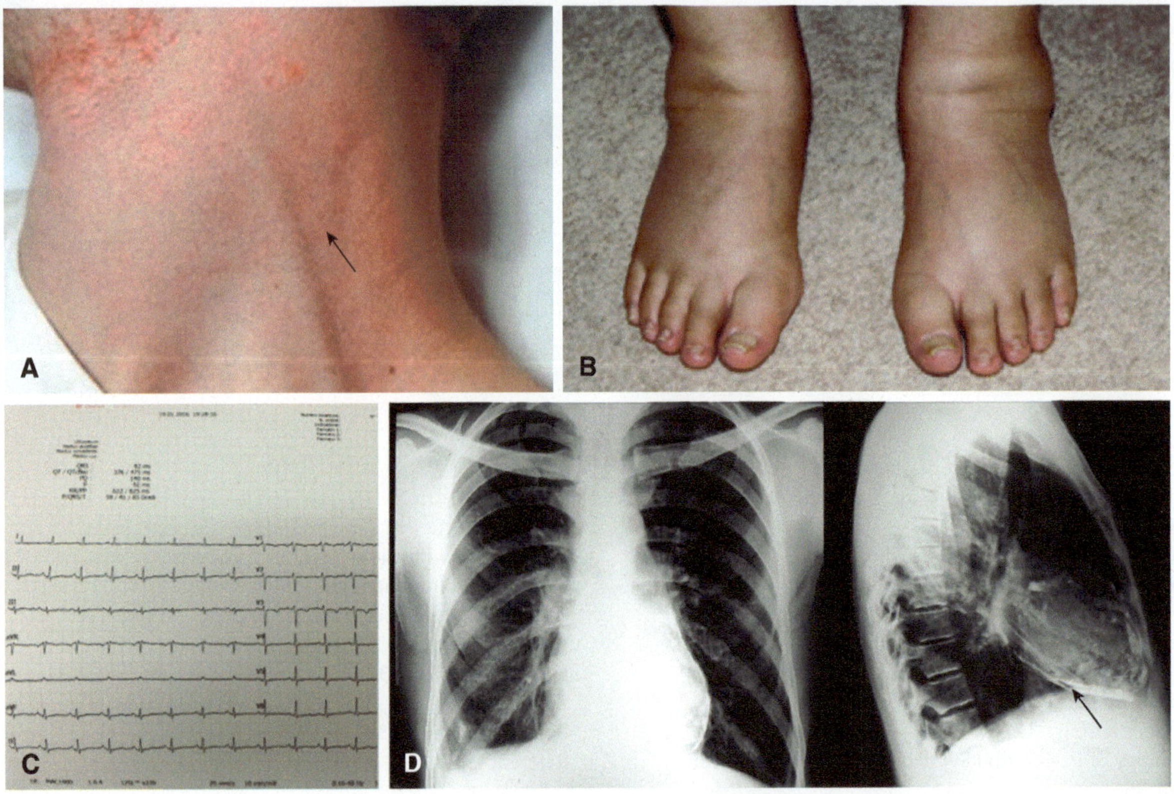

Fig. 3.1 A case of incessant pericarditis with signs of right heart failure with distended jugular veins (A), peripheral edema (B), nonspecific ST/T changes on the ECG (C), and pericardial calcifications (D).

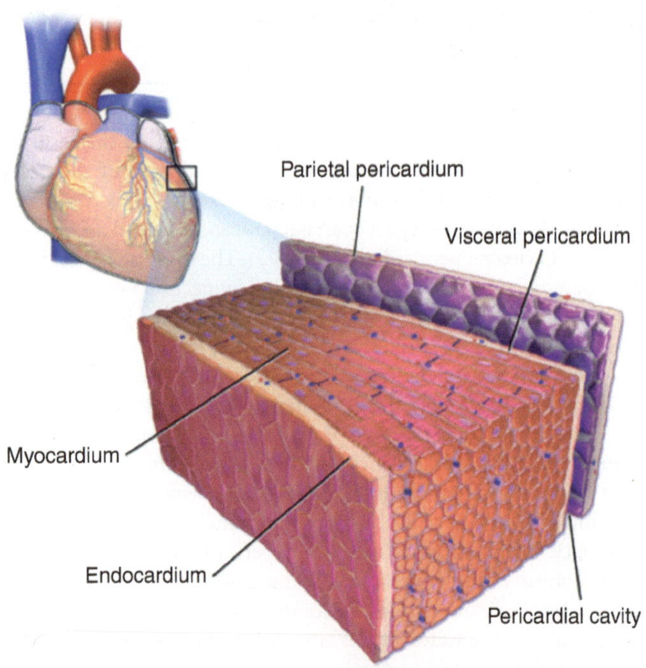

Fig. 3.2 The pericardium as the external envelope of the heart, including the visceral pericardium (epicardium) and parietal pericardium (see text for additional explanation).

Fat is present under the epicardium (epicardial fat) and in connection with the parietal pericardium (epipericardial fat).[18] Fat tissue provides mechanical, immunologic protection of the heart and serves as a source of fatty acids and thus energy; it may also have endocrine functions by cytokines that act through paracrine mechanisms on myocardial and endocardial cells.[19,20]

The pericardium is fixed to the surrounding anatomic structures by ligaments: anteriorly to the sternum by the sternopericardial ligaments, posteriorly to the vertebral column, and inferiorly to the diaphragm.

The thickness of the normal pericardium is less than 3 mm by imaging studies and less than 1 to 2 mm on autopsy and surgical specimens.[1,13]

The pericardium has an extensive network of lymphatics that drain substances from pericardial space and allows the spread of pathologic process from and to the pericardium in case of mediastinal and pulmonary pathology. The anterior part of the pericardium is drained either upwards to anterior mediastinal lymph nodes or downwards to the diaphragm; the posterior part drains into paraesophageal and tracheobronchial lymph nodes; the inferior part drains into prepericardial, lateropericardial, paraesophageal, and tracheobronchial lymph nodes; the lateral part drains into mediastinal, tracheobronchial, lateropericardial, prepericardial, and paraesophageal lymph nodes.[14]

The arterial blood supply of the pericardium is provided by the descending aorta, branches of the mammary arteries, and musculophrenic arteries.

The pericardium has both sympathetic (first dorsal ganglion, stellate ganglion, aortic, and cardiac plexuses) and parasympathetic innervation (vagus, left recurrent laryngeal nerve, esophageal plexus).[18]

The pericardium acts as a relatively inelastic sac because of its high content of collagen fibers, enveloping the heart and providing mechanical protection to the heart, thus allowing movement of cardiac chambers without attrition and limiting their distension. This effect is especially evident on right cardiac chambers.

This effect explains the exaggerated interventricular interdependence that can be observed in pathologic conditions (e.g., cardiac tamponade and constrictive pericarditis), as well as how rapidly accumulating pericardial fluid may be responsible for cardiac tamponade

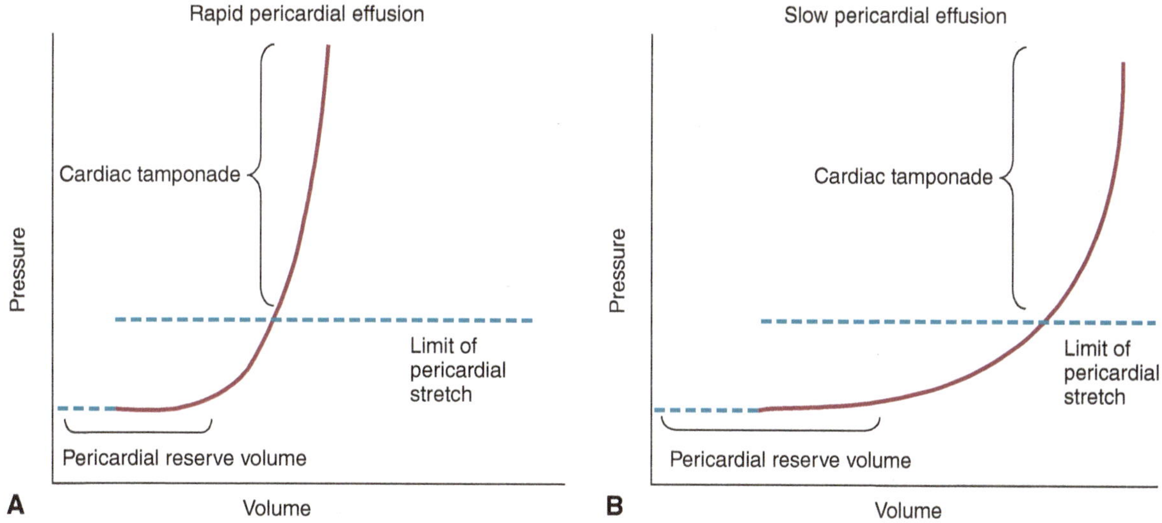

Fig. 3.3 Pressure/volume curve of the pericardium. The pericardium acts as a rather inelastic sac due to its high content of collagen fibers. On this basis, rapid changes of the volume of the pericardial space will soon reach the limit of pericardial stretch with a sudden rise of intrapericardial pressure (this explains the quick development of cardiac tamponade in these settings [e.g., aortic dissection with hemopericardium]). On the other hand, slowly accumulating pericardial fluid can reach high volumes (1–2 L) without the development of cardiac tamponade (e.g., idiopathic chronic pericardial effusions). (From Imazio M, Adler Y. Management of pericardial effusion. *Eur Heart J.* 2013;34[16]:1186–1197.)

BOX 3.1 Physiologic Functions of the Pericardium

Mechanical functions
Reduction of the friction between the myocardium and surrounding structures
Limitation of the distension of cardiac chambers
Limitation of the regurgitation of cardiac valves
Barrier to mechanical and infections noxa
Immunologic and additional functions
Protection from infectious agents
Production of factors that modulate sympathetic tone
Endocrine and metabolic functions of the epicardial fat
Fibrinolytic activity of pericardial mesothelial cells
Lymphatic drainage of the heart

with limited amount of fluid, such as 200 to 300 mL in hemopericardium. On the other hand, slowly accumulating pericardial fluid can allow the generation of large pericardial effusions as 1 to 2 L without the development of cardiac tamponade (e.g., large chronic pericardial effusions). This is well explained by the pressure-volume curve of the pericardium (Fig. 3.3).[19]

The pericardium is not simply a mechanical barrier but also has an active immunologic role that is very relevant in inflammatory conditions such as pericarditis and myocarditis.

Although the pericardium has several important functions (Box 3.1), its absence (total agenesis) or surgical removal (e.g., pericardiectomy) has limited consequences for life, and it is absolutely compatible with a normal life.[14,18]

NONINVASIVE IMAGING OF THE PERICARDIUM

Multimodality imaging of the pericardium is an integral part of contemporary management of pericardial diseases that is recommended in all patients with suspected pericardial disease.[12] The main imaging modalities include chest x-ray, echocardiography, computed tomography (CT), and cardiovascular magnetic resonance imaging (cardiac MRI).[21]

In 2013, the American Society of Echocardiography issued a consensus statement on multimodality cardiovascular imaging of pericardial diseases that has been endorsed by the Society of Cardiovascular Magnetic Resonance and Society of Cardiovascular Computed Tomography.[1] In 2014, a European position paper was published by the European Association of Cardiovascular Imaging and European Society of Cardiology (ESC) Working Group on myocardial and pericardial diseases,[13] and multimodality imaging has been revised and recommendations issued in 2015 ESC guidelines on pericardial diseases.[12] A detailed description of the imaging findings in specific pathologic conditions (e.g., cardiac tamponade and constrictive pericarditis) will be provided in subsequent chapters.

X-ray

Chest x-ray is a first-level imaging modality in patients with a suspected pericarditis or pericardial effusion to detect the presence of a cardiomegaly (may suggest a pericardial effusion), pericardial calcifications (chronic and constrictive pericarditis), and/or concomitant pleuropulmonary disease as first screening (e.g., pleural effusion, pneumonia, tuberculosis, lung cancer, and hilar and mediastinal enlargement) (Fig. 3.4).

In a patient with pericarditis and without significant structural heart diseases, the chest x-ray may be absolutely normal. A pericardial effusion greater than 300 mL is able to increase the size of the cardiac silhouette. This one assumes a bottle shape in the presence of large pericardial effusions, especially when chronic and slowly accumulating.

In our patient, pericardial calcifications were detected (see Fig. 3.1). Pericardial calcifications have been reported in 30% to 40% of patients with chronic constrictive pericarditis.[22]

Echocardiography

Transthoracic echocardiography is the first-line imaging test in patients with suspected pericardial disease (Class I indication, Level of Evidence [LOE] C).[12] One of the first applications of echocardiography was the

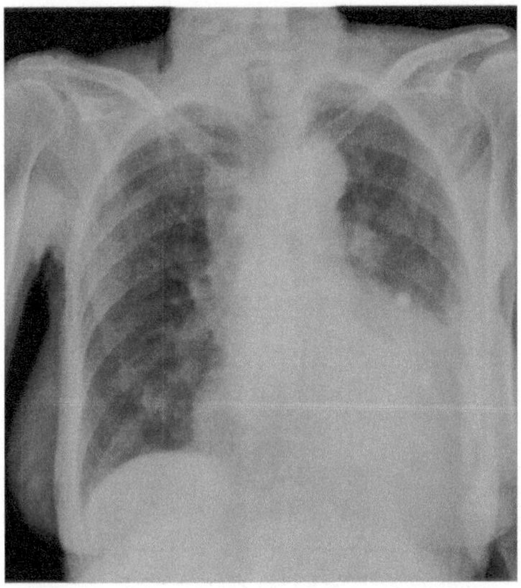

Fig. 3.4 A patient with pleuropericarditis and pneumonia. Cardiomegaly is also evident due to pericardial effusion. A concomitant left pleural effusion was noted.

detection of pericardial effusion. Even nowadays, echocardiography represents the simplest and most economical diagnostic option to detect the presence of a pericardial effusion, providing a semiquantitative assessment of the size that can be easily performed even at bedside and in urgent/emergency settings.

In clinical practice, the size of pericardial effusion on M mode and two-dimensional (2D) echocardiography is qualitatively assessed by the end-diastolic distance of the echo-free space between the epicardium and parietal pericardium: trivial (only seen in systole), small (<10 mm), moderate (10–20 mm), large (>20 mm, very large > 2.5 mm)). Pericardial fluid accumulates following available spaces and gravity forces. On left lateral decubitus, the fluid starts accumulating posteriorly (mild effusions); then, after the complete filling of anterior posterior space, pericardial effusions become circumferential. On this basis, an isolated anterior pericardial echo-free space should be considered as evidence of increased epicardial fat instead of pericardial fluid, especially in the absence of previous cardiac surgery, trauma, or pericarditis with or without interventional procedures. CT and cardiac MRI may provide better tissue characterization of pericardial content.

Cardiac Magnetic Resonance Imaging

Cardiac MRI is a useful second-level imaging technique for the study of pericardial and myopericardial diseases. Similar to CT, the normal pericardium appears on T1-weighted imaging as a thin hypointense (dark) curvilinear structure surrounded by hyperintense (bright) mediastinal and epicardial fat. Normal pericardial thickness is less than 3 mm.[23,24] Our patient had increased thickness of the pericardium. Irregular areas of increased thickness caused by calcifications appeared on cardiac MRI as signal losses (Fig. 3.5). Possible evidence of pericardial inflammation can be seen on short-tau inversion-recovery (STIR) T2-weighted images providing evidence of pericardial edema and as pericardial late gadolinium enhancement providing evidence of inflammatory pericarditis. The presence and extent of pericardial inflammation on cardiac MRI may be helpful for the diagnosis and to guide the duration and intensification of medical therapy.[25–27]

Additional contributions of cardiac MRI[28] may include:

a. Characterization of pericardial fluid
b. Assessment of concomitant constrictive physiology (pericardial thickening, adhesions on tagging, septal bounce on cine real-time images)
c. Assessment of concomitant myocarditis
d. Study of pericardial masses and cysts
e. Study of congenital abnormalities of the pericardium
f. Evaluation of concomitant heart and pleuropulmonary diseases

The main limitation of cardiac MRI is the limited availability in many clinical settings, the costs, the need of breath-holding, and regular cardiac rhythms to achieve better image quality.[1,12–14]

Computed Tomography

The normal pericardium is visible as a thin curvilinear structure surrounded by the hypodense mediastinal and epicardial fat, and has a thickness ranging between 0.7 and 2 mm. The pericardial sinuses and their respective recesses are well visualized on CT.

CT is a second-level complementary imaging modality that is especially useful for the study of pericardial calcifications as well as concomitant pleuropulmonary diseases. In addition, CT may be helpful to provide some tissue characterization of pericardial fluid. Attenuation values of pericardial fluid measured in Hounsfield units (HU) yield information with regard to the nature of fluid: low attenuation values (e.g., 0–20 HU) indicate a simple effusion and a transudate; intermediate values (e.g., 20–60 HU) are suggestive of a proteinaceous, exudative effusion; high attenuation values (>60 HU) suggest hemorrhage.[1,12–14]

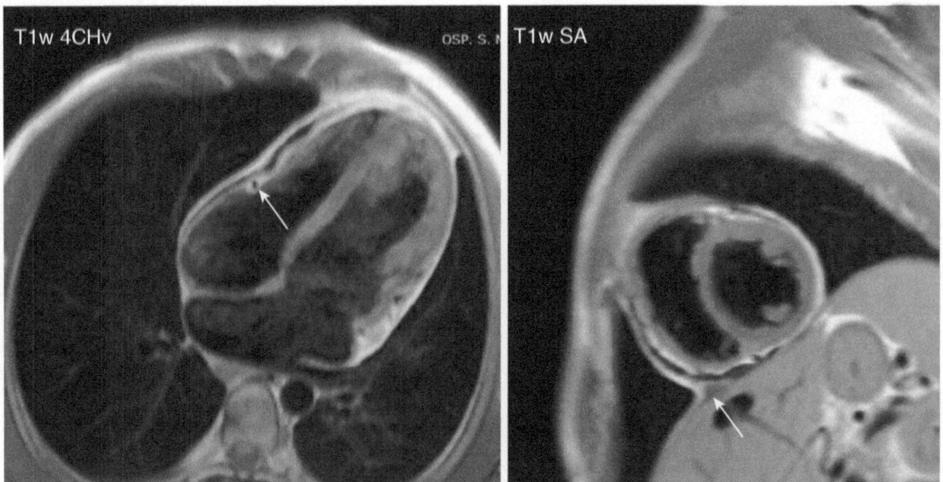

Fig. 3.5 Evidence of pericardial thickening greater than 3 mm on cardiac MRI from the introductory descriptive case.

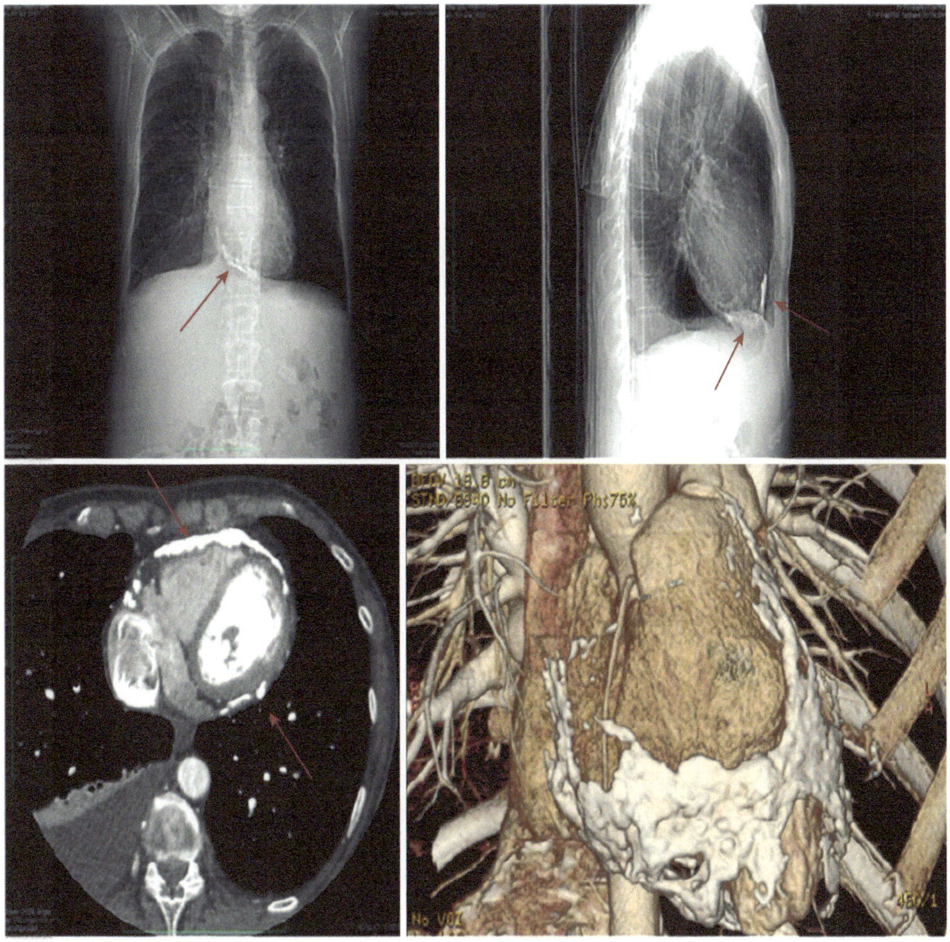

Fig. 3.6 Evidence of extensive calcifications on CT scan with 3D reconstruction of the calcifications of the patient from the introductory case.

CT is the most accurate technique to image calcified tissue, and it is especially helpful to depict the extension of calcifications allowing a better surgical plan for pericardiectomy (Fig. 3.6). Nowadays modern multidetector CT scanners combine both acquisition speed, high contrast and spatial resolution providing excellent anatomic details. Low-radiation cardiac CT is feasible using prospective electrocardiographic triggering. Intravenous administration of iodinated contrast material is able to detect pericardial inflammation since the inflamed pericardium is enhanced after contrast injection.

Additional contribution of CT studies includes the evaluation and diagnosis of pericardial masses and cysts and the congenital partial or complete absence of the pericardium. The added value of CT is also the assessment of concomitant pleuropulmonary diseases, which is valuable for the etiologic screening of pericardial diseases.[29,30]

Although cine CT is feasible, in clinical practice CT provides limited contribution to the functional study of the heart and pericardium since images are acquired under a single breath-hold.

Nuclear Scintigraphy

Nuclear medicine imaging techniques have specific indication in selected cases to assess the metabolic activity of the pericardium, especially in suspected neoplastic pericardial disease or infectious pericarditis, such as tuberculous pericarditis. Positron emission tomography (PET) alone, or preferably in combination with CT (PET/CT), is commonly utilized for this diagnostic application. Pericardial uptake of ^{18}F-fluorodeoxyglucose (FDG) tracer in patients with solid cancers and lymphoma is indicative of (malignant) pericardial involvement. The clinical application of this technique ranges from diagnosis to staging, and assessment of therapeutic response.[28,31]

The different main imaging techniques should be considered as complimentary modalities to be considered according to clinical judgment. Second-level imaging is usually recommended for complicated cases (Fig. 3.7).

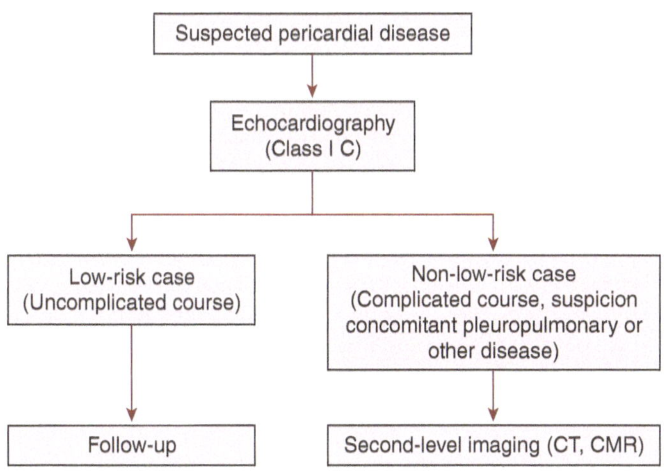

Fig. 3.7 The different main imaging techniques should be considered as complimentary modalities to be considered according to clinical judgment. Second-level imaging is usually recommended for complicated cases.

TABLE 3.1 Indications, Strengths, and Weaknesses of Imaging Techniques for Pericardial and Pericardial Diseases

	Echocardiography	Computed Tomography	Cardiac Magnetic Resonance Imaging
Indications	First-level assessment and follow-up study for pericardial diseases	Second-level imaging technique (best for assessment of calcifications)	Second-level imaging technique (best for tissue characterization and assessment of inflammation)
Main strengths	Widely available Inexpensive Use in urgent/emergency settings and bedside Safe and repeatable	Better anatomic study Evaluation of concomitant pleuropulmonary diseases Evaluation of calcifications	Better anatomic study Evaluation of concomitant pleuropulmonary diseases Assessment of pericardial and myocardial inflammation
Main weaknesses	Limited windows Operator dependent Limited tissue characterization Poor-quality imaging	Use of ionizing radiation Use of iodinated contrast Limited functional study Difficult in cardiac arrhythmias Need for breath-hold Only stable patients	Time consuming Limited availability High costs Not good for pericardial calcifications Difficult in cardiac arrhythmias Need for breath-hold Only stable patients

Indications, strengths, and weaknesses of imaging techniques for pericardial and pericardial diseases are summarized in Table 3.1.

PATHOPHYSIOLOGY OF PERICARDIAL SYNDROMES AFFECTING DIASTOLIC FUNCTION

The main pericardial syndromes include pericarditis, pericardial effusion, cardiac tamponade, and constrictive pericarditis. The pathophysiologic features of the pericardium that may affect diastolic function are summarized in this section.

Acute/Recurrent Pericarditis

In the setting of pericarditis, inflammation may be responsible for an excess of pericardial fluid that may impair diastolic filling when the accumulation is fast or very large leading to cardiac tamponade in the most dramatic scenario. Pericardial edema and fibrosis may also be responsible for increased stiffness of the pericardium due to a constrictive pathophysiology or effusive-constrictive pathophysiology in the setting of a concomitant pericardial effusion. Such changes may be reversible with resolution of inflammation, explaining the syndrome of transient pericardial constriction in up to 10% of cases with pericarditis.[32–35]

Pericardial Effusion

An isolated pericardial effusion may be asymptomatic or have symptoms related to the underlying disease or related to the effusion itself, if moderate to large. Moreover, a pericardial effusion may be an isolated process, but often (50%–60% of cases) it is associated and related to a systemic or underlying disease.[36,37] The speed of its accumulation is critical for the time course of symptoms. Since the pericardium is rather inelastic (as witnessed by a steep relationship between pressure and volume), a rapid accumulating pericardial effusion reaches the limit of pericardial stretch very soon with low volumes, while a slowly accumulating fluid reaches the limit of pericardial stretch only for volumes as big as 1 to 2 L without the development of cardiac tamponade (see Fig. 3.3).[8,19]

Cardiac Tamponade

Cardiac tamponade is the pericardial syndrome occurring when pericardial effusion impairs diastolic filling of the heart leading to a symptomatic reduction in cardiac output. The impairment of diastolic filling is continuous through the entire diastole.[38,39] The size of the effusion as well as its distribution may be variable. Since the pericardium is relatively stiff, if a pericardial fluid collects quickly, such as in hemopericardium, the limit of pericardial stretch is reached soon with volumes of 200 to 300 mL. On the other hand, a slowly accumulating pericardial effusion may reach 1 to 2 L before the development of cardiac tamponade. This pathophysiology explains that cardiac tamponade is a last drop phenomenon. Thus a small increase of pericardial volume may precipitate the syndrome, and the aspiration of small amounts of pericardial fluid may greatly improve the clinical condition in urgent pericardiocentesis.[14,40]

Usually pericardial effusions are circumferential, but after trauma or cardiac surgery they may be loculated and even be responsible for localized compression and the development of cardiac tamponade. The classic presentation of cardiac tamponade has been described by the thoracic surgeon Beck in 1935. Beck identified a triad, including hypotension, increased jugular venous pressure, and a small and quiet heart. This triad was classically identified in "surgical tamponade" with acute cardiac tamponade due to intrapericardial hemorrhage because of trauma, myocardial rupture, or aortic rupture. The Beck triad may be lacking in patients with "medical tamponade" with slowly accumulating pericardial fluid. Hypotension is absolute or relative. Acute cardiac tamponade is usually associated with low blood pressure (<90 mmHg) but only slightly reduced in subacute, chronic tamponade. Hypertensive patients may have normal to mildly elevated blood pressure concomitant to cardiac tamponade.[14,40,41]

On physical examination, classic signs include neck vein distention with elevated jugular venous pressure at bedside examination, pulsus paradoxus, and diminished heart sounds on cardiac auscultation. Pulsus paradoxus was first described by Kussmaul in 1873 as a palpable reduction of radial pulse on inspiration in patients with cardiac tamponade. The so-called paradox was the "waxing and waning" of the peripheral pulse, in contrast to the unvarying strength of the apical cardiac impulse. Pulsus paradoxus is classically defined as an inspiratory reduction of at least 10 mmHg of the systolic blood pressure. It can be easily detected recording the systolic pressure at which Korotkoff sounds are first audible and the systolic pressure at which they are audible through the whole respiratory cycle.[14,42]

Pulsus paradoxus is due to exaggerated ventricular interdependence occurring in cardiac tamponade when overall volume of cardiac chambers becomes fixed and any change in the volume of one side of the heart causes the opposite changes in the other side (i.e., inspiratory increase of venous return and right chambers with decreased left chamber volume and reduced systemic blood pressure). On ECG, the patient usually shows tachycardia, low QRS voltages, and electrical alternans. Both ECG signs are nonspecific and considered related to the damping effect of pericardial fluid and swinging heart.[43]

Constrictive Pericarditis

Constrictive pericarditis is a syndrome where the pericardium becomes relatively rigid and inelastic, may be thickened and calcified or not, and impairs mid to late diastolic filling. Constrictive pericarditis is the final pathway of several different diseases or causes, usually causing pericarditis and pericardial effusion and progressing toward pericardial fibrosis and calcification.[44–46]

In constrictive pericarditis the typical impairment of diastolic filling is mid to late diastolic with a suddenly blocked early diastolic filling causing several signs on physical examination (pericardial knock) and echocardiography (septal notch on M mode, 2D echo recordings). In addition, the fibrotic evolution of the pericardium is responsible for the obliteration of pericardial space with dissociation of intrathoracic pressures from intracardiac pressures as in cardiac tamponade. On this basis the overall pericardial volume becomes fixed, and the increase of one ventricle (e.g., right ventricle during inspiration due to increased venous return) can only occur with the decrease of the other (e.g., left ventricle). This causes an exaggerated interventricular interdependence with inspiratory decrease of the left ventricular volume and flow and contemporary increase in right ventricle volume and flow with septal bulging that can be seen on echocardiography.[44–46] The typical presentation of a patient with constrictive pericarditis includes signs and symptoms of right heart failure usually with preserved right and left ventricular function in the absence of previous or concomitant myocardial disease or advanced forms. Patients complain about dyspnea, fatigue, peripheral edema, breathlessness, hepatomegaly, pleural effusions, ascites, and abdominal swelling. The delay between the initial pericardial inflammation and the onset of constriction is variable and possibly a direct evolution from subacute/chronic pericarditis to constrictive pericarditis.[44–46] In specific forms as in tuberculous pericarditis or effusion the evolution usually occurs within 3 to 6 months.[47]

In advanced cases, pericardial fibrosis and scarring may extend into the myocardium, thus causing myocardial fibrosis and dysfunction. In specific forms (e.g., radiation pericarditis), the same etiologic agent (radiation) affecting the pericardium also affects the myocardium (as well as valves and coronary arteries), thus causing ventricular dysfunction as well.

Effusive Constrictive Pericarditis

Effusive constrictive pericarditis is caused especially by tuberculosis in developing countries.[35,48] Most cases of effusive constrictive pericarditis are idiopathic in developed countries, reflecting the frequency of idiopathic pericardial disease in general. Other reported causes include radiation, neoplasia, chemotherapy, infections (especially tuberculosis and purulent forms), and postsurgical pericardial disease. Patients with effusive constrictive pericarditis have both a fibrotic and scarred pericardium (only with special involvement of the epicardium) plus pericardial effusion.[35,48,49] Patients with effusive constrictive pericarditis usually have clinical features of pericardial effusion, constrictive pericarditis, or both. The constrictive physiology is often masked by cardiac tamponade, and right atrial pressure is persistently elevated after pericardiocentesis. The classic hemodynamic criterion is the failure of the right atrial pressure to fall by 50% or to a level below 10 mmHg after pericardiocentesis.[35] Although the traditional diagnosis is made by invasive measurement of right atrial pressure, nowadays it may also be well diagnosed by noninvasive imaging.[50]

FUTURE DIRECTIONS

The pericardium as an external envelope of the heart may affect the diastolic filling of the heart mainly in two ways that can be combined (e.g., pericarditis with effusion, effusive constrictive pericarditis): (1) Pericardial inflammation with pericardial edema and fibrosis may increase the stiffness of the normal pericardium leading to constriction with mid to late impairment of diastolic filling and dissociation of intrathoracic pressures from intracardiac pressures; and (2) increased production of pericardial fluid that, if it is sufficiently fast, may lead to increased intrapericardial pressure with cardiac tamponade. In the second case the impairment of diastolic filling is continuous through the entire diastole.

Multimodality imaging has greatly improved the understanding of the pathophysiology of pericardial syndromes allowing to reach a definite diagnosis without cardiac catheterization and invasive assessment for most cases by means of noninvasive multimodality imaging (echocardiography, cardiac MRI, CT) guided by clinical evaluation.

Future directions are developing to improve either the understanding of the etiopathogenesis of pericardial syndromes or the use of imaging to tailor treatments on the basis of the individual response by the assessment of pericardial inflammation by imaging.

KEY POINTS

- The pericardium is composed by an outer parietal fibroserosal layer (parietal pericardium) and an inner serosal visceral layer (visceral pericardium or epicardium). The normal thickness of the pericardium is less than 3 mm in imaging studies. A pericardial space is contained within the two layers and filled by 20 to 30 mL of plasma ultrafiltrate (pericardial fluid).
- The pericardium acts as a rather inelastic sac surrounding and protecting the heart allowing myocardial contraction without attrition and regulating the expansion of cardiac chambers thus affecting diastolic function.
- The pericardium is rather stiff, which means that it is not able to allow rapid changes of volume without a sudden increase of intrapericardial pressure. This leads to cardiac tamponade for small, rapidly increasing pericardial effusions but also allows the formation of a large, slowly accumulating pericardial effusion such as a chronic idiopathic pericardial effusion.
- In constrictive pericarditis, a fibrotic pericardium impairs diastolic filling in mid to late diastole and dissociates intrathoracic pressures from intracardiac pressures, thus generating an exaggerated interventricular interdependence. The clinical picture is that of right heart failure with a preserved ventricular function if cases are not advanced or complicated by concomitant myocardial dysfunction.

REVIEW QUESTIONS

1. Cardiac tamponade
   a. is characterized by impairment of diastolic filling in mid to late diastole.
   b. is always associated with large pericardial effusions.
   c. can be caused by a quickly accumulating mild pericardial effusion.
2. Constrictive pericarditis
   a. is always associated with increased pericardial thickness.
   b. is characterised by impairment of diastolic filling in mid to late diastole.
   c. is characterised by impairment of diastolic filling through all the diastole.
3. Impairment of diastolic function in pericardial diseases
   a. can occur only with large pericardial effusions.
   b. can occur only if the pericardium is thickened.
   c. is associated with exaggerated interventricular interdependence.

REFERENCES

1. Klein AL, Abbara S, Agler DA, et al. American Society of Echocardiography clinical recommendations for multimodality cardiovascular imaging of patients with pericardial disease: endorsed by the Society for Cardiovascular Magnetic Resonance and Society of Cardiovascular Computed Tomography. *J Am Soc Echocardiogr.* 2016;26(9). 965–1012.e15.
2. Cremer PC, Kumar A, Kontzias A, et al. Complicated pericarditis: understanding risk factors and pathophysiology to inform imaging and treatment. *J Am Coll Cardiol.* 2016;68(21):2311–2328.
3. Imazio M, Cecchi E, Demichelis B, et al. Indicators of poor prognosis of acute pericarditis. *Circulation.* 2007;115(21):2739–2744.
4. Imazio M, Brucato A, Maestroni S, et al. Prevalence of C-reactive protein elevation and time course of normalization in acute pericarditis: implications for the diagnosis, therapy, and prognosis of pericarditis. *Circulation.* 2011;123(10):1092–1097.
5. Imazio M, Brucato A, Maestroni S, et al. Risk of constrictive pericarditis after acute pericarditis. *Circulation.* 2011;124(11):1270–1275.
6. Imazio M, Brucato A, Barbieri A, et al. Good prognosis for pericarditis with and without myocardial involvement: results from a multicenter, prospective cohort study. *Circulation.* 2013;128(1):42–49.
7. Imazio M, Lazaros G, Picardi E, et al. Incidence and prognostic significance of new onset atrial fibrillation/flutter in acute pericarditis. *Heart.* 2015;101(18):1463–1467.
8. Imazio M, Lazaros G, Valenti A, et al. Outcomes of idiopathic chronic large pericardial effusion. *Heart.* 2019:105(6):477–481. doi:10.1136/heartjnl-2018-313532. [Epub ahead of print].
9. Imazio M, Brucato A, Cemin R, et al. A randomized trial of colchicine for acute pericarditis. *N Engl J Med.* 2013;369(16):1522–1528.
10. Imazio M, Belli R, Brucato A, et al. Efficacy and safety of colchicine for treatment of multiple recurrences of pericarditis (CORP-2): a multicentre, double-blind, placebo-controlled, randomised trial. *Lancet.* 2014;383(9936):2232–2237.
11. Brucato A, Imazio M, Gattorno M, et al. Effect of anakinra on recurrent pericarditis among patients with colchicine resistance and corticosteroid dependence: the AIRTRIP randomized clinical trial. *JAMA.* 2016;316(18):1906–1912.
12. Adler Y, Charron P, Imazio M, et al. 2015 ESC guidelines for the diagnosis and management of pericardial diseases: the Task Force for the Diagnosis and Management of Pericardial Diseases of the European Society of Cardiology (ESC) endorsed by: European Association for Cardio-Thoracic Surgery (EACTS). *Eur Heart J.* 2015;36(42):2921–2964.
13. Cosyns B, Plein S, Nihoyanopoulos P, et al. European Association of Cardiovascular Imaging (EACVI); European Society of Cardiology Working Group (ESC WG) on myocardial and pericardial diseases. European Association of Cardiovascular Imaging (EACVI) position paper: multimodality imaging in pericardial disease. *Eur Heart J Cardiovasc Imaging.* 2015;16(1):12–31.
14. Imazio M. *Myopericardial Diseases.* Switzerland: Springer International Publishing; 2016.
15. Little WC, Freeman GL. Pericardial diseases. *Circulation.* 2006;113(12): 1622–1632.
16. LeWinter MM. Clinical practice. Acute pericarditis. *N Engl J Med.* 2014;371(25):2410–2416.
17. Lachman N, Syed FF, Habib A, et al. Correlative anatomy for the electrophysiologist, part I: the pericardial space, oblique sinus, transverse sinus. *J Cardiovasc Electrophysiol.* 2010;21(12):1421–1426.
18. Peebles CR, Shambrook JS, Harden SP. Pericardial disease—anatomy and function. *Br J Radiol.* 2011;84(3):S324–S337.
19. Imazio M, Adler Y. Management of pericardial effusion. *Eur Heart J.* 2013;34(16):1186–1197.
20. Bertaso AG, Bertol D, Duncan BB, Foppa M. Epicardial fat: definition, measurements and systematic review of main outcomes. *Arq Bras Cardiol.* 2013;101(1):e18–e28.
21. Imazio M, Pedrotti P, Quattrocchi G, et al. Multimodality imaging of pericardial diseases. *J Cardiovasc Med (Hagerstown).* 2016;17(11):774–782.
22. Senapati A, Isma'eel HA, Kumar A, et al. Disparity in spatial distribution of pericardial calcifications in constrictive pericarditis. *Open Heart.* 2018;5(2):e000835. doi:10.1136/openhrt-2018-000835.
23. Bogaert J, Francone M. Cardiovascular magnetic resonance in pericardial diseases. *J Cardiovasc Magn Reason.* 2009;11:14.
24. Bogaert J, Francone M. Pericardial disease: value of CT and MR imaging. *Radiology.* 2013;267:340–356.
25. Feng D, Glockner J, Kim K, et al. Cardiac magnetic resonance imaging pericardial late gadolinium enhancement and elevated inflammatory markers can predict the reversibility of constrictive pericarditis after anti-inflammatory medical therapy: a pilot study. *Circulation.* 2011;124: 1830–1837.
26. Cremer PC, Tariq MU, Karwa A, et al. Quantitative assessment of pericardial delayed hyperenhancement predicts clinical improvement in patients with constrictive pericarditis treated with anti-inflammatory therapy. *Circ Cardiovasc Imaging.* 2015;8(5):e003125.
27. Alraies MC, AlJaroudi W, Yarmohammadi H, et al. Usefulness of cardiac magnetic resonance-guided management in patients with recurrent pericarditis. *Am J Cardiol.* 2015;115(4):542–547.
28. Alter P, Figiel JH, Rupp TP, Bachmann GF, Maisch B, Rominger MB. MR, CT, and PET imaging in pericardial disease. *Heart Fail Rev.* 2013;18(3):289–306.
29. Maggiolini S, De Carlini CC, Ferri LA, et al. The role of early contrast-enhanced chest computed tomography in the aetiological diagnosis of patients presenting with cardiac tamponade or large pericardial effusion. *Eur Heart J Cardiovasc Imaging.* 2016;17(4):421–428.
30. Kligerman S. Imaging of pericardial disease. *Radiol Clin North Am.* 2019;57(1):179–199.
31. Makis W, Ciarallo A, Hickeson M, et al. Spectrum of malignant pleural and pericardial disease on FDG PET/CT. *AJR Am J Roentgenol.* 2012;198(3):678–685.
32. Mittal SR. Transient pericardial constriction. *J Assoc Physicians India.* 2013;61(3):205–206.
33. Gentry J, Klein AL, Jellis CL. Transient constrictive pericarditis: current diagnostic and therapeutic strategies. *Curr Cardiol Rep.* 2016;18(5):41.
34. Paiardi S, Pellegrino M, Cannata F, Bocciolone M, Voza A. Transitory effusive-constrictive pericarditis. *Am J Emerg Med.* 2018;36(3):524.e1–524.e6.
35. Sagrista-Sauleda J, Angel J, Sanchez A, Permanyer-Miralda G, Soler-Soler J. Effusive-constrictive pericarditis. *N Engl J Med.* 2004;350:469–475.
36. Sagristà-Sauleda J, Mercé J, Permanyer-Miralda G, Soler-Soler J. Clinical clues to the causes of large pericardial effusions. *Am J Med.* 2000;109(2):95–101.
37. Sagristà-Sauleda J, Mercé AS, Soler-Soler J. Diagnosis and management of pericardial effusion. *World J Cardiol.* 2011;3(5):135–143.

38. Asher CR, Klein AL. Diastolic heart failure: restrictive cardiomyopathy, constrictive pericarditis, and cardiac tamponade: clinical and echocardiographic evaluation. *Cardiol Rev.* 2002;10(4):218–229.
39. Appleton C, Gillam L, Koulogiannis K. Cardiac tamponade. *Cardiol Clin.* 2017;35(4):525–537.
40. Shabetai R. Pericardial effusion: haemodynamic spectrum. *Heart.* 2004;90(3):255–256.
41. Hoit BD. Pericardial effusion and cardiac tamponade in the new millennium. *Curr Cardiol Rep.* 2017;19(7):57.
42. Kearns MJ, Walley KR, Tamponade: hemodynamic and echocardiographic diagnosis. *Chest.* 2018;153(5):1266–1275.
43. Roy CL, Minor MA, Brookhart MA, Choudhry NK. Does this patient with a pericardial effusion have cardiac tamponade? *JAMA.* 2007;297(16):1810–1818.
44. Syed FF, Schaff HV, Oh JK. Constrictive pericarditis—a curable diastolic heart failure. *Nat Rev Cardiol.* 2014;11(9):530–544.
45. Welch TD, Oh JK. Constrictive pericarditis. *Cardiol Clin.* 2017;35(4):539–549.
46. Miranda WR, Oh JK. Constrictive pericarditis: a practical clinical approach. *Prog Cardiovasc Dis.* 2017;59(4):369–379.
47. Imazio M, Brucato A, Mayosi BM, et al. Medical therapy of pericardial diseases: part II: noninfectious pericarditis, pericardial effusion and constrictive pericarditis. *J Cardiovasc Med (Hagerstown).* 2010;11:785–794.
48. Noubiap JJ, Agbor VN, Ndoadoumgue AL, et al. Epidemiology of pericardial diseases in Africa: a systematic scoping review. *Heart.* 2018;105(3):180–188. doi:10.1136/heartjnl-2018-313922. [Epub ahead of print.]
49. Syed FF, Ntsekhe M, Mayosi BM, Oh JK. Effusive-constrictive pericarditis. *Heart Fail Rev.* 2013;18(3):277–287.
50. Kim KH, Miranda WR, Sinak LJ, et al. Effusive-constrictive pericarditis after pericardiocentesis: incidence, associated findings, and natural history. *JACC Cardiovasc Imaging.* 2018;11(4):534–541.

4

Left Atrial Function: Basic Physiology

Brian D. Hoit

OUTLINE

Case Study

DL is a 75-year-old white male with a history of hypertension who presented with a 6-month history of reduced exercise tolerance, dyspnea on exertion, and occasional palpitations. The patient was scheduled for an exercise test but was noted to be in atrial fibrillation (AF). His physical examination was normal except for a blood pressure of 150/98 mmHg and an irregularly irregular pulse at 73 bpm. He underwent an unsuccessful cardioversion and was referred for cryoablation of his arrhythmia. The preablation transesophageal echocardiogram revealed normal left ventricular (LV) size and systolic function, restrictive LV filling, biatrial enlargement, mild mitral regurgitation, and normal sinus rhythm (Fig. 4.1A). There was spontaneous echo contrast in the left atrial (LA) appendage, but no thrombus (see Fig. 4.1B). Transmitral, pulmonary venous, and LA appendage velocities (Fig. 4.2A–C) were consistent with LA systolic failure. A transthoracic echocardiogram 6 weeks later showed a pseudonormal transmitral filling pattern with a return of atrial systolic activity (see Fig. 4.2D), leading to the diagnosis of atrial stunning. Symptomatically, the patient was improved.

Atrial stunning is a transient (minutes to weeks) mechanical dysfunction of the body and appendage of the atrium that is reported to occur with all methods of cardioversion (including spontaneous) of AF and flutter. Postulated mechanisms include tachycardia-induced atrial cardiomyopathy and abnormal calcium homeostasis.[1]

INTRODUCTION

A resurgence of interest in atrial function has enhanced our understanding of the atrial contributions to cardiovascular (CV) performance in health and disease. The reasons responsible for this renaissance are multifactorial and include (1) the recognition that atrial function is an important, at times critical, determinant of LV filling; (2) the increasing number of drugs, devices, ablative procedures, and surgery available for the treatment of AF[2,3]; (3) the considerable interest in dual and three-chamber pacemakers that maintain atrioventricular and biventricular synchrony, respectively[4]; (4) the growing number of transcatheter procedures for mitral valve repair, atrial septal defect closure, and LA appendage occlusion[5–7]; (5) the pathophysiologic and clinical relevance of chamber-specific structural, electrical, and ionic remodeling[8]; (6) the availability of newer techniques to accurately measure atrial size and function[9]; (7) the clinical impact of atrial stiffness and stunning, particularly post cardioversion and ablation[10]; and (8) the increasing data that support the use of atrial size and function to assist in risk stratification and the prediction of CV outcomes.[11] Despite this attention, quantifying atrial function is difficult, in part because the atria are geometrically complex.

ANATOMIC AND HISTOLOGIC CONSIDERATIONS

Because of the obliquity of the atrial septum, the right atrium projects anteriorly, inferiorly, and to the right of the left atrium (LA). The broad, triangular, muscular right atrial appendage protrudes anteriorly, the superior vena cava opens into the dome of the right atrium, and the inferior vena cava opens into its inferior and posterior portion. The body of the left atrium is smaller and thicker than the right atrium. The chamber has been modeled as a sphere, cube, or ellipse. The LA appendage is longer, narrower, and more tortuous than the right appendage and contains all the pectinate muscles of the left atrium. The four pulmonary veins, upper and lower from each lung (the left pair frequently opening via a common channel), enter the posterior aspect of the left atrium.[12]

The atrial walls consist of two muscular layers, the fascicles of which both originate and terminate at an atrioventricular ring and follow nearly perpendicular courses. Fascicles in the inner layer ascend vertically through a pectinate muscle, change depth and course circumferentially in the outer layer, encircle the atrium, dive into the inner layer, and descend vertically within a pectinate muscle. While some fascicles are intrinsic to one atrium, others are shared. The muscular terminations of the veins are also composed of two layers, the inner longitudinal and the outer circular.[13]

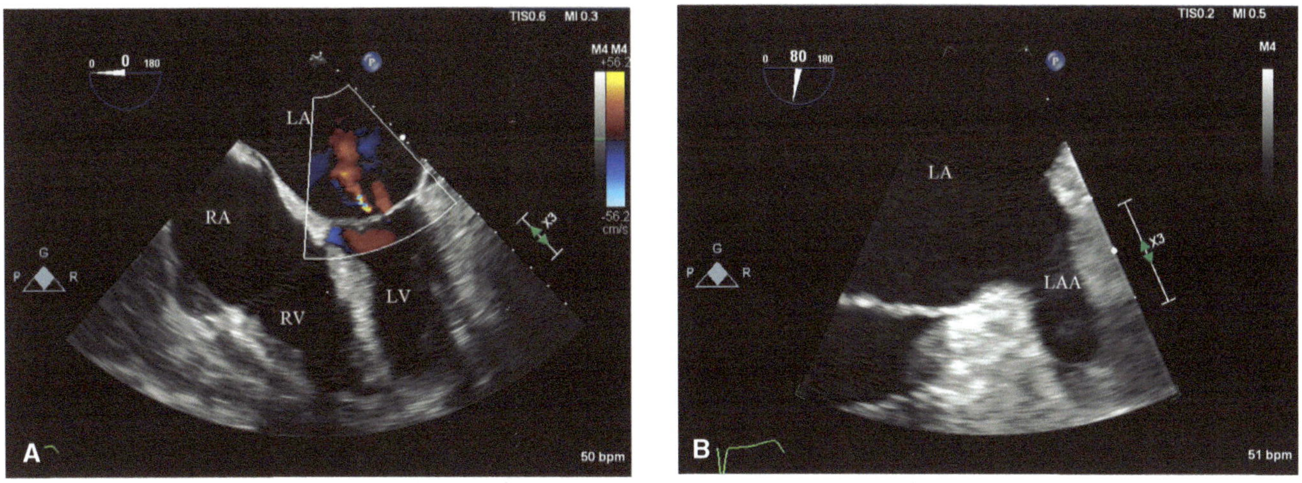

Fig. 4.1 (A) Apical four-chamber Transesophageal echocardiography (TEE) view with color flow Doppler demonstrates normal left ventricular *(LV)* systolic function, left *(LA)* and right atrial *(RA)* enlargement, and mitral regurgitation. Note P waves on the accompanying electrocardiogram. *RV,* Right ventricle. (B) Two-chamber TEE view of the left atrial appendage *(LAA)* with spontaneous echocontrast, indicating stasis of appendage flow.

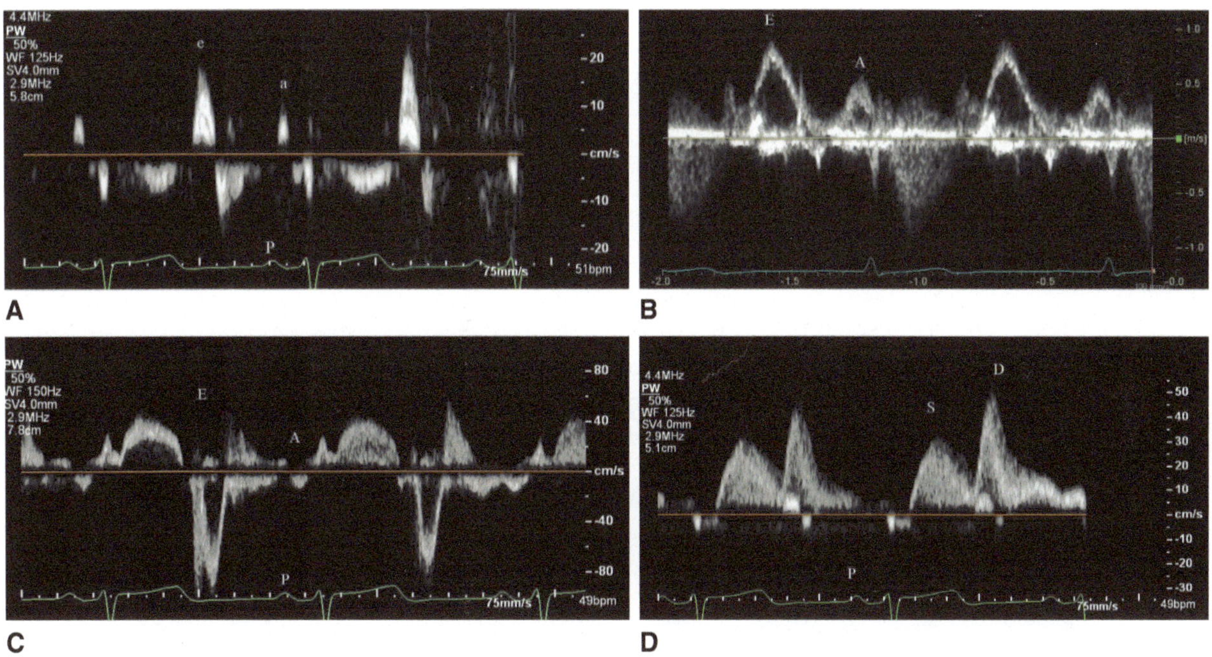

Fig. 4.2 (A) TEE spectral Doppler of left atrial appendage flow with markedly reduced late diastolic emptying velocity *(a)* and increased early velocity *(e)*. (B) TEE spectral Doppler of transmitral flow with high early diastolic velocity *(E)* and virtually no flow in late diastole *(A)* after the electrocardiographic P wave. (C) Transthoracic echocardiography (TTE) of transmitral flow 4 weeks after radiofrequency (RF) ablation demonstrates a return of the late diastolic *(A)* velocity. (D) TEE spectral Doppler of pulmonary venous flow with decreased systolic *(S)*, increased diastolic *(D)* flow and absent reversed flow after the electrocardiographic P wave.

Ultrastructurally, atrial myocardium differs significantly from ventricular myocardium. For example, myocytes are smaller in diameter, have fewer T tubules, and have more abundant Golgi apparatus in the atrium than ventricle.[14] Rates of contraction and relaxation, and conduction velocity and anisotropy, differ, as do their respective biophysical underpinnings (i.e., myosin isoform composition and qualitative and quantitative differences in a wide assortment of ion transporters, channels, and gap junctional proteins).[15,16]

Atrial interstitium contains cellular and extracellular components. The cellular elements are comprised of fibroblasts/myofibroblasts, adipocytes, and undifferentiated mesenchymal cells. The extracellular components include primarily collagen (mostly type I) fibers, which form the largest part of the myocardial skeleton, and proteoglycans, matrix vesicles, and lipidic debris.[17]

While there are important differences between left and right atrial structure and function at various organizational hierarchies, function of the left atrium at the organ level will be used in this chapter to illustrate the atrial contributions to ventricular filling. The discussion is drawn largely from studies our group has performed over the past three decades.

PATHOPHYSIOLOGY

Atrial Function in Health

The primary mechanical function of the left atrium is to modulate LV filling and CV performance; this task is accomplished by its interrelated roles as a reservoir for pulmonary venous flow during ventricular systole, as a conduit for pulmonary venous flow during early ventricular diastole, and as a booster pump that increases ventricular filling during late ventricular diastole. There is a critical interplay between these cardiac cycle-dependent atrial functions and ventricular performance. For example, while reservoir function is most strictly defined by the atrial compliance (or its inverse, stiffness), it is influenced by systolic ventricular function and atrial contraction and relaxation. Conduit function is affected by atrial compliance during ventricular diastole but is closely related to LV relaxation and stiffness. Finally, atrial booster pump function is largely due to the magnitude and timing of atrial contractility but is also determined by the degree of venous return (atrial preload), LV end-diastolic pressures (atrial afterload), and LV systolic reserve.[11]

Although atrial function can be evaluated with a number of imaging modalities, including echocardiography, cardiac computed tomography (CCT), cardiac magnetic resonance imaging (cardiac MRI), angiography, and sonomicrometry, echocardiography is arguably best suited for this task because of its availability, safety, versatility, and ability to image in real time with high temporal and spatial resolution. LA function is assessed using volumetric analysis (maximum, minimum, and pre-A wave LA volumes and their derived functions [total, passive, and active emptying fractions and expansion index]); transmitral, pulmonary venous, and LA appendage flow analysis; and deformational imaging (strain and strain rate).[9]

Left Atrial Booster Pump Function

The importance of the atrial booster pump function (i.e., the augmented ventricular filling resulting from active atrial contraction) has been estimated by measurements of (1) cardiac output and LV diastolic volume both with and without effective atrial systole[18]; (2) relative LV filling (e.g., early to late [E/A] filling ratios) using steady-state Doppler echocardiographic transmitral flow or radionuclide angiography[19]; (3) atrial shortening using methods such as two-dimensional (2D) and three-dimensional (3D) echocardiography, CCT, cardiac MRI, angiography, and sonomicrometry[9]; (4) by estimating the kinetic energy and force generated with atrial contraction[20,21]; and (5) strain and strain rates during atrial systole, which represent the magnitude and rate of myocardial deformation, respectively, that are measured using either echocardiographic (color tissue Doppler imaging or 2D speckle tracking) techniques or cardiac MRI (feature tracking or tagged MRI) (Figs. 4.3 and 4.4).[9] LA appendage pump function is assessed by late emptying spectral and tissue Doppler velocities. However, measurements of atrial systolic function and the importance of the atrial booster pump are dependent on a multiplicity of factors, including the timing of atrial systole, vagal stimulation, and (as noted) the magnitude of venous return, LV end-diastolic pressures, and LV systolic reserve. Not surprisingly, despite considerable study, the magnitude and relative importance of the atrial contribution to LV filling and cardiac output remain controversial.

Analogous to end-systolic elastance measurements in the left ventricle (where end-systolic elastance is calculated as the slope of the ventricular end-systolic pressure-volume [P-V] relation), a load-independent index of atrial contraction based on the instantaneous atrial P-V relation has the potential to explain and minimize the discrepancies and confusion that exist in the literature. Accordingly,

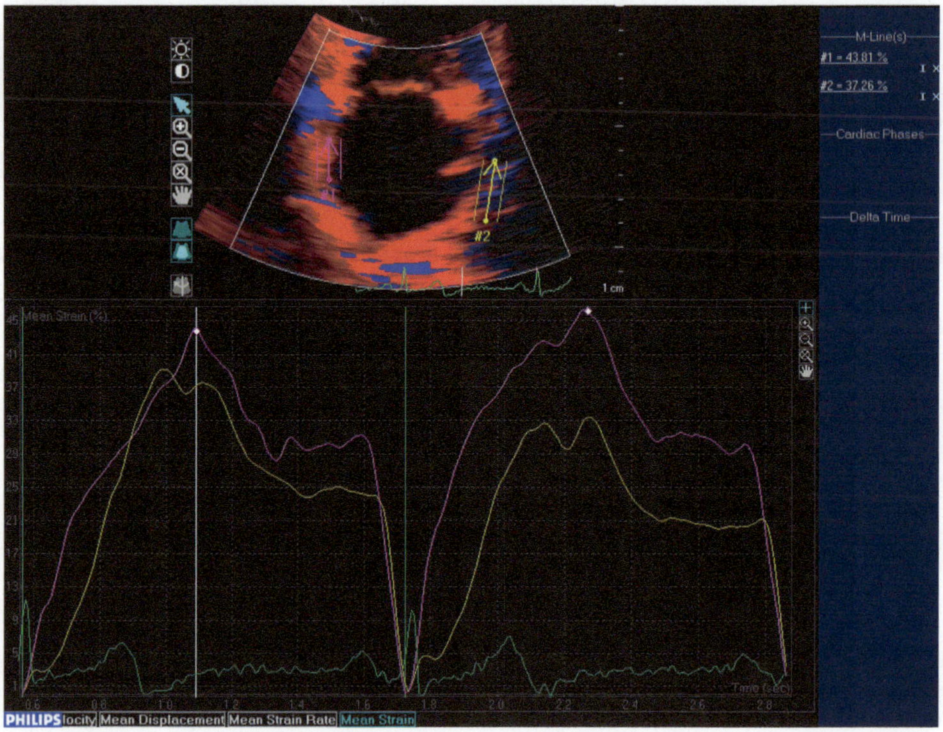

Fig. 4.3 Example of tissue Doppler imaging LA strain. Strain curves for the inferior *(purple)* and anterior segments *(yellow)* are shown. Peak systolic strain is represented by the white circles. (Reproduced with permission from Hoit BD. *J Am Coll Cardiol.* 2014;63:493–505.)

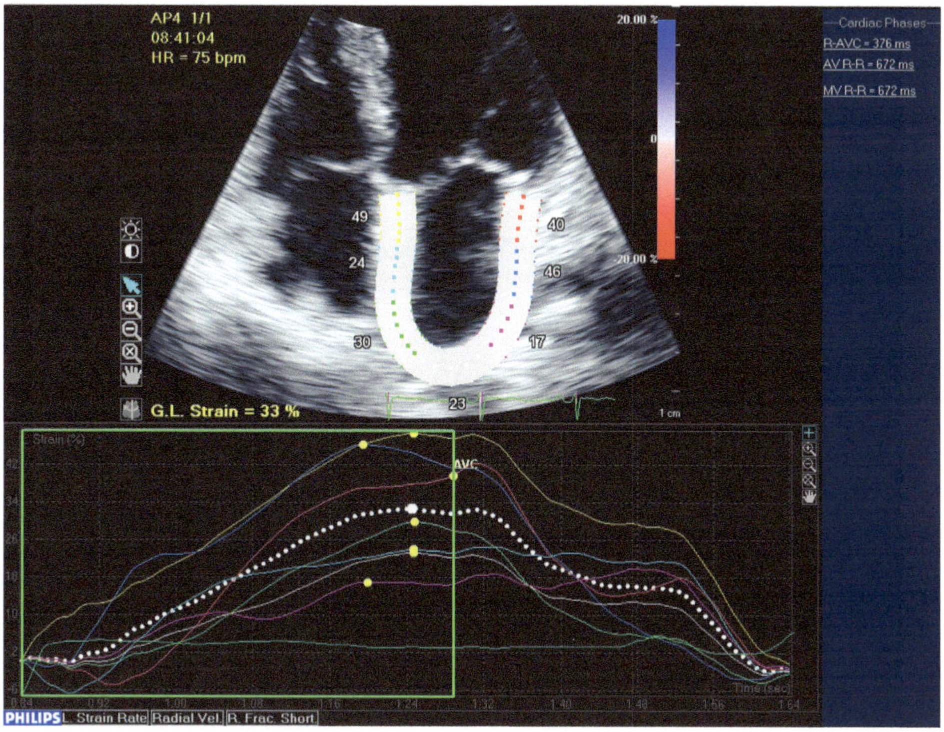

Fig. 4.4 Example of speckle tracking echo-derived LA strain. Regional strains are denoted by the colored lines, global longitudinal *(GL)* strain by the white dotted line. The closed circles on each regional strain-time curve identify peak systolic strain. *AVC,* Aortic valve closure. (Reproduced with permission from Hoit BD. *J Am Coll Cardiol.* 2014;63:493–505.)

understanding and deriving atrial elastance require a consideration of the relation between instantaneous atrial pressure and volume.

Pressure-volume relations of the atrium. A time-independent representation of the atrial events during the cardiac cycle can be obtained by plotting instantaneous atrial pressure and volume (Fig. 4.5). During ventricular systole, atrial relaxation and descent of the ventricular base lower atrial pressure (the x descent) and assist in atrial filling; the latter results in a v wave on the atrial pressure tracing. Thus, during ventricular systole, the atrium operates as a reservoir, storing systemic and pulmonary venous return. When the atrioventricular valves open, blood stored in the atria empties into the ventricles and atrial pressure falls (the y descent), during which time the atria act as conduits for venous blood flow into the ventricles. Atrial contraction, denoted by an a wave on the atrial pressure tracing, actively assists ventricular filling. The resultant P-V loop inscribes a figure-8 path that consists of a clockwise V loop due to atrial filling and passive emptying and a counterclockwise A loop due to active atrial contraction.

Although Alexander et al. described instantaneous LA pressure-volume relations by a time-varying elastance in the isolated LA using computer-simulated LA loading conditions,[22] assessment of atrial systolic elastance in vivo was hampered by the lack of an accurate measurement of LA volume with an adequate sampling frequency. Therefore, as a critical initial step, we demonstrated that cast-validated LA volumes could be estimated accurately with high temporal resolution sonomicrometry using two nearly orthogonal atrial dimensions.[23,24] The LA was assumed to be a general ellipsoid of revolution (LA volume = $\pi/6(SAX)^2(LAX)$, where SAX is the short or mediolateral, and LAX is the long or anteroposterior axis) and coupled with high-fidelity micromanometers, instantaneous P-V loops of the intact left atrium were generated (Fig. 4.6). The maximum slope of the isochronal P-V relation was measured every 10 ms during the A loop (from atrial diastasis to atrial end systole) from five variably loaded beats and were fitted to a time-varying elastance model: $E_{(t)} = P_{(t)}/[V_{(t)} - V_{(o)}]$, where $E_{(t)}$ is time-varying elastance, $V_{(o)}$ is the volume axis intercept, and $P_{(t)}$ and $V_{(t)}$ are instantaneous isochronal pressure and volume, respectively. Loading conditions were altered with either phenylephrine boluses or vena caval occlusions. Time-dependent changes in $E_{(t)}$ and maximal atrial systolic elastance (E_{max}) were found to be highly linear and sensitive to pharmacologically induced changes in inotropic state. In addition, LA systolic P-V relations using either the nonisochronal maximal P-V ratio ($E_{max\ P/V}$) or end systole (E_{es}) were shown to be useful estimates of E_{max}.

In addition to assisting the quantitation of ejection phase (i.e., ejection fraction, stroke volume, mean normalized systolic ejection rate [MNSER], and velocity of circumferential shortening [Vcf]) and load-independent indices of contraction (i.e., E_{max}, E_{es}, $E_{max\ P/V}$), P-V loops of the left atrium offered the potential to begin studying atrial energetics in vivo. Specifically, the planimetered A loop P-V area (total mechanical work done *by* the atrium) minus the V loop P-V area (work done *on* the atrium by pulmonary venous blood flow during ventricular systole) represents the net atrial mechanical work. In a study using normal, open chest dogs, A and V loop areas were similar and did not change with increased atrial preload, suggesting that booster pump and reservoir functions of the atrium were balanced over a wide range of LA pressures. However, calcium-induced increases in contractility and subsequent volume loading produced significant increases in the A but not V loop area, indicating that net atrial mechanical work was greater and load dependent after calcium infusion. Calcium infusion was also associated with a change in the trajectory of the A loop resulting in a decrease in the time from E_{max} to end systole; thus the atrial A loop, which resembled a right ventricular P-V loop before, looked like the LV pressure-volume loop after calcium infusion, suggesting an effect of calcium on ventricular input impedance.

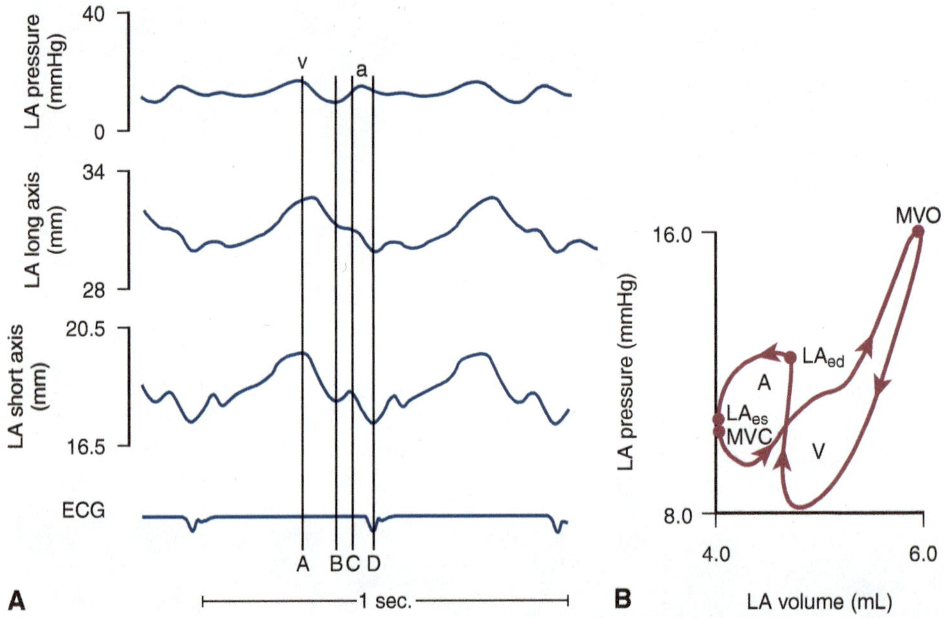

Fig. 4.5 (A) Analog recording of left atrial *(LA)* pressure and dimensions in the time domain. The vertical lines indicate times of mitral valve opening *(A)*, end of passive atrial emptying and onset of atrial diastasis *(B)*, atrial end diastole *(C)*, and atrial end systole *(D)*. Labels a and v represent respective venous pressure waves. (B) Left atrial pressure-volume loop from a single beat illustrating the characteristic figure-8 configuration. Arrows indicate direction of loop as a function of time. The A loop represents active atrial contraction. The V loop represents passive filling and emptying of the left atrium. *LA_{ed}*, Left atrial end diastole; *LA_{es}*, left atrial end systole; *MVO*, mitral valve opening. (Reprinted with permission from Hoit BD, Shao Y, Gabel M, Walsh RA *Circulation.* 1994;89:1829–1838.)

While atrial P-V loops can be generated in humans using invasive and semiinvasive means,[25–27] these methods are cumbersome, time consuming, and difficult to apply. Clearly there is a need for an objective, noninvasive measurement of atrial myocardial performance and contractility. Measurement of myocardial strain and especially strain rate during atrial systole are indices that have the potential to overcome these limitations. In addition, these indices can assist risk stratification and predict CV events. For example, LA booster pump strain rate predicted a composite of all-cause death and CV hospitalization in patients with either heart failure with preserved ejection fraction (HFpEF) or heart failure with reduced ejection fraction (HFrEF)[28]; and abnormal atrial booster pump strain was associated with increased CV events in 308 HFpEF patients prospectively enrolled and followed longitudinally for a median 13.8 months.[29]

Atrial booster pump function is also assessed by (late) diastolic emptying velocities of the left atrial appendage (LAA). Using sonomicrometer pairs on the LAA and LV and transesophageal echo, we showed that in dogs with normal LAA function, the major determinants of late emptying velocities were isovolumic and ejection phase indices of LV systolic function (i.e., peak positive dP/dt and LV fractional shortening, respectively)[30]; as expected, velocities decreased markedly when atrial systolic failure was produced by 1 week of rapid (400 bpm) atrial pacing.[31]

Left Atrial Reservoir Function

Grant et al. estimated that 42% of the LV stroke volume and its associated energy are stored in the left atrium during LV systole.[32] The subsequent dissipation of this energy during the reservoir phase acts as a ventricular restoring force during the ensuing LV diastole. Reservoir function is governed by atrial distensibility during ventricular systole, but has been shown to be related to LA contraction and descent of the LV base during systole,[33] LA systolic shortening, and LV end-systolic volume.[34] Atrial distensibility is measured most rigorously by fitting atrial pressures and dimensions, taken either at the time of mitral valve opening over a range of atrial pressures and volumes or from one of the limbs of the V loop in a static P-V loop, to an exponential equation.[35]

Suga et al. showed that atrial compliance was a significant determinant of cardiac performance in a circulatory analog model.[36] Specifically, decreased atrial compliance was associated with greater phasic and mean atrial pressures, but a lower mean level of atrial pressure during ventricular filling; this resulted in a smaller LV end-diastolic volume and decreased venous return. We confirmed earlier mathematical predictions that early LV filling (i.e., Doppler mitral E velocity) increases directly with operative atrial compliance.[37] Thus it is interesting to speculate that regions of increased distensibility in the left atrium may facilitate early diastolic filling of the left ventricle. One such region of the left atrium with increased distensibility is the atrial appendage.

In isolated canine atria, the slope of the P-V relation for the left atrium without the appendage is significantly greater than with the appendage intact.[38] We subsequently showed that in the intact dog, the pressure-strain relation is steeper (i.e., stiffer or less distensible) in the body than in the appendage of the left atrium (Fig. 4.7). Atrial systolic shortening and reservoir capacity (measured as the change in dimension during atrial systole and the maximum minus minimum dimension, respectively), increased in both the body and appendage during volume infusion and were greater in the appendage than body of the left atrium. Thus, for a given increase in LA pressure, there was a greater increase in the end-diastolic atrial dimension, with greater utilization of the Frank-Starling mechanism by the appendage than the body of the left atrium. Interestingly, biochemical studies indicate that atrial natriuretic factor is concentrated in the LA appendage,[39] which may, by virtue of its increased distensibility, be better suited for

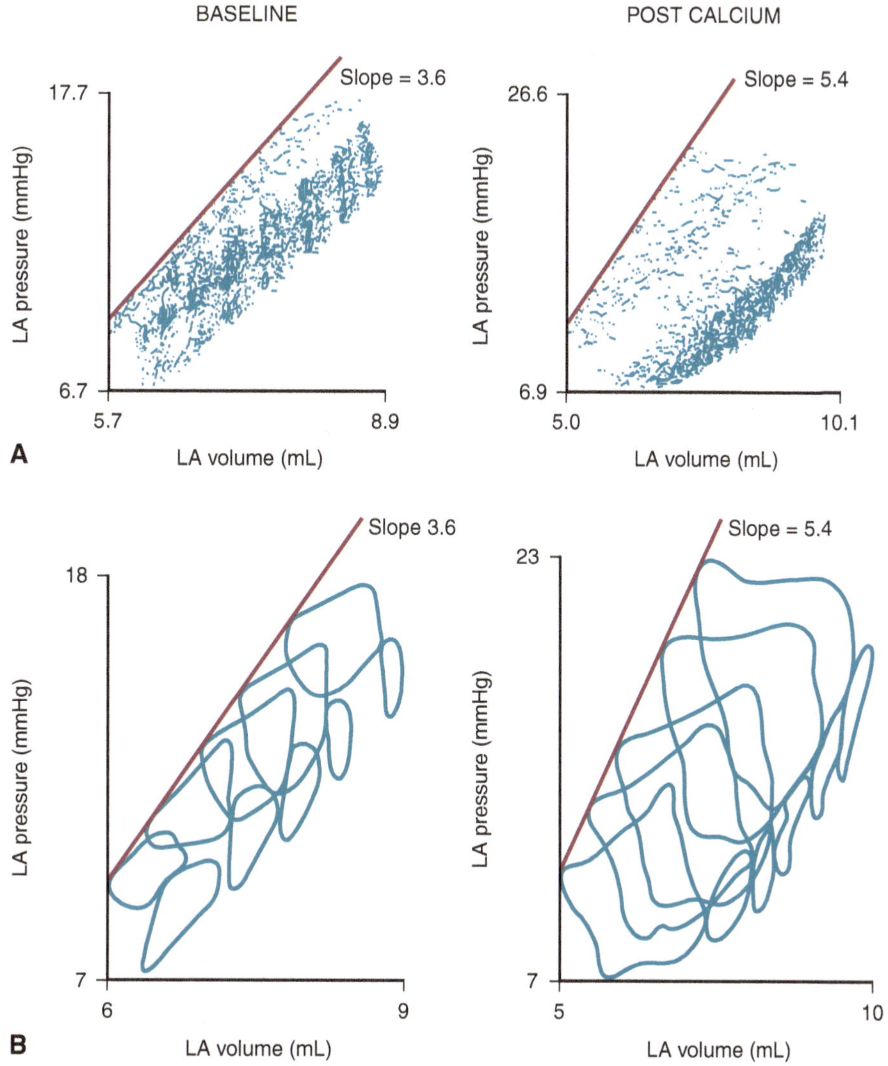

Fig. 4.6 Five left atrial *(LA)* pressure-volume loops at baseline (A) and after calcium infusion (B). Note the linearity of the end-systolic pressure volume relations, and the greater extent of atrial systolic shortening and the increase in the end-systolic pressure volume slope after calcium infusion (the latter indicating a positive inotropic effect). Loops are computer smoothed for clarity. (Reprinted with permission from Hoit BD, Shao Y, Gabel M, Walsh RA. *Circulation.* 1994;89:1829–1838.)

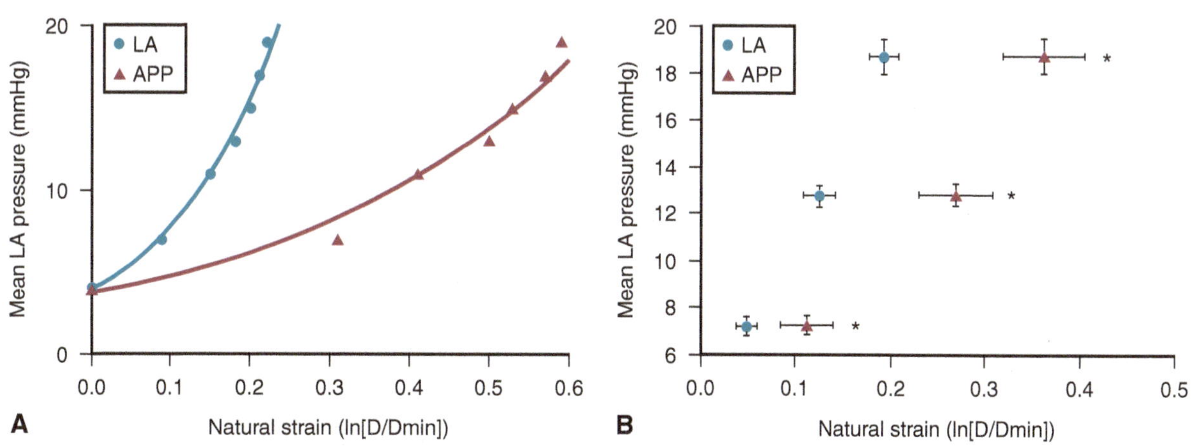

Fig. 4.7 (A) Representative mean left atrial *(LA)* pressure-natural strain relationships for the LA body and appendage *(APP)* from a single dog. Data are fitted to an exponential function. Pressure-strain relationship of appendage is shifted to the right of the body. (B) Mean pressure-natural strain data for 12 dogs. Error bars represent SE. Data indicate that the appendage is more distensible than the body of the left atrium. (Reprinted with permission from Hoit BD, Walsh RA. *Am J Physiol.* 1992;262:H1356–1360.)

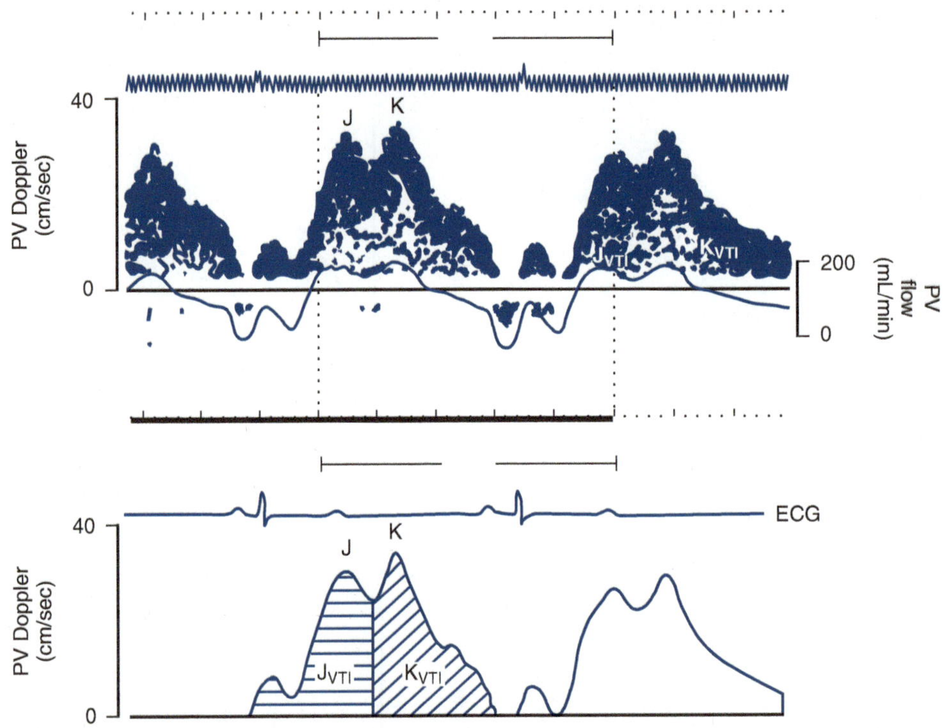

Fig. 4.8 Representative pulmonary vein *(PV)* Doppler with flow-probe waveform superimposed *(top panel)* and a schematic of the pulmonary venous flow velocity *(bottom panel)*. J and K are peak systolic and diastolic velocities; J_{VTI} and K_{VTI} are systolic and diastolic integrals, respectively. The ratio of systolic to diastolic velocities (and integrals) represents the relative reservoir to conduit function of the left atrium. (Reprinted with permission from Hoit BD, Shao Y, Gabel M, Walsh RA. *Circulation.* 1992;86:651–659.)

the regulation of intravascular volume. In addition, greater distensibility of the appendage than body of the left atrium would be potentially beneficial in the context of increased LV filling pressures and decreased global atrial distensibility. It is interesting that relative blood flow to the LA appendage was increased with experimental LA hypertrophy,[40] and the appendage-to-nonappendage LA blood flow ratio was increased during severe exercise in dogs, further suggesting that the LA appendage may become functionally important during stress. These data suggest that the substantial contributions of the appendage to overall LA compliance may have important negative implications for routine atrial appendectomy at the time of mitral valve surgery and for the use of percutaneous appendage exclusion devices.[41,42]

Although atrial dimensions and pressures are required for measurement of atrial distensibility, the relative reservoir function can be estimated simply with pulmonary vein Doppler (Fig. 4.8). Thus the proportion of LA inflow during ventricular systole provides an index of the reservoir capacity of the atrium.[43] In this regard, we showed that LA compliance is an important independent determinant of the pattern of pulmonary venous flow using an experimental protocol that excluded the LA appendage and produced an isolated decrease in atrial compliance and relative reservoir to conduit flow.[44] As a consequence, alterations in atrial compliance in various disease stages should be considered when the pattern of pulmonary venous flow is used to estimate LA pressure, assess LV diastolic function, or quantify mitral regurgitation.

Clinically, atrial reservoir function is estimated by volumetry using echocardiography, CCT, or cardiac MRI, and deformational imaging using echocardiography or cardiac MRI. The total LA emptying fraction $[(LA_{max} - LA_{min})/LA_{max})]$ and the LA expansion index $[(LA_{max} - LA_{min})/LA_{min})]$, where max and min refer to maximum and minimum LA volumes, approximate reservoir function. Myocardial strains are obtained using tissue Doppler imaging, 2D speckle tracking echocardiography, or feature tracking cardiac MRI.[9] A large body of data demonstrate that decreases in total atrial emptying indices and atrial strain and strain rates during ventricular systole (peak longitudinal systolic or reservoir strains) are common in CV diseases and their risk factors, are powerful predictors of CV events, and can stratify risk in general and referral populations as well as in a wide variety of CV diseases.[11] Moreover, coupled with an estimate of atrial pressure,[45,46] strain has the potential to estimate the atrial stiffness constant noninvasively.

The biophysical underpinning of atrial stiffness and impaired reservoir capacity of the atrium is atrial fibrosis, which may be interstitial or adventitial.[17] Replacement atrial fibrosis is detected with late gadolinium-enhanced cardiac MRI, and diffuse interstitial fibrosis is detected with postcontrast cardiac MRI T1 mapping.[17] Both techniques, which require specialized postprocessing, correlate well with result of voltage mapping. Importantly, LA reservoir strain correlates with both the amount of cardiac MRI–quantified replacement fibrosis and bipolar voltage during invasive mapping and predicts the recurrence after radiofrequency (RF) ablation of AF.[47]

Left Atrial Conduit Function

Atrial conduit function occurs primarily but not exclusively during ventricular diastole and represents the volume of blood that passes through the left atrium that cannot be attributed to reservoir or booster pump functions; in a well-characterized animal model, atrial conduit function accounted for 35% ± 8% of all flow through the atrium.[48] Volumetric measures of conduit function include the transmitral E velocity, the E/A ratio, diastolic pulmonary venous flow velocity, and the passive emptying fraction [$(LA_{max} - LA_{preA})/LA_{max}$)], where preA denotes the pre-A wave LA volume. Atrial conduit strain and strain rates are those that occur in early LV diastole, during passive LV filling. A reciprocal relation exists between conduit and reservoir functions of the left atrium. Indeed, the redistribution of atrial functions was reported as an important compensatory mechanism that facilitates LV filling in patients with myocardial ischemia, acute myocardial infarction, hypertensive heart disease, and mitral stenosis.[49–52]

Although it has been postulated that a more distensible atrium reduces atrial conduit flow, we showed that, while pericardiectomy decreased the atrial stiffness constant (increased distensibility), the relative conduit function, measured as the ratio of flow probe–determined systolic to diastolic pulmonary vein flow, actually increased.[43] However, it should be noted that the LA reservoir volume (max-min LA volume) and absolute systolic pulmonary venous flow also increased postpericardiectomy. In addition, removal of the pericardium was associated with an increase in the peak early velocity and deceleration time of transmitral diastolic flow, consistent with the increase in LV compliance after pericardiectomy. Thus it is possible that the decreased systolic to diastolic PV ratio reflects a greater change in compliance of the left ventricle than atrium. Irrespective of the mechanisms, these data underscore the complexity of pericardial influences on atrial and ventricular filling and the multifactorial determinants of P-V relations.

LA Function and Dyssynchrony

Regional strains have not been as rigorously studied as global strains but are potentially useful to quantify LA dyssynchrony. Atrial dyssynchrony has been defined by both the maximal time to peak delay of opposing atrial walls[53] and the mechanical dispersion, the standard deviation of contraction durations; the latter is defined as the time from the peak electrocardiographic P wave to maximal atrial systolic (booster pump) shortening in each segment. Atrial dyssynchrony reflects a heterogeneous pattern of LA fibrosis and dysfunction and predicts recurrence of AF after RF ablation.[54] In another prospective study of 130 patients undergoing cardioversion for AF, atrial dyssynchrony (quantified as mechanical dispersion) was an independent predictor of recurrence of AF, whereas LA volume was not.[55] Hemodynamic abnormalities may result from dyssynchrony and interatrial conduction delay. For example, atrial contraction may occur after mitral valve closure, with a resultant loss of atrial contribution to ventricular filling and an increase in LA pressure during ventricular systole.

LEFT ATRIAL FUNCTION IN DISEASE

The European Heart Rhythm Association, the Heart Rhythm Society, the Asia Pacific Heart Rhythm Society, and Sociedad Latinoamericana de Estimulacíon Cardíaca y Electrofisiología (EHRA/HRS/APHRS/SOLAECE) expert consensus on atrial cardiomyopathies defines atrial cardiomyopathy as "any complex of structural, architectural, contractile, or electrophysiological changes affecting the atrium with the potential to produce clinically-relevant manifestations." Nonspecific changes from hypertension, heart failure, diabetes, and myocarditis, and conditions such as aging or endocrine abnormalities, can result in atrial cardiomyopathy. The Working Group proposed the following descriptive histopathophysiologic classification scheme: primarily cardiomyocyte dependent (Class I [e.g., genetic diseases]), primarily fibroblast dependent (Class II [e.g., stiff LA syndrome]), mixed cardiomyocyte-fibroblast dependent (Class III [e.g., heart failure]), and primarily noncollagen deposits (Class IV [e.g., isolated atrial amyloidosis]).[17]

Atrial systolic failure may result from stunning (Class I), as occurred in the case presentation, or from an injury to the atrium that influences atrial contraction and compliance. Loss of contraction may be due to abnormalities at the cardiomyocyte level or from atrial scarring; abnormal atrial compliance is generally the result of fibrosis. Loss of atrial contraction leads to absent atrial booster pump function in the presence of an electrocardiographic P wave. Reduced atrial compliance results in increased LA pressure during ventricular systole (V wave); increased transmitral E wave and decreased A wave velocities, shortened mitral deceleration time, decreased pulmonary vein systolic/diastolic ratio, and decreased reservoir (systolic) atrial strain are characteristic echo Doppler findings.

A cause of atrial systolic failure once considered rare, the stiff LA syndrome (Class II) is reported to complicate up to 1% to 2% RF ablations of AF.[42,56] It is likely underdiagnosed, and its true prevalence underestimated. The stiff LA syndrome should be considered in the evaluation of dyspnea after an RF ablation when there are disproportional increases in the LA V wave relative to left ventricular end-diastolic pressure (LVEDP) (after excluding other causes of large V waves [e.g., mitral regurgitation and pulmonary vein stenosis]). Noninvasively, a large transmitral E wave and short deceleration time coupled with decreased reservoir strain should raise one's suspicion and justify a catheterization. However, the majority of atrial cardiomyopathies are mixed cardiomyocyte-fibroblast dependent and are associated with abnormal loading conditions.

Although LV adaptation to chronic hemodynamic loading has been studied extensively, the mechanisms by which the LA compensates for sustained increases in pressure and volume are less clear. We considered that adaptation may be due to the addition of contractile units (hypertrophy), an alteration in the molecular composition of the contractile machinery (e.g., protein isoform transitions), or a reduction of atrial systolic stress by structural remodeling. In pathologic studies of human atria, increases in the amount of the slow, β myosin isoform were correlated with the severity and duration of pressure and volume overload. In this context, a switch from the fast (α) to slow (β) myosin heavy chain (MHC) isoform in the ventricles of small mammals is accompanied by decreased myosin ATPase activity and velocity of contraction, reduced oxygen consumption, and a greater efficiency of contraction.[57] Thus these isoform switches are likely to represent adaptations to the functional requirements imposed by sustained hemodynamic loads in a chamber such as the LA, which contains predominantly α MHC.

Left Atrial Function and Systolic LV Dysfunction

Experimental studies that examine atrial adaptation use models of mitral regurgitation,[58] myocardial infarction,[59] LV diastolic dysfunction,[60] and pacing-induced myocardial failure (ventricular and atrial tachypacing).[57,61] In the ventricular tachypacing model of heart failure, we found a significant upregulation of β MHC in the LA body that was associated with LA hypertrophy, increased atrial mechanical work (A loop area) (Fig. 4.9), maintained force generation (E_{max} and E_{es}), and decreased velocity of LA contraction. Another important finding of that study was that atrial MHC isoform switches vary by region. Despite hypertrophy of the appendage, the percent β MHC did not increase in comparison to controls, suggesting that adaptation to hemodynamic overload includes differentially determined quantitative (e.g., hypertrophy) and qualitative (e.g., isoform switch) components, and that there are fundamental differences in the atrial response to stress hypertrophy that occurs in the body versus strain hypertrophy that occurs in the appendage.[57]

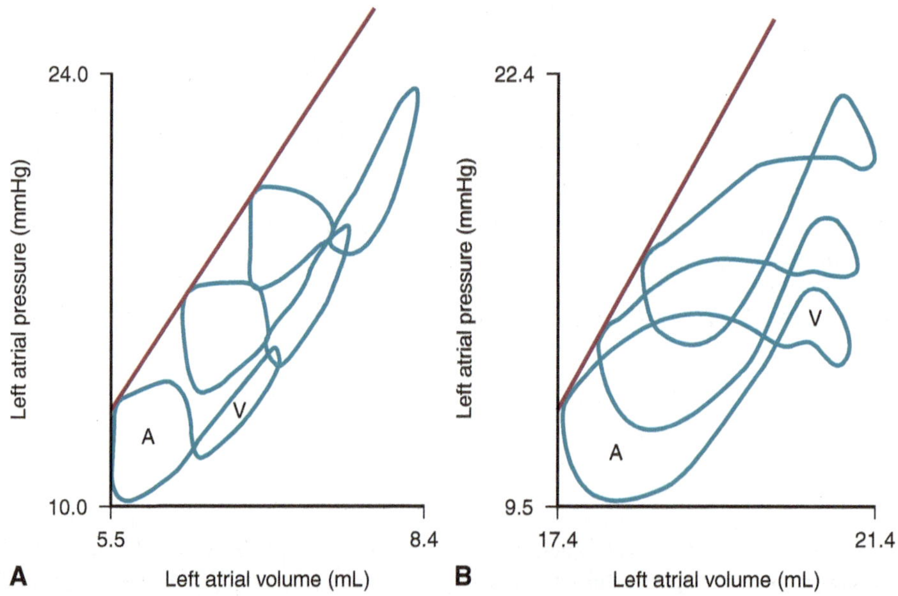

Fig. 4.9 Left atrial pressure-volume loops from three variably loaded beats in a control dog (A) and in a dog with pacing induced heart failure (B). The A loop represents active atrial contraction; the V loop represents passive filling and emptying of the left atrium. The increase in A loop area after pacing indicates increased atrial systolic work. Loops are computer smoothed for clarity. (Reprinted with permission from Hoit BD, Shao Y, Gabel M, Walsh RA. *Cardiovasc Res.* 1995;29:469–474.)

Left Atrial Function and Diastolic LV Dysfunction

In carefully studied animal models, the improvement in systolic function that occurs after cessation of tachypacing is associated with residual abnormalities of LV isovolumic relaxation and chamber compliance, and in some instances the development of LV hypertrophy. Since LV diastolic dysfunction represents a source of excess afterload on the left atrium, we examined the gravimetric, myosin biochemical, and functional changes in the left atrium that accompany regression of pacing-induced heart failure. Animals were rapidly paced for 3 weeks to produce heart failure, and hemodynamic and functional studies were performed 3 weeks after pacing cessation.[61] We showed that improvement of LV systolic dysfunction was associated with persistent LV diastolic dysfunction and normalization of both atrial E_{es} and net atrial work despite the persistent abnormalities of load-dependent indices of LA systolic function (e.g., ejection fraction, systolic ejection rate). LA stiffness and reservoir volumes also remained abnormal. Atrial stiffness constants were greatest in systolic and diastolic heart failure compared to control dogs, and numerically greater in systolic than diastolic failure, a finding consistent with Kurt et al. using the ratio of pulmonary capillary wedge pressure (PCWP) or E/e′ to LA reservoir strain.[46] Changes in systolic and diastolic function of the left atrium were accompanied by persistent upregulation of the atrial β-myosin heavy chain isoform and incomplete regression of LA hypertrophy, indicating an apparent dissociation of myosin isoform shifts, myocardial hypertrophy, and atrial work.

Left Atrial Function in a Model of Atrial Systolic Failure

We examined global and regional LA pump functions after 1 week of isolated atrial flutter (atrial pacing at 400 bpm) in closed chest, sedated dogs.[31] LV function, as assessed by the echocardiographic LV area shortening fraction, was preserved. Global and regional atrial pump functions were determined by mitral and LA appendage waveform analysis, and relative conduit and reservoir functions by pulmonary venous waveform analysis with Doppler velocimetry. We found that after 1 week of rapid atrial pacing, global and regional atrial booster pump functions (i.e., body and appendage) were reversibly impaired and relative reservoir to conduit function of the LA reduced (Fig. 4.10), findings identical to those in the case presentation. Potential mechanisms responsible for this model of atrial failure include atrial stunning, impaired calcium homeostasis, and neurohormonal and ultrastructural changes. Interestingly, similar mechanical changes in the absence of atrial hypertrophy were noted in a highly instrumented preparation treated with similar atrial tachypacing for 6 weeks. In that study,[61] the normalized atrial stiffness constant was increased, the response to calcium infusion attenuated, and atrial efficiency reduced compared to controls.

Importance of LA Function and Their Interplay in LV Systolic Dysfunction

The redistribution of atrial reservoir and conduit functions and augmented booster pump function are important compensatory mechanisms that facilitate LV filling in patients with myocardial ischemia, acute myocardial infarction, and hypertensive heart disease. However, considerably less is known how these mechanisms operate in the setting of LV dysfunction. Therefore we tested the hypothesis that in contrast to dogs with a normal left ventricle, cardiac output falls with the loss of atrial systolic contraction in dogs with concomitant LV dysfunction because atrial compensatory mechanisms fail.

Chronic atrial and ventricular dysfunction (both singly and in combination) were modeled with rapid pacing in dogs with RF AV nodal ablation and implantation of right atrial and ventricular pacing catheters.[62] Serial echocardiographic analysis of global and regional LA pump function were estimated from mitral and LA appendage Doppler velocimetry, and relative reservoir and conduit functions of the LA were determined from pulmonary venous Doppler. Right heart catheterization studies were performed simultaneously to assess right heart pressures and cardiac output. Isolated atrial systolic failure was produced by 1 week of rapid atrial pacing (400 bpm), and moderate LV dysfunction was produced by 2 weeks of rapid right ventricular pacing (220 bpm). Two weeks of rapid ventricular pacing superimposed on

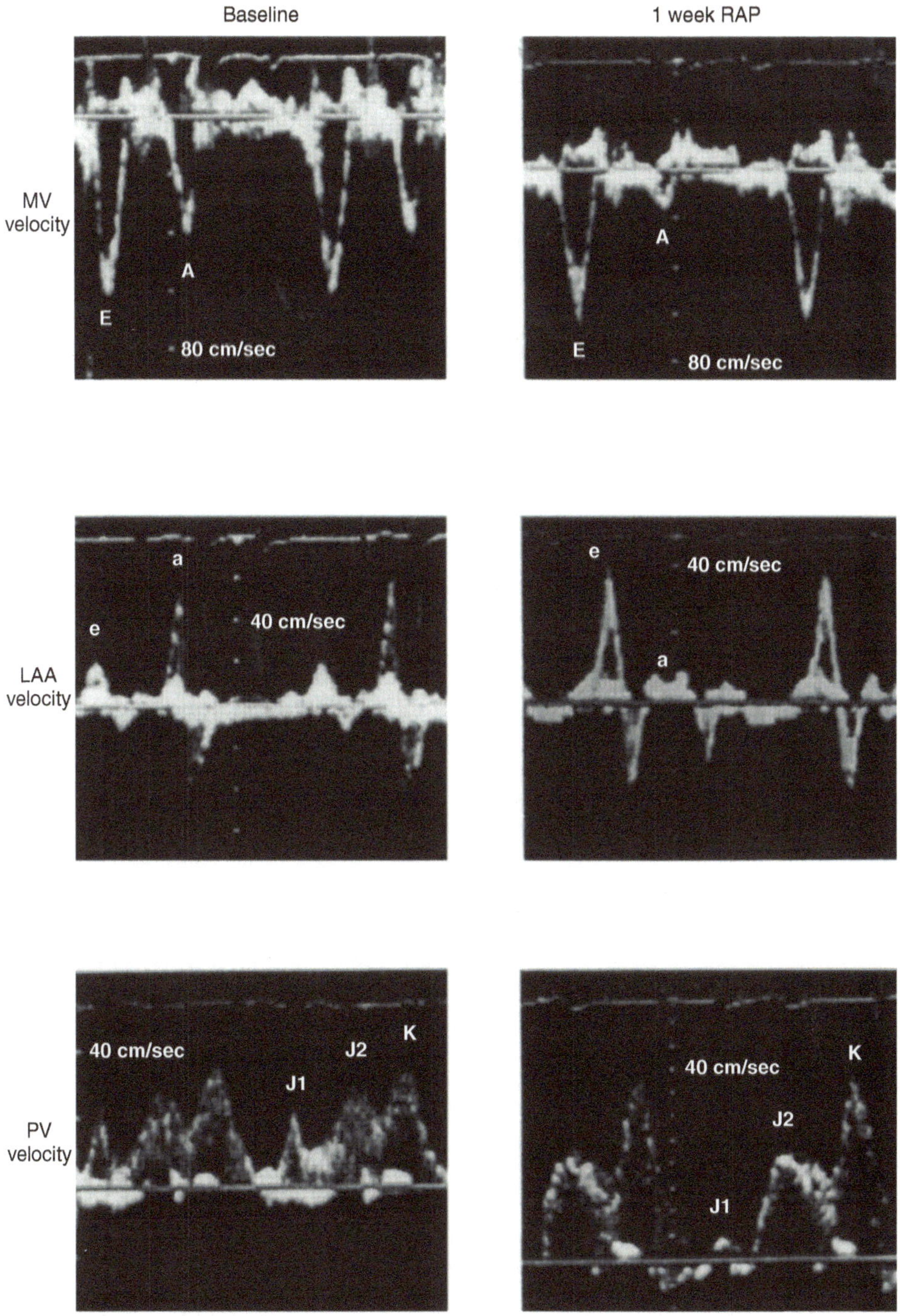

Fig. 4.10 Doppler waveforms of transmitral ((*MV, top panel*), left atrial appendage (*LAA, middle panel*), and pulmonary vein *(PV, bottom panel)* flows at baseline and after 1 week of rapid atrial pacing *(RAP)*. *A,* Late transmitral diastolic velocity; *a,* late LAA emptying velocity; *E,* early transmitral diastolic velocity; *e,* early LAA emptying velocity; *J1* and *J2,* systolic velocities; *K,* diastolic PV velocities. The corresponding electrocardiogram is shown in each panel. (Reprinted with permission from Hoit BD, Shao Y, Gabel M *J Am Soc Echo.* 1997;10:805–810.)

rapid atrial pacing during the second week produced combined LA and LV dysfunction. As previously noted, isolated LV dysfunction resulted in increased atrial booster pump and reservoir functions, whereas isolated rapid atrial pacing resulted in decreased atrial booster pump and increased relative conduit function of the LA. In contrast, the decreased atrial booster pump function in animals with combined atrial and ventricular dysfunction was incompletely compensated by the redistribution of the reservoir and conduit functions of the LA. As a result, cardiac output decreased and right heart pressures increased only after superimposed atrial and ventricular pacing.

FUTURE DIRECTIONS

While knowledge of atrial function lags considerably behind that of the ventricle, the chasm continues to close. The studies discussed herein describe the role of atrial function to ventricular filling in normal physiology and provide a framework for understanding mechanical, energetic, and biochemical mechanisms responsible for atrial adaptation to chronic hemodynamic loading. Important future directions include distinguishing the role of atrial function in early versus late LV systolic dysfunction, investigating the role of fibrosis and matrix metalloproteinases (and other molecules) in structural remodeling of the atria, characterizing the biochemical and molecular biologic changes that accompany atrial adaptation and failure, and identifying the relation between structural and electrical remodeling of the LA. Additional studies are needed to validate the EHRA/HRS/APHRS/SOLAECE classification of atrial cardiomyopathies and assess their value in the management of both heart failure and AF. These goals are likely to be met with the development of novel techniques to evaluate atrial reservoir, conduit, and booster pump functions of the atrium.

ACKNOWLEDGMENTS

This work was supported in part by a Grant in Aid award from the American Heart Association Ohio Valley Affiliate (0355198B).

KEY POINTS

- The primary mechanical function of the left atrium is to modulate left ventricular filling by its interrelated roles as a reservoir, conduit, and booster pump.
- Echocardiography is best suited for the evaluation of LA function because of its availability, safety, versatility, and ability to image in real time with high temporal and spatial resolution.
- Echocardiographically derived LA booster pump strain rate predicts all-cause death and CV hospitalization in patients with either HFpEF or HFrEF.
- The total LA emptying fraction calculated from 2D or 3D echocardiographically derived volumes approximates LA reservoir function.
- LA reservoir strain correlates with both the amount of cardiac MRI–quantified replacement fibrosis and bipolar voltage during invasive mapping and predicts the recurrence after radiofrequency ablation of atrial fibrillation.
- The redistribution of atrial reservoir and conduit functions and augmented booster pump function are important compensatory mechanisms that facilitate LV filling in patients with myocardial ischemia, acute myocardial infarction, and hypertensive heart disease.

REVIEW QUESTIONS

1. Which of the following can be determined from the atrial pressure-volume loop?
   a. Net atrial mechanical work
   b. Atrial conduit volume
   c. Atrioventricular coupling
   d. Peak atrial longitudinal strain
2. Maximal atrial systolic elastance
   a. is estimated by fitting atrial pressures and volumes at the time of mitral valve opening.
   b. is a load-independent index of atrial contraction.
   c. has only been measured in experimental animals.
   d. is used as a measure of atrial reservoir function.
3. Which of the following is most associated with atrial reservoir function?
   a. LV end-diastolic volume
   b. Vagal tone
   c. The timing of atrial systole
   d. Descent of the LV base
4. The stiff LA syndrome
   a. is suspected by a disproportionately large atrial V wave in the absence of mitral regurgitation.
   b. is characterized by increased atrial compliance.
   c. may complicate as many as 10% RF ablations for atrial fibrillation.
   d. is associated with decreased early diastolic transmitral (E wave) velocity.
5. An LA adaptation to chronic hemodynamic loading is
   a. increased myosin ATPase activity.
   b. myosin heavy chain isoform switches.
   c. decreased LA stiffness.
   d. downregulation of LA mechanical work.
6. Rapid (400 bpm) atrial pacing for 6 weeks results in
   a. a compensatory increase in relative reservoir/conduit function.
   b. LA hypertrophy.
   c. attenuated LA response to calcium infusion.
   d. reduced LA stiffness.

REFERENCES

1. Khan IA. Atrial stunning: basics and clinical considerations. *Int J Cardiol.* 2003;92:113–128.
2. Hersi A, Wyse DG. Management of atrial fibrillation. *Curr Prob Cardiol.* 2005;30:175–233.
3. Gillinov AM, Wolf RK. Surgical ablation of atrial fibrillation. *Progr Cardiov Dis.* 2005;48:169–177.
4. Frielingsdorf J, Gerber AE, Hess OM. Importance of maintained atrio-ventricular synchrony in patients with pacemakers. *Eur Heart J.* 1994;15:1431–1440.
5. Nyman CB, Mackensen GB, Jelacic S, Little SH, Smith TW, Mahmood F. Transcatheter mitral valve repair using the edge-to-edge clip. *J Am Soc Echocardiogr.* 2018;31:434–453.
6. Wiktor DM, Carrol JD. ASD closure in structural heart disease. *Curr Cardiol Reports.* 2018;20:37. doi: 10.1007/s11886-018-0983-x.
7. Bergmann MW. LAA occlude device for stroke prevention: data on WATCHMAN and other LAA occluders. *Trends Cardiovasc Med.* 2017;27:435–446.
8. Nattel S, Shiroshita-Takeshita A, Cardin S, Pelletier P. Mechanisms of atrial remodeling and clinical relevance. *Curr Opin Cardiol.* 2005;20:21–25.
9. Hoit BD. Evaluation of left atrial function: current status. *Struct Heart.* 2017;1(3–4):109–120. doi: 10.1080/24748706.2017.1353718.
10. Grimm RA, Leung DY, Black IW, Thomas JD. Left atrial appendage "stunning" after spontaneous conversion of atrial fibrillation demonstrated by transesophageal Doppler echocardiography. *Am Heart J.* 1995;130:174–176.
11. Hoit BD. Left atrial size and function: role in prognosis. *J Am Coll Cardiol.* 2014;63:493–505.
12. Strandring S, ed. *Gray's Anatomy.* London: Elsevier; 2005.

13. Thomas CE. The muscular architecture of the atria of hog and dog hearts. *Am J Anat.* 1959;104:207–236.
14. McNutt NS, Fawcett DW. The ultrastructure of the cat myocardium. II. Atrial muscle. *J Cell Biol.* 1969;42:46–67.
15. Li GR, Lau CP, Shrier A. Heterogeneity of sodium current in atrial vs epicardial ventricular myocytes of adult guinea pig hearts. *J Mol Cell Cardiol.* 2002;34:1185–1194.
16. Tuteja D, Xu D, Timofeyev V, et al. Differential expression of small-conductance Ca2+-activated K+ channels SK1, SK2, and SK3 in mouse atrial and ventricular myocytes. *Am J Physiol. Heart Circ Physiol.* 2005;289:H2714–H2723.
17. Goette A, Kalman JM, Aguinaga L, Akar J, Cabrera JA, Chen SA. EHRA/HRS/APHRS/SOLAECE expert consensus on atrial cardiomyopathies: definition, characterization, and clinical implication. *Heart Rhythm.* 2017;14:e3–e40.
18. Mitchell JH, Gupta DN, Payne RM. Influence of atrial systole on effective ventricular stroke volume. *Circ Res.* 1965;17:11–18.
19. Hoit BD, Rashwan M, Verba J, Pretorius T, Sahn DJ, Bhargava V. Instantaneous transmitral flow using Doppler and M-mode echocardiography: comparison with radionuclide ventriculography. *Am Heart J.* 1989;118:308–314.
20. Stefanadis C, Dernellis J, Lambrou S, Toutouzas P. Left atrial energy in normal subjects, in patients with symptomatic mitral stenosis, and in patients with advanced heart failure. *Am J Cardiol.* 1998;82:1220–1223.
21. Manning WJ, Silverman DI, Katz SE, Douglas PS. Atrial ejection force: a noninvasive assessment of atrial systolic function. *J Am Coll Cardiol.* 1993;22:221–225.
22. Alexander J, Sunagawa K, Chang N, Sagawa K. Instantaneous pressure-volume relation of the ejecting canine left atrium. *Circ Res.* 1987;61:209–219.
23. Hoit BD, Shao Y, McMannis K, Gabel M, Walsh RA. Determination of left atrial volume using sonomicrometry: a cast validation study. *Am J Physiol.* 1993;264:H1011–H1016.
24. Hoit BD, Shao Y, Gabel M, Walsh RA. In vivo assessment of left atrial contractile performance in normal and pathological conditions using a time-varying elastance model. *Circulation.* 1994;89:1829–1838.
25. Stefanadis C, Dernellis J, Stratos C, et al. Assessment of left atrial pressure-area relation in humans by means of retrograde left atrial catheterization and echocardiographic automatic boundary detection: effects of dobutamine. *J Am Coll Cardiol.* 1998;31:426–436.
26. Dernellis JM, Stefanadis CI, Zacharoulis AA, Toutouzas PK. Left atrial mechanical adaptation to long-standing hemodynamic loads based on pressure-volume relations. *Am J Cardiol.* 198;81:1138–1143.
27. Tse HF, Hettrick DA, Mehra R, Lau CP. Improved atrial mechanical efficiency during alternate- and multiple-site atrial pacing compared with conventional right atrial appendage pacing: implications for selective site pacing to prevent atrial fibrillation. *J Am Coll Cardiol.* 2006;47:209–212.
28. Sanchis L, Andrea R, Falces C, et al. Prognostic value of left atrial strain in outpatients with de novo heart failure. *J Am Soc Echocardiogr.* 2016;29(11):1035–1042.
29. Freed BH, Daruwalla V, Cheng JY, et al. Prognostic utility and clinical significance of cardiac mechanics in heart failure with preserved ejection fraction: importance of left atrial strain. *Circ Cardiovasc Imaging.* 2016;9(3):e003754.
30. Hoit BD, Shao Y, Gabel M. Influence of acutely altered loading conditions on left atrial appendage flow velocities. *J Am Coll Cardiol.* 1994;24:1117–1123.
31. Hoit BD, Shao Y, Gabel M. Global and regional atrial function after rapid atrial pacing: an echo Doppler study. *J Am Soc Echocardiogr.* 1997;10:805–810.
32. Grant C, Bunnell IL, Green DG. The reservoir function of the left atrium during ventricular systole. *Am J Med.* 1964;37:36–43.
33. Barbier P, Solomon SB, Schiller NB, Glantz SA. Left atrial relaxation and left ventricular systolic function determine left atrial reservoir function. *Circulation.* 1999;100:427–436.
34. Hoit BD, Shao Y, Gabel M, Walsh RA. Influence of loading conditions and contractile state on pulmonary venous flow. Validation of doppler velocimetry. *Circulation.* 1992;86:651–659.
35. Hoit BD, Walsh RA. Regional atrial distensibility. *Am J Physiol.* 1992;262:H1356–H1360.
36. Suga H. Importance of atrial compliance in cardiac performance. *Circ Res.* 1974;35:39–43.
37. Hoit BD, LeWinter M, Lew WY. Independent influence of left atrial pressure on regional peak lengthening rates. *Am J Physiol.* 1990;259:H480–H487.
38. Davis CA, Rembert JC, Greenfield JC. Compliance of the left atrium with and without left atrium appendage. *Am J Physiol.* 1990;259:H1006–H1008.
39. Hintze TH, McIntyre JJ, Patel MB, et al. Atrial wall function and plasma atriopeptin during volume expansion in conscious dogs. *Am J Physiol.* 1989;256:H713–H719.
40. Bauman RP, Rembert JC, Greenfield JC. Regional atrial blood flow in dogs. Effect of hypertrophy on coronary flow reserve. *J Clin Invest.* 1989;83:1563–1569.
41. Bergmann MW. LAA occluder device for stroke prevention data on WATCHMAN and other LAA occluders. *Trends Cardiovasc Med.* 2017;27:435–446.
42. Reddy YNV, El Sabbagh A, Packer D, Nishimura RA. Evaluation of shortness of breath after atrial fibrillation ablation–is there a stiff left atrium?. *Heart Rhythm.* 2018;15:930–935.
43. Hoit BD, Shao Y, Gabel M, Walsh RA. Influence of pericardium on left atrial compliance and pulmonary venous flow. *Am J Physiol.* 1993;264:H1781–H1787.
44. Hoit BD, Shao Y, Tsai LM, Patel R, Gabel M, Walsh RA. Altered left atrial compliance after atrial appendectomy. Influence on left atrial and ventricular filling. *Circ Res.* 1993;72:167–175.
45. Nagueh SF. Non-invasive assessment of left ventricular filling pressure. *Eur J Heart Failure.* 2018;20:38–48.
46. Kurt M, Wang J, Torre-Amione G, Nagueh SF. Left atrial function in diastolic heart failure. *Circ Cardiovasc Imag.* 2009;2:10–15.
47. Kuppahally SS, Akoum N, Burgon NS, et al. Left atrial strain and strain rate in patients with paroxysmal and persistent atrial fibrillation: relationship to left atrial structural remodeling detected by delayed-enhancement MRI. *Circ Cardiovasc Imag.* 2010;3:231–239.
48. Hitch DC, Nolan SP. Descriptive analysis of instantaneous left atrial volume—with special reference to left atrial function. *J Surg Res.* 1981;30:110–120.
49. Sigwart U, Grbic M, Goy JJ, Kappenberger L. Left atrial function in acute transient left ventricular ischemia produced during percutaneous transluminal coronary angioplasty of the left anterior descending coronary artery. *Am J Cardiol.* 1990;65:282–286.
50. Matsuda Y, Toma Y, Moritani K, et al. Assessment of left atrial function in patients with hypertensive heart disease. *Hyperten Dallas.* 1986;8:779–785.
51. Matsuda Y, Toma Y, Ogawa H. Importance of left atrial function in patients with myocardial infarction. *Circulation.* 1983;65:566–571.
52. Triposkiadis F, Wooley CF, Boudoulas H. Mitral stenosis: left atrial dynamics reflect altered passive and active emptying. *Am Heart J.* 1990;120:124–132.
53. Loghin C, Karimzadehnajar K, Ekeruo IA, Mukerji SS, Memon NB, Kantharia BK. Outcome of pulmonary vein isolation ablation for paroxysmal atrial fibrillation: predictive role of left atrial mechanical dyssynchrony by speckle tracking echocardiography. *J Intervent Card Electrophysiol.* 2014;39(1):7–15.
54. Sarvari SI, Haugaa KH, Stokke TM, et al. Strain echocardiographic assessment of left atrial function predicts recurrence of atrial fibrillation. *Eur Heart J Cardiovasc Imag.* 2016;17(6):660–667.
55. Rondano E, Dell'Era G, De Luca G, Piccinino C, Bellomo G, Marino PN. Left atrial asynchrony is a major predictor of 1-year recurrence of atrial fibrillation after electrical cardioversion. *J Cardiovasc Med (Hagerstown).* 2010;11(7):499–506.
56. Gibson DN, Di Biase L, Mohanty P, et al. Stiff left atrial syndrome after catheter ablation for atrial fibrillation: clinical characterization, prevalence, and predictors. *Heart Rhythm.* 2011;8:1364–1371.

57. Hoit BD, Shao Y, Gabel M, Walsh RA. Left atrial mechanical and biochemical adaptation to pacing induced heart failure. *Cardiovasc Res.* 1995;29:469–474.
58. Kihara Y, Sasayama S, Miyazaki S, et al. Role of the left atrium in adaptation of the heart to chronic mitral regurgitation in conscious dogs. *Circ Res.* 1988;62:543–553.
59. Kono T, Sabbah HN, Rosman H, Alam M, Stein PD, Goldstein S. Left atrial contribution to ventricular filling during the course of evolving heart failure. *Circulation.* 1992;86:1317–1322.
60. Hoit BD, Shao Y, Gabel M, Pawloski-Dahm C, Walsh RA. Left atrial systolic and diastolic function after cessation of pacing in tachycardia-induced heart failure. *Am J Physiol.* 1997;273:H921–H927.
61. Hoit BD, Shao Y, Gabel M. Left atrial systolic and diastolic function accompanying chronic rapid pacing-induced atrial failure. *Am J Physiol.* 1998;275:H183–H189.
62. Hoit BD, Gabel M. Influence of left ventricular dysfunction on the role of atrial contraction: an echocardiographic-hemodynamic study in dogs. *J Am Coll Cardiol.* 2000;36:1713–1719.

5

Physical Determinants of Diastolic Flow

Zoran B. Popović and James D. Thomas

OUTLINE

Comprehensive assessment of ventricular diastolic function is a complex process. Full elucidation generally requires invasive measurements, such as left ventricular end-diastolic pressure (EDP), the time constant of isovolumic left ventricular (LV) relaxation (τ), the pressure-volume (P-V) relationship of the ventricle at end diastole, and mean left atrial pressure. Such invasive measurements are inappropriate for routine clinical purposes and thus diastolic function is generally assessed using Doppler echocardiography, largely through the observation of transmitral and pulmonary venous flow, supplemented by myocardial velocity and color M mode Doppler information. To intelligently use these noninvasive indices to infer actual diastolic function of the heart, however, it is critical that a conceptual framework be in place that reflects the physical and physiologic determinants of intracardiac blood flow. In this chapter we will attempt to outline in both basic physical principles and computer simulations the relationship between basic parameters of diastolic function and the intracardiac flow patterns that can be obtained clinically.

PATHOPHYSIOLOGY

Mechanical Properties of Left Ventricular Chamber During Diastole

The major function of the heart in diastole is to let the blood column flow from the antechambers (left atrium [LA] and pulmonary veins [PV]) into LV, while keeping filling pressures to a minimum. During exercise, this task is compounded by shortening of time allowed for filling and increase of volume needed to get into the LV. Out of various chamber wall properties that affect this process, we will briefly cover three: chamber stiffness, relaxation, and early diastolic suction.

Chamber Stiffness

Chamber stiffness can be defined as the instantaneous change of pressure for a given volume increment, mathematically the first derivative of LV pressure by volume (dP/dV). LV pressure is a complex nonlinear function of LV volume, meaning that stiffness changes with diastolic volume. Although the LV P-V relationship was initially considered to be exponential in shape (concave upward),[1] more recent work suggests that it is sigmoidal in shape (Fig. 5.1), with a concave downward portion to the left of the usual rising exponential.[2,3] This sigmoidal curve can be expressed as:

$$P = A \times e^{(V - V_{d0})Kp^{+}} + P_b^{+} \qquad V \geq V_{d0}$$

$$P = -B \times e^{(V_{d0} - V)Kp^{-}} + P_b^{-} \qquad V < V_{d0}$$

where V_{d0} is the inflection point, A and B are the exponential curve multipliers of the upper and lower part, P_{b^+} and P_{b^-} are pressure offsets of the upper and lower part, while K_{p^+} and K_{p^-} are the diastolic chamber stiffness indices, determining the overall steepness of the end-diastolic P-V relationship (EDPVR) above and below the inflection volume. Frequently, EDPVR is conceptually simplified by assuming that V_{d0} equals 0,[1] and even further simplified by neglecting P_b^+, leaving us with the equation $P = Ae^{K \times EDV}$, or in other words $\text{LnP} = a + K \times \text{EDV}$ (see also chapter 2).[1] By differentiating this equation, we see that end-diastolic stiffness dP/dV is $K \times Ae^{K \times EDV}$ or $K \times P_{EDV}$. Another parameter of note is the average stiffness[4] (i.e., the stroke volume divided by the LV pressure increment during diastole), a simple measure that gives the clinician an overall measure of how stiff the patient's LV is during diastole over a given (working) set of conditions.[5] The fact that myocardial relaxation is a continuous process throughout diastole results in changing relationships between pressure and volume from very stiff end-systole P-V relationships to much more compliant EDPVR.

Relaxation

Myocardial relaxation occurs due to calcium reuptake at the end of systole, producing a shift downward and rightward, leading to a fall in LV pressure (at a given volume). The rate of pressure decrease during relaxation depends on the velocity of calcium reuptake and on the LV volume: The smaller the volume, the lower the potential for pressure to fall,[2] limited by the EDP curve shown in Fig. 5.1. Rate of calcium reuptake is further modified by LV lengthening during relaxation, so true relaxation can be measured only during the isovolumic period.[6]

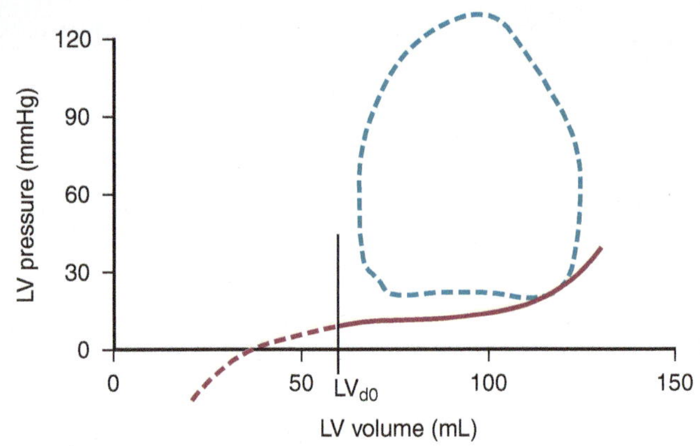

Fig. 5.1 The diagram of passive P-V loop relationships. The thick continuous and thick dotted line represent the upper and lower part of the sigmoid end-diastolic pressure volume relationship, respectively. The curvature of the upper part is determined by chamber stiffness index, which can be interpreted as the inverse of the volume needed to increase the steepness of the PV curve by a factor of 2.72.

Several equations have been proposed to describe the rate of isovolumic pressure decay,[7] the most general being:

$$P(t) = (P_0 - P_b) \times e^{-t/\tau} + P_b$$

which can be, with some caveats, simplified to:

$$P(t) = P_0 \times e^{-t/\tau}$$

and further to[8,9]:

$$\tau \approx \text{IVRT}/(\ln P_{AVC} - \ln P_{MVO}),$$

where IVRT is the isovolumic relaxation time (the time between aortic valve closure and mitral valve opening), and P_{AVC} and P_{MVO} are LV pressure at aortic valve closure and mitral valve (MV) opening, respectively, which can be approximated noninvasively by systolic blood pressure and an estimate of left atrial pressure.

Importantly, LV relaxation is a never-ending process, which critically impacts the end-diastolic pressure that the patient achieves, particularly during exercise. Consider Fig. 5.2A, showing a series of PV curves, representing successive intervals of τ, and Fig. 5.2B, the same curves zoomed on diastolic pressures. Note that after 6τ, the filling curve is virtually indistinguishable from the end-diastolic PV curve, as relaxation is 99.8% complete. When relaxation rate is normal the end-diastolic filling curve is completely relaxed at normal heart rates (12.5τ) (see Fig. 5.2C) and almost complete during exercise (5τ) (see Fig. 5.2D); with delayed relaxation, however, while the EDPV curve is fully relaxed at rest (6.25τ) (see Fig. 5.2E), it becomes stiff with exercise (3τ) (see Fig. 5.2F).

The combination of relaxation and the EDPVR results in a dynamic PV relationship, represented by the round dots in Fig. 5.2A. Note that in early diastole LV pressure continues to fall even though volume is increasing, meaning that the instantaneous stiffness is actually negative, which some consider diastolic suction. Two other definitions of diastolic suction are also relevant. Consider ventricular filling from a very low end-systolic volume (where the EDPVR is concave downward). If relaxation is very rapid or filling delayed (by mitral stenosis or experimentally with a mitral occluder[2]), then LV pressure can fall below atmospheric pressure.[2,10] Alternatively, suction has been used to refer to the small (1–3 mmHg) differences in pressure between the base and the apex, which assist in the low pressure filling of the ventricle, particularly with exercise, and which will be discussed later.[11]

Determinants of Intracardiac Blood Flow

In the most general sense, the motion of blood inside the heart, as the motion of any fluid, is determined by the Navier-Stokes equation, a complex set of four multidimensional partial differential equations, which must be solved simultaneously at every point in space and moment in time:

$$\nabla \cdot v = 0$$

and:

$$\rho \frac{Dv}{Dt} = -\nabla P + B + \mu \nabla^2 v$$

These equations appear deceptively simple but contain such complex mathematical concepts that, except in the simplest of geometries, can never be solved either analytically or with powerful supercomputers. Fortunately, considerable simplifications can be made to these equations that will allow a much simpler conceptual and computational approach. The most important simplification is to take the distribution of blood throughout the heart and replace it with just a few measurements at specific points inside the heart. For instance, instead of describing pressure in every cubic millimeter inside the left ventricle, we assume that left ventricular pressure can be approximated by an average of these and give a single number for LV pressure, which is precisely how we measure and report left ventricular pressure in practice. Similarly, instead of describing the direction and speed of blood flow at every point within the heart, we focus on points where blood velocity is maximum, such as the tips of the mitral leaflets and the pulmonary vein orifices. Finally, we assume fluid incompressibility and zero viscosity and heat conduction losses. In this way, the thousands of partial differential equations that would have to be solved simultaneously throughout the heart are replaced by a few ordinary differential equations that can be solved quite easily on a personal computer.

To understand how these equations can model the flow within the heart, we first start by replacing the Navier-Stokes equations with the well-known Bernoulli equation that applies to flow across discrete points such as valves. Here we present it with its inertial and convective terms (we still omit the viscous term since it is negligible in almost every intracardiac situation):

$$\Delta p = M\frac{dv}{dt} + \tfrac{1}{2}\rho\Delta(v^2)$$

where Δp is the pressure difference between two points, M is the inertial constant and represents the so-called effective mass being accelerated, dv/dt is the instantaneous temporal acceleration of flow through the region, ρ is blood density, and $\Delta(v^2)$ is the change in the square of velocity from one point to another (with pressure in mmHg and velocity in m/sec, $\frac{1}{2}\rho v^2$ reduces to $4v^2$ in the simplified Bernoulli equation). The first product is the **inertial** term of the Bernoulli equation, and corresponds to the energy used accelerating and decelerating flow; the second term is the **convective** term and represents kinetic energy of flow. The effective mass of blood in a narrow orifice is small and thus M is a negligible quantity in, for example, valve stenosis, but the dominant term when flow is not obstructed, such as the normal mitral valve. For constant flow through an orifice of minimal diameter D, the inertial constant M varies approximately in proportion to D, while the kinetic term $\frac{1}{2}\rho v^2$ varies inversely to D^4.

For nonobstructive flow through the body of heart chambers, where pressure changes gradually over a distance, not at a discrete

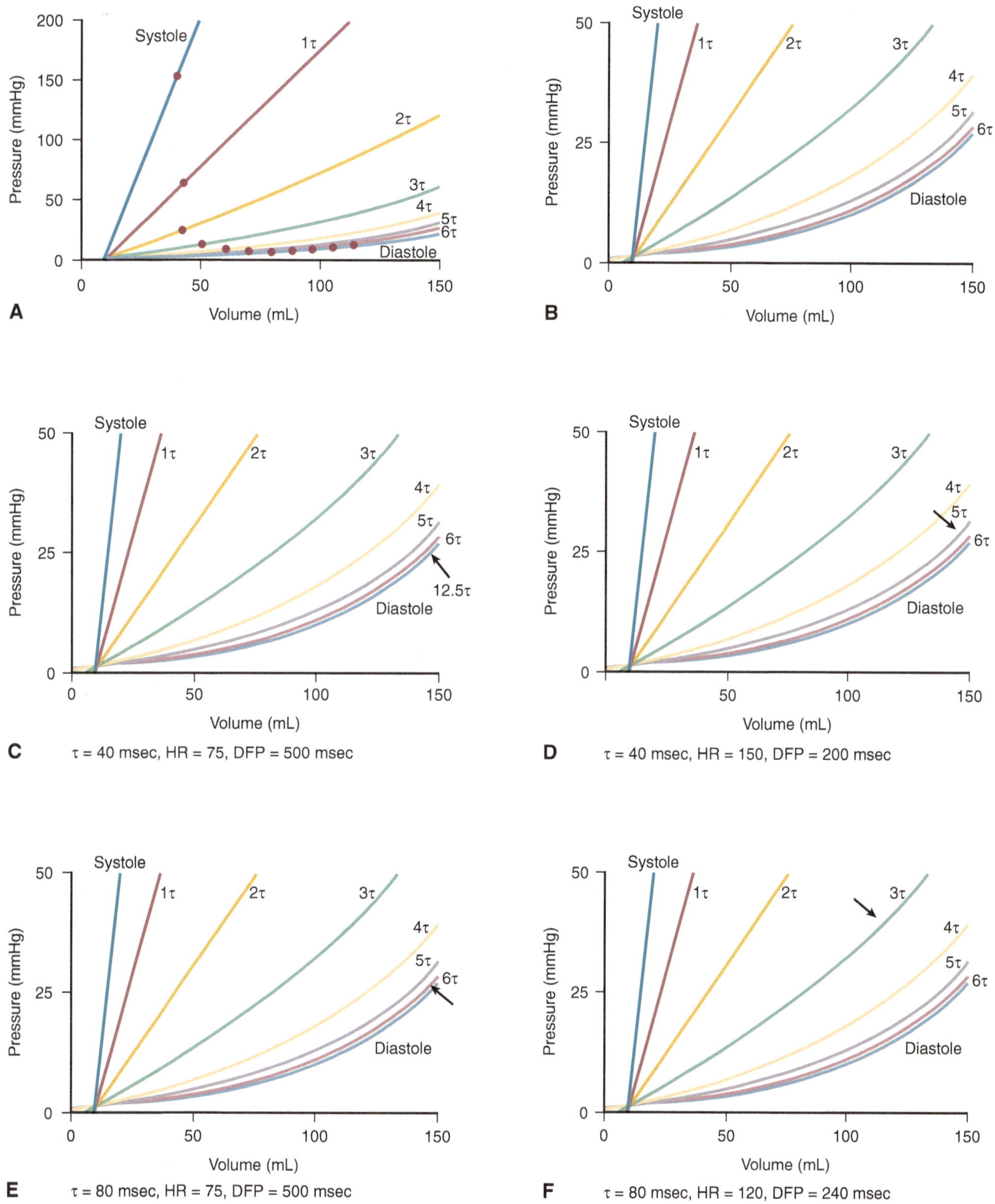

Fig. 5.2 Diastolic P-V relationships shown as a function of the duration of diastole. Duration of diastole is measured by the multiples of a time constant of relaxation (τ). (A) shows series of P-V relationships that occur after successive intervals of τ, while (B) shows the same curves zoomed on diastolic pressures. The combination of relaxation and the EDPVR results in a dynamic diastolic part of P-V loop represented by the round dots in (A). Note that in early diastole LV pressure continues to fall even though volume is increasing, meaning that the instantaneous stiffness is actually negative, which some consider diastolic suction. When relaxation rate is normal the end-diastolic filling curve is completely relaxed at normal heart rates [*arrow* 12.5τ, (C)] and almost complete during exercise [*arrow* 5τ, (D)]; with delayed relaxation, however, while the EDPV curve is fully relaxed at rest [*arrow* 6.25τ, (E)], it becomes stiff with exercise [*arrow* 3τ, (F)].

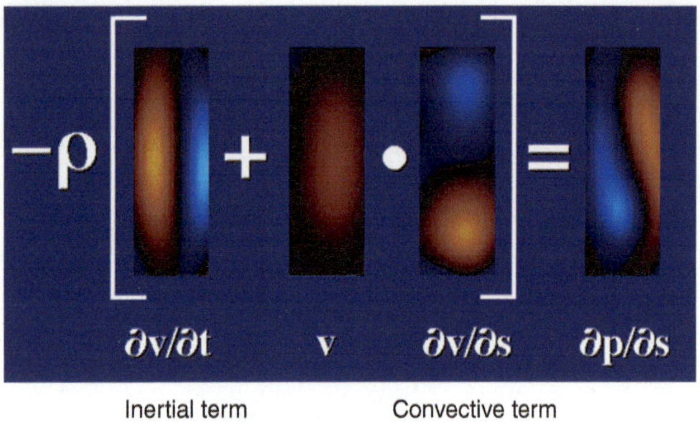

Fig. 5.3 Illustration of the way convective *(right)* and inertial *(left)* terms combine to produce intraventricular pressure gradient. (Adapted from Thomas JD, Popovic ZB. Intraventricular pressure differences: a new window into cardiac function. *Circulation.* 2005;112:1684–1686 [fig. 1].)

point, we must use the Euler equation, a differential version of the Bernoulli equation for pressure change along a streamline of flow:

$$\frac{\partial p}{\partial s} = -\rho \cdot \left(\frac{\partial v}{\partial t} + v \cdot \frac{\partial v}{\partial s} \right)$$

where the inertial and convective terms are in the same order as the Bernoulli equation, but the discrete terms [Δp and $\Delta(v^2)$] have been replaced by their spatial derivatives, yielding the rate of pressure change per centimeter of distance along the streamline. To return the total pressure drop between points *A* and *B* along the streamline, this equation must be integrated numerically:

$$\Delta p = -\rho \cdot \int_A^B \left(\frac{\partial v}{\partial t} + v \cdot \frac{\partial v}{\partial s} \right) ds.$$

Fig. 5.3 shows schematically how these partial derivatives are summed together to produce the pressure gradient map.[12] Another, practical, fact is that we can obtain the same map by applying the Euler equation to a color Doppler M mode tracing.

CLINICAL RELEVANCE

In this part of the chapter we will demonstrate how interaction of solid and fluid mechanics determines intracardiac flow within three specific regions of the heart: mitral valve, pulmonary vein, and the left ventricle.

Physical Factors Governing LV Filling Velocities

To describe flow mathematically through the mitral valve, we first consider a very simplified construct, consisting of the left ventricle, which has pressure as a function of time $p_V(t)$, the left atrium, which has a pressure as a function of time [$p_A(t)$], and the mitral valve, which has an area A_{MV} and contains a mass of blood *M* that is accelerating in passing from the left atrium to the left ventricle, which, to a first approximation, is the blood within a cylinder that can fit inside the narrowest portion of the mitral leaflet tips and whose length is approximately the diameter of the valve. In reality though, since pressure is applied across the mitral valve, the most relevant hydrodynamic concept is the length of this cylinder, termed the mitral inertance, related linearly to the diameter of that structure. We will use this construct to discuss three parameters of transmitral flow: mitral acceleration, peak mitral flow, and mitral deceleration.

Acceleration of Mitral Flow

To understand the acceleration of blood across the mitral valve, we apply Newton's second law of motion that the rate at which an object accelerates is given by the force exerted on that object divided by its mass. In this case, the acceleration would be recorded by Doppler echocardiography as the velocity acceleration detected for mitral inflow, while the force is the difference in pressure on either side of the mitral valve multiplied by the area of the valve[13]:

$$a = \frac{F}{m} = \frac{\Delta pA}{\rho M} \approx \frac{\Delta p}{\rho L}$$

Here we have taken advantage of the fact that valve area appears in both the numerator and the denominator (through the definition of inertial mass) to simplify the relationship. Clearly the higher the pressure difference across the valve and the smaller the length of blood column within the mitral valve, the more rapidly the velocity will accelerate. This is why mitral velocity increases almost instantaneously in mitral stenosis, which has a very high-pressure gradient across the valve and a very small blood mass due to the small diameter of the mitral orifice. If the blood within the mitral valve was subject to an instantaneously applied pressure difference (as if the relaxation of the LV occurred suddenly), mitral velocity would start to rise linearly. In the physiologic situation, the pressure gradient is not abruptly applied but rather increases gradually (roughly linearly) with time as the ventricle relaxes, resulting in a roughly parabolic mitral velocity acceleration curve.[14]

Peak E Wave Velocity and Conservation of Energy

Mitral valve acceleration eventually decreases with time because the maximal velocity generated by a pressure difference is limited by conservation of energy (expressed in the Bernoulli equation). Within the heart, energy in the blood takes on three principal forms: pressure (a form of potential energy), kinetic energy, and heat; the total energy in the system must remain constant. In the left atrium, where blood velocity is low, most of the energy is in the form of pressure, but as it moves toward the mitral valve, its velocity rises and it acquires a kinetic energy ($\frac{1}{2}\rho v^2$), which causes the local blood pressure to fall. If no energy losses appear, pressure difference and velocity are related by the simplified Bernoulli relation, which becomes roughly $\Delta p = 4v^2$ when pressure is measured in mmHg and velocity in meters per second. While the velocity reaches asymptotically the target gradient, reaching of this asymptote is delayed by the amount of inertance present. Reaching the asymptote can be even further delayed by gradient not being imposed abruptly, but slowly, as seen in a normally relaxing LV.

Deceleration of Mitral Flow

Returning to our general model of the mitral valve, once flow has been accelerated to maximal velocity by the pressure difference across the mitral valve, it begins falling as the pressure difference between the left atrium and left ventricle equilibrates. This is analogous to flow between two tanks stopping when the level of water in the two tanks becomes the same. When we speak of the change in pressure with a change in volume, we are dealing with the concept of compliance or its inverse, stiffness, the change in pressure for a given change in volume, which is a major determinant of the deceleration of flow across the mitral valve. Since the stiffer the ventricle, the more rapidly the pressure equilibrates across the mitral valve to decelerate the flow, we can understand why short deceleration time across the mitral valve is associated with increased ventricular stiffness. Note that in this situation, we must place atrial and ventricular stiffness together, since both chambers are involved in determining how quickly pressure equilibrates across the mitral valve. For ventricular stiffness S_V and atrial stiffness S_A, the net atrioventricular stiffness S_n is simply $S_A + S_V$. To obtain a mathematical expression for mitral velocity deceleration rate, we first note that for a restrictive mitral valve with area *A* (i.e., mitral stenosis, though even for a normal mitral valve, the overall principle holds):

$$\Delta p = {}^1/_2 \rho v^2$$

which simplifies to $4v^2$ when Δp is in mmHg and *v* in m/sec. Differentiating this yields

$$d\Delta p/dt = \rho v\, dv/dt$$

But $d\Delta p/dt$ can also be expressed in terms of flow across the mitral valve (*Av*) and net A-V stiffness:

$$d\Delta p/dt = -Av S_n$$

Substituting for $d\Delta p/dt$ yields

$$\rho v\, dv/dt = -Av S_n$$

or, rearranging,

$$dv/dt = AS_n/\rho$$

Thus the stiffer the ventricle (or atrium) and the larger the valve area, the faster the deceleration.

Alternatively, one can represent this as a purely inertial system (with a nonrestrictive orifice), which yields a simple harmonic motion in which case the velocity across the valve is described roughly by a sine wave:

$$v(t) = v_0 \sin\left(\frac{t}{\sqrt{m/k}}\right)$$

where v_0 is the peak E wave velocity, *m* is mitral inertance, and *k* is the stiffness constant of the ventricle. The deceleration time (time for the E wave to fall from its peak to zero velocity) can be solved for as:

$$t_{dec} = \frac{\pi}{2}\sqrt{\frac{\rho \cdot L}{A} \cdot \frac{1}{k}}$$

where ρ, *L*, and *A* are blood viscosity, mitral valve length, and mitral valve area, respectively. To sum it up, the stiffer the ventricle, the shorter the deceleration time. This is intuitively very understandable: Tighter springs oscillate fast. Note that in this simplification, one assumes that active relaxation is complete at the time of interest.[13]

Modeling of mitral valve flow. Until now, we have been discussing specific features of the transmitral E wave through significant simplifications that allow closed-form mathematical solution. To permit more realistic modeling of transmitral flow, however, one needs more general equations that can only be solved numerically. A generalized equation for blood flow through the mitral valve and its interaction with the transmitral gradient is the equation[15]:

$$dv/dt = (P_A - P_V - {}^1\!/_2 \rho v^2)/M$$

where *v* is velocity, *t* is time, P_A and P_V are instantaneous atrial and ventricular pressures, and *M* is mitral inertance. Conversely, the impact of mitral flow on LA and LV pressures is expressed through the equations:

$$dP_A/dt = -Av/C_A$$

$$dP_V/dt = Av/C_V + \partial P_V/dt$$

where *A* is mitral valve area, and C_A and C_V atrial and ventricular compliance (inverse of stiffness). By solving these three differential equations, we can assess how changing the parameters of the equation that represent passive diastolic properties, LV relaxation, mitral inertance, and preload can affect transmitral flow. We start with a preliminary discussion of these interactions before presenting an even more detailed model that includes pulmonary vein flow in addition to transmitral flow.

Impact of Relaxation

Changes in relaxation affect the earliest part of the mitral flow (Fig. 5.4A and B). They have a profound effect on the peak values of E wave velocity. The overall effect of relaxation on the descending phase of the E wave is more complex: When *t* is very short, relaxation is essentially complete by the time the E wave peaks, and small changes in *t* have little effect on deceleration; on the other hand, if *t* is significantly longer, the relaxation remains an important aspect of the deceleration phase and further lengthening of *t* will cause a decrease in the deceleration rate (i.e., prolongation in deceleration time).

Passive Diastolic Properties of the Left Ventricle

Increasing the steepness of the diastolic PV curve affects primarily deceleration time (i.e., the operative chamber stiffness) (see Fig. 5.4C and D). However, a caveat has to be introduced. The ventricular PV curve (as well as atrial PV curve) is exponential in shape. Since operative chamber stiffness is equal to the slope of these curves, stiffness and mitral deceleration rise when operative chamber volumes increase. This change is indistinguishable from the change that may arise from a change of material properties of the ventricle leading to steeper curves at all pressures (i.e., a true change in the diastolic properties of the ventricle).

Preload Alterations

Preload affects all components of the mitral velocity curve (see Fig. 5.4E and F). However, its most prominent effect is on the E wave. For mitral deceleration, the effects depend on the initial position of the PV curve. If the preload increase does not move the PV loop too much into the steeper portion of EDPVR, the effects may be negligible. It is not so in the severely diseased ventricles operating close to the limit of the preload reserve.

Mitral Inertance

Mitral inertance affects both MV acceleration and deceleration. It changes acceleration of MV inflow and leads to flattening of the parabolic curve of velocity rise. Mitral inertance essentially acts by introducing the time lag between transmitral pressure gradient and mitral velocity curve: It makes the peak of velocity curve to occur after the peak of transmitral pressure gradient curve (Fig. 5.5). It also introduces the difference between true MV pressure gradient and pressure gradient calculated from application of the simplified Bernoulli equation to transmitral velocity (see Fig. 5.5). As it correlates with the mitral valve area, it can be largely neglected in patients with mitral stenosis, but it is an important factor in nonstenotic valve. We have shown, by using the combination of echocardiography and direct pressure recordings, that average values of mitral inertance in humans are

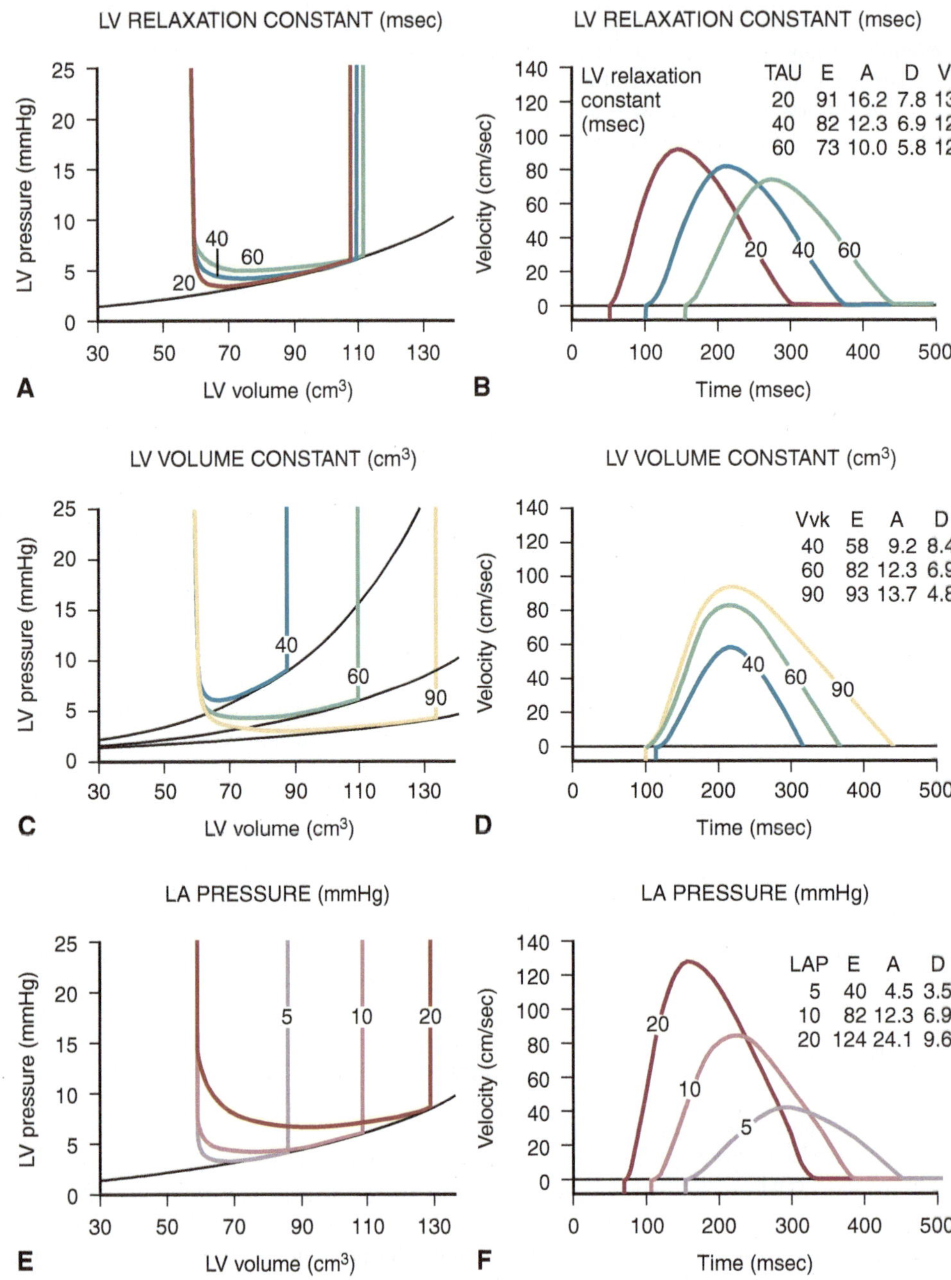

Fig. 5.4 Impact of relaxation *(t)*, chamber stiffness (inverse of chamber stiffness index) and LA pressure (preload) on MV velocity profile. (Adapted from Thomas JD, Weyman AE. Echocardiographic Doppler evaluation of left ventricular diastolic function. Physics and physiology. *Circulation.* 1991;84:977–990 [fig. 2].)

3.82 ± 1.22 g/cm^2, corresponding to an effective length of the blood column of about 3.6 cm within the mitral valve.[16] Future research may allow direct estimation of inertance from echocardiography data alone.

Interaction of Ventricular Compliance and Relaxation: Importance of Heart Rate

During early filling, relaxation is not yet complete. This means that filling occurs while the dynamic PV curve continuously shifts downward and toward the right. Thus, as the ventricle fills, it moves to the steeper part of the EDPVR, which in turn is becoming progressively flatter. These two trends may offset each other with a result of diastolic pressures being constant or falling despite an increase in LV volume, giving the impression of negative stiffness in early diastole. Fig. 5.4A and B shows how τ impacts MV flow and end-diastolic P-V relationships.[15] We reiterate here that while τ affects the early part of the diastolic PV curve, τ effects end-diastolic volume only when dramatically prolonged. The situation is different during exercise, where shortening of the diastolic interval and the increase of arterial blood pressures produce incomplete relaxation (with a rise in end-diastolic pressure) rather than simply delayed relaxation (which has little impact on left ventricular end-diastolic pressure [LVEDP]).[17]

Understanding Pulmonary Vein Flow Through Computer Modeling of the Heart

Such conceptual thought experiments as those already presented can be helpful in understanding general trends in the relationship between the invasive parameters and noninvasive measurements, but a more

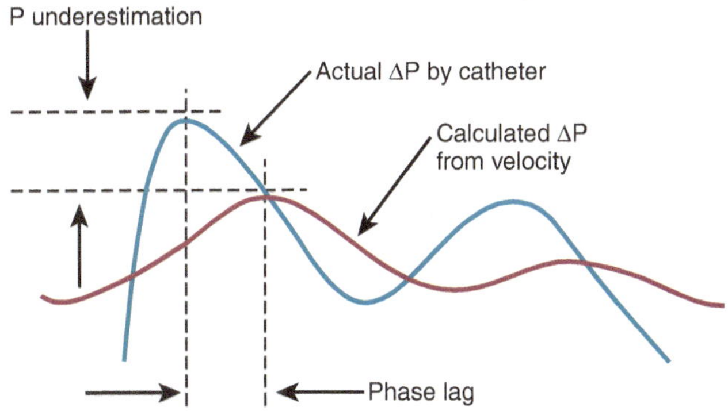

Fig. 5.5 Impact of mitral inertance: transmitral velocities lag behind transmitral pressure differences. (Adapted from Nakatani S, Firstenberg MS, Greenberg NL, Vandervoort PM, Smedira NG, McCarthy PM, et al. Mitral inertance in humans: critical factor in Doppler estimation of transvalvular pressure gradients. *Am J Physiol Heart Circ Physiol.* 2001;280:H1340–H1345 [fig. 2].)

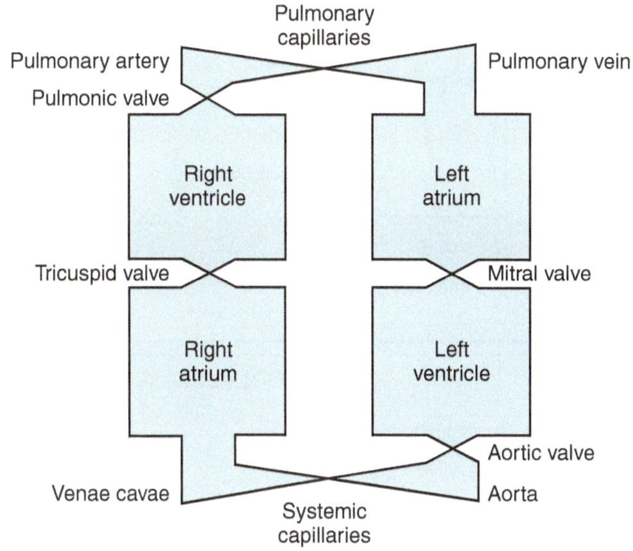

Fig. 5.6 A lumped parameter model of the heart. (From Thomas JD, Zhou J, Greenberg N, Bibawy G, McCarthy PM, Vandervoort PM. Physical and physiological determinants of pulmonary venous flow: numerical analysis. *Am J Physiol.* 1997;272:H2453–H2465 [fig. 1].)

comprehensive approach can be obtained with a computer model that invokes realistic descriptions of chamber and valvular function. The reason for this is that the blood flows through different parts of the circulatory system are interdependent. A change in a single parameter (e.g., resistance in systemic arterioles) affects flow throughout the system. Thus changes in the pulmonary circulation affect systemic circulation even if not assuming any ventricular-ventricular interactions.

Lumped Parameter Model of the Heart and Circulation

Over the past 20 years, the authors and colleagues have worked to develop models of the heart with increasing complexity, beginning from a very simple isolated model of the mitral valve used to understand the mitral pressure halftime, to ones incorporating more realistic diastolic characteristics of the ventricle and atrium, to one that simulated all the cardiac chambers and valves, as well as the peripheral and pulmonary vasculature, and to a simulation that links knowledge of basic myocyte and fiber function to the gross architecture of the heart. We will use a lumped parameter model to explore some of the determinants of transmitral and pulmonary venous flow inside the heart.[3]

The lumped parameter approach assumes that blood flow is similar to a flow of a current through an electric circuit, which can be represented at specific nodes of the circuit (left atrium, left ventricle, aortic valve, etc.). Each of these nodes is represented by a specific ordinary differential equation. The principle of the conservation of flow (Kirchoff's first law) is applied throughout the circuit, and the parameters of the system are obtained by simultaneously solving all differential equations. Our model consists of 24 coupled differential equations representing eight different chambers (the right atrium and ventricle, pulmonary arteries and veins, left atrium and ventricle, aorta, and systemic veins) as well as the valves and vascular beds connecting them (Fig. 5.6), giving time-varying flows and pressures throughout the model. Fig. 5.7 displays normal Doppler velocity tracing of PV and transmitral flow recorded in the normal subject by transesophageal echocardiography (left) and a model output of corresponding pulmonary vein and transmitral flow velocities, along with simulated pressure curves. Starting from this normal shape of velocity and pressure tracings, we first modeled delayed relaxation pattern, by increasing *t* from 50 to 120 ms. Then, to model restrictive filling, we shifted ESPVR by 10 mL toward right and decreased contractility from 4 to 2.5 mmHg/mL, thus moving the PV loop toward the steeper part of EDPVR. The model outputs are displayed in the figure along with actual Doppler and pressure tracings of a representative patient with delayed relaxation (see Fig. 5.7B) and restrictive filling (see Fig. 5.7C). One can observe a close correspondence between the modeled and actual shapes, with a correlation coefficient approaching 1.

Fig. 5.8 shows impact of some of the model parameters on PV and MV flow. LA systolic and diastolic function had the opposing effects on PV S and AR waves, with minimal effect on the D wave (see Fig. 5.8A–D). Finally, all waveforms showed strong positive response to preload (see Fig. 5.8E and F). Worse LV relaxation decreases MV E/A ratio and blunts diastolic waves of PV flow (see Fig. 5.8G and H). These observations are analyzed in depth in Table 5.1 (an abbreviated table 7 from Thomas et al.[3]), by showing the sensitivities of peak velocity of the three PV flow waves and of two mitral inflow waves on model parameters. The sensitivities represented here were obtained by calculating a normalized Jacobian matrix, showing the proportional change in an output index for a given incremental change in an input parameter. A sensitivity of 1 means that for each 1% change of a model parameter value, the output variable will change by 1%. A value of 2 indicates a 2% change for a 1% increase. Negative numbers indicate inverse relationships. Because of the highly nonlinear nature of the model, these observations are only relevant to very small increments, but do provide an overall sense of the dependency of Doppler indices on hemodynamic parameters. For example, one can readily observe the dramatic effect of preload on all three PV flow waves, in particular AR, which increases almost sixfold the increment in blood volume. Furthermore, one can observe that LA diastolic and systolic functions have opposite effects. MV regurgitation (through the parameter MV ERO) has its effect mostly on the systolic waveform, while *Kp*+ and τ have the effect mostly on AR. These sensitivity analysis results illustrate the complexities of these relationships, which are not intuitively apparent. In contrast, for the mitral inflow, as expected, the greatest influence was exerted by preload. Importantly, τ showed the opposite effects on E and A waves, in congruence to the E/A ratio being reversed in the setting of impaired relaxation. This table should be kept in mind as, very often, PV flow is used as a surrogate marker of LA function, with S, D, and AR reflecting LA reservoir, conduit, and pump function, respectively. Our table indicates that for none of these is there a straightforward

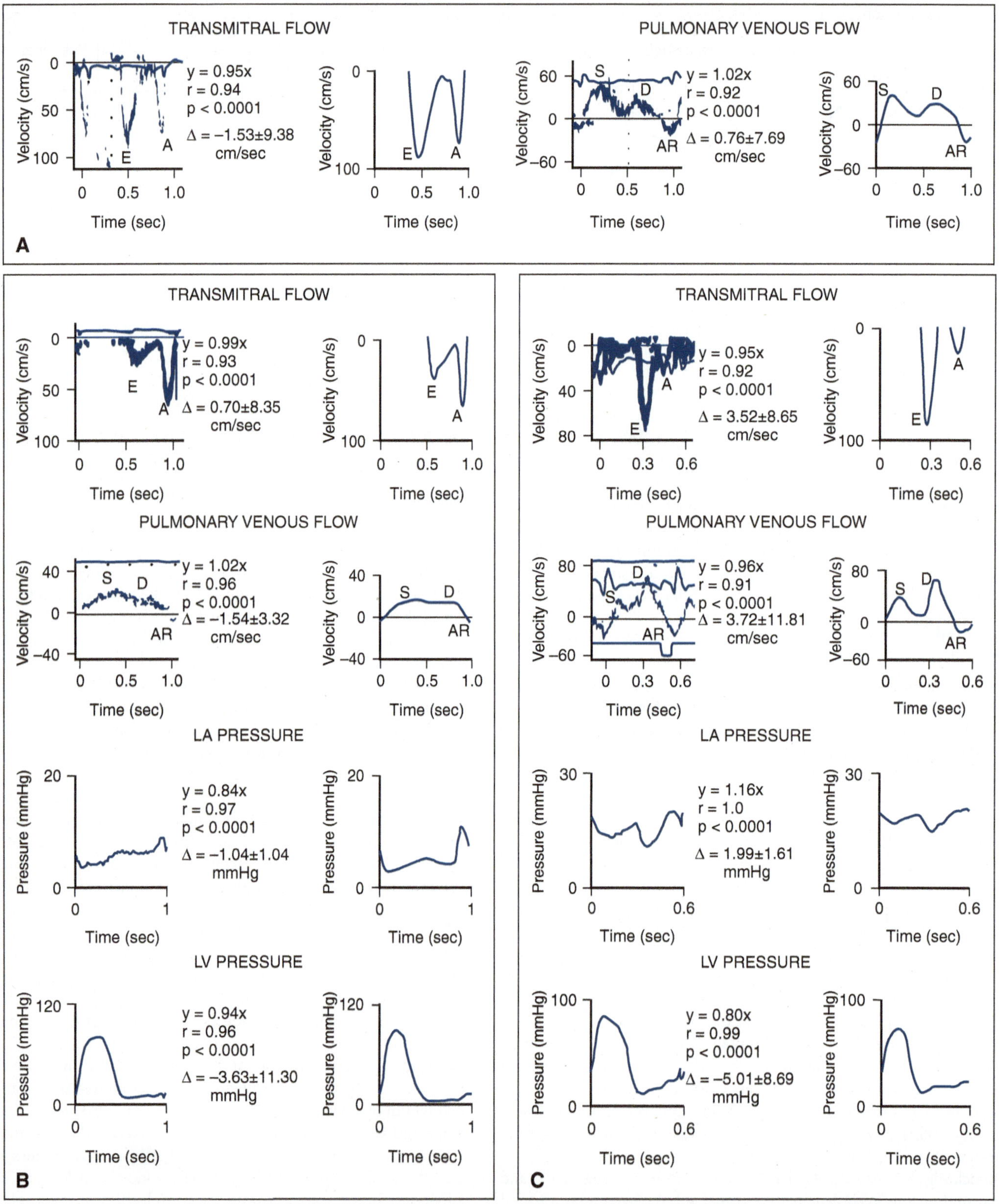

Fig. 5.7 Actual and modeled pressures and filling patterns in a normal subject (A), patient with delayed relaxation (B), and patient with restrictive filling (C). (From Thomas JD, Zhou J, Greenberg N, Bibawy G, McCarthy PM, Vandervoort PM. Physical and physiological determinants of pulmonary venous flow: numerical analysis. *Am J Physiol.* 1997;272:H2453–H2465 [figs. 4 to 6].)

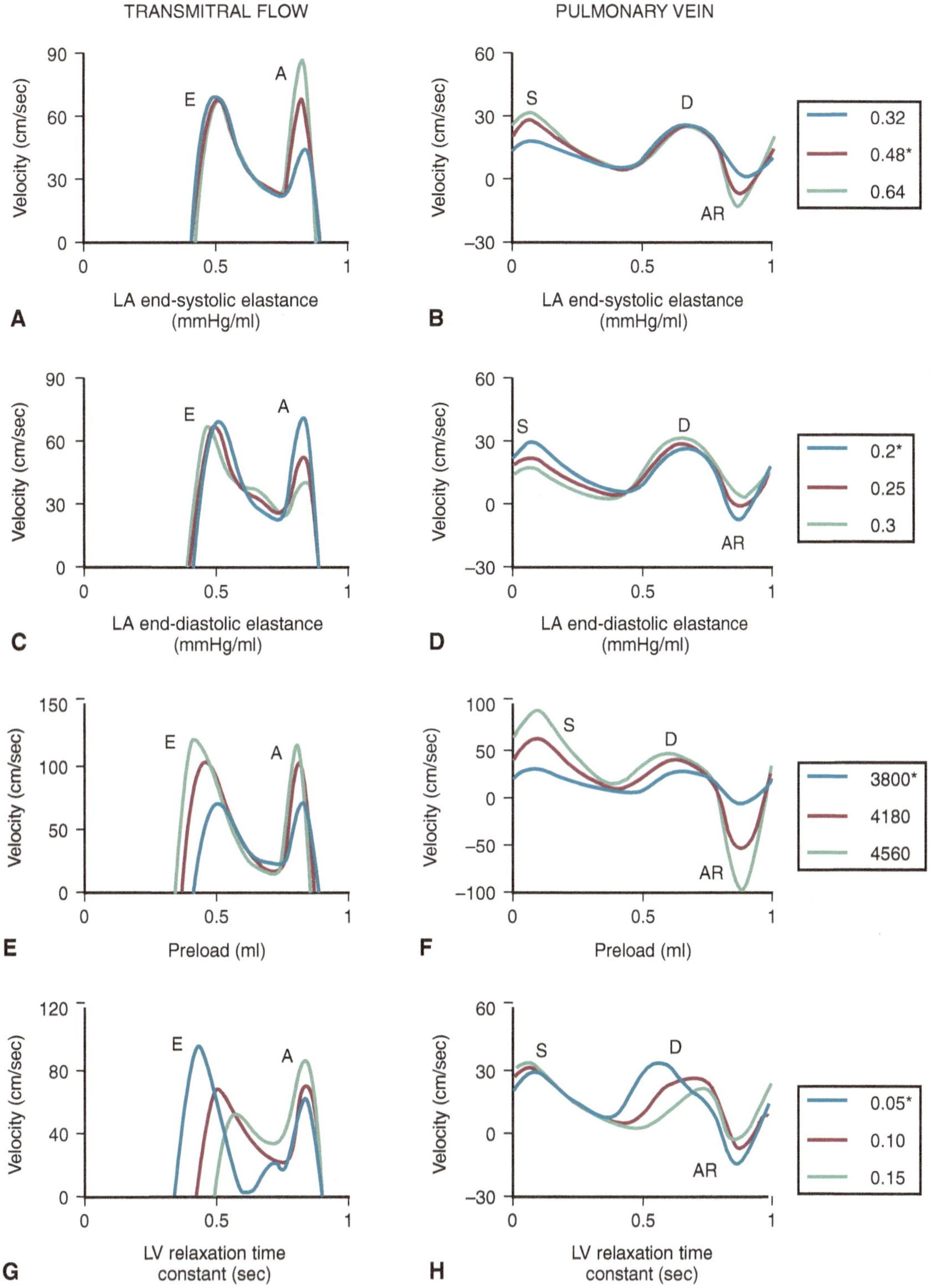

Fig. 5.8 Simultaneous modeling of pulmonary vein and transmitral velocities using lumped-parameter approach. Impact of left atrial systolic (A and B) and diastolic properties (C and D), preload (E and F), and relaxation (G and H). (From Thomas JD, Zhou J, Greenberg N, Bibawy G, McCarthy PM, Vandervoort PM. Physical and physiological determinants of pulmonary venous flow: numerical analysis. *Am J Physiol.* 1997;272:H2453–H2465 [fig. 9].)

TABLE 5.1 Results of Sensitivity Analysis for the Pulmonary Vein and Transmitral Flow

	Pulmonary Vein Flow			Transmitral Flow	
	S	D	AR	E	A
Parameters:					
Preload	2.38	2.33	5.88	1.53	1.9
LV compliance index	−0.45	−0.12	−1.15	−0.24	−0.04
LV systolic elastance	−0.2	0.05	−0.44	−0.09	−0.19
LV τ	0.05	−0.19	−1.76	−0.33	0.16
LA systolic elastance	0.8	−0.14	0.97	−0.38	−0.25
LA diastolic stiffness	−0.79	0.6	−1.27	−0.11	0.97
Mitral valve area	−0.06	0.12	−0.16	0.07	−1.02
MV ERO	−2.73	0.17	−0.18	0.32	−0.11

A, Atrial wave; *AR,* atrial reversal wave; *D,* diastolic wave; *E,* early wave; *ERO,* effective regurgitant orifice; *LA,* left atrial; *LV,* left ventricular; *MV,* mitral valve; *S,* systolic wave.

From Thomas JD, Zhou J, Greenberg N, Bibawy G, McCarthy PM, Vandervoort PM. Physical and physiological determinants of pulmonary venous flow: numerical analysis. *Am J Physiol.* 1997;272:H2453–H2465 [table 7].

relationship between the specific waveform and specific material parameter of the PV flow waveform.

Impact of Pulmonary Vein–LA Pressure Gradient and LA Size

Similar to mitral valve inertance, there is also pulmonary vein inertance. Its effect on pulmonary vein flow is similar to its effect on transmitral flow. Inertance leads to a lag of pulmonary vein flow behind the pulmonary vein–LA pressure gradient. This is intuitively understandable: The pressure is needed to push the blood column, which then keeps moving because of its kinetic energy.[18] Another interesting observation is the impact of the change of LA size induced by clipping of LA appendage on PV flow. The only affected PV flow wave was the S wave, indicating that LA size affects primarily LA reservoir function.[19]

Understanding Intraventricular Flow

The previous model formulations seem like child's play when confronted with the task of simulating intraventricular flow, with its demands for representing pressure and velocity throughout the chamber. Three major phenomena develop simultaneously during filling: An intraventricular gradient appears at the beginning of LV filling, the blood column slows after exiting the MV while continuing as laminar flow toward the apex, and finally vortices start appearing due to propagation of the blood column past the tips of the mitral leaflets, while the LV continually changes its size.

It is well documented that a small LV base-to-apex pressure gradient develops in early diastole (Fig. 5.9A). We have already discussed that this gradient is of utmost importance for the low pressure filling of the ventricle and is commonly termed *diastolic suction.* However, the exact mechanisms causing it are unclear. The most probable mechanisms are isovolumic conformational changes in LV shape that are driven by elastic forces within the myocyte and/or the myocardial interstitium, explored in greater depth later in the chapter.

As blood emerges from the mitral valve, it slows as the flow stream expands to fill the left ventricle. Interestingly, within the first 4 cm of the LV, the velocity of propagation of the blood column is fairly constant, despite the dramatic change of the chamber size, but is generally less than the actual velocities within the bolus of blood traversing the mitral valve. For example, pulsed-wave Doppler may record a velocity of 100 cm/sec while the normal propagation velocity will be only 60 or 70 cm/sec, and even lower in diseased hearts due to the bleeding off of vortices at the front of the bolus of blood. We and others have shown that in heart disease, the amount of slowing of blood column relative to the component velocity (i.e., so-called E/v_p ratio) is related to LV filling pressures,[20,21] though the exact mechanistic relationship between these two phenomena is unclear (see Fig. 5.9B).

As noted, intraventricular flow during diastole characteristically forms circular eddies lateral to the main flow, which can be seen when the heart is imaged by echocardiography with high-frequency transducers, or after the contrast injection, and can be quantified by magnetic resonance velocity mapping (see Fig. 5.9C).[22] Creation of vortices plays a crucial role in mitral valve closure, and in the transfer of blood toward the apex and then into the LV outflow tract. Again, full elucidation of vortex generation and movement is unclear.

Modeling of the Intraventricular Flow by Fluid-Mechanical Computer Models

Modeling of the intraventricular flow is demanding because ventricular motion impacts blood flow, but blood flow itself impacts ventricular motion. Some simplification is possible with computational fluid dynamics (CFD) models, where LV motion is prescribed based on images from echocardiography or magnetic resonance imaging, but these models lack fluid feedback on the myocardium. Full fluid-structure interaction (FSI) models are being developed where movement of the blood and muscle is not known a priori but is computed during the simulation on a ~mm three-dimensional grid at ~msec intervals, an extraordinary computational challenge. Furthermore, most commercially available software only allow small strain deformations (up to 5%) and are inadequate for cardiac modeling where strains may exceed 50%. Fortunately, large strain solvers have recently been implemented in commercial codes, which enabled several authors to begin true fluid-solid interaction modeling of LV function.[23–25] Although these models have simplified geometry and muscle properties, they give us insight into flow propagation in the normal heart.

Flow propagation inside the ventricle. We will first discuss the filling modeled by an axisymmetric thin-walled FSI model of the LV containing both LV outflow and inflow.[26] During the rapid filling phase, a jet starts its propagation through the mitral valve into the ventricular chamber. Driven by this jet, a doughnut-shaped vortex is formed around the jet just downstream from the mitral orifice. During filling, the vortex ring travels toward the middle of the expanding ventricle, while a weak vortex is formed within the aortic outflow tract, which dissipates late during in diastasis. After the vortex ring reaches the middle of the ventricle, its anterior part becomes stationary while the posterior part continues forward. During the atrial contraction, a new, weaker vortex ring that encompasses a part of the outflow tract is formed, while the posterior side of the initial vortex ring continues to

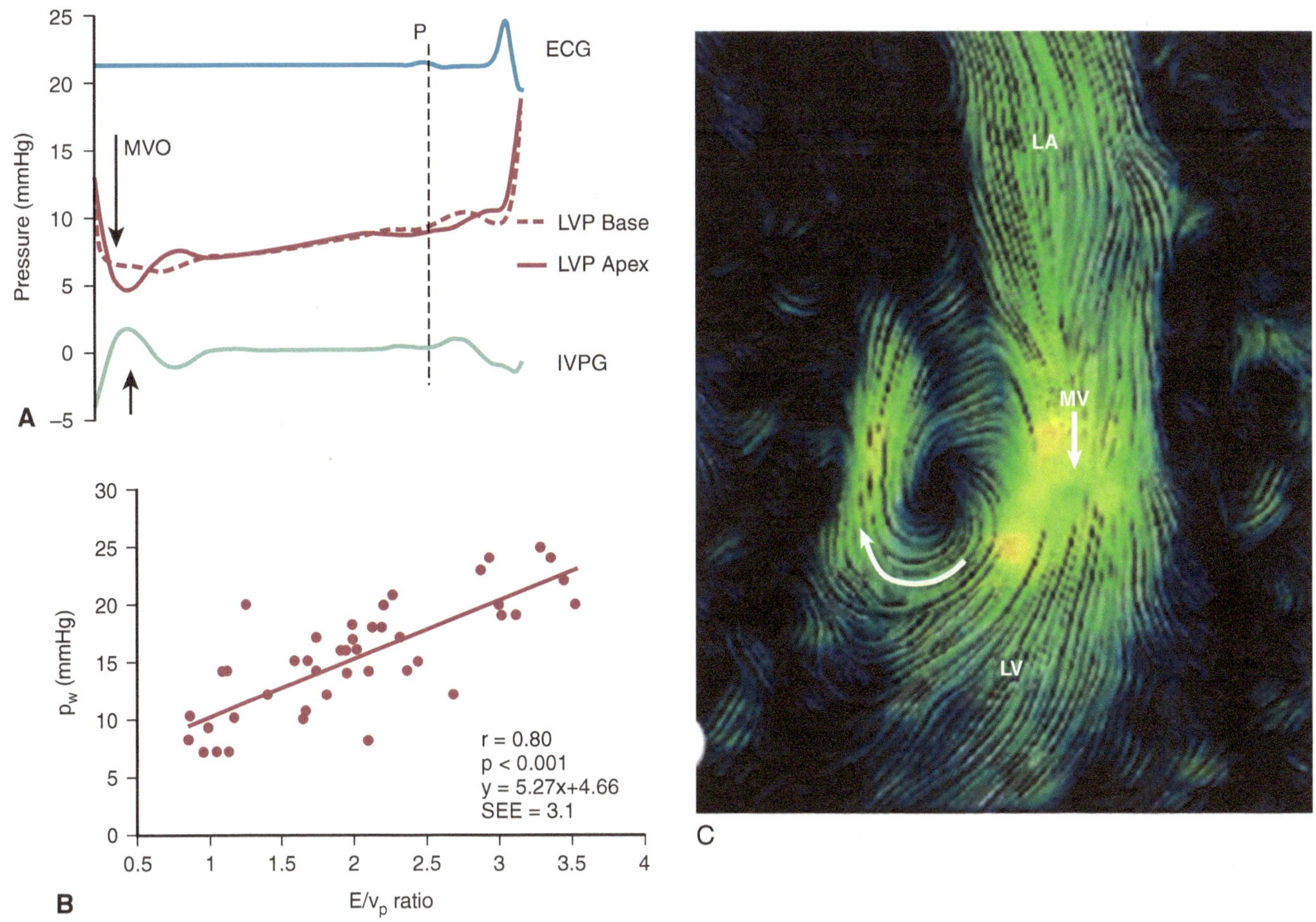

Fig. 5.9 Three consecutive early diastolic intraventricular phenomena: Intraventricular pressure gradient formation in early diastole (A), relationship between the slowing of the blood column in the early diastole with preload (B), and formation of vortices (C). (A, B: From Garcia MJ, Ares MA, Asher C, Rodriguez L, Vandervoort P, Thomas JD. An index of early left ventricular filling that combined with pulsed Doppler peak E velocity may estimate capillary wedge pressure. *J Am Coll Cardiol.* 1997;29:448–454 [fig. 4]; C: Kilner PJ, Yang GZ, Wilkes AJ, Mohiaddin RH, Firmin DN, Yacoub MH. Asymmetric redirection of flow through the heart. *Nature.* 2000;404:759–761 [fig. 1].)

move into the posterior apical region of the ventricle. In the end of the filling, the posterior part of the second vortex ring merges with the first one, forming a large vortex in the posterior apex (Fig. 5.10).

Impact of ventricular dilation on flow. A fascinating conundrum in the echocardiography is the possibility to have very high velocities of the MV inflow, while the flow propagation velocity (velocity of the blood column inside the LV) may be several times slower. Baccani et al. did a simple CFD simulation of this problem in dilated cardiomyopathy.[27] They showed that LV dilation slows flow propagation velocity, which is consistent with our data showing that hypertrophic cardiomyopathy patients with narrow left ventricle have higher flow propagation velocities than the ones with dilated cardiomyopathy.[28] Furthermore, they have shown that this is associated with the initial vortex staying attached to the mitral valve (Fig. 5.11).

Pressure propagation inside the ventricle. Flow and velocity propagation, though tightly linked, are separate phenomena. To analyze this relationship, we developed a two-dimensional axisymmetric, thick-walled FSI model. The fluid domain was represented by 6321 triangular elements, while the solid domain was represented by 1206 bricklike quadrilateral elements. The time-varying pressure at the mitral valve opening was generated by the numerical simulations of the lumped parameter model. The fluid domain was represented by incompressible Navier-Stokes equations. The LV wall was given time-varying stiffness properties, with strains calculated using a large strain deformation code. Finally, the decrease in stiffness of the wall during ventricular relaxation was modeled as an exponential decay from systolic stiffness to diastolic stiffness.[29,30]

The baseline ventricular filling pattern is illustrated in Fig. 5.12 showing the E wave entering the cavity, with formation of a vortex off the tips of the mitral valve that then pinches off[31] and propagates alongside the E wave into the ventricle. The ventricle expands under the influence of decreased elasticity and increased strain due to LV filling. As the relaxation finishes after about 200 ms, the E wave loses strength, and velocity slowly decreases as the expansion of the ventricle ceases. After the E wave ends, atrial pressure increases, and the A wave enters the ventricular cavity, forming another vortex off the mitral valve. As the A wave propagates toward the apex, this vortex is taken up by the first vortex that is still present. By now, ventricular stresses have significantly increased, raising LV pressure and slowing filling. The filling behavior described here corresponds with clinically observed behavior.

Using this fluid-structure interaction model, we have investigated the influence of changes in relaxation (τ) and end-diastolic stiffness. Color Doppler M mode images from four different conditions are

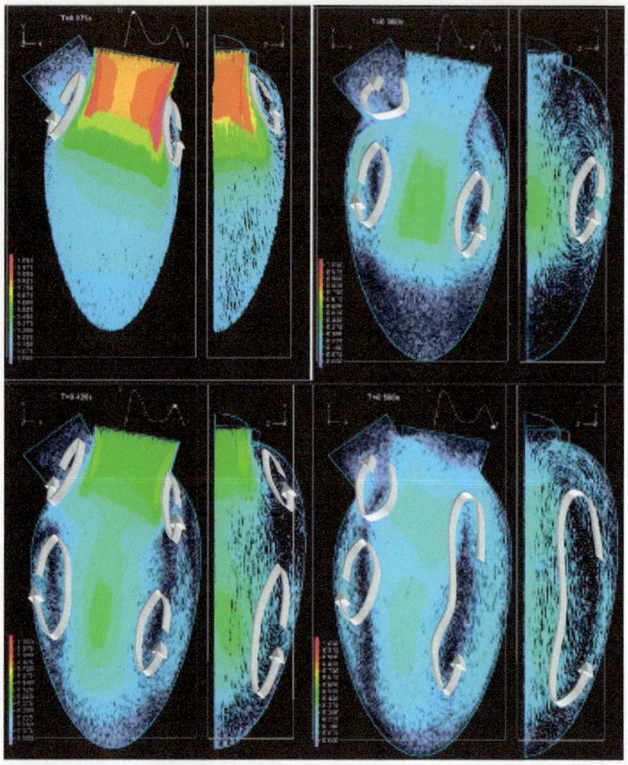

Fig. 5.10 Computer modeling of vortices during left ventricular filling. During the rapid filling phase, initial inflow through the mitral valve forms a doughnut-shaped vortex downstream from the mitral orifice. This vortex ring then travels toward the middle of the expanding ventricle, while a weak vortex of brief duration is formed within the aortic outflow tract. After initial vortex ring reaches the middle of the ventricle, its anterior part becomes stationary while the posterior part continues forward. During the atrial contraction, a new, weaker vortex ring that encompasses a part of the outflow tract is formed, while the posterior side of the initial vortex ring continues to move into the posterior apical region of the ventricle. In the end of the filling, the posterior part of the second vortex ring merges with the first one, forming a large vortex in the posterior apex. (From Cheng Y, Oertel H, Schenkel T. Fluid-structure coupled CFD simulation of the left ventricular flow during filling phase. *Ann Biomed Eng.* 2005;33:567–576 [fig. 7].)

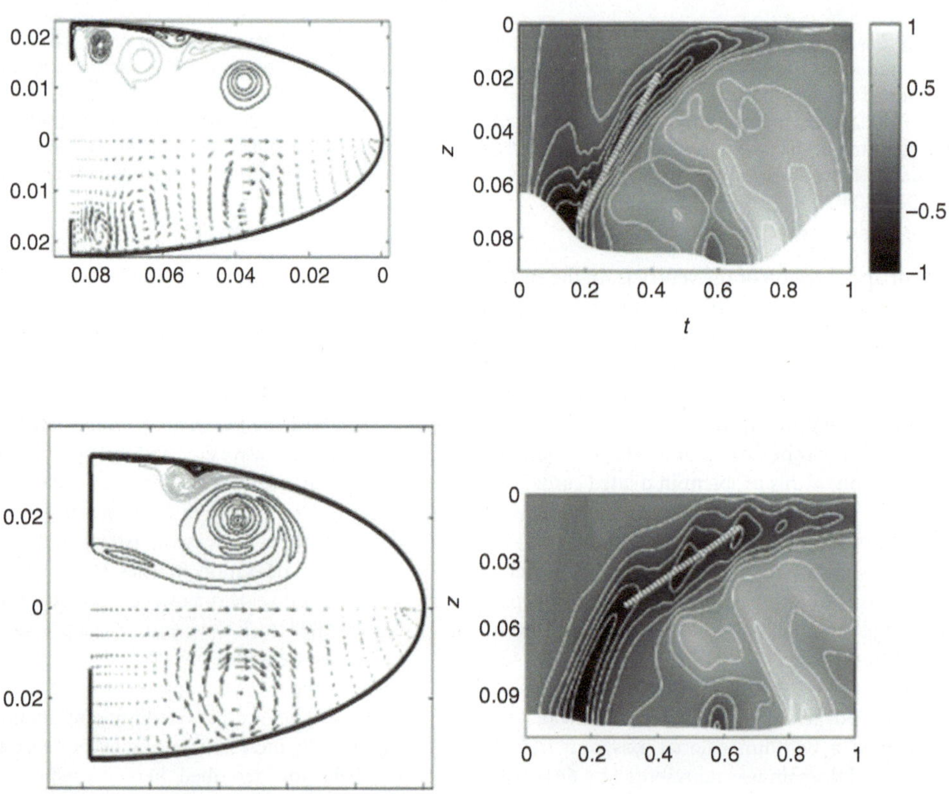

Fig. 5.11 Impact of ventricular dilation on flow. Images represent a computer model of left ventricular (LV) flow in mid-diastole. In a normal ventricle *(upper left panel)*, proximal vortex becomes unattached and freely moves toward the apex, enabling prompt filling of the ventricle as evidenced by high flow propagation velocity *(upper right panel)*. In contrast, left ventricular dilation prohibits the movement of vortices toward the *(lower left panel)*, and slows flow propagation velocity *(lower right panel)*. (From Baccani B, Domenichini F, Pedrizzetti G, Tonti G. Fluid dynamics of the left ventricular filling in dilated cardiomyopathy. *J Biomech.* 2002;35:665–671 [figs. 2, 4, 5].)

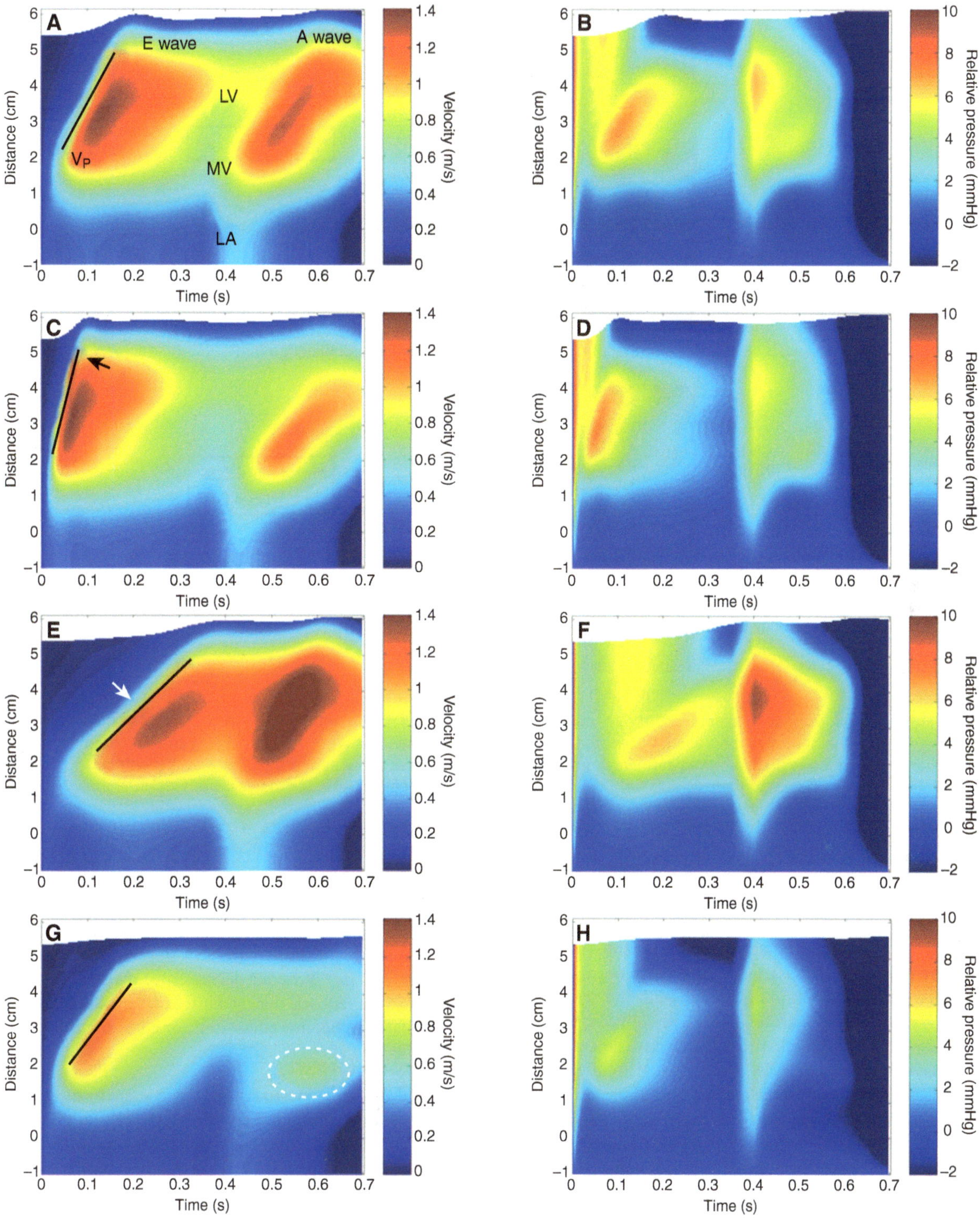

Fig. 5.12 Modeling of fluid-structure interaction model showing influence of changes in relaxation (τ) and end-diastolic stiffness. Pseudo-M mode images of time-velocity *(left panels)* and time-pressure data from four different conditions: (A and B) baseline, (C and D) shorter τ, (E and F) longer τ, and (G and H) increased ventricular diastolic stiffness, are shown. At baseline, the E and A waves are roughly balanced (equal color mapped peak velocities). IVPGs are slightly above normal due to the mild mitral stenosis inherent in the model. With shorter τ, the E wave velocity, Vp, and IVPG increase, while with longer τ, the classic appearance of delayed relaxation (low E velocity, slow propagation, large A wave, and reduced IVPG) appears. Because of the mild mitral stenosis, E wave deceleration time is prolonged and for very large time constants no longer fully separated from the A wave. With a stiffer ventricle, velocities and IVPG are reduced, reflecting lower stroke volume, the expected behavior when atrial pressure is held at baseline so no pseudonormalization will occur. The A wave is particularly blunted, reflecting ineffective filling of the stiff ventricle.

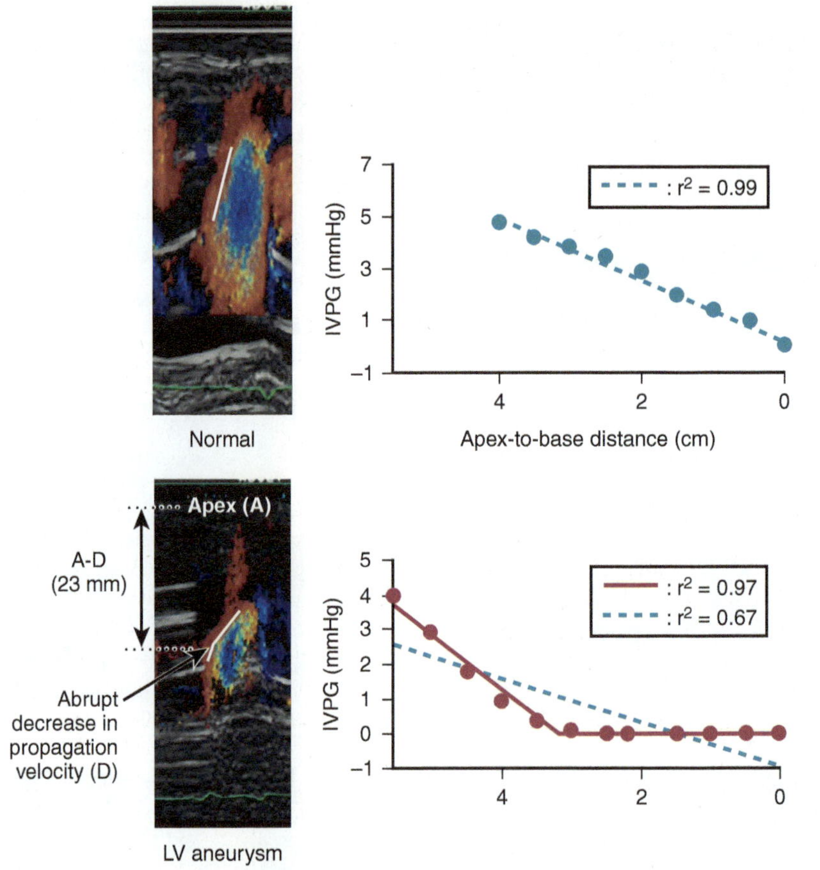

Fig. 5.13 Impact of apical aneurysm on intraventricular flow propagation. Flow propagation velocity decreases abruptly when blood enters the aneurysm. This sudden deceleration coincided with the loss of intraventricular pressure gradient. (From Asada-Kamiguchi J, Jones M, Greenberg NL, et al. Intraventricular pressure gradients in left ventricular aneurysms determined by color M-mode Doppler method: an animal study. *J Am Soc Echocardiogr.* 2006;19:1112–1118 [fig. 3].)

shown: baseline (see Fig. 5.12A and B), shorter τ (see Fig. 5.12C and D), longer τ (see Fig. 5.12E and F), and increased ventricular diastolic stiffness (see Fig. 5.12G and H). At baseline, the E and A waves are roughly balanced (equal color mapped peak velocities). Intraventricular pressure gradients (IVPGs) are slightly above normal due to the mild mitral stenosis inherent in the model. With shorter τ, the E wave velocity (Vp) and IVPG increase, while with longer τ, the classic appearance of delayed relaxation (low E velocity, slow propagation, large A wave, and reduced IVPG) is evident.[30,32–34] Because of the mild mitral stenosis, E wave deceleration time is prolonged and for very large time constants no longer fully separated from the A wave.[30] With a stiffer ventricle, velocities and IVPG are reduced, reflecting lower stroke volume, the expected behavior when atrial pressure is held at baseline so no pseudonormalization will occur. The A wave is particularly blunted, reflecting ineffective filling of the stiff ventricle.[33,35] As a support of these findings, we have shown that in humans, IVPG in the elderly becomes blunted with worsened relaxation.[9] Interestingly, elderly with preserved ventricular compliance (i.e., less stiff ventricle) still had worsened IVPG, reflecting the dependence of IVPG on intact relaxation, without an impact of compliance.

Insights From Experimental Studies

Currently no model can predict the impact of structural changes of LV shape on flow propagation within the LV. In that situation, we are left with some experimental studies. We will discuss briefly some of them.

Presence of Ischemia

Acute ischemia delays apical filling[36,37] and is associated with the loss of intraventricular pressure gradients.[38,39] Beppu et al. described the altered apical blood flow pattern in dogs with apical akinesis after coronary ligation.[40] Ischemia decreases the maximal distance of mitral inflow into the ventricle during diastole, when blood flow in the region of the infarction became either static or eddied.[40,41]

Distorted LV Geometry

We a used a sheep model to create LV aneurysm by the ligation of coronary arteries subtending LV apex.[42] We showed that flow propagation velocity abruptly decreases when blood flow column enters LV aneurysms, and that the point of this deceleration coincided with the edge of the aneurysm (Fig. 5.13). The infarct size correlated with the distance from the apex to the point of the deceleration of flow propagation. However, no point of abrupt decrease was detected when myocardial infarct was induced by circumflex occlusion. Also, significantly, presence of breakpoint coincided to loss of intraventricular pressure gradient. In a clinical study that is congruent with these findings, we have shown that removal of the aneurysm by infarct exclusion surgery improves intraventricular pressure gradients.[43] These data show that, for flow to enter the heart cavity, heart walls have to be compliant.

Impact of Isovolumic Processes

During the isovolumic period of LV relaxation, LV changes its shape in the absence of any change of volume. The most dramatic aspect of this is LV untwisting, a process that is linked to the elastic elements of the ventricle that induce early LV suction. Untwisting is a necessary successor of systolic torsion (twist). Systolic torsion and diastolic untwisting occur because myocardial fibers form a leftward helix in the subepicardium.[44] The contraction of these fibers rotates base and apex of the left ventricle clockwise and counterclockwise, respectively. However, unlike systolic torsion that increases proportional to systolic volume change, untwisting is a phenomenon that peaks prior to the opening of the mitral valve.[11,45] The reason why this occurs is that systolic torsion builds potential energy within the elastic elements of the heart.[46] With relaxation, energy is released, and elastic elements promptly restore original, untwisted LV shape. It is of no surprise that untwisting is inversely related to t, and its magnitude may be used as a surrogate measure of relaxation.

We can thus summarize events during early diastole in a normal left ventricle in the following way: Relaxation leads to prompt LV untwisting whose peak coincides with mitral valve opening; this is immediately followed by peak early mitral annulus velocity; finally, formation of IVPG facilitates early LV filling. Interestingly, we have shown a strong correlation between untwisting and IVPG at rest and during exercise.[11] Furthermore, we have shown that essentially the same slope of untwisting-IVPG relationship exists in patients with severe hypertrophic cardiomyopathy (Fig. 5.14). This indicates that untwisting and IVPG are tightly coupled, and that either untwisting is necessary to produce IVPG or some strong third factor binds them, expressed simultaneously by untwisting and IVPG. Thus it seems that three major factors determine flow propagation and intraventricular pressure gradients: chamber dilation, worsened relaxation, and loss of compliance.

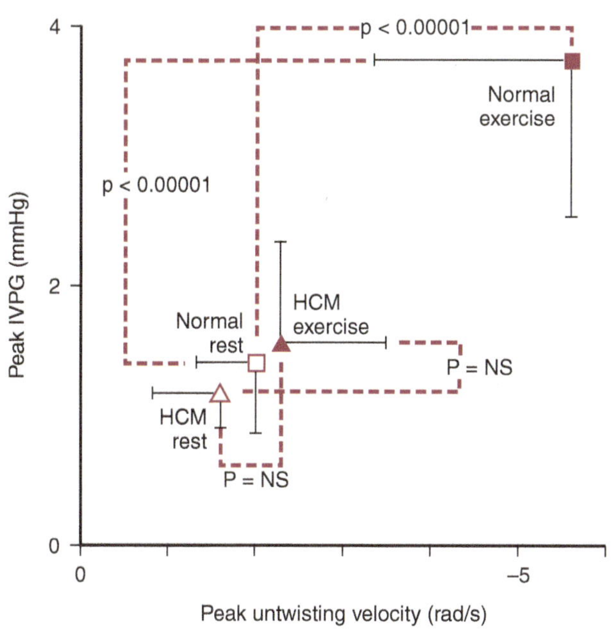

Fig. 5.14 Relationship between left ventricular untwisting and intraventricular pressure gradients *(IVPGs)* at rest *(open markers)* and during exercise *(closed markers)*. Normal subjects are marked by squares, while hypertrophic cardiomyopathy patients are marked by triangles. While the same slope of untwisting-IVPG relationship exists in normals and in patients with severe hypertrophic cardiomyopathy, patients with hypertrophic cardiomyopathy cannot generate the increase of untwisting during the exercise, leading to smaller IVPG increase. (From Notomi Y, Martin-Miklovic MG, Oryszak SJ, et al. Enhanced ventricular untwisting during exercise: a mechanistic manifestation of elastic recoil described by Doppler tissue imaging. *Circulation.* 2006;113:2524–2533 [fig. 6].)

FUTURE DIRECTIONS

The number of flow-based diastolic parameters that are proposed to be helpful in clinical practice is staggering and increasing.[47] Some kind of synthesis of the patient-level data that is not empirical but based on principles of physics would be worthwhile, since recently novel approaches in quantitating diastolic function have been proposed that move from enumerating individual diastolic parameters to incorporating them into personalized models of cardiac function. While the field is expanding, we will focus on two of them, analysis of mitral inflow and quantitation of vorticeal formation.

Kovács et al. developed a model-based approach to assess early LV filling, where they use model-based image processing to obtain patient-specific parameters of diastolic function.[48] In the most simple terms, imagine that the bolus of a blood is represented as a solid ball that falls into the vessel full of thick, viscous fluid (i.e., left ventricle). The force that drives the ball into the fluid is atrioventricular pressure gradient. The force that resists it is the LV viscosity with, by default, resistive force always smaller than driving force. Kovács's work showed that in patients with diastolic dysfunction, with increasing preload, resistive force increases to a higher degree than driving force. The novelty of Kovács's findings is that these forces can be quantified from the analysis of a simple mitral inflow profile,[49] provided that some preload variability (whether induced simply by breathing, provocation maneuvers, or saline bolus) is available. Fig. 5.15A shows mitral inflow velocities of a patient with initially asymptomatic resistant hypertension, and with subsequent development of overt heart failure in the context of worsening systolic and diastolic dysfunction several years later; Fig. 5.15B shows the relationships between peak resistive and driving forces at these two points. As can be noted, with development of heart failure, forces not only both became higher (due to increase in atrioventricular gradients and E wave velocities) but also the relationship became less steep, indicating development of higher resistance at higher preload. In sum, while lumped parameter in silico modeling can predict Doppler flows from the model input of physical determinants of cardiovascular system, this type of analysis goes in the opposite direction, deriving physical determinants from flow data.

Another fascinating topic emerged with recent availability to quantitate vorticeal contribution to diastolic inflow by combined analysis of color Doppler and grayscale imaging data. Vortex formation is linked to flow propagation velocity—they appear once flow propagation velocity starts decelerating.[31] As noted, flow propagation velocity is impaired and thus starts decelerating later in the setting of LV eccentric remodeling.[27,28] Modeling vortices still necessitate powerful computers needed to solve complex fluid-solid boundary problems. On the other hand, recently developed echocardiography techniques that combine high frame rate color Doppler and grayscale imaging can provide these data in vivo.[50] It appears that with eccentric remodeling the impairment in LV filling is counterbalanced by creation of vortices, which contribute to ~19% of LV filling in dilated cardiomyopathy (DCM) (compared to 12% in healthy subjects) (Fig. 5.16).[50] In contrast, wall constraints in hypertrophic cardiomyopathy (HCM) are associated with very rapid flow propagation velocity but decreased vortex formation—again, something to be expected when a narrow ventricle impedes vortex formation. In sum, these findings further illustrate profound differences in the patterns of LV diastolic dysfunction seen in HCM and DCM, despite similar diastolic function parameters such as E/E′, E/A ratio, and left atrial dimensions.[28]

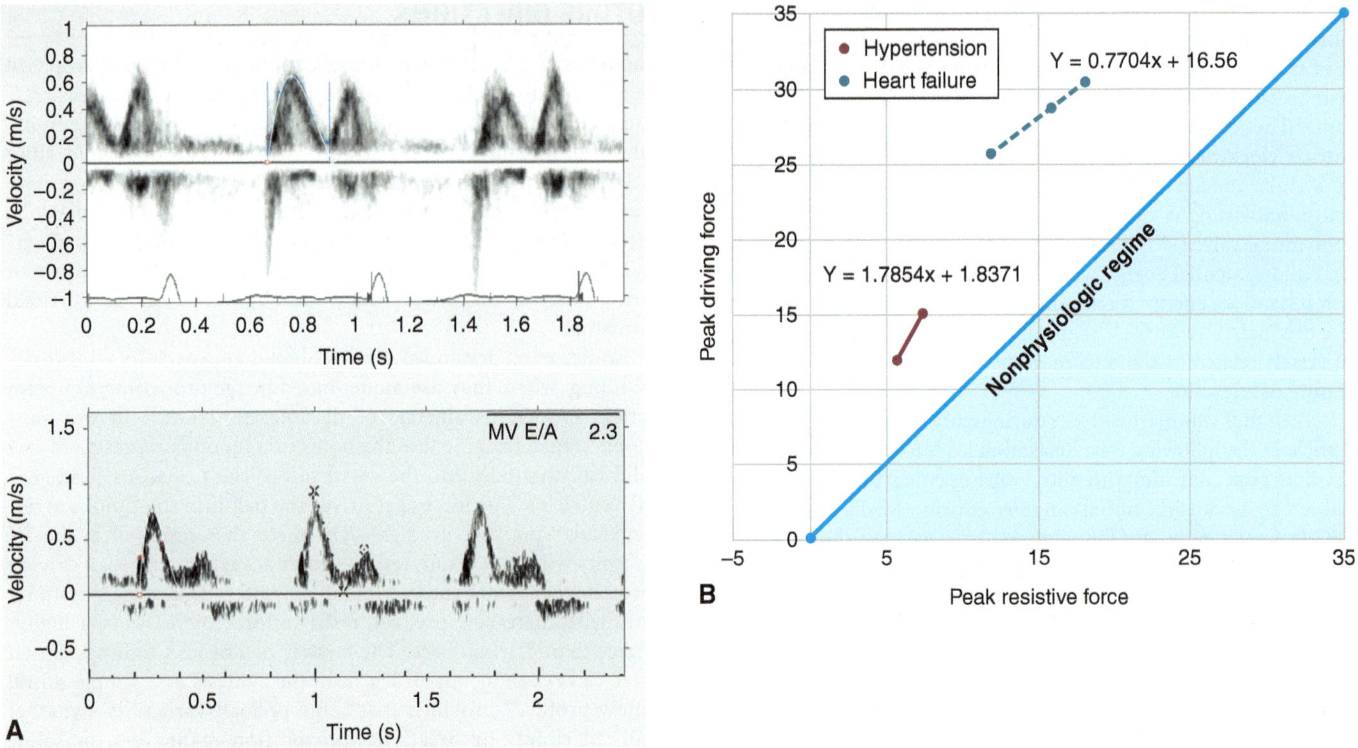

Fig. 5.15 Mitral inflow of a patient with resistant hypertension at baseline (A) and several years later after development of heart failure (B), superimposed by a computer-detected velocity profile *(thin white line)*; (C) shows corresponding relationships between resistive and driving force. Note the less steep slope of resistive/driving force relationships once heart failure is developed. (Data from Shmuylovich L, Kovacs SJ. Load-independent index of diastolic filling: Model-based derivation with in vivo validation in control and diastolic dysfunction subjects. *J Appl Physiol.* 2006;101:92–101)

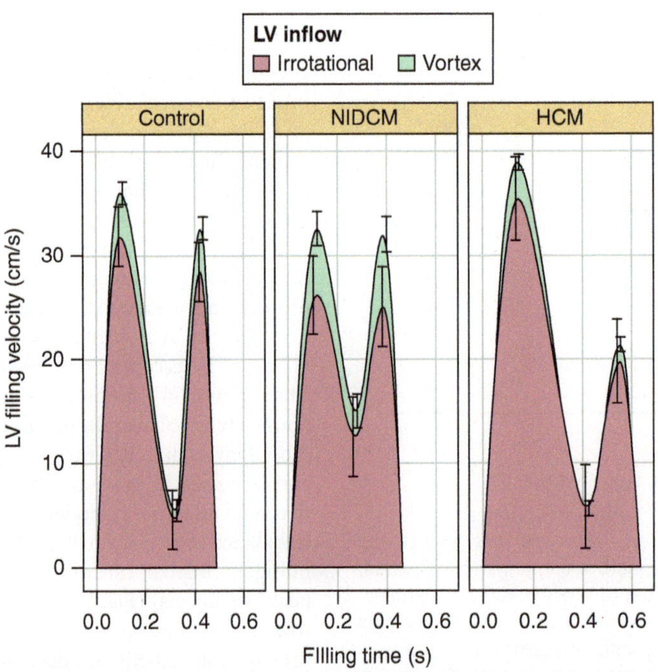

Fig. 5.16 Contribution of vorticeal flow to left ventricular filling in normal subjects, patients with dilated cardiomyopathy and hypertrophic cardiomyopathy. (From Martínez-Legazpi P, Bermejo J, Benito Y, et al. Contribution of the diastolic vortex ring to left ventricular filling. *J Am Coll Cardiol.* 2014;64:1711–1721.)

KEY POINTS

- The major function of the heart in diastole is to let the blood column flow from the antechambers into the main chambers, while keeping filling pressures to a minimum. During exercise, this task is compounded by shortening of time allowed for filling and increase of volume needed to enter into the cardiac chambers. The three major parameters that define diastole are chamber stiffness, relaxation, and early diastolic suction.
- Chamber stiffness is the instantaneous change of pressure for a given volume increment. Higher stiffness results mean less blood volume can enter the left ventricle at a given filling pressure. Chamber stiffness is not constant during diastole, but changes depending on chamber size and completeness of relaxation.
- Myocardial relaxation is a process of pressure decay that is necessary to chamber filling and thus restarts another cardiac cycle. Relaxation is a time-dependent process, which means that it may impact end-diastolic pressure when time available for relaxation is short (i.e., during exercise).
- The relationship between relaxation, chamber stiffness, chamber geometry, and intracardiac blood flow is determined by the complex Navier-Stokes equation. Based on these equations, one can demonstrate the presence of diastolic suction (negative intracavitary pressure) that facilitates early left ventricular filling.
- Chamber filling is associated with formation of vortices, which help the entrance of fluid column from atria to the ventricles.
- Current research is focused on developing personalized, patient-based computer models of diastolic function from noninvasive data.

REVIEW QUESTIONS

1. An otherwise healthy patient undergoes a resection of intramyocardial tumor. Because of the size of the tumor, the left ventricle is reconstructed with use of a large patch. Compared to a normal heart, one can expect that
   a. deceleration time will increase.
   b. deceleration time will decrease.
   c. deceleration time will stay the same, but time constant of relaxation (τ) will increase.
2. Assuming normal heart rate, increase of time constant of relaxation (τ) will
   a. increase left ventricular end-diastolic pressure (LVEDP).
   b. decrease LVEDP.
   c. increase early LV diastolic pressure.
   d. decrease early LV diastolic pressure.
3. High E wave velocity, but slow flow propagation velocity, is a characteristic of
   a. nonischemic dilated cardiomyopathy.
   b. hypertrophic cardiomyopathy.
   c. constrictive pericarditis.
4. The chronological events of left ventricular relaxation are
   a. peak left ventricular (LV) untwisting, peak intraventricular pressure gradient, peak E wave velocity.
   b. peak LV untwisting, peak E wave velocity, peak intraventricular pressure gradient.
   c. peak E wave velocity, peak LV untwisting, peak intraventricular pressure gradient.

REFERENCES

1. Glantz SA, Parmley WW. Factors which affect the diastolic pressure-volume curve. *Circ Res.* 1978;42:171–180.
2. Nikolic S, Yellin EL, Tamura K, et al. Passive properties of canine left ventricle: diastolic stiffness and restoring forces. *Circ Res.* 1988;62:1210–1222.
3. Thomas JD, Zhou J, Greenberg N, Bibawy G, McCarthy PM, Vandervoort PM. Physical and physiological determinants of pulmonary venous flow: numerical analysis. *Am J Physiol.* 1997;272:H2453–H2465.
4. Ohno M, Cheng CP, Little WC. Mechanism of altered patterns of left ventricular filling during the development of congestive heart failure. *Circulation.* 1994;89:2241–2250.
5. Matsubara H, Nakatani S, Nagata S, et al. Salutary effect of disopyramide on left ventricular diastolic function in hypertrophic obstructive cardiomyopathy. *J Am Coll Cardiol.* 1995;26:768–775.
6. Nikolic S, Yellin EL, Tamura K, Tamura T, Frater RW. Effect of early diastolic loading on myocardial relaxation in the intact canine left ventricle. *Circ Res.* 1990;66:1217–1226.
7. Senzaki H, Fetics B, Chen CH, Kass DA. Comparison of ventricular pressure relaxation assessments in human heart failure: quantitative influence on load and drug sensitivity analysis. *J Am Coll Cardiol.* 1999;34:1529–1536.
8. Scalia GM, Greenberg NL, McCarthy PM, Thomas JD, Vandervoort PM. Noninvasive assessment of the ventricular relaxation time constant (tau) in humans by Doppler echocardiography. *Circulation.* 1997;95:151–155.
9. Popovic ZB, Prasad A, Garcia MJ, et al. Relationship between diastolic intraventricular pressure gradients, relaxation, and preload: impact of age and fitness. *Am J Physiol Heart Circ Physiol.* 2006; 290:H1454–9.
10. Nikolic SD, Yellin EL, Dahm M, Pajaro O, Frater RW. Relationship between diastolic shape (eccentricity) and passive elastic properties in canine left ventricle. *Am J Physiol.* 1990;259:H457–H463.
11. Notomi Y, Martin-Miklovic MG, Oryszak SJ, et al. Enhanced ventricular untwisting during exercise: a mechanistic manifestation of elastic recoil described by Doppler tissue imaging. *Circulation.* 2006;113:2524–2533.
12. Thomas JD, Popovic ZB. Intraventricular pressure differences: a new window into cardiac function. *Circulation.* 2005;112:1684–1686.
13. Thomas JD, Weyman AE. Echocardiographic Doppler evaluation of left ventricular diastolic function. Physics and physiology. *Circulation.* 1991;84:977–990.
14. Courtois M, Kovacs Jr SJ, Ludbrook PA. Transmitral pressure-flow velocity relation. Importance of regional pressure gradients in the left ventricle during diastole. *Circulation.* 1988;78:661–671.
15. Thomas JD, Newell JB, Choong CY, Weyman AE. Physical and physiological determinants of transmitral velocity: numerical analysis. *Am J Physiol.* 1991;260:H1718–H1731.
16. Nakatani S, Firstenberg MS, Greenberg NL, et al. Mitral inertance in humans: critical factor in Doppler estimation of transvalvular pressure gradients. *Am J Physiol Heart Circ Physiol.* 2001;280:H1340–1345.
17. Hay I, Rich J, Ferber P, Burkhoff D, Maurer MS. Role of impaired myocardial relaxation in the production of elevated left ventricular filling pressure. *Am J Physiol Heart Circ Physiol.* 2005;288:H1203–H1208.
18. Firstenberg MS, Greenberg NL, Smedira NG, et al. Doppler echo evaluation of pulmonary venous-left atrial pressure gradients: human and numerical model studies. *Am J Physiol Heart Circ Physiol.* 2000;279:H594–H600.
19. Kamohara K, Fukamachi K, Ootaki Y, et al. Evaluation of a novel device for left atrial appendage exclusion: the second-generation atrial exclusion device. *J Thorac Cardiovasc Surg.* 2006;132:340–346.
20. Garcia MJ, Ares MA, Asher C, Rodriguez L, Vandervoort P, Thomas JD. An index of early left ventricular filling that combined with pulsed Doppler peak E velocity may estimate capillary wedge pressure. *J Am Coll Cardiol.* 1997;29:448–454.

21. Firstenberg MS, Vandervoort PM, Greenberg NL, et al. Noninvasive estimation of transmitral pressure drop across the normal mitral valve in humans: importance of convective and inertial forces during left ventricular filling. *J Am Coll Cardiol.* 2000;36:1942–1949.
22. Kilner PJ, Yang GZ, Wilkes AJ, Mohiaddin RH, Firmin DN, Yacoub MH. Asymmetric redirection of flow through the heart. *Nature.* 2000;404: 759–761.
23. Vierendeels JA, Dick E, Verdonck PR. Hydrodynamics of color M-mode Doppler flow wave propagation velocity V(p): a computer study. *J Am Soc Echocardiogr.* 2002;15:219–224.
24. Vierendeels JA, Riemslagh K, Dick E, Verdonck PR. Computer simulation of intraventricular flow and pressure gradients during diastole. *J Biomech Eng.* 2000;122:667–674.
25. Verdonck P, Vierendeels J, Riemslagh K, Dick E. Left-ventricular pressure gradients: a computer-model simulation. *Med Biol Eng Comput.* 1999;37:511–516.
26. Cheng Y, Oertel H, Schenkel T. Fluid-structure coupled CFD simulation of the left ventricular flow during filling phase. *Ann Biomed Eng.* 2005;33:567–576.
27. Baccani B, Domenichini F, Pedrizzetti G, Tonti G. Fluid dynamics of the left ventricular filling in dilated cardiomyopathy. *J Biomech.* 2002;35: 665–671.
28. Buakhamsri A, Popovic ZB, Lin J, et al. Impact of left ventricular volume/mass ratio on diastolic function. *Eur Heart J.* 2009;30:1213–1221.
29. Mirsky I. Assessment of diastolic function: suggested methods and future considerations. *Circulation.* 1984;69:836–841.
30. Thomas JD, Zhou J, Greenberg N, Bibawy G, McCarthy PM, Vandervoort PM. Physical and physiological determinants of pulmonary venous flow: numerical analysis. *Am J Physiol.* 1997;272:H2453–H2465.
31. Stewart KC, Charonko JC, Niebel CL, Little WC, Vlachos PP. Left ventricular vortex formation is unaffected by diastolic impairment. *Am J Physiol Heart Circ Physiol.* 2012;303:H1255–H1262.
32. Lemmon JD, Yoganathan AP. Computational modeling of left heart diastolic function: examination of ventricular dysfunction. *J Biomech Eng.* 2000;122:297–303.
33. Takatsuji H, Mikami T, Urasawa K, et al. A new approach for evaluation of left ventricular diastolic function: spatial and temporal analysis of left ventricular filling flow propagation by color M-mode Doppler echocardiography [see comments]. *J Am Coll Cardiol.* 1996;27:365–371.
34. Garcia MJ, Smedira NG, Greenberg NL, et al. Color M-mode Doppler flow propagation velocity is a preload insensitive index of left ventricular relaxation: animal and human validation. *J Am Coll Cardiol.* 2000;35: 201–208.
35. Appleton CP, Hatle LK, Popp RL. Relation of transmitral flow velocity patterns to left ventricular diastolic function: new insights from a combined hemodynamic and Doppler echocardiographic study. *J Am Coll Cardiol.* 1988;12:426–440.
36. Stugaard M, Smiseth OA, Risoe C, Ihlen H. Intraventricular early diastolic filling during acute myocardial ischemia. *Circulation.* 1993;88:2705–2713.
37. Steine K. Mechanisms of retarded apical filling in acute ischemic left ventricular failure. *Circulation.* 1999;99:2048–2054.
38. Steine K, Stugaard M, Smiseth OA. Mechanisms of retarded apical filling in acute ischemic left ventricular failure. *Circulation.* 1999;99:2048–2054.
39. Steine K, Flogstad T, Stugaard M, Smiseth OA. Early diastolic intraventricular filling pattern in acute myocardial infarction by color M-mode Doppler echocardiography. *J Am Soc Echocardiogr.* 1998;11: 119–125.
40. Beppu S, Izumi S, Miyatake K, et al. Abnormal blood pathways in left ventricular cavity in acute myocardial infarction. Experimental observations with special reference to regional wall motion abnormality and hemostasis. *Circulation.* 1988;78:157–164.
41. Delemarre BJ, Visser CA, Bot H, Dunning AJ. Prediction of apical thrombus formation in acute myocardial infarction based on left ventricular spatial flow pattern. *J Am Coll Cardiol.* 1990;15:355–360.
42. Asada-Kamiguchi J, Jones M, Greenberg NL, et al. Intraventricular pressure gradients in left ventricular aneurysms determined by color M-mode Doppler method: an animal study. *J Am Soc Echocardiogr.* 2006;19:1112–1118.
43. Firstenberg MS, Smedira NG, Greenberg NL, et al. Relationship between early diastolic intraventricular pressure gradients, an index of elastic recoil, and improvements in systolic and diastolic function. *Circulation.* 2001;104:1330–1335.
44. Ingels Jr NB, Hansen DE, Daughters GT, Stinson EB, Alderman EL, Miller DC. Relation between longitudinal, circumferential, and oblique shortening and torsional deformation in the left ventricle of the transplanted human heart. *Circ Res.* 1989;64:915–927.
45. Gibbons Kroeker CA, Ter Keurs HE, Knudtson ML, Tyberg JV, Beyar R. An optical device to measure the dynamics of apex rotation of the left ventricle. *Am J Physiol.* 1993;265:H1444–H1449.
46. Bell SP, Nyland L, Tischler MD, McNabb M, Granzier H, LeWinter MM. Alterations in the determinants of diastolic suction during pacing tachycardia. *Circ Res.* 2000;87:235–240.
47. Popovic ZB, Sato K, Desai MY. Is universal grading of diastolic function by echocardiography feasible? *Cardiovasc Diagn Therapy.* 2018;8:18–28.
48. Shmuylovich L, Kovács SJ. Load-independent index of diastolic filling: model-based derivation with in vivo validation in control and diastolic dysfunction subjects. *J Appl Physiol. (Bethesda, MD).* 2006;101:92–101.
49. Sundqvist MG, Salman K, Tornvall P, Ugander M. Kinematic analysis of diastolic function using the freely available software Echo E-waves—feasibility and reproducibility. *BMC Med Imaging.* 2016;16:60.
50. Martínez-Legazpi P, Bermejo J, Benito Y, et al. Contribution of the diastolic vortex ring to left ventricular filling. *J Am Coll Cardiol.* 2014;64:1711–1721.

6

Ventricular–Arterial Interaction in Patients With Heart Failure and a Preserved Ejection Fraction

Yogesh N.V. Reddy, Barry A. Borlaug, and Vojtech Melenovsky

OUTLINE

Case Study

A 79-year-old obese male (body mass index 33 kg/m^2) with prior history of coronary bypass grafting, hypertension, and diabetes presented with New York Heart Association functional class III dyspnea progressive over 1 year. Vitals included a blood pressure of 162/90 mmHg and heart rate of 55 bpm. Jugular venous pressure and cardiac auscultation was normal, and there was no edema. Stress echocardiogram demonstrated no ischemia with a normal ejection fraction (60%), estimated right ventricular systolic pressure of 24 mmHg, and an E/e′ ratio of 8. Due to persistent unexplained dyspnea, hemodynamic exercise catheterization was pursued, which demonstrated a high pulmonary capillary wedge pressure (PCWP) at rest along with central aortic hypertension (Fig. 6.1). With exercise, there was a pathologic increase in left-sided filling pressures and impaired cardiac output response consistent with underlying heart failure with preserved ejection fraction (HFpEF).

As we will explain in this chapter, these central hemodynamic derangements were coupled with abnormal pulsatile, reflective, and steady-state load that failed to demonstrate the normal expected degree of reduction in arterial load during exercise. Abnormalities in vascular stiffness and their coupling with ventricular systolic and diastolic performance during rest and exercise contribute to exercise intolerance and symptom manifestation in HFpEF.

INTRODUCTION

The mammalian cardiovascular system evolved to provide adequate flow at physiologic pressures both at rest and under a broad range of demands. Since blood flow is pulsatile, changes in cardiac output are accompanied by alterations in the arterial pulse wave amplitude and peak systolic pressure. To prevent wide fluctuations in blood pressure that otherwise can lead to vascular and end-organ damage, the heart and arteries are compliant so that pulse and peak pressures can be buffered, while systemic diastolic pressures are augmented. For the vasculature, this compliance is largely contained within the proximal conduit vessels, while within the heart it is described by the end-systolic stiffness (elastance, inverse of compliance) that is achieved during contraction. The normal heart develops a ventricular systolic stiffness of about 2.0 mmHg/mL of ventricular end-systolic volume, while arterial stiffness is about 1.5 mmHg/mL.[1,2] These low values allow relatively large changes in volume in both the heart and the vascular bed to be achieved with only modest changes in ejected pressures.

With advancing age, both ventricular and arterial stiffness increase, and these changes may be further exacerbated by common disorders such as hypertension, obesity, diabetes mellitus, and renal disease.[3–7] Since the heart and arterial systems are coupled, such stiffening results in amplification of systolic and pulse pressures during ejection, faster pressure decay during diastole, and enhanced cardiac systolic loading. Stiff arteries facilitate rapid transit of the flow and pressure pulse through the vasculature, increasing the velocity at which these waves encounter regions of impedance mismatch (e.g., distal arteriolar narrowings), which then increases the amplitude of reflected pressure waves, further exacerbating systolic load. The net effect is an adverse impact on cardiac systolic and diastolic function, with increased myocardial oxygen consumption required to provide the body with blood flow, impaired cardiovascular reserve function, labile systemic blood pressures, and diminished coronary flow reserve.[1,7–9] Aging is also associated with endothelial dysfunction,[10] which may in part relate to mechanical stiffening, as reduced wall distensibility can itself compromise endothelial-dependent responses to shear stress stimulation[11,12] and vasorelaxation. One can consider this adverse interaction between heart and arteries as a form of coupling disease that ultimately limits the ability of the integrated cardiovascular system to respond to stress.

Abnormal ventricular-arterial stiffening and thus coupling may play an important role in patients with heart failure symptoms but with apparent preservation of systolic function. Such patients are typically older and female, with histories of chronic hypertension and a

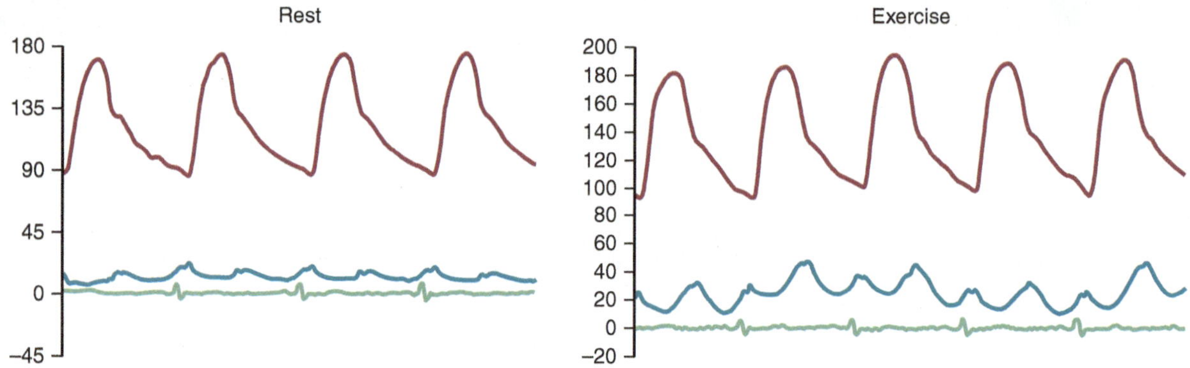

Rest	Hemodynamics	Exercise
177/99/130	Aortic BP (S/D/M), mmHg	197/102/145
4.9	Cardiac output, L/min	6
85	Stroke volume, ml/min	75
60	Heart rate, bpm	80
1.1	Total arterial compliance, ml/mmHg	0.8
1.9	Effective arterial elastance, mmHg/ml	2.4
21	Augmentation index, %	17
2012	Systemic vascular resistance, dyn s cm^{-5}	1680
20 (25)	PCWP, mean (v wave)	37 (55)

Fig. 6.1 Rest and exercise hemodynamics in a patient with HFpEF and increased arterial load with exercise.

high prevalence of diabetes, obesity, and renal dysfunction. They often develop marked systolic hypertension under conditions of stress, and both their arterial and ventricular systolic pressures are very sensitive to blood volume status. While abnormal diastolic function is thought to contribute to heart failure symptoms by increasing congestion, it cannot explain the observed increases in systemic pressures, nor does it fully underlie limitations of cardiac reserve. Here, we review the pathophysiology of ventricular-arterial stiffening and its role in the syndrome of heart failure with a preserved ejection fraction (HFpEF).

PATHOPHYSIOLOGY OF LEFT VENTRICULAR-ARTERIAL COUPLING

The influence of increases in ventricular systolic and vascular stiffness on net cardiovascular function is best depicted in the pressure-volume (P-V) plane. Ventricular end-systolic chamber stiffness is expressed as end-systolic elastance (Ees) (Fig. 6.2), defined by the slope of the end-systolic P-V relationship.[13] Ventricular afterload can be represented as aortic input impedance, derived from Fourier analysis of aortic pressure and flow waves.[14,15] Impedance is expressed in the frequency domain and thus is more difficult to match with optimal measures of ventricular systolic function, which are typically determined in the time domain. One approach to this problem involves the development of a vascular parameter that shares units applicable to the heart, namely effective arterial elastance (Ea).[16,17] Ea combines both mean and pulsatile loading, providing a lumped parameter that reflects the net impact of arterial vascular load on the heart. This index was developed and validated by Sunagawa et al. in the −1980s, and then applied and verified in humans by Kelly et al.[16] The latter group confirmed that the simple ratio of end-systolic pressure to stroke volume (Pes/SV) could serve to estimate Ea in both hypertensive and normal humans. Graphically, Ea can be depicted as the absolute value of the slope of a line linking the coordinate points of end-systolic volume [Ves], Pes, and end-diastolic volume [Ved], $P = 0$ (see Fig. 6.2).

Coupling of heart and artery is often then depicted by the interaction of these two relations and expressed as a ratio of Ea/Ees.[18–20] The intersection of these lines determines Pes and Ves (see Fig. 6.2). As shown in Fig. 6.3, the Ea/Ees ratio is fairly preserved with normal aging to maintain optimal efficiency, declining somewhat in women, while both the numerator (vascular load) and the denominator (ventricular stiffness) increase.[2] Ea is dominated by mean ventricular load, namely systemic vascular resistance (SVR),[17,18] but it is also altered by artery stiffening to increase pulse pressure. Blood pressure pulsatility rises with aging, and this is reflected in the P-V diagram in the elderly individual (see Fig. 6.2B) and the HFpEF patient (see Fig. 6.2C) by the rise in systolic pressure throughout ejection *((arrows)*.[1,21,22] Since Ea is determined by the ratio Pes/SV, the greater the disparity between Pes and mean arterial pressure (i.e., the more pulsatile or stiff the arterial system), the higher Ea will be relative to mean resistance load. Ea also varies directly with heart rate, since for any given cardiac SV, the systolic pressure will increase or decrease proportionally with the number of strokes (i.e., cardiac output). It is important to keep these factors in mind when interpreting data reporting on Ea and Ea/Ees coupling.

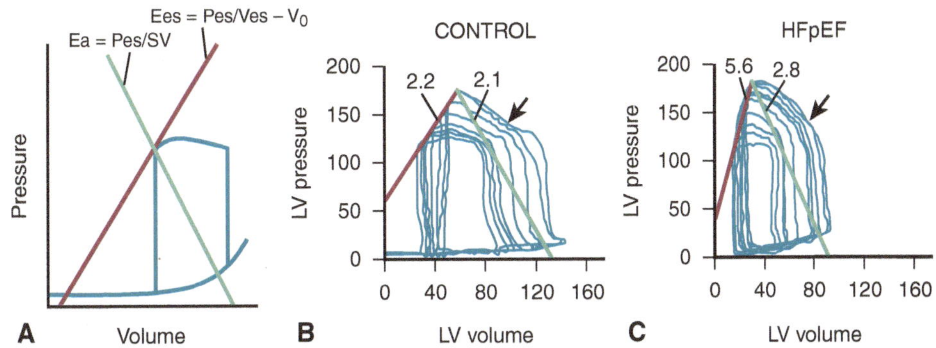

Fig. 6.2 (A) Idealized pressure-volume loop in a young person. Contractility is expressed as end-systolic elastance *(Ees)*, the slope of the end-systolic pressure-volume relationship. Afterload is defined by effective arterial elastance *(Ea)*, the negative slope passing through the end-systolic and end-diastolic pressure-volume points. Note the loop's rectangular shape, with little increase in pressure during systole. (B) Typical pressure-volume loops obtained from a normal 65-year-old man during preload reduction. Note that the coupling ratio (Ea/Ees) is close to unity. (C) Example loops from a subject with heart failure with preserved ejection fraction *(HFpEF)*. Ea and Ees are elevated, the coupling ratio is lower, and the loops have a more trapezoidal shape due to the gradual increase in systolic pressure during ejection (reflecting increased arterial pulse pressure), related to a decrease in arterial compliance and increase in wave reflections *(arrow)*. *Pes,* End-systolic pressure; *SV,* stroke volume; *Ves,* end-systolic volume; *V_0,* volume intercept. (Modified from Kawaguchi M, Hay I, Fettics B, Kass DA. Combined ventricular systolic and arterial stiffening in patients with heart failure and preserved ejection fraction: implications for systolic and diastolic reserve limitations. *Circulation.* 2003;107:714–720.)

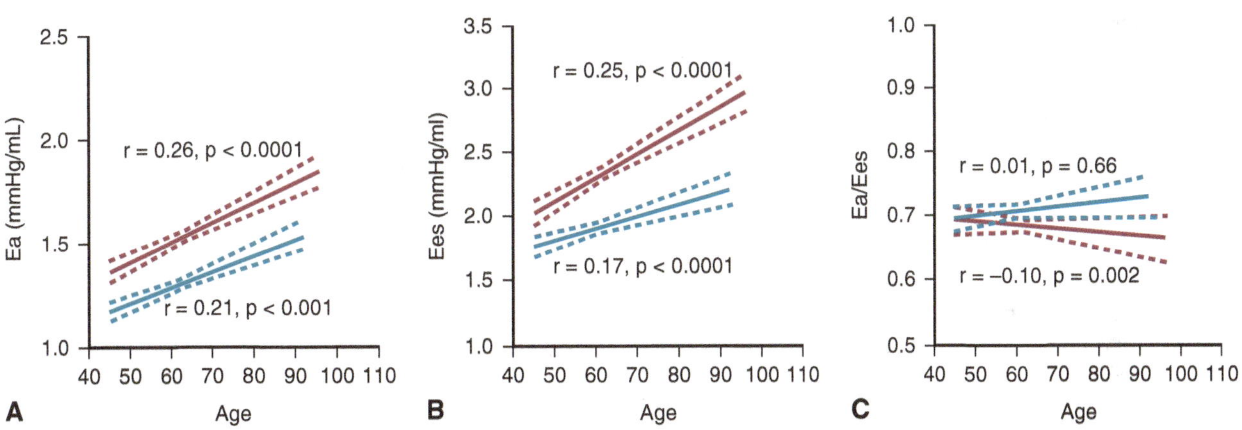

Fig. 6.3 (A, B) Arterial and ventricular systolic stiffness increase with aging in both men *(blue)* and women *(red)*. At each age level, stiffness is higher in women, in whom the age-dependent increase in ventricular-arterial stiffness is accentuated. (C) The increase in ventricular and arterial stiffness is matched with aging in men, resulting in stable coupling ratio, while in women this ratio decreases with age. (Modified from Redfield MM, et al. Age and gender related ventricular-vascular stiffening: a community based study. *Circulation.* 2005;112:2554–2262.)

Effective coupling of heart to artery can be defined in several ways. One is the optimal transfer of blood from heart to periphery without excessive increases in pulse or systolic pressures. One can mathematically express optimal coupling as the interaction that best enhances the work performed by the heart on the body (i.e., optimal external work). Lastly, one must consider the efficiency of the heart in performing this work—the energy consumption required to effect this external work. All of these are reasonable definitions, although prior experimental and clinical studies have tended to focus on the latter two: optimizing external work and efficiency. For this, one can both predict[23] and observe experimentally[20,23] that an Ea/Ees coupling ratio of 0.6 to 1.2 achieves near optimal work and efficiency. This range is normally maintained under various physiologic stresses, as shown elegantly some years back in exercising animals.[24] It can become very high, particularly in dilated cardiomyopathy, where depressed heart function (low Ees) is coupled to a high arterial impedance (high Ea).[25]

Methods to evaluate arterial stiffness

Measurement of a vascular load is complex and not easily summarized by instantaneous single values of peak systolic and nadir diastolic pressures as is commonly used in clinical practice. Arterial pressures oscillate in a time-varying pulsatile fashion around a mean arterial blood pressure, and therefore a time-varying pulsatile load is more difficult to quantify by such static pressure measurements. In addition, arterial stiffness and pulsatile load are dynamic measures that vary with both heart rate and baseline ambient pressure in the systemic circulation. Furthermore, in terms of quantifying the vascular load on the left ventricle, measuring the central aortic pressure is more important than brachial blood pressure (which is subject to pulse pressure amplification of brachial systolic pressure).

For accurate measurement of pulsatile hemodynamics, pressure waveforms over time must be recorded with high fidelity. The gold standard measure is by invasive arterial pressure measurement, but this is obviously not practical for routine use. Applanation tonometry has enabled high-quality noninvasive measurement of radial or carotid arterial waveforms (although calibration to absolute pressures using independently measured brachial blood pressure is necessary). Since the carotid artery is anatomically close to the central aorta, carotid tonometry derived pressure can be used as a direct surrogate of central aortic pressure, whereas radial tonometry requires a mathematical transfer function to derive central aortic pressure from validated algorithms.[26,27]

Once central aortic pressure is obtained, the pulse pressure (systolic-diastolic pressure) and stroke volume can be used to estimate total arterial compliance (TAC) (stroke volume/pulse pressure) as a measure of pulsatile load.[28] This is the simplest and most commonly used method to estimate compliance, but it remains an estimate as the arterial circulation is not truly a chamber, and there is continuous outflow from the arterial capacitor during systole.[29] Alternate methods of calculating TAC include: (1) an iterative pulse pressure method, where compliance is altered until the derived pulse pressure from a two-element Windkessel model matches measured pulse pressure[30] and (2) analysis of the diastolic decay (during which there is no arterial inflow), which can be fit to an exponential curve to derive the Resistance*Compliance (RC) constant. Since SVR can be readily calculated by modeling the circulation as a steady-state resistor [SVR = mean arterial − atrial pressure/cardiac output], TAC can therefore be solved from this measured RC time constant. However, the stroke volume/pulse pressure estimate remains a widely used approximation of these more complex methods and has been validated.[28,29]

As mentioned, effective arterial elastance provides a lumped measure of steady-state and pulsatile arterial load derived in the pressure volume plane and is also dependent on heart rate.[16] This can be calculated by end-systolic pressure/stroke volume, with end-systolic pressure often approximated by 0.9 *systolic pressure.[16] It is important to note that although Ea is inversely proportional to TAC, it is not merely the simple inverse of TAC but in fact incorporates the principal elements of vascular load, including peripheral resistance, total arterial compliance, characteristic impedance, and systolic and diastolic time intervals.[16,23] In other words, Ea is affected by TAC (and varies inversely with it), but Ea is not in itself equal to 1/TAC.[31]

Although the three-element Windkessel model is useful to study the arterial circulation, reflected waves also contribute to arterial load but are not well represented by such modeling. Pulse wave analysis can estimate augmentation of systolic pressure by reflected waves based on the initial inflection point in the systolic arterial pressure tracing from which the augmentation index can be calculated (augmentation pressure/pulse pressure). Wave separation analysis can further quantify the reflected load by separating the time-varying central aortic waveform into a forward wave and backward wave to calculate the reflection index (backward wave/forward wave). This wave separation can be done using either directly measured aortic flow in the ascending aorta (measured either invasively by a Doppler flow wire or noninvasively by echocardiographic Pulsed-wave Doppler or phase contrast magnetic resonance imaging [MRI]) or most commonly by estimation/modeling of flow patterns from the pressure tracing configuration alone.[32] Such flow patterns when combined with instantaneous pressure also allow more complex measures of aortic characteristic impedance, which is typically represented in the frequency domain, and therefore is less intuitive to relate to existing pressure measures in the time domain.

Another commonly used measure of arterial stiffness that is widely utilized is measurement of pulse wave velocity (which should increase as arterial stiffness worsens). This can be measured from knowledge of the time delay of pressure wave onset between the carotid and radial/femoral artery sites measured by applanation tonometry. The distance between the two measurement sites, along with the time delay of onset, can be used to directly calculate pulse wave velocity as distance/time.

Ventricular-Arterial Stiffening in Heart Failure With a Preserved Ejection Fraction

In patients with HFpEF, the Ea/Ees ratio falls compared with younger individuals but is similar to that of nonsymptomatic hypertensive elderly patients.[1,21] Importantly, it still falls in a range where external work and efficiency are not likely compromised. However, while the ratio itself is reduced, the absolute values of both numerator and denominator are significantly elevated (Fig. 6.4). Thus HFpEF patients have elevated vascular stiffness,[1,33] as well as increased ventricular stiffness in both systole[1] and diastole.[34,35] The net interaction of ventricular and arterial stiffness is important because it can significantly affect the first two components of what we can consider optimal coupling—blood pressure homeostasis and preservation of adequate cardiovascular reserve. As displayed in Fig. 6.5, an increase in both Ea and Ees means that systolic pressures are much more sensitive to changes in cardiac preload and thus central vascular blood volume.[36] Small changes in volume that might accompany dietary indiscretion or diuretic usage will translate to more exaggerated changes in arterial pressure.[21] This also predicts higher pressures during stress, which in addition to requiring a greater amount of energy to deliver a given SV, can also alter both ejection and relaxation. A higher resting Ees means that there can be less effective contractile reserve to call upon during stress demands (Fig. 6.6A). Higher combined ventricular and vascular stiffening leads to greater cardiac energy demands to provide the body with a given amount of blood flow (see Fig. 6.6B).[1] Lastly, increased vascular stiffness and thus pulsatile loading can affect vascular homeostasis, coronary perfusion, and flow reserve.[7] We next discuss each of these mechanisms in more detail.

Mechanisms of Ventricular-Vascular Stiffening

Ventricular stiffening is a product of both passive and active muscle properties. Passive behavior is somewhat of a misnomer, since diastolic tone is regulated in part by calcium and also by the phosphorylation state and isoforms of various sarcomeric proteins.[37,38] Nonetheless, we can ascribe diastolic stiffening to properties of muscle cell size, wall geometry, intrasarcomeric protein composition, cytosolic and membrane distensibility, extracellular matrix composition, fibrillar crosslinking, and biophysical properties. These are discussed in detail in Chapter 2. Systolic ventricular stiffness is related to the same determinants of stiffness in diastole, as well as activated myofilament properties, changes in structural protein behavior shortened to smaller lengths, and interactions of the activated myocytes with the matrix. As mentioned, the latter is typically measured as chamber stiffness or elastance (pressure/volume), but has also been assessed invasively by transverse indentation methods or estimated based on stress-strained analysis.[39,40] Vascular stiffening also stems from structural and muscle tone–dependent factors. Smooth muscle tone plays an important role, as does the geometry of the vessel (e.g., dilation), elastin and collagen content, crosslinking of matrix components, and other factors. This has been reviewed in detail.[41]

How do these mechanisms relate to patients with HFpEF? Many HFpEF patients have left ventricular hypertrophy (LVH), concentric

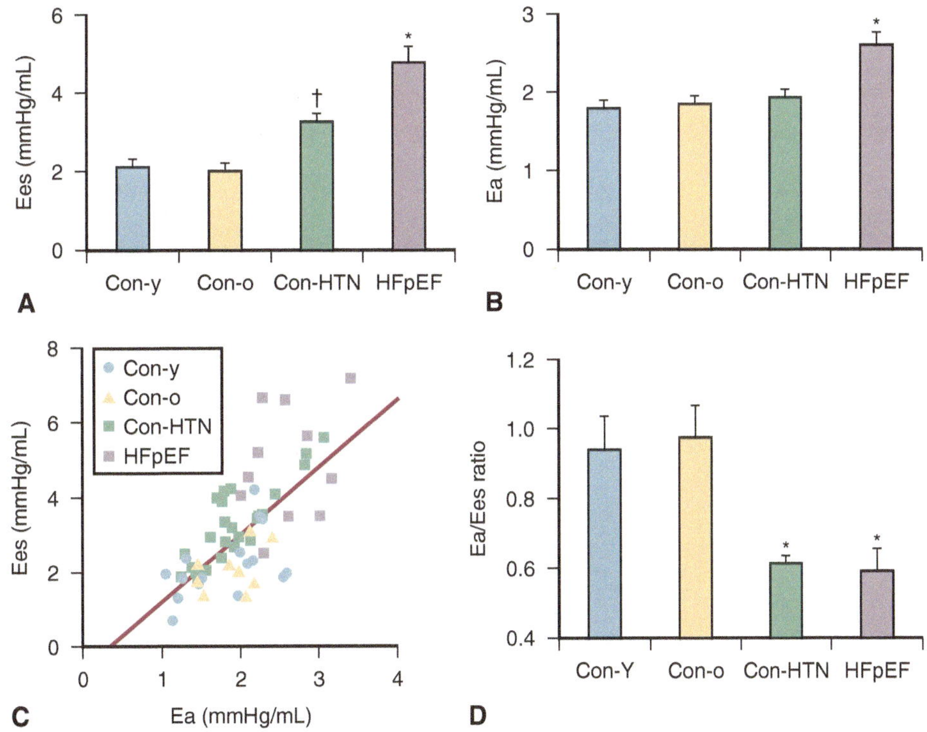

Fig. 6.4 (A) Ventricular systolic stiffness is elevated in hypertensive patients compared with younger and age-matched controls, but significantly higher in heart failure with preserved ejection fraction *(HFpEF)*. (B) Arterial elastance is higher in HFpEF patients than in both hypertensive and nonhypertensive controls. (C) Increases in vascular stiffness are correlated with increased ventricular systolic stiffness in all groups, with HFpEF showing an exaggerated increase in ventricular stiffness. (D) Coupling ratio is lower to a similar extent in both hypertensive patients and HFpEF patients compared with controls. HFpEF is thus distinguished from hypertension by the extent of ventricular and arterial stiffening, not simply by the ratio of Ea/Ees. *Con-HTN,* Hypertensive-matched controls; *Con-o,* older age-matched controls; *Con-y,* young controls. (Modified from Miho Kawaguchi, MD; Ilan Hay, MD; Barry Fetics, MSE; David A. Kass, MD. Combined Ventricular Systolic and Arterial Stiffening in Patients With Heart Failure and Preserved Ejection Fraction Implications for Systolic and Diastolic Reserve Limitations. DOI: 10.1161/01.CIR.0000048123.22359.A0)

chamber remodeling, or both.[42–45] While in some HFpEF mimics this may develop from a primary sarcomeric protein defect (as with genetic hypertrophic cardiomyopathies), this cause is uncommon compared with the maladaptive response to chronically increased ventricular load, and we will focus on the latter here. In a large observational study of consecutive patients presenting with HFpEF, the mean LV mass index was 66.5 g/m$^{2.7}$, well above cutoff partition values for defining LVH (46.7 g/m$^{2.7}$ in women and 49.2 g/m$^{2.7}$ in men).[43] Myocyte hypertrophy has been documented, along with a modest rise in myofibrillar content and increases in passive myocyte stiffness in triton-skinned cells.[46,47] Myocardial fibrosis is also frequently observed, although this is only modestly different from hearts displaying dilated cardiomyopathy[47] or hypertensive controls.[48,49] Ventricular cellular passive stiffness has been found to correlate with estimates of diastolic chamber differences[46] in HFpEF subjects, and indeed, diastolic stiffening is reported in these patients.[35] Not all diastolic stiffening is intrinsic to the chamber, however, as external loading factors also appear to contribute importantly to observed diastolic stiffening, as indicated by invasive pressure-volume analysis.[1,50]

Diastolic stiffening alone can contribute to fluid redistribution into the lungs and limit net cardiac filling, but it cannot explain why patients with HFpEF typically present with severe, uncontrolled hypertension when they develop pulmonary edema[51] and often display marked blood pressure sensitivity to vasodilator or diuretic therapy. The latter more directly relates to increased left ventricular systolic stiffening (Ees).[1,21] In addition to arterial systolic pulse pressure and stiffness, which are known to increase with age,[2,4,22,52] Ees also has been shown to rise in tandem with Ea (see Fig. 6.3).[2,21] In subjects who develop hypertension and cardiac hypertrophy, and those who further develop HFpEF, this stiffening is more pronounced over age-matched controls (see Figs. 6.2B and 6.4). Since Ees also has been viewed as a measure of systolic contractile function, one might conclude that this reflects enhanced contractility. However, this seems unlikely, as other parameters less dependent on chamber geometry do not increase with aging.

In addition to being older and often hypertensive, the majority of HFpEF patients are female.[43–45] Women develop concentric LVH in the setting of pressure overload more often compared with men.[2,53,54] In addition, in a large population-based study of largely asymptomatic individuals, age-dependent increases in ventricular systolic and arterial stiffness were found to be more marked in women compared with men (see Fig. 6.3). This may underlie part of the increased prevalence of HFpEF in older women.[2] The precise cause for this remains unknown but may in part relate to hormonal factors and differences in ventricular and aortic size and length. In contrast to vascular and ventricular systolic stiffening, mean peripheral vascular resistance does not show this age-dependent rise and is greater in men. Thus women are more likely to display accentuated increases in pulsatile loading with age, associated with greater coupled ventricular-arterial stiffening.[55]

Pathophysiology of Ventricular-Arterial Stiffening

There are several important physiologic consequences of combined ventricular and arterial stiffening, as summarized in Table 6.1, and

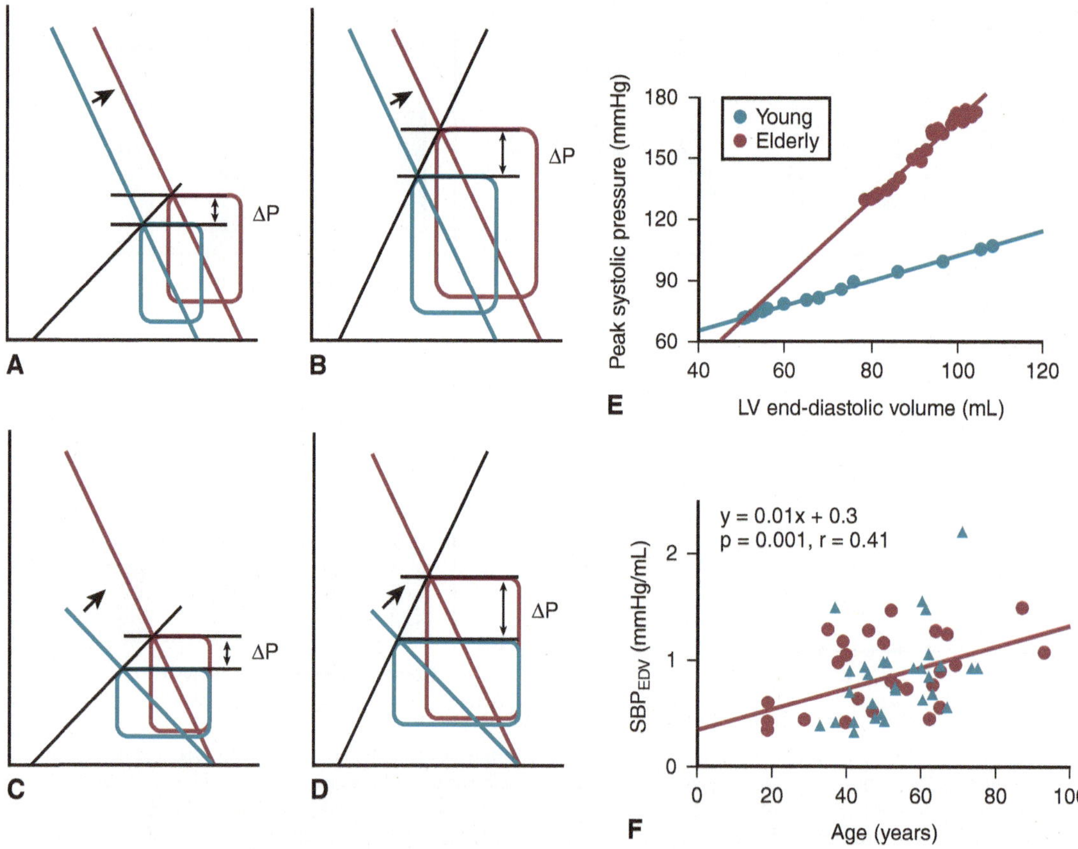

Fig. 6.5 Effects of varying preload and afterload on systolic blood pressure (SBP) in the presence or absence of increased ventricular systolic stiffening. (A) In a normal patient, an increase in end-diastolic volume (EDV) (arterial elastance [Ea] constant) leads to a corresponding increase in SBP (ΔP). (B) In a typical patient with heart failure with preserved ejection fraction with increased end-systolic elastance (Ees), the same increase in preload causes a much greater increase in SBP. Similarly, while an increase in Ea causes an increase in SBP (C), this increase is amplified in the setting of elevated Ees (D), causing a much greater increase in SBP. With normal aging, the dependence of SBP on preload becomes increased, as shown by a typical younger and older patient (E). The slope of the SBP-preload relation plotted in (E) increases significantly with aging (F), related to increases in ventricular and arterial stiffness. *LV,* Left ventricular. (Modified from Chen C-H, Nakayama M, Nevo E, Fetics BJ, et al: Coupled systolic-ventricular and vascular stiffening with age: implications for pressure regulation and cardiac reserve in the elderly. *J Am Coll Cardiol.* 1998;32:1221–1227.)

while each of the two components confers morbidity, the combination of both leads to synergistic effects. One major repercussion is increased blood pressure lability and sensitivity to volume and vascular loading.[1,21] In a normal heart-artery system, a rise in Ved results in a given rise in Pes (see Fig. 6.5A). However, in a typical HFpEF patient, even if the coupling ratio is normal, the same increase in Ved will lead to an accentuated increase in systolic pressure (see Fig. 6.5B). The pressure-volume area or stroke work to achieve this given SV therefore also is higher in the HFpEF patient. Conversely, a given decrease in Ved will also lead to exaggerated drops in systolic pressure in this stiffly coupled system. Similarly, an isolated increase in afterload (Ea) in a HFpEF patient will lead to a much more exaggerated increase in blood pressure because of the higher baseline Ees (see Fig. 6.5C and D). Increased ventricular-arterial stiffening explains why systolic blood pressure is much more preload-dependent in older versus younger patients (see Fig. 6.5E and F).

In addition to increased preload and afterload sensitivity, systolic reserve also becomes limited with increased stiffening. A high basal Ees means that there is less effective change in systolic performance for a given percent rise in Ees during stress demands. Increases in Ees reflect contractility reserve, but the effect of a change in Ees on net cardiac output is nonlinear, being much greater when the starting value is low than when it rises (see Fig. 6.6). If you link a heart with a high Ees to a stiff arterial system, the net effect of systolic pressure is exacerbated,[21] and thus ejection is further compromised. Since exercise duration is determined predominantly by cardiac output reserve,[56] combined systolic ventricular and vascular stiffening can be an important contributor to exertional incapacity.

A third consequence of combined arterial-ventricular systolic stiffening is that the cardiac work required to deliver a given cardiac output increases. As shown in Fig. 6.6B, using a previously validated model, one can estimate the required rise in cardiac work to achieve a given change in SV (heart rate constant) as a function of ventricular (Ees) and arterial (Ea) properties.[1] This is depicted as a three-dimensional surface, with the lowest cost to the heart when both ventricular and arterial net elastances are low and increasing cost as these rise. Mean values for both parameters are depicted for four patient groups, including subjects with HFpEF, who have double or more the energetic cost to the heart compared with younger controls, and age-matched hypertensive subjects without LVH. Patients with chronic LVH and hypertension but without heart failure symptoms had elevation of both[33] and an increased energy cost to the heart.

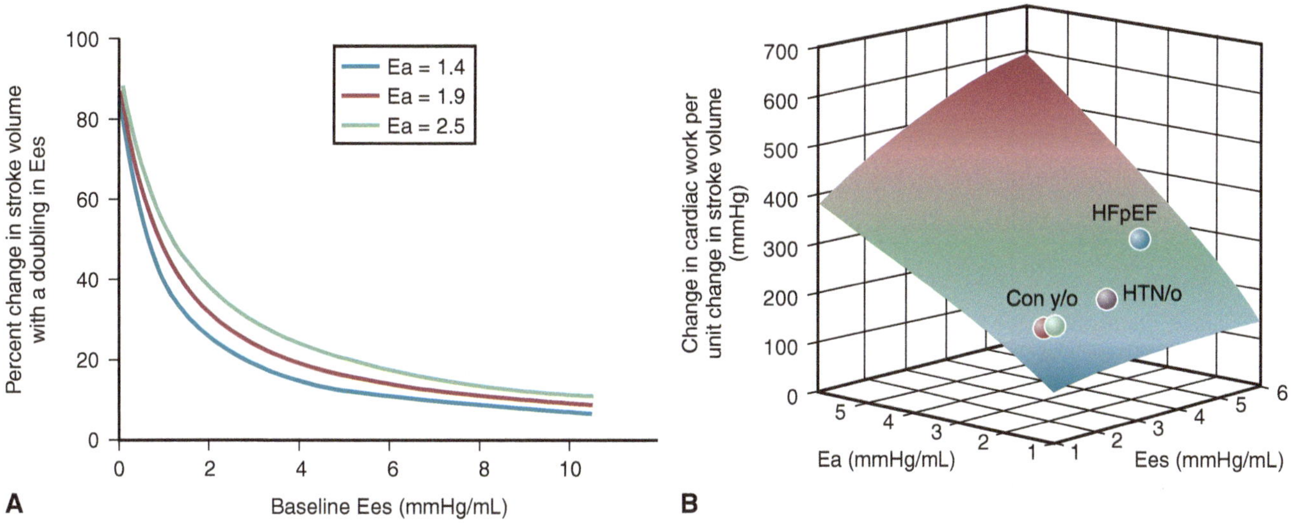

Fig. 6.6 The effects of basal end systolic elastance (Ees) on cardiovascular reserve function. (A) The percent increase in stroke volume for a 100% increase in Ees (i.e., contractility increase) is quite low when the baseline Ees is high. This hyperbolic relationship shifts in parallel with changes in arterial load (arterial elastance, Ea), but this shift is modest compared to the effect of the baseline Ees value. (B) The energetic cost for a given increase in cardiac stroke volume is greatly increased in the setting of increased ventricular-arterial stiffness, as is seen in HFpEF. This increased myocardial oxygen demand may promote ischemia in addition to reducing reserve capacity. HTN/o refers to older-aged hypertensives, and Con y/o refers to young and old nonhypertensive, healthy controls, respectively. For this prediction model, oxygen consumption is estimated based on the total pressure-volume area [PVA = stroke work + potential area = SV × ESP + 0.5 × (ESV − V0) × ESP], and this equation is resolved in terms of Ees, Ea by using two additional primary equations, one for the end-systolic elastance: ESP = Ees (ESV − V0), and the other for effective arterial elastance: Ea = ESP/SV. *Ees,* End-systolic elastance; *ESP,* end-systolic pressure; *ESV,* end-systolic volume; *SV,* stroke volume; *V0,* volume axis intercept of the end-systolic pressure-volume relationship. More complete details of the mathematics can be found in Suga H. Ventricular energetics. *Physiol Rev.* 1990;70:247–277. (Modified from Kawaguchi M, Hay I, Fetics B, Kass DA. Combined ventricular systolic and arterial stiffening in patients with heart failure and preserved ejection fraction: implications for systolic and diastolic reserve limitations. *Circulation.* 2003;107:714–720.)

TABLE 6.1 Pathophysiology of Ventricular-Arterial Stiffening

Underlying Abnormality	Hemodynamic Consequences	Clinical Relevance
Increased ventricular systolic stiffness	1. Amplified change in blood pressure for a given change in preload or afterload	1. Hypotension and oliguria with slight overdiuresis or the addition of a new vasodilator agent
	2. Lower contractile reserve	2. Modest volume infusion leads to hypertension and/or acute pulmonary edema
	3. Lower stroke volume reserve	3. Impaired exercise tolerance and functional disability
	4. Greater energetic cost to eject a given stroke volume	4. Increased myocardial oxygen demand and ischemia
Increased arterial stiffness	1. Amplified change in blood pressure for a given change in preload or contractility	1. Hypotension and oliguria with slight overdiuresis or the addition of a new vasodilator agent
	2. Greater dependence on systolic pressure for coronary flow	2. Modest volume infusion leads to hypertension and/or acute pulmonary edema
	3. Increase wave reflections and late systolic load	3. Greater degree of ischemia and larger infarct size for given decrease in systolic blood pressure
	4. Abnormal endothelial mechanotransduction	4. Prolonged systole, abbreviated diastole, impaired relaxation
		5. Endothelial dysfunction, further limiting vasodilation in response to stress

The heart normally depends on diastolic arterial pressure as the driving force for coronary artery perfusion, with more than 70% of coronary flow provided during diastole. However, when the heart ejects into a stiff vasculature, it becomes more dependent on flow entering the circulation during systole.[9,57] Animal studies have revealed that this change in pulse perfusion pattern has consequences, as it can render the heart more sensitive to declines in systolic performance. Consider a heart exposed to coronary artery occlusion to induce acute ischemia (Fig. 6.7). When the heart ejects into a compliant arterial system, the occlusion is well compensated for by moderate chamber dilation, and there is little decline in systolic pressure. However, when the same heart ejects into a stiff system by means of an in vivo aortic bypass tube,[9] the results are markedly different. In this case, the heart dilates much more with the same occlusion, and the magnitudes of

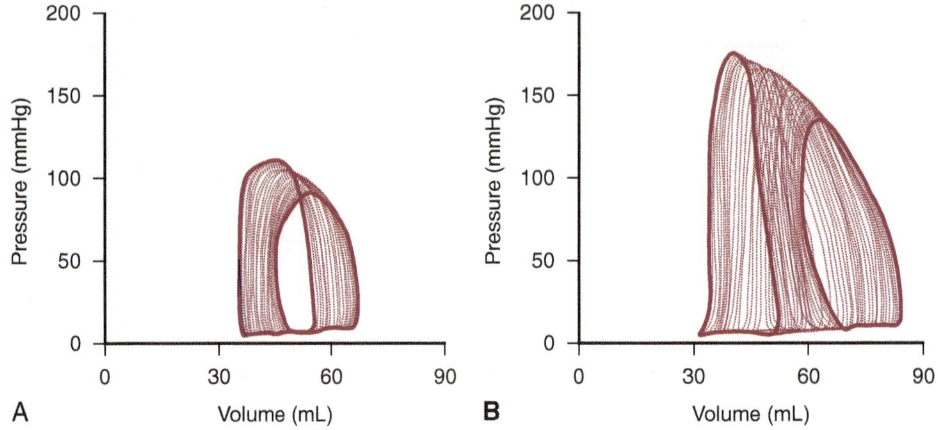

Fig. 6.7 The effects of acute ischemia in the setting of increased arterial stiffening. (A) If the heart ejects into a normally compliant system, acute occlusion of the left anterior descending induces a rightward shift in the pressure-volume loop, with an increase in end-diastolic and systolic volumes and a slight decrease in systolic pressure. (B) If the same experiment is performed with the heart ejecting into a stiff vasculature, the heart dilates more, end-systolic volume shifts more to the right, and there is greater diminution in the systolic blood pressure developed. (From Miho Kawaguchi, MD; Ilan Hay, MD; Barry Fetics, MSE; David A. Kass, MD. Combined Ventricular Systolic and Arterial Stiffening in Patients With Heart Failure and Preserved Ejection Fraction Implications for Systolic and Diastolic Reserve Limitations. DOI: 10.1161/01.CIR.0000048123.22359.A1)

both the ischemic bed size and the resulting decline in function are exacerbated.

Cardiac interaction with a stiff arterial system also amplifies late systolic pressure loading, and this can affect both the net amount of volume ejected and diastolic processes.[58] Elevation of afterload prolongs relaxation,[59–62] an effect that can be mitigated in the setting of β-adrenergic activation.[63] Progressive increases in late systolic load, induced by timed inflation of intraaortic balloons in animal models, have been shown to prolong LV relaxation.[59] The increase in loading required to elicit a prolongation was rather marked, at nearly 80% of maximum (i.e., isovolumic contraction). However, we have found that in patients with HFpEF, acute increases in afterload induced by the isometric handgrip can also slow isovolumic relaxation rate,[1] and this could contribute to elevated diastolic pressures and disease pathophysiology.

A sixth mechanism, whereby loss of arterial compliance and thus distensibility with vascular stiffening may contribute to disease pathophysiology, lies in endothelial mechanosignaling. The endothelium is a major physical force transducer that registers local changes in shear stress (flow) and vessel distension (stretch), and translates these signals to alterations in endothelial function and vascular tone. Pulsatile perfusion combines both stimuli, and studies from our laboratory have revealed that these two signals combined provide additive stimulation for nitric oxide synthase (NOS), a primary upstream kinase activator (Akt), and cytoprotective effects against oxidant stress.[11,12] The latter appear mediated primarily by the augmented rise in Akt activation. However, pulse perfusion in the relative absence of wall cyclic distension yields a different response. Here, Akt activation is blunted, and there is correspondingly less rise in NOS activation and substantial blunting of the protection to oxidant stress. This signaling appears specifically coupled to stretch stimulation (rather than shear), and although the exact cascade responsible remains to be elucidated, it has intriguing implications. One is that reduced arterial compliance can blunt the normal flow-mediated dilatory response that is a central component of vasodilator reserve under stress. While this direct link has yet to be proven in vivo in HFpEF, it has been suggested to contribute to vascular stiffening in continuous-flow left ventricular assist devices where there is loss of pulsatilily.[64,65] Therefore it may indeed contribute to vasodilator reserve limitations in the elderly, and in particular in individuals with HFpEF, who require such reserve as a compensation for the loss of other cardiovascular mechanisms.[66]

Relationship Between Ventricular-Arterial Stiffening and Exercise Reserve

Increases in ventricular and vascular stiffness affect cardiovascular reserve function with exercise stress. Warner et al. studied the effects of losartan on exercise performance in 20 asymptomatic hypertensive subjects with echo-Doppler diastolic dysfunction and a hypertensive response to exercise, suggesting increased ventricular-vascular stiffness.[67] While losartan had no effect on resting blood pressure, it decreased peak systolic pressure during exercise, increased the time for blood pressure to exceed 190 mmHg, and was associated with an approximately 10% increase in peak oxygen consumption. In another study from this group, 6 months of losartan compared with hydrochlorothiazide treatment found similar reductions in exercise-induced hypertension in this population, while only losartan improved exercise performance and quality of life measures, suggesting that direct ventricular and vascular effects, rather than blood pressure change per se, are critical in determining cardiovascular reserve function.[68] However, these results have not been reproduced with alternative antihypertensives,[69–71] with in fact a trend toward worse activity and exercise capacity.[70,71]

Hundley et al. studied the relationship between proximal aortic distensibility derived from MRI and exercise performance in 10 young, 10 older, and 10 HFpEF subjects.[72] They demonstrated that aortic distensibility is highest in the young and most compromised in HFpEF patients, even compared with healthy older subjects (although the HFpEF group was significantly older than the healthy older volunteers). The authors went on to show that changes in aortic distensibility and cross-sectional area strongly predict exercise performance (peak oxygen consumption) (Fig. 6.8), even after adjusting for age and gender in multivariate regression analysis. Aortic wall thickness was significantly greater in HFpEF subjects compared with both groups, supporting the notion that exaggerated vascular remodeling contributes to increased arterial stiffening in these patients, independent of or in addition to normal aging. Similarly, Tartière-Kesri et al. demonstrated that proximal aortic impedance worsened

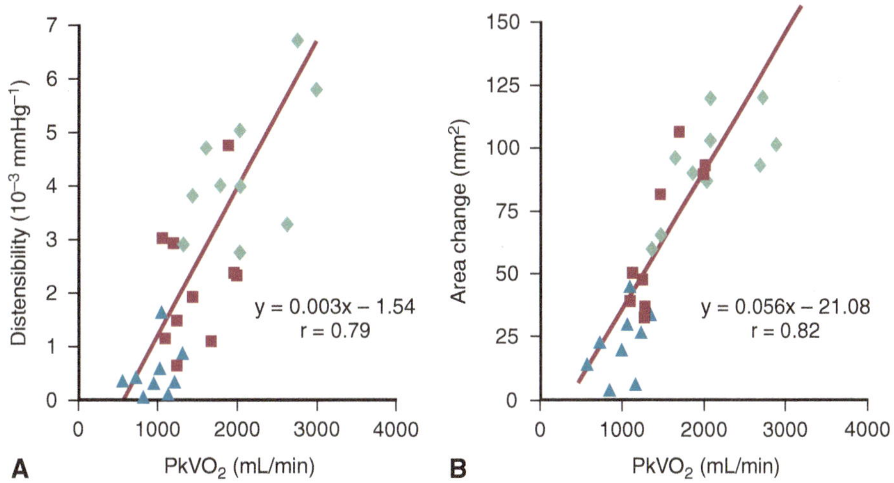

Fig. 6.8 Increased vascular stiffness impairs metabolic exercise performance in heart failure with preserved ejection fraction (HFpEF). Both (A) aortic distensibility and (B) change in cross-sectional area correlate strongly with peak oxygen consumption *($PkVO_2$)* during metabolic exercise testing in young *(green diamonds)*, older *(red squares)*, and HFpEF subjects *(blue triangles)*. (Modified from Hundley WG, Kitzman DW, Morgan TM, et al. Cardiac cycle-dependent changes in aortic area and distensibility are reduced in older patients with isolated diastolic heart failure and correlate with exercise intolerance. *J Am Coll Cardiol.* 2001;38:796–802.)

during exercise, which was associated with decreased 6-minute walk distance and a trend to reduced peak exercise capacity.[73]

We have previously shown that compared with hypertensive subjects with LVH, patients with HFpEF display a markedly blunted ability to augment cardiac output with upright exercise, despite a similar increase in LV Ved.[66] Their inability to increase cardiac output with stress correlated with chronotropic incompetence and an inability to properly vasodilate and reduce SVR during exercise. Baseline blood pressure and vascular stiffness were similarly elevated in both groups, and only by measuring changes with exercise was the deficit in vasodilator reserve function observed.

Abnormal Ventricular-Arterial Stiffening During Exercise in Heart Failure With Preserved Ejection Fraction

Many patients with HFpEF remain compensated at rest but show marked derangements in central hemodynamics during exercise, culminating in exertional pulmonary venous hypertension and dyspnea.[74,75] Therefore although some HFpEF patients may have abnormal ventricular-vascular coupling and pulsatile loading at rest,[72,76] many demonstrate arterial reserve limitations only during exercise[77] with impaired vasodilatory and contractile reserve, resulting in impaired reduction in exertional Ea/Ees.[78] HFpEF patients have been demonstrated to have worse exertional wave reflections,[77,79] central aortic stiffness,[73,77] pulse wave velocity,[73] and arterial compliance reserve[77] compared to controls. We recently demonstrated using gold standard invasive arterial pressure measurements that compared to hypertensive controls, HFpEF patients with exertional dyspnea have comparable central aortic blood pressure and arterial load at rest[77] (Fig. 6.9), similar to prior investigations.[33,78,80–83] However, in response to the increased flow and tachycardia during submaximal exercise, pulsatile load as assessed by TAC and Ea were worse in HFpEF despite matched heart rates and mean arterial pressure compared to hypertensive controls. With peak exercise, in addition to augmented pulsatile load, reflected waves became more prominent in HFpEF.[77] These abnormalities were associated with worse cardiac output and filling pressure during exercise (Figs. 6.10 and 6.11). Therefore measurement of the arterial load at rest may underestimate dynamic arterial stiffening and reserve limitations that contribute to exercise intolerance in HFpEF.

Such abnormal arterial loading contributes to the increase in pulmonary capillary wedge pressure and cardiac output reserve limitations in HFpEF through multiple mechanisms, including (1) worsening of early active diastolic relaxation from late pulsatile loading,[84] which during the tachycardia and shortened diastolic filling period of exercise can cause incomplete relaxation and dynamic increase in end-diastolic pressure,[85,86] (2) a direct afterload-mediated worsening of myocardial end-diastolic stiffness and pressure,[1,87] (3) impaired ventricular-vascular coupling with worse systolic myocardial performance during exercise,[77,78,83,88–90] and (4) abnormal ventricular-vascular-atrial coupling, resulting in decreased atrial emptying with worse atrial operating compliance and atrial dysfunction.[91–94] Therefore efforts to target vascular stiffness during exercise, such as with inorganic nitrite oral administration, are currently undergoing investigation and have been preliminarily shown to decrease invasively measured pulsatile load during exercise coupled with improved cardiac output and filling pressures.[77] The clinical implications of these changes are being investigated in multiple ongoing clinical trials.

CLINICAL RELEVANCE: THERAPEUTIC STRATEGIES TARGETING STIFFNESS

Ventricular-vascular stiffening can be treated with agents that acutely modulate ventricular systolic and diastolic performance, vascular smooth muscle tone, and endothelial function. Interventions such as verapamil that acutely reduce ventricular and vascular stiffness have been shown to improve exercise capacity in patients with HFpEF[95] and hypertrophic cardiomyopathy[96,97] and in elderly patients with hypertension and hypertrophy.[98] A large part of the mechanistic benefit has been believed to be related to improvements in ventricular peak filling rate (PFR), assessed by nuclear gated blood pool study.[95–97] However, a more recent trial in older hypertensive patients found that

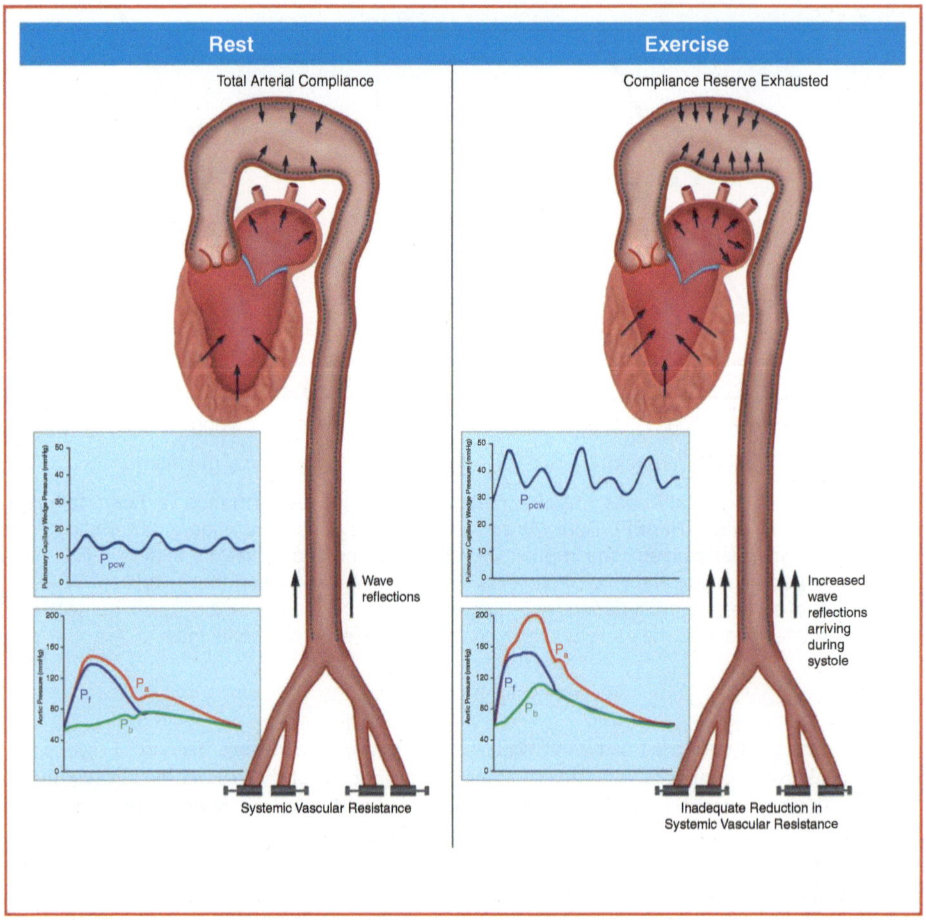

Fig. 6.9 With exercise, arterial reserve is exhausted with impaired arterial compliance, systemic vasodilation, and increased wave reflection. At rest *(left panel)*, the aortic pressure waveform, Pa *(red)* is shown as a composite of the forward wave, Pf *(blue)* and reflected wave, Pb *(green)*. Wave reflections, which develop at the points of impedance mismatch along the arterial tree, are reflected back to the aorta causing systolic pressure augmentation. Total arterial compliance, which reflects the ability of the arteries to store blood during systole without untoward elevation in pressure, is not significantly compromised, and PCWP is near normal. During exercise *(right panel)*, venous return and cardiac output increase. Stiffening of the aorta, along with a lack of small vessel vasodilation in the periphery (inadequate reduction in systemic vascular resistance), augments pressure wave reflections, Pb *(green)* and pressure augmentation of the central aorta during mid to late systole. Total arterial compliance reserve becomes saturated, such that increases in stroke volume cause greater elevation in aortic pulse pressure, further augmenting left ventricular load. These changes are then correlated with pathologic increases in PCWP that promote symptoms of dyspnea, and impairment in forward cardiac output reserve, limiting oxygen transfer to the body. Ppcw = pulmonary capillary wedge pressure. (Modified from Reddy YN, Andersen MJ, Obokata M, et al. Arterial stiffening with exercise in patients with heart failure and preserved ejection fraction. *J Am Coll Cardiol.* 2017;70:136–148.)

verapamil did not produce a consistent increase in PFR.[98] In contrast, it was associated with significant reductions in ventricular systolic stiffness (contractility/peak cardiac power index) and vascular stiffness (Ea, pulse wave velocity, augmentation index), and these changes were in turn associated with a 50% improvement in aerobic exercise performance. In subjects with lower resting PFR, verapamil tended to increase it, but if PFR was higher at rest, verapamil tended to diminish it. However, it is important to note that exercise performance improved similarly in both groups of patients. In a previous study of HFpEF subjects, we found that resting PFR was elevated compared with hypertensive/LVH controls because of volume overload, suggesting that verapamil may have less benefit in this population.[66] It is noteworthy that all of these trials were limited by relatively small sample sizes and did not involve chronic administration of study drug, and definitive clinical trials for efficacy are lacking. Nonpharmacologic therapies such as low-salt diets[99] or prolonged exercise training[100] are also promising and merit further investigation.

Pure vasodilators may have more variable effects. Two weeks and 6 months of treatment with the angiotensin receptor antagonist losartan improved exercise performance in subjects with a hypertensive response to exercise,[67,68] while acute vasodilation with sodium nitroprusside did not share such beneficial effects.[101] The latter is somewhat predictable, since a given reduction in Ea results in more exaggerated decreases in blood pressure with relatively less increase in stroke volume in the setting of high baseline Ees (see Fig. 6.5D). Propranolol, which decreases Ees, but increases Ea, also does not improve net exercise performance.[102] However, none of these small trials were performed in patients with HFpEF. In cohorts with clinical HFpEF, the results have been disappointing using either enalapril,[69] hydralazine/isosorbide dinitrate,[71] or organic nitrates,[70] with a trend

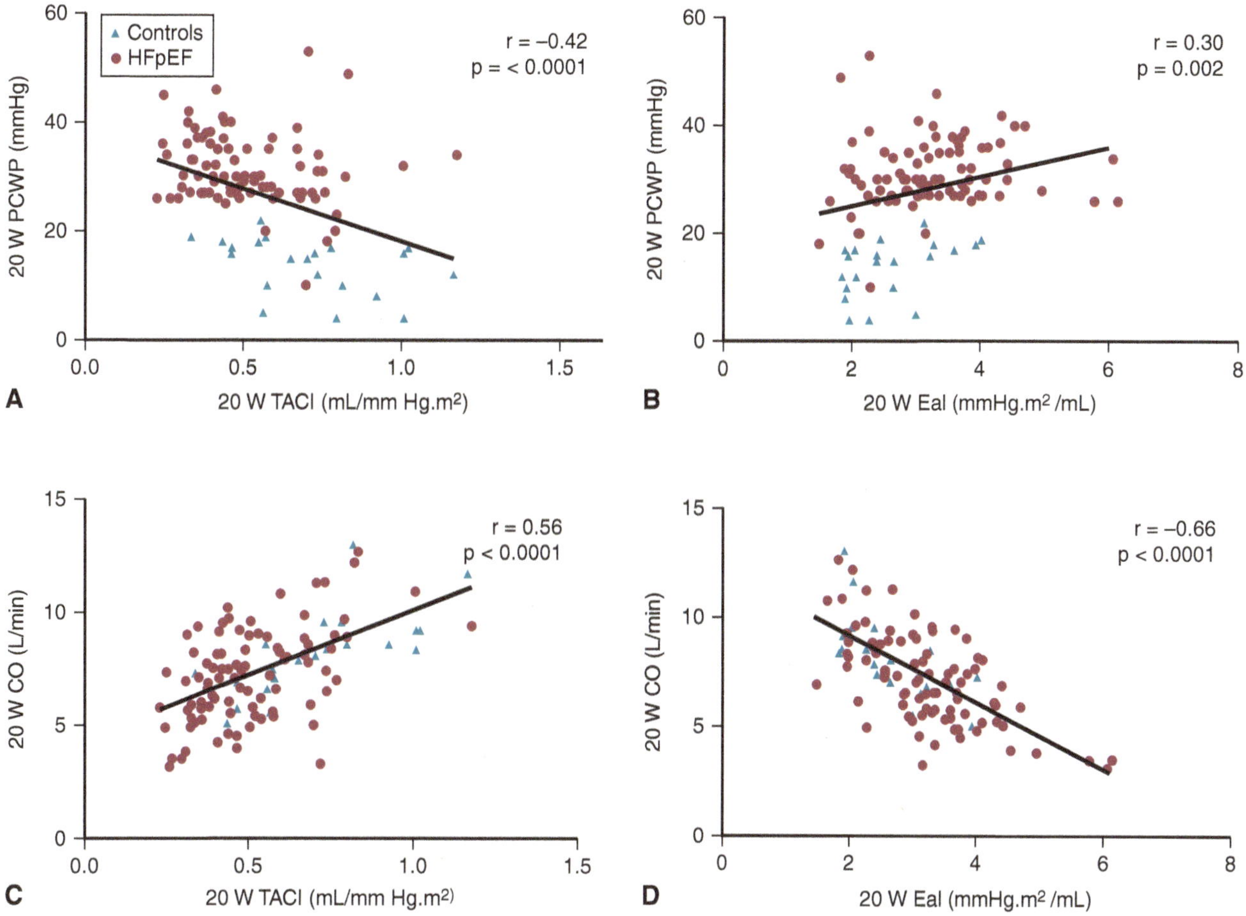

Fig. 6.10 Pulmonary capillary wedge pressure *(PCWP)* during exercise is associated with (A) impaired total arterial compliance index *(TACI)* and (B) effective arterial elastance index *(Eal)*. Impaired cardiac output *(CO)* is similarly associated with (C) decreased TACI and (D) increased Eal. (Modified from Reddy YN, Andersen MJ, Obokata M, et al. Arterial stiffening with exercise in patients with heart failure and preserved ejection fraction. *J Am Coll Cardiol.* 2017;70:136–148.)

toward worse activity and exercise capacity.[70,71] Given the extent of chronotropic incompetence in HFpEF patients,[66,103] drugs, such as calcium channel antagonists and beta blockers require further study to compare offsetting effects on ventricular and arterial stiffness and heart rate. Although heart rate reduction can result in a decrease in Ea and TAC as shown by the benefit of ivabradine in systolic heart failure,[104] results with ivabradine in HFpEF have been mixed.[105–107]

One reason for potential inefficacy of systemic vasodilators may relate to excessive vasodilation and blood pressure reduction at rest in subjects with high ventricular-vascular stiffness, resulting in intolerable side effects.[36] Inorganic nitrite has greater efficacy during hypoxia and acidosis of exercise while remaining minimally active at rest, raising hope that it may provide the best balance between efficacy during exercise to improve exercise capacity while minimizing hemodynamic embarrassment during rest.[108] Although initial hemodynamic studies have been promising,[77,109,110] definitive outcome trials are ongoing.

FUTURE DIRECTIONS

Many of the increases in ventricular-arterial stiffness in HFpEF are chronic in nature due to changes in the material properties of the cardiovascular system.[7] In the largest randomized trial of heart failure with near-normal EF (Candesartan in Heart Failure: Assessment of Reduction in Mortality and Morbidity [CHARM]-Preserved), there was a borderline-significant treatment effect driven by a reduction in hospitalizations for heart failure.[111] However, this trial enrolled subjects with heart failure and EF greater than 40%, therefore including HFpEF subjects who are not typical of the garden-variety with LVH and LV ejection fraction greater than 60%.[43–45] Other therapies targeting these chronic changes include aldosterone,[112,113] transforming growth factor-β,[114] and chymase antagonists,[115] but a large-scale randomized trial funded by the National Institutes of Health to test the efficacy of the aldosterone antagonist spironolactone in HFpEF was similarly negative.[116]

Drugs specifically targeting ventricular hypertrophy may also prove very useful. An emerging player in hypertrophy signaling, rho kinase,[117] is a key downstream effector of G_q-protein–coupled angiotensin-II signaling. Rho kinase increases vascular smooth muscle cell tone, and the rho kinase inhibitor fasudil is being evaluated as an antianginal drug. Fasudil also attenuates angiotensin-II–induced cardiac hypertrophy, thus therapies interfering with rho kinase may prove synergistically useful relative to its vasodilatory and antihypertrophic properties.[118] Intriguingly, hydroxymethylglutaryl coenzyme-A (HMG-CoA) reductase inhibitors (statins), which are known to inhibit rho kinase activation,[119] have also been shown to be associated with improved survival in a retrospective analysis of patients with HFpEF.[120]

As basic research continues to define more of the cellular mechanisms contributing to increases in ventricular and arterial stiffness, remodeling, and hypertrophy, we will increasingly be able to target HFpEF more specifically and efficaciously at its pathophysiologic

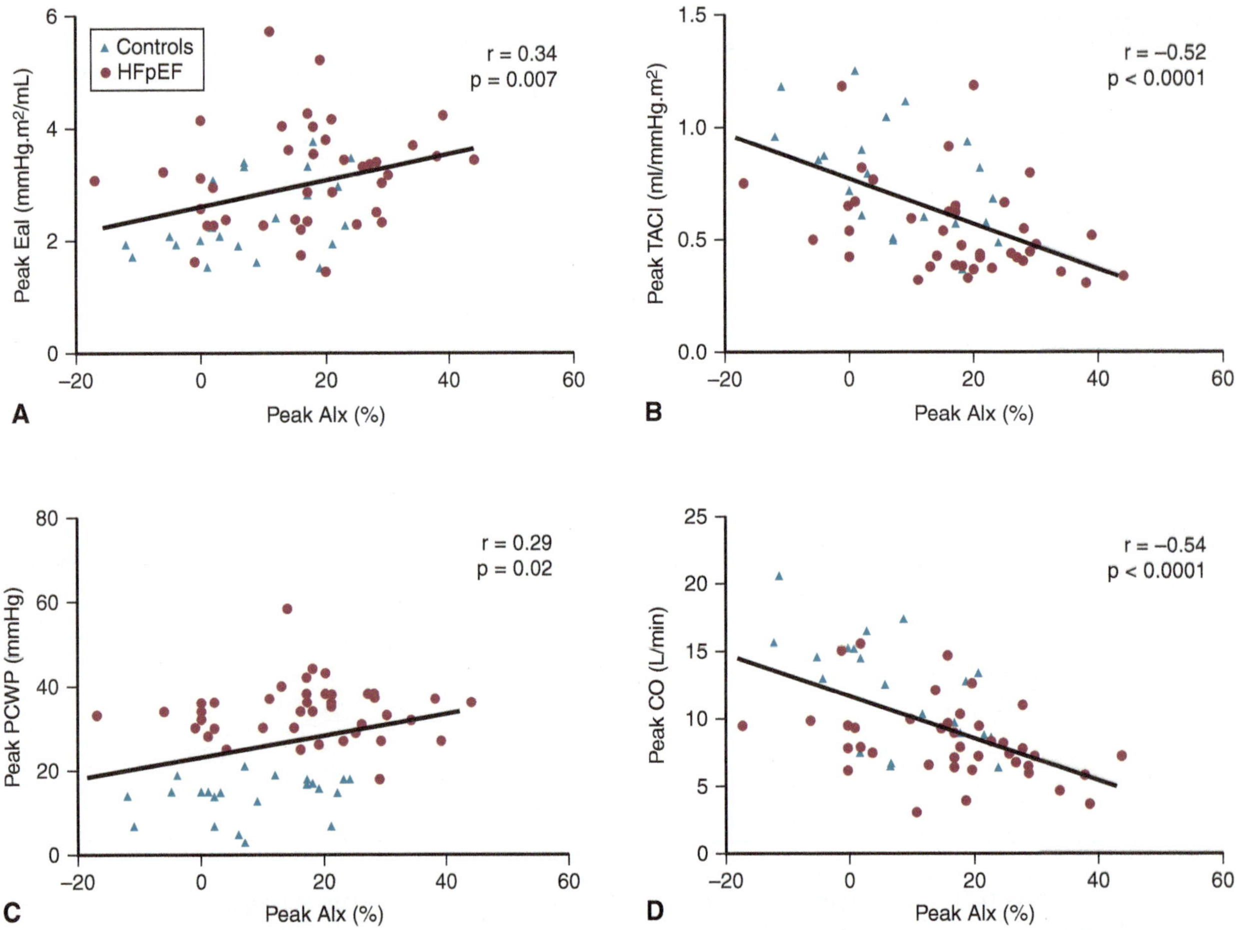

Fig. 6.11 Worsening augmentation index (Aix) is associated with (A) increased peak effective arterial elastance index *(EaI)*, (B) decreased peak total arterial compliance index *(TACI)*, (C) higher peak pulmonary capillary wedge pressure *(PCWP)*, and (D) lower peak cardiac output *(CO)*. (Modified from Reddy YN, Andersen MJ, Obokata M, et al. Arterial stiffening with exercise in patients with heart failure and preserved ejection fraction. *J Am Coll Cardiol*. 2017;70:136–148.)

foundations. Such basic findings will be more effectively translated to the bedside as additional clinical hemodynamic studies are performed to distill how each component of ventricular-arterial stiffening specifically modifies systolic and diastolic performance in patients with HFpEF. The role of traditional vasodilator therapy in HFpEF has so far been disappointing, and investigation of inorganic nitrite therapy has shown some promise but remains to be validated in controlled clinical trials.

KEY POINTS

- Ventricular afterload can be represented as aortic input impedance, derived from Fourier analysis of aortic pressure and flow waves, but this remains cumbersome for clinical use.
- In contrast, effective arterial elastance (Ea) can be more easily calculated as end-systolic pressure/stroke volume. This combines both mean and pulsatile loading, providing a lumped parameter that reflects the net impact of arterial vascular load on the heart.
- Relating Ea to end-systolic elastance of the ventricle (Ees) (as a load-independent measure of contractility), allows understanding of the ventricular-vascular coupling relationships of the heart.
- An Ea/Ees coupling ratio of 0.6 to 1.2 achieves near optimal work and efficiency.
- An increase in this ratio implies ventricular-vascular uncoupling that contributes to the pathogenesis of heart failure with preserved ejection fraction (HFpEF), particularly during exertion.
- Wave reflections are also important determinants of vascular load and contribute to the pathogenesis of exercise intolerance in HFpEF.
- Future therapies targeting reduction of vascular stiffness in HFpEF during exertion are undergoing ongoing investigation.

REVIEW QUESTIONS

1. Which of the following is an afterload-independent measure of ventricular function?
   a. Effective arterial elastance
   b. End-systolic elastance
   c. Total arterial compliance
   d. Augmentation index
   e. Systemic vascular resistance

2. Patients with HFpEF would be expected to demonstrate which of the following responses to sodium nitroprusside infusion?
   a. Large improvement in stroke volume with minimal drop in blood pressure
   b. Small improvement in stroke volume with large drop in blood pressure
   c. Minimal change in stroke volume with minimal change in blood pressure
3. Which of the following is true regarding vascular stiffness in HFpEF?
   a. Patients with HFpEF always have higher resting measures of afterload compared to controls without heart failure.
   b. Control of blood pressure and resting vascular afterload has not been demonstrated to improve symptoms in HFpEF.
   c. Vasodilator therapy causes smaller drops in blood pressure in HFpEF compared to heart failure with reserved ejection fraction (HFrEF).
   d. During exercise, pulsatile and reflected wave load is similar in HFpEF compared to controls.

REFERENCES

1. Kawaguchi M, Hay I, Fetics B, Kass DA. Combined ventricular systolic and arterial stiffening in patients with heart failure and preserved ejection fraction: implications for systolic and diastolic reserve limitations. *Circulation.* 2003;107(5):714–720.
2. Redfield MM, Jacobsen SJ, Borlaug BA, Rodeheffer RJ, Kass DA. Age- and gender-related ventricular-vascular stiffening: a community-based study. *Circulation.* 2005;112(15):2254–2262.
3. Avolio AP, Chen SG, Wang RP, Zhang CL, Li MF, O'Rourke MF. Effects of aging on changing arterial compliance and left ventricular load in a northern Chinese urban community. *Circulation.* 1983;68(1):50–58.
4. Avolio AP, Deng FQ, Li WQ, et al. Effects of aging on arterial distensibility in populations with high and low prevalence of hypertension: comparison between urban and rural communities in China. *Circulation.* 1985;71(2):202–210.
5. Fernandes-Silva MM, Shah AM, Claggett B, et al. Adiposity, body composition and ventricular-arterial stiffness in the elderly: the atherosclerosis risk in communities study. *Eur J Heart Fail.* 2018;20(8):1191–1201.
6. Kass DA. Age-related changes in venticular-arterial coupling: pathophysiologic implications. *Heart Fail Rev.* 2002;7(1):51–62.
7. Kass DA. Ventricular arterial stiffening: integrating the pathophysiology. *Hypertension.* 2005;46(1):185–193.
8. Kelly RP, Tunin R, Kass DA. Effect of reduced aortic compliance on cardiac efficiency and contractile function of in situ canine left ventricle. *Circ Res.* 1992;71(3):490–502.
9. Kass DA, Saeki A, Tunin RS, Recchia FA. Adverse influence of systemic vascular stiffening on cardiac dysfunction and adaptation to acute coronary occlusion. *Circulation.* 1996;93(8):1533–1541.
10. Najjar SS, Scuteri A, Lakatta EG. Arterial aging: is it an immutable cardiovascular risk factor? *Hypertension.* 2005;46(3):454–462.
11. Peng X, Haldar S, Deshpande S, Irani K, Kass DA. Wall stiffness suppresses Akt/eNOS and cytoprotection in pulse-perfused endothelium. *Hypertension.* 2003;41(2):378–381.
12. Li M, Chiou KR, Bugayenko A, Irani K, Kass DA. Reduced wall compliance suppresses Akt-dependent apoptosis protection stimulated by pulse perfusion. *Circ Res.* 2005;97(6):587–595.
13. Suga H, Sagawa K. Instantaneous pressure-volume relationships and their ratio in the excised, supported canine left ventricle. *Circ Res.* 1974;35(1):117–126.
14. Nichols WW, Pepine CJ, Geiser EA, Conti CR. Vascular load defined by the aortic input impedance spectrum. *Fed Proc.* 1980;39(2):196–201.
15. Murgo JP, Westerhof N, Giolma JP, Altobelli SA. Aortic input impedance in normal man: relationship to pressure wave forms. *Circulation.* 1980;62(1):105–116.
16. Kelly RP, Ting CT, Yang TM, Liu CP, Maughan WL, Chang MS, et al. Effective arterial elastance as index of arterial vascular load in humans. *Circulation.* 1992;86(2):513–521.
17. Sunagawa K, Maughan WL, Burkhoff D, Sagawa K. Left ventricular interaction with arterial load studied in isolated canine ventricle. *Am J Physiol.* 1983;245(5 Pt 1):H773–H780.
18. Kass DA, Kelly RP. Ventriculo-arterial coupling: concepts, assumptions, and applications. *Ann Biomed Eng.* 1992;20(1):41–62.
19. Asanoi H, Sasayama S, Kameyama T. Ventriculoarterial coupling in normal and failing heart in humans. *Circ Res.* 1989;65(2):483–493.
20. De Tombe PP, Jones S, Burkhoff D, Hunter WC, Kass DA. Ventricular stroke work and efficiency both remain nearly optimal despite altered vascular loading. *Am J Physiol.* 1983;264(6 Pt 2):H1817–H1824.
21. Chen CH, Nakayama M, Nevo E, Fetics BJ, Maughan WL, Kass DA. Coupled systolic-ventricular and vascular stiffening with age: implications for pressure regulation and cardiac reserve in the elderly. *J Am Coll Cardiol.* 1998;32(5):1221–1227.
22. Nichols WW, O'Rourke MF, Avolio AP, et al. Effects of age on ventricular-vascular coupling. *Am J Cardiol.* 1985;55(9):1179–1184.
23. Sunagawa K, Maughan WL, Sagawa K. Optimal arterial resistance for the maximal stroke work studied in isolated canine left ventricle. *Circ Res.* 1985;56(4):586–595.
24. Little WC, Cheng CP. Effect of exercise on left ventricular-arterial coupling assessed in the pressure-volume plane. *Am J Physiol.* 1983;264(5 Pt 2):H1629–H1633.
25. Feldman MD, Pak PH, Wu CC, et al. Acute cardiovascular effects of OPC-18790 in patients with congestive heart failure. Time- and dose-dependence analysis based on pressure-volume relations. *Circulation.* 1996;93(3):474–483.
26. Pauca AL, O'Rourke MF, Kon ND. Prospective evaluation of a method for estimating ascending aortic pressure from the radial artery pressure waveform. *Hypertension.* 2001;38(4):932–937.
27. Chen CH, Nevo E, Fetics B, et al. Estimation of central aortic pressure waveform by mathematical transformation of radial tonometry pressure. Validation of generalized transfer function. *Circulation.* 1997;95(7):1827–1836.
28. Chemla D, Hébert JL, Coirault C, et al. Total arterial compliance estimated by stroke volume-to-aortic pulse pressure ratio in humans. *Am J Physiol.* 1998;274(2):H500–H505.
29. Stergiopulos N, Meister JJ, Westerhof N. Evaluation of methods for estimation of total arterial compliance. *Am J Physiol.* 1995;268(4 Pt 2):H1540–H1548.
30. Stergiopulos N, Segers P, Westerhof N. Use of pulse pressure method for estimating total arterial compliance in vivo. *Am J Physiol.* 1999;276(2 Pt 2):H424–428.
31. Segers P, Stergiopulos N, Westerhof N. Relation of effective arterial elastance to arterial system properties. *Am J Physiol. Heart Circ Physiol.* 2002;282(3):H1041–H1046.
32. Hametner B, Wassertheurer S, Kropf J, et al. Wave reflection quantification based on pressure waveforms alone—methods, comparison, and clinical covariates. *Comput Meth Prog Bio.* 2013;109(3):250–259.
33. Melenovsky V, Borlaug BA, Rosen B, et al. Cardiovascular features of heart failure with preserved ejection fraction versus nonfailing hypertensive left ventricular hypertrophy in the urban Baltimore community: the role of atrial remodeling/dysfunction. *J Am Coll Cardiol.* 2007;49(2):198–207.
34. Liu CP, Ting CT, Lawrence W, Maughan WL, Chang MS, Kass DA. Diminished contractile response to increased heart rate in intact human left ventricular hypertrophy. Systolic versus diastolic determinants. *Circulation.* 1993;88(4 Pt 1):1893–1906.
35. Zile MR, Baicu CF, Gaasch WH. Diastolic heart failure—abnormalities in active relaxation and passive stiffness of the left ventricle. *N Eng J Med.* 2004;350(19):1953–1959.
36. Schwartzenberg S, Redfield MM, From AM, Sorajja P, Nishimura RA, Borlaug BA. Effects of vasodilation in heart failure with preserved or

reduced ejection fraction implications of distinct pathophysiologies on response to therapy. *J Am Coll Cardiol.* 2012;59(5):442–451.

37. Granzier HL, Labeit S. The giant protein titin: a major player in myocardial mechanics, signaling, and disease. *Circ Res.* 2004;94(3):284–295.
38. Kass DA, Bronzwaer JG, Paulus WJ. What mechanisms underlie diastolic dysfunction in heart failure? *Circ Res.* 2004;94(12):1533–1542.
39. Halperin HR, Chew PH, Weisfeldt ML, Sagawa K, Humphrey JD, Yin FC. Transverse stiffness: a method for estimation of myocardial wall stress. *Circ Res.* 1987;61(5):695–703.
40. Miyaji K, Sugiura S, Omata S, Kaneko Y, Ohtsuka T, Takamoto S. Myocardial tactile stiffness: a variable of regional myocardial function. *J Am Coll Cardiol.* 1998;31(5):1165–1173.
41. Zieman SJ, Melenovsky V, Kass DA. Mechanisms, pathophysiology, and therapy of arterial stiffness. *Arterioscl Throm Vas.* 2005;25(5):932–943.
42. Devereux RB, Roman MJ, Liu JE, et al. Congestive heart failure despite normal left ventricular systolic function in a population-based sample: the Strong Heart Study. *Am J Cardiol.* 2000;86(10):1090–1096.
43. Klapholz M, Maurer M, Lowe AM, et al. Hospitalization for heart failure in the presence of a normal left ventricular ejection fraction: results of the New York Heart Failure Registry. *J Am Coll Cardiol.* 2004;43(8):1432–1438.
44. Owan TE, Redfield MM. Epidemiology of diastolic heart failure. *Prog Cardiovasc Dis.* 2005;47(5):320–332.
45. Owan TE, Hodge DO, Herges RM, Jacobsen SJ, Roger VL, Redfield MM. Trends in prevalence and outcome of heart failure with preserved ejection fraction. *N Engl J Med.* 2006;355(3):251–259.
46. Borbély A, van der Velden J, Papp Z, et al. Cardiomyocyte stiffness in diastolic heart failure. *Circulation.* 2005;111(6):774–781.
47. van Heerebeek L, Borbély A, Niessen HW, et al. Myocardial structure and function differ in systolic and diastolic heart failure. *Circulation.* 2006;113(16):1966–1973.
48. Mohammed SF, Hussain S, Mirzoyev SA, Edwards WD, Maleszewski JJ, Redfield MM. Coronary microvascular rarefaction and myocardial fibrosis in heart failure with preserved ejection fraction. *Circulation.* 2015;131(6):550–559.
49. Zile MR, Baicu CF, Ikonomidis JS, et al. Myocardial stiffness in patients with heart failure and a preserved ejection fraction: contributions of collagen and titin. *Circulation.* 2015;131(14):1247–1259.
50. Dauterman K, Pak PH, Maughan WL, et al. Contribution of external forces to left ventricular diastolic pressure. Implications for the clinical use of the Starling law. *Ann Intern Med.* 1995;122(10):737–742.
51. Gandhi SK, Powers JC, Nomeir AM, et al. The pathogenesis of acute pulmonary edema associated with hypertension. *N Eng J Med.* 2001;344(1):17–22.
52. Kelly R, Hayward C, Avolio A, O'Rourke M. Noninvasive determination of age-related changes in the human arterial pulse. *Circulation.* 1989;80(6):1652–1659.
53. Carroll JD, Carroll EP, Feldman T, et al. Sex-associated differences in left ventricular function in aortic stenosis of the elderly. *Circulation.* 1992;86(4):1099–1107.
54. Villari B, Campbell SE, Schneider J, et al. Sex-dependent differences in left ventricular function and structure in chronic pressure overload. *Eur Heart J.* 1995;16(10):1410–1419.
55. Beale AL, Meyer P, Marwick TH, Lam CSP, Kaye DM. Sex differences in cardiovascular pathophysiology: why women are overrepresented in heart failure with preserved ejection fraction. *Circulation.* 2018;138(2):198–205.
56. Franciosa JA, Leddy CL, Wilen M, Schwartz DE. Relation between hemodynamic and ventilatory responses in determining exercise capacity in severe congestive heart failure. *Am J Cardiol.* 1984;53(1):127–134.
57. Saeki A, Recchia F, Kass DA. Systolic flow augmentation in hearts ejecting into a model of stiff aging vasculature. Influence on myocardial perfusion-demand balance. *Circ Res.* 1995;76(1):132–141.
58. Nichols WW, O'Rourke MF, Avolio AP, Yaginuma T, Pepine CJ, Conti CR. Ventricular/vascular interaction in patients with mild systemic hypertension and normal peripheral resistance. *Circulation.* 1986;74(3):455–462.
59. Leite-Moreira AF, Correia-Pinto J, Gillebert TC. Afterload induced changes in myocardial relaxation: a mechanism for diastolic dysfunction. *Cardiovasc Res.* 1999;43(2):344–353.
60. Leite-Moreira AF, Correia-Pinto J. Load as an acute determinant of end-diastolic pressure-volume relation. *Am J Physiol. Heart Circ Physiol.* 2001;280(1):H51–H59.
61. Gillebert TC, Leite-Moreira AF, De Hert SG. Load dependent diastolic dysfunction in heart failure. *Heart Fail Rev.* 2000;5(4):345–355.
62. Borlaug BA, Kass DA. Mechanisms of diastolic dysfunction in heart failure. *Trends Cardiovasc Med.* 2006;16(8):273–279.
63. Takimoto E, Soergel DG, Janssen PML, Stull LB, Kass DA, Murphy AM. Frequency- and afterload-dependent cardiac modulation in vivo by troponin I with constitutively active protein kinase A phosphorylation sites. *Circ Res.* 2004;94(4):496–504.
64. Ambardekar AV, Hunter KS, Babu AN, Tuder RM, Dodson RB, Lindenfeld J. Changes in aortic wall structure, composition, and stiffness with continuous-flow left ventricular assist devices: a pilot study. *Circ Heart Fail.* 2015;8(5):944–952.
65. Purohit SN, Cornwell WK III, Pal JD, Lindenfeld J, Ambardekar AV. Living without a pulse: the vascular implications of continuous-flow left ventricular assist devices. *Circ Heart Fail.* 2018;11(6):e004670.
66. Borlaug BA, Melenovsky V, Russell SD, et al. Impaired chronotropic and vasodilator reserves limit exercise capacity in patients with heart failure and a preserved ejection fraction. *Circulation.* 2006;114(20):2138–2147.
67. Warner JG Jr, Metzger DC, Kitzman DW, Wesley DJ, Little WC. Losartan improves exercise tolerance in patients with diastolic dysfunction and a hypertensive response to exercise. *J Am Coll Cardiol.* 1999;33(6):1567–1572.
68. Little WC, Zile MR, Klein A, Appleton CP, Kitzman DW, Wesley-Farrington DJ. Effect of losartan and hydrochlorothiazide on exercise tolerance in exertional hypertension and left ventricular diastolic dysfunction. *Am J Cardiol.* 2006;98(3):383–385.
69. Kitzman DW, Hundley WG, Brubaker PH, et al. A randomized double-blind trial of enalapril in older patients with heart failure and preserved ejection fraction: effects on exercise tolerance and arterial distensibility. *Circ Heart Fail.* 2010;3(4):477–485.
70. Redfield MM, Anstrom KJ, Levine JA, et al. Isosorbide mononitrate in heart failure with preserved ejection fraction. *N Eng J Med.* 2015;373(24):2314–2324.
71. Zamani P, Akers S, Soto-Calderon H, et al. Isosorbide dinitrate, with or without hydralazine, does not reduce wave reflections, left ventricular hypertrophy, or myocardial fibrosis in patients with heart failure with preserved ejection fraction. *J Am Heart Assoc.* 2017;6(2):e004262.
72. Hundley WG, Kitzman DW, Morgan TM, et al. Cardiac cycle-dependent changes in aortic area and distensibility are reduced in older patients with isolated diastolic heart failure and correlate with exercise intolerance. *J Am Coll Cardiol.* 2001;38(3):796–802.
73. Tartière-Kesri L, Tartière JM, Logeart D, Beauvais F, Cohen Solal A. Increased proximal arterial stiffness and cardiac response with moderate exercise in patients with heart failure and preserved ejection fraction. *J Am Coll Cardiol.* 2012;59(5):455–461.
74. Obokata M, Olson TP, Reddy YNV, Melenovsky V, Kane GC, Borlaug BA. Haemodynamics, dyspnoea, and pulmonary reserve in heart failure with preserved ejection fraction. *Eur Heart J.* 2018;39(30):2810–2821.
75. Reddy YNV, Carter RE, Obokata M, Redfield MM, Borlaug BA. A simple, evidence-based approach to help guide diagnosis of heart failure with preserved ejection fraction. *Circulation.* 2018;138:861–870.
76. Weber T, Wassertheurer S, O'Rourke MF, et al. Pulsatile hemodynamics in patients with exertional dyspnea: potentially of value in the diagnostic evaluation of suspected heart failure with preserved ejection fraction. *J Am Coll Cardiol.* 2013;61(18):1874–1883.
77. Reddy YNV, Andersen MJ, Obokata M, et al. Arterial stiffening with exercise in patients with heart failure and preserved ejection fraction. *J Am Coll Cardiol.* 2017;70(2):136–148.
78. Borlaug BA, Olson TP, Lam CS, et al. Global cardiovascular reserve dysfunction in heart failure with preserved ejection fraction. *J Am Coll Cardiol.* 2010;56(11):845–854.
79. Holland DJ, Sacre JW, Leano RL, Marwick TH, Sharman JE. Contribution of abnormal central blood pressure to left ventricular filling pressure during exercise in patients with heart failure and preserved ejection fraction. *J Hypertens.* 2011;29(7):1422–1430.
80. Lam CS, Roger VL, Rodeheffer RJ, et al. Cardiac structure and ventricular-vascular function in persons with heart failure and preserved

ejection fraction from Olmsted County, Minnesota. *Circulation.* 2007;115(15):1982–1990.
81. Borlaug BA, Lam CS, Roger VL, Rodeheffer RJ, Redfield MM. Contractility and ventricular systolic stiffening in hypertensive heart disease insights into the pathogenesis of heart failure with preserved ejection fraction. *J Am Coll Cardiol.* 2009;54(5):410–418.
82. Fujimoto N, Prasad A, Hastings JL, et al. Cardiovascular effects of 1 year of progressive endurance exercise training in patients with heart failure with preserved ejection fraction. *Am Heart J.* 2012;164(6):869–877.
83. Kosmala W, Rojek A, Przewlocka-Kosmala M, Mysiak A, Karolko B, Marwick TH. Contributions of nondiastolic factors to exercise intolerance in heart failure with preserved ejection fraction. *J Am Coll Cardiol.* 2016;67(6):659–670.
84. Borlaug BA, Melenovsky V, Redfield MM, et al. Impact of arterial load and loading sequence on left ventricular tissue velocities in humans. *J Am Coll Cardiol.* 2007;50(16):1570–1577.
85. Hay I, Rich J, Ferber P, Burkhoff D, Maurer MS. Role of impaired myocardial relaxation in the production of elevated left ventricular filling pressure. *Am J Physiol Heart Circ Physiol.* 2005;288(3):H1203–H1208.
86. Borlaug BA, Jaber WA, Ommen SR, Lam CS, Redfield MM, Nishimura RA. Diastolic relaxation and compliance reserve during dynamic exercise in heart failure with preserved ejection fraction. *Heart.* 2011;97(12):964–969.
87. Perez Del Villar C, Savvatis K, López B, et al. Impact of acute hypertension transients on diastolic function in patients with heart failure with preserved ejection fraction. *Cardiovasc Res.* 2017;113(8):906–914.
88. Phan TT, Abozguia K, Nallur Shivu G, et al. Heart failure with preserved ejection fraction is characterized by dynamic impairment of active relaxation and contraction of the left ventricle on exercise and associated with myocardial energy deficiency. *J Am Coll Cardiol.* 2009;54(5):402–409.
89. Wachter R, Schmidt-Schweda S, Westermann D, et al. Blunted frequency-dependent upregulation of cardiac output is related to impaired relaxation in diastolic heart failure. *Eur Heart J.* 2009;30(24):3027–3036.
90. Borlaug BA, Kane GC, Melenovsky V, Olson TP. Abnormal right ventricular-pulmonary artery coupling with exercise in heart failure with preserved ejection fraction. *Eur Heart J.* 2016;37(43):3293–3302.
91. Zakeri R, Moulay G, Chai Q, et al. Left atrial remodeling and atrioventricular coupling in a canine model of early heart failure with preserved ejection fraction. *Circ Heart Fail.* 2016;9(10):e003238.
92. Sugimoto T, Bandera F, Generati G, Alfonzetti E, Bussadori C, Guazzi M. Left atrial function dynamics during exercise in heart failure: pathophysiological implications on the right heart and exercise ventilation inefficiency. *JACC Cardiovasc Imag.* 2017;10(10 Pt B):1253–1264.
93. von Roeder M, Rommel KP, Kowallick JT, et al. Influence of left atrial function on exercise capacity and left ventricular function in patients with heart failure and preserved ejection fraction. *Circ Cardiovas Imag.* 2017;10(4):e005467.
94. Chirinos JA, Phan TS, Syed AA, et al. Late systolic myocardial loading is associated with left atrial dysfunction in hypertension. *Circ Cardiovasc Imag.* 2017;10(6):e006023.
95. Setaro JF, Zaret BL, Schulman DS, Black HR, Soufer R. Usefulness of verapamil for congestive heart failure associated with abnormal left ventricular diastolic filling and normal left ventricular systolic performance. *Am J Cardiol.* 1990;66(12):981–986.
96. Bonow RO. Effects of calcium-channel blocking agents on left ventricular diastolic function in hypertrophic cardiomyopathy and in coronary artery disease. *Am J Cardiol.* 1985;55(3):172B–178B.
97. Bonow RO, Rosing DR, Bacharach SL, et al. Effects of verapamil on left ventricular systolic function and diastolic filling in patients with hypertrophic cardiomyopathy. *Circulation.* 1981;64(4):787–796.
98. Chen CH, Nakayama M, Talbot M, et al. Verapamil acutely reduces ventricular-vascular stiffening and improves aerobic exercise performance in elderly individuals. *J Am Coll Cardiol.* 1999;33(6):1602–1609.
99. Hummel SL, Seymour EM, Brook RD, et al. Low-sodium DASH diet improves diastolic function and ventricular-arterial coupling in hypertensive heart failure with preserved ejection fraction. *Circ Heart Fail.* 2013;6(6):1165–1171.
100. Shibata S, Fujimoto N, Hastings JL, et al. The effect of lifelong exercise frequency on arterial stiffness. *J Physiol.* 2018;596(14):2783–2795.
101. Nussbacher A, Gerstenblith G, O'Connor FC, et al. Hemodynamic effects of unloading the old heart. *Am J Physiol.* 1999;277(5 Pt 2):H1863–H1871.
102. Fleg JL, Schulman S, O'Connor F, et al. Effects of acute beta-adrenergic receptor blockade on age-associated changes in cardiovascular performance during dynamic exercise. *Circulation.* 1994;90(5):2333–2341.
103. Brubaker PH, Joo KC, Stewart KP, Fray B, Moore B, Kitzman DW. Chronotropic incompetence and its contribution to exercise intolerance in older heart failure patients. *J Cardiopulm Rehabil.* 2006;26(2):86–89.
104. Reil JC, Tardif JC, Ford I, et al. Selective heart rate reduction with ivabradine unloads the left ventricle in heart failure patients. *J Am Coll Cardiol.* 2013;62(21):1977–1985.
105. Kosmala W, Holland DJ, Rojek A, et al. Effect of If-channel inhibition on hemodynamic status and exercise tolerance in heart failure with preserved ejection fraction: a randomized trial. *J Am Coll Cardiol.* 2013;62(15):1330–1338.
106. Pal N, Sivaswamy N, Mahmod M, et al. Effect of selective heart rate slowing in heart failure with preserved ejection fraction. *Circulation.* 2015;132(18):1719–1725.
107. Komajda M, Isnard R, Cohen-Solal A, et al. Effect of ivabradine in patients with heart failure with preserved ejection fraction: the EDIFY randomized placebo-controlled trial. *Eur J Heart Fail.* 2017;19(11):1495–1503.
108. Reddy YNV, Lewis GD, Shah SJ, et al. INDIE-HFpEF (inorganic nitrite delivery to improve exercise capacity in heart failure with preserved ejection fraction): rationale and design. *Circ Heart Fail.* 2017;10(5):e003862.
109. Borlaug BA, Koepp KE, Melenovsky V. Sodium nitrite improves exercise hemodynamics and ventricular performance in heart failure with preserved ejection fraction. *J Am Coll Cardiol.* 2015;66(15):1672–1682.
110. Borlaug BA, Melenovsky V, Koepp KE. Inhaled sodium nitrite improves rest and exercise hemodynamics in heart failure with preserved ejection fraction. *Circ Res.* 2016;119(7):880–886.
111. Yusuf S, Pfeffer MA, Swedberg K, et al. Effects of candesartan in patients with chronic heart failure and preserved left-ventricular ejection fraction: the CHARM-Preserved Trial. *Lancet.* 2003;362(9386):777–781.
112. Pitt B, Zannad F, Remme WJ, et al. The effect of spironolactone on morbidity and mortality in patients with severe heart failure. Randomized aldactone evaluation study investigators. *N Eng J Med.* 1999;341(10):709–717.
113. Pitt B, Reichek N, Willenbrock R, et al. Effects of eplerenone, enalapril, and eplerenone/enalapril in patients with essential hypertension and left ventricular hypertrophy: the 4E-left ventricular hypertrophy study. *Circulation.* 2003;108(15):1831–1838.
114. Kuwahara F, Kai H, Tokuda K, et al. Transforming growth factor-beta function blocking prevents myocardial fibrosis and diastolic dysfunction in pressure-overloaded rats. *Circulation.* 2002;106(1):130–135.
115. Matsumoto T, Wada A, Tsutamoto T, Ohnishi M, Isono T, Kinoshita M. Chymase inhibition prevents cardiac fibrosis and improves diastolic dysfunction in the progression of heart failure. *Circulation.* 2003;107(20):2555–2558.
116. Pitt B, Pfeffer MA, Assmann SF, et al. Spironolactone for heart failure with preserved ejection fraction. *N Engl J Med.* 2014;370(15):1383–1392.
117. Brown JH, Del Re DP, Sussman MA. The Rac and Rho hall of fame: a decade of hypertrophic signaling hits. *Circ Res.* 2006;98(6):730–742.
118. Higashi M, Shimokawa H, Hattori T, et al. Long-term inhibition of Rho-kinase suppresses angiotensin II-induced cardiovascular hypertrophy in rats in vivo: effect on endothelial NAD(P)H oxidase system. *Circ Res.* 2003;93(8):767–775.
119. Liao JK. Statin therapy for cardiac hypertrophy and heart failure. *J Invest Med.* 2004;52(4):248–253.
120. Fukuta H, Sane DC, Brucks S, Little WC. Statin therapy may be associated with lower mortality in patients with diastolic heart failure: a preliminary report. *Circulation.* 2005;112(3):357–363.

7

General Principles, Clinical Definition, Epidemiology, and Pathophysiology

Edlira Tam, Sandhya Murthy, and Ileana Piña

OUTLINE

Case Study

A 63-year-old woman has the following past medical history:

1. Coronary artery disease (drug-eluting stents placed in the right carotid artery [RCA] 3 years prior)
2. Hypertension diagnosed 20 years prior
3. Obesity with a body mass index (BMI) of 39 kg/m^2
4. Type 2 diabetes mellitus with an A1C of 8.2%

She presents with complaints of dyspnea on exertion, which has worsened over several months. She denies chest pain, palpitations, or syncope. She is sleeping on three pillows and complains of frequent nighttime waking—gasping for air. Additionally, she notes increased leg swelling over the last month. She reports difficulty breathing with minimal exertion and has not been able to take care of her activities of daily living during the last 2 weeks.

Current medications include aspirin 81 mg daily, metoprolol tartrate 25 mg twice daily (BID), lisinopril 20 mg daily, atorvastatin 40 mg daily, and metformin 1000 mg BID. She reports strict compliance with all of her medications.

On presentation vital signs are as follows: blood pressure 162/84 mmHg, heart rate 84 bpm, saturating 96% oxygen on 2-L nasal cannula. Her electrocardiogram showed normal sinus rhythm at 82 bpm with no significant ST-T wave changes. An echocardiogram was obtained, which showed mild left ventricular hypertrophy, LV end-diastolic diameter of 4.8 cm, and an ejection fraction of 60%. Mitral inflow pattern showed an E:A ratio of 1.4 that decreased to 0.7 with Valsalva maneuver. Septal E/e′ ratio was measured at 26 and peak tricuspid regurgitation (TR) velocity at 3.6 m/s. Lab work showed an elevated NT-proBNP at 2310 pg/mL, with normal CBC and chemistry.

INTRODUCTION

Heart failure with preserved ejection fraction (HFpEF) is emerging as a global epidemic. Since its recognition some 50 years ago, there have been countless controversies in relation to terminology, mechanism, and treatment. Owing partly to improved diagnostics and treatment of comorbid conditions, prevalence is increasing over time, without improved survival. This is in stark contrast to heart failure with reduced ejection fraction (HFrEF), whose survival is improving over time with the widespread application of effective medical and device therapies. HFpEF remains an extremely complex syndrome involving an intricate interplay of cellular, vascular, and inflammatory pathways. It is increasingly evident that HFpEF and HFrEF are distinguished phenotypic entities with widely divergent therapeutic targets.

HFpEF Versus HFrEF

Heart failure is a clinical spectrum with a similar presentation regardless of ejection fraction. To add historical perspective, the recognition of diastolic dysfunction as a distinct clinical entity is roughly 50 years old.[1] Over the years, it has become apparent that both HFpEF and HFrEF are equally prevalent and carry similar risks of morbidity and mortality.[2] Knowledge of the fundamental pathophysiologic differences and overlaps between the two syndromes has progressed greatly in the recent past. Nomenclature has changed dramatically over the last 20 years, thus highlighting the evolving understanding of the syndrome. Originally called diastolic heart failure, it was soon appreciated that the mechanism of impaired relaxation was much more than the single descriptive term. In fact, it encompasses a syndrome of maladaptive changes that are more accurately encapsulated with the broad descriptor of heart failure with preserved ejection fraction, hence HFpEF.

Nonetheless, practical questions remain with this current terminology. It is still unclear what the exact EF partition value should be when categorizing between the two syndromes. It is gathered from available data that there is an ejection fraction cutoff in which traditional neurohormonal blockade is much more effective in treatment. This observation underscores the vastly different mechanisms of HFrEF and HFpEF. The Treatment of

Preserved Cardiac Function Heart Failure with an Aldosterone Antagonist (TOPCAT) trial data perfectly summarize this point. This was a large trial of spironolactone in HFpEF that failed to show an improvement in the primary end point of cardiovascular death, HF hospitalization, or aborted cardiac arrest in people with HF and an EF greater than or equal to 45%.[3] However, Solomon et al. elegantly analyzed this data and found that the efficacy of spironolactone was apparent in reducing the primary end point in patients with a lower EF range, and essentially of no benefit in those with a higher EF range (>55%). This supports the proposition that neurohormonal blockade may still be effective in the so-called mildly depressed EF with the range of 45% to 55%. It is hypothesized that perhaps this group should be treated as HFrEF patients.[4] Thus the EF can be an important tool to distinguish separate biologic mechanisms of disease that would warrant separate therapies. It is important to note that although ejection fraction is used as one of the distinguishing features between HFrEF and HFpEF, there have been recent data demonstrating an impairment in systolic function in the HFpEF population. It is quite apparent that there is a complex interaction among several pathways, which fall under the umbrella of HFpEF. Recent insights in microvascular inflammation, pulmonary vascular dysfunction, cellular and structural changes, and the involvement of left atrial hypertension only add to the complexity of the syndrome; thus nomenclature will also likely evolve to reflect the growing sophistication in the pathophysiology of the disease.[5]

Prevalence and Economic Burden

Based on data from National Health and Nutrition Examination Survey (NHANES) 2009–2012, an estimated 5.7 Americans suffer from heart failure. In 2030, it is projected that more than 8 million people in America will carry the diagnosis of heart failure.[6] It has been very difficult to accurately estimate the true prevalence of HFpEF among this HF population. Historically this has been attributed to a lack of standardized criteria and an inclusion based on arbitrary ejection fraction cutoffs, as well as complex comorbid conditions in the elderly populations that may cloud diagnosis. Echocardiographic techniques add some level of precision, thereby circumventing the historic selection biases. There are several large community-based echocardiographic studies that have given us important insight into the true prevalence of the disease. Taken together, these provide our best estimate of the prevalence of HFpEF among all HF patients, which ranges from 40% to 71% (average 56%).[7–10] An important large population-based study from Olmsted County (Minnesota) demonstrates that there has been an observed temporal increase in the prevalence of HFpEF yet a relatively stable survival. Global experience mirrors this finding, along with the observation that trends of hypertension, obesity, diabetes, and atrial fibrillation are also increasing. This underscores the importance of HFpEF as a worldwide public health issue. HFrEF survival, conversely, has increased during the same time period. Based on data from the American Heart Association's Get With the Guidelines–Heart Failure (GWTG-HF) registry, the proportion of hospitalized HF patients classified as HFpEF is growing and may exceed that of HFrEF in the future (Fig. 7.1).[11]

Although there seems to be an increased prevalence of HF over time, there does not seem to be an increase in incidence. Several studies suggest that this rate is stable or even decreasing over time, especially in women. Many factors have been attributed to this observation, notably improved treatment strategies especially in the realm of acute coronary syndromes. There are a few large community-based studies that provide vital incidence data. The range of incidence in these groups was 1.5% to 4.7% over a period of 7 to 11 years of follow-up. Every year in the United States there are still 915,000 new cases of HF, leading to an incidence of 10 per 1000 after age 65 years. The lifetime risk at age 40 is one in five, while at age 80, despite limited life expectancy, this rate remains high at 20%.[6] As the population ages and survival improves even further, we can certainly expect a dramatic increase in cases of HF despite relatively stable incidence rates (Fig. 7.2).[12]

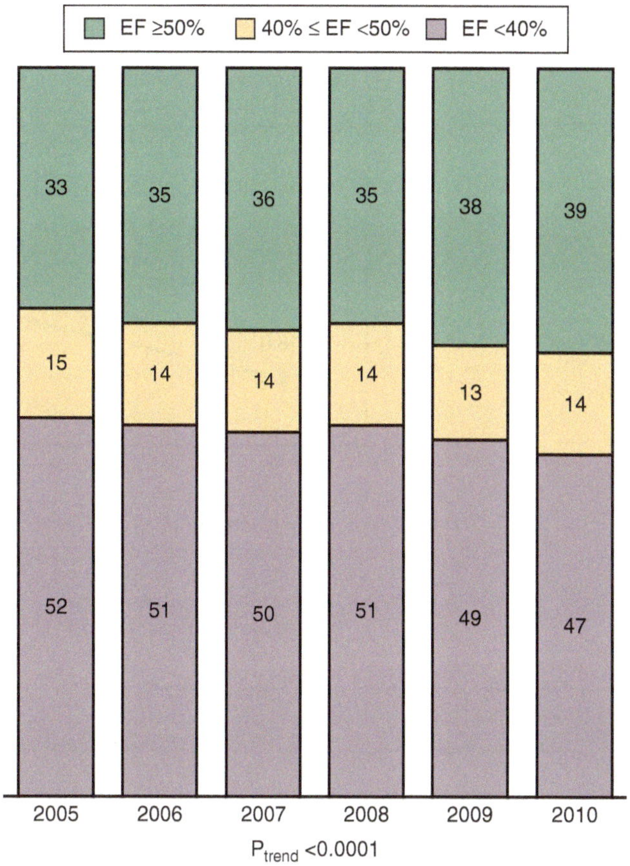

Fig. 7.1 Breakdown of patients by EF over time. The percentage of patients with preserved ejection fraction (EF) has gradually increased during the enrollment period of the Get With the Guidelines–Heart Failure (GWTG-HF) registry. (From Steinberg BA, Zhao X, Heidenreich PA, et al. Trends in patients hospitalized with heart failure and preserved left ventricular ejection fraction: prevalence therapies and outcomes. *Circulation.* 2012;126:65–75.)

Demographics vary considerably in HFpEF and HFrEF. In particular, HFpEF patients are more likely to be older, obese, female gender, and with worse functional capacity. In addition, these patients have a higher incidence of cardiovascular and noncardiovascular comorbidities (atrial fibrillation, chronic kidney disease, chronic pulmonary disease, anemia). Conversely, males with coronary artery disease are more prevalent in the HFrEF population.[2]

Mode of death in HFpEF is neither well understood nor well characterized. Several studies suggest mortality rates are just below that of systolic dysfunction. One of the most comprehensive meta-analyses on the topic suggests a few salient points: The majority of patients die of cardiovascular death; however, this definition is somewhat loose and arbitrary among the largest clinical trials. Next, sudden cardiac death makes up 30% to 40% of the cardiovascular death, which is somewhat surprising given that ventricular arrhythmia has not been shown to be a major issue in preserved systolic function. Finally, noncardiac death makes up roughly 30% to 40% of the cases. Admittedly, the data regarding specific cause of death are sparse and difficult to ascertain in many cases in this analysis; based on available information, however, noncardiac death includes cancer, infections, and respiratory causes. This is a direct reflection of the highly comorbid elderly population dying with HFpEF rather than of HFpEF (Fig. 7.3).[13]

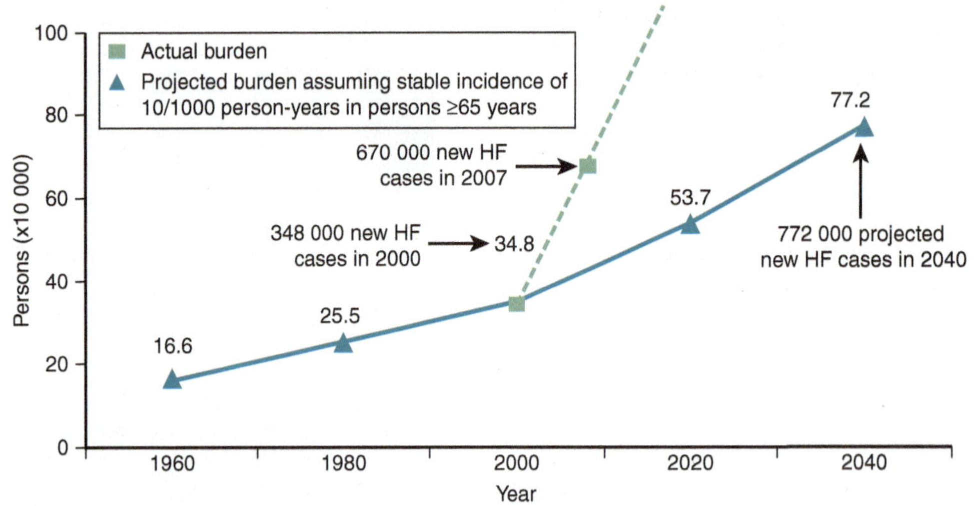

Fig. 7.2 Burden of heart failure *(HF)*. The actual annual incidence of heart failure reported in the United States *(squares and dotted line)* exceed the projected annual incidence *(triangle and solid line)* calculated based on a stable incidence of 10 per 1000 person-years in persons aged 65 years and older. (From Lam CSP, Donal E, Kraigher-Krainer E, Vasan RS. Epidemiology and clinical course of heart failure with preserved ejection fraction. *Eur J Heart Fail.* 2011;13 [1]:18–28.)

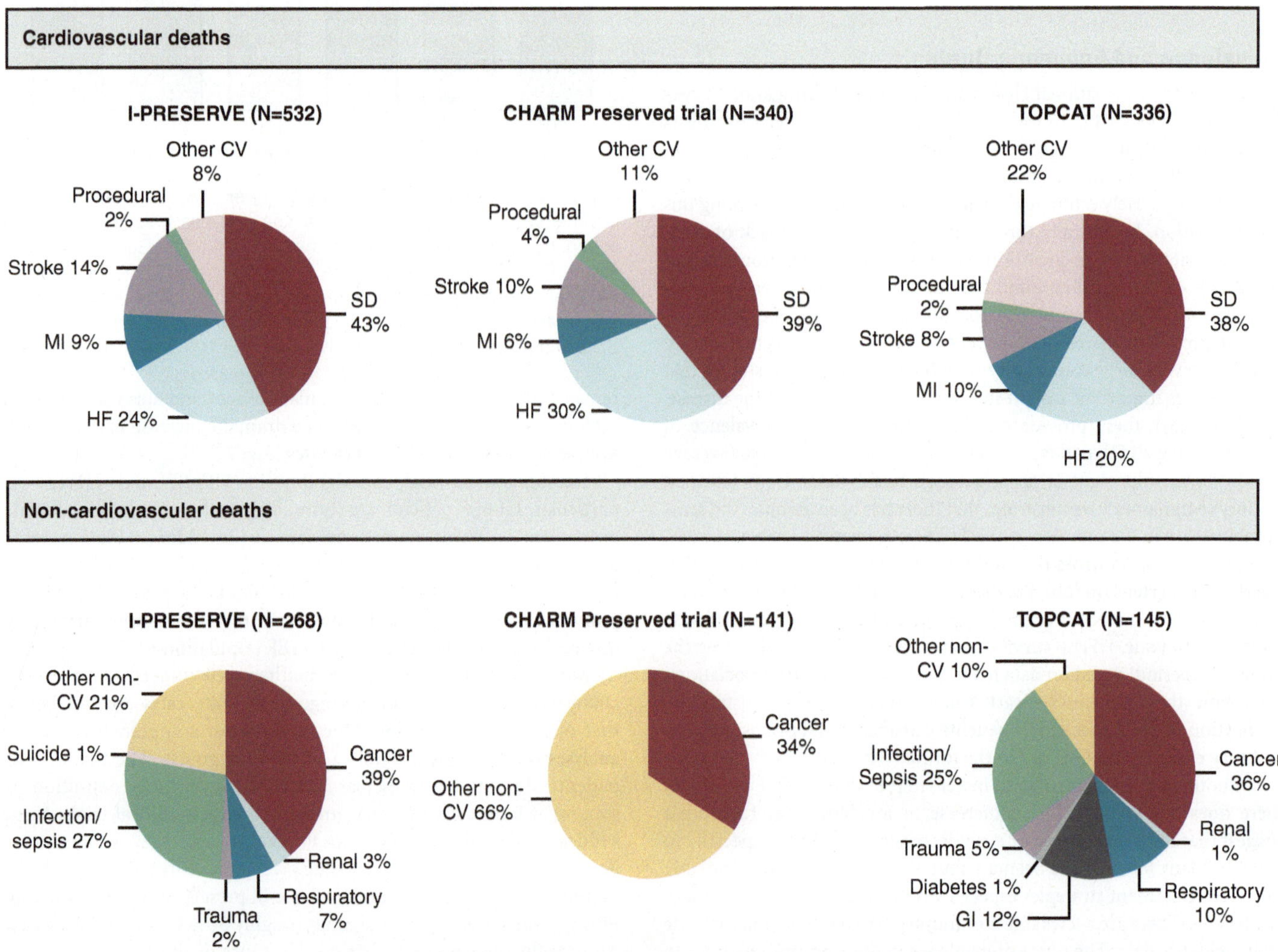

Fig. 7.3 Cause-specific mortality in random controlled trials of heart failure with preserved ejection fraction (HFpEF). Mode of death was stratified into cardiovascular *(CV) (top)* and noncardiovascular *(non-CV) (bottom)* deaths. The N reported refers to the total number of CV or non-CV deaths in each individual trial. *GI,* Gastrointestinal; *HF,* heart failure; *MI,* myocardial infarction; *SD,* sudden deaths. (From Vaduganathan M, Patel RB, Michel A, et al. Mode of death in heart failure with preserved ejection fraction. *J Am Coll Cardiol.* 2017;69 [5]:556–569.)

Several important limitations in the modern trial era of HFpEF are apparent. The definition of HFpEF itself varies considerably among trials, thus incorrect adjudication of patients may be an inherent flaw.[14] In addition, important exclusions of malignancy and advanced renal and pulmonary disease will bias the mode of death in this elderly HFpEF population.

Hospitalization rates can speak to the morbidity of the disease. Arora et al. used the National Readmissions database to approximate the rate of readmissions in patients with HFpEF. Around 20% were readmitted within the first 30 days, and 28% of those readmitted were within 2 weeks. Age and the presence of comorbidities such as renal disease and pulmonary disease were among the most important predictors of readmissions.[15]

The cause of readmission has been dissected in several large trials. The I-PRESERVE cohort has been explored in detail with regard to hospitalization. A total of 5863 hospitalizations occurred in 2278 patients during a mean follow-up of 49.5 months. The cause of the first hospitalization was found to be worsening HF in 54% of the patients. Readmissions were consistently found to confer a worse survival compared to patients who were never hospitalized (hazard ratio 8.53 in hospitalized vs. never hospitalized patients).[16]

Diastolic Dysfunction in HFpEF

The term *diastole* stems from Greek, and literally means "to send apart." On a cellular level, diastole begins as calcium is taken back into the sarcoplasmic reticulum (SR), thus myocyte relaxation becomes the dominant process within the cycle. A complete description of the cellular and physical determinants of diastolic function is provided in Chapters 1 through 6.

In normal hearts, relaxation and recoil properties are sufficient for maintaining a normal left atrial pressure. On the contrary, diastolic dysfunction is characterized by impaired relaxation and recoil—the end result being a rise in left atrial pressure to maintain adequate LV filling. The biochemical and physical mechanisms in diastolic dysfunction contribute to the overall syndrome but are certainly not specific to HFpEF. The same pathophysiology can be seen in a wide variety of disease states, including coronary artery disease, heart failure with and without systolic dysfunction, hypertrophic cardiomyopathy, hypertension, and in healthy elderly subjects as part of the aging of the heart. Initial studies from the 1980s noted the presence of diastolic dysfunction in subjects with seemingly normal LV systolic function. These included patients with constrictive pericarditis, restrictive and hypertrophic cardiomyopathy, and a large proportion with concentric ventricular hypertrophy. The most common etiologies for the development of concentric hypertrophy are hypertension and coronary artery disease. The process by which pressure overload–induced concentric hypertrophy leads to diastolic dysfunction at a cellular level is described in detail inChapter 20.

It has long been hypothesized that microvascular dysfunction plays an important role in the pathophysiology of HFpEF.[17] In 2018 the largest prospective trial to date was published and has provided some insight into the prevalence of coronary microvascular dysfunction (CMD) in HFpEF. Of the 202 HFpEF patients, 75% were found to have CMD, as defined by abnormal Doppler echo coronary flow reserve during adenosine challenge. This finding was correlated with increased HF biomarkers (NT-proBNP), increased systemic endothelial dysfunction, and increased cardiac dysfunction (echo strain patterns, etc.). Thus coronary microvascular dysfunction may also be an attractive target for therapeutic intervention.[18]

One of the major reasons the term *diastolic dysfunction* is no longer used to describe the HFpEF syndrome is that it was recognized that systolic dysfunction is also quite abnormal in these patients. Seminal works in 2002 reported that regional systolic function as measured by tissue Doppler imaging in HFpEF patients was impaired, despite the global ejection fraction being preserved.[19] Larger scale and more recent studies mirror this finding; contractile dysfunction in HFpEF patients was shown to correlate with increased mortality and may serve as a marker for disease severity.[20]

A hallmark in HFpEF is ventricular and vascular stiffening (see Chapter 6). This can also be seen in aging, hypertension, and diabetes and is a leading contributor of exercise intolerance in these disease states. Unique to HFpEF, at the onset of exercise, there is an impaired systemic vasodilatory response, which leads to an acutely high afterload. This is compounded by the ventricle's inability to augment contractility in the face of an increased pressure. These blunted responses further amplify exercise intolerance in this population (the so-called arterial elastance–end-systolic elastance coupling).[21]

There are several physiologic consequences of exercise that work in parallel to provide adequate output for the body's higher metabolic demands. This includes augmentation of cardiac output through higher venous return, increased heart rate, increased contractility, and peripheral vasodilation. Dysfunction in any part of this intricate system will compromise exercise tolerance. It is important to note that most HFpEF patients do not have rest symptoms, yet obvious exercise limitations. Normal hearts have the ability to quickly accommodate larger preload by increasing diastolic reserve rather quickly. This is blunted in HFpEF patients, and the consequence is a marked rise in filling pressure.[22]

Chronotropic reserve is abnormal in HFpEF patients in comparison to normal age-matched controls. Compounding this is the finding that autonomic dysfunction is also abnormal and may contribute further to the inability to augment heart rate. The precise mechanism of impaired autonomic dysfunction in HFpEF is not fully understood; however, some proposed theories evolve around blunted baroreflex control secondary to reduced arterial compliance, impaired central reflex regulation, and a decrease in end-organ responsiveness.[23] Heart rate recovery is also impaired in a significant number of patients with HFpEF, which suggests an imbalance of the parasympathetic system.[24] These changes seen are more pronounced than what is seen in a normally aging heart. All of these abnormalities combined point to the notion of HFpEF as a fundamental disease of global cardiovascular dysfunction, including impairments in contraction, relaxation, peripheral vascular tone, and reflex pathways.

COMORBID CONDITIONS

The comorbid conditions in HFpEF appear to be more severe and frequent than in HFrEF. This may simply be a reflection of the older population, but it is also possible that these comorbidities contribute to the underlying pathophysiology of the disease. Given a dearth of specific treatment options for HFpEF, oftentimes the clinician is left to focus on the prevalent comorbidities as a target for therapy. At one time HFpEF was viewed simply as a collection of separate comorbidities. Through recent meta-analyses, it is now understood to be a separate clinical entity and, when combined with comorbid conditions, carries a worse prognosis.

Age: The speed of LV relaxation declines with age even in the absence of cardiovascular disease. These mechanical changes can be correlated with those found on a cellular level: increased cardiomyocyte size, increased apoptosis, and increased collagen deposition. The resulting phenotype is increased ventricular and vascular stiffness. Thus diastolic function is expected to decline with age, as the prevalence of the HFpEF syndrome increases.[25] It is important to note, however, that the presence of diastolic dysfunction alone is not synonymous with the HFpEF syndrome.

Female gender: The reasons for the increased sex-based predominance of HFpEF are still unclear. Women certainly have higher vascular and LV wall stiffness compared to men, and this rises exponentially with age.[26] The reproductive hormones do have some bearing on LV function by the way of the response of the vasculature to abrupt changes in afterload.[27]

Hypertension: Hypertension is by far the most commonly associated comorbid condition in patients with HFpEF. One of the largest meta-analyses reported the prevalence of hypertension to be 51% among HFpEF patients.[28] Chronically high afterload induces important structural changes in the myocardium, namely left ventricular hypertrophy. These factors are tightly linked to the development of the HFpEF syndrome. Some of the pathologic findings in left ventricular hypertrophy include perivascular and myocardial fibrosis, medial thickening of the coronary arteries, and myocyte hypertrophy.[29] Left ventricular hypertrophy in isolation does not equate HFpEF. There is additional neurohormonal activation that, in conjunction with the maladaptive structural changes, needs to be present to trigger the acute decompensation episode. Nonetheless, blood pressure control has been the cornerstone of HFpEF treatment. In a study from 2007, it was shown that treating hypertension (regardless of agent used) improved diastolic function.[30] More recently, the Systolic Blood Pressure Intervention Trial (SPRINT) study randomized nondiabetic patients to intensive blood pressure control (defined as a systolic target < 120 mmHg) versus the standard goal of less than 140 mmHg, and found that there was a 38% lower relative risk of the development of heart failure.[31] Current hypertension guidelines advocate for aggressive early control of blood pressure (systolic goal < 120 mmHg), given the plethora of data strongly correlating hypertension to adverse cardiovascular events.[32] To date, no specific antihypertensive agents have been shown to reduce morbidity or mortality in patients with HFpEF; however, there may be some incremental benefit in certain classes. Diuretics certainly improve symptoms,[33] and mineralocorticoid receptor antagonists have been shown to reduce hospitalizations.[3]

Obesity: Obesity has been shown to be more prevalent in both types of heart failure, although more common in HFpEF. A recent review by Packer highlighted the two main abnormalities that occur in obese individuals with HFpEF: sodium retention and an inflammatory state caused by the presence of adiposity. The increased plasma volume caused by this retention is not able to be accommodated due to the inflammatory induced vascular and ventricular stiffness. Therefore the end result is a marked rise in intracardiac pressures and thus the HFpEF syndrome of obesity.[34] Interestingly the subgroup analysis from the TOPCAT trial of aldosterone antagonism in HFpEF seems to suggest that individuals with a higher BMI respond better to RAAS blockade than the rest of the cohort. This provocative observation begins to shift the idea of obesity-inflammation from a comorbid bystander to a veritable target for existing therapy. To further support this idea is that dramatic weight loss through bariatric surgery has been shown to improve LV diastolic dysfunction.[35]

Diabetes mellitus: Diabetes is associated with the development of HFrEF and HFpEF, even in the absence of significant coronary artery disease or hypertension. Hyperglycemia seems to be central to the pathogenesis of diabetic cardiomyopathy and triggers a series of maladaptive stimuli, including mitochondrial dysfunction, abnormal calcium homeostasis, renin-angiotensin-aldosterone system (RAAS) activation, oxidative stress, and deposition of advanced glycation end products (AGE). In particular, accumulation of AGE directly results in increased stiffness via collagen deposition.[36–39] Functionally this manifests as impaired endothelial vasodilation and subtle contractile dysfunction. Improved glycemic control in turn has been shown to improve echocardiographic parameters of diastolic function.[40]

Atrial fibrillation: Atrial fibrillation (AF) is a common impetus for decompensation in patients with HFpEF. Studies have shown that AF is independently associated with an increased risk for all-cause mortality during long-term follow-up in HFpEF.[41,42] Importantly, the relationship between HF and AF is bidirectional, with HF also increasing the risk for subsequent AF. This is at least partly because diastolic dysfunction directly leads to left atrial enlargement, which portends AF occurrence.

Coronary artery disease: Coronary artery disease and acute myocardial ischemia are precursors to the development of diastolic dysfunction. This is mediated through mechanisms involving impaired calcium ion sequestration in the sarcoplasmic reticulum, increased scarring, fibrosis, and compensatory hypertrophy of noninfarcted myocardium.[43,44] Ischemia in the presence of hypertensive heart disease leads to an exaggerated rise in filling pressures. Coronary revascularization in this population has been shown to improve overall LV diastolic function.[45] The transition from ischemic heart disease to the HFpEF syndrome is a poorly understood phenomenon that warrants further research.

Infiltrative heart disease/restrictive cardiomyopathy: Heart failure is the most common initial presentation of restrictive cardiomyopathy (RCM). It is approximated that 10% to 15% of the patients with HFpEF have some form of RCM or chronic pericardial disease. Histologically, RCM is characterized by abnormalities of the myocyte and intercellular matrix that lead to increased myocardial stiffness and impaired relaxation.[46] Primary RCM is often idiopathic, although familial inheritance has been described as mutations in desmin or troponin I formation.[47] Secondary etiologies of RCM include amyloidosis, radiation heart disease, eosinophilic endomyocardial disease, storage diseases (e.g., Anderson-Fabry, Pompe), sarcoidosis, scleroderma, chemotherapy induced, and carcinoid.[45,48] Early diagnosis and disease-directed therapy can positively impact prognosis, thus these entities are important to consider in the differential of new onset HFpEF.

FUTURE DIRECTIONS

HFpEF is indeed a global epidemic, with rising prevalence as the population ages. In stark contrast to HFrEF, there is a paucity of outcome-driven therapies approved for treatment of this syndrome. This highlights the divergent pathophysiologic mechanisms of the two conditions and thus a need for novel therapies. These therapies should target the well-understood maladaptive changes (i.e., impaired relaxation and increased stiffness). On a cellular level, this could mean manipulation of calcium homeostasis, disruption of extracellular matrix fibrosis, modulation of natriuretic peptides, and reversing hypertrophy. On a broader view, the syndrome as a whole contains several processes in disarray: abnormal vascular tone, endothelial dysfunction, and exercise intolerance. All distinct pathways are interwoven to manifest as the breathless patient who is acutely decompensated. Given the complexities of the concomitant abnormalities, there must be therapies that address all of these together. That is, simply focusing on treating fibrosis and not the neurohormonal milieu will surely lead to clinical futility. A major barrier in the effective clinical trial process has been a lack of uniform diagnostic criteria for HFpEF, thus prior participant recruitment following loose criteria may have led to erroneous results. It is imperative that future trials follow rigorous inclusion criteria to ensure the validity of data. Lastly, comorbid conditions remain a high-yield target for therapy. Aggressive blood pressure and diabetes control can prevent the adverse remodeling associated with the development of HFpEF. At this current state, the goals of therapy should be multipronged with a focus on the patient condition as a whole, including management of comorbidities and amelioration of the systemic and cellular disarray associated with HFpEF.

KEY POINTS

- Heart failure with preserved ejection fraction (HFpEF) is a distinct clinical entity with a unique and complex pathophysiology.
- Traditional neurohormonal blockade has had a neutral effect on survival in all available clinical trials.
- The prevalence of HFpEF has been steadily rising, while survival remains stable.
- The mechanism of death in HFpEF is not well understood, but it appears that more than half the deaths are attributed to cardiovascular causes.
- The treatment of comorbidities such as hypertension, coronary artery disease, and diabetes is a cornerstone in the management of HFpEF.
- HFpEF is a global epidemic with rising prevalence as the population ages, thus new mechanisms of treatment are desperately needed that focus on the complex interplay between the vascular bed, the periphery, and the neurohormonal disarray.

REVIEW QUESTIONS

1. Which of the following statements regarding HFpEF is correct?
   a. The majority of elderly patients with heart failure have reduced LVEF.
   b. Diabetes mellitus has the highest population attributable risk for the development of heart failure.
   c. Five-year mortality rate in patients with newly diagnosed heart failure is 20% to 30%.
   d. Natriuretic peptides are lower in women and renal failure patients.
   e. Morbidity and mortality are similar in patients with heart failure with reduced and preserved ejection fraction (HFrEF and HFpEF).
2. Which of the following hemodynamic sequelae is characteristic of HFpEF during exercise?
   a. Systemic hypotension
   b. Increase in mixed venous saturation
   c. Decrease in pulmonary capillary wedge pressure
   d. Exaggerated increase in pulmonary artery pressures
   e. Inappropriate increase in heart rate
3. Which management strategies have been shown to improve outcomes in HFpEF?
   a. Renin-angiotensin-aldosterone system (RAAS) blockade
   b. ICD therapy
   c. Treatment of risk factors (i.e., hypertension, coronary disease, diabetes)
   d. Avoidance of exercise
   e. All of these

REFERENCES

1. Dock E. How some hearts age. *JAMA.* 1996;195(6):442–444.
2. Bursi F, Weston SA, Redfield MM, et al. Systolic and diastolic heart failure in the community. *JAMA.* 2006;296:2209–2216.
3. Pitt B, Pfeffer MA, Assmann SF, et al. Spironolactone for heart failure with preserved ejection fraction. *N Engl J Med.* 2014;370:1383–1392.
4. Solomon SD, Claggett B, Lewis EF, et al. Influence of ejection fraction on outcomes and efficacy of spironolactone in patients with heart failure and reserved ejection fraction. *Eur Heart J.* 2016;37:455–462.
5. Lam CSP, Voors AA, de Boer RA, Solomon SD, van Veldhuisen DJ. Heart failure with preserved ejection fraction: from mechanisms to therapies. *Eur Heart J.* 2018;39:2780–2792.
6. Mozaffarian D, Benjamin EJ, Go AS, et al. Heart disease and stroke statistics—2016 update. *Circulation.* 2015;133:e38–e360.
7. Redfield MM, Jacobsen SJ, Burnett Jr JC, Mahoney DW, Bailey KR, Rodeheffer RJ. Burden of systolic and diastolic ventricular dysfunction in the community: appreciating the scope of the heart failure epidemic. *JAMA.* 2003;289(2):194–202.
8. Kitzman DW, Gardin JM, Gottdiener JS, et al. Importance of heart failure with preserved systolic function in patients > or = 65 years of age. CHS Research Group. Cardiovascular Health Study. *Am J Cardiol.* 2001;87(4):413–419.
9. Ceia F, Fonseca C, Mota T, et al. Prevalence of chronic heart failure in Southwestern Europe: the EPICA study. *Eur J Heart Fail.* 2002;4(4):531–539.
10. Mosterd A, Hoes AW, de Bruyne MC, et al. Prevalence of heart failure and left ventricular dysfunction in the general population. *Eur Heart J.* 1999;20(6):447–455.
11. Steinberg BA, Zhao X, Heidenreich PA, et al. Trends in patients hospitalized with heart failure and preserved left ventricular ejection fraction: prevalence therapies and outcomes. *Circulation.* 2012;126:65–75.
12. Lam CSP, Donal E, Kraigher-Krainer E, Vasan RS. Epidemiology and clinical course of heart failure with preserved ejection fraction. *Eur J Heart Fail.* 2011;13(1):18–28.
13. Vaduganathan M, Patel RB, Michel A, et al. Mode of death in heart failure with preserved ejection fraction. *J Am Coll Cardiol.* 2017;69(5):556–569.
14. Kelly JP, Mentz RJ, Mebazaa A, et al. Patient selection in heart failure with preserved ejection fraction clinical trials. *J Am Coll Cardiol.* 2015;65(16):1668–1682.
15. Arora S, Patel P, Lahewala S, et al. Etiologies, trends, and predictors of 30-day readmission in patients with heart failure. *Am J Cardiol.* 2017;119(5):760–769.
16. Carson PE, Anand IS, Win S, et al. The hospitalization burden and post-hospitalization mortality risk in heart failure with preserved ejection fraction. *JACC. Heart Fail.* 2015;3:429–441.
17. Franssen C, Chen S, Unger A, et al. Myocardial microvascular inflammatory endothelial activation in heart failure with preserved ejection fraction. *JACC Heart Fail.* 2016;4(4):312–324.
18. Shah SJ, Lam CSP, Svedlund S, Saraste A, Hage C, Tan R. Prevalence and correlates of coronary microvascular dysfunction in heart failure with preserved ejection fraction: PROMIS-HFpEF. *Eur Heart J.* 2018;39:3439–3450.
19. Yu CM, Lin H, Yang H, Kong SL, Zhang Q, Lee SW. Progression of systolic abnormalities in patients with "isolated" diastolic heart failure and diastolic dysfunction. *Circulation.* 2002;105:1195–1201.
20. Borlaug BA, Lam CS, Roger VL, Rodeheffer RJ, Redfield MM. Contractility and ventricular systolic stiffening in hypertensive heart disease

insights into the pathogenesis of heart failure with preserved ejection fraction. *J Am Coll Cardiol.* 2009;54(5):410–418.
21. Phan TT, Abozguia K, Nallur Shivu G, et al. Heart failure with preserved ejection fraction is characterized by dynamic impairment of active relaxation and contraction of the left ventricle on exercise and associated with myocardial energy deficiency. *J Am Coll Cardiol.* 2009;54:402–409.
22. Borlaug BA, Melenovsky V, Russell SD, et al. Impaired chronotropic and vasodilator reserves limit exercise capacity in patients with heart failure with a preserved ejection fraction. *Circulation.* 2006;114:2138–2147.
23. Mancia G, Seravalle G, Giannattasio C, et al. Reflex cardiovascular control in congestive heart failure. *Am J Cardiol.* 1992;69:17G.
24. Phan TT, Shivu GN, Abozguia K, et al. Impaired heart rate recovery and chronotropic incompetence in patients with heart failure with preserved ejection fraction. *Circ Heart Fail.* 2010;3(1):29–34.
25. Van Heerebeek L, Franssen CP, Hamdani N, Verheugt FW, Somsen GA, Paulus WJ. Molecular and cellular basis for diastolic dysfunction. *Curr Heart Fail Rep.* 2012;9:293.
26. Redfield MM, Jacobsen SJ, Borlaug BA, Rodeheffer RJ, Kass DA. Age- and gender-related ventricular–vascular stiffening a community-based study. *Circulation.* 2005;112(15):2254–2262.
27. Little WC, Lam C, Little WC. Sex and cardiovascular risk: are women advantaged or men disadvantaged?. *Circulation.* 2012;5:710.
28. Berry C, Doughty RN, Granger C, et al. The survival of patients with heart failure with preserved ejection fraction: a 5 year prospective population-based study. *Eur Heart J.* 2008;29(3):339–347.
29. Gradman AH, Alfayoumi F. From left ventricular hypertrophy to congestive heart failure: management of hypertensive heart disease. *Prog Cardiovasc Dis.* 2006;48(5):326–341. 2006.
30. Solomon SD, Janardhanan R, Verma A, et al. Effect of angiotensin receptor blockade and antihypertensive drugs on diastolic function in patients with hypretnsion and diastolic dysfunction: a randomized trial. *Lancet (London, England).* 2007;369(9579):2079–2087.
31. Wright JT, Williamson JD, Whelton PK, et al. A randomized trial of intensive versus standard blood-pressure control. *N Engl J Med.* 2015;373(22):2103–2116.
32. Whelton PK, Carey RM, Aronow WS, et al. Guideline for the prevention, detection, evaluation, and management of high blood pressure in adults: a report of the American College of Cardiology/American Heart Association Task Force on Clinical Practice Guidelines. *J Am Coll Cardiol.* 2018;71:e127–e248.
33. Faris R, Flather M, Purcell H, Henein M, Poole-Wilson P, Coats A. Current evidence supporting the role of diuretics in heart failure: a meta analysis of randomised controlled trials. *Int J Cardiol.* 2002;82:149–158.
34. Packer M, Kitzman DW. Obesity-related heart failure with a preserved ejection fraction. *JACC Heart Fail.* 2018;6:633–639.
35. Vest AR, Heneghan HM, Schauer PR, Young JB. Surgical management of obesity and the relationship to cardiovascular disease. *Circulation.* 2013;127:945.
36. Boudina S, Abel ED. Diabetic cardiomyopathy revisited. *Circulation.* 2007;115:3213–3223.
37. Aneja A, Tang WH, Bansilal S, Garcia MJ, Farkouh ME. Diabetic cardiomyopathy: insights into pathogenesis, diagnostic challenges, and therapeutic options. *Am J Med.* 2008;121:748–757.
38. Liu JE, Palmieri V, Roman MJ, et al. The impact of diabetes on left ventricular filling pattern in normotensive and hypertensive adults: the Strong Heart Study. *J Am Coll Cardiol.* 2001;37:1943–1949.
39. Schannwell CM, Schneppenheim M, Perings S, Plehn G, Strauer BE. Left ventricular diastolic dysfunction as an early manifestation of diabetic cardiomyopathy. *Cardiology.* 2002;98:33–39.
40. Van Heerebeek L, Hamdani N, Handoko ML, et al. Diastolic stiffness of the failing diabetic heart: importance of fibrosis, advanced glycation end products, and myocyte resting tension. *Circulation.* 2008;117:43.
41. Cheng M, Lu X, Huang J, Zhang J, Zhang S, Gu D. The prognostic significance of atrial fibrillation in heart failure with a preserved and reduced left ventricular function: insights from a meta-analysis. *Eur J Heart Fail.* 2014;16(12):1317–1322.
42. Jobs A, Schwind J, Katalinic A, et al. Prognostic significance of atrial fibrillation in acute decompensated heart failure with reduced versus preserved ejection fraction. *Clin Res Cardiol.* 2018;108:74–82.
43. Choudhury L, Gheorghiade M, Bonow RO. Coronary artery disease in patients with heart failure and preserved systolic function. *Am J Cardiol.* 2002;89:719–722.
44. Bonow RO, Udelson JE. Left ventricular diastolic dysfunction as a cause of congestive heart failure: mechanisms and management. *Ann Int Med.* 1992;117:502–510.
45. Gorcsan J, Diana P, Lee J, Katz WE, Hattler BG. Reversible diastolic dysfunction after successful coronary artery bypass surgery: assessment by transesophageal Doppler echocardiography. *Chest.* 1994;106:1364–1369.
46. Garcia MJ. Constrictive pericarditis versus restrictive cardiomyopathy? *J Am Coll Cardiol.* 2016;67:2061–2076.
47. Zhang J, Kumar A, Stalker HJ, et al. Clinical and molecular studies of a large family with desmin-associated restrictive cardiomyopathy. *Clin Genet.* 2001;59:248–256.
48. Kushwaha DD, Fallon JT, Fuster V. Restrictive cardiomyopathy. *N Engl J Med.* 1997;336:267–276.

8

Invasive Hemodynamic Assessment in Heart Failure With Preserved Ejection Fraction

Masaru Obokata and Barry A. Borlaug

OUTLINE

INTRODUCTION

Assessment of left ventricular (LV) systolic and diastolic function is fundamental to understanding cardiovascular pathophysiology and guiding accurate diagnosis, especially for patients with heart failure (HF). Invasive hemodynamic assessment was the standard for almost all patients in the 1950s to 1970s, but subsequently waned with development of echocardiography and a shift in the catheterization laboratory from diagnostics to intervention (percutaneous coronary intervention). Noninvasive imaging has emerged as a useful test for evaluating diastolic function (and by extension, heart failure with preserved ejection fraction [HFpEF]), mainly by analyzing mitral inflow Doppler and mitral annulus tissue Doppler.[1] Contemporary guidelines emphasize echocardiography and natriuretic peptide testing rather than invasive means for the diagnosis of HFpEF.[2] However, recent studies have shown how noninvasive hemodynamic assessments may have inadequate sensitivity to identify HFpEF.[3,4]

Invasive hemodynamic assessment is often required to quantify ventricular systolic and diastolic properties. Recently there has been a significant increase in usage of invasive procedures for hemodynamic assessment, particularly in the evaluation of exertional dyspnea.[3–7]

Cardiac catheterization provides direct measures of left-sided filling pressure, which is the fundamental hemodynamic abnormality in patients with HFpEF.[3–7] Right heart catheterization further allows for assessment of pulmonary artery (PA) and right atrial (RA) pressures, pulmonary artery resistance (PVR), and cardiac output (CO). These parameters are frequently impaired in HFpEF. The role of invasive hemodynamic assessment is now expanding from a research tool to the diagnostic area, and it enables a robust, sensitive, and specific way to diagnose or exclude HFpEF. This chapter summarizes basic invasive assessments of systolic and diastolic properties and how these relate to the pathophysiology of HFpEF, discusses concerns about current diagnostic approaches for patients with HFpEF, and extends to the reemerging role of invasive hemodynamics in the evaluation of HFpEF.

Case Study

A 56-year-old woman presented with unexplained dyspnea, which had become progressively more severe over the last few years. She had a history of chronic systemic hypertension. Jugular venous pressure was normal, S3 was not audible, and there was no peripheral edema. Electrocardiogram revealed normal sinus rhythm without abnormalities, and N-terminal pro-B-type natriuretic (NT-proBNP) was 26 pg/mL. Echocardiography demonstrated normal LVEF (54%) and there was no evidence of LV hypertrophy (LV mass index 78 g/m^2). Mitral inflow pattern showed an E/A ratio of 1.3. Average E/e′ ratio of 9.5, left atrial (LA) volume index of 21 ml/m^2, and tricuspid regurgitant velocity of 2.1 cm/sec were all within the normal range. Despite her severe exertional dyspnea, her diastolic function by echocardiography was inconsistent with diagnosis of HFpEF. Can we exclude HFpEF based on these noninvasive findings?

INVASIVE ASSESSMENT OF SYSTOLIC FUNCTION

Ejection fraction is the most common noninvasive measure of systolic function in standard clinical practice; however, EF is not a pure measure of LV contractile function. It is highly sensitive to loading conditions

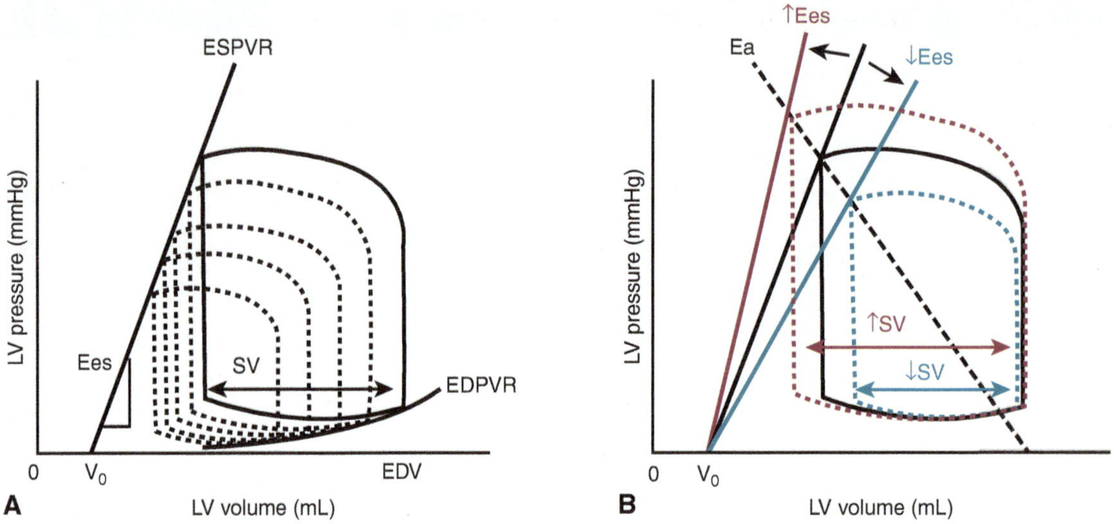

Fig. 8.1 (A) Pressure-volume (P-V) loops obtained at baseline *(solid loop)* and during transient reduction in preload *(dotted loops)* with a constant inotropic state and afterload. By connecting end-systolic P-V points, the linear end-systolic P-V relationship (ESPVR) is obtained. The slope of the ESPVR defines end-systolic elastance *(Ees)*, which reflects load-independent measure of contractility. In contrast, the end-diastolic P-V relationship *(EDPVR)*, which represents passive chamber stiffness, is nonlinear. (B) Isolated increase in contractility with inotropic agents (e.g., catecholamines) increases the ESPVR slope (increases Ees, *red slope*) while negative inotropic agents (e.g., acute β-blocker) decrease its slope (decrease Ees, *blue slope*), with little change in V_0. *Ea,* Effective arterial elastance; *EDV,* end-diastolic volume; *LV,* left ventricular; *SV,* stroke volume; *V_0,* LV volume at LV pressure is 0 mmHg.

(both preload and afterload) and is more accurately conceptualized as a measure of ventricular-arterial coupling.[5,8,9] Ejection fraction is also influenced by chamber remodeling because its denominator is end-diastolic volume. To quantify myocardial contractility, ideally a parameter should reflect inotropic state and should be independent of loading conditions, heart rate, and chamber geometry. LV contractility can be assessed invasively by use of a conductance catheter, which provides high fidelity pressure data and time-varying assessment of chamber volume to derive pressure-volume (P-V) loops.[5,8,9] Micromanometers and conductance catheter-based analyses enable assessment of the maximal rate of pressure increase (dP/dt_{max}), preload recruitable stroke work (PRSW), and LV end-systolic elastance (Ees). Ees is defined by the linear slope of the end-systolic pressure-volume relationship (ESPVR) that is obtained from multiple PV loops during acute preload reduction (Fig. 8.1A).[10,11] End-systolic elastance is commonly examined in the context of effective arterial elastance (Ea) to assess ventricular-arterial coupling and myocardial efficiency.[8] As shown in Fig. 8.1B, the ESPVR increases its slope (↑Ees) with positive inotropic interventions and decreases its slope (↓Ees) with negative inotropic interventions, with little change in V_0.

With this PV relationship, one can graphically understand how changes in contractility and loading influence ventricular mechanics. Although Ees is independent of preload and afterload, it is influenced by chamber remodeling. There is a well-known dissociation between Ees and contractility in patients with HFpEF, in which Ees can be elevated owing to increased passive chamber stiffness even when LV contractile function is depressed.[9] Basic tenets of ventricular-arterial coupling are discussed in Chapter 6. The dP/dt_{max} is an isovolumic index of contractility, and as such is relatively insensitive to changes in afterload; however, it is highly dependent on preload and heart rate.[5,8] The end-diastolic volume-dP/dt_{max} relationship is potentially more sensitive to changes in contractile state than Ees.[12] The PRSW has advantages that it is independent of preload, cardiac geometry, and heart rate, and insensitive to afterload.[13] Each of these approaches is limited in research by their complex measurements and invasive nature, particularly for those that rely on the conductance catheter, which requires additional expertise and calibration to measure chamber volumes.

Systolic function is profoundly impaired in patients with HF and reduced EF (HFrEF), and verification of depressed ejection properties in the cath lab is usually not needed because of clear reduction in EF on echocardiography. Despite relatively preserved EF, it is also known that patients with HFpEF display subtle abnormalities in systolic function. This finding is evident when systolic function is assessed by load-independent contractile parameters (e.g., PRSW) and particularly longitudinal shortening using tissue Doppler or strain imaging.[9,14,15] The subtle impairments in systolic function become dramatic during physiologic stress such as exercise.[14,16,17] Impaired LV contractile function is associated with worse outcomes in HFpEF.[9,15] Because these deficits are readily identifiable using imaging, invasive assessment is rarely used to assess systolic ventricular properties in clinical practice.

INVASIVE ASSESSMENT OF DIASTOLIC FUNCTION

Myocardial Relaxation

Diastole is defined as the period between aortic valve closure and mitral valve closure (diastole is considered to start with the onset of relaxation of ventricular muscle contraction just proceeding the closure of the aortic valve), which consists of four phases: isovolumic relaxation, rapid filling, diastasis, and atrial systolic phases.[18] Physiologically, diastolic function is determined from active relaxation and passive chamber stiffness. During isovolumic relaxation, there is rapid decline in LV pressure, which is primarily caused by active relaxation, a process that requires adenosine triphosphate hydrolysis to release tightly bound actin-myosin bonds and to take calcium back into the sarcoplasmic reticulum. Myocardial relaxation is measured by the rate of pressure decay that is often modeled by a monoexponential decay. However, this model fit may not describe the course of pressure decay in some diseases such as dilated cardiomyopathy, leading to erroneous conclusions.[19] Other alternative mathematical models have been developed such as a logistic equation.[19–21] The time constant of LV relaxation (tau) can be accurately determined from a high-fidelity micromanometer catheter placed within the LV cavity and is considered to be the gold standard for assessment of myocardial relaxation. The rate of LV pressure decline is influenced by several physiologic factors, including elastic recoil (the heart restores energy that is generated during contraction and releases it during relaxation), arterial afterload, and loading sequence.[18,22–24] Because elastic recoil depends on the extent of systolic function (i.e., end-systolic volume), LV pressure decay is also influenced by cardiac contractility. Other invasively obtained parameters quantifying myocardial relaxation include the isovolumic relaxation time (IVRT) and the maximal rate of pressure decline (dP/dt_{min}). Abnormal relaxation results in prolongation of the IVRT, decrement of dP/dt_{min}, and longer tau.

Passive Chamber Stiffness

Passive ventricular stiffness can be assessed on the basis of the LV end-diastolic P-V relationship (EDPVR). Unlike the ESPVR, the EDPVR is intrinsically nonlinear and is often modeled by a monoexponential function and quantified by the exponential stiffness coefficient (β) as well as a fitting constant (α). In the low P-V range, there is a small increase in pressure for a given increment in volume. As volume increases to a higher range, pressure rises more steeply. The EDPVR can be estimated from a single heartbeat, though it is limited by the impact of external forces (pericardial restraint, right heart compression).[20,25] Given the nonlinear relationship, these approximations must be compared within similar loading conditions. Multibeat EDPVR is a more accurate approach to assess passive chamber stiffness, where multiple PV loops are obtained during acute preload reduction, usually achieved by transient inferior vena caval occlusion, and end-diastolic points in each cycle are connected.[20,25] An increase in passive chamber stiffness is represented by a shift up and to the left in the EDPVR (*red line* in Fig. 8.2). This increased passive chamber stiffness can lead to an elevation in LV end-diastolic pressure (LVEDP), which is a fundamental hemodynamic abnormality in HFpEF.[26,27] It is important to remember that LVEDP may be elevated even in the absence of increased chamber stiffness. Volume overload (high preload) can increase LVEDP by simply increasing end-diastolic volume on a normal EDPVR *(dotted black line)*. Increased external forces that stem from right heart loading and pericardial restraint can shift the entire EDPVR upward, which results in elevation in LVEDP *(blue line)*. The curvature of the EDPVR (stiffness) is similar to that in normal subjects. In contrast, a rightward shift of the EDPVR indicates myocardial remodeling, which is often observed in patients with dilated cardiomyopathy.[20,25]

Although these invasive hemodynamic assessments serve as the gold standards for the assessment of myocardial relaxation and passive chamber stiffness, these rarely are performed in clinical practice, owing to requirement of high-fidelity micromanometer and conductance catheters and the need to manipulate preload as with transient caval occlusion techniques.

Left Ventricular Filling Pressure

In everyday practice, left-sided filling pressures (either LVEDP or pulmonary capillary wedge pressure [PCWP]) are the most common measure of diastolic dysfunction and central to current invasive hemodynamic assessments of HFpEF. One cannot determine whether

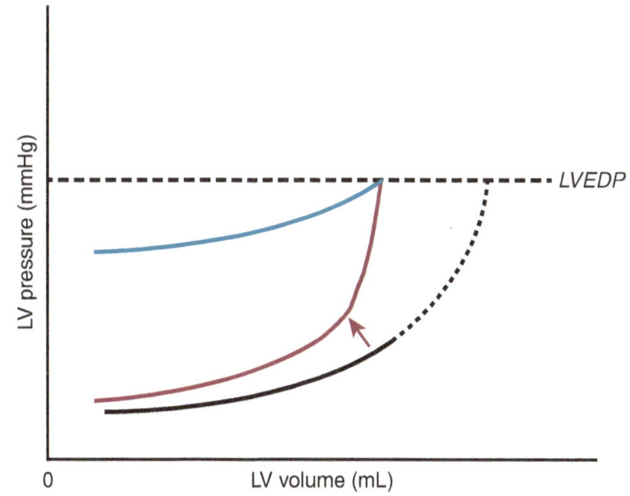

Fig. 8.2 The solid black line shows the end-diastolic P-V relationship (EDPVR) in a healthy subject. The curve shifts up and to the left means, as indicated by the red arrow, an increase in passive chamber stiffness *(red line)*. Left ventricular end-diastolic pressure *(LVEDP)* may be elevated even in the absence of increased chamber stiffness. Volume overload (higher preload) can increase LVEDP on the normal EDPVR *(dotted black line)*. Increased external forces (e.g., right heart loading and pericardial restraint) can shift the entire EDPVR upward, which results in elevation in LVEDP *(blue line)*. The curvature of the EDPVR (stiffness) in this latter case is similar to that in the normal subject. *LV,* Left ventricular.

elevation in filling pressures reflects increased chamber stiffness, larger preload, or increased external forces without additional data (see earlier discussion). The LVEDP is considered to be the gold standard of LV filling pressure that reflects diastolic dysfunction in subjects with HFpEF because it is directly measured in the left ventricle. However, this assessment requires arterial puncture and insertion of a catheter into the left ventricle. In contrast, in the absence of lesions in the pulmonary venules, veins, left atrium, and mitral valve, the PCWP obtained by right heart catheterization provides an accurate measurement of LA pressure and LVEDP. It is increasingly recognized that a high-quality PCWP via right heart catheterization is just as robust as directly measured LVEDP, and elevated PCWP at rest or during exercise is now used as a gold standard metric to definitively establish the diagnosis of HFpEF.[3,4]

In addition to its role in diagnosis, elevated PCWP identifies HFpEF patients at increased risk of death,[28] and lowering PCWP and PA pressures reduces HF hospitalizations in patients with HFpEF.[29] As such, a number of interventions targeting PCWP elevation have been tested in people with HFpEF.[30–33] LV filling pressures can be estimated noninvasively through echocardiography, radiography, physical examination, or by measuring plasma natriuretic peptide levels. However, these estimates have limitations compared to the gold standard of invasive hemodynamic evaluation and are sometimes insufficient to make the clinical diagnosis of HFpEF.[4]

Differences in LVEDP and PCWP

It is possible that there is disagreement between PCWP and LVEDP measurements. Any lesions that lie between the pulmonary capillaries and left ventricle can influence the relationship between PCWP and LVEDP, such as mitral stenosis, LA dysfunction, and pulmonary venous stenosis.[34] It has recently become clear that many people with HFpEF display pathology in these domains, including structural and functional changes in the left atrium, the lung parenchyma, and the

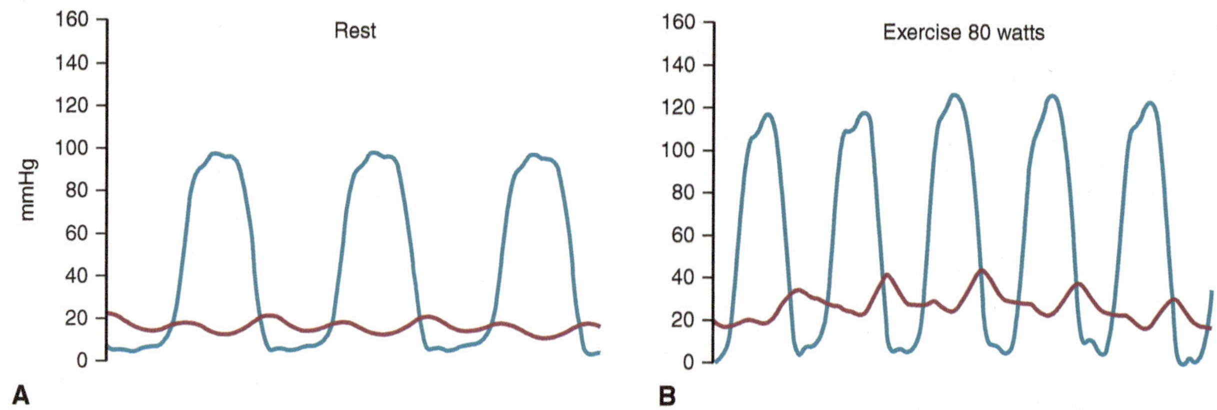

Fig. 8.3 Left ventricular (LV, *blue*) and pulmonary capillary wedge pressures (PCWP, *red*) in a patient who has history of mitral valve repair presenting with severe dyspnea. Echocardiography demonstrates a normal LV ejection fraction (LVEF, 61%) and mild diastolic doming of mitral leaflets with acceleration of inflow velocity (mean pressure gradient 7 mmHg). (A) At rest, left ventricle end-diastolic pressure (LVEDP) is 6 mmHg and PCWP is 14 mmHg with a pressure gradient of 9 mmHg. (B) During exercise, the LVEDP remains stable (8 mmHg) but PCWP increases to 25 mmHg. There is an increase in the pressure gradient between the PCWP and LVEDP to 17 mmHg. These findings indicate that functional mitral valve stenosis across previous mitral valve repair, not heart failure with preserved ejection fraction (HFpEF), is the cause of this patient's symptoms.

pulmonary vasculature.[35–37] Beyond the deleterious effects of LV diastolic dysfunction alone, accumulation of these impairments can make PCWP higher than LVEDP. In addition, PCWP correlates best with mean LA pressure and pre-A wave pressure in the LV tracing. Often LVEDP is significantly higher than pre-A wave pressure in patients with decreased LV compliance in sinus rhythm. Importantly, elevated PCWP has been shown to be more closely related to adverse outcome in HFpEF rather than LVEDP.[28]

A simultaneous recording of LV and PCWP is sometimes necessary when a patient presenting unexplained dyspnea has known abnormalities between the pulmonary capillaries and left ventricle (e.g., mitral valve disease, excessive LA stiffness or dysfunction). This helps determine whether LV diastolic dysfunction contributes to patient symptoms of dyspnea or not (Fig. 8.3). An abnormal PCWP with a proportionally elevated LVEDP is indicative of HFpEF. If there is an elevation in PCWP but no elevation in LVEDP, this indicates that the cause is not simply due to left ventricular diastolic dysfunction. The PCWP should be obtained from both the right and the left lung if one needs to exclude pulmonary vein stenosis. In some cases, transseptal puncture is necessary to directly measure LA pressure together with PCWP and LVEDP.

Pitfalls in PCWP Measurements

Measuring an accurate PCWP requires attention to detail and careful assessment. Wedge position should be verified by typical waveforms, appearance on fluoroscopy, and ideally confirmed by oximetry (blood saturation ≥94%). The correct measurements should be made mid-A wave during end expiration because negative intrathoracic pressures with inspiration frequently cause large decreases in intrathoracic pressure, which tethers down all intracardiac pressures especially during exercise (even as transmural pressures remain stable). This respiratory variation in intracardiac filling pressures can occur even at resting conditions and are often prominent in obese subjects in the supine position, where large negative intrathoracic pressures are required to elevate the abdominal pannus and inflate the lungs (Fig. 8.4).

The average PCWP during the respiratory cycle, which is reported automatically by most recording systems, is often used in practice. However, the values obtained in this way are systematically lower than end-expiratory pressures (usually by ~20%), and this may result in underrecognition of disease. One exception to the preferred use of end-expiratory pressures is the patients with obstructive lung disease, where there may be intrinsic positive end-expiratory pressure due to air trapping, especially with exercise when inadequate expiratory time is available due to tachypnea.

Most laboratories measure pressures using standard fluid-filled catheter systems, which have relatively low frequency response. Use of a high-fidelity micromanometer-tipped catheter provides greater accuracy and precision but is limited by cost and the need for additional monitoring equipment. This greater cost needs to be weighed against the reduction in data quality that may occur with standard

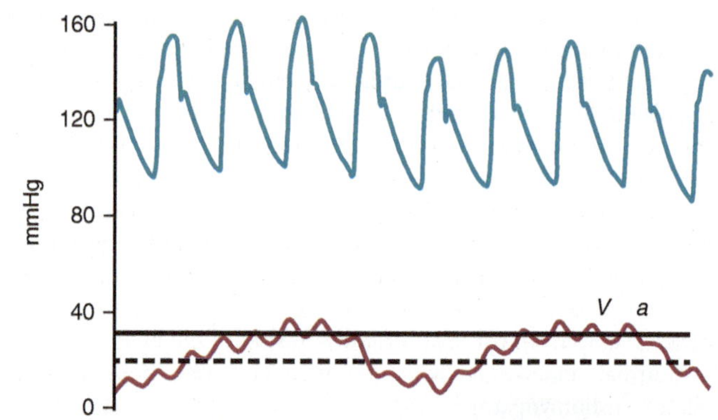

Fig. 8.4 Respiratory variation in cardiac filling pressure in an obese patient. Radial artery pressure *(blue)* and pulmonary capillary wedge pressure (PCWP) *(red)* tracings at rest from a 46-year-old obese man presenting progressive shortness of breath over a period of months (body weight 145 kg, body mass index 40 kg/m^2) and preserved EF (60%) on echocardiography. The PCWP at end-expiration of 32 mmHg (measured at mid-A wave) is severely elevated *(solid line)*, suggesting that heart failure with ejection fraction (HFpEF) is the cause of the patient's symptoms. Note that there is a significant respiratory variation in PCWP even at rest, and the average PCWP during the respiratory cycle (reported automatically by most recording systems) is substantially lower (19 mmHg, *dashed line*) due to the large negative intrathoracic pressures with inspiration.

fluid-filled catheter systems. The practice of the Mayo Clinic hemodynamic laboratory has evolved to use micromanometer catheters for all hemodynamic cases for this reason. If micromanometers cannot be used, the operator should choose the stiffest, shortest catheter system with the widest inner lumen to achieve greater frequency response.

Right Heart Catheterization

In addition to measurement of PCWP to estimate LV filling pressures, right heart catheterization allows for assessment of PA, right ventricular (RV), and RA pressures; PVR and compliance; and CO. Studies have shown that a significant number of HFpEF patients display pulmonary hypertension (PH) and impaired RV-PA coupling, and patients with this phenotype suffer from high morbidity and mortality.[17,38–43] Right heart catheterization can be useful in the evaluation in HFpEF in this regard. The importance of invasive hemodynamic assessment of PA and right heart in HFpEF is appreciated increasingly and discussed later in this chapter. Exercise intolerance is a cardinal feature of HFpEF. In addition to elevation in filling pressures, patients with HFpEF frequently display significant limitations in the ability to augment cardiac output in response to exercise.[17,44] Afflicted patients also have multiple impairments that contribute to reduced exercise capacity (i.e., reduced peak oxygen consumption), such as impaired lung diffusion and abnormalities in peripheral oxygen extraction and utilization.[36,45,46] Using simultaneous expired gas analysis and arterial and mixed venous blood sampling, right heart catheterization also provides information to identify the defective steps that impair each one's exercise capacity. It will be useful in the future to better phenotype patients to individualize therapy.[44,45]

THE PATHOPHYSIOLOGY OF HFpEF

Heart failure is defined hemodynamically as an inability of the heart to pump blood to the body at a rate commensurate with its needs, or to do so only at the cost of elevated filling pressures.[44] LV diastolic dysfunction was formerly conceptualized as the sole pathophysiologic contributor of HFpEF. Invasive hemodynamic studies reported that patients with HFpEF had impaired relaxation and left upward shift of EDPVR (increased LV stiffness) compared to controls.[26,27,47] In contrast, another invasive study using multiple PV loops at varying preloads has shown no differences in relaxation (tau) or diastolic stiffness (β) between subjects with HFpEF and controls.[48] This discrepancy can be related to heterogeneity in HFpEF or different stage of disease. Indeed, many patients with earlier stage of HFpEF display normal filling pressure when assessed at rest in a well-compensated state, but develop abnormal elevation in filling pressure during physical stress such as exercise.[3,4,49] This elevation in filling pressure is caused by diastolic reserve limitation: acute increase in chamber stiffness (EDPVR), inadequate relaxation response, and impaired suction (see Chapters 2, 18).[50] Identification of elevation in filling pressure at rest and/or during exercise is important especially from the diagnostic viewpoint, and this topic is discussed in the next section.

Research in the past decade has made it clear that, rather than being solely caused by abnormal LV diastolic function and reserve, HFpEF is caused by multiple impairments in the cardiovascular system, including LV diastolic and systolic dysfunction, chronotropic incompetence, abnormal vasorelaxation, deranged ventricular-arterial coupling, PH and right heart dysfunction, impaired endothelial dysfunction, and abnormalities in the periphery.[50] Importantly, many of these abnormalities are not always apparent at rest, but noted when the cardiovascular system is stressed, such as during exercise.[17] It is also likely that different factors contribute to the global cardiovascular reserve dysfunction in HFpEF, including cardiac senescence, inflammation, microvascular endothelial dysfunction and rarefaction, and abnormalities in nitric oxide signaling.[16,51]

DIAGNOSIS OF HFpEF

Invasive Hemodynamic Assessment in HFpEF

The diagnosis of HFpEF is more challenging than the diagnosis of HFrEF. In HFrEF, clinicians only need to demonstrate the presence of LV systolic dysfunction, which is often accompanied by LV dilation. However, LV systolic function (i.e., EF) and size are normal in most patients with HFpEF. Thus the clinician requires objective evidence of congestion or inadequate output, and the most direct and conspicuous finding in this regard is elevated LV filling pressure. Diagnosis of HFpEF is straightforward when patients display congestive findings at the bedside, such as jugular distention, bilateral peripheral edema, and pulmonary congestion on chest x-ray. These findings are often absent among stable outpatients presenting with chronic dyspnea. Invasive hemodynamic testing remains the gold standard for making this assessment. Demonstration of an elevation in PCWP or LVEDP (>15 mmHg at rest or ≥25 mmHg during exercise) provides sufficient evidence to establish or refute HFpEF among patients with exertional dyspnea of unclear etiology.[3,4,49,52,53] Given the robust discriminative ability, this approach is applied as one of the eligibility criteria for recent large HFpEF clinical trials.[30,54–56] Beyond the role in diagnosis, elevated PCWP provides both risk stratification and a potential therapeutic target for novel treatment in patients with HFpEF.[17,32,57,58]

Controversy in the Current Guidelines for Diagnosis of HFpEF

The European Society of Cardiology (ESC) guidelines for the diagnosis of HFpEF have proposed a combination of elevated natriuretic peptide and echocardiography as objective evidence of diastolic dysfunction.[59] The latter requires LA volume index greater than 34 mL/m^2, LV mass index 115 g/m^2 and above for men or 95 g/m^2 and above for women, or E/e′ ratio 13 and above, and a mean e′ septal and lateral wall less than 9 cm/sec. The American Society of Echocardiography/European Association of Cardiovascular Imaging (ASE/EACVI) guidelines require LA volume index greater than 34 mL/m^2, average E/e′ greater than 14, septal e′ less than 7 cm/sec or lateral e′ less than 10 cm/sec, and tricuspid regurgitation velocity greater than 2.8 cm/sec.[60] On the other hand, the American College of Cardiology Foundation/American Heart Association guidelines do not refer to specific parameters and their cutoffs.[61] Importance of the role of noninvasive estimates of LV filling pressure in clinical practice cannot be overstated, but recent data validating the former two guidelines against the gold standard assessment have raised questions regarding their diagnostic accuracy. Data on accuracy, sensitivity, and specificity of the guidelines specific to patients with preserved EF are available in three studies, in which echocardiographic data were obtained simultaneously or just before invasive assessment.[4,62,63]

The Euro-Filling study included 159 subjects with and without HF who underwent clinically indicated coronary angiography due to ascertained or suspected coronary artery disease, of whom 120 (75%) had EF at or more than 50%. This study has found that the 2016 ASE/EACVI guidelines are poorly sensitive (10%) but fairly specific (78%) for diagnosing elevated LV filling pressures in patients with preserved EF.[62] The other study examining 90 patients with various cardiac diseases (of whom 50 [56%] had EF ≥ 50%) has also shown that the 2016 ASE/EACVI recommendations have poor sensitivity (57%) for detecting elevated filling pressure even after excluding the 10%

indeterminate cases although specificity is high (90%).[63] A previous study pooled together both HFpEF and HFrEF patients and demonstrated high sensitivity (87%), specificity (88%), and diagnostic accuracy (87%) of the 2016 ASE/EACVI guidelines to identify elevated filling pressure after excluding 7% indeterminate cases, but it did not report sensitivity and specificity specific to HFpEF.[64]

Case Study

Although the patient's natriuretic peptide levels and echocardiography were inconsistent with elevated LV filling pressure, given the clinical suspicion for HFpEF, invasive hemodynamic testing was performed at rest and during exercise. Right-sided and left-sided filling pressures in this patient were slightly elevated at rest (mean RA pressure 10 mmHg and mean PCWP 16 mmHg) (Fig. 8.5A).

As shown in the patient in the case study, many patients with HFpEF will be missed if the diagnosis exclusively relies on noninvasive estimates such as natriuretic peptides and echocardiography. Each of the echocardiographic parameters that are currently considered to be central in the guidelines has been shown to correlate with invasively measured filling pressure, but weakly.[62] The ratio of early diastolic transmitral inflow velocity to mitral annular tissue velocity (E/e′) is probably the most extensively used parameter for estimate of filling pressure in clinical practice.[1] However, the diagnostic accuracy of E/e′ ratio has been recently questioned in a meta-analysis of HFpEF reporting a modest correlation of E/e′ ratio with invasive filling pressure ($r = 0.56$).[65] The low sensitivity for the ASE/EACVI algorithm is also caused by a significant proportion of indeterminate cases, which means that filling pressures cannot be estimated by echocardiography.[4,62,63] Application of the algorithm is limited to subjects with atrial fibrillation, mitral annular calcification, mitral valve disease, or paced rhythm though the guidelines recommend complicated cutoffs for each disease.[60] This limitation is especially problematic in atrial fibrillation, which occurs in two-thirds of patients at some point during the course of HFpEF and is associated with increased mortality.[66]

The Importance of Exercise Stress Testing

Many patients with HFpEF have normal filling pressure when they are assessed at rest, in a fasted, well-compensated state, but with abnormalities that develop only during physiologic stresses such as exercise.[3,4,53] A recent study examining exclusively patients with suspected HFpEF at rest and during exercise has demonstrated low sensitivities for the ASE/EACVI algorithm (34% and specificity 83%) and for the ESC guidelines (60% and specificity 75%) to diagnose HFpEF.[4] The most important finding is that resting invasive hemodynamic assessment resulted in 56% sensitivity for diagnosing HFpEF, and 44% of the patients had normal filling pressure at rest. In other words, these patients developed abnormal increases in filling pressure only during exercise. Collectively, in addition to the inaccuracy of noninvasive estimates of LV filling pressure, the absence of elevation in filling pressure at rest lowers sensitivity for diagnosis of HFpEF.

Case Study

The same patient exercised to exhaustion on a supine cycle ergometer achieving a peak workload of just 100 watts. Right atrial pressure (13 mmHg) and mean PA pressure (41 mmHg) increased during exercise. PCWP further increased to 28 mmHg, with V wave to 50 mmHg (see Fig. 8.5B). Based on the findings, the diagnosis of HFpEF was confirmed.

If a patient with many features of HFpEF (e.g., older age, obesity, atrial fibrillation, and specific physical examinations such as jugular distention and peripheral edema) displays structural remodeling and diastolic dysfunction indicating high filling pressure at rest, clinicians can conclude that a patient has HFpEF with reasonably high probability. However, the clinicians cannot exclude possibility of having HFpEF if the patient has no signs of elevated filling pressure on the basis of echocardiography or natriuretic peptides.[3,4,53] The diagnosis of HFpEF could only be made using provocative maneuvers in such a patient. Exercise provides the most robust and physiologically relevant stressor and can be performed safely in the supine or upright positions in virtually all patients. Invasive right heart catheterization during exercise allows the unmasking of occult abnormalities in hemodynamics and the enhancement to diagnose or exclude HFpEF, which has emerged as the gold standard test. An increase in PCWP (or LVEDP) to greater than or equal to 25 mmHg during exercise is sufficient evidence to make the diagnosis of HFpEF. Because not all laboratories have the equipment and expertise to perform invasive exercise testing, other alternative provocative maneuvers have been investigated. Rapid saline infusion can be used although it is not as sensitive or specific of a stressor as exercise.[49]

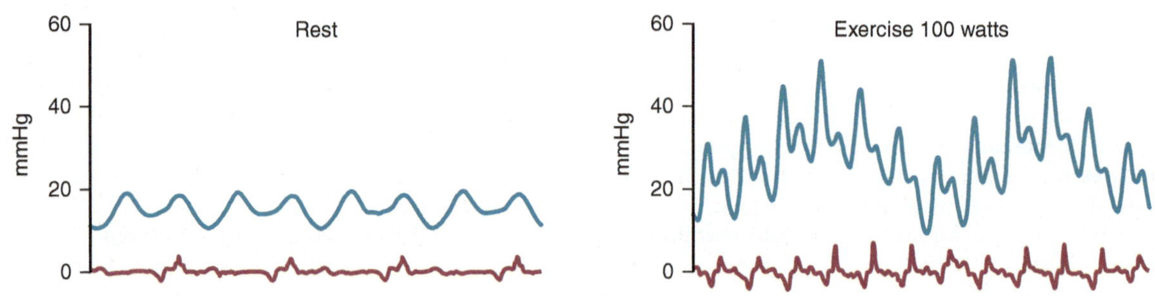

Fig. 8.5 (A) Pulmonary capillary wedge pressure *(blue)* at rest in a patient who has severe symptoms of dyspnea and normal left ventricular ejection fraction (LVEF). Despite normal N-terminal pro-B-type natriuretic (NT-proBNP) levels and normal diastolic function on echocardiography, left-sided filling pressure is mildly elevated (16 mmHg). (B) During peak exercise on supine ergometer (100 watts), PCWP further increases to 28 mmHg, with a marked V wave (50 mmHg). There is also an increase in mean pulmonary artery (PA) pressure from 21 to 41 mmHg, without deterioration in mitral regurgitation (MR) with exercise (mild). This is evidence of severely elevated left heart filling pressure and secondary postcapillary exercise-induced pulmonary hypertension (PH) and underlying heart failure with ejection fraction (HFpEF).

Noninvasive Diastolic Stress Test

Some data suggest that noninvasive diastolic stress echocardiography may be useful to improve sensitivity for the diagnosis of HFpEF.[4] However, a primary limitation of the diastolic stress test is lack of evidence-based agreement concerning the diagnostic variables to be recorded and their cutoff points.[67] Exercise stress echocardiography is often performed to assess new regional wall motion abnormality or dynamic increase in severity of valvular heart disease during exercise. The objective of diastolic stress testing for HFpEF is to detect abnormal increases in LV filling pressure during exercise. However, like echocardiographic parameters at rest, there is little consensus on the noninvasive definition of elevated filling pressure during exercise. E/e′ is used as an estimate of LV filling pressure during exercise. However, studies have called into question its ability to track changes in filling pressure during exercise.[68,69]

The 2016 ASE/EACVI guidelines require the following three criteria to diagnose elevated filling pressures: average E/e′ ratio greater than 14 or septal E/e′ ratio greater than 15 with exercise, peak tricuspid regurgitant (TR) velocity over 2.8 m/sec with exercise, and septal e′ velocity less than 7 cm/sec (if only lateral e′ velocity is acquired, values <10 cm/sec at baseline) (see Chapter 18).[60] While this kind of algorithm may allow for greater specificity, the sensitivity to detect filling pressure, which is actually the primary aim of the stress test, will be reduced. At higher workloads, the feasibility of obtaining diagnostic-quality images is sometimes limited. Volume loading is more feasible to acquire good-quality echocardiographic imaging during volume loading and it might be an alternative to exercise.[70] If echocardiographic imaging is of poor quality or is equivocal, invasive exercise testing should also be performed. Further study is clearly needed to establish diastolic stress echocardiography for HFpEF.

Strength of Invasive Exercise Hemodynamic Assessment With Simultaneous Echocardiography

Although an invasive exercise hemodynamic testing is optimal to diagnose HFpEF, like other modalities, it has limitations. An invasive hemodynamic testing does not provide visual assessment of systolic function, wall motion abnormalities, or valvular heart disease. Echocardiography obtained simultaneously with invasive exercise catheterization (right heart catheterization) with expired gas analysis (cardiopulmonary exercise testing) provides the strongest data regarding aerobic capacity, cardiac function, and hemodynamics.

Fig. 8.6 shows hemodynamics from a 68-year-old man who has exertional dyspnea, normal EF (63%), grade I diastolic dysfunction, and mild mitral valve regurgitation on resting echocardiography. Right heart catheterization demonstrates normal PCWP (12 mmHg at mid A wave) with a V wave of 14 mmHg (see Fig. 8.6A). During low workload, PCWP increases to 33 mmHg, with an increase in the V wave amplitude to 78 mmHg (see Fig. 8.6B). This is associated with a simultaneous reduction in arterial blood pressure. Echocardiography reveals severe mitral regurgitation with the development of LV basal inferolateral hypokinesis (see Fig. 8.6C), indicating that the patient's symptoms may be caused primarily by exercise-induced mitral regurgitation. Here the combination of hemodynamics and echocardiography was essential to reach the correct diagnosis.

Fig. 8.7 demonstrates invasive exercise hemodynamics in a 73-year-old woman presenting with paroxysmal atrial fibrillation and shortness of breath. Transthoracic echocardiography demonstrates normal EF (57%), LA enlargement (indexed LA volume 43 mL/m^2), and mild mitral regurgitation. Right heart catheterization reveals moderately elevated LVEDP (25 mmHg) and PCWP (26 mmHg) with a large V wave (56 mmHg) at rest. With supine exercise up to 20 watts, there are increases in LVEDP to 32 mmHg and PCWP to 34 mmHg with a prominent V wave to 69 mmHg (see Fig. 8.7A). Simultaneous echocardiographic imaging reveals development of sonographic lung B-lines, but only mild mitral regurgitation, unchanged from rest (see Fig. 8.7B). The findings are consistent with HFpEF and large V waves due to poor left atrial operating compliance. While invasive exercise hemodynamic testing with simultaneous echocardiography is not necessary for routine evaluation, it provides a robust approach to understand the pathophysiology underlying a patient's symptom of dyspnea in more challenging clinical scenarios.

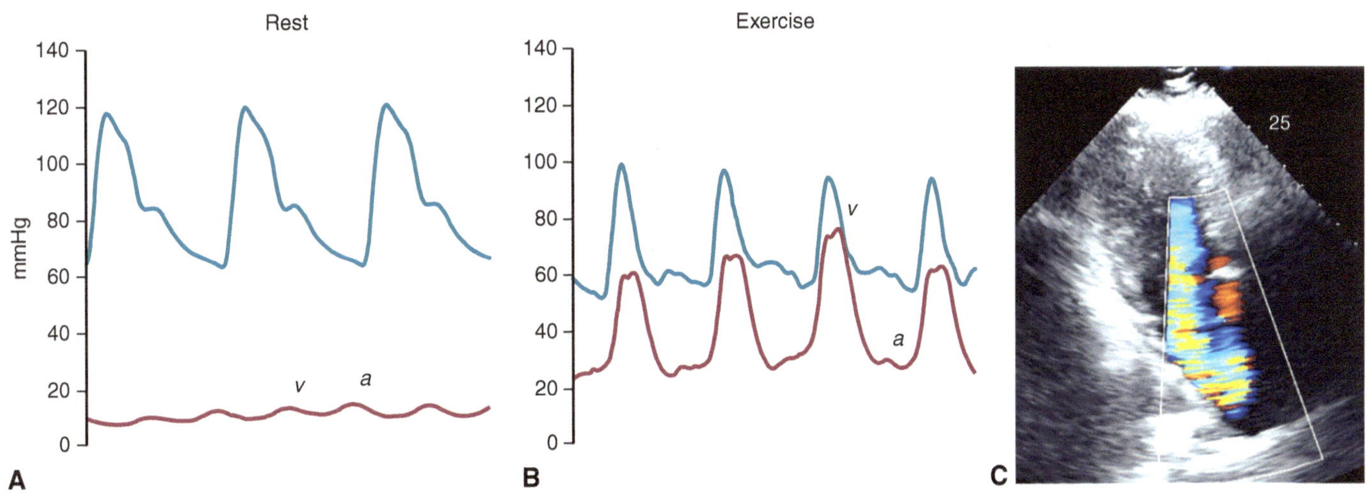

Fig. 8.6 Exercise hemodynamics and echocardiography in a patient presenting exertional dyspnea and normal ejection fraction (EF). (A) Radial artery pressure *(blue)* and pulmonary capillary wedge pressure (PCWP) *(red)* are normal at rest (PCWP, 12 mmHg at mid-A wave and 14 mmHg at V wave). (B) However, PCWP increases to 33 mmHg during low-level exercise, with a dramatic increase in the V wave amplitude to 78 mmHg. This is associated with a simultaneous drop in arterial blood pressure. (C) Echocardiography reveals severe mitral regurgitation (MR) with development of LV basal inferolateral hypokinesis, indicating that the patient's symptoms may be caused primarily by exercise-induced MR.

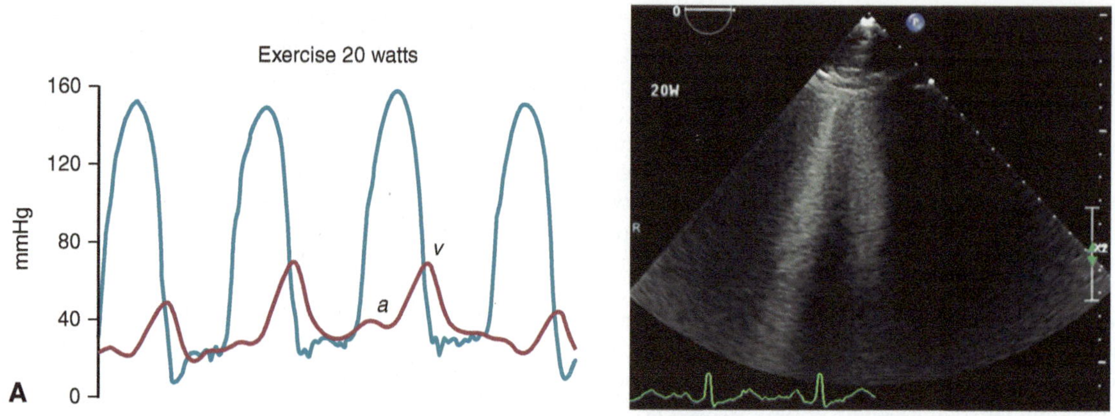

Fig. 8.7 Left ventricular *(blue)* and pulmonary capillary wedge *(red)* pressures during 20 watts exercise in a patient with shortness of breath and a history of paroxysmal atrial fibrillation. Resting echocardiography demonstrates left atrial enlargement and mild mitral regurgitation (MR). (A) During exercise, left ventricular end-diastolic pressure (LVEDP) and pulmonary capillary wedge pressure (PCWP) are severely elevated (32 and 34 mmHg), with a large V wave (69 mmHg). (B) Simultaneous lung ultrasound shows prominent B-lines. The findings are consistent with heart failure with ejection fraction (HFpEF) and large V waves due to poor atrial operating compliance.

BEYOND THE LEFT HEART

Pulmonary Hypertension and Pulmonary Vascular Disease

Pulmonary hypertension is very common in patients with HFpEF and associated with adverse clinical outcomes.[38] Pulmonary hypertension in HFpEF may be caused by a reflection of passive elevation in PCWP, increased impedance to flow through the pulmonary vessels, or both. The former has been termed isolated postcapillary PH (IpcPH) and the latter combined postcapillary and precapillary PH (CpcPH, or out-of-proportional PH).[40,41] The identification of HFpEF patients who have CpcPH is important because they have worse hemodynamic response to exercise and poorer prognosis than those with IpcPH.[71] Although PA pressures can be estimated by Doppler echocardiography, invasive hemodynamic assessment is clinically useful for definitive diagnosis and identification of this phenotype as well as a therapeutic guide. Fig. 8.8A shows resting hemodynamics from a 71-year-old man who has normal EF (67%), severe PH (estimated RV systolic pressure 84 mmHg), and RV enlargement (RV basal and mid-diameters 60 mm and 56 mm) and dysfunction (RV fractional area change 20%) on echocardiography. Right-sided and left-sided filling pressures are severely elevated at rest with severe PH. Pulmonary vascular resistance and diastolic pressure gradient (DPG), defined as diastolic PA pressure minus PCWP, are also elevated, indicative of severe CpcPH due to HFpEF.

Current guidelines stipulate the presence of CpcPH by either an elevation in the PVR or the DPG.[41,72] There is increasing controversy about using DPG as an estimation of CpcPH. The DPG does not have major advantages over transpulmonary pressure gradient in distinguishing between CpcPH and IpcPH.[73] A recent study has shown that all of the patients with HFpEF who have CpcPH display elevated PVR, yet only a minority demonstrated an elevated DPG.[71] Previous studies have also demonstrated that DPG does not have prognostic values.[74] These imply that PVR rather than DPG may be an optimal index to distinguish these groups. Given the hyperbolic relationship between resistance and compliance,[75] PA compliance may be a more sensitive predictor of both the presence of CpcPH and outcomes in earlier stage patients' HFpEF.[43] Further research is needed to investigate whether other hemodynamic parameters such as PA compliance may provide added value in this regard.

In normal adults, there is pulmonary vasodilation and reduction in PVR during exercise.[76] However, even in the earliest stage of HFpEF, there is failure of PVR reduction or even an apparent increase in PVR with exercise, with drop in PA compliance.[17] Fig. 8.8B shows increases in PA pressures caused by increases in left heart filling pressure and PVR during 20-watts exercise from the same patient. Patients with HFpEF and elevated PVR display a unique pathophysiology characterized by greater inability to enhance pulmonary blood flow and greater right heart congestion, which reduces LV transmural filling pressures during exercise, limiting left heart output according to the Frank-Starling relationship.[71]

Since the hemodynamic feature that differentiates primary PH (World Health Organization Group 1 PH) from HFpEF is PCWP at the time of evaluation, accurate assessment of the latter is crucial in that it guides most subsequent treatment decisions, and it is often difficult to know how to interpret borderline abnormal values.[40,77,78] A recent registry has shown that roughly 20% of patients with primary arterial PH who had intermediate PCWP of 13 to 15 mmHg at diagnosis catheterization have elevated PCWP ($\geq$16 mmHg) at second catheterization.[77] To complicate matters further, many patients with HFpEF have normal PAWP when they are assessed at rest in a compensated state. In this regard, invasive hemodynamic testing with provocative maneuver (exercise, saline infusion) can be useful to distinguish these groups.[40,78,79]

The Right Heart and Right Ventricular-Pulmonary Artery Coupling

RV systolic dysfunction is common in HFpEF and an important predictor of adverse outcomes.[39,80] Invasive hemodynamic assessment of the RV is used principally in research to help in understanding the pathophysiology. Because the RV ejects blood into the low resistive and high compliant pulmonary vascular circuit, peak RV pressure occurs before end-systolic ejection, and ejection continues beyond end systole. As a result, in striking contrast to the LV, the RV P-V loop normally is triangular (it becomes more rectangular like the LV in patients who have PH).[81] A shallower RV end-systolic P-V relationship than the LV results in less increase in end-systolic pressure but greater decrease in end-systolic volume for a given change in afterload. This can explain why RV systolic function is highly sensitive to changes in afterload. The afterload sensitivity in the RV makes it difficult to determine whether alterations in RV function are reflective of true impaired intrinsic RV function, solely the consequence of increased RV afterload, or both. In addition, assessment of RV function is affected by pericardial restraint and biventricular remodeling.

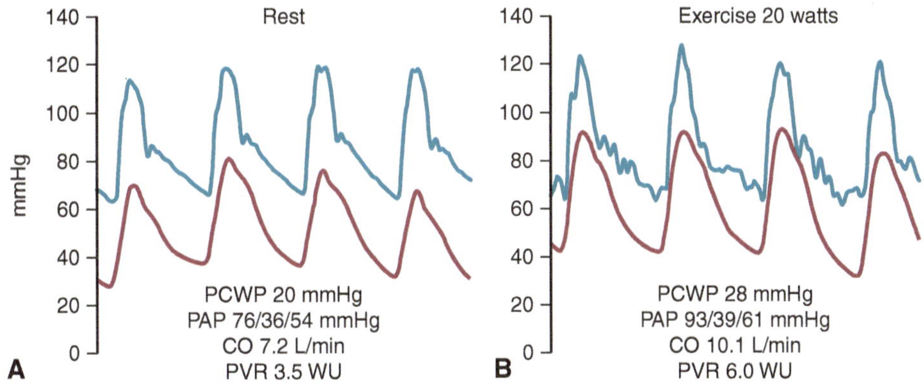

Fig. 8.8 Arterial *(blue)* and pulmonary artery (PAP, *red)* pressures at rest and during 20 watts exercise in a patient with severe pulmonary hypertension (PH) due to heart failure with ejection fraction (HFpEF). (A) At rest, there are severely elevated biventricular filing pressures (right atrial pressure 16 mmHg and pulmonary capillary wedge pressure *(PCWP)* 20 mmHg) with severe PH (mean PA 54 mmHg) due to high left heart pressures and coexisting high pulmonary vascular resistance (*PVR* 3.5 WU) and diastolic pressure gradient (16 mmHg). Cardiac output is normal (2.93 L/min/m^2). (B) With exercise, right (24 mmHg) and left heart filling pressures (28 mmHg) become severely elevated. PA mean pressure further increases to 61 mmHg with increase in PVR to 6.0 WU. These findings are diagnostic of severe combined precapillary and postcapillary PH due to HFpEF, with impaired PA vasodilation during exercise.

Like the LV, the interaction of the RV and pulmonary vascular (RV-PA coupling) is important in patients with HFpEF in view of the frequent presence of RV dysfunction and PH (see Chapter 6 for discussion about ventricular-arterial coupling in the LV).[17,82,83] Invasive RV P-V loop assessment is a gold standard, yet previous data in subjects with HFpEF are quite limited. A recent study has revealed elevated RV end-systolic P-V relationship (RV-Ees) and arterial load (RV-Ea), and diastolic abnormalities (prolonged RV relaxation and elevated intrinsic RV stiffness and RV end-diastolic pressure) even in patients with early stage HFpEF who have preserved RVEF compared to controls without HF.[84] The leftward shift of the RV end-systolic P-V relationship (or RV-Ees) is considered to be a response of the RV to increased vascular load (RV-Ea) to maintain flow (stroke volume).

In a compensated stage, the RV adapts with a roughly fivefold increase in myocardial contractility (i.e., RV end-systolic slope or RV-Ees).[85] Mechanisms to achieve this enhanced contractility include myocardial hypertrophy leading to an increase in wall thickness, but this hypertrophic change itself makes the RV stiffer with diastolic dysfunction, as observed in the study in HFpEF.[39,84,86] As the disease advances, the RV becomes dilated to maintain stroke volume, and the RV end-systolic PV relationship shifts to the right, resulting in decreased RV contractility (RV-Ees) and increased RV-Ea/Ees ratio (RV-PA uncoupling). Importantly, even in the earlier disease stage, RV-PA uncoupling can occur during exercise. The abnormality is associated with cardiac output limitation and high filling pressure.[17]

The Pericardium and Ventricular Interaction

The LV and RV share the common interventricular septum, and this interdependence influences pressure and volume on one side of the heart by the other. Approximately 40% of a measured LV cavity pressure stems from the external forces by the right heart compression and pericardial pressure, and thus a LVEDP is not equal with increased LV diastolic stiffness.[87] The pericardial pressure can be estimated by RA pressure,[88] and thus patients with tightly coupled increases in RA pressure and PCWP may experience enhanced pericardial restraint and ventricular interaction. The phenomenon of diastolic ventricular interaction due to increased pericardial restraint becomes more important as total heart size increases (i.e., as pericardial space decreases). Even though the LV cavity volume is normal in HFpEF, right heart dilation, biventricular hypertrophy, and LA enlargement can lead to a marked increase in cardiac volume. This effect is supported by invasive data from patients with obese HFpEF who have larger heart volume in which both RA (i.e., pericardial pressure) and PCWP are increased and the interventricular septum shifted to the LV cavity.[89] Importantly, this diastolic ventricular interaction can be enhanced during exercise, which further contributes to elevation in filling pressures and limits enhancement in stroke volume owing to the effects that prevent additional preload recruitment (Fig. 8.9). The same phenomenon is observed in patients with HFpEF and pulmonary vascular disease (see earlier discussion), advanced HFrEF, and in those with severe tricuspid regurgitation who often develop increase in LV filling pressures owing to right heart overload.[71,90,91]

Recent studies have shown how diastolic ventricular interaction and pericardial restraint may be therapeutic targets for HFpEF.[31,92] In fact, a recent study has demonstrated that anterior pericardial resection mitigates the increase in LV filling pressures with volume loading in a HFpEF pig model, suggesting that direct interventions to reduce pericardial restraint through surgical modification can be a therapeutic target for HFpEF.[31] Thus even as diastolic chamber stiffness remains elevated, filling pressures may be reduced owing to lesser restraint. In patients with dilated hearts, removal of external constraint could be harmful because it might promote even greater eccentric remodeling.[93]

FUTURE DIRECTIONS

Over the past 30 years hemodynamic assessments shifted away from the catheterization laboratory to the echocardiography lab, but recent studies have highlighted the important role for invasive assessment in the diagnosis and management of patients with HF, particularly HFpEF. Invasive hemodynamic assessment provides not only robust diagnosis but also insights into the mechanisms of this complex disorder, in which there are few effective therapies. In the near future, invasive hemodynamic assessment, in tandem with imaging and biomarker assessments, may allow more careful phenotyping to individualized therapy and hold promise to improve morbidity and mortality in the growing population of patients suffering from HFpEF.

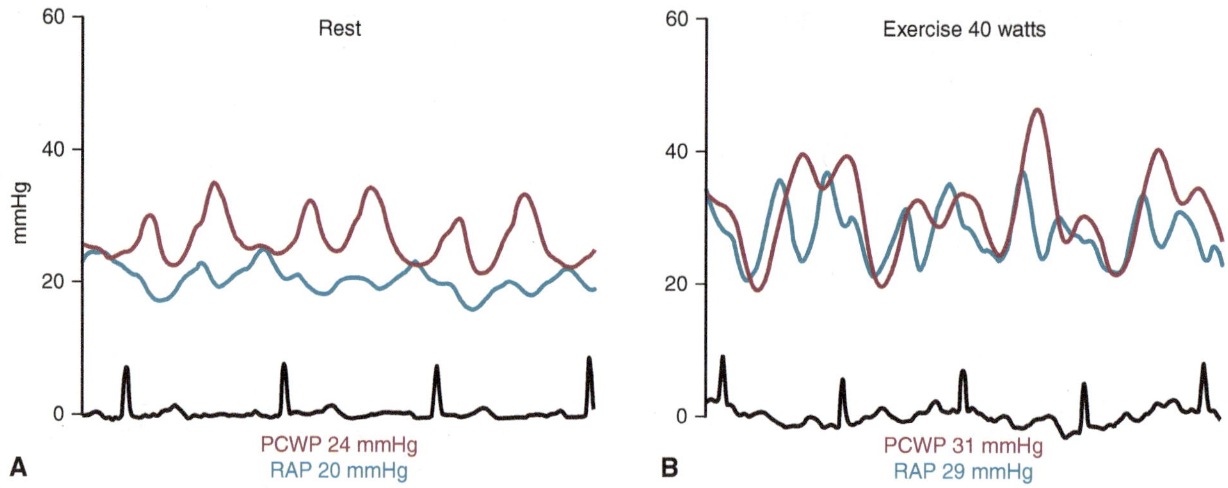

Fig. 8.9 Right atrial *(RAP, blue)* and pulmonary capillary wedge *(PCWP, red)* pressure tracings in a patient with obese heart failure with ejection fraction (HFpEF) (body mass index 43 kg/m^2) at rest (A) and during 40 watts exercise (B). At rest, RAP (which approximates pericardial pressure) and PCWP are severely elevated (24 and 24 mmHg), indicative of heightened ventricular interaction and pericardial restraint. During exercise, biventricular filing pressures are increased and become near equalization, suggesting that diastolic ventricular interaction is further enhanced during exercise.

KEY POINTS

- Diastolic function is determined by active relaxation and passive chamber stiffness. While invasive hemodynamic evaluation serves as the gold standard to make this assessment, it is used primarily for research.
- Elevated left heart filling pressure, either PCWP or LVEDP, represents the final common effect of diastolic dysfunction upon which much of the pathophysiology of HFpEF is based.
- Diagnosis of HFpEF is often challenging because left-sided pressure can be normal and develop abnormally only during exercise.
- Noninvasive estimates of filling pressure such as echocardiography or natriuretic peptides (NP) may be useful to include HFpEF, but the absence of echocardiographic and NP abnormalities cannot be used to exclude the disease.
- Invasive hemodynamic exercise testing has been emerging as a gold standard to establish or refute HFpEF when clinical evaluation and echocardiography are not diagnostic.
- Right heart catheterization allows for assessment of pulmonary artery and right atrial pressures, pulmonary artery resistance, and cardiac output.
- Echocardiography obtained simultaneously with catheterization may be a useful approach in the evaluation of patients with unexplained dyspnea and HFpEF.
- In the near future, invasive hemodynamic profiling may more rigorously phenotyped to patients, to individualize therapy for those with HFpEF.

REVIEW QUESTIONS

1. A 72-year-old man is referred for evaluation of a 2-year history of progressive exertional dyspnea with fatigue. He is obese (body mass index [BMI]: 36.2 kg/m^2) and has history of chronic systemic hypertension and atrial fibrillation. Jugular venous pressure is 8 cm, and there is no lower edema. N-terminal pro-B-type natriuretic peptide is 80 pg/mL. Transthoracic echocardiography reveals normal LVEF (62%), LV size (LV end-diastolic dimension 51 mm), LA volume (LA volume index 22 mL/m^2), and RV size, with normal systolic function. Transmitral inflow Doppler shows an E/A ratio of 1.0 with medial E/e′ of 12.9 and estimated RV systolic pressure is 36 mmHg (peak TR velocity 2.8 m/sec). Which of the following is the most appropriate step in the diagnostic evaluation of this case?
   a. He does not have apparent physical sign of congestion. We can probably exclude the possibility of HFpEF.
   b. The normal natriuretic peptide levels and echocardiographic findings (E/e′ and LA volume index) can exclude the possibility of HFpEF. Thus workup for other etiology will be required.
   c. Despite the normal natriuretic peptide levels and echocardiographic data, the patient has typical comorbidities of HFpEF, and the diagnosis of HFpEF cannot be excluded. Noninvasive diastolic stress echocardiography is the best subsequent test to establish HFpEF.
   d. Diagnosis of HFpEF cannot be excluded because normal natriuretic peptide levels and echocardiography at rest have poor sensitivity to identify HFpEF. Invasive right heart catheterization during exercise should be performed to bring out abnormalities in hemodynamics and to enhance diagnosis or exclude HFpEF.
   e. All of these are correct.
2. A 65-year-old obese woman (BMI 50 kg/m^2) is referred for cardiac catheterization for evaluation of exertional dyspnea. Which of the following is the correct explanation regarding invasive hemodynamic evaluation?
   a. Wedge position should be verified by typical waveforms, appearance on fluoroscopy, and ideally confirmed by oximetry (blood saturation ≥94%).
   b. The average PCWP reported automatically by recording systems demonstrates 10 mmHg in a supine position. However, measurements should be made mid-A wave during end expiration because negative intrathoracic pressures with inspiration

frequently cause large decreases in intrathoracic pressure especially in obese subjects in the supine position and thus cause underestimation of filling pressure.
   c. Standard fluid-filled catheter systems are relatively low frequency response. Use of a high-fidelity micromanometer-tipped catheter provides greater accuracy and precision.
   d. A simultaneous recording of LV and PCWP will be required if this patient has known abnormalities in mitral valve disease, excessive left atrial stiffness, or dysfunction.
   e. All of these are correct.
3. Which of the following is the correct statement about the pathophysiology of HFpEF?
   a. In addition to LV diastolic dysfunction, HFpEF patients display multiple impairments in cardiovascular system, including LV systolic dysfunction, chronotropic incompetence, abnormal vasorelaxation, deranged ventricular-arterial coupling, pulmonary hypertension and right heart dysfunction, impaired endothelial dysfunction, and abnormalities in the periphery.
   b. Pulmonary hypertension in HFpEF may be caused by a reflection of passive elevation in PCWP, pulmonary vascular remodeling, or both. The identification of HFpEF patients with pulmonary vascular remodeling (combined postcapillary and precapillary PH) is important, since they have worse hemodynamic response to exercise and poorer prognosis than those with isolated postcapillary PH.
   c. RV systolic dysfunction is common in HFpEF. The interaction of the RV and pulmonary vascular (RV-PA coupling) is important in patients with HFpEF, and RV-PA coupling can be assessed by the ratio of RV function and PA systolic pressure.
   d. LV filling pressures can be elevated from enhanced diastolic ventricular interdependence. The same phenomenon is observed in HFpEF patients with pulmonary vascular disease or obesity, advanced HFrEF, and severe tricuspid regurgitation.
   e. All of these are correct.

REFERENCES

1. Nagueh SF, Middleton KJ, Kopelen HA, Zoghbi WA, Quiñones MA. Doppler tissue imaging: a noninvasive technique for evaluation of left ventricular relaxation and estimation of filling pressures. *J Am Coll Cardiol.* 1997;30(6):1527–1533.
2. Ponikowski P, Voors AA, Anker SD, et al. 2016 ESC Guidelines for the diagnosis and treatment of acute and chronic heart failure: the task force for the diagnosis and treatment of acute and chronic heart failure of the European Society of Cardiology (ESC) developed with the special contribution of the Heart Failure Association (HFA) of the ESC. *Eur Heart J.* 2016;37(27):2129–2200.
3. Borlaug BA, Nishimura RA, Sorajja P, Lam CS, Redfield MM. Exercise hemodynamics enhance diagnosis of early heart failure with preserved ejection fraction. *Circ Heart Fail.* 2010;3(5):588–595.
4. Obokata M, Kane GC, Reddy YN, Olson TP, Melenovsky V, Borlaug BA. Role of diastolic stress testing in the evaluation for heart failure with preserved ejection fraction: a simultaneous invasive-echocardiographic study. *Circulation.* 2017;135(9):825–838.
5. Borlaug BA, Kass DA. Invasive hemodynamic assessment in heart failure. *Cardiol Clin.* 2011;29(2):269–280.
6. Andersen MJ, Borlaug BA. Invasive hemodynamic characterization of heart failure with preserved ejection fraction. *Heart Fail Clin.* 2014;10(3):435–444.
7. Reddy YN, Olson TP, Obokata M, Melenovsky V, Borlaug BA. Hemodynamic correlates and diagnostic role of cardiopulmonary exercise testing in heart failure with preserved ejection fraction. *JACC Heart Fail.* 2018;6:665–675. doi: 10.1016/j.jchf.2018.03.003.
8. Borlaug BA, Kass DA. Ventricular-vascular interaction in heart failure. *Cardiol Clin.* 2011;29(3):447–459.
9. Borlaug BA, Lam CS, Roger VL, Rodeheffer RJ, Redfield MM. Contractility and ventricular systolic stiffening in hypertensive heart disease insights into the pathogenesis of heart failure with preserved ejection fraction. *J Am Coll Cardiol.* 2009;54(5):410–418.
10. Kass DA, Maughan WL, Guo ZM, Kono A, Sunagawa K, Sagawa K. Comparative influence of load versus inotropic states on indexes of ventricular contractility: experimental and theoretical analysis based on pressure-volume relationships. *Circulation.* 1987;76(6):1422–1436.
11. Kass DA, Maughan WL. From 'Emax' to pressure-volume relations: a broader view. *Circulation.* 1988;77(6):1203–1212.
12. Little WC. The left ventricular dP/dtmax-end-diastolic volume relation in closed-chest dogs. *Circ Res.* 1985;56(6):808–815.
13. Glower DD, Spratt JA, Snow ND, et al. Linearity of the Frank-Starling relationship in the intact heart: the concept of preload recruitable stroke work. *Circulation.* 1985;71(5):994–1009.
14. Tan YT, Wenzelburger F, Lee E, et al. The pathophysiology of heart failure with normal ejection fraction: exercise echocardiography reveals complex abnormalities of both systolic and diastolic ventricular function involving torsion, untwist, and longitudinal motion. *J Am Coll Cardiol.* 2009;54(1):36–46.
15. Shah AM, Claggett B, Sweitzer NK, et al. Prognostic importance of impaired systolic function in heart failure with preserved ejection fraction and the impact of Spironolactone. *Circulation.* 2015;132(5):402–414.
16. Borlaug BA, Olson TP, Lam CS, et al. Global cardiovascular reserve dysfunction in heart failure with preserved ejection fraction. *J Am Coll Cardiol.* 2010;56(11):845–854.
17. Borlaug BA, Kane GC, Melenovsky V, Olson TP. Abnormal right ventricular-pulmonary artery coupling with exercise in heart failure with preserved ejection fraction. *Eur Heart J.* 2016;37(43):3293–3302.
18. Borlaug BA, Kass DA. Mechanisms of diastolic dysfunction in heart failure. *Trends Cardiovasc Med.* 2006;16(8):273–279.
19. Kass DA. Assessment of diastolic dysfunction: invasive modalities. *Cardiol Clin.* 2000;18(3):571–586.
20. Borlaug BA, Kass DA. Invasive hemodynamic assessment in heart failure. *Heart Fail Clin.* 2009;5(2):217–228.
21. Senzaki H, Kass DA. Analysis of isovolumic relaxation in failing hearts by monoexponential time constants overestimates lusitropic change and load dependence: mechanisms and advantages of alternative logistic fit. *Circ Heart Fail.* 2010;3(2):268–276.
22. Opdahl A, Remme EW, Helle-Valle T, et al. Determinants of left ventricular early-diastolic lengthening velocity: independent contributions from left ventricular relaxation, restoring forces, and lengthening load. *Circulation.* 2009;119(19):2578–2586.
23. Borlaug BA, Melenovsky V, Redfield MM, et al. Impact of arterial load and loading sequence on left ventricular tissue velocities in humans. *J Am Coll Cardiol.* 2007;50(16):1570–1577.
24. Yano M, Kohno M, Kobayashi S, et al. Influence of timing and magnitude of arterial wave reflection on left ventricular relaxation. *Am J Physiol Heart Circ Physiol.* 2001;280(4):H1846–H1852.
25. Pak PH, Maughan L, Baughman KL, et al. Marked discordance between dynamic and passive diastolic pressure-volume relations in idiopathic hypertrophic cardiomyopathy. *Circulation.* 1996;94(1):52–60.
26. Westermann D, Kasner M, Steendijk P, et al. Role of left ventricular stiffness in heart failure with normal ejection fraction. *Circulation.* 2008;117(16):2051–2060.
27. Borlaug BA, Jaber WA, Ommen SR, et al. Diastolic relaxation and compliance reserve during dynamic exercise in heart failure with preserved ejection fraction. *Heart (British Cardiac Society).* 2011;97(12):964–969.

28. Mascherbauer J, Zotter-Tufaro C, Duca F, et al. Wedge pressure rather than left ventricular end-diastolic pressure predicts outcome in heart failure with preserved ejection fraction. *JACC Heart Fail.* 2017;5(11):795–801.
29. Adamson PB, Abraham WT, Bourge RC, et al. Wireless pulmonary artery pressure monitoring guides management to reduce decompensation in heart failure with preserved ejection fraction. *Circ Heart Fail.* 2014;7(6):935–944.
30. Feldman T, Mauri L, Kahwash R, et al. Transcatheter interatrial shunt device for the treatment of heart failure with preserved ejection fraction (REDUCE LAP-HF I [reduce elevated left atrial pressure in patients with heart failure]): a phase 2, randomized, sham-controlled trial. *Circulation.* 2018;137(4):364–375.
31. Borlaug BA, Carter RE, Melenovsky V, et al. Percutaneous pericardial resection: a novel potential treatment for heart failure with preserved ejection fraction. *Circ Heart Fail.* 2017;10(4):e003612.
32. Borlaug BA, Melenovsky V, Koepp KE. Inhaled sodium nitrite improves rest and exercise hemodynamics in heart failure with preserved ejection fraction. *Circ Res.* 2016;119(7):880–886.
33. Borlaug BA, Koepp KE, Melenovsky V. Sodium nitrite improves exercise hemodynamics and ventricular performance in heart failure with preserved ejection fraction. *J Am Coll Cardiol.* 2015;66(15):1672–1682. 2015.
34. Luchsinger PC, Seipp Jr HW, Patel DJ. Relationship of pulmonary artery-wedge pressure to left atrial pressure in man. *Circ Res.* 1962;11:315–318.
35. Fayyaz AU, Edwards WD, Maleszewski JJ, et al. Global pulmonary vascular remodeling in pulmonary hypertension associated with heart failure and preserved or reduced ejection fraction. *Circulation.* 2018;137(17):1796–1810.
36. Olson TP, Johnson BD, Borlaug BA. Impaired pulmonary diffusion in heart failure with preserved ejection fraction. *JACC Heart Fail.* 2016;4(6):490–498.
37. Melenovsky V, Hwang SJ, Redfield MM, Zakeri R, Lin G, Borlaug BA. Left atrial remodeling and function in advanced heart failure with preserved or reduced ejection fraction. *Circ Heart Fail.* 2015;8(2):295–303.
38. Lam CS, Roger VL, Rodeheffer RJ, Borlaug BA, Enders FT, Redfield MM. Pulmonary hypertension in heart failure with preserved ejection fraction: a community-based study. *J Am Coll Cardiol.* 2009;53(13):1119–1126.
39. Melenovsky V, Hwang SJ, Lin G, Redfield MM, Borlaug BA. Right heart dysfunction in heart failure with preserved ejection fraction. *Eur Heart J.* 2014;35(48):3452–3462.
40. Borlaug BA, Obokata M. Is it time to recognize a new phenotype? Heart failure with preserved ejection fraction with pulmonary vascular disease. *Eur Heart J.* 2017;38(38):2874–2878.
41. Hoeper MM, Lam CSP, Vachiery JL, et al. Pulmonary hypertension in heart failure with preserved ejection fraction: a plea for proper phenotyping and further research. *Eur Heart J.* 2017;38(38):2869–2873.
42. Vanderpool RR, Saul M, Nouraie M, Gladwin MT, Simon MA. Association between hemodynamic markers of pulmonary hypertension and outcomes in heart failure with preserved ejection fraction. *JAMA Cardiol.* 2018;3(4):298–306.
43. Al-Naamani N, Preston IR, Paulus JK, Hill NS, Roberts KE. Pulmonary arterial capacitance is an important predictor of mortality in heart failure with a preserved ejection fraction. *JACC Heart Fail.* 2015;3(6): 467–474.
44. Abudiab MM, Redfield MM, Melenovsky V, et al. Cardiac output response to exercise in relation to metabolic demand in heart failure with preserved ejection fraction. *Eur J Heart Fail.* 2013;15(7):776–785.
45. Houstis NE, Eisman AS, Pappagianopoulos PP, et al. Exercise intolerance in heart failure with preserved ejection fraction: diagnosing and ranking its causes using personalized O2 pathway analysis. *Circulation.* 2018;137(2):148–161.
46. Dhakal BP, Malhotra R, Murphy RM, et al. Mechanisms of exercise intolerance in heart failure with preserved ejection fraction: the role of abnormal peripheral oxygen extraction. *Circ Heart Fail.* 2015;8(2):286–294.
47. Zile MR, Baicu CF, Gaasch WH. Diastolic heart failure—abnormalities in active relaxation and passive stiffness of the left ventricle. *N Engl J Med.* 2004;350(19):1953–1959.
48. Kawaguchi M, Hay I, Fetics B, Kass DA. Combined ventricular systolic and arterial stiffening in patients with heart failure and preserved ejection fraction: implications for systolic and diastolic reserve limitations. *Circulation.* 2003;107(5):714–720.
49. Andersen MJ, Olson TP, Melenovsky V, Kane GC, Borlaug BA. Differential hemodynamic effects of exercise and volume expansion in people with and without heart failure. *Circ Heart Fail.* 2015;8(1):41–48.
50. Borlaug BA. The pathophysiology of heart failure with preserved ejection fraction. *Nat Rev Cardiol.* 2014;11(9):507–515.
51. Shah SJ, Kitzman DW, Borlaug BA, et al. Phenotype-specific treatment of heart failure with preserved ejection fraction: a multiorgan roadmap. *Circulation.* 2016;134(1):73–90.
52. Givertz MM, Fang JC, Sorajja P, et al. Executive summary of the SCAI/HFSA clinical expert consensus document on the use of invasive hemodynamics for the diagnosis and management of cardiovascular disease. *J Cardiac Fail.* 2017;23(6):487–491.
53. Maron BA, Cockrill BA, Waxman AB, Systrom DM. The invasive cardiopulmonary exercise test. *Circulation.* 2013;127(10):1157–1164.
54. Reddy YNV, Lewis GD, Shah SJ, et al. INDIE-HFpEF (inorganic nitrite delivery to improve exercise capacity in heart failure with preserved ejection fraction): rationale and design. *Circ Heart Fail.* 2017;10(5):e003862.
55. Redfield MM, Borlaug BA, Lewis GD, et al. PhosphdiesteRasE-5 inhibition to improve clinical status and exercise capacity in diastolic heart failure (RELAX) trial: rationale and design. *Circ Heart Fail.* 2012;5(5):653–659.
56. Zakeri R, Levine JA, Koepp GA, et al. Nitrate's effect on activity tolerance in heart failure with preserved ejection fraction trial: rationale and design. *Circ Heart Fail.* 2015;8(1):221–228.
57. Reddy YNV, Olson TP, Obokata M, Melenovsky V, Borlaug BA. Hemodynamic correlates and diagnostic role of cardiopulmonary exercise testing in heart failure with preserved ejection fraction. *JACC Heart Fail.* 2018;6(8):665–675.
58. Obokata M, Olson TP, Reddy YNV, Melenovsky V, Kane GC, Borlaug BA. Haemodynamics, dyspnoea, and pulmonary reserve in heart failure with preserved ejection fraction. *Eur Heart J.* 2018;39(30):2810–2821.
59. Ponikowski P, Voors AA, Anker SD, et al. 2016 ESC Guidelines for the diagnosis and treatment of acute and chronic heart failure: the task force for the diagnosis and treatment of acute and chronic heart failure of the European Society of Cardiology (ESC) developed with the special contribution of the Heart Failure Association (HFA) of the ESC. *Eur Heart J.* 2016;37(27):2129–2200.
60. Nagueh SF, Smiseth OA, Appleton CP, et al. Recommendations for the evaluation of left ventricular diastolic function by echocardiography: an update from the American Society of Echocardiography and the European Association of Cardiovascular Imaging. *J Am Soc Echocardiogr.* 2016;29(4):277–314.
61. Yancy CW, Jessup M, Bozkurt B, et al. ACC/AHA/HFSA focused update of the 2013 ACCF/AHA guideline for the management of heart failure: a report of the American College of Cardiology/American Heart Association task force on clinical practice guidelines and the Heart Failure Society of America. *Circulation.* 2017;136:e137–e161.
62. Lancellotti P, Galderisi M, Edvardsen T, et al. Echo-Doppler estimation of left ventricular filling pressure: results of the multicentre EACVI Euro-filling study. *Eur Heart J Cardiovasc Imag.* 2017;18(9):961–968.
63. Balaney B, Medvedofsky D, Mediratta A, et al. Invasive validation of the echocardiographic assessment of left ventricular filling pressures using the 2016 diastolic guidelines: head-to-head comparison with the 2009 guidelines. *J Am Soc Echocardiogr.* 2018;31(1):79–88.
64. Andersen OS, Smiseth OA, Dokainish H, et al. Estimating left ventricular filling pressure by echocardiography. *J Am Coll Cardiol.* 2017;69(15): 1937–1948.
65. Nauta JF, Hummel YM, van der Meer P, Lam CSP, Voors AA, van Melle JP. Correlation with invasive left ventricular filling pressures and prognostic relevance of the echocardiographic diastolic parameters used in the 2016 ESC heart failure guidelines and in the 2016 ASE/EACVI recommendations: a systematic review in patients with heart failure with preserved ejection fraction. *Eur J Heart Fail.* 2018;20:1303–1311.
66. Zakeri R, Chamberlain AM, Roger VL, Redfield MM. Temporal relationship and prognostic significance of atrial fibrillation in heart failure patients with preserved ejection fraction: a community-based study. *Circulation.* 2013;128(10):1085–1093.

67. Erdei T, Smiseth OA, Marino P, Fraser AG. A systematic review of diastolic stress tests in heart failure with preserved ejection fraction, with proposals from the EU-FP7 MEDIA study group. *Eur J Heart Fail.* 2014;16(12):1345–1361.
68. Bhella PS, Pacini EL, Prasad A, et al. Echocardiographic indices do not reliably track changes in left-sided filling pressure in healthy subjects or patients with heart failure with preserved ejection fraction. *Circ Cardiovasc Imag.* 2011;4(5):482–489.
69. Maeder MT, Thompson BR, Brunner-La Rocca HP, Kaye DM. Hemodynamic basis of exercise limitation in patients with heart failure and normal ejection fraction. *J Am Coll Cardiol.* 2010;56(11):855–863.
70. Obokata M, Borlaug BA. Stress imaging in heart failure: physiologic, diagnostic, and therapeutic insights. *Circ Cardiovasc Imag.* 2018;11(5):e007785.
71. Gorter TM, Obokata M, Reddy YNV, Melenovsky V, Borlaug BA. Exercise unmasks distinct pathophysiologic features in heart failure with preserved ejection fraction and pulmonary vascular disease. *Eur Heart J.* 2018;39(30):2825–2835.
72. Galie N, Humbert M, Vachiery JL, et al. 2015 ESC/ERS guidelines for the diagnosis and treatment of pulmonary hypertension: the Joint Task Force for the Diagnosis and Treatment of Pulmonary Hypertension of the European Society of Cardiology (ESC) and the European Respiratory Society (ERS): endorsed by: Association for European Paediatric and Congenital Cardiology (AEPC), International Society for Heart and Lung Transplantation (ISHLT). *Eur Heart J.* 2016;37(1):67–119.
73. Handoko ML, De Man FS, Oosterveer FP, Bogaard HJ, Vonk-Noordegraaf A, Westerhof N. A critical appraisal of transpulmonary and diastolic pressure gradients. *Physiol Rep.* 2016;4(17):e12910.
74. Tampakakis E, Leary PJ, Selby VN, et al. The diastolic pulmonary gradient does not predict survival in patients with pulmonary hypertension due to left heart disease. *JACC Heart Fail.* 2015;3(1):9–16.
75. Tedford RJ, Hassoun PM, Mathai SC, et al. Pulmonary capillary wedge pressure augments right ventricular pulsatile loading. *Circulation.* 2012;125(2):289–297.
76. Lewis GD, Bossone E, Naeije R, et al. Pulmonary vascular hemodynamic response to exercise in cardiopulmonary diseases. *Circulation.* 2013; 128(13):1470–1479.
77. Frost AE, Farber HW, Barst RJ, Miller DP, Elliott CG, McGoon MD. Demographics and outcomes of patients diagnosed with pulmonary hypertension with pulmonary capillary wedge pressures 16 to 18 mm Hg: insights from the REVEAL registry. *Chest.* 2013;143(1):185–195.
78. Robbins IM, Hemnes AR, Pugh ME, et al. High prevalence of occult pulmonary venous hypertension revealed by fluid challenge in pulmonary hypertension. *Circ Heart Fail.* 2014;7(1):116–122.
79. Maor E, Grossman Y, Balmor RG, et al. Exercise haemodynamics may unmask the diagnosis of diastolic dysfunction among patients with pulmonary hypertension. *Eur J Heart Fail.* 2015;17(2):151–158.
80. Mohammed SF, Hussain I, AbouEzzeddine OF, et al. Right ventricular function in heart failure with preserved ejection fraction: a community-based study. *Circulation.* 2014;130(25):2310–2320.
81. Maughan WL, Shoukas AA, Sagawa K, Weisfeldt ML. Instantaneous pressure-volume relationship of the canine right ventricle. *Circ Res.* 1979;44(3):309–315.
82. Hussain I, Mohammed SF, Forfia PR, et al. Impaired right ventricular-pulmonary arterial coupling and effect of sildenafil in heart failure with preserved ejection fraction: an ancillary analysis from the phosphodiesterase-5 inhibition to improve clinical status and exercise capacity in diastolic heart failure (RELAX) trial. *Circ Heart Fail.* 2016;9(4):e002729.
83. Guazzi M, Dixon D, Labate V, et al. RV contractile function and its coupling to pulmonary circulation in heart failure with preserved ejection fraction: stratification of clinical phenotypes and outcomes. *JACC Cardiovasc Imag.* 2017;10(10 Pt B):1211–1221.
84. Rommel KP, von Roeder M, Oberueck C, et al. Load-independent systolic and diastolic right ventricular function in heart failure with preserved ejection fraction as assessed by resting and handgrip exercise pressure-volume loops. *Circ Heart Fail.* 2018;11(2):e004121.
85. Vonk Noordegraaf A, Westerhof BE, Westerhof N. The relationship between the right ventricle and its load in pulmonary hypertension. *J Am Coll Cardiol.* 2017;69(2):236–243.
86. Rain S, Handoko ML, Trip P, et al. Right ventricular diastolic impairment in patients with pulmonary arterial hypertension. *Circulation.* 2013; 128(18):2016–2025.
87. Dauterman K, Pak PH, Maughan WL, et al. Contribution of external forces to left ventricular diastolic pressure. Implications for the clinical use of the Starling law. *Ann Int Med.* 1995;122(10):737–742.
88. Tyberg JV, Taichman GC, Smith ER, Douglas NW, Smiseth OA, Keon WJ. The relationship between pericardial pressure and right atrial pressure: an intraoperative study. *Circulation.* 1986;73(3):428–432.
89. Obokata M, Reddy YNV, Pislaru SV, Melenovsky V, Borlaug BA. Evidence supporting the existence of a distinct obese phenotype of heart failure with preserved ejection fraction. *Circulation.* 2017;136(1):6–19.
90. Janicki JS. Influence of the pericardium and ventricular interdependence on left ventricular diastolic and systolic function in patients with heart failure. *Circulation.* 1990;81(2):SIII15–SIII20.
91. Andersen MJ, Nishimura RA, Borlaug BA. The hemodynamic basis of exercise intolerance in tricuspid regurgitation. *Circ Heart Fail.* 2014;7(6): 911–917.
92. Borlaug BA, Schaff HV, Pochettino A, et al. Pericardiotomy enhances left ventricular diastolic reserve with volume loading in humans: implications for the surgical management of heart failure with preserved ejection fraction. *Circulation.* 2018;138:2295–2297.
93. Tischler MD, Rowan M, LeWinter MM. Increased left ventricular mass after thoracotomy and pericardiotomy. A role for relief of pericardial constraint? *Circulation.* 1993;87(6):1921–1927.

9

Two-Dimensional and Doppler Evaluation of Left Ventricular Filling, Including Pulmonary Venous Flow Velocity

Christopher P. Appleton, M.D.

OUTLINE

ABBREVIATIONS

2-D	two-dimensional (echo)
A-fib	atrial fibrillation
A-wave	flow velocity due to atrial contraction
BPM	beats per minute
CMM	color M-mode (Doppler)
CV	cardiovascular
CW Doppler	continuous wave Doppler (technique)
DHF	diastolic heart failure
E-wave	ventricular inflow velocity in early diastole
HF	heart failure
HFpEF	heart failure with preserved ejection fraction
HFrEF	heart failure with reduced ejection fraction
HT	hypertension
HV	hepatic vein
IR	impaired relaxation (LV filling)
IVRT	isovolumic relaxation time
LA	left atrial
LBBB	left bundle branch block
LV	left ventricular
LVEF	LV ejection fraction
LV EDP	LV end-diastolic pressure
LVOT	LV outflow tract
LA A-wave	LV pressure rise due to atrial contraction
LVH	LV hypertrophy
MAM	mitral annular motion
Mitral Adur	duration if mitral A-wave velocity
Mitral DT	mitral deceleration time
MR	mitral regurgitation
MS	mitral stenosis
PA	pulmonary artery
PN	pseudonormal (LV filling)
Pre-A	mitral velocity or LV pressure at the start of atrial contraction
PV	pulmonary venous
PVd	pulmonary venous diastolic flow velocity
PVs	pulmonary venous systolic flow velocity
PVs1	PV flow velocity in early systole

PVs2	PV flow velocity in middle and late systole
PVa	reverse pulmonary flow at atrial contraction
PV Adur	reverse PV flow velocity at atrial contraction
PW Doppler	pulsed-wave Doppler (technique)
RST	restrictive (LV filling)
RV	right ventricular
SHF	systolic heart failure
TDI	tissue Doppler imaging
TMPG	transmitral pressure gradient
TR	tricuspid regurgitation

INTRODUCTION

The cardiac cycle is continuous. The filling of the ventricle (diastole) is followed by ventricular contraction (systole) to provide an adequate cardiac output during both rest and exercise to meet the body's metabolic demands. Both systole and diastole affect each other in an intimate manner to accomplish this goal. The normal elastic recoil after left ventricular (LV) contraction aids early filling of the ventricle with the late diastolic atrial contraction ensuring that the myocardial sarcomeres are adequately stretched to optimize contractile force. Exercise tests the health of this integrated system by shortening the time for filling and myocardial perfusion, and a normally functioning cardiac electrical system is also needed for optimal performance.

- Systole and diastole are inextricably linked, with ventricular contraction compressing elastic elements whose recoil augments early diastolic filling.
- This interrelation helps ensure adequate diastolic time for cardiac filling and myocardial perfusion.
- Loading conditions, inotropic stimulation, and neurohumoral factors generally affect both systolic and diastolic function in parallel fashion.

The so-called new epidemiology of LV diastolic dysfunction has been discussed in Chapter 7. Diastolic heart failure or heart failure with preserved ejection fraction (HFpEF) is now recognized as a major national health problem, especially in the elderly who have a high incidence of LV hypertrophy (LVH). These patients present with symptomatic heart failure (HF) despite a normal LV ejection fraction (LVEF) and have morbidity and mortality nearly equal to that of patients with reduced systolic function. They are also at risk for first onset atrial fibrillation and a higher incidence of stroke. Although the LVEF is normal in HFpEF, ventricular contractile mechanics have been altered in a way that lengthens the isovolumic contraction and relaxation period so that the period for diastolic filling becomes shorter and may be inadequate. With both heart failure with reduced ejection fraction (HFrEF) and HFpEF the degree of diastolic dysfunction is a powerful predictor of prognosis.

Despite this new appreciation of the importance of both systole and diastole in maintaining normal cardiovascular (CV) physiology, the role of LV diastolic function in health and disease is incompletely understood and underappreciated by many primary care physicians and cardiologists. As discussed in Chapters 1 - 6, diastole is a complex phenomenon with many determinants that are difficult to study individually and with several phases that encompass both the relaxation and then filling of the ventricle. Physical examination, electrocardiogram (ECG), chest radiographs, and laboratory studies are unreliable in diagnosing diastolic HF in many individuals, and invasive measurements of LV diastolic properties and pressures are impractical in clinical practice. Therefore, at present, assessing the type and degree of LV diastolic dysfunction relies on evaluating the pattern of LV filling. Although this can be assessed by radionuclide, computed tomography (CT), and magnetic resonance imaging (MRI) techniques, cardiac echocardiography, because of its noninvasive and portable nature, is currently the method of choice. Evaluating LV filling, two-dimensional (2-D) anatomic findings, and Doppler flow and tissue Doppler imaging (TDI) variables have emerged as powerful predictors of adverse CV events such as new onset atrial fibrillation (Afib) and HF, as well as mortality, regardless of LVEF.

- The symptoms of LV systolic (HFrEF) and diastolic (HFpEF) HF are often identical.
- Almost half the patients over 70 years old with HF have HFpEF, and females predominate.
- Long-term hypertension (HNT), obesity, sleep apnea, diabetes, and atherosclerosis are risk factors.
- The incidence of elderly HFpEF patients is rapidly increasing and expected to equal patients with HFrEF in the near future.
- The morbidity and mortality of HFrEF and HFpEF are similar, although currently only therapies for HFrEF have been shown to be effective.
- Echo Doppler technique is the only practical and accepted method for diagnosing and staging both types of HF.

The purpose of this chapter will be to describe the various LV filling patterns encountered in clinical practice, and what these patterns and their measurable variables reveal about LV diastolic function in both HFrEF and especially HFpEF. In cases of possible ambiguity ancillary variables such as left atrial (LA) volume, pulmonary venous (PV) flow velocity, and TDI that help in interpreting mitral flow velocity patterns will be discussed.

LEFT VENTRICULAR FILLING: A HISTORICAL PERSPECTIVE

In 100 BC Galen proposed that the heart is filled by dilation of the right ventricle. Sixteen hundred years later, in 1628, William Harvey described the heart as a central pump in a circulatory system with both arteries and veins. This was followed by recognition that most cases of HF were due to damage or weakening of the heart muscle and a decrease in the pumping function of the heart. Ventricular filling was considered simply as the interval in which the cardiac chambers filled passively between each pumping cycle and therefore was largely ignored.

Gradually, evidence emerged that abnormalities of ventricular filling could cause symptoms, and that diastolic and systolic LV function were interrelated. About 1915, Wiggers described the phases of the entire cardiac cycle, and the Frank-Starling mechanism was described, whereby LV end-diastolic volume helps regulate LV stroke volume on a beat-to-beat basis. In 1930 Katz recognized the role of LV relaxation in the filling of the ventricle suggesting that the normal heart acts like a "suction" pump, a concept proven 60 years later.[1] A limitation in cardiac filling, not pumping function, with resultant reduced cardiac output was recognized as the cardinal feature of constrictive pericarditis further emphasizing that disorders of filling could also cause cardiac symptoms and disease.

In the 1960s, the study of ventricular biomechanics accelerated. Although most research continued to focus on LV contractile function, cardiac diseases with thickened and noncompliant ventricles such as restrictive[2] and hypertrophic[3] cardiomyopathies were described. Angiographic differences in LV filling patterns between normals and patients with various heart diseases were reported even when the LVEFs were similar,[4] and these were subsequently studied by M mode echocardiography.[5,6] At the same time, the importance of LV systolic function in determining diastolic restoring forces and rate of LV relaxation was appreciated. Our current view that systole and diastole are an intertwined continuum, with each part affecting the other, gradually began to be accepted.

In the mid-1980s, echocardiographic studies showed that 20% to 40% of elderly patients with HF symptoms had a normal LVEF and therefore presumably isolated diastolic dysfunction causing pulmonary congestion.[7,8] However, because of the difficulties in quantitating individual LV diastolic properties,[9] the clinical study of LV diastolic dysfunction proceeded slowly. LV filling patterns were analyzed by digitized M mode,[10] angiographic,[11] or radionuclide[12] methods. In 1982 pulsed-wave (PW) Doppler study of mitral flow velocities to study LV filling was reported.[13,14] Because of its ease of use, noninvasive nature, and ability to determine dynamic changes in LV filling after interventions and over time, this technique revolutionized the study of LV diastolic function. Age-related changes in LV filling were recognized early.[15–18] Three basic abnormal LV filling patterns were then described using Doppler mitral flow velocity, and correlation was made with LV diastolic variables and filling pressures that were found to be independent of disease state.[19] This suggested that different pathologies altered common diastolic properties.[19] The three abnormal filling patterns were soon found to have clinical significance and prognostic value regardless of cardiac disease type.[20–23] Pulmonary venous flow velocity helped assess the filling of the left atrium, and variables were found to aid the interpretation of LV filling patterns and pressures.[24–27] Using the two flow velocities a so-called natural history of LV filling in normals and with disease patterns was described.[24–27] In addition, manipulation of preload and afterload showed that LV filling patterns changed in response to loading conditions,[28–30] and that these changes had prognostic significance in patients with cardiac disease.[31,32] Additional Doppler methods followed, such as the rate of color Doppler mitral inflow propagation velocity (Vp), TDI of mitral annular motion (MAM), and model-based image processing, which continued to improve diagnostic accuracy and advance the new field of diastology.[33–46]

Although all echo Doppler variables have limitations in interpreting diastolic function, the aggregate sum of the 2-D echo findings and multiple Doppler variables provides a practical way to noninvasively assess LV diastolic function and to objectively follow serial changes after medical intervention or with disease progression.[47–49] These methods have now been shown to have prognostic value in asymptomatic patients[50] as well as those with HFrEF and HFpEF from various diseases.[21,31,51] As a result, the clinical syndrome of HFpEF is now more readily recognized, and studies on improved diagnosis and the best treatment strategies for both symptomatic and asymptomatic patients are being studied.

- The strengths of echo Doppler technique in diagnosing diastolic abnormalities, filling pressures, and prognosis are the numerous variables available for analysis.
- Attempts to simplify this complex physiology to a few variables has resulted in confusion, most notably that elevated pressures are equivalent to diastolic dysfunction, or the reverse, that normal filling pressures mean normal diastolic function.
- The result has been fewer individuals receiving the correct assessment of their diastolic function, a prerequisite for studying possible interventions to reduce future adverse events.

LEFT VENTRICULAR FILLING

Assessment by Doppler Mitral Flow Velocity Patterns and Variables

Because of its noninvasive nature and ease of use, echo Doppler technique has become the accepted clinical standard for assessing LV diastolic function. LV filling is assessed with both continuous wave (CW) and PW Doppler technique. Fig. 9.1 shows the mitral flow velocity obtained with PW Doppler technique and the variables that are measured.[52] These include LV isovolumic relaxation time (IVRT), peak mitral flow velocity in early diastole (E wave) and at atrial contraction (A wave), the mitral deceleration time (mitral DT), the E wave velocity just before atrial contraction (E/A, also sometimes referred to as pre-A velocity), and the duration of mitral A wave velocity (Adur). An E/A wave velocity of more than 20 cm/sec results in a peak A wave velocity that is larger than it would have been at a slower heart rate when mitral flow velocity has time to fall to a lower level before atrial contraction.[53] In these cases, the E/A wave ratio will be reduced compared to values obtained at a slower heart rate, so that more reliance on other echo Doppler variables may be appropriate when interpreting the LV filling pattern.

- Besides the simple E/A wave velocity ratio, valuable information is present in the mitral recording, including LV IVRT, mitral DT, and A wave duration.

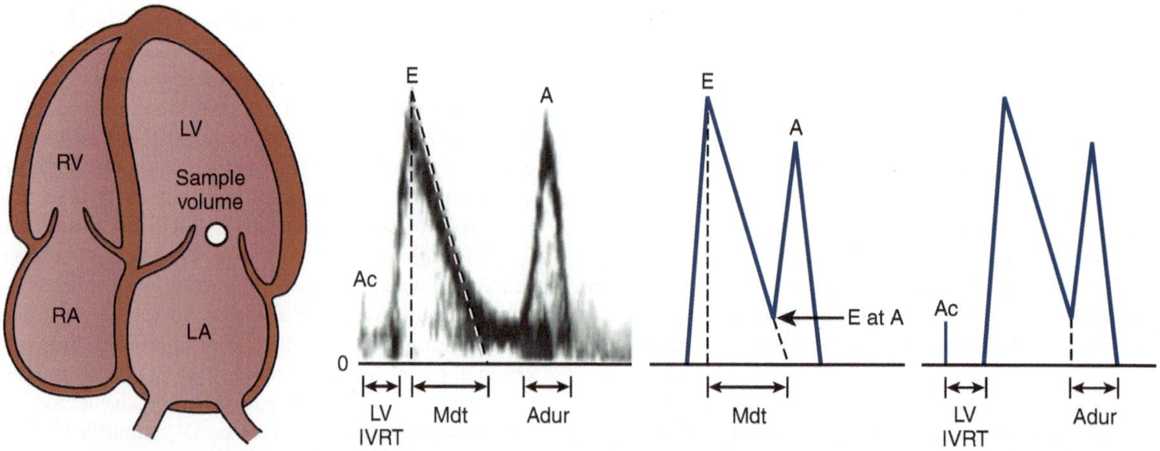

Fig. 9.1 Mitral flow velocity variables. These are obtained with PW Doppler by placing a 1–3-mm sample volume between the mitral leaflet tips as shown. Variables measured include peak E and A wave velocities as well as the E wave velocity just prior to atrial contraction (E/A velocity). The LV isovolumic relaxation time (IVRT) is the time interval from aortic valve closure (Ac) to mitral valve opening. Mitral deceleration time (Mdt or DT) is from peak E wave velocity to a line extrapolated down the decreasing velocity to the zero baseline. The duration of mitral A wave (Adur) is from the E/A (pre-A) velocity to the time the A wave returns to the zero baseline.

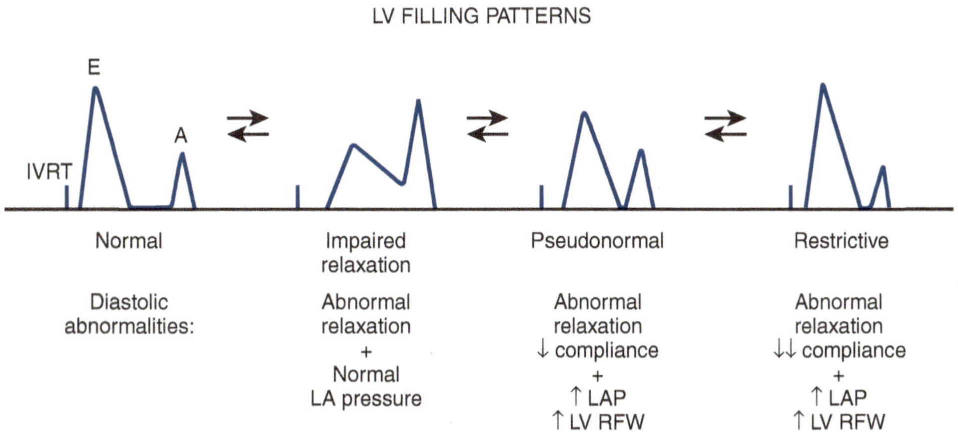

Fig. 9.2 Normal and abnormal LV filling patterns and their associated LV diastolic abnormalities. The degree of abnormality increases from left to right. The arrows indicate their dynamic nature in response to loading conditions and other variables.

Normal and Abnormal LV Filling Patterns at Rest and During Exercise and Their Associated Diastolic Properties

The normal and abnormal LV filling patterns at rest and during exercise, and their associated diastolic properties, are shown in Fig. 9.2. The numerous factors that affect LV diastolic properties and the filling of the left ventricle are described in Chapters 1 through 6. Although the interaction of these is complex, their sum reflects the diastolic transmitral pressure gradient (TMPG), which ultimately determines mitral inflow and the LV filling pattern[54] (Fig. 9.3). A positive LA to LV pressure gradient in diastole results in flow across the mitral valve, while negative gradients decelerate, stop, or reverse flow.

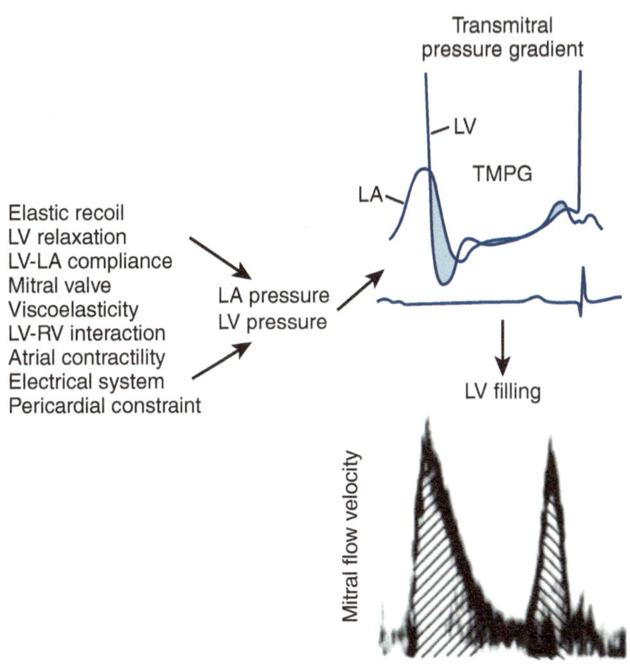

Fig. 9.3 The major determinants of LV filling are shown. In sum they affect the transmitral pressure gradient (TMPG), which determines the LV filling pattern. When LV pressure falls below LA pressure a positive pressure gradient occurs and early diastolic filling begins (hatching). Pressure in the ventricle rises and then briefly exceeds LA pressure, which decelerates mitral flow velocity. A positive pressure gradient occurs again at atrial contraction and results in flow in late diastole just before systole begins.

Two key diastolic properties, the rate of LV relaxation (diastolic pressure fall) and LV compliance throughout diastole, are especially important in understanding pressures and LV filling.[55] Normal LV contraction and relaxation are vigorous and rapid, with diastolic elastic recoil augmenting early diastolic filling through a suction effect,[56,57] meaning initially LV volume increases while pressure is still decreasing. This promotes an early mitral valve opening and helps maximize the diastolic filling period and the time available for myocardial perfusion. At normal resting heart rates (<75 bpm) rapid ejection and a predominance of early diastolic filling leaves a period of diastasis before atrial contraction as a reserve that can help maintain adequate LV filling when exercise shortens cardiac cycle length.

The first hemodynamic abnormality seen in nearly all cardiac diseases is a slower rate of LV relaxation.[58,59] This is most commonly associated with hypertension or LV hypertrophy. Both systole and diastole are affected even when the LVEF remains normal. In systole the LV isovolumic contraction and ejection times become prolonged. In diastole the impaired LV relaxation causes a slower fall in LV pressure after aortic valve closure. This causes the mitral valve to open later and the early diastolic TMPG and proportion of filling to decline.[59] The diastasis period often disappears, and a greater proportion of filling at atrial contraction is needed to reach an optimal end-diastolic volume. These changes shorten the time available for diastolic filling and alter the LV filling pattern (Fig. 9.4). Patients who have this impaired relaxation (IR) filling pattern most often have normal filling pressures and are asymptomatic, although a few may show a blunted cardiac output and functional limitation with exercise.[60]

- Numerous factors affect LV diastolic properties, but their sum defines the transmitral pressure gradient, which determines mitral inflow and the LV filling pattern.
- The two most important diastolic properties are the rate of relaxation and LV compliance, the latter affecting LA and LV filling pressures.
- The most common cause of early LV diastolic dysfunction is LV hypertrophy due to HTN heart disease, which slows relaxation and reduces early diastolic filling.
- However, in IR patients, pressures remain normal and the patients asymptomatic, sometimes for decades in this largest group of patients with early diastolic dysfunction.

With more advanced disease LV relaxation remains abnormal, but a decrease in LV compliance occurs first in late diastole after atrial

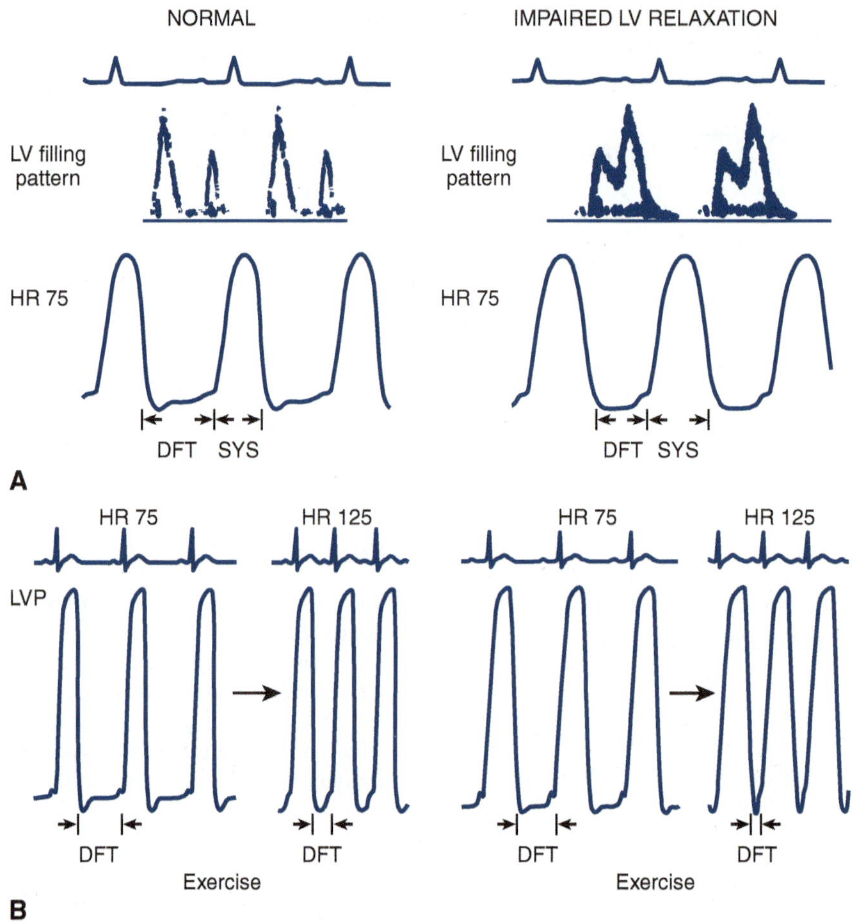

Fig. 9.4 The effect of impaired LV relaxation on LV diastolic filling time (DFT) and LV filling patterns. (A) ECG, PW Doppler of mitral flow velocity, and high-fidelity LV pressure recordings are shown in two individuals at rest. Both individuals have heart rates of 75 bpm and a normal LV ejection fraction. In the normal subject LV pressure increases and decreases rapidly so that the DFT is longer than systole (SYS) with a period of diastasis in mid-diastole. In contrast *(top right),* with impaired LV relaxation longer isovolumic contraction and relaxation times result in the DFT being longer than systole. As a result the LV filling pattern is markedly altered to achieve the same end-diastolic volume, with less filling in early diastole, a disappearance of diastasis, and a larger contribution of filling at atrial contraction. (B) The effect of increased heart rates on diastolic filling time LV pressure (LVP) is shown in the same two individuals at rest and with exercise. At 125 bpm the DFT with impaired LV relaxation is markedly abbreviated compared to normal and only 25% as long as systole making it difficult to maintain adequate LV filling. The result is a reduced end-diastolic volume, blunted cardiac output, and reduced functional aerobic capacity.

contraction and then throughout diastole, which increases mean LA pressure and size and begins to result in symptomatic HF. The increased LA pressure will oppose the effect of a slower rate of LV relaxation, causing an earlier mitral valve opening and higher TMPG so the LV filling pattern appears like normal. However, in this case the increase in early diastolic LV filling is due to increased driving (LA) pressure rather than suction created by normal ventricular elastic recoil. Patients with this pseudonormal LV filling[19] begin to have HF symptoms and show moderate functional limitation.[48,49,61,62]

With a severe decrease in LV compliance the marked elevation in LA pressure causes atrial dilation and failure, and early diastolic filling predominates with only a small and abbreviated amount of late diastolic filling. This third and most abnormal LV filling pattern is termed restrictive (RST). Patients with RST filling patterns still have impaired LV relaxation, but the severe decrease in LV compliance and marked elevation of LA result in an increased proportion of early diastolic filling that has an abrupt, premature termination (short mitral DT) with little filling at atrial contraction. Patients with this pattern are markedly symptomatic, demonstrate severe functional impairment, and have a poor prognosis.[21,31,51]

- LV chamber compliance includes myocardial stiffness as well as elements such as volume, which stretch the myocardium or the pericardium and thus constrain cardiac dilation.
- Intrinsic myocardial stiffness is affected by cardiac interstitial elements such as collagen and by myocardial elements such as titin.
- Although LA and LV filling pressures may increase with volume overload, diastolic dysfunction is only present when myocardial stiffness is increased, first only near maximum end-diastolic volume, which elevates LV end-diastolic pressure (EDP).
- With progressive increase in stiffness LV filling pressures are elevated throughout diastole and raise mean LA pressure, an advanced stage of disease.

An increase in heart rate as with exercise is the heart's diastolic stress test. As heart rate increases, the diastolic filling time shortens. In normal individuals a coordination of the electrical and mechanical systems provides for increased filling and cardiac output without an elevation of diastolic pressures.[56,60] These include shortening of the PR interval,[53] as well as faster heart rates triggering the treppe (or staircase) effect, which increases LV contractility and rate of relaxation. LVEF increases and end-systolic volume decreases. The overall effect is an earlier mitral valve opening, increased elastic recoil, and a larger early diastolic TMPG. LV contractility is also increased by sympathetic tone, while systemic vascular resistance falls.

Impaired relaxation may reduce the cardiac output achieved by reducing the diastolic filling time below that needed for optimal LV filling[63] and myocardial perfusion. A premature fusion of early and late diastolic filling often occurs (see Fig. 9.4), and atrial contraction may occur into an incompletely relaxed left ventricle. The inability to increase LV end-diastolic volume with exercise leads to a blunted increase in cardiac output and reduced exercise capacity. Patients with pseudonormal and RST filling patterns also have a significant decrease in exercise capacity, but in these individuals it is more likely an increase in mean LA pressure due to reduced LV compliance that limits exercise than an inability to increase LV end-diastolic volume.

Changes in Mitral Flow Velocity Patterns With Aging Together With Disease States

The Natural History of LV Filling

Elastic recoil and rapid LV relaxation in adolescents and young adults result in a predominance of early diastolic filling (E wave) with much less filling (10–15%) due to atrial contraction. With normal aging LVEF changes little, but LV relaxation slows in most individuals. The slower relaxation appears to be largely due to a gradual increase in systolic blood pressure (BP) and LV mass. The result is reduced LV filling in early diastole and increased filling at atrial contraction.[16–18] In most individuals, the peak E and A wave velocities become approximately equal during the sixth and seventh decades of life, with atrial filling contributing up to 35% to 40% of LV diastolic stroke volume. In individuals who maintain lower BPs and have no increase in LV mass, the age-related changes of decreasing E/A wave ratio in asymptomatic normal patients used in most reference studies are less pronounced, and normal E wave predominance can occasionally be seen into the seventh decade of life. In these individuals, normal 2-D findings, LA size, and annular TDI variables confirm that diastolic function is normal. Normal age-related values for mitral flow variables are listed in Table 9.1.

- With aging LV relaxation slows in most individuals causing a reduced E/A wave ratio, which appears to be largely due to a gradual increase in systolic BP and LV mass.
- Published normal values for diastolic variables in the over 70 years age group are difficult to define because few studies have convincing data that the asymptomatic patients used were truly normal.

The three basic abnormalities of LV filling patterns were discussed previously and shown in Fig. 9.2. The arrows in the figure indicate that abnormal mitral filling patterns are a dynamic continuum and may worsen or become more normal with changes in loading conditions. Common usage describes the three abnormal filling patterns as IR, pseudonormal, and RST. Impaired LV relaxation is present in all patterns; the difference being that with pseudonormal and RST filling, mean LA pressure is abnormal and progressively higher as LV compliance becomes more reduced and abnormal.

The changes in LV filling with normal aging and the changes with cardiac disease states can be combined into a natural history of LV filling, which is shown together with their corresponding pulmonary venous flow velocities (Fig. 9.5). Although theoretical when proposed in 1992,[24] the progression of abnormalities in LV filling patterns with disease states (from IR to pseudonormal to RST), together with changes in LV relaxation and compliance, has been documented in experimental models of congestive HF[64] and clinically observed in patients with restrictive cardiomyopathies.[20] Gradations in LV filling patterns between the three basic abnormal patterns are common due to the multiple variations of the degree of LV relaxation and compliance abnormalities. However, the abnormal LV filling patterns remain specific to the alterations in diastolic properties rather than the type of cardiac disease, with all three patterns, depending on disease stage, being seen in disorders as diverse as restrictive and dilated cardiomyopathies.

This natural history of LV filling explains how both young normal individuals and patients with severe disease and a restrictive filling pattern can have a high proportion of filling in early diastole and an audible S_3 gallop.[65] It also shows that pulmonary flow velocity has its own changes that occur with normal aging and in cardiac disease states (discussed later in the chapter), and that these associated PV filling patterns are more distinctive than some similar appearing normal and abnormal mitral flow velocity patterns.[26]

- Three basic abnormal LV filling patterns exist, which are descriptively called impaired relaxation, pseudonormal, and restrictive.
- All have slowed LV relaxation, the difference being pseudonormal and restrictive have an elevated LA pressure, which increases early diastolic filling and thus masks the slowed relaxation.
- Restrictive LV filling occurs with markedly abnormal myocardial stiffness, which terminates filling abruptly and has a poor prognosis.
- Changes in PV patterns follow changes in the abnormal mitral filling patterns and provide valuable information on identifying increased mean LA pressure as well as helping stratify patients with pseudonormal filling patterns.

TABLE 9.1 MITRAL FLOW VELOCITY IN NORMALS: AGE-RELATED CHANGES

AGE (yr)	*n*	IVRT (msec)	E (mmHg)	A (mmHg)	MDT (msec)	ADUR (msec)
2–20	46	50 ± 9	88 ± 14	49 ± 12	142 ± 19	113 ± 17
21–40	51	67 ± 8	75 ± 13	51 ± 11	166 ± 14	127 ± 13
41–60	33	74 ± 7	71 ± 13	57 ± 13	181 ± 19	133 ± 13
>60	10	87 ± 7	71 ± 11	75 ± 12	200 ± 29	138 ± 19

Normal age-related values for mitral E and A wave velocities, and mitral E/A wave ratios are shown ± SD. All individuals were free of cardiac disease, and had a normal blood pressure, physical exam, ECG and treadmill ECG with >100% functional aerobic capacity for age, normal BP response and no ECG abnormalities. LV hypertrophy was excluded, and all E at A velocities were less than 20 cm/sec so that the peak A wave velocity was not increased above that expected for the aging process.

Adur, Duration of mitral A wave; *IVRT,* isovolumic relaxation time; *Mdt,* mitral deceleration time.

All measured by LK Hatle; unpublished data; used with permission.

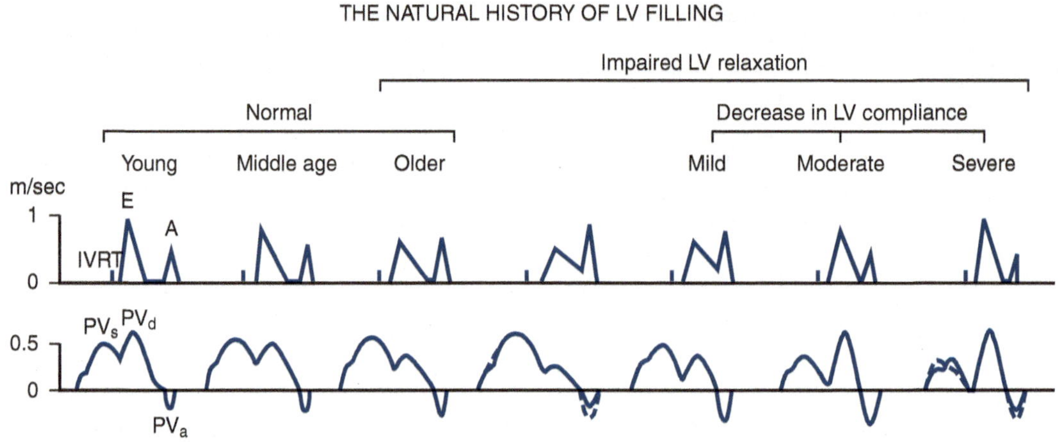

Fig. 9.5 The natural history of LV filling patterns with normal aging and with progressive diastolic dysfunction as assessed by PW Doppler mitral and pulmonary venous flow velocity recordings. Several abnormal LV filling patterns have E/A wave velocity ratios, which are similar to those seen in normal individuals. This can occur because different combinations of LV relaxation and LA pressure may result in the same early diastolic TMPG and hence a similar mitral flow velocity pattern. For this reason, additional data, such as pulmonary venous flow velocity, is often helpful in distinguishing normal and abnormal mitral filling patterns, especially of the pseudonormal type. *A,* Peak mitral flow velocity at atrial contraction; *E,* peak mitral flow velocity in early diastole; *IVRT,* LV isovolumic relaxation time; *PVa,* reverse pulmonary venous flow at atrial contraction; *PVd,* pulmonary venous flow velocity in diastole; *PVS,* pulmonary venous flow velocity in systole.

LV Filling and Changing Cardiac Loading Conditions

Simple maneuvers in the echo laboratory to reduce (Valsalva) or increase (leg raising) venous return demonstrate that mitral flow velocity patterns are a dynamic continuum.[28–30] During the strain phase of a Valsalva maneuver, preload (mean LA pressure) is reduced and alters the LV filling pattern that is present (Fig. 9.6). In normals, peak mitral E wave velocity decreases by at least 20% during maximum strain with a smaller decrease in peak A wave velocity. Similarly, in patients with IR filling pattern, mean LA pressure is normal so that with preload reduction the TMPG decreases and both E and A wave velocities decrease. In patients with reduced systolic function and IR pattern, increasing preload by leg raising may result in no change in the filling pattern. However, if a pseudonormal mitral flow velocity pattern results, it indicates a higher cardiovascular morbidity than if the E/A ratio remains less than 1.[28]

With pseudonormal mitral flow patterns, the Valsalva strain lowers the elevated LA pressure and unmasks the underlying impaired LV relaxation.[29] A notable feature of this change is the increase in mitral A wave velocity and duration as the left atrium ejects into a ventricle that has less volume and a lower pressure. In patients with RST filling patterns, preload-sensitive individuals will revert to a pseudonormal filling pattern. If a RST pattern does not improve with an adequate Valsalva manuever, LV stiffness is markedly increased even when LA pressure is lowered or normalized, and these patients have a very poor prognosis.[32]

- LV filling patterns are dynamic and change with loading conditions that affect the transmitral pressure gradient.
- By reducing venous return and LA pressure the Valsalva maneuver is especially helpful in unmasking a pseudonormal filling pattern to its underlying IR pattern.
- As loading conditions affect LV filling the most accurate assessment of cardiac diastolic properties in all individuals occurs when both the central venous pressure (CVP) and BP are normal.

Grading the Degree of LV Diastolic Dysfunction by Mitral Flow Velocity Pattern Alone

A simplified grading system for diastolic function based on the three abnormal mitral flow velocity patterns has been proposed[48] and is shown in Fig. 9.7. Grades Ia and Ib are both IR patterns with normal mean LA pressure and LA size. The difference is whether LV filling pressures are normal (Ia) or LV EDP is elevated (Ib). This is important because an elevated LV EDP is the first hemodynamic abnormality of diastolic dysfunction, and these patients, although usually asymptomatic, have a significant increase in future cardiovascular events. Grade II indicates mean LA pressure is increased with pseudonormal filling, and Grade III is restrictive LV filling. Grade IV is RST filling that does not become pseudonormal with preload reduction indicating the most advanced LV diastolic dysfunction and the worst prognosis.

Although grading LV diastolic dysfunction by mitral flow velocity pattern alone can be helpful, many patients (especially the elderly) may be misclassified. The degree of abnormality in LV relaxation and the LV compliance and filling pressures are a continuum, and similar LV filling patterns are possible with different combinations of these two diastolic properties.[48,49] Later sections will emphasize a major area of misinterpretation is patients with markedly impaired LV relaxation, where LA pressure is elevated with an increase in E wave velocity, yet the filling pattern appears to be impaired (E/A ratio <1) because of partial fusion of early and late diastolic filling.

Fig. 9.8 shows an extreme example of how different combinations of the speed of LV relaxation and LA pressure may result in similar looking normal LV filling patterns. In this case three individuals with hypertrophic cardiomyopathy have E/A wave ratios of approximately 2, yet their mean LA pressure varies threefold because of the markedly different rates of LV relaxation.[66] In these cases ancillary data such as 2-D anatomic abnormalities, reduced LVEF, LVH, LA enlargement, altered PV flow, or annular TDI velocities are indicators that abnormal diastolic function and pressures are present.[47–49,67] Also some mitral filling patterns are atypical, meaning that a biphasic mitral deceleration time, mid-diastolic filling hump, or some other unusual feature is present. These less common LV filling patterns do not fit well into the simplified grading schemes for diastolic HF (DHF) that use only the mitral flow velocity pattern, and are best understood by evaluating the abnormal diastolic properties and physiology that the altered LV filling reflect.

- Since the LV filling pattern reflects the transmitral pressure gradient, the more impaired the LV relaxation the higher the LA filling pressure will need to be to exhibit a pseudonormal pattern.

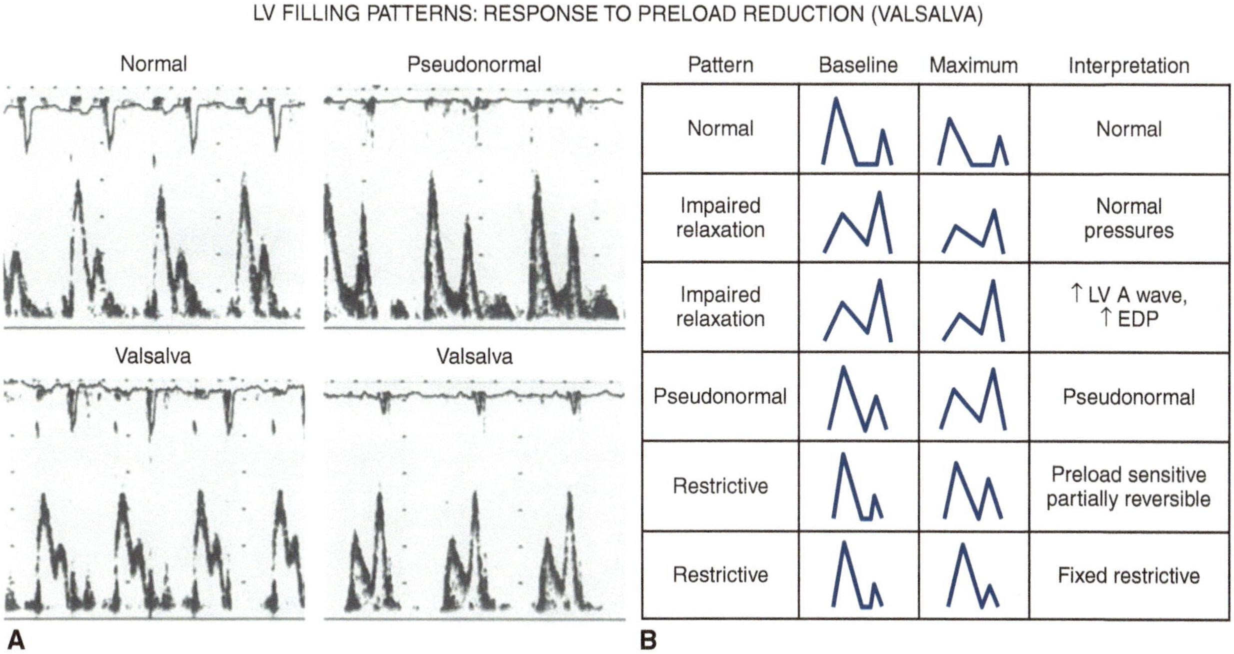

Fig. 9.6 Changes in mitral flow velocity patterns to preload reduction using the Valsalva maneuver. The left panel shows PW mitral flow velocity recordings from a normal individual and a patient with pseudonormal LV filling. After Valsalva the normal has both E and A wave velocity decrease with little change in E/A ratio, while the lowering of LA pressure in the pseudonormal patient unmasks an IR LV relaxation pattern. The right panel shows in tabular form the different responses seen in mitral LV filling patterns with a Valsalva maneuver after ~10 sec of strain. In all but fixed restrictive the E wave velocity should decrease at least 20%. When mean LA pressure is normal the mitral A wave velocity also decreases. No A wave change with an IR filling pattern suggests an elevated LV end-diastolic pressure. With mean LAP increased pesudonormal filling reverts to IR filling, and most RST patterns to pseudonormal. The exception is irreversibly RST where advanced disease results in no change in filling even with a moderate decrease in mean LA pressure.

- In these cases, which usually have a nonlinear mitral deceleration decay, ancillary variables such as LV IVRT, mitral A wave duration, and PV flow velocity pattern are used to reach a conclusion regarding diastolic properties and filling pressures.

Grading the Degree of LV Diastolic Dysfunction in Epidemiology Studies

Recent landmark studies show that many asymptomatic individuals with a normal LVEF have abnormal diastolic function, which is a risk factor for future development of adverse CV events such as new onset HF, first episode of Afib, stroke, and increased death.[50,68] In an effort to improve predictive value above that by analyzing mitral flow velocity alone, classifying the degree of LV diastolic abnormality in these studies included mitral inflow velocity variables (especially the E/A wave ratio), their response to Valsalva maneuver, PV flow velocity, and TDI of the mitral annulus. Fig. 9.9 shows the multiple echo Doppler criteria for grading diastolic dysfunction in these epidemiologic studies and provides a preview of the ancillary variables that aid in this interpretation that will be discussed in the next section.

Interpretation of Individual Mitral Flow Velocity Variables

Left Ventricular IVRT Interval

This is the interval from aortic valve closure to mitral valve opening and the start of mitral inflow (see Fig. 9.1). This interval can be a powerful tool in patients with heart disease in helping to evaluate diastolic

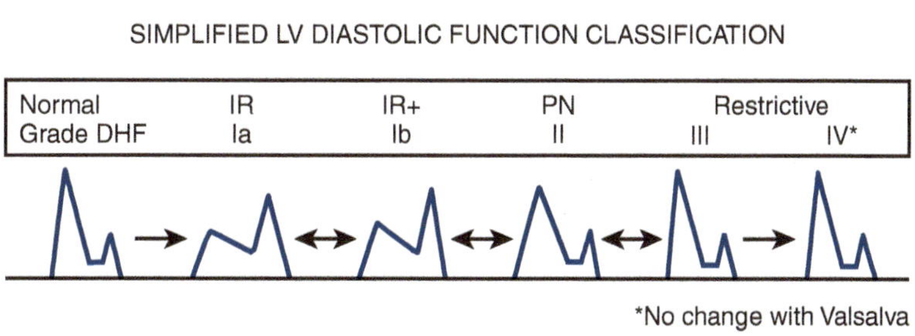

Fig. 9.7 A simplified grading system for diastolic dysfunction is shown, which assigns each abnormal mitral flow velocity pattern to a progressively more advanced grade of diastolic HF. Impaired relaxation (IR) Ia has normal filling pressures, while IR+ Ib has an increase in LV EDP, the first hemodynamic abnormality that occurs in diastolic dysfunction. Grade III is restrictive (RST), which will revert to a pseudonormal (PN) pattern with Valsalva maneuver and LA pressure (preload) reduction, while Grade IV DHF will not, an ominous prognostic sign.

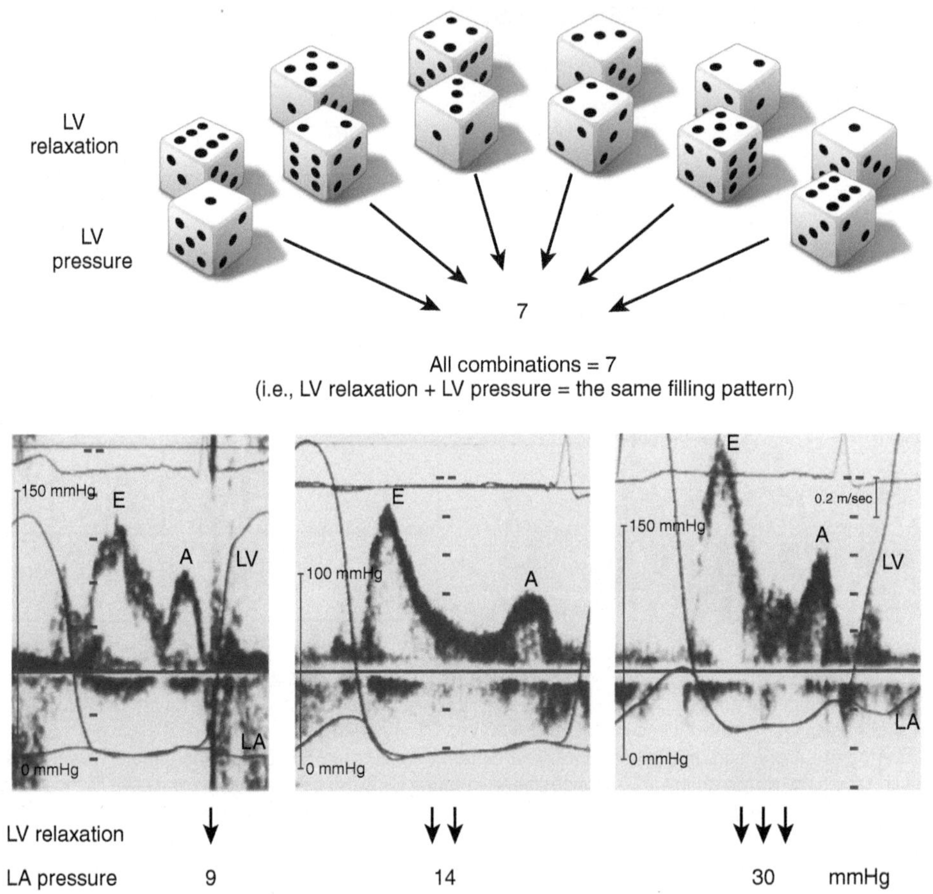

Fig. 9.8 An illustration of how different combinations of impaired LV relaxation and LA pressure can result in mitral flow velocity patterns with similar E/A ratios but markedly different filling pressures. The PW mitral recordings shown are from three patients with hypertrophic cardiomyopathy. The patient on the left is the most normal, with the least impaired LV relaxation and a normal mean LAP. The patient on the right has a similar LV filling pattern but marked diastolic dysfunction, with severely impaired LV relaxation and a mean LA pressure of 30 mmHg. In these cases, the simplified grading system of diastolic dysfunction in Fig. 8 would be misleading, and other ancillary variables would indicate the degree of diastolic HF.

dysfunction and especially LA filling pressure. We suggest it be measured on all echo Doppler studies.

In normals, IVRT varies with age, being shorter in the young who have rapid LV relaxation that results in an earlier mitral valve opening and then lengthening as relaxation slows with age (see Fig. 9.3 and Table 9.1). Fig. 9.10 shows the effect of changes in the rate of LV relaxation and LA pressure on the IVRT interval, timing of mitral valve opening, and LV filling pattern in a middle-age subjects.

The IVRT interval is most easily interpreted when at its extremes, meaning furthest from expected norms, being either short (<60 msec) or long (>110 msec). When between these values, interpretation requires correlation along with other echo Doppler variables. A normal IVRT for a middle-aged adult is approximately 80 msec. A short IVRT (<60 msec) indicates an early mitral valve opening, a long IVRT (>100 msec) delayed LV relaxation, usually with a normal LA pressure, and a late valve opening. In patients with IR filling and normal pressures, a prolonged IVRT is an early indicator of LV diastolic dysfunction.[59,69] If mean LA pressures remain normal, extremely slow LV relaxation can result in IVRT values that may approach 200 msec. The higher LA pressure in pseudonormal filling patterns causes the mitral valve to open earlier, so the IVRT shortens back to more normal values of 60 to 100 msec, and the IVRT value is less useful than other assessed variables. A short IVRT of 40 to 60 msec is seen in young, healthy, normal individuals or in patients with very high mean LA pressure and RST filling. This clinical distinction is easily made by the normal versus abnormal 2-D anatomic findings, especially LA size and contractile function.

A common instance that IVRT duration can be very helpful is when heavy mitral annular calcification is present and there is a question of mild calcific mitral stenosis versus LV diastolic dysfunction. The mitral annular narrowing may increase E wave velocity, the E/A wave ratio, and LA size, making the assessment of LV diastolic dysfunction difficult. If the pressure half-time is normal or borderline but the IVRT is short (20 msec less than that expected for age) LA pressure is likely elevated. Conversely, if E wave velocity is increased but the IVRT is normal, the annular narrowing is likely the cause for the increased velocity. A significant transmitral gradient and markedly prolonged pressure half-time indicate calcific mitral stenosis, in which case a short IVRT would also indicate increased mean LA pressure similar to the auscultatory findings of a short opening snap interval.

- The LV IVRT directly reflects LA pressure, but age and an expected rate of LV relaxation for the findings present have to be assessed.
- When the IVRT is markedly prolonged, LA pressure is very likely normal.
- With advanced cardiac pathology a short LV IVRT indicates LA pressure is elevated.

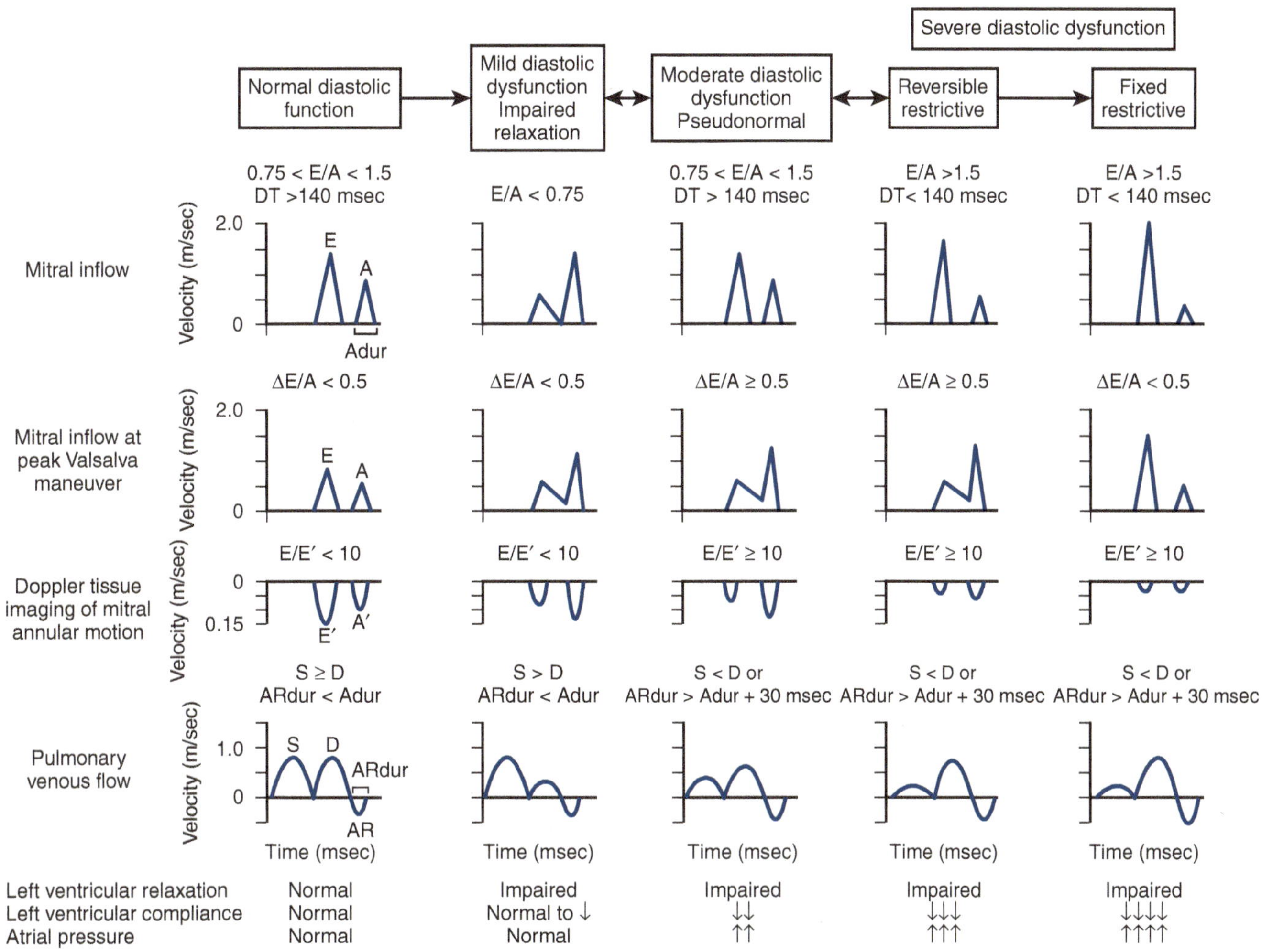

Fig. 9.9 A more complicated grading system for LV diastolic dysfunction that incorporates multiple mitral flow velocity variables, their response to Valsalva maneuver, PV flow velocity variables, and TDI of the septal mitral annulus. These criteria have been used in epidemiologic studies to assess the asymptomatic prevalence of diastolic dysfunction in the community and to understand how LV diastolic dysfunction increases the risk for future adverse cardiac events.

IVRT Flow

IVRT flow refers to flow, usually apically directed, from one part of the ventricle to another that occurs during the IVRT period when both aortic and mitral valves are closed.[70] The importance of recognizing IVRT flow is twofold: It indicates abnormal dyssynchronous LV relaxation is present between apex and base, and it should not be confused with the mitral E wave velocity that immediately follows it. In the normal situation no significant LV flow is detected during the IVRT period. When present, IVRT flow is most easily detected from an apical transducer position with CW or color M mode (CMM) Doppler because both techniques scan the long axis of the ventricle. PW Doppler can then be used for better velocity definition. IVRT flow is usually 20 to 60 cm/sec but can occasionally be as high as 1 to 2 m/sec (Fig. 9.11).

When IVRT flow is present, the most common cause is late systolic LV narrowing and increased flow velocities at the papillary muscle level, either due to LV hypertrophy or hyperdynamic systolic function. The increased mid-systolic or late systolic load placed on the LV apical segments due to the mid-systolic LV narrowing causes the apex to relax prematurely before the basal myocardial segments, with blood flow moving toward the lower pressure in the apex before the mitral valve opens. Bidirectional IVRT flow is occasionally seen when apical flow is followed by flow reversing and flowing back toward the LV base as basilar relaxation reduces pressure below that in the apex. IVRT flow can also be observed in the left ventricle with dyssynchronous LV relaxation due to coronary artery disease (CAD) or left bundle branch block (LBBB) and in the right ventricular (RV) apex when it is hyperdynamic and exhibits cavity obliteration.

- IVRT flow reflects dyssynchrous LV relaxation as is best seen by CMM or CW Doppler from an apical four-chamber view.
- The most common cause is a small LV cavity with a late peaking dagger-shaped increase in velocity in the midventricle in late systole, with IVRT flow seen just below that level.

Mitral Time Velocity Integral

Though rarely considered when discussing the assessment of LV diastolic function, the absolute value of the mitral time velocity integral (TVI) is often helpful in interpreting mitral flow velocity patterns. In the absence of significant mitral (MR) or aortic (AR) regurgitation, mitral TVI multiplied by mitral valve cross-sectional orifice area represents the LV stroke volume. Cardiac output is this stroke volume times the heart rate. Since the mitral orifice is larger than the aortic

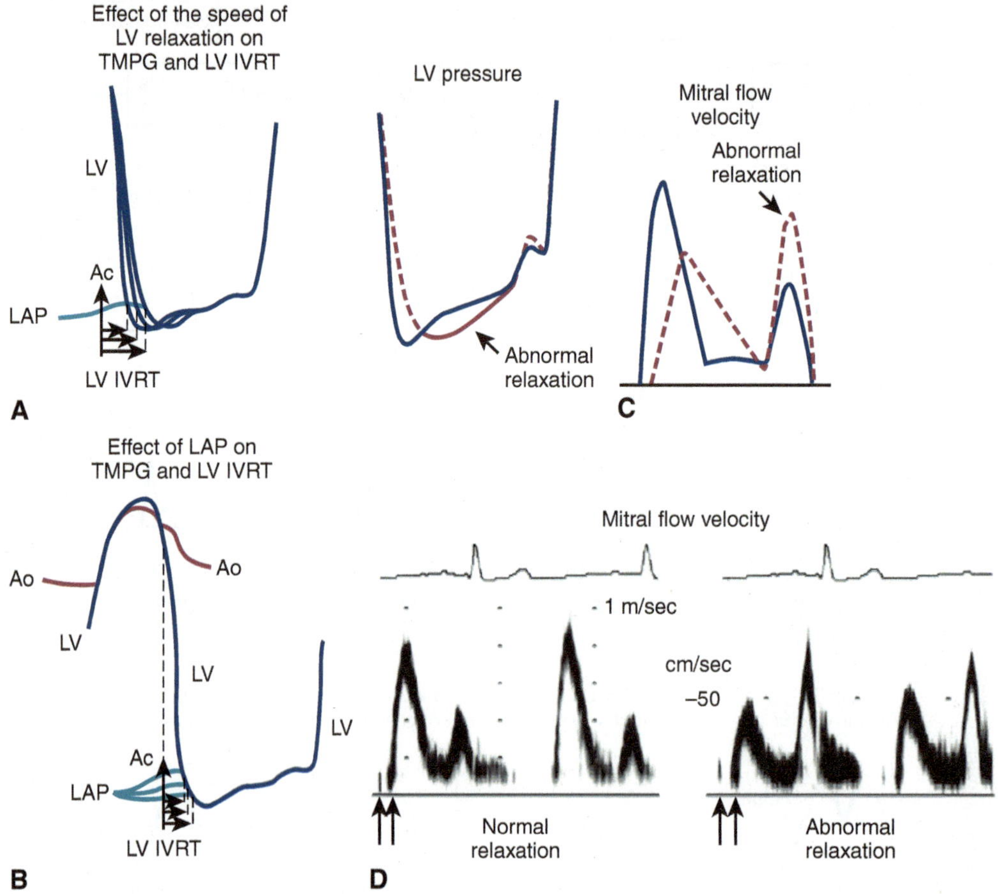

Fig. 9.10 The isovolumic relaxation time (IVRT). *(Top left)* The effect of the speed of LV relaxation on early diastolic (E wave) transmitral pressure gradient (TMPG) and IVRT with constant LA pressure. The slower the LV relaxation the longer the IVRT interval and smaller the TMPG (E wave). *(Top right)* The effect of different LA pressures (LAP) on LV IVRT with a constant rate of LV relaxation. The higher the LA pressure the shorter the IVRT and the earlier the mitral valve opening. *(Bottom)* Three middle-aged subjects illustrating the principles above. PW Doppler mitral flow velocity is shown with a mid-left ventricular M mode recording. The normal subject *(left)* shows normal LV thickness, rapid relaxation, a normal LV filling pattern, and normal IVRT of 70 msec. With mild LVH *(middle panel)* LV relaxation is slower. The longer IVRT (110 msec), lower E wave, increased A wave velocity, and A wave duration suggest uncomplicated IR filling pattern with normal pressures. The patient on the right has more extensive LVH and the slowest LV relaxation *(small arrow)*. However, a decrease in LV compliance and increase in LA pressure result in an earlier mitral valve opening, a shorter IVRT than the middle panel, and pseudonormal filling. The shorter A wave duration also suggests reduced LV compliance and higher filling pressures.

annulus the mitral TVI should be smaller than the LV outflow tract (LVOT) TVI by about 30%.

If cardiac output is either elevated or decreased the mitral to LVOT TVI ratio should remain normal. With significant MR or mitral stenosis (MS), the mitral TVI will increase and be nearly as large or larger than the LVOT TVI. With isolated AR the reverse will be true in relation to its severity. As early and late diastolic mitral TVIs represent the sum of LV filling, an inverse relation exists. A large early diastolic mitral TVI will be associated with a smaller TVI at atrial contraction. Conversely, when the E wave TVI is decreased, the ventricle can only reach a normal end-diastolic volume if there is a corresponding increase in A wave TVI. If mitral E and A waves are partially fused at rest due to impaired LV relaxation, a LBBB, or first-degree AV block (prolonged PR interval), a low proportion of E wave versus A wave TVI may be present. These patients often have a reduced functional aerobic capacity because of an inability to increase LV diastolic volume (their mitral TVI) adequately with exercise.

- In the absence of significant MR the mitral TVI reflects LV filling and stroke volume.
- Fused LV inflow patterns often have reduced mitral TVIs, which may limit cardiac filling and output, especially with exercise.
- When LV filling occurs only with LA contraction, the ability to increase ventricular filling and output with exercise is markedly reduced even if LA pressure is normal at rest.

Peak Mitral E Wave Velocity

This is determined by the early diastolic TMPG[58] (Fig. 9.3). Values for peak E wave velocity in normals of various ages (usually meaning asymptomatic) have been published but unsurprisingly have wide confidence limits.[16–18] These studies were also performed before additional variables such as LA volume or TDI annular velocities were routinely performed, which would verify that normal cardiac physiology was present. Table 9.1 lists E wave velocities in individuals of various ages without a history of cardiac disease, in whom these newer

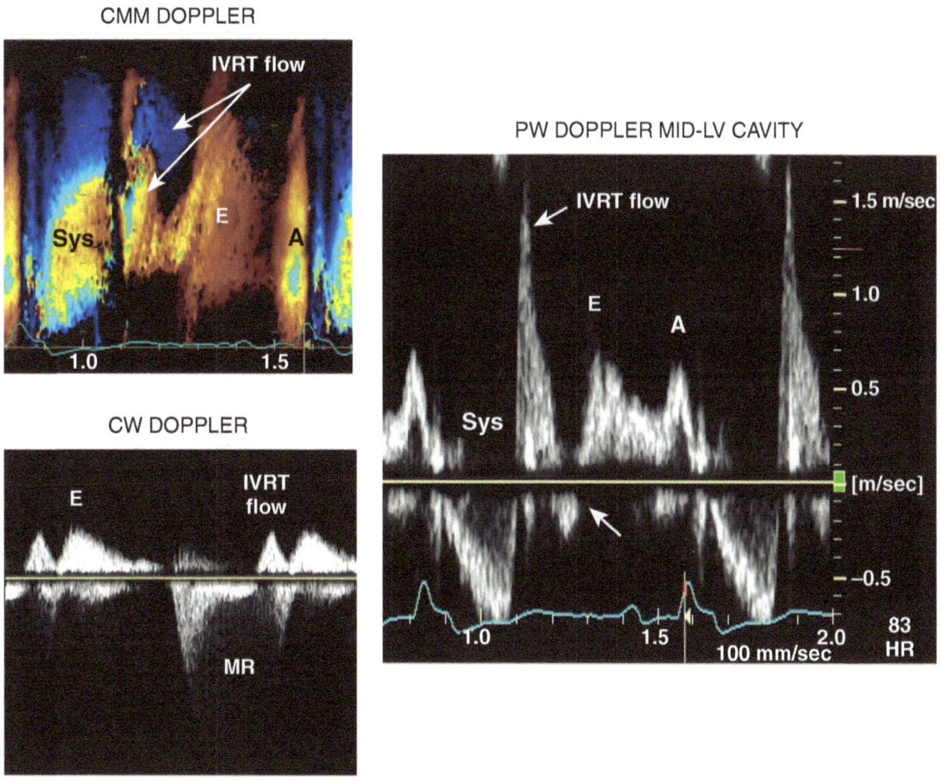

Fig. 9.11 IVRT flow in the mid-LV cavity in a patient with LV hypertrophy and near systolic cavity obliteration. All recordings are from an apical transducer position. The color M mode *(top left)* is directed through the mitral valve. Midcavity systolic flow *(Sys)* is followed by bidirectional IVRT flow, first toward the apex *(orange)* and then a shorter period toward the base *(blue, arrows)*. This is followed by mitral E and A waves. CW Doppler shows the apically directed IVRT flow, followed by mitral E wave and mild mitral regurgitation. PW Doppler at the mid-LV cavity shows late peaking systolic flow acceleration at the area of LV narrowing (papillary muscles), and then very prominent IVRT flow first toward the apex (1.6 m/sec, *arrow above baseline*) and then lower velocity toward the base (0.3 m/sec, *arrow below baseline*).

variables were included, and who also had normal BP, ECG and echo-derived LV mass. Therefore, although much smaller in terms of absolute patient numbers, the confidence limits are smaller and the values more likely to represent true normal values. Newer normal values that include TDI MAM measurements have been published but do not include large numbers of older subjects or variables such as IVRT, mitral DT, A wave duration, or PV velocities.[71]

Since E wave and LVOT velocities are related to stroke volume and orifice area, a predictable ratio between these variables exists in normals regardless of heart rate and cardiac output. The normal LVOT velocity is approximately 1 m/sec. Table 9.1 shows the mitral/LVOT velocity ratio is about 80% in younger individuals, decreasing to 70% in middle-age patients and 60% in the elderly as LV relaxation slows slightly and E wave velocity decreases. Routinely checking this E wave/LVOT velocity ratio improves the assessment of LV filling patterns and diastolic function. An E wave/LVOT velocity ratio lower than expected indicates impaired LV relaxation and normal mean LA pressure. A normal ratio with increased or decreased E and A wave velocities is seen with reduced or increased cardiac output. Higher than expected ratios indicate that peak E wave velocity is elevated, which may occur for several reasons. These include MS, MR, or increased filling pressures.

Patients with MS or MR have increased E wave velocities that may not reflect diastolic dysfunction. Mean transvalvular gradient and pressure half-time help assess the severity of MS, while the IVRT reflects mean LA pressure. Significant MR increases E wave velocity due to the regurgitant volume recrossing the mitral valve in early diastole. Normally the ventricle and left atrium become more compliant (a rightward shift in the pressure-volume [P-V] relation) as reflected by mitral DT and pulmonary artery (PA) pressures remaining normal despite the volume overload and chamber enlargement. A shortening of mitral DT or increased PA pressures suggest acute MR or a decrease in LV compliance.

Many elderly patients with HTN and LVH have an elevated E wave velocity of 1 m/sec or greater with a mitral E/A wave ratio of less than 1. Using a diastolic function assessment by mitral filling pattern alone frequently underestimates the degree of LV diastolic dysfunction in these patients. The increased E wave velocity is due to increased mean LA pressure, while the higher A wave velocity reflects LA hypertrophy. With a small LV cavity volume, relative tachycardia is present with partial fusion of E and A wave velocities. Clues that these patients with an IR pattern actually have moderate diastolic dysfunction and elevated mean LA pressure are marked LV hypertrophy, LA enlargement, and a pre-A velocity greater than 20 cm/sec.

The differentiation between a normal and pseudonormal filling pattern can be made by 2-D findings (vigorous LV and RV contraction, normal LA size) or other ancillary variables such as PV systolic fraction, CMM mitral inflow propagation velocity, and mitral annular TDI. The change to a less abnormal LV filling pattern with a Valsalva maneuver (see Fig. 9.6) reveals the preload sensitivity of the abnormal diastolic function. Fig. 9.12 shows increased E wave velocities from expected values in several patients illustrating the concepts discussed earlier in the chapter.

- Comparing E wave and LVOT velocities is helpful in identifying when the E velocity is abnormally elevated.
- When the E wave velocity is increased possibilities include increased cardiac output, MS, MR, or an elevated LA pressure.
- In the case of high cardiac output both the E wave LVOT velocities will also be elevated in their normal relation (LVOT > E wave).

Mitral Deceleration Time

Mitral DT is arguably the most important mitral variable for prognosis when heart disease is present regardless of LVEF.[21,32,72,73] In cardiac patients mitral DT relates to LV chamber stiffness[74]; that is, the shorter the mitral DT, and the more restrictive the LV filling pattern, the higher the mortality.

The acceleration of E wave mitral flow velocity is related to the maximum early diastolic TMPG. The deceleration of this flow, the mitral DT, is related to how fast (or slow) LV pressure increases in early diastolic as volume enters the ventricle (the rapid filling wave shown in Figs. 9.3 and 9.10). As with other mitral flow velocity variables mitral DT changes with age, lengthening as the rate of LV relaxation slows and less volume is transferred to the ventricle in early diastole (see Table 9.1). A short mitral DT (140–160 msec) is normal in healthy, young individuals due to the high proportion of filling in early diastole that occurs because of LV elastic recoil. As E wave velocity and the proportion of early diastolic filling declines with age, DT increases to about 200 msec by age 65 (see Table 9.1).

With impaired LV relaxation and normal mean LA pressure, early diastolic filling is reduced (E/A wave ratio <1) and mitral DT is prolonged roughly in proportion to the slowing in the rate of LV relaxation.[75] With pseudonormal mitral filling, the elevated mean LA pressure increases filling in early diastole into a noncompliant ventricle; the steeper rapid filling wave shortens the DT, with values that appear more normal for age. More advanced disease and further decreases in LV compliance cause such high LA pressure that blood is forced rapidly into a stiff ventricle in early diastole, which causes an early mitral valve opening and then a very rapid rise in LV pressure that abruptly stops mitral inflow.[19] A mitral DT of less than 140 msec characterizes this RST filling, which is most commonly seen in advanced dilated or restrictive cardiomyopathies. In these cases, and despite the widely variable LVEF, mitral DT is strongly related to both the elevated filling pressures[51] and survival,[21] even in Afib.[73]

Mitral DT is dynamic and will change with alterations in preload and afterload that change the TMPG. Patients who are volume overloaded may lengthen their deceleration time with diuresis. Similarly, the mitral DT may lengthen and become less restrictive in response to a Valsalva maneuver (see Fig. 9.6) that lowers preload.[30] Persistence of a restrictive LV filling pattern in a cardiomyopathy despite Valsalva maneuver or after maximum medical therapy is the most severe form of diastolic dysfunction (Grade IV) (see Fig. 9.7), an ominous prognostic sign that indicates very high mortality.[32]

Mitral DT is also useful in patients with mitral regurgitation, where the well-adapted ventricle will retain a normal deceleration time. Shortening of the mitral DT from expected normal values for age indicates increased ventricular stiffness and is a better indicator of myocardial abnormality than the peak E wave velocity (see Fig. 9.12).

- In patients with cardiac disease mitral DT reflects how rapid LV pressure increases with early diastolic filling.
- A high E wave velocity and short DT indicate a very stiff ventricle, restrictive physiology, and a poor prognosis unless loading conditions are markedly abnormal.

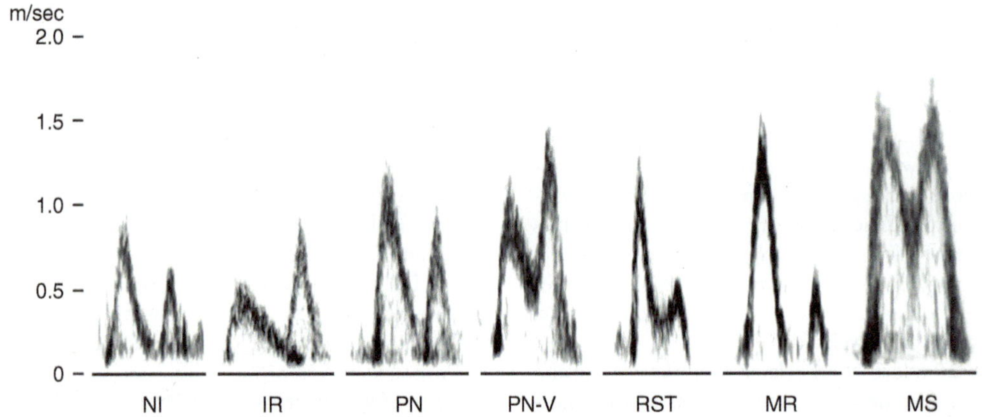

Fig. 9.12 PW Doppler recordings of mitral flow velocity in seven individuals *(left to right panels)* illustrating how different E wave velocities compared to expected values aid in the interpretation of LV filling patterns, some of which might be misdiagnosed by a simplified scheme of grading diastolic dysfunction by E/A wave ratio alone. All individuals had a LVOT velocity of approximately 1 m/sec. The last two subjects have mitral valve disease. The 35-year-old normal (Nl) has a mitral E wave/LVOT velocity ratio of 85%. This ratio is reduced to 50% in the second patient who has impaired LV relaxation (IR). The patient with PN filling has a normal appearing E/A wave ratio, but the E wave velocity of 1.2 m/sec is 20% higher than LVOT velocity indicating the increase in mean LA pressure. The next patient appears to have an IR filling pattern with an E/A wave ratio less than 1, but really has a PN pattern variant (PN-V) caused by the partial fusion of early and late diastolic filling. PN abnormalities present include an E wave velocity elevated at 1 m/sec and an A wave that would be much smaller (with a higher E/A ratio) if the heart rate was slower and atrial contraction had occurred after the mitral flow velocity had fallen below 20 cm/sec. The next patient has a dilated cardiomyopathy and RST filling with a short mitral DT (130 msec) and diminished atrial contribution. The last two patients have an increased E wave velocity due to mitral valve disease. The sixth has severe MR with an E wave of 1.4 m/sec, 40% higher than LVOT velocity. A shorter than expected mitral DT (170 msec) indicates reduced LV compliance, in this case from CAD and diabetes. The last patient has rheumatic MS, a high E wave velocity, increased mean gradient, and prolonged pressure half-time.

- Mitral DT has consistently been a major prognostic factor in patients with both HFrEF and HFpEF because it represents an advanced stage of disease, which is often irreversible.

Mitral Flow Velocity at the Start of Atrial Contraction (E/A Wave or Pre-A Velocity)

This value (see Fig. 9.1), rarely measured or even considered, is important because it affects peak mitral A wave velocity, mitral E/A wave ratio, and mitral A wave duration. Therefore we encourage its routine measurements along with the other mitral flow velocity variables to improve the accuracy of assessing LV diastolic function.

In normal individuals the heart rate at rest is slow enough to keep this velocity at less than 20 cm/sec. This maximizes early and mid-diastolic ventricular filling and minimizes the proportion of filling associated with the booster pump function of atrial contraction. With exercise, fusion of early and late diastolic filling will occur, but only at relatively rapid heart rates because of the mitigating effects of shortening of the PR interval and faster LV relaxation (see Fig. 9.4).

If mitral flow velocity does not have sufficient time to fall below 20 cm/sec before atrial contraction, early and late diastolic filling (E and A waves) begin to merge (Fig. 9.13). This decreases filling efficiency and may increase the workload and size of the left atrium. The fusion of early and late diastolic filling most often occurs when the heart rate is too fast for a diastolic filling period that is shortened by impaired LV relaxation from LVH, a LBBB, or CAD. First-degree AV block may also cause mitral E and A wave fusion due to atrial contraction occurring too soon after ventricular systole. Depending on the physiology and ECG variables fusion of early and late diastolic filling can occur at heart rates as low as 70 to 80 bpm. In both cases the A velocity generated by atrial contraction added to a higher starting velocity will make peak A wave velocity higher than if no fusion were present, which decreases the E/A ratio reduced compared to if early and late diastolic filling were separated (see Fig. 9.13).

The consequences of resting or premature fusion of early and late diastolic filling are frequently a limited ability to increase mitral TVI (the LV stroke volume) and LV end-diastolic volume during exercise, with associated decrease in exercise capacity.[60,63] The ability to see if the resting heart rate is well matched to the E and A wave filling pattern in individual patients is one of great strengths of echo Doppler technique that cannot be determined by physical exam. If possible, altering

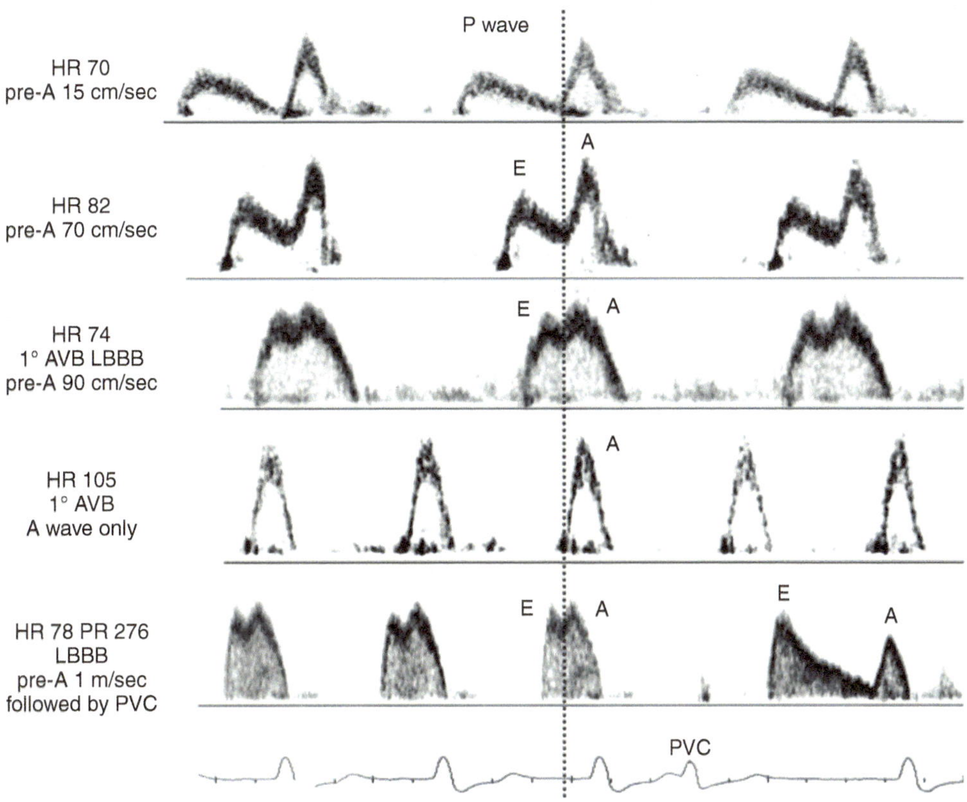

Fig. 9.13 Variable mitral E wave velocity at the start of atrial contraction (pre-A velocity, *dotted vertical line*) and how it affects the LV filling pattern and especially E/A wave ratio and A wave duration. PW Doppler recordings of mitral flow velocity in five separate patients are shown and referred to from top to bottom. The ECG at bottom relates to the final patient only. These fused patterns make assessment of diastolic dysfunction more challenging. Only the top patient with an IR mitral pattern has a pre-A velocity below 20 cm/sec, the cutoff value at which E/A ratio, peak A velocity, and A wave duration are unaffected by partial fusion of early and late diastolic LV filling. Patients 2 and 3 are in their 70s and have a history of hypertension. They have higher E wave velocities than expected for age, yet the high pre-A velocity increases the peak A wave velocity and makes the E/A ratio less than 1. Since the mitral TVI represents LV filling volume the higher pre-A also results in a larger A wave TVI and A wave duration. Slower heart rates would decrease peak A wave velocity and increase the E/A wave ratio. Patient 4 has sinus tachycardia so that only an A wave is present. The A wave velocity is high (1.6 m/sec) because all LV filling must occur during the PR interval. Finally, patient 5 shows how after a PVC and compensatory pause, the longer R-R interval markedly changes the LV filling pattern.

the heart rate to restore a normal separation between early and late diastolic filling frequently improves patient symptoms and exercise capacity.

- In patients whose atrial contraction occurs when the mitral velocity decay is still above 20 cm/sec the A wave is larger than if diastole was longer, and the E/A wave ratio will then be reduced.
- This is a common pitfall seen in elderly patients with HFpEF and short diastolic filling periods.
- The resultant E/A ratio is less than 1 and is then thought to represent IR filling when other variables clearly indicate LA pressure is elevated.

Peak Mitral A Wave Velocity

The mitral A wave velocity is determined by the late diastolic TMPG (see Fig. 9.3) and varies from 50 cm/sec in younger individuals to 75 cm/sec in normals over 60 years of age (see Table 9.1). In patients with IR filling and reduced E wave velocity an increased A wave velocity and TVI are expected and necessary to maintain a normal LV end-diastolic volume and cardiac output. When LV relaxation is slowed, the reduced filling in early diastole results in less LV pressure increase after LV minimum pressure, so that the atrium contracts into a relatively low-pressure, compliant chamber. By 2-D echo, the left atrium is usually normal in size and appears hypercontractile with exaggerated annular movement superiorly toward the pulmonary veins. The A wave peak velocity is increased, the A wave TVI is relatively large, and the flow duration is increased (usually >140 msec). If A wave velocity is above 1 m/sec or the atrial deceleration time unusually short (<110 msec), this may indicate a decrease in late diastolic LV chamber compliance and increase in LV end-diastolic pressure as long as a short PR interval is not present.

- A large mitral A wave with long duration (>140 msec) is often a compensatory mechanism for reduced E wave flow in early diastole that helps preserve a normal LV end-diastolic volume.

Mitral A Wave Duration

The importance of mitral A wave duration is what it reveals about late diastolic LV compliance. It is best used in comparison with pulmonary venous A wave duration. Like all mitral variables, A wave duration varies with age in normals, being about 120 msec in the young and 140 msec in individuals over 60 years (see Table 9.1). In general, when viewed in patients with CV disease, the longer the mitral A wave duration the more likely filling pressures are normal, while a shortened A wave duration indicates increased LV end-diastolic pressure.

Mitral A wave duration, like peak A wave velocity, is determined by the TMPG at atrial contraction (Fig. 9.14). Under normal circumstances the pressure increase in the atrium is larger than the ventricle. In pseudonormal or RST LV filling patterns, the mitral A wave duration is shortened because the reduced LV compliance results in an excessive rise in LV pressure with atrial contraction, which abruptly terminates transmitral flow.[76] The reduced time of a positive TMPG is indicated by a shorter mitral A wave duration, whose deceleration time is shorter than acceleration time.[77] When a normal PR interval is present, a mitral A wave duration that stops before the peak QRS complex indicates that the pressure rise in the ventricle at atrial contraction terminated mitral flow rather than ventricular contraction, a reliable sign that an elevated LV EDP is present[76] (Fig. 9.16).

Conditions that affect mitral A wave duration and make it more difficult for use in assisting the evaluation of LV diastolic function include partial fusion of early and late diastolic filling[78] (see Fig. 9.13), variation in cardiac cycle length due to sinus arrhythmia, premature atrial or ventricular beats, second-degree or third-degree AV block, or a short (<120 msec) PR interval. Longer cycles result in more mid-diastolic LV filling and pressure increase so that when the atrium finally contracts, A-wave velocity, velocity integral, and duration may be reduced. Conversely, shorter R-R intervals result in longer A wave durations. A short PR interval (<120 ms) will have a reduced A wave duration because the rise in LV pressure soon after atrial contraction will result in mitral valve closure and abrupt termination of A wave flow. Advanced degrees of heart block continually change the relation between early and late diastolic filling so that virtually every A wave has a different velocity and duration.

Observing changes in A wave duration over time, or after changes in loading conditions or medical therapy (see Fig. 9.14), may confirm that LV diastolic function is improving more easily than examining other Doppler variables. For instance, in patients with hypertensive heart disease and an impaired LV relaxation filling pattern, a lengthening of A wave duration after medical therapy is helpful in confirming if an increase in peak E wave velocity represents improved LV relaxation versus increased left atrial pressure.[79]

- The A wave duration reflects the relation between the amount of late diastolic filling and LA and LV pressure rise.
- A short A wave duration (<120 msec) suggests an abnormal rise in LV pressure with A wave filling that terminates forward A wave flow.
- If the PR interval is normal, termination of the mitral A wave before peak QRS is an indication of an increased LV EDP.

PULMONARY VENOUS FLOW VELOCITY

Pulmonary venous flow velocity, usually obtained with PW Doppler from the right upper pulmonary vein during transthoracic apical imaging, reflects the filling dynamics of the left atrium. With experience, high-quality PW Doppler transthoracic recordings can be obtained in approximately 85% to 90% of patients.[52] Within a short time after mitral flow velocity patterns were correlated with hemodynamics, it became apparent that pulmonary venous flow velocity could be of additional help in assessing LV filling patterns,[26] especially IR filling with increased LV EDP and pseudonormal LV filling.[80–83] While there are now several additional echo Doppler variables to help identify pseudonormal filling (LA size, CMM inflow propagation velocity, mitral annular TDI), PV flow velocity analysis remains unique and indispensable to identify an abnormal increase in LV pressure at atrial contraction and prognosis in patients with pseudonormal filling patterns.

The various components of PV flow velocity change with age, mitral flow velocity, and disease states and can be matched to their corresponding mitral Doppler patterns (see Fig. 9.5). The hemodynamic determinants of PV flow velocity have been studied in vivo[83–86] and clinically[26,87–89] and related to individual variables (Fig. 9.15). These include peak forward flow velocity in early systole (PVs1), late systole (PVs2), early diastole (PVd), and peak reverse flow velocity at atrial contraction (PVa), and its duration (PVa dur). A dip or notch between PVs1 and PVs2 in early LV systole represents the C wave seen in LA pressure recordings at the time of mitral valve closure. PVs1 blends with PVs2 velocity, and this notch is not distinctly seen in about 70% of transthoracic flow velocity recordings[52] but is observed in virtually all transesophageal echocardiography (TEE) recordings in patients in sinus rhythm.[88,89]

PVs1 occurs in early ventricular systole as a result of LA relaxation and a decrease in downstream LA pressure at a time when PV pressure is relatively constant.[85] PVs2 peaks later in systole and is due to the increase in PV flow and pressure that results from systolic RV stroke volume. Maximal PVs2 velocity, its TVI, and deceleration of flow reflect the pressure difference between PV and downstream LA pressure as blood fills both vascular systems. Pulmonary venous diastolic flow velocity (PVd) initially follows early diastolic mitral flow velocity, but in mid-diastole LV filling slows, while PVd flow continues with ongoing

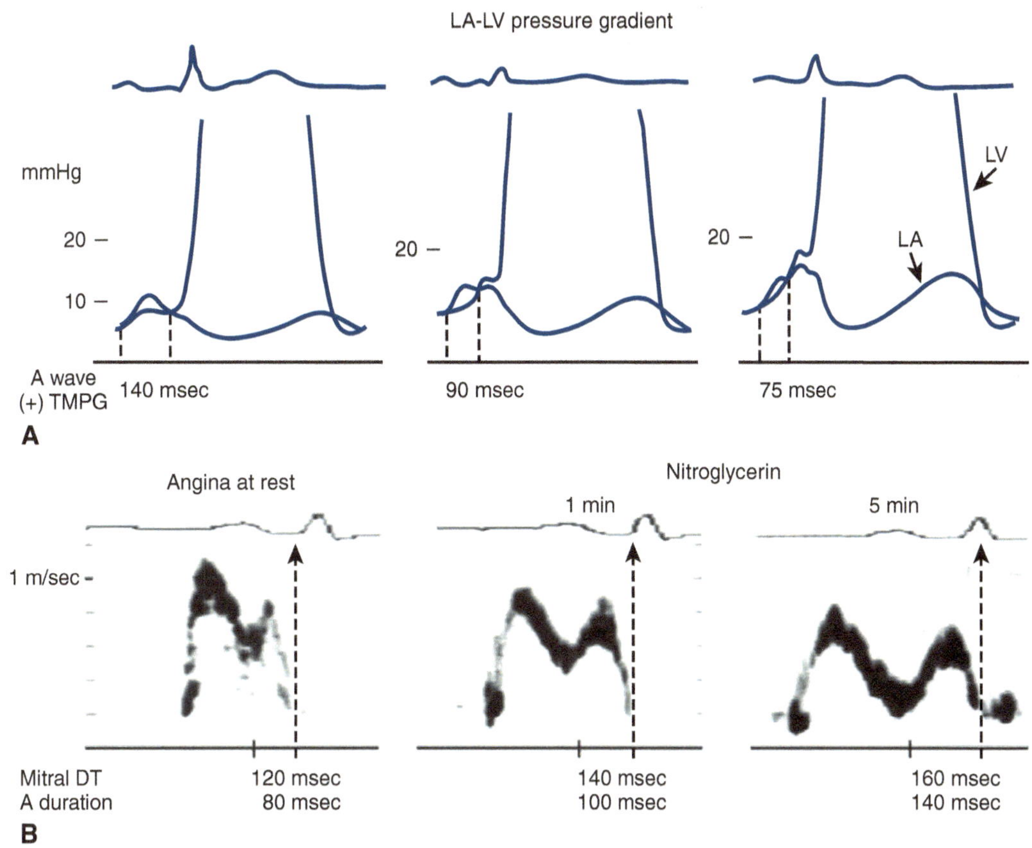

Fig. 9.14 The hemodynamic determinants of peak mitral A wave velocity and duration (A), and an example of their dynamic variation in a patient with rest angina treated with sublingual nitroglycerin therapy (B). In (A) high-fidelity recordings of LV and LA pressure show the positive late diastolic TMPG associated with LA contraction *(dotted lines)* in three individuals (0). In the normal subject *(left)* LA pressure rise at atrial contraction exceeds that seen in the ventricle so that the positive (+) A wave TMPG goes on until LA pressure falls below LV pressure during atrial relaxation. The patient in the middle panel has a decrease in LV compliance. The maximal LA-LV pressure gradient at atrial contraction is approximately the same, but the rise in LV pressure exceeds LA pressure at 90 msec, shortening the (+) A wave TMPG and A wave duration but not its peak velocity. The patient on the right has a marked decrease in LV compliance. LV pressure increases rapidly after LA contraction so the maximum (+) TMPG and duration is further shortened resulting in a lower peak A wave velocity with a shorter duration. The patient at the bottom is having angina at rest. The PW mitral flow velocity showing a high E wave velocity, a short, restrictive-like mitral DT, and a low A wave velocity and duration, which are partially masked by some fusion of early and late diastolic filling (velocity at the start of atrial contraction >20 cm/sec). One minute after taking sublingual nitroglycerine LV hemodynamics are improving as evidenced by a longer diastolic filling period, lower E wave velocity, longer mitral DT, and wider A wave duration. By 5 minutes the improvement in mitral filling variables are even more obvious.

LA enlargement. Pulmonary venous flow reversal due to atrial contraction (PVa) is determined by LA contractility and LV compliance, with more and longer reverse flow seen as LV compliance decreases.

Changes in PV flow velocity and their relation to LV compliance and LA pressures are shown in Fig. 9.16. In patients with IR filling, decreased LV compliance and normal mean LA pressure, early diastolic filling (mitral E wave) is reduced. In these cases, LA hypertrophy provides a sufficient atrial kick to fill the LV to its optimal end-diastolic volume. An important benefit of LA hypertrophy is that it confines the abnormal pressure rise in atrium, ventricle, and pulmonary veins to the short period associated with atrial contraction so that mean LA pressure remains normal (see Fig. 9.12). PVs1 is increased so the PV systolic to diastolic flow velocity ratio remains above 50%. If LV compliance decreases further, the atrium may begin to decompensate, enlarge, and have contractile dysfunction. A reduced systolic fraction of PV antegrade flow (<40%) indicates LA systolic dysfunction (decline in PVs1) and has a high specificity for an increased mean LA pressure[27,89] (see Fig. 9.16). In addition, regardless of LVEF, adult cardiac patients with a pseudonormal or RST filling pattern who have blunted peak systolic flow velocity that decreases below peak PVd flow velocity have a marked increase in mortality compared to patients who have PVs flow velocity dominance[90,91] (Fig. 9.17). Pulmonary venous A wave and its relation to mitral A wave duration are of special importance in diagnosing an abnormal rise in LV pressure at atrial contraction, as discussed in detail later in the chapter.

- PVs flow velocity occurs when the mitral valve is closed and therefore reflects the PV-LA pressure gradient during this time.
- PVs flow has an early component due to atrial relaxation and a later component due to LV systole. Both events decrease LA pressure, which increases the PV-LA pressure gradient.
- Adults with well-compensated heart disease have a PVs > PVd velocity.
- With LA or LV systolic failure, systolic LA pressure fall is reduced so that PVs flow becomes blunted.

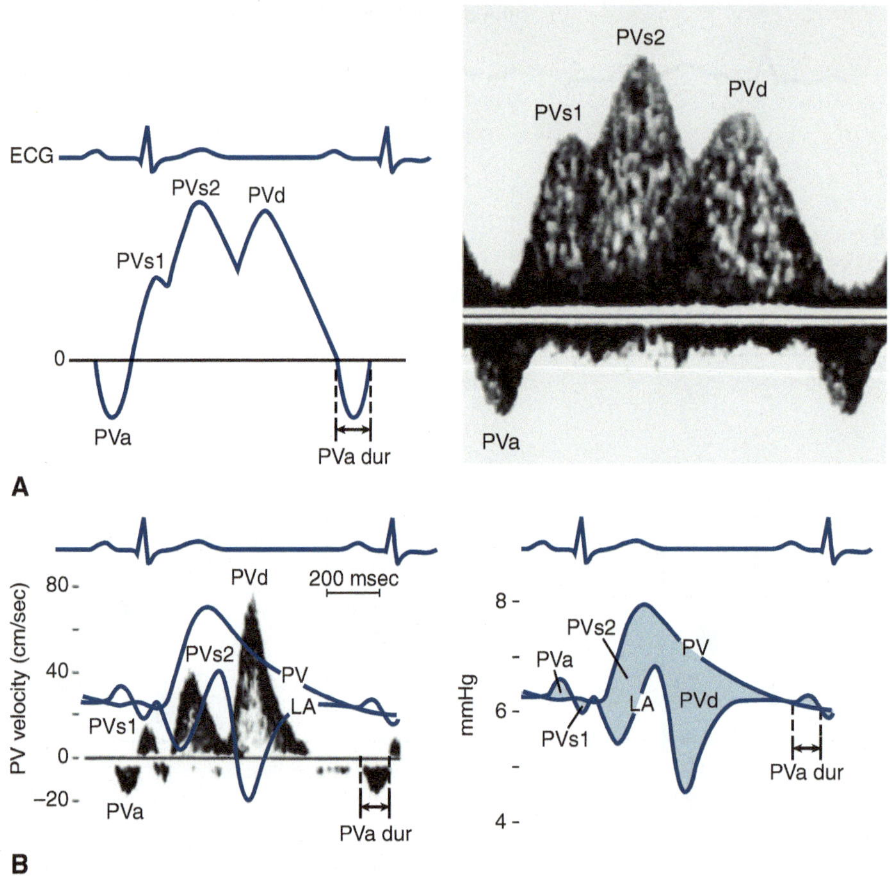

Fig. 9.15 (A) Pulmonary venous variables obtained with the pulse wave Doppler technique include peak flow velocity and early systole (PVs1), late systole (PVs2), and early diastole (PVd), peak reverse flow velocity (PVa), and its duration (PVa dur) at atrial contraction. (B) The left panel shows simultaneously recording of pulmonary venous flow velocity together with pulmonary venous (PV) and left atrial (LA) pressures. The right panel is a schematic drawing of PV and LA pressures showing the different hemodynamic pressure gradients *(hatched areas)* that determine the four individual pulmonary venous flow velocity components. These components are described in the text.

- This blunting of PVs flow is one of the best signs of an elevated LA pressure in cardiac patients in normal sinus rhythm.
- In patients with a pseudonormal filling pattern, PVs dominance means the LA remains well compensated despite the elevated LA pressure, and the prognosis is nearly the same as an IR filling pattern.
- With pseudonormal filling and a blunted PVs < PVd velocity, the prognosis is poor and nearly equal to that of a RST filling pattern.

Relation of Mitral to Pulmonary Venous A Wave Duration and Termination

When both A wave flow velocity durations are accurately recorded, this relation is an important indication of LV A wave pressure increase and LV end-diastolic pressure,[80–82,92,93] even in the pediatric age group.[94] Laboratories that do not routinely record pulmonary venous flow velocity will miss the unique aspects of this derived variable. Unlike other Doppler variables the relation is independent of age, meaning that mitral A wave duration remains equal to or longer than pulmonary venous A wave (PVa) duration throughout life in normal individuals. Secondly, this time interval relation is our only echo Doppler variable that directly relates to the rise in LV pressure at atrial contraction (Fig. 9.20), thereby separating patients with impaired relaxation that have normal filling pressures from those who have an increased LV EDP (>12 mmHg), the first hemodynamic abnormality seen with diastolic dysfunction (see Fig. 9.12) and one that confers increased future CV risk even in asymptomatic patients.

Under normal circumstances, when the left atrium contracts, the net volume and duration of flow should be greater forward into the left ventricle than backward into the pulmonary veins. If PVa is either increased in velocity (>35 cm/sec) or duration (>30 msec longer than mitral A wave), LV A wave pressure is increased and LV EDP is elevated. Even in cases where the atrium is enlarged, markedly hypokinetic, and failing, the pulmonary venous A wave duration of reverse flow continues to be longer than the abbreviated mitral A wave inflow duration (see Fig. 9.17). The uncertainty of accuracy of a PVa measurement by transthoracic echocardiography (TTE) has contributed to the greater than 30-msec longer duration cutoff, as it is likely PV flow duration is abnormal if it exceeds that of the mitral A wave by any amount.[85] When the pulmonary venous A wave duration is difficult to measure by TTE due to a suboptimal recording, referencing the end of both A wave flows to the QRS complex is then helpful and frequently easier to see if PVa duration is prolonged compared to the mitral A wave, which indicates EDP is elevated. The start of PVs is a surrogate for the end of the PVa reversal, as the two flows are continuous, and is often an easier way to decide where the PVa reversal ends, which then can be compared to the end of mitral A wave flow in relation to the ECG recording. A detailed guide to obtaining high-quality PW Doppler pulmonary venous flow velocity recordings has been published.[52]

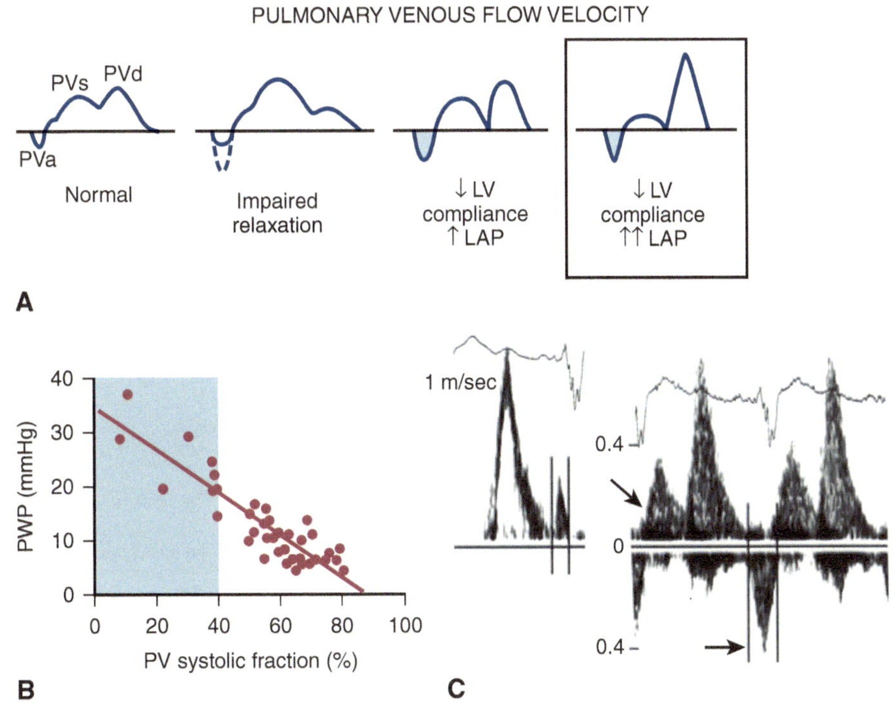

Fig. 9.16 (Top) Pulmonary venous (PV) flow velocity patterns obtained with PW Doppler from normal to most abnormal *(left to right)*. With impaired relaxation the proportion of PV systolic flow (PVs) increases as PV diastolic flow (PVd) decreases, paralleling the decrease in mitral E wave velocity. Reverse flow back into the pulmonary veins with atrial contraction (PVa) is variable, being increased in velocity (>30 cm/sec) and duration (>30 msec greater than mitral A wave duration) if LV end-diastolic pressure is elevated. As LV compliance decreases and LA pressure (LAP) increases the proportion of PVs flow decreases. At the same time PVd and E wave velocity increase with PN and RST LV filling being seen. All mitral and their corresponding PV patterns are shown together in Fig. 6. (Bottom left) The relation of pulmonary venous systolic fraction (in % of total forward flow) to pulmonary wedge pressure (PWP). When PVs is less than 40% in a patient with heart disease PWP is elevated. (Bottom right) PW Doppler mitral and pulmonary venous flow velocity in a patient with PN to RST filling who has an enlarged left atrium whose contractile function is failing. PVs is decreased with a systolic fraction less than 40%, PVd is increased, and the velocity and duration of PVa exceed that of the mitral A wave.

The interpretation of mitral versus pulmonary venous A wave duration may not be reliable if the mitral velocity at the start of atrial contraction is greater than 20 cm/sec[89] or if atrial contraction occurs when PVd has not fallen to the zero velocity baseline.[49] In the first case, the peak mitral A wave velocity, TVI, and A wave duration are longer than normal to accommodate the increased atrial stroke volume that is present, and in the latter the PV A wave duration is shorter because it started above the conventional measuring point of the zero velocity baseline.

- With LA contraction, flow duration forward into the left ventricle should be the same or longer than flow backward into the pulmonary vein at all ages.
- When flow backward into the pulmonary vein is longer than forward, an abnormal rise in LV pressure occurred shortening the mitral A wave duration, which indicates LV EDP is elevated.
- This is the first hemodynamic abnormality that occurs with diastolic dysfunction and can only be diagnosed by comparing the mitral and PV A wave durations.
- When PVa is difficult to measure, the ending of mitral and PVa flow referenced to the QRS can be used to obtain the same information.

E/A Wave Ratio

The E/A wave ratio has been the single most important variable used to help characterize the overall mitral flow velocity pattern[47–49,67,95–98] and define diastolic function patient groups in previous research studies[68,99] (see Figs. 9.7 and 9.9). In patients with systolic HF the E/A ratio is related to filling pressures and prognosis. While this diastolic function evaluation by E/A ratio pattern recognition is quick and has yielded useful data, using it without consideration of the individual variables for mitral velocities described earlier, other 2-D findings, and ancillary Doppler variables may lead to misinterpretation of LV diastolic function and filling pressures. The E/A ratio is most helpful when the mitral DT is linear and pre-A velocity is below 20 cm/sec. If mitral DT is curved, biphasic, or if there is partial fusion of E and A wave velocities, then the LV filling pattern needs a careful assessment in relation to the other echo Doppler findings and variables.

ANCILLARY DATA THAT HELPS THE INTERPRETATION OF MITRAL FLOW VELOCITY PATTERNS

M Mode and 2-D Echocardiography

There is considerable information about LV diastolic function and filling pressures available from M mode and 2-D cardiac ultrasound recordings to complement Doppler variables.[5,100] With practice, the visual interpretation of these anatomic findings will usually suggest what Doppler LV filling patterns are present. From the parasternal long axis view, observing the movement at the atrioventricular groove helps

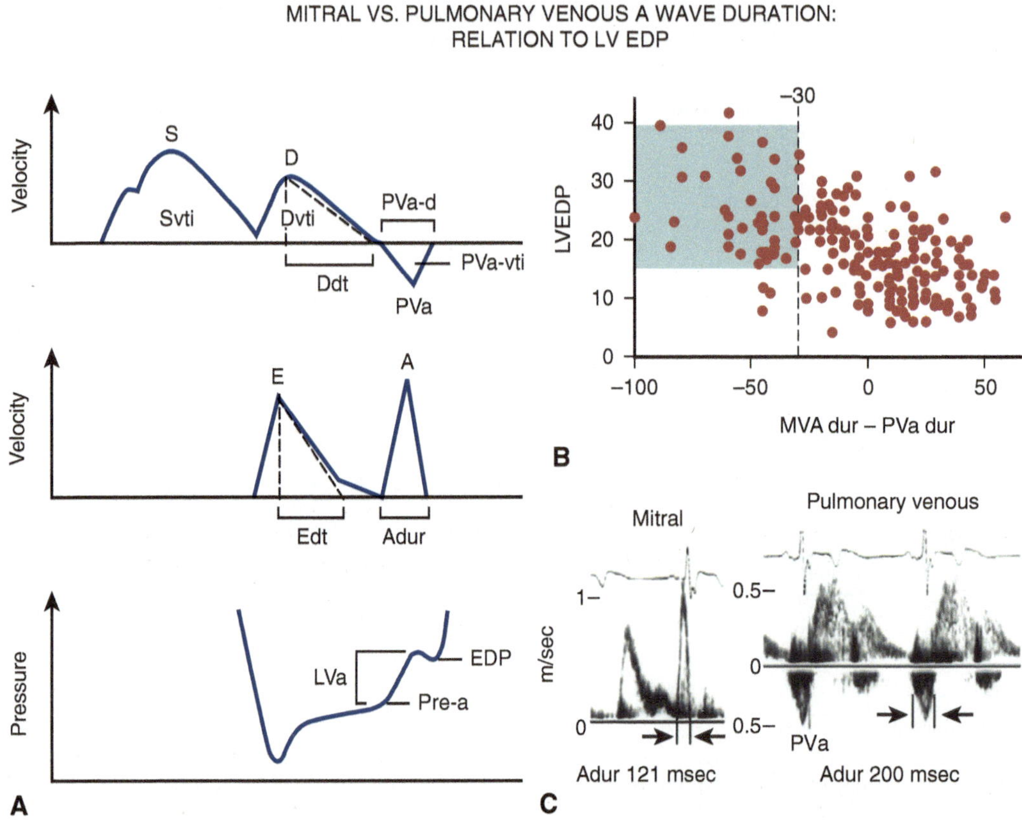

Fig. 9.17 (A) Schematic diagram of the relation of PV and mitral flow velocity A wave duration, which relates to the LV pressure rise at atrial contraction (LVa). The graph combines Doppler data from three separate studies and shows that when the reverse duration of PV compared to mitral A wave flow exceeds 30 msec, LV end-diastolic pressure is usually above 15 mmHg (B). (C) PW Doppler mitral and PV flow velocity from a patient with LV hypertrophy and IR filling. The mitral A wave duration is 121 msec and PV A wave duration 200 msec so that flow backwards into the pulmonary vein continues for 80 msec after flow into the LV stops. This indicates LV A wave pressure increases and LV EDP is elevated.

identify the cardiac rhythm, LA size, and contractility. In the parasternal short axis, the normal left atrium appears approximately the same size or slightly larger than the aorta. From apical views the sizes of both atria in relation to their respective ventricles can be made, as well as comparing the size and contractility of each other. Differences are usually obvious. A normal-sized left atrium that appears hypercontractile indicates reduced LV filling in early diastole, increased filling at atrial contraction, and an IR pattern. LA enlargement and reduced contractility are often associated with elevated pressures and pseudonormal or RST mitral filling patterns as long as there have been no recent atrial arrhythmias. At the same time, noting asymmetry in the rate of LV and RV contractility and relaxation, and the excursion of AV longitudinal plane movement, often indicates the abnormalities of ventricular diastolic filling that will be seen on Doppler exam.

Left ventricular hypertrophy slows LV relaxation independent of other cardiac abnormalities and results in an impaired relaxation that is often obvious in M mode LV recordings (see Fig. 9.18). In the absence of MR, arrhythmias, or cardiac conduction system disease, LA enlargement usually indicates an elevated mean LA pressure associated with pseudonormal and restrictive mitral flow velocity patterns.[93,99,101] Because maximal LA volume is strongly associated with adverse cardiac events such as new onset Afib, congestive HF, and stroke[99,101–103] we agree that it should be measured according to American Society of Echocardiography (ASE)/European Society of Cardiology (ESC) guidelines[104] in all patients. Conversely, normal LA size suggests mean LA pressure is normal. LA minimum volume is related to pulmonary wedge pressure with a correlation coefficient equal to that of most other Doppler variables.[93]

- The M mode of LV wall motion in diastole is an easy way to assess LV relaxation.
- An enlarged LA, out of proportion to the other cardiac chambers, may indicate elevated pressure and is associated with increased risk for future Afib and HF.

Tricuspid Flow Velocity

Tricuspid and mitral flow velocity patterns are normally qualitatively similar, and with RV pathology the alterations are similar to those seen on the left side of the heart. Tricuspid valve opening normally occurs before mitral valve opening, which is easily assessed visually from the stand apical four-chamber view. If mitral valve opening occurs at the same time, or before tricuspid opening, this is abnormal and reflects altered physiology that needs investigation. Since the tricuspid leaflet orifice is larger, tricuspid velocities are slightly lower. Tricuspid flow velocity increases significantly with respiration; this aspect, which differs from left heart filling, will be discussed in the section on assessing RV diastolic function.

Normally, mitral and tricuspid inflow patterns appear similar. Significant differences between the two indicate cardiac pathology is present. Since most cardiac diseases affect the left heart, the more abnormal filling pattern is usually seen in LV filling, although the right heart is also affected through the involvement of the intraventricular septum. For instance, in an individual with an ischemic

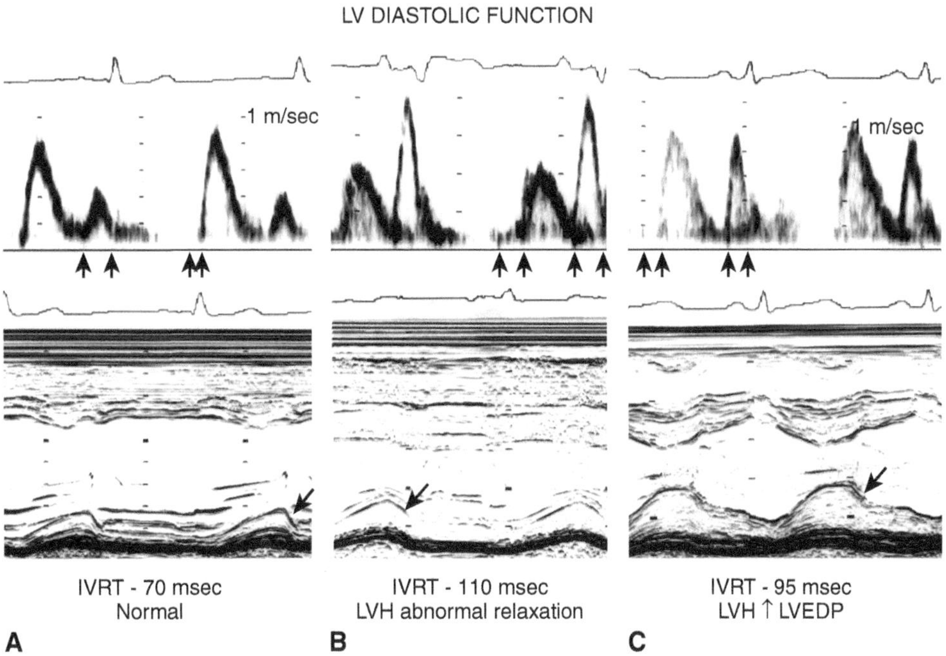

Fig. 9.18 PW mitral flow velocity together with M mode recordings of the LV cavity in three individuals illustrating how the diastolic wall motion helps in interpreting the LV filling pattern. Compared to the normal subject *(left)* the patient in the middle panel with LVH has IR filling. Their longer IVRT and reduced E wave velocity matches the slower rate of early diastolic LV filling seen in the LV posterior wall *(arrow)*. The patient on the right has a mitral pattern, which may be difficult to interpret without additional data. However, the M mode recording shows marked LVH, very delayed early diastolic filling with relaxation, and mid-diastolic LV cavity expansion continuing to occur up to the time of atrial contraction. These findings, along with the increased E wave velocity (1m/sec) indicate PN LV filling and moderate diastolic dysfunction.

cardiomyopathy who has a pseudonormal LV filling pattern, the tricuspid filling often lags behind showing an IR pattern.

Tissue Doppler Imaging of Mitral Annular Motion

This recently developed ultrasound imaging modality discussed in detail in Chapter 10 has underlying physics and principles similar to those of conventional PW spectral Doppler. From the apical views the velocities are related to LV contraction and relaxation. In interpreting LV filling patterns TDI MAM has its greatest use in distinguishing normal and pseudonormal LV filling. The ratio peak mitral E wave velocity to MAM e′ velocity is used to estimate mean LA pressure.[80,105]

The normal diastolic velocity pattern of MAM obtained from TDI is similar to that of transmitral flow in patients in sinus rhythm, except inverted.[39,104–111] There is positive (above the zero velocity baseline) movement toward the apex with systolic contraction and negative movement back toward the pulmonary veins with LV filling in early (e′) and late diastole (a′). In patients with normal ventricular diastolic function the e′/a′ and mitral E/A flow velocity wave ratios are similar. Patients with IR filling have a MAM e′/a′ ratio less than 1, again mirroring the findings seen with mitral flow velocity. However, in pseudonormal mitral flow velocity patterns, a MAM e′/a′ ratio less than 1, rather than more than 1, is present, reflecting the impaired LV relaxation that separates these patients from true normals. This is similar to the relaxation abnormality seen in the myocardial M mode in Fig. 9.19 despite the normal appearing Doppler LV filling pattern. With RST LV filling the e′/a′ ratio frequently is greater than 1 because the majority of filling occurs in early diastole with little contribution due to atrial contraction. Fig. 9.19 shows a schematic diagram of abnormal LV filling patterns together with TDI MAM and pulmonary venous flow velocity patterns for reference.

The interpretation of TDI MAM is enhanced by an awareness of the factors that influence these annular movements. The e′/a′ ratio is higher in the lateral as compared to the septal annulus because the septal is tethered to the right ventricle and other structures in the middle of the heart. The e′ diastolic annular movement predominates in normals because LV longitudinal movement at the base in both systole and diastole is greater than displacement in a radial direction. In patients with a normal LVEF and pseudonormal filling, a reduced e′ is present because LVH causes an increase in systolic radial movement that is reversed (outward LV motion) in early diastole. The e′/a′ ratio will be less abnormal if there is another reason for the reduced LV compliance than LVH or if the LVEF is decreased. Regardless of LVH a large volume of blood flow across the mitral valve in early diastole due to MR will fill the ventricle and increase upward annular movement and e′ velocity.

- DTI MAM is a widely accepted part of modern diastolic function exams that has often replaced other Doppler variables.
- Comparing the DTI MAM pattern of e′/a′ to mitral E and A wave pattern helps distinguish pseudonormal from normal LV filling patterns.
- The commonly used E/e′ ratio, when elevated, has been found to be a powerful predictor of adverse outcomes in large studies in cardiac patients.
- However, the use of E/e′ ratio in individual patients for predicting filling pressures is less useful than commonly believed because of a lack of sensitivity and specificity.

Exercise as a Diastolic Stress Test

As shown in Fig. 9.4, impaired relaxation reduces the time available for diastolic filling and myocardial perfusion. With the increase in heart rate with exercise, some individuals with LVH, LV systolic dysfunction

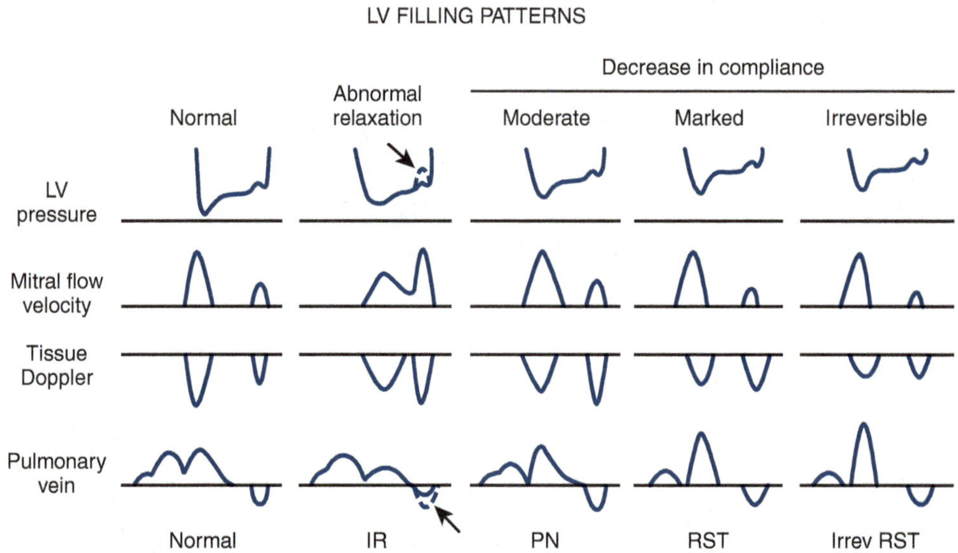

Fig. 9.19 Schematic diagram showing the correlation of tissue Doppler imaging (TDI) recordings of the mitral annulus with normal and abnormal LV filling patterns. TDI is especially helpful in distinguishing Nl from PN LV filling. Also shown are corresponding LV pressures, abnormal diastolic properties, and PV flow velocity. Note that in Nl filling the mitral and TDI patterns are inverted but similar in terms of early and late diastolic ratios. In contrast, PN filling has a markedly disparate TDI with reduced longitudinal movement in early diastole and increased movement at atrial contraction. In IR filling the arrows in LV pressure and pulmonary venous flow refer to patients with decreased LV compliance in late diastole who have an increase in LV end-diastolic pressure. *IR,* Impaired relaxation; *Irrev RST,* irreversibly restrictive; *Nl,* normal; *PN,* pseudonormal; *RST,* restrictive.

of cardiac conduction system disease, and IR filling may have premature fusion of early and late diastolic filling and be unable to increase LV end-diastolic volume normally so that a limitation in cardiac output occurs[60,63] (Fig. 9.20). Complaints of a reduced aerobic capacity with exertional dyspnea are common. Patients with pseudonormal and RST filling patterns also have a significant decrease in exercise capacity. However, in these individuals it is the increase in mean LA pressure due to reduced LV compliance that limits exercise rather than a blunted increase in LV end-diastolic volume.

In patients presenting with exertional dyspnea, examining changes in the ratio of mitral E wave and TDI e′ velocity at rest and exercise has been proposed as a diastolic stress.[112] Using supine bicycle exercise and classifying patients by E/e′ above 10, exercise duration was significantly longer in patients whose E/e′ ratios were 10 or less and did not increase with exercise. These preliminary results suggest the hemodynamic consequences of exercise-induced increase in diastolic filling pressure may be possible noninvasively with exercise Doppler echocardiography, an area that needs further study that includes more diastolic variables.

Pulmonary Artery Pressures

The estimation of PA systolic and diastolic pressures is a valuable adjunct to assessing LV filling patterns. Using the modified Bernoulli equation, this can be accomplished in a high percentage of patients with right-sided valvular regurgitation. The velocity of pulmonary regurgitation at end diastole together with an estimate of central venous pressure at the same time (physical exam, inferior vena cava [IVC] size and degree of respiratory collapse, hepatic venous Doppler pattern) is used to estimate PA end-diastolic pressure. In the absence of pulmonary vascular disease this is a surrogate estimate of mean LA pressure. Similarly, peak TR velocity together with central venous pressure at the same time during systole (again best evaluated by the HV = hepatic vein or hepatic venous [HV] Doppler pattern) helps estimate PA systolic pressure.

Patients with IR LV filling are expected to have normal or at worst borderline increases in PA pressure in the absence of pulmonary parenchymal or vascular disease. Pseudonormal filling is associated with elevated mean LA pressure and so PA pressures are passively elevated, usually in the range of 30 to 45 mmHg. With the higher left heart pressures seen in RST filling, PA systolic pressure can be quite elevated, in the range of 50 to 70 mmHg.

PERFORMING AN ECHO DOPPLER EVALUATION OF LV DIASTOLIC FUNCTION

The assessment of LV diastolic function requires high-quality 2-D images and Doppler recordings of mitral, pulmonary venous, and TDI flow velocities. Guides for optimizing these recordings and avoiding pitfalls with many examples are available.[110] Techniques for optimizing CMM mitral inflow velocity propagation and TDI of the mitral annulus are also covered in chapters in this book on these techniques.

Organizing an echo Doppler assessment of LV diastolic function into a standard routine helps both the sonographer and the physician improve their technical and interpretative skills.[62,113–115] We recommend starting with M mode and 2-D anatomic imaging to obtain measurements of chamber sizes, maximal LA volume, and LV diastolic and systolic volumes. LV mass, relative wall thickness,[116] and LVEF are then calculated. The measurement techniques and normal values are published regularly in ASE standardized guidelines. Variables of special importance include LV absolute mass and relative wall thickness, and maximal LA size (normal <32 mL/m^2).

After the 2-D exam is finished, an apical four-chamber color Doppler screen is performed to check for significant valvular regurgitation. CMM of mitral inflow and LV outflow is then used to preview the LV filling pattern, mitral E wave flow velocity propagation, and whether systolic LV intracavitary gradients or IVRT flow is present. Continuous wave Doppler is activated to profile the LV filling and

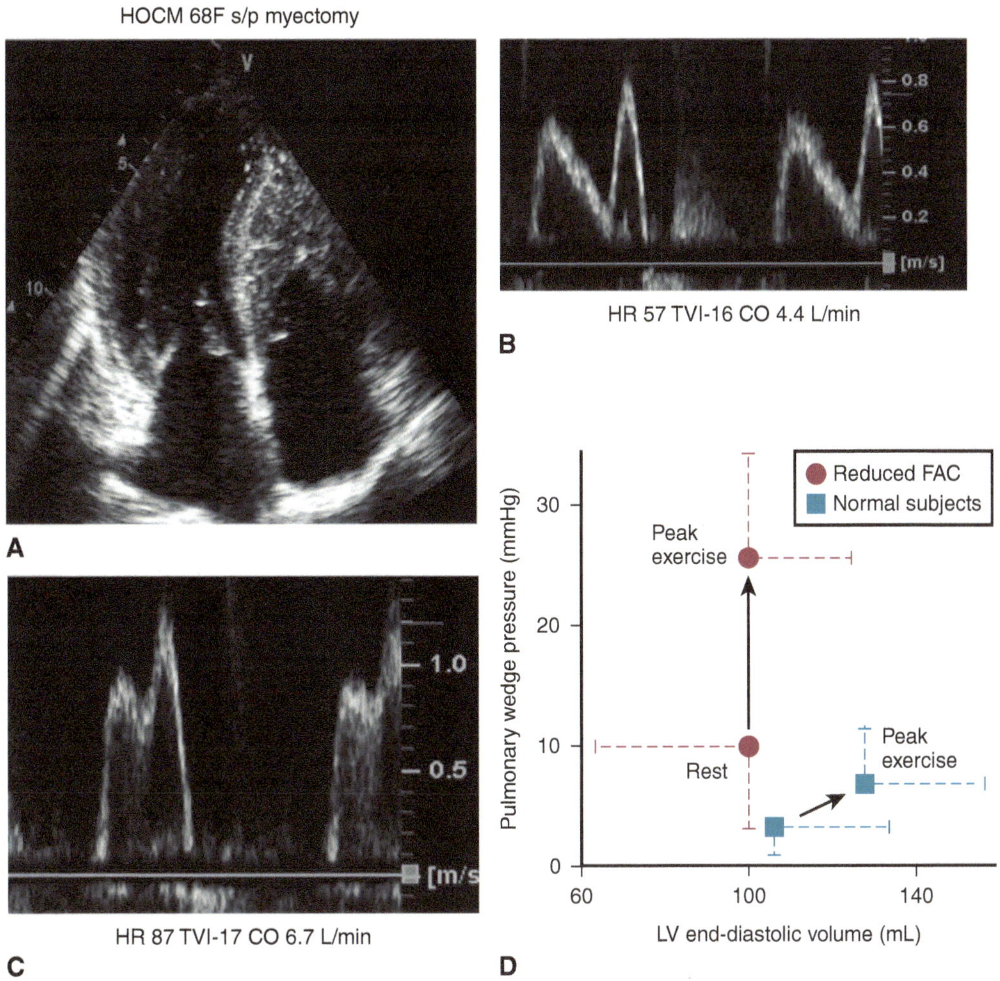

Fig. 9.20 An example of a patient with a reduced functional aerobic capacity due to markedly impaired LV relaxation and a LBBB. The patient has hypertrophic obstructive cardiomyopathy (HOCM) and is status post septal myectomy with resultant gradient reduction and surgically induced LBBB. At rest an IR pattern is present *(lower left)*. With exercise *(lower right)* an increase in HR to only 87 bpm results in premature fusion of early and late diastolic filling with a minimal increase in mitral TVI. As shown in the graph the inadequate diastolic filling period blunts the normal increase in end-diastolic volume, reducing cardiac output while at the same time causing an increase in pulmonary congestion.

ejection velocities throughout the ventricle. CW technique is used before PW Doppler because it profiles the mitral inflow pattern, provides a reference for the peak E and A wave velocities that will be obtained during the subsequent PW Doppler interrogation, and displays IVRT flow and the magnitude of any systolic intracavitary gradients. PW Doppler mitral inflow velocity, mitral velocity response to Valsalva maneuver, and PW Doppler of pulmonary venous flow is then performed. If confusion still exists regarding the normalcy of LV filling pattern, TDI spectral Doppler of mitral annular motion (lateral, medial, or both) will usually help make this distinction and, together with peak mitral E wave velocity, may indicate whether normal or increased mean LA pressure is present. Before leaving the left side of the heart, any LV intracavitary gradients or IVRT flow seen on the CMM screen are located and quantified by PW Doppler. The transducer is then moved medially toward the sternum, and PW Doppler of tricuspid inflow along with estimation of PA systolic pressures using peak tricuspid regurgitant velocity by CW Doppler is performed. Finally, PW analysis of Doppler hepatic veins and superior vena cava (SVC) flow throughout respiration is recorded.[117]

With practice and performing a complete diastolic function exam on every patient, the components listed earlier can be completed with only an additional 5 to 10 minutes of scanning time. The information derived not only helps assess LV diastolic function, filling pressures, and future possible adverse CV events, but also aids patient management decisions.

MITRAL FLOW VELOCITY PATTERNS: INTERPRETIVE CHALLENGES

Mitral E/A Ratio

The most common mitral filling pattern is also the one most frequently underinterpreted or misinterpreted and therefore deserves special mention. The true IR filling pattern is due to slow LV relaxation with normal mean LA pressure. Criteria include normal LA volume, with hypercontractile-appearing LA systolic function (especially in the parasternal long axis view) due to ejection into a ventricle with a lower than normal pre-A pressure. Compared to normal age-related values the LV IVRT should be prolonged, mitral E wave velocity lower than expected for age and LVOT velocity, mitral DT prolonged, and the pre-A velocity less than 20 cm/sec. If the analysis stops here the interpretation is incomplete, for it has not been determined if LV end-diastolic compliance and pressure are normal or abnormal, the latter being the first indication of elevated LV filling pressures (see Fig. 9.12). This can only be determined by comparing the duration of mitral and pulmonary venous flow velocity A waves as previously described. If PVa duration is more than 30 msec longer than mitral A wave duration, then LV EDP is elevated and reduced LV compliance indicating early diastolic dysfunction is present (see Fig. 9.17).

There are two common instances where the E/A wave velocity ratio is less than 1, implying an IR filling pattern, and yet the diastolic abnormalities are more severe and closer to pseudonormal with decreased LV compliance and increased mean LA pressure. The first occurs when the mitral velocity at atrial contraction is more than 20 cm/sec and there is fusion of early and late diastolic LV filling (see Figs. 9.13). In this case the A wave velocity is higher than it would be at a slower heart rate or shorter PR interval, which reduces the E/A wave ratio to below 1. A premature beat or slower heart rate will reveal the pseudonormal filling pattern. An E/A ratio less than 1 with increased filling pressures can also be seen in patients with marked LVH and severely impaired LV relaxation. In these cases, a markedly elevated LA pressure may be needed before the filling pattern appears pseudonormal (see Fig. 9.8). In both instances the presence of moderate or severe LVH, increased LA volume, and E wave velocity that approaches or exceeds LVOT velocity are clues that despite the E/A wave ratio of less than 1 mean LA pressure is elevated.

Mitral Regurgitation and Stenosis

Hemodynamically significant MR will increase the volume returning through the mitral valve in early diastole and increase the mitral E wave velocity. Left atrial size and the mitral E wave/LVOT velocity ratio will both be increased. However, LV diastolic dysfunction and filling pressures are not necessarily abnormal since the normal adaptation of the left atrium and ventricle to chronic volume overload is a rightward shift in the P-V relation, which makes both chambers more compliant. A normal mitral DT is the best indicator of a healthy adaptation to the chronic volume overload of MR. Conversely, a shortened mitral DT indicates an abnormal rise in early diastolic LV pressure from reduced LV chamber compliance. This finding is expected in acute MR because of a lack of time for the ventricle to adapt, but in chronic regurgitation it signifies an increase in myocardial stiffness from a process unrelated to the valve disease. A shortened mitral IVRT, decrease in PV systolic fraction, and increase in TR velocity are other indicators of increased left heart filling pressures.

Mitral stenosis increases E wave velocity by reducing orifice size and is associated with a prolonged mitral pressure half-time as well as LA enlargement. Impaired LV relaxation may prolong the mitral DT, while reduced LV myocardial compliance may shorten it independent of valve area. When MS is present a clinically useful approach is to measure the LV IVRT (whose shortening indicates the degree of mean LA pressure elevation), calculate the mean mitral gradient while noting the heart rate, estimate the mitral valve area by the pressure half-time method, and estimate the PA pressure by TR velocity. If mitral pre-A velocity is more than 20 cm/sec, slowing the heart rate may improve the hemodynamic abnormalities and patient symptoms. In patients with mixed MS and MR, the focus is on the valve disease and its consequences rather than LV diastolic dysfunction. The LV IVRT, mitral valve area, and PA pressures become important objective data to relate to patient symptoms.

Sinus Tachycardia and Effect on LV Filling at Rest and During Exercise

Previous animal studies link the normal cardiac pathophysiology that occurs as heart rate increases with changes in mitral flow velocity.[10–14] The method by which heart rate is increased (withdrawal of parasympathetic tone, increase in sympathetic tone or exercise) markedly affects when mitral E and A waves begin to fuse and when complete fusion (A wave flow only) occurs. For example, in normal dogs, withdrawal of parasympathetic tone with atropine administration results in complete fusion of E and A waves at 160 bpm, while with isoproterenol infusion this is not observed until a heart rate of 220 bpm. These differences are related to the effect of each intervention on LV contractility and the degree of shortening of the PR interval. Increased contractility shortens the LV isovolumic contraction, ejection, and relaxation times so that diastolic filling time is maximized, while shortening of the PR interval provides for more diastolic filling before atrial contraction. With exercise, increased venous return and LA pressure also result in an earlier mitral valve opening, which also helps keep early and late diastolic filling separated. LVH, systolic dysfunction, increased wall stress, and cardiac conduction system disease (first degree or LBBB) prolong systolic periods and shorten the diastolic filling time so that E and A wave fusion occur at lower heart rates (see Fig. 9.4). This may limit LV filling and result in a reduced exertional cardiac output and functional aerobic capacity as previously discussed (see Fig. 9.20).

Uncommon Mitral Flow Velocity Patterns

Variations in LV filling patterns are seen where impaired LV relaxation persists into mid-diastole or altered compliance is present only in early diastole rather than throughout the diastolic filling period. This physiology is most commonly present with marked LVH, especially in the elderly with severe and long-standing HTN[118] or patients with hypertrophic cardiomyopathy. Fig. 9.21 shows examples of variations of these unusual mitral patterns. Most typically the initial mitral E wave velocity is increased compared to LVOT velocity, and there is a short initial mitral DT. The predominant abnormality present is markedly impaired LV relaxation, which causes a severe decrease in LV compliance (the short initial mitral DT), but one that is confined to early diastole, perhaps because of delayed actin-myosin cross-bridge detachment. In mid-diastole there is continued LV relaxation and a fall in pressure so that the mitral DT markedly slows (is biphasic) or a mid-diastolic filling hump is seen. The width of the A wave is then seen to vary, which may indicate whether LV compliance is reduced once relaxation is finally finished. Because of the profound relaxation abnormality these patients often do well with very slow (45–55 bpm) resting heart rates while faster heart rates result in exercise intolerance and pulmonary congestion.

Increased Mitral Respiratory Flow Velocity Variation

Increased mitral respiratory flow velocity variation can be seen in a number of important conditions to diagnose, and it will be missed in laboratories that do not record mitral flow velocity initially at the slower sweep speed of 50 cm/sec to observe if exaggerated respiratory variation is present. Although respiratory variation in tricuspid E wave flow velocity is expected and is often 15% to 25%, the change in mitral E wave velocity in normals is less than 5%.[119] Increased changes in both mitral and tricuspid inflow velocities with respiration can be seen in patients with acute or chronic pulmonary disease[120] or pericardial abnormalities, including tamponade,[121,122] constriction,[119,120,123] and pericardial restraint due to acute cardiac dilation from RV infarction, pulmonary embolus, or acute valvular regurgitation.

So that abnormal respiratory mitral changes are not overlooked, we recommend recording mitral flow velocity using CW Doppler technique from the apical transducer position at a sweep speed of 50 mm/sec. Any variation greater than 10% with a regular heart rate is considered abnormal. Accompanying changes in the LV IVRT verify that the alterations in velocity are due to alterations in LA pressure and the

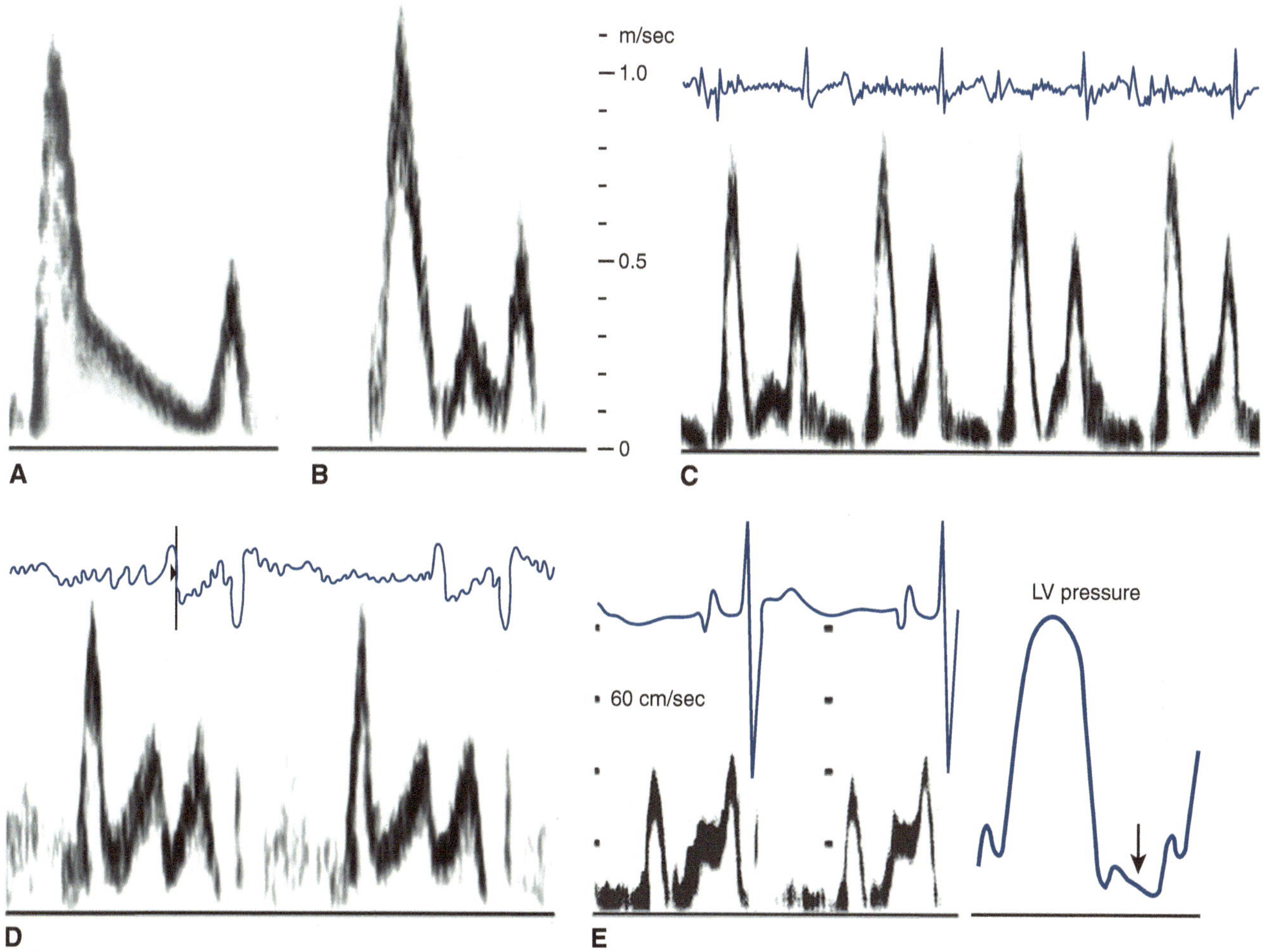

Fig. 9.21 Five patients (A–E) with markedly impaired LV relaxation that result in unusual PW Doppler mitral flow velocity recordings that do not fit conventional LV filling patterns of diastolic dysfunction. All patients are in normal sinus rhythm. Each peak E wave velocity is followed by an initial restrictive-like mitral DT and then variable degrees of additional filling in mid-diastole and with atrial contraction. Patient A has marked LVH from long-standing HTN and a normal LVEF. The initial mitral DT is 100 msec, which then changes to 280 msec in mid-diastole with A wave duration of 100 msec. LV posterior wall M mode motion showed continuous filling throughout mid-diastole. Patient B is a 35-year-old on dialysis with LVH and normal LVEF. Without the abnormal mid-diastolic filling the mitral pattern might be mistaken for normal. Patient C is elderly with HTN and slight sinus arrhythmia. With a slower heart rate, the filling pattern would be similar to patient B, but the slightly faster heart rate results in the mid-diastolic filling blending into the A wave making its true duration difficult to measure except on the first beat. Patient D has a 50-year history of nonobstructive hypertrophic cardiomyopathy with a giant left atrium. The initial mitral DT is only 80 msec, with over two-thirds of LV filling occurring in mid-diastole and at atrial contraction. The patient reports feeling best with a resting heart rate of 40 to 45 bpm. Functional aerobic capacity is severely reduced. Patient E has a mitral flow velocity somewhat similar to patient D. The LV pressure recording shows an initial rapid filling wave correlating with the restrictive early diastolic mitral DT, but then LV pressure declines in mid-diastole with reestablishment of transmitral flow. The cellular mechanisms that result in these marked derangements of LV relaxation and early diastolic restrictive physiology, which is transient rather than fixed, are under investigation.

timing of mitral valve opening. A PW Doppler exam of mitral flow velocity with respirometer is then performed. The clinical history and the characteristic 2-D findings (such as an inspiratory septal shift) are noted along with the exact timing of the flow velocity changes. This will help determine if pulmonary or pericardial disease is present. The hepatic venous Doppler is especially important and should always be recorded because in primary pericardial disease the heart is having difficulty filling, while with pulmonary disease the heart is overfilling due to the excessive swings in intrathoracic pressure and RV minimum pressure.[120]

- Increased mitral respiratory flow velocity variation of greater than 5% is abnormal and suggests increased LV and RV interaction in a fixed pericardial space.
- Recording mitral flow with CW Doppler technique ensures the respiratory variation is real and not due to cardiac movement changing the position of the mitral valve in relation to a fixed sample volume location.
- Venous Doppler is key to determining whether the variation is due to a constrictive process versus overfilling the heart due to dyspnea where pericardial restraint occurs.

Atrial Flutter and Fibrillation

Regardless of whether there is 2:1 or higher degree AV block, almost no assessment on LV diastolic function can be made from mitral flow velocity when atrial flutter is present. All LV filling is due to atrial contractions so that no E velocity, E/A wave ratio, or mitral DT is available for measurement. If 3:1 or 4:1 AV block is present, multiple filling waves are seen with diastolic mitral regurgitation interspersed between each. Pulmonary artery pressure calculated from peak TR velocity may be the best indicator of increased left heart filling pressures if no lung disease is present.

New onset coarse Afib may resemble atrial flutter in that multiple pulses of blood flow from atrial contraction enter the ventricle in diastole. This makes the interpretation of peak E wave velocity and mitral DT difficult to relate to LV diastolic properties. Chronic Afib, when LA mechanical function is negligible and the rate is less than 100 bpm, is easier to interpret. In patients with heart disease LV IVRT is a good indicator of whether filling pressures are elevated. Since all LV filling must occur without an atrial booster pump, mean LA pressure and peak E wave velocity are usually slightly higher than normal for age, except in young patients with lone Afib and vigorous elastic recoil. Mitral DT is generally about 20 msec shorter than expected, and PV flow should have a reduced but not absent systolic fraction since the PV S1 component due to atrial relaxation is absent. In adult cardiac patients a short LV IVRT (<60 msec), mitral E wave velocity equal to LVOT velocity, short mitral DT (<160 msec), and reduced (<25%) PV systolic fraction all suggest reduced LV compliance and increased filling pressures. The ratio of mitral E wave to TDI e′ (E/e′) velocity may also indicate elevated pressures,[124] while a mitral DT of less than 140 msec has been shown to have the same unfavorable prognosis as that for patients in sinus rhythm.[72]

When recording Afib, CW technique is again suggested first to display the maximum velocities and measure the LV IVRT. PW Doppler is used for mitral DT, and five beats are averaged to assess mitral variables. Beats with short R-R intervals should be excluded, especially if systole causes an abrupt cessation of mitral inflow. Examples of atrial flutter and Afib are shown in Fig. 9.22.

Diastolic Mitral and Tricuspid Regurgitation

Diastolic mitral and tricuspid regurgitation can be seen when there is a reverse diastolic TMPG, where LV pressure exceeds LA pressure in diastole. Although the magnitude of the reverse TMPG can exceed the normal forward flow gradient, the amount of regurgitation is hemodynamically insignificant because it is limited by a small AV valve orifice area.[125]

There are several situations in which diastolic MR and AR can be seen. By far the most common is with first-degree, second-degree, or third-degree AV block,[126] or with atrial flutter and greater than 2:1 AV block (see Fig. 9.22). In these cases the atrium contracts, and atrial and ventricular pressure both increase. However, in the absence of a normal PR interval and properly timed ventricular systole, atrial relaxation causes its pressure to fall below ventricular pressure, and diastolic regurgitation occurs. Diastolic MR due to first-degree AV block is usually not seen until the PR interval exceeds 280 msec. It is worth noting especially if it is causing partial fusion of early and late diastolic filling.

Diastolic MR is more pathologic when associated with advanced RST LV filling. After filling in mid-diastole or after atrial contraction there is a marked increase in LV pressure that not only decelerates but transiently reverses transmitral flow. AR with marked bradycardia or Afib and a very slow ventricular rate is an additional uncommon etiology.

RIGHT VENTRICULAR DIASTOLIC FUNCTION

The same Doppler analysis and variables used for mitral flow velocity can be applied to tricuspid inflow and RV filling.[113,127] Because inspiration increases RV filling, changes in tricuspid flow velocity are seen throughout

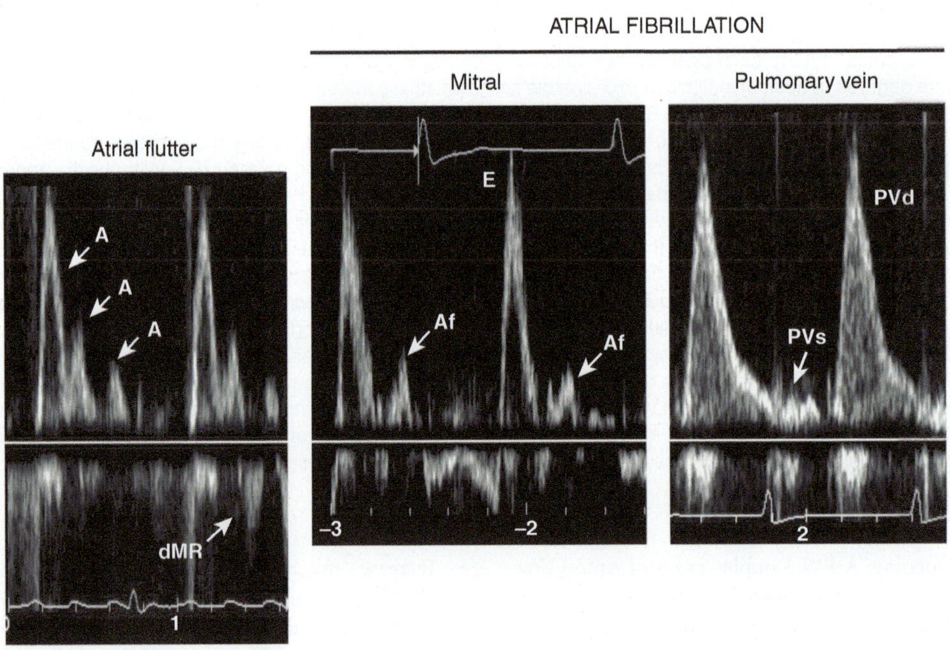

Fig. 9.22 PW Doppler mitral flow velocity in a patient with atrial flutter and atrial fibrillation. In A-flutter LV filling is a regular pulsation of A waves *(arrows)*, often with mild diastolic MR (dMR) during atrial relaxation. LA size is often enlarged from the arrhythmia, the IVRT is affected by the atrial contractions, and there is no E wave or mitral DT to measure making the assessment of diastolic function problematic. In Afib peak E wave velocity and mitral DT can be measured but can also be affected by the fibrillatory contractions of the atrium (Af flow, *arrows*). It is likely that this patient does have an increase in mean LA pressure because the IVRT was short (50 msec) and PV systolic (PVs) filling is negligible, a sign of reduced LA compliance.

the respiratory cycle, while on the left side of the heart Doppler mitral variables vary only about 5%.[120] This increase in inspiratory RV filling can be used, in conjunctive with hepatic and superior vena cava flow velocities, to assess the diastolic properties of the right ventricle.

PW Doppler tricuspid DT is about 25 msec longer than its mitral counterpart. With normal RV diastolic function this value changes little with the increased flow during inspiration, and hepatic A wave reversals decrease in velocity and duration. With a decrease in late diastolic RV compliance, hepatic venous A wave velocity and duration increase with inspiration. An inspiratory shortening of tricuspid DT, diastolic predominance of hepatic venous flow with prominent V and A wave reversals are signs of a marked decrease in RV compliance and increased diastolic filling pressures.[127] The early diastolic slope and A wave decrease in velocity in pulmonary regurgitation Doppler signals can also be used to assess early and late diastolic RV compliance. The assessment of right heart pressures from IVC size[128] and systemic venous flow (hepatic vein and SVC) has also been described.[129,130]

USING LV FILLING PATTERNS FOR PATIENT MANAGEMENT

If the only information available from examining LV filling patterns was whether the patient had an elevated LA pressure, this can often be ascertained from the patient's history, physical examination, chest x-ray, and natriuretic peptide levels. Unique information available from an echo Doppler study is the identification of early diastolic dysfunction (IR filling pattern with or without elevated LV EDP), the relation of LV systolic to diastolic function, identifying which diastolic property (relaxation or compliance) is most abnormal, and which parts of diastole are most affected by these abnormalities. In addition, seeing whether the patient's heart rate at rest is well matched to the cardiac physiology present is a great strength of echo Doppler technique. Using this information is a powerful tool for intervening to prevent progression of diastolic abnormalities and treat patients with symptoms of HFpEF to improve their functional status and prognosis.

After the echo Doppler study is completed, the first question is, What is the main cardiac abnormality present—systolic dysfunction, diastolic dysfunction, or valvular heart disease? In patients with a reduced LVEF, diastolic dysfunction is expected and is usually matched to the reduction in LVEF. For example, patients with a moderate reduction in LVEF (30–35%) often have a pseudonormal (Grade II) abnormal mitral filling pattern, while patients with severe reduction in LVEF (<20%) commonly demonstrate RST filling. A mismatch between these expected relations is notable. Better diastolic function than systolic function suggests a well-adapted, compliant ventricle despite their marked reduction in systolic function. Such individuals often have a good functional capacity and a favorable prognosis.[28] Conversely, a pseudonormal or RST mitral filling pattern with mild systolic function suggests volume overload (easily detected by IVC imaging) or pathology, which increases myocardial stiffness. Why patients with LV systolic dysfunction have such variability in LV compliance remains a key enigma that requires further investigation.

In patients with normal LV systolic function and HFpEF, questions to be answered include whether abnormalities of LV relaxation or compliance predominate, and during what part(s) of diastole are the abnormalities present. This gives an idea of the best approach for short-term therapy and whether altering the heart rate is likely to improve patient symptoms. Although classifying patients as having one of the three abnormal filling patterns is often useful for this purpose, enough variations in LV filling patterns and combinations of LA pressure and rates of LV relaxation exist that what treatments might benefit the patient are still best available by carefully examining the mitral flow velocity pattern and its individual Doppler variables. Examining the magnitudes of PVs and PVd velocity in patients has special importance because of the elevated LA pressure and failing LA contractility indicated by PVs decreasing below PVd and the poor prognosis it confers[90,91] (Fig. 9.17).

LIMITATIONS

The greatest limitation to the echo Doppler assessment of LV diastolic dysfunction by mitral and pulmonary venous patterns is understanding the physiology that results in the wide variety of patterns seen and how to interpret them. Assuming high-quality recordings are available the principles illustrated in this chapter can then be used to decide which of the key diastolic properties (LV relaxation or compliance) is most abnormal, how these are related to LV systolic function, and how both interact to affect the overall LV and pulmonary venous filling patterns. In some cases, the anatomic findings with only a few variables can be used for diagnosis, while in others several ancillary variables are needed to increase diagnostic certainty. When first learning to interpret LV diastolic function there is a tendency to try to make all variables fit into one abnormal LV filling pattern or another, when in reality there are nearly endless variations and exceptions to defined criteria. Also there is now confusion from these algorithms that increased filling pressures indicate diastolic dysfunction is present, which is not always true. Conversely, patients with abnormal relaxation for their age most often have normal filling pressures. This is why we believe examining the mitral filling pattern and variables together with all available 2-D and Doppler information is the most helpful for patient management. This approach acknowledges that the variables used are imperfect indicators of individual diastolic filling properties or pressures and can sometimes appear contradictory, but in aggregate they usually provide sufficient information to be clinically useful in the great majority of patients.

A common limitation is the lack of technical experience in acquiring high-quality Doppler recordings so that all variables are accurately measured. It can be expected that even when performing a routine diastolic function examination on every patient undergoing echocardiography, it could take at least 6 months for sonographers and physicians to master these skills. With the advent of Doppler annular TDI the number of labs that routinely obtain PV flow velocity recordings has likely declined. Additional ways to identify reduced LV compliance in its earliest and most treatable stages are therefore needed.

Atrial fibrillation is becoming increasingly prevalent. More research is needed on ways to assess LV diastolic dysfunction and filling pressures in this important group, despite the fact that LV IVRT, mitral DT, and the amount of pulmonary venous systolic flow are often indicators of filling pressures or LV compliance in this group.

Pediatric patients present their own challenges. Isolated diastolic dysfunction is rare in this group, and there is much less literature available to establish when abnormal diastolic properties are present.

FUTURE DIRECTIONS

Over the last several years new technological advances in noninvasive imaging have been applied to the study of diastolic function. Nevertheless, pulsed Doppler techniques remain the cornerstone of any diastology study. Even in the most difficult to image patients, pulsed Doppler information can be easily recorded with high reliability and reproducibility. Pulsed Doppler velocities have a solid foundation on well-established physical and mathematical principles. Accordingly, future research should be focused on the use of artificial intelligence for automated analysis and interpretation.

KEY POINTS

- The greatest limitation to interpreting diastolic function is understanding the complex physiology of LV filling and the lack of accurate normal ranges for various echo Doppler variables in the elderly who have a high incidence of HFpEF.
- A second limitation is the technical experience required in acquiring high-quality Doppler recordings so that variables can be accurately measured and used for interpretation and serial studies.
- Other current challenges include recent attempts at using simplified algorithms with only a few Doppler variables. These have been predictably inadequate to assess the wide variety of clinical diastolic abnormalities seen in practice.
- Increased confusion about the diagnosis of diastolic dysfunction has been another consequence as elevated filling or PA pressures are often equated with diastolic dysfunction when simple volume overload or pulmonary disease may be present.
- Studies that show effective therapies for patients with HFpEF may make laboratories more inclined to devote a greater portion of the echo Doppler exam to the many variables that help identify abnormal diastolic properties and filling pressures.
- Systolic and diastolic function are inextricably linked and affected in parallel fashion by loading conditions, inotropic stimulation, and neurohumoral factors.
- The morbidity and mortality of HFrEF and HFpEF is similar. The incidence of elderly HFpEF patients is rapidly increasing and is expected to equal patients with HFrEF in the near future.
- Echo Doppler technique is the only practical method for diagnosing, staging, and following patients with both types of HF.
- Elevated filling pressures can exist without diastolic abnormalities under various clinical conditions such as volume overload or increased cardiac output.
- Conversely, the earliest diastolic abnormality, impaired LV relaxation, most often has normal filling pressures for some time, even though it confers an increased long-term risk of adverse CV events.
- Identifying the presence of LV diastolic function requires considering multiple echo Doppler parameters and an estimated CVP in the context of clinical data and patient age.
- Key diastology parameters include the transmitral and pulmonary venous flow velocities as well as LA volume, DTI mitral annular velocities, and peak TR velocity.
- Assessing the degree of underlying diastolic abnormalities in relaxation and compliance is most accurate when preload and afterload are normal.
- Algorithms, with concordance between two or more parameters, can sometimes be applied to determine filling pressures or diastolic abnormalities in patients, but they frequently lack sensitivity or specificity in the diverse group of patients encountered in clinical medicine.
- The strength of echo Doppler technique in diagnosing diastolic abnormalities, filling pressures, and prognosis is using the numerous variables available for analysis, with IVRT, pulmonary venous flow velocity, and preload reduction with Valsalva being the most valuable underused variables.
- Suggested Doppler flow velocities and variables are listed in the chapter, with an explanation of their physiology, what they specifically indicate in regard to diastolic properties and filling pressures, and interpretive pitfalls.

REVIEW QUESTIONS

A 27-year-old patient with end-stage renal disease on dialysis undergoes a transthoracic echo. The patient has the following vitals: BMI 26, pulse 78, BPM 135/85, a mild four-chamber enlargement, mild LVH with LVEF 65%, cardiac index 4 L/m^2/min.

Echo Variables

LA volume: 37 mL/m^2
LV IVRT: 50 msec
E wave: 110 cm/sec
A wave: 40 cm/sec
E/A ratio: 2.75
Mitral DT: 170 msec
Mitral A-dur: 130 msec
PVs: 70 cm/sec
PVd: 70 cm/sec
PVa: 40 cm/sec
PVa dur: 160 msec
DTI MAM
  e′ average: 12
  a′ average: 5
  E/e′ average: 9.2
PAS: 38 mmHg
IVC: normal diameter

1. Which LV filling pressure is increased?
   a. None
   b. LV EDP
   c. Mean LA pressure
2. What is the filling pattern?
   a. Normal
   b. IR
   c. Pseudonormal
   c. RST
3. Which early diastolic property is abnormal?
   a. None
   b. Slowed relaxation
   c. Reduced LV compliance

A 52-year-old executive undergoes echo for white coat HTN. The patient has the following vitals: BMI 33, pulse 70, BPM 129/82, all chamber sizes normal, borderline LVH, no valve disease, normal cardiac output.

Echo Variables

LA volume: 25 mL/m^2
LV IVRT: 110 msec
E wave: 50 cm/sec
A wave: 95 cm/sec
E/A ratio: 0.5
Mitral DT: 230 msec
Mitral A-dur: 140 msec
PVs: 60 cm/sec
PVd: 30 cm/sec
PVa: 25 cm/sec
PVa dur: 140 msec
DTI MAM
  e′ average: 5
  a′ average: 10
  E/e′ average: 10
PAS: 28 mmHg
IVC: normal

4. Which LV filling pressure is increased?
   a. None
   b. LV EDP
   c. Mean LA pressure
5. What is the filling pattern?
   a. Normal
   b. IR
   c. Pseudonormal
   d. RST
6. Which diastolic property is abnormal?
   a. None
   b. Slowed relaxation
   c. Reduced LV compliance

A 72-year-old male with CAD, HTN, and diabetes undergoes TTE echocardiography. The patient has the following vitals: BMI 28, pulse 70; BPM 148/82, estimated GFR 30 mL/m^2/min, both ventricles normal in size with normal EFs, moderate LV hypertrophy present, no valve disease except aortic sclerosis and mild MAC, cardiac output normal.

Echo Variables

LA volume: 39 mL/m^2
LV IVRT: 65 msec
E wave: 90 cm/sec
A wave: 45 cm/sec
E/A ratio: 2
Mitral DT: 170 msec
Mitral A-dur: 120 msec
PVs: 60 cm/sec
PVd: 40 cm/sec
PVa: 45 cm/sec
PVa dur: 155 msec
DTI MAM
  e′ average: 4
  a′ average: 10
  E/e′ average: 22
PAS: 42 mmHg
IVC: markedly dilated
E/A ratio with Valsalva: 0.9

7. Which LV filling pressure is increased?
   a. None
   b. LV EDP
   c. Mean LA pressure
   d. Both
8. What is the filling pattern?
   a. Normal
   b. IR
   c. Pseudonormal
   d. RST
9. Which diastolic properties are abnormal?
   a. None
   b. Slowed relaxation
   c. Reduced LV chamber compliance
   d. Both

An 82-year-old female is admitted to the hospital with HFpEF. She has a 30-year history of medical noncompliance and poorly controlled HTN. The patient has the following vitals: BMI 27.5, pulse 78, BPM 158/68, estimated GFR 50 mL/m^2/min, NT-proBNP moderately elevated, small hyperdynamic LV cavity with marked LVH and near systolic cavity obliteration, no significant valvular heart disease present, cardiac output normal.

Echo Variables

LA volume: 45 mL/m^2
LV IVRT: 55 msec
E wave: 90 cm/sec
A wave: 30 cm/sec
E/A ratio: 3
Mitral DT: 175 msec
Mitral A-dur: 110 msec
PVs: 35 cm/sec
PVd: 70 cm/sec
PVa: 35 cm/sec
PVa dur: 150 msec
DTI MAM
  e′ average: 5
  a′ average: 10
  E/e′ average: 18
PAS: 50 mmHg
IVC: normal
E/A ratio with Valsalva: 2.6

10. Which LV filling pressure is increased?
    a. None
    b. LV EDP
    c. Mean LA pressure
    d. Both
11. What is the filling pattern?
    a. Normal
    b. IR
    c. Pseudonormal
    d. RST
12. Which diastolic properties are abnormal?
    a. None
    b. Slowed relaxation
    c. Reduced LV chamber compliance
    d. Both
13. By pulmonary venous variables what is the patient's CV mortality risk?
    a. Unknown
    b. Low
    c. Medium
    d. High

REFERENCES

1. Ingels Jr NB, Daughters II GT, Nikolic SD, et al. Left atrial pressure-clamp servomechanism demonstrates LV suction in canine hearts with normal mitral valves. *Am J Physiol.* 1994;267:H354–H362.
2. Child JS, Perloff JK. The restrictive cardiomyopathies. *Cardiol Clin.* 1988;6:289–316.
3. Braunwald E. Hypertrophic cardiomyopathy—continued progress. *N Engl J Med.* 1989;320:800–802.
4. Hammermeister KE, Warbasse JR. The rate of change of left ventricular volume in man. II. Diastolic events in health and disease. *Circulation.* 1974;49:739–747.
5. Gibson DG, Brown DJ. Measurement of peak rates of left ventricular wall movement in man. Comparison of echocardiography with angiography. *Br Heart J.* 1975;37:677–683.
6. Upton MT, Gibson DG, Brown DJ. Echocardiographic assessment of abnormal left ventricular relaxation in man. *Br Heart J.* 1976; 38:1001–1009.

7. Soufer R, Wohlgelernter D, Vita NA, et al. Intact systolic left ventricular function in clinical congestive heart failure. *Am J Cardiol.* 1985;55: 1032–1036.
8. Topol EJ, Traill TA, Fortuin NJ. Hypertensive hypertrophic cardiomyopathy of the elderly. *N Engl J Med.* 1985;312:277–283.
9. Little WC DT, Applegate RJ. Invasive evaluation of left ventricular diastolic performance. *Herz.* 1990;15:362–376.
10. Hanrath P, Mathey DG, Siegert R, Bleifeld W. Left ventricular relaxation and filling pattern in different fore of left ventricular hypertrophy: an echocardiographic study. *Am J Cardiol.* 1980;45:15–23.
11. Rokey R, Kuo LC, Zoghbi WA, Limacher MC, Quinones MA. Determination of parameters of left ventricular diastolic filling with pulsed Doppler echocardiography: comparison with cineangiography. *Circulation.* 1985;71:543–550.
12. Spirito P, Maron BJ, Bonow RO. Noninvasive assessment of left ventricular diastolic function: comparative analysis of Doppler echocardiographic and radionuclide angiographic techniques. *J Am Coll Cardiol.* 1986;7:518–526.
13. Kitabatake A, Inoue M, Asao M, et al. Transmitral blood flow reflecting diastolic behavior of the left ventricle in health and disease—a study by pulsed Doppler technique. *Jpn Circ J.* 1982;46:92–102.
14. Tanouchi J, Kitabatake A, Asao M, et al. [Role of left ventricular relaxation on transmitral flow dynamics during early diastole: pulsed Doppler flowmetry]. *J Cardiogr.* 1983;13:301–307.
15. Kuo LC, Quinones MA, Rokey R, Sartori M, Abinader EG, et al. Quantification of atrial contribution to left ventricular filling by pulsed Doppler echocardiography and the effect of age in normal and diseased hearts. *Am J Cardiol.* 1987;59:1174–1178.
16. Gardin JM, Drayer JI, Weber M, et al. Doppler echocardiographic assessment of left ventricular systolic and diastolic function in mild hypertension. *Hypertension.* 1987;9:II90–II96.
17. Klein AL, Burstow DJ, Tajik AJ, Zachariah PK, Bailey KR, et al. Effects of age on left ventricular dimensions and filling dynamics in 117 normal persons. *Mayo Clin Proc.* 1994;69:212–224.
18. Miyatake K, Okamoto M, Kinoshita N, Owa N, Nakasone I, et al. Augmentation of atrial contribution to left ventricular inflow with aging as assessed by intracardiac Doppler flowmetry. *Am J Cardiol.* 1984;70:586–589.
19. Appleton CP, Hatle LK, Popp RL. Relation of transmitral flow velocity patterns to left ventricular diastolic function: new insights from a combined hemodynamic and Doppler echocardiographic study. *J Am Coll Cardiol.* 1988;12:426–440.
20. Klein AL, Taliercio CP, Oh JK, Kyle RA, Gertz MA, et al. Prognostic significance of diastolic function in cardiac amyloidosis. A Doppler echocardiographic study. *Circulation.* 1991;83:808–816.
21. Pinamonti B, Di Lenarda A, Sinagra G, Camerini F. Restrictive left ventricular filling pattern in dilated cardiomyopathy assessed by Doppler echocardiography: clinical, echocardiographic and hemodynamic correlations and prognostic implications. Heart Muscle Disease Study Group. *J Am Coll Cardiol.* 1993;22:808–815.
22. Rich MW, Stitziel NO, Kovacs SJ. Prognostic value of diastolic filling parameters derived using a novel image processing technique in patients > or = 70 years of age with congestive heart failure. *Am J Cardiol.* 1999;84:82–86.
23. Xie GY, Berk MR, Smith MD, Gurley JC, DeMaria AN. Prognostic value of Doppler transmitral flow patterns in patients with congestive heart failure [see comments]. *J Am Coll Cardiol.* 1994;24:132–139.
24. Appleton CP. The natural history of left ventricular filling abnormalities: assessment by two-dimensional and Doppler echocardiography. *Echocardiography.* 1992;9:437–457.
25. Keren G, Pardes A, Miller HI, Scherez J, Laniado S. Pulmonary venous flow determined by Doppler echocardiography in mitral stenosis. *Am J Cardiol.* 1990;65:246–249.
26. Klein AL. Doppler assessment of pulmonary venous flow in healthy subjects and patients with heart disease. *J Am Soc Echocardiogr.* 1991;4:379–392.
27. Kuecherer HF, Muhiudeen IA, Kusumoto FM, et al. Estimation of mean left atrial pressure from transesophageal pulsed Doppler echocardiography of pulmonary venous flow. *Circulation.* 1990;82:1127–1139.
28. Pozzoli M, Traversi E, Cioffi G, Stenner R, Sanarico M, et al. Loading manipulations improve the prognostic value of Doppler evaluation of mitral flow in patients with chronic heart failure. *Circulation.* 1997;95(5):1222–1230.
29. Dumesnil JG, Gaudreault G, Honos GN, Kingma Jr JG. Use of Valsalva maneuver to unmask left ventricular diastolic function abnormalities by Doppler echocardiography in patients with coronary artery disease or systemic hypertension. *Am J Cardiol.* 1991;68:515–519.
30. Hurrell DG, Nishimura RA, Ilstrup DM, Appleton CP. Utility of preload alteration in assessment of left ventricular filling pressure by Doppler echocardiography: a simultaneous catheterization and Doppler echocardiographic study. *J Am Coll Cardiol.* 1997;30:459–467.
31. Klein AL, Hatle LK, Taliercio CP, et al. Prognostic significance of Doppler measures of diastolic function in cardiac amyloidosis. A Doppler echocardiography study. *Circulation.* 1991;83:808–816.
32. Pinamonti B, Zecchin M, Di Lenarda A, Gregori D, Sinagra G, et al. Persistence of restrictive left ventricular filling pattern in dilated cardiomyopathy: an ominous prognostic sign. *J Am Coll Cardiol.* 1997;29:604–612.
33. Brun P, Tribouilloy C, Duval AM, et al. Left ventricular flow propagation during early filling is related to wall relaxation: a color M-mode Doppler analysis. *J Am Coll Cardiol.* 1992;20:420–432.
34. Garcia MJ, Rodriguez L, Ares M, Griffin BP, Thomas JD, et al. Differentiation of constrictive pericarditis from restrictive cardiomyopathy: assessment of left ventricular diastolic velocities in longitudinal axis by Doppler tissue imaging. *J Am Coll Cardiol.* 1996;27:108–114.
35. Garcia MJ, Smedira NG, Greenberg NL, et al. Color M-mode Doppler flow propagation velocity is a preload insensitive index of left ventricular relaxation: animal and human validation. *J Am Coll Cardiol.* 2000;35:201–208.
36. Garcia MJ, Thomas JD, Klein AL. New Doppler echocardiographic applications for the study of diastolic function. *J Am Coll Cardiol.* 1998;32:865–875.
37. Kovacs Jr SJ, Barzilai B, Perez JE. Evaluation of diastolic function with Doppler echocardiography: the PDF formalism. *Am J Physiol.* 1987;252:H178–H187.
38. Kovacs SJ, Meisner JS, Yellin EL. Modeling of diastole. *Cardiol Clin.* 2000;18:459–487.
39. Sohn DW, Chai IH, Lee DJ, et al. Assessment of mitral annulus velocity by Doppler tissue imaging in the evaluation of left ventricular diastolic function. *J Am Coll Cardiol.* 1997;30:474–480.
40. Yellin EL, Meisner JS. Physiology of diastolic function and transmitral pressure-flow relations. *Cardiol Clin.* 2000;18:411–433. vii.
41. Thomas JD, Newell JB, Choong CY, Weyman AE. Physical and physiological determinants of transmitral velocity: numerical analysis. *Am J Physiol.* 1991;260:H1718–H1731.
42. Choong CY, Abascal VM, Thomas JD, Guerrero JL, McGlew S, et al. Combined influence of ventricular loading and relaxation on the transmitral flow velocity profile in dogs measured by Doppler echocardiography. *Circulation.* 1988;78:672–683.
43. Greenberg NL, Vandervoort PM, Firstenberg MS, Garcia MJ, Thomas JD. Estimation of diastolic intraventricular pressure gradients by Doppler M-mode echocardiography. *Am J Physiol Heart Circ Physiol.* 2001;280:H2507–H2515.
44. Greenberg NL, Vandervoort PM, Thomas JD. Automated assessment of color Doppler M-mode flow velocity propagation features. *Comput Cardiol.* 1996;201–204.
45. Riordan MM, Kovacs SJ. Quantitation of mitral annular oscillations and longitudinal "ringing" of the left ventricle: a new window into longitudinal diastolic function. *J Appl Physiol.* 2006;100:112–119.
46. Riordan MM, Kovacs SJ. Absence of diastolic mitral annular oscillations is a marker for relaxation-related diastolic dysfunction. *Am J Physiol Heart Circ Physiol.* 2007;292(6):H2952–H2958.
47. Garcia MJ. Comprehensive echocardiographic assessment of diastolic function. *Heart Fail Clin.* 2006;2:163–178.
48. Oh JK, Hatle L, Tajik AJ, Little WC. Diastolic heart failure can be diagnosed by comprehensive two-dimensional and Doppler echocardiography. *J Am Coll Cardiol.* 2006;47:500–506.
49. Appleton CP, Firstenberg MS, Garcia MJ, Thomas JD. The echo-Doppler evaluation of left ventricular diastolic function. A current perspective. *Cardiol Clin.* 2000;18:513–546. ix.

50. Bursi F, Weston SA, Redfield MM, et al. Systolic and diastolic heart failure in the community. *JAMA*. 2006;296:2209–2216.
51. Giannuzzi P, Temporelli PL, de Vito F, Silva PL, Scapellato F, et al. Doppler-derived mitral deceleration time of early filling as a strong predictor of pulmonary wedge pressure in postinfarction patients with left ventricular dysfunction. *J Am Coll Cardiol*. 1994;23:1630–1637.
52. Jensen JL, Williams FE, Beilby BJ, et al. Feasibility of obtaining pulmonary venous flow velocity in cardiac patients using transthoracic pulsed wave Doppler technique. *J Am Soc Echocardiogr*. 1997;10:60–66.
53. Appleton CP. Influence of incremental changes in heart rate on mitral flow velocity: assessment in lightly sedated, conscious dogs. *J Am Coll Cardiol*. 1991;17:227–236.
54. Courtois M, Kovacs Jr SJ, Ludbrook PA. Transmitral pressure-flow velocity relation. Importance of regional pressure gradients in the left ventricle during diastole. *Circulation*. 1988;78:661–671.
55. Nishimura RA, Housmans PR, Hatle LK, Tajik AJ. Assessment of diastolic function of the heart: background and current applications of Doppler echocardiography. Part I. Physiologic and pathophysiologic features. *Mayo Clin Proc*. 1989;64:71–81.
56. Cheng CP, Igarashi Y, Little WC. Mechanism of augmented rate of left ventricular filling during exercise. *Circ Res*. 1992;70:9–19.
57. Ingels Jr NB, Daughters GT, Nikolic SD, et al. Left ventricular diastolic suction with zero left atrial pressure in open-chest dogs. *Am J Physiol*. 1996;270:H1217–H1224.
58. Ishida Y, Meisner JS, Tsujioka K, et al. Left ventricular filling dynamics: influence of left ventricular relaxation and left atrial pressure [published erratum appears in Circulation 1986 Sep;74(3):462]. *Circulation*. 1986;74:187–196.
59. Nishimura RA, Abel MD, Hatle LK, Tajik AJ. Assessment of diastolic function of the heart: background and current applications of Doppler echocardiography. Part II. Clinical studies. *Mayo Clin Proc*. 1989;64:181–204.
60. Kitzman DW, Higginbotham MB, Cobb FR, Sheikh KH, Sullivan MJ. Exercise intolerance in patients with heart failure and preserved left ventricular systolic function: failure of the Frank-Starling mechanism [see comments]. *J Am Coll Cardiol*. 1991;17:1065–1072.
61. Vanoverschelde JL, Raphael DA, Robert AR, Cosyns JR. Left ventricular filling in dilated cardiomyopathy: relation to functional class and hemodynamics. *J Am Coll Cardiol*. 1990;15:1288–1295.
62. Rakowski H, Appleton C, Chan KL, et al. Canadian consensus recommendations for the measurement and reporting of diastolic dysfunction by echocardiography: from the Investigators of Consensus on Diastolic Dysfunction by Echocardiography. *J Am Soc Echocardiogr*. 1996;9:736–760.
63. Cuocolo A, Sax FL, Brush JE, Maron BJ, Bacharach SL, et al. Left ventricular hypertrophy and impaired diastolic filling in essential hypertension. Diastolic mechanisms for systolic dysfunction during exercise. *Circulation*. 1990;81:978–986.
64. Ohno M, Cheng CP, Little WC. Mechanism of altered patterns of left ventricular filling during the development of congestive heart failure. *Circulation*. 1994;89:2241–2250.
65. Manson AL, Nudelman SP, Hagley MT, Hall AF, Kovacs SJ. Relationship of the third heart sound to transmitral flow velocity deceleration. *Circulation*. 1995;92:388–394.
66. Nishimura RA, Schwartz RS, Tajik AJ, Holmes Jr DR. Noninvasive measurement of rate of left ventricular relaxation by Doppler echocardiography. Validation with simultaneous cardiac catheterization. *Circulation*. 1993;88:146–155.
67. Nishimura RA, Tajik AJ. Evaluation of diastolic filling of left ventricle in health and disease: Doppler echocardiography is the clinician's Rosetta Stone. *J Am Coll Cardiol*. 1997;30:8–18.
68. Redfield MM, Jacobsen SJ, Burnett Jr JC, Mahoney DW, Bailey KR, et al. Burden of systolic and diastolic ventricular dysfunction in the community: appreciating the scope of the heart failure epidemic. *JAMA*. 2003;289:194–202.
69. Snider AR, Gidding S, Rocchini AP, Rosenthal A, Dick M, et al. Doppler evaluation of left ventricular diastolic filling in children with systemic hypertension. *Am J Cardiol*. 1985;56:921–926.
70. Sasson Z, Hatle L, Appleton CP, Jewett M, Alderman EL, et al. Intraventricular flow during isovolumic relaxation: description and characterization by Doppler echocardiography. *J Am Coll Cardiol*. 1987;10:539–546.
71. Caballero L, et al. Echocardiographic reference ranges for normal cardiac Doppler data: results from the NORRE Study. *Eur Heart J Cardiovasc Imag*. 2015;16(9):1031–1041. doi: 10.1093/ehjci/jev083.
72. Klein AL, Hatle LK, Taliercio CP, et al. Serial Doppler echocardiographic follow-up of left ventricular diastolic function in cardiac amyloidosis. *J Am Coll Cardiol*. 1990;16:1135–1141.
73. Hurrell DG, Oh JK, Mahoney DW, Miller Jr FA, Seward JB. Short deceleration time of mitral inflow E velocity: prognostic implication with atrial fibrillation versus sinus rhythm. *J Am Soc Echocardiogr*. 1998;11:450–457.
74. Little WC, Ohno M, Kitzman DW, Thomas JD, Cheng CP. Determination of left ventricular chamber stiffness from the time for deceleration of early left ventricular filling. *Circulation*. 1995;92:1933–1939.
75. Hirota Y. A clinical study of left ventricular relaxation. *Circulation*. 1980;62:756–763.
76. Matsuda Y, Toma Y, Matsuzaki M, et al. Change of left atrial systolic pressure waveform in relation to left ventricular end-diastolic pressure. *Circulation*. 1990;82:1659–1667.
77. Tenenbaum A, Motro M, Hod H, Kaplinsky E, Vered Z. Shortened Doppler-derived mitral A wave deceleration time: an important predictor of elevated left ventricular filling pressure. *J Am Coll Cardiol*. 1996;27:700–705.
78. Sohn DW, Choi YJ, Oh BH, Lee MM, Lee YW. Estimation of left ventricular end-diastolic pressure with the difference in pulmonary venous and mitral A durations is limited when mitral E and A waves are overlapped. *J Am Soc Echocardiogr*. 1999;12:106–112.
79. Nishimura RA, Schwartz RS, Holmes Jr DR, Tajik AJ. Failure of calcium channel blockers to improve ventricular relaxation in humans. *J Am Coll Cardiol*. 1993;21:182–188.
80. Ommen SR, Nishimura RA, Appleton CP, et al. Clinical utility of Doppler echocardiography and tissue Doppler imaging in the estimation of left ventricular filling pressures: a comparative simultaneous Doppler-catheterization study. *Circulation*. 2000;102:1788–1794.
81. Rossvoll O, Hatle LK. Pulmonary venous flow velocities recorded by transthoracic Doppler ultrasound: relation to left ventricular diastolic pressures. *J Am Coll Cardiol*. 1993;21:1687–1696.
82. Yamamoto K, Nishimura RA, Burnett Jr JC, Redfield MM. Assessment of left ventricular end-diastolic pressure by Doppler echocardiography: contribution of duration of pulmonary venous versus mitral flow velocity curves at atrial contraction. *J Am Soc Echocardiogr*. 1997;10:52–59.
83. Hoit BD, Shao Y, Gabel M, Walsh RA. Influence of loading conditions and contractile state on pulmonary venous flow. Validation of Doppler velocimetry. *Circulation*. 1992;86:651–659.
84. Basnight MA, Gonzalez MS, Kershenovich SC, Appleton CP. Pulmonary venous flow velocity: relation to hemodynamics, mitral flow velocity and left atrial volume, and ejection fraction. *J Am Soc Echocardiogr*. 1991;4:547–558.
85. Appleton CP. Hemodynamic determinants of Doppler pulmonary venous flow velocity components: new insights from studies in lightly sedated normal dogs. *J Am Coll Cardiol*. 1997;30:1562–1574.
86. Smiseth OA, Thompson CR, Lohavanichbutr K, et al. The pulmonary venous systolic flow pulse--its origin and relationship to left atrial pressure. *J Am Coll Cardiol*. 1999;34:802–809.
87. Keren G, Sherez J, Megidish R, Levitt B, Laniado S. Pulmonary venous flow pattern—its relationship to cardiac dynamics. A pulsed Doppler echocardiographic study. *Circulation*. 1985;71:1105–1112.
88. Bartzokis T, Lee R, Yeoh TK, Grogin H, Schnittger I. Transesophageal echo-Doppler echocardiographic assessment of pulmonary venous flow patterns. *J Am Soc Echocardiogr*. 1991;4:457–464.
89. Kuecherer HF, Kusumoto F, Muhiudeen IA, Cahalan MK, Schiller NB. Pulmonary venous flow patterns by transesophageal pulsed Doppler echocardiography: relation to parameters of left ventricular systolic and diastolic function. *Am Heart J*. 1991;122:1683–1693.
90. Dini FL, Dell'Anna R, Micheli A, et al. Impact of blunted pulmonary venous flow on the outcome of patients with left ventricular systolic

dysfunction secondary to either ischemic or idiopathic dilated cardiomyopathy. *Am J Cardiol.* 2000;85:1455–1460.
91. Buffle E, Kramarz J, Elazar E, et al. Added value of pulmonary venous flow Doppler assessment in patients with preserved ejection fraction and its contribution to the diastolic grading paradigm. *Eur Heart J Cardiovasc Imag.* 2015;16:1191–1197.
92. Klein AL, Abdalla I, Murray RD, et al. Age independence of the difference in duration of pulmonary venous atrial reversal flow and transmitral A-wave flow in normal subjects. *J Am Soc Echocardiogr.* 1998;11:458–465.
93. Appleton CP, Galloway JM, Gonzalez MS, Gaballa M, Basnight MA. Estimation of left ventricular filling pressures using two-dimensional and Doppler echocardiography in adult patients with cardiac disease. Additional value of analyzing left atrial size, left atrial ejection fraction and the difference in duration of pulmonary venous and mitral flow velocity at atrial contraction. *J Am Coll Cardiol.* 1993;22:1972–1982.
94. O'Leary PW, Durongpisitkul K, Cordes TM, et al. Diastolic ventricular function in children: a Doppler echocardiographic study establishing normal values and predictors of increased ventricular end-diastolic pressure. *Mayo Clin Proc.* 1998;73:616–628.
95. Appleton CP. Doppler assessment of left ventricular diastolic function: the refinements continue. *J Am Coll Cardiol.* 1993;21:1697–1700.
96. Garcia MJ. Diastolic dysfunction and heart failure: causes and treatment options. *Cleve Clin J Med.* 2000;67:727–729. 733–738.
97. Nishimura RA, Appleton CP. Diastology": beyond E and A. *J Am Coll Cardiol.* 1996;27:372–374.
98. Quinones MA. Assessment of diastolic function. *Prog Cardiovasc Dis.* 2005;47:340–355.
99. Tsang TS, Barnes ME, Gersh BJ, Bailey KR, Seward JB. Left atrial volume as a morphophysiologic expression of left ventricular diastolic dysfunction and relation to cardiovascular risk burden. *Am J Cardiol.* 2002;90:1284–1289.
100. Gibson DG, Prewitt TA, Brown DJ. Analysis of Left ventricular wall movement during isovolumic relaxation and its relation to coronary artery disease. *Brit Heart J.* 1976;38:1010–1019.
101. Abhayaratna WP, Seward JB, Appleton CP, et al. Left atrial size: physiologic determinants and clinical applications. *J Am Coll Cardiol.* 2006;47:2357–2363.
102. Tsang TS, Miyasaka Y, Barnes ME, Gersh BJ. Epidemiological profile of atrial fibrillation: a contemporary perspective. *Prog Cardiovasc Dis.* 2005;48:1–8.
103. Tsang TS, Petty GW, Barnes ME, et al. The prevalence of atrial fibrillation in incident stroke cases and matched population controls in Rochester, Minnesota: changes over three decades. *J Am Coll Cardiol.* 2003;42:93–100.
104. Lang RM, Bierig M, Devereux RB, et al. Recommendations for chamber quantification. *Eur J Echocardiogr.* 2006;7:79–108.
105. Nagueh SF, Middleton KJ, Kopelen HA, Zoghbi WA, Quinones MA. Doppler tissue imaging: a noninvasive technique for evaluation of left ventricular relaxation and estimation of filling pressures. *J Am Coll Cardiol.* 1997;30:1527–1533.
106. Alam M, Wardell J, Andersson E, Samad BA, Nordlander R. Characteristics of mitral and tricuspid annular velocities determined by pulsed wave Doppler tissue imaging in healthy subjects. *J Am Soc Echocardiogr.* 1999;12:618–628.
107. Garcia MJ, Rodriguez L, Ares M, et al. Myocardial wall velocity assessment by pulsed Doppler tissue imaging: characteristic findings in normal subjects. *Am Heart J.* 1996;132:648–656.
108. Garcia MJ, Thomas JD. Tissue Doppler to assess diastolic left ventricular function. *Echocardiography.* 1999;16:501–508.
109. Oki T, Tabata T, Mishiro Y, et al. Pulsed tissue Doppler imaging of left ventricular systolic and diastolic wall motion velocities to evaluate differences between long and short axes in healthy subjects. *J Am Soc Echocardiogr.* 1999;12:308–313.
110. Oki T, Tabata T, Yamada H, et al. Clinical application of pulsed Doppler tissue imaging for assessing abnormal left ventricular relaxation. *Am J Cardiol.* 1997;79:921–928.
111. Rodriguez L, Garcia M, Ares M, Griffin BP, Nakatani S, et al. Assessment of mitral annular dynamics during diastole by Doppler tissue imaging: comparison with mitral Doppler inflow in subjects without heart disease and in patients with left ventricular hypertrophy. *Am Heart J.* 1996;131:982–987.
112. Ha JW, Oh JK, Pellikka PA, et al. Diastolic stress echocardiography: a novel noninvasive diagnostic test for diastolic dysfunction using supine bicycle exercise Doppler echocardiography. *J Am Soc Echocardiogr.* 2005;18:63–68.
113. Appleton CP, Jensen JL, Hatle LK, Oh JK. Doppler evaluation of left and right ventricular diastolic function: a technical guide for obtaining optimal flow velocity recordings. *J Am Soc Echocardiogr.* 1997;10:271–292.
114. Cohen GI, Pietrolungo JF, Thomas JD, Klein AL. A practical guide to assessment of ventricular diastolic function using Doppler echocardiography. *J Am Coll Cardiol.* 1996;27:1753–1760.
115. Oh JK, Appleton CP, Hatle LK, Nishimura RA, Seward JB, et al. The noninvasive assessment of left ventricular diastolic function with two-dimensional and Doppler echocardiography. *J Am Soc Echocardiogr.* 1997;10:246–270.
116. Koren MJ, Casale PN, Savage DD, Laragh JH. Relation of left ventricular mass and geometry to morbidity and mortality in uncomplicated essential hypertension. *Ann Intern Med.* 1991;114:345–352.
117. Appleton CP, Hatle LK, Popp RL. Superior vena cava and hepatic vein Doppler echocardiography in healthy adults. *J Am Coll Cardiol.* 1987;10:1032–1039.
118. Ha JW, Oh JK, Redfield MM, Ujino K, Seward JB, et al. Triphasic mitral inflow velocity with middiastolic filling: clinical implications and associated echocardiographic findings. *J Am Soc Echocardiogr.* 2004;17:428–431.
119. Hatle LK, Appleton CP, Popp RL. Differentiation of constrictive pericarditis and restrictive cardiomyopathy by Doppler echocardiography. *Circulation.* 1989;79:357–370.
120. Boonyaratavej S, Oh JK, Tajik AJ, Appleton CP, Seward JB. Comparison of mitral inflow and superior vena cava Doppler velocities in chronic obstructive pulmonary disease and constrictive pericarditis. *J Am Coll Cardiol.* 1998;32:2043–2048.
121. Burstow DJ, Oh JK, Bailey KR, Seward JB, Tajik AJ. Cardiac tamponade: characteristic Doppler observations. *Mayo Clin Proc.* 1989;64:312–324.
122. Appleton CP, Hatle LK, Popp RL. Cardiac tamponade and pericardial effusion: respiratory variation in transvalvular flow velocities studied by Doppler echocardiography. *J Am Coll Cardiol.* 1988;11:1020–1030.
123. McCully RB, Higano ST, Oh JK. Diagnosis of constrictive pericarditis. *Circulation.* 1999;99:2476.
124. Nagueh SF, Kopelen HA, Quinones MA. Assessment of left ventricular filling pressures by Doppler in the presence of atrial fibrillation. *Circulation.* 1996;94:2138–2145.
125. Appleton CP, Basnight MA, Gonzalez MS. Diastolic mitral regurgitation with atrioventricular conduction abnormalities: relation of mitral flow velocity to transmitral pressure gradients in conscious dogs. *J Am Coll Cardiol.* 1991;18:843–849.
126. Schnittger I, Appleton CP, Hatle LK, Popp RL. Diastolic mitral and tricuspid regurgitation by Doppler echocardiography in patients with atrioventricular block: new insight into the mechanism of atrioventricular valve closure. *J Am Coll Cardiol.* 1988;11:83–88.
127. Klein AL, Hatle LK, Burstow DJ, et al. Comprehensive Doppler assessment of right ventricular diastolic function in cardiac amyloidosis. *J Am Coll Cardiol.* 1990;15:99–108.
128. Simonson JS, Schiller NB. Sonospirometry: a new method for noninvasive estimation of mean right atrial pressure based on two-dimensional echographic measurements of the inferior vena cava during measured inspiration. *J Am Coll Cardiol.* 1988;11:557–564.
129. Nagueh MF, Kopelen HA, Zoghbi WA, Quinones MA, Nagueh SF. Estimation of mean right atrial pressure using tissue Doppler imaging. *Am J Cardiol.* 1999;84:1448–1451. A8.
130. Nagueh SF, Kopelen HA, Zoghbi WA. Relation of mean right atrial pressure to echocardiographic and Doppler parameters of right atrial and right ventricular function. *Circulation.* 1996;93:1160–1169.

10

Evaluation of Diastolic Function by Tissue Doppler, Strain, and Torsion Analysis

Mohammed Makkiya and Mario J. Garcia

OUTLINE

INTRODUCTION

Early Doppler echocardiographic indices of left ventricular (LV) diastolic function have studied the mechanics of left atrial (LA) and ventricular filling. These filling indices have been proven to be useful in providing prognostic information in heart failure patients.[1–3] However, filling indices have limited accuracy predicting intrinsic parameters of diastolic function due to the confounding effects of extrinsic loading conditions and intrinsic cardiac performance. Tissue Doppler imaging (TDI) overcame some of the disadvantages of pulse wave Doppler, but it is angle-dependent and still faces several important limitations. Recently, two-dimensional (2-D) and three-dimensional (3-D) speckle tracking has been applied to study LV myocardial mechanics. Compared to Doppler imaging, they provide mechanical analysis of the whole thickness of myocardium seen in one echocardiographic view or the entire myocardium with the introduction of 3-D speckle tracking. Since myocardial mechanical events precede left atrial and ventricular filling, they may be potentially less dependent on extrinsic variables, and therefore more accurate characterizing intrinsic myocardial properties.

In this chapter, we will review the role of 2-D and 3-D speckle tracking echocardiography (STE) and their derivatives for the assessment of LV diastolic function.

Case Study

A 62-year-old obese man with a past medical history significant for hypertension has been complaining of chronic shortness of breath and fatigue mostly with exertion. He went to see his primary care medical doctor and a diagnosis of asthma was made. He was started on bronchodilators, but his symptoms did not improve. Physical examination was notable for obesity. The remainder of his examination was unremarkable. His electrocardiogram (ECG) showed sinus rhythm with normal voltage. The patient underwent a complete 2-D transthoracic echocardiogram, which revealed normal LV ejection fraction (EF). There was grade I diastolic dysfunction (a mitral inflow pattern revealed abnormal relaxation with a normal range of early filling velocity/early filling contraction E/e′). There was no significant valvular disease. 2-D speckle tracking global longitudinal strain was obtained from apical windows. It was noted to be reduced (Fig. 10.1). Based on these findings, the patient was sent for a bicycle exercise stress echocardiogram. At 50 watts, the exercise mitral inflow pattern dramatically changed from normal to restrictive physiology with a significantly elevated E/e′. A diagnosis of diastolic heart failure was made (Fig. 10.2).

TECHNICAL CONSIDERATIONS

Measurements of Myocardial Deformation

Myocardial Velocities

Myocardial velocities can be obtained from multiple locations of the myocardium using TDI.

In technical terms, to display the velocities of the myocardium, TDI differs from standard Doppler by eliminating the high pass filter and using low gain amplification. TDI velocities may be displayed in spectral pulsed mode or in color encoded 2-D maps superimposed over structural images.

In a typical spectral display, the myocardial velocity waveform displays a positive wave representing ventricular systole (s′) and two waves corresponding to early filling (e′) and atrial contraction (a′). From the apical acoustic windows, the diastolic myocardial velocities obtained from any of the LV myocardial segments appear as a mirror image of the mitral inflow early (E) and atrial (A) filling velocities. In normal humans, the peak of e′ precedes the peak of LV filling E velocity, suggesting that active relaxation of the myocardium generates negative pressures in the LV cavity that initiate LV filling.

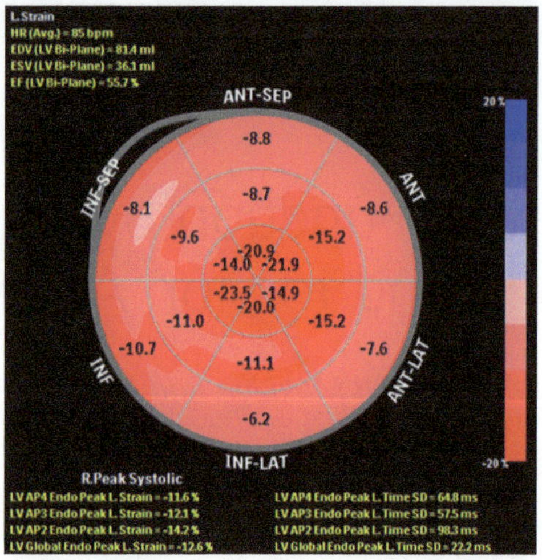

Fig. 10.1 Bull's eye image of peak systolic global longitudinal strain. The GLS is reduced −12.6%. LVEF is preserved 55.7%.

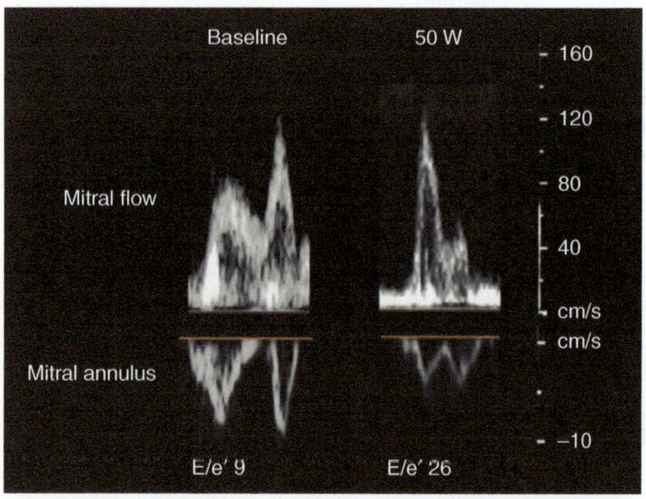

Fig. 10.2 Mitral flow and annular velocity at rest and during supine bicycle exercise. Mitral inflow pattern dramatically changed at 50 W of supine bicycle exercise from normal to restrictive physiology, with significantly elevated E/e′ consistent with diastolic heart failure.

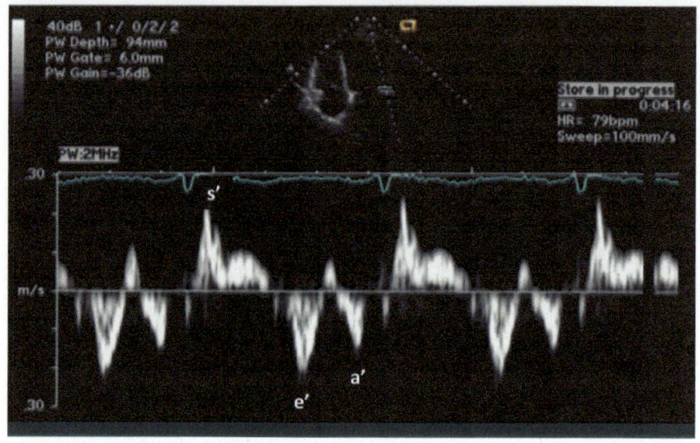

Fig. 10.3 Longitudinal axis tissue Doppler velocities obtained using spectral Doppler from the basal lateral left ventricular segment. *a′*, Atrial contraction velocity; *e′*, early diastolic velocity; *s′*, systolic velocity.

TDI velocities are influenced not only by regional LV mechanical events but also by global translation and rotation of the heart. Since LV longitudinal velocities are less affected by translational motion, they are usually obtained from the apical acoustic window (Figs. 10.3 and 10.4).

Alternatively, translational motion may be corrected by off-line analysis from color-encoded tissue Doppler echocardiography (TDE) velocities. One method plots the velocity of each adjacent scan line from the distance from epicardium to endocardium. From a parasternal color M mode image, the rates of circumferential fiber shortening and lengthening are proportional to the slope of the velocity/distance regression line. The value of this slope has been referred to as the myocardial velocity gradient (MVG).

Strain

The term *deformation* refers to the myocardium changing shape and dimensions during the cardiac cycle. Strain is a unitless measurement of deformational change of the myocardium and is often expressed as a percentage. It is well known that the spiral architecture of the myocardial fiber bundles deforms in multiple directions; strain imaging can identify and measure that deformation. Thus changes in LV geometry during LV systole relate primarily to radial (short axis), longitudinal (long axis), circumferential, and torsional strain. Lengthening or thickening of the myocardium is represented by positive strain values, whereas negative values represent shortening or thinning.

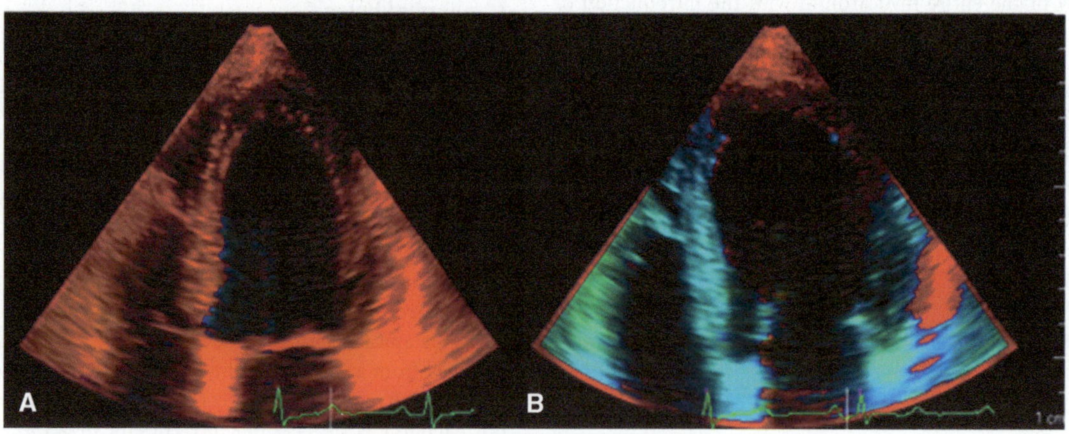

Fig. 10.4 Color-encoded tissue Doppler velocities obtained from the four-chamber view during (A) systole and (B) diastole.

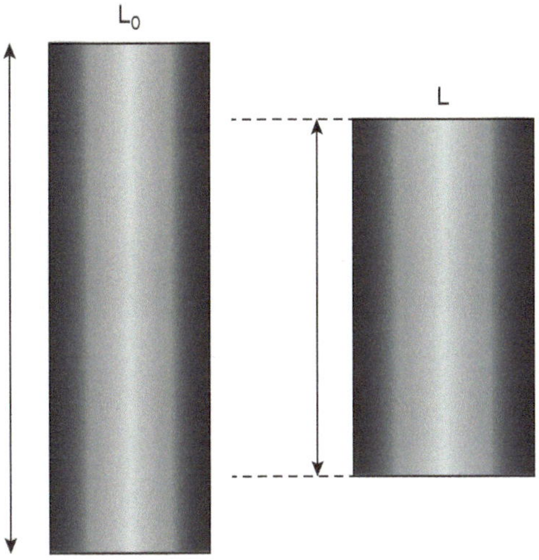

Fig. 10.5 Strain in three dimensions. The cylinder shows longitudinal strain, which can be described as Lagrangian strain from L_0 to L. The figure also shows simultaneous thickening or expansion in the two transverse directions. (From Støylen A. *Strain Rate Imaging of the Left Ventricle by Ultrasound. Feasibility, Clinical Validation and Physiological Aspects*. Trondheim, Norway: Norwegian University of Science and Technology; 2001.)

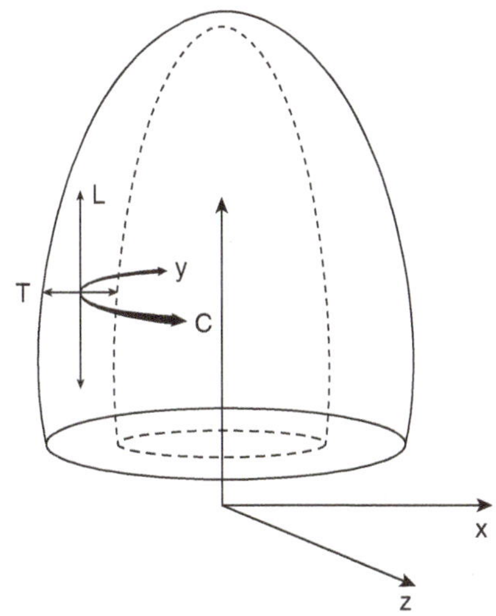

Fig. 10.6 The three main directions of the left ventricle: longitudinal *(L)*, transverse/transmural or radial *(T)*, and circumferential *(C)*. (From Støylen A. *Strain Rate Imaging of the Left Ventricle by Ultrasound. Feasibility, Clinical Validation and Physiological Aspects*. Trondheim, Norway: Norwegian University of Science and Technology; 2001.)

The concept of strain is complex, but linear strain can be defined by the Lagrangian formula:

$$\varepsilon = L - L_0/L_0 = \Delta L/L_0,$$

where ε is strain, L_0 is baseline length, and L is the instantaneous length at the time of measurement (Figs. 10.5 and 10.6).[4]

Multiple noninvasive techniques can quantify myocardial strain, including using magnetic resonance imaging (MRI), TDI, or high frame rate 2-D echocardiography with speckle tracking.

The first ultrasound-based strain measurements were derived from TDI but were limited to the interrogation of a few segments aligned with the Doppler beam. With the introduction of speckle tracking imaging, interrogation from all strain components became feasible from most myocardial segments, becoming as of today the preferred method. Global longitudinal strain can be calculated from apical views, while radial and circumferential strain are calculated from short axis views (Figs. 10.7 and 10.8). With the introduction of 3-D speckle tracking imaging, regional and global mechanics may be obtained in the full thickness of myocardium. 3-D provides assessment of area strain that represents a combination of longitudinal and circumferential strain. However, one of the major limitations in 3-D strain is lower temporal and spatial resolution, thus in the clinical setting strain is obtained from multiple 2-D views.[5–7]

Strain Rate

The strain rate (SR) is the instantaneous strain (or change in strain) per time unit.

$$\varepsilon = \Delta\varepsilon/\Delta t$$

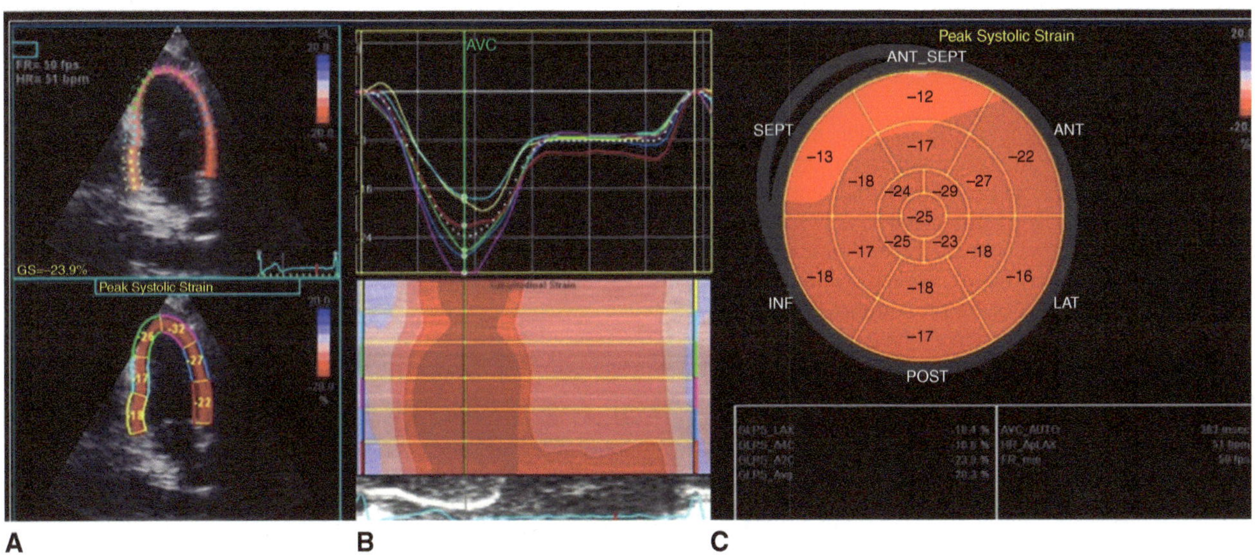

Fig. 10.7 (A) Global longitudinal strain, which is calculated from apical views from most commercial available systems. (B) Deformation curves and curved anatomic M mode mapping were also provided by the software. (C) Bull's eye of peak systolic strain. (Courtesy of PrivaCors.)

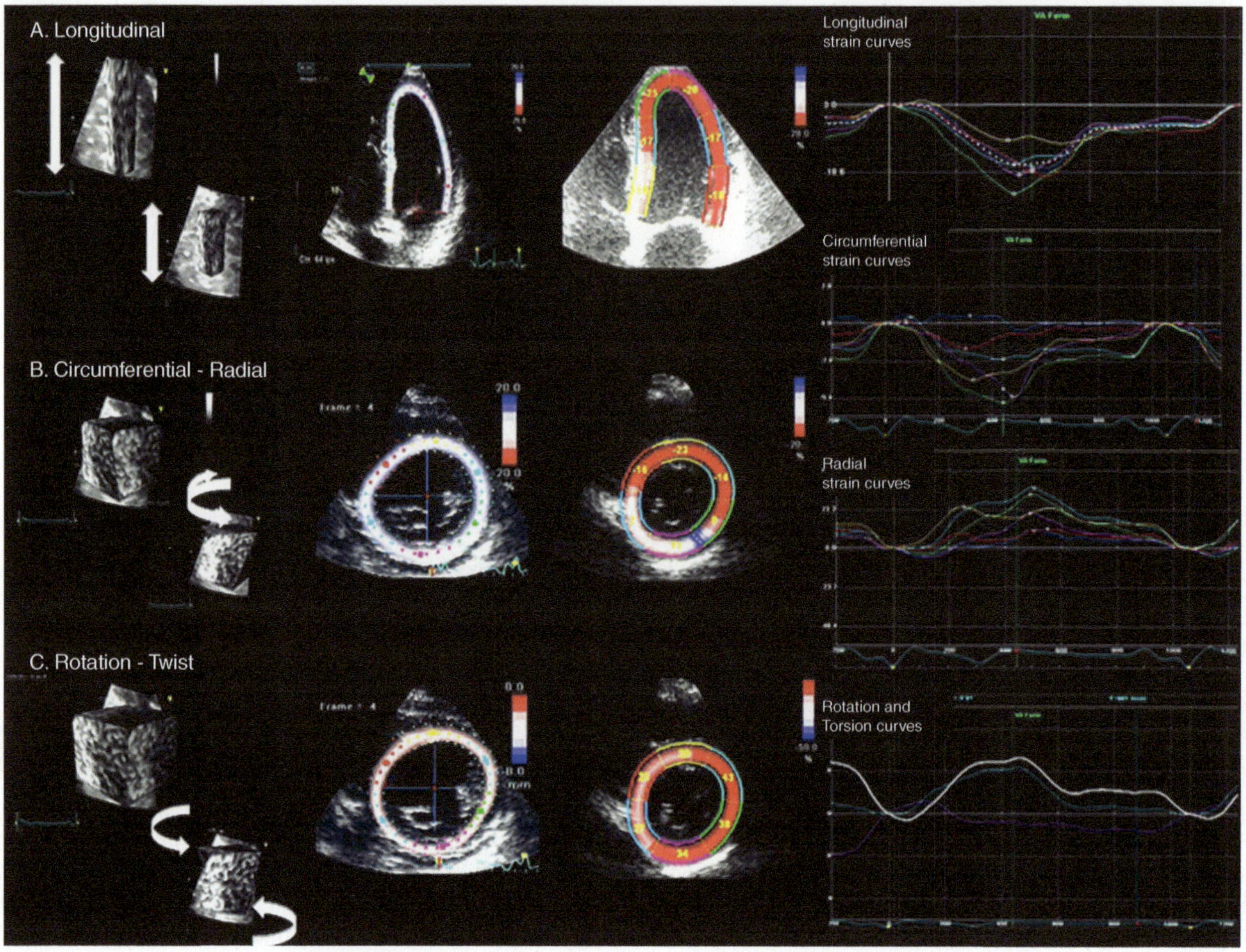

Fig. 10.8 Longitudinal, radial, circumferential strains curves with torsion.

The unit of strain rate is cm/s, or s^{-1}. The strain rate has the same direction as strain (i.e., negative strain rate during shortening, positive strain during elongation). SR corresponds to the velocity profile of a myocardial segment through the cardiac cycle. SR reflects the shortening/lengthening rate of the studied myocardial segment relatively independently of possible tethering or whole-body effects, an advantage over simple velocity measurements (Fig. 10.9).[8]

Twist and Torsion

In addition to radial and longitudinal deformation, there is twist and torsional deformation of the LV, which play an important role in LV filling. There is a systolic twist and an early diastolic untwist of the LV of oppositely directed apical and basal rotations, which is expressed in degrees. The term *torsion* is the twist normalized value to the distance between the LV apex and base and refers to the base-to-apex gradient in rotation angle, expressed in degrees per centimeter (°/cm).

During initial isovolumic contraction, the apex and the base both rotate in a counterclockwise direction when viewed from apex to base. Subsequently, during systole, the base changes direction and starts to rotate in a clockwise direction, while the apex continues to rotate in a counterclockwise direction.[9]

LV torsion is followed by rapid untwisting, which contributes to ventricular filling. Because LV torsion is directly related to fiber orientation, it might reflect subclinical abnormalities in heart function, especially diastolic dysfunction. Initially, LV twist and torsion were measured invasively using implanted sonomicrometer units. Later, for LV deformation and rotation, tissue tagging cardiac magnetic

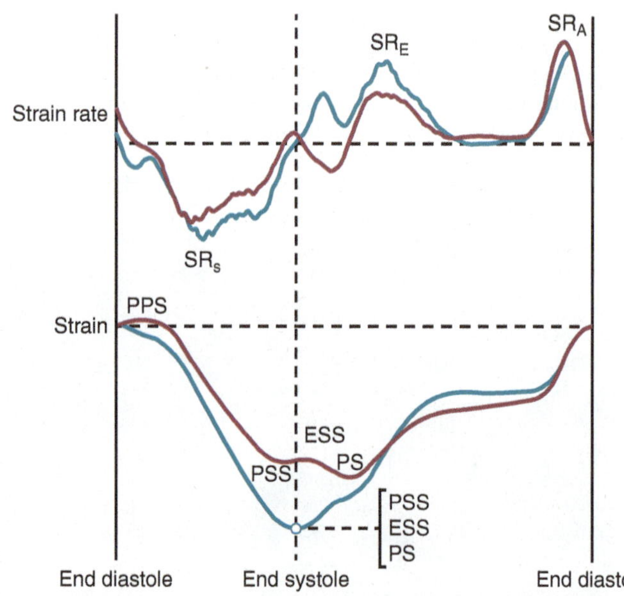

Fig. 10.9 Strain and strain rate from normal *(blue)* and ischemic myocardium *(red)*. There is an early peak positive strain *(PPS)* in ischemic myocardium, and peak systolic strain *(PSS)* is typically lower than end-systolic strain *(ESS)*. A postsystolic shortening is often seen, and peak strain *(PS)* therefore occurs after end systole. The thicker and thinner tracings are obtained from ischemic and normal myocardium, respectively. (© 2011 Gjesdal O, Edvardsen T. Published in [short citation] under CC BY 3.0 license. Available from: http://dx.doi.org/10.5772/24458.)

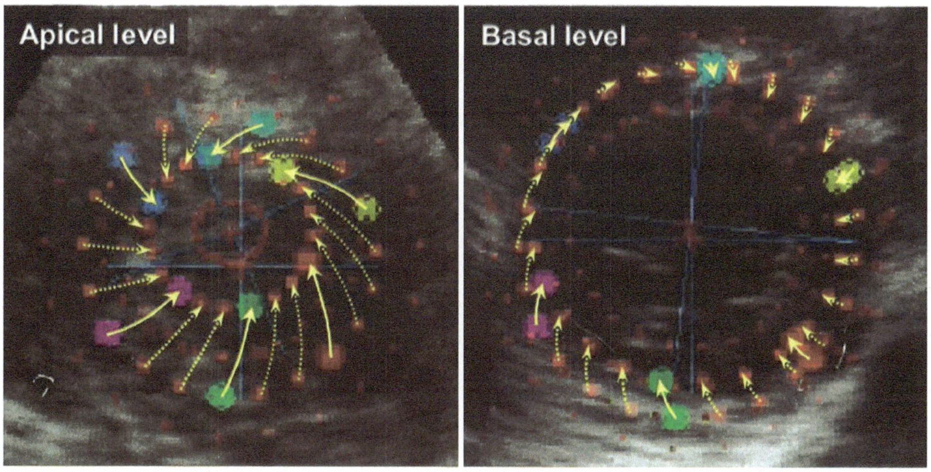

Fig. 10.10 Diagram indicating the vectors of apical counterclockwise and basal clockwise twist. Torsion is the sum of both components. (From Notomi Y, Shiota T, Popovic ZB, et al. Measurement of ventricular torsion by two-dimensional ultrasound speckle tracking imaging. *J Am Coll Cardiol.* 2005;45:2034–2041.)

resonance was regarded as the noninvasive reference standard. Recently, speckle tracking echocardiography was introduced for quantification of LV twist and torsion, providing higher spatial and temporal resolution compared to MRI. STE measurements of LV twist and torsional deformation have been tested and validated with sonomicrometry in animal models and with MRI tagging in humans (Fig. 10.10).[10] However, 2-D echocardiography does not provide an accurate determination of the distance between the two image planes required for quantification of torsional deformation. Because of this 2-D limitation, recent investigational efforts have shifted to speckle tracking analysis using real-time 3-D echocardiographic data sets. Validation of 3-D STE has been performed in animal studies using sonomicrometry as the reference standard and in simulated models and in vitro as well.[11]

Doppler Versus B-Mode Methods

Tissue Doppler imaging was the first method used for directly measuring myocardial deformation by echocardiography. Since a regional velocity gradient is analytically identical with the temporal derivative of a change in length, strain rate can be directly calculated from two velocity samples at a known distance apart. Integrating strain rate over time results in strain (Fig. 10.11). TDI-derived strain quantifies tissue deformation based on Doppler velocity shifts. Unlike tissue Doppler velocities, TDI-derived strain is less affected by segmental tethering and translational motion; therefore it primarily reflects the intrinsic deformation of the myocardial segment within the sample region. However, tissue Doppler-based strain is still limited by angle dependency.

STE is based on B mode gray scale tracking of 2-D speckles. Speckles are small dots or groups of myocardial pixels that are routinely created by the interaction of ultrasonic beams and the myocardium. A kernel is a number of adjacent speckles clumped together with unique arrangements. This unique signature kernel is easy to track, just like a fingerprint that identifies the unique myocardial segment. Using the end-diastolic dimensions as a surrogate for original length and reference point, these speckles can be tracked on frame-by-frame units as they move through the cardiac cycle (Fig. 10.12).

2-D STE-derived strain estimates myocardial velocities at a 2-D level (rather than TDI 1-D transducer-tissue velocities), which allows discrimination between normal, active myocardial segmental deformation versus passive displacement of a dysfunctional myocardial segment due to adjacent segment tethering and global cardiac motion. Also, in contrast to TDI-based strain, which measures deformations between time points (so-called natural strains), STE lends itself more readily to Lagrangian strain, which compares deformation to original length.

2-D speckle tracking–derived strain is angle-independent and provides mechanical analysis of the whole thickness of myocardium seen in one echocardiographic view.[12]

NORMAL PHYSIOLOGY

Myocardial Fiber Orientation

In describing LV anatomic structure, many theories arise. One widely accepted theory is the helical ventricular myocardial band (HVMB) model. It recognizes three LV myocardial layers: endocardial, midmyocardial (not present at the apex), and epicardial. There is no sharp border between these different layers. Subepicardial fibers are lying at an angle about −60 degrees to the horizontal plane, making a right-handed (clockwise) helix, the midwall fibers are practically horizontal, whereas the subendocardial myocytes lay with an angle of nearly +60 degrees to the horizontal plane from the left-handed (counterclockwise) helix. Together, they are forming LV free wall and interventricular septum; the subepicardial clockwise helix is forming the right half of the septum, whereas the counterclockwise right-handed helix forms the left septal half. Both epicardial and endocardial layers consist of clockwise and counterclockwise helix segments (Fig. 10.13).[13]

The myocyte fibers' angular arrangement is very important to LV function. It has been shown that normal contraction of purely longitudinally or circumferentially arranged myocytes would yield mathematically an ejection fraction of 15% to 25%, respectively, whereas fibers aligned at 60-degree angles are needed to achieve EF of more than 60%.[14]

LV twist and rotation can be evaluated noninvasively by using MRI and advanced echocardiography techniques. The two most common MRI methods for measuring myocardial motion are tagging and phase contrast velocity mapping. Given the multiple known limitations of MRI, STE has gained ground and become clinically most useful. Modern STE techniques measure LV rotation and twist by quantifying apical and basal twist rotation followed by the calculation of LV torsion from short axis projections. These speckles are cross-correlated and tracked on a frame-by-frame basis, and average angular motion can be quantified as average rotation. The accuracy of speckle tracking imaging has been validated, but this method is still limited for quantitative torsional measurements as previously mentioned.[15,16]

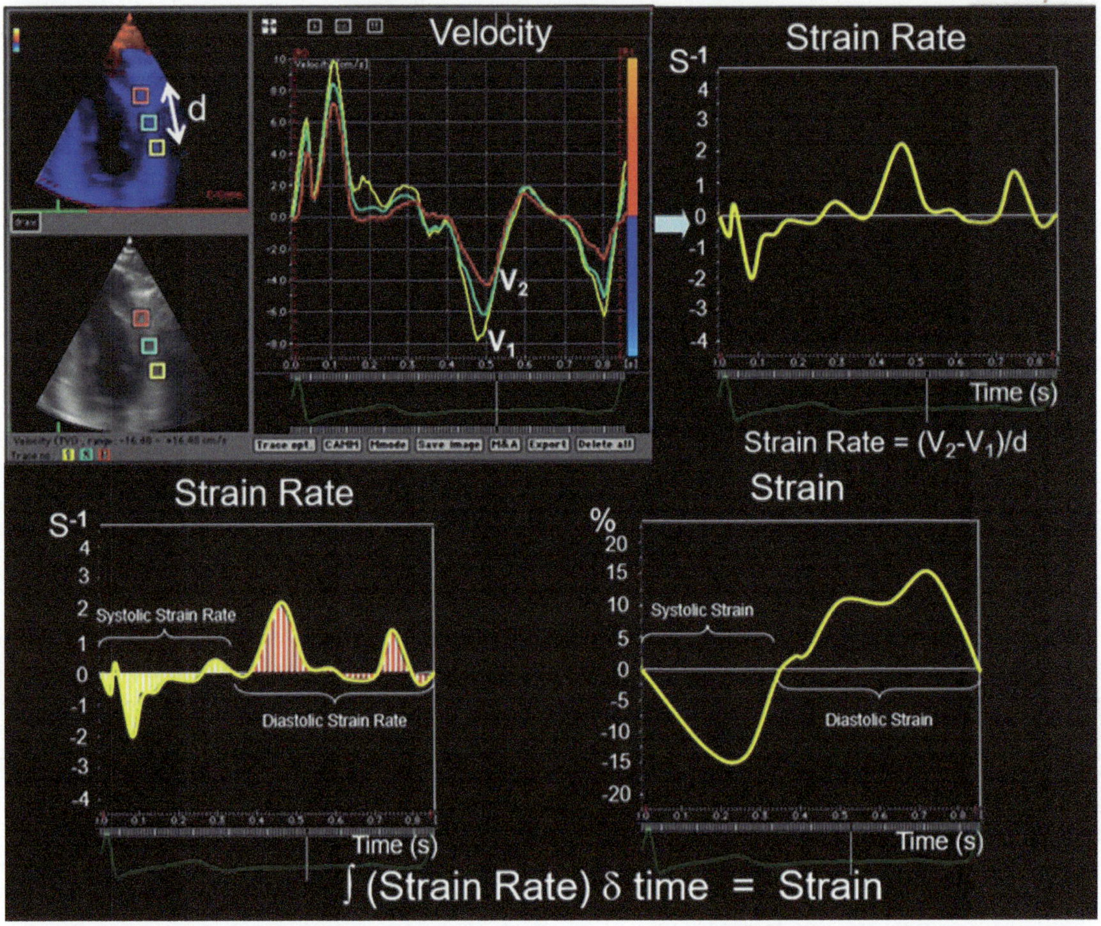

Fig. 10.11 Diagram indicating the mathematical steps used to derive strain rate and strain from tissue velocities. *d*, Distance; *V*, velocity.

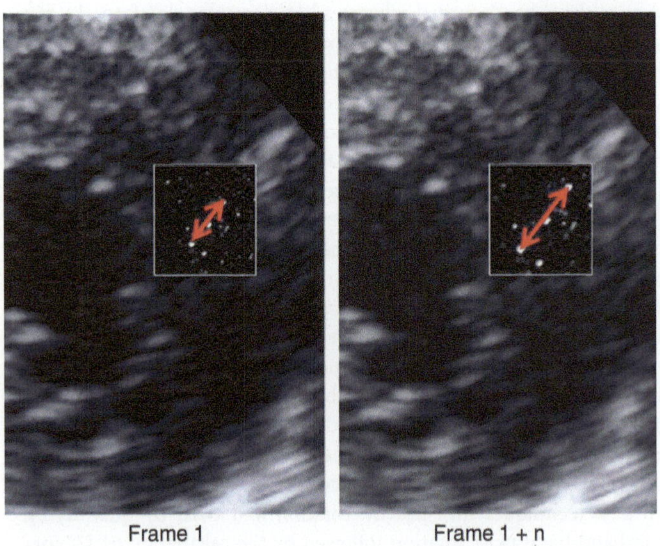

Fig. 10.12 STE is based on the identification and on the tracking of speckles (spots generated by the interaction between the ultrasound beam and myocardial fibers) on routine 2-D ultrasonic-derived images. (From Gorcsan J 3rd, Tanaka H. Echocardiographic assessment of myocardial strain. *J Am Coll Cardiol.* 2011;58(14):1401–1413. doi:10.1016/j.jacc.2011.06.038.)

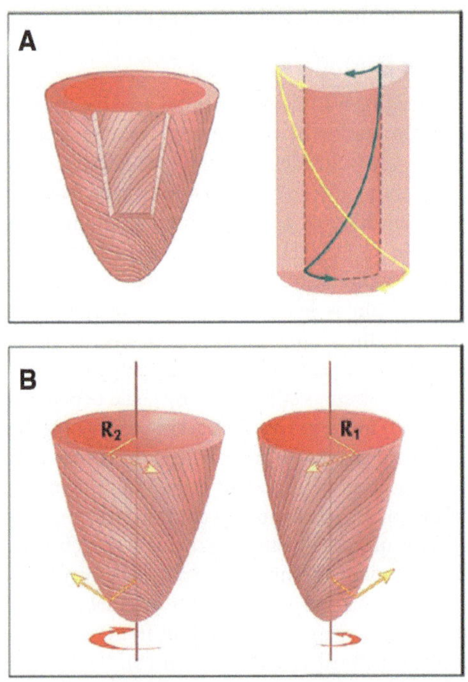

Fig. 10.13 Myofiber orientation in the LV changes smoothly from a left-handed helix in the subepicardium to a right-handed helix in the subendocardium (A), showing (B) the subendocardial fiber wrapped in a right-handed helix and a subepicardial fiber wrapped in a left-handed helix. (From Sengupta PP, Tajik AJ, Chandrasekaran K, Khandheria BK. Twist mechanics of the left ventricle: principles and application. *JACC Cardiovasc Imag.* 2008;1(3):366–376.)

Electromechanical Activation

The normal electromechanical activation sequence of the LV is an intricate process that involves the interaction of multiple elements, from the ultrastructural level of the myocytes and specialized conduction system to the macroscopic complex arrangement of myofibers.[17]

As the cardiac electromechanical activation occurs, first to become excited are the subendocardial fibers near the mid- and apical septal walls with an apex-to-base sequence of activation. First there will be a subendocardial shortening and subepicardial stretch, which contribute to a brief clockwise rotation of the LV apex. As there are no Purkinje cells in the mid- and epicardial layers, there is a delay in the transmural spread of electrical activation, resulting in sequential subendocardial-to-subepicardial fiber shortening. Together, these are responsible for pressure buildup in the LV chamber. Direction of rotation is dominated by the higher torque produced by the larger radius of the subepicardial region despite the higher forces generated by the subendocardium. This results in global counterclockwise LV rotation near the apex and clockwise rotation near the LV base during ejection. In the subepicardium, this twist aids contraction in the principal fiber direction. In the midwall, this torque enhances shortening in the circumferential direction. In the subendocardium, it causes fiber rearrangement such that subendocardial fibers are sheared toward the LV cavity for LV wall thickening, whereas the LV base is pulled toward the apex, shortening the longitudinal axis of the LV.[18] As the matrix deforms from the twisting and shearing of the subendocardial fibers, storage of potential energy ensues, which is subsequently utilized for diastolic recoil. The torsional recoil during isovolumic relaxation and early diastole releases the potential energy stored in the deformed matrix of the subendocardium. This process is facilitated by the presence of lengthening-shortening gradients in the LV wall, which hasten lengthening of relaxed segments.

During isovolumic relaxation (IVR), the subepicardium lengthens from the base toward the apex and the subendocardium from the apex toward the base. The subsequent period of diastole is characterized by relaxation in both layers with minimum untwisting. Recognizing and evaluating the normal propagation of this electromechanical activation is important and can be applied in the evaluation of cardiac dyssynchrony and response to chronic resynchronization therapy (CRT).

STE has emerged as a method for assessing dyssynchrony in potential candidates for CRT by measuring the maximum time delay between the peak systolic strain of two segments (usually between the anteroseptal and posterolateral walls) and the desynchrony index of the LV taken from the standard deviation of time to peak systolic strain.[19] One of the limitations of 2-D STE is that it follows motion (speckles) occurring within the 2-D imaging plane. The inability of 2-D STE to measure one of the three components of the local displacement vector, which is 3-D as some speckles may be lost in through-plane motion during the cardiac cycle, is an important limitation that affects its accuracy. According to the American Society of Echocardiography Consensus Statement, ventricular dyssynchrony is a 3-D phenomenon.[20] Recently an activation imaging system has been developed that uses 3-D STE, particularly 3-D strain or areas strain, to define the onset of deformation in individual segments using a color-coded system. The algorithm uses a threshold for differentiating between varying physiologic onset of deformation and distinct delay of mechanical activation. It can be plotted on dynamic polar plot images and may be superimposed onto short and long axis planes. It provides better overview of the extension of dyssynchrony, as it has the ability to perform frame-by-frame analysis of the distribution of delayed activation (Fig. 10.14).[21]

Myocardial Deformation and LV Hemodynamics

Measurement of LV hemodynamics is best performed invasively; however, noninvasive estimations are important due to easier feasibility and lower complications rates. With the recent introduction of 2-D STE, studies tested their application for the evaluation of LV hemodynamics. Some studies showed that global longitudinal strain (GLS), longitudinal systolic strain rate, radial and circumferential systolic strain rate, torsion, and torsional rate significantly correlate to invasively measured LV filling pressures. One study reported that GLS, global circumferential strain (GCS), global radial strain (GRS), and torsion deteriorated in heart failure with preserved ejection fraction (HFpEF) patients with LV filling pressures greater than 15 mmHg compared to those patients with filling pressures less than 15 mmHg.[22]

It has been suggested that strain deterioration first starts in the longitudinal direction, and then when HFpEF becomes more advanced it affects the radial and circumferential direction, too.[23]

Impaired GLS identifies patients with low exercise capacity in HFpEF. One study showed that GLS and peak pulmonary arterial systolic pressures were independently associated with peak oxygen uptake (VO_2) in HFpEF individuals. Reduced GLS proved to be superior to EF and E/e′ in detection of patients with impaired functional capacity (peak VO_2 <20 mL/kg/min). Furthermore, in HFpEF patients, GLS was lower and correlated with LA volume index and E/e′ while EF did not, indicating tight coupling of systolic and diastolic function in HFpEF patients despite normal EF.[24]

Dysfunction of the left atrium is highly associated with HFpEF (see chapters 4 and 12). There are three major components of LA function: reservoir (LA expansion), conduit (passive emptying), and booster pump (active emptying). With recent advances in myocardial deformation imaging, 2-D STE can be applied in their evaluation. In a study on 229 patients, the LA peak reservoir strain correlated well with invasively measured LV filling pressures. LA reservoir strain decreases sequentially and significantly with rising diastolic dysfunction grades, and cutoff values were able to discriminate grades with excellent accuracy.[25]

LV diastolic time constant (tau) is an important index of LV relaxation, which is measured invasively by left heart catheterization. Tau is reported to be deteriorated even in the early stages of hypertension (HTN). However, reliable echocardiographic parameters to estimate tau have not yet been elucidated. In a recent study of 164 patients to develop a novel index based on the combination of left atrial volume (LAV) and LA function evaluated by the time–LA volume curve using speckle tracking echocardiography to estimate pulmonary capillary wedge pressure (PCWP) compared to the invasively measured PCWP by right heart catheterization, it was shown that a novel index (kinetics tracking [KT] index: log10 active LAEF/minimum LA volume index) could be a more accurate and useful predictor of PCWP than E/e′, LA volume, function, or other combinations of LA function and volume. PCWP can be estimated from 10.8 to 12.4 × KT index.[26]

ABNORMAL MYOCARDIAL DEFORMATION IN HFpEF

Aging

The aging population with heart failure is increasing worldwide. It has been shown that HTN is the driver for most aging-related changes that can contribute to adverse cardiac remodeling, myocardial fibrosis (MF), and HFpEF. Aging and concomitant HTN or myocardial infarction (MI) accelerates the march to heart failure. Identifying early age-related changes is thought to help in prognosis and tailoring medical

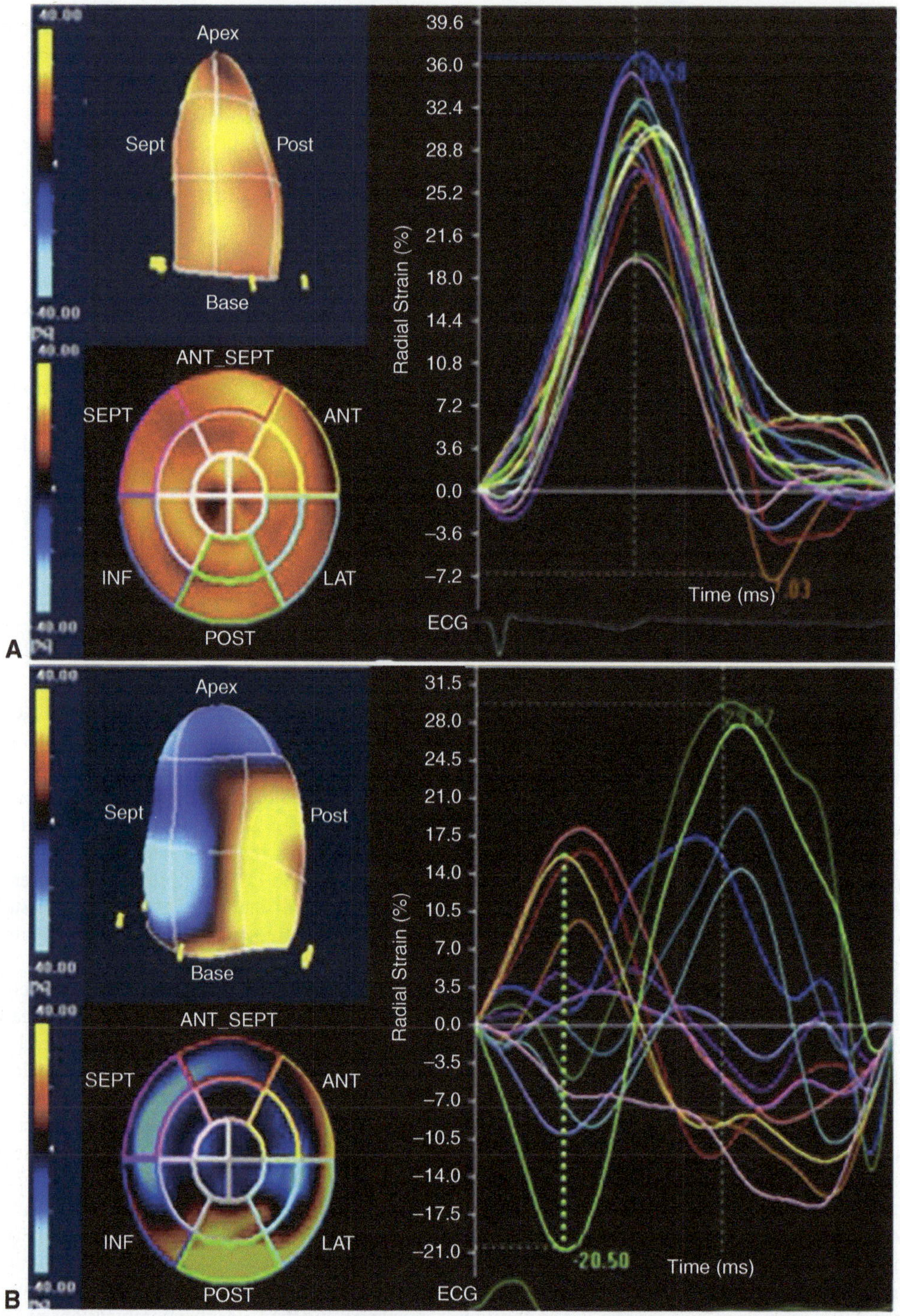

Fig. 10.14 (A) The color-coded 3-D LV display *(top left)* and bull's eye plot image *(bottom left)* and corresponding time-to-strain curves from 16 LV sites *(right panel)* from a normal control, demonstrating synchronous time-to-peak strain curves represented by homogeneous coloring at end systole. (B) The color-coded 3-D LV display *(top left)* and bull's eye plot image *(bottom left)* and corresponding time-to-strain curves from 16 LV sites *(right panel)* from a heart failure patient with left bundle branch block, demonstrating dyssynchronous time-to-peak strain curves represented by heterogeneous coloring at end systole, with early peak strain in septal segments and delayed peak strain in posterior lateral segments. (From Tanaka H, Hara H, Saba S, Gorcsan J III. Usefulness of three-dimensional speckle tracking strain to quantify dyssynchrony and the site of latest mechanical activation. *Am J Cardiol.* 2010;105:235–242.)

treatment.[27] Echocardiography has been used in basic and translational research for several years to study age-related cardiac dysfunction. Recent studies paid substantial attention to the measurement of global myocardial strain as a sensitive and strong marker of subclinical myocardial dysfunction. It showed that aging is associated in a decrease in GLS.[28] In a recent study done to determine the aging effect on cardiac morphology and function in horses, age had a significant influence on the LV free wall systolic radial strain rate and early diastolic relaxation. In the interventricular septum, systolic and late diastolic contraction velocities also increased with aging.[29] Another study showed a gradual decline in the LV regional contractility in aging mice, depicted in a decrease in both radial and longitudinal strains. Furthermore, LV segmental desynchrony in longitudinal axis reliably differentiated between aged and young mice.[30] In another human study, systolic strain rate remained unchanged (corresponding to the reservoir function) with respect to controls; early diastolic strain rate (correlated with conduit phase) decreased, whereas late diastolic strain rate (corresponding to the contractile function) increased to compensate the age-dependent LV diastolic dysfunction, and thus the reservoir function is maintained.[31]

Pressure Overload and Hypertrophy

Echocardiography plays a vital role in providing differential diagnosis, prognosis, and management of hypertrophic cardiomyopathy (HCM). Hypertrophy and fibrosis progress despite a preservation in EF. Myocardial deformation imaging can be utilized to evaluate the etiology of increased LV wall thickness whether due to HTN, infiltration, or physiologic adaptation (so-called athlete's heart). Measurement of GLS using speckle tracking echocardiography is typically reduced in patients with HCM and fibrosis. Reduction of GLS to 15% in an HCM patient cohort with preserved LV EF was associated with fibrosis.[32] GLS was the strongest independent predictor of fibrosis assessed by late gadolinium enhancement on cardiac MRI. Furthermore, there is a prognostic significance in HCM with preserved LV EF in patients who have reduced GLS.[33]

GLS can also help in characterizing infiltrative cardiac disease. In cardiac amyloidosis early diagnosis is crucial, specifically in AL amyloid as early treatment has implications on mortality (see chapter 23). In 60% of amyloid patients, there is a reduction of strain globally, but the apex tends to be spared (Fig. 10.15).[34] In Fabry disease an early systolic peak followed by a rapid fall and a second peak during the isovolumic relaxation phase indicative of postsystolic shortening is characteristic on the strain rate curves (Fig. 10.16).[35] In asymmetric septal HCM, there is reduced septal strain (Fig. 10.17).

Myocardial Ischemia

Measurement of GLS or segmental strain at rest is a helpful tool in the evaluation and detection of ischemic heart disease (IHD), especially when the LVEF is preserved and there are no apparent wall motion abnormalities. In evaluating myocardial deformation in IHD, an important marker is postsystolic shortening, so the use of end systole rather than peak strain is more helpful.

In animal models of induced coronary ischemia, there was a strong direct correlation between the spatial distributions of postsystolic shortening measured by strain rate imaging and myocardium at risk.[36] In patients with ischemic cardiomyopathy, an increase of peak systolic strain rate from rest to dobutamine stimulation by more than $-0.23\ s^{-1}$ allowed accurate discrimination of viable from nonviable myocardial segments, as determined by 18-fluorodeoxyglucose positron emission tomography with a sensitivity of 83% and a specificity of 84%. In this study, strain imaging was superior to TDE and 2-D wall thickening subjective assessment.

It has been shown that both lesion-specific regional strain and GLS are reduced in patients with stable coronary artery disease (CAD). Basal segment involvement with relatively apical sparing is seen more in left main or three vessel disease with a sensitivity of 79%.[37,38] Although CAD is inherently a regional disease, abnormal GLS detects moderate to severe CAD with 74% sensitivity and 72% specificity. Measuring GLS during exercise test can provide a prediction for CAD and thus has a role in work.

In a study of 64 patients presenting to the emergency room (ER) with suspected non-ST elevation myocardial infraction (NSTEMI), a GLS below 21% had a negative predictive value of 92% for exclusion of significant CAD.[39]

GLS may play a role in detecting infarct burden and size. In a study of 38 patients, reduced GLS less than 15% independently predicted infarct masses larger than 30 g with sensitivity and specificity of 83% and 93%, respectively.[40] Another study evaluated 111 patients with suspected NSTEMI 1 hour after admission to the ER; in this study, lesion-specific regional circumferential strain was the best parameter for predicting acute coronary occlusion. A territorial circumferential strain value greater than −10% had 90% sensitivity and 88% specificity.[41]

Interstitial Fibrosis

Myocardial fibrosis is a common early morphologic alteration in different cardiac pathologies associated with abnormal cardiac remodeling. Fibrosis is associated with both diastolic and systolic LV dysfunction from increased wall stiffness and stress and, ultimately, the

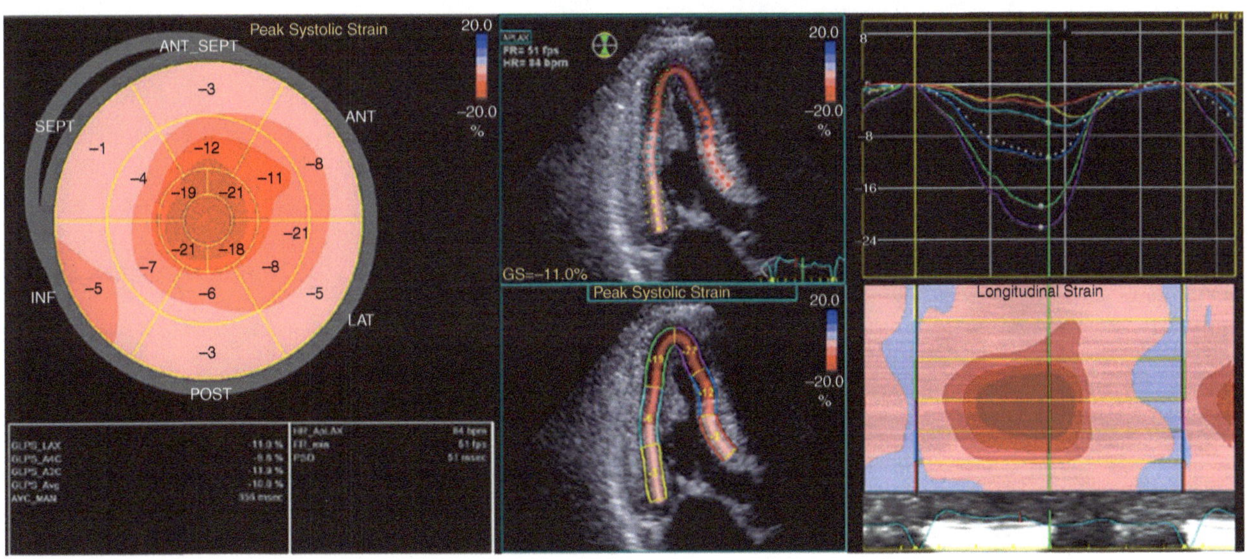

Fig. 10.15 Speckle tracking echocardiographic example of impaired peak systolic strain and the typical bull's eye showing relative apical sparing. (From Brouwers S, Laptseva N, Gerber B, Schwotzer R, Ruschitzka F, Flammer AJ. Cardiac amyloidosis. *Cardiovasc Med.* 2018;21(11):282–289.)

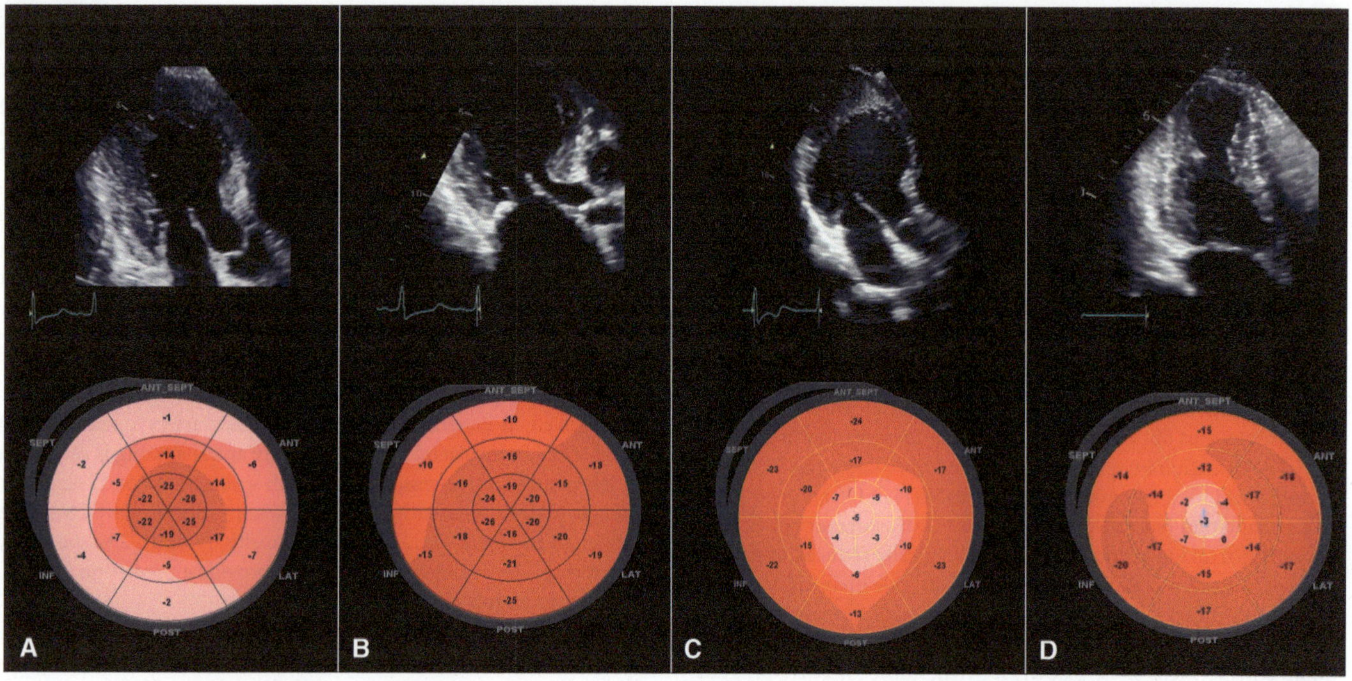

Fig. 10.16 Two-dimensional images (top panels) and bull's eye plots (bottom panels) show (A) an apical sparring pattern in cardiac amyloidosis vs (B) reduced septal strain in asymmetric obstructive hypertrophic cardiomyopathy; (C) reduced apical strain in apical hypertrophic cardiomyopathy; and (D) reduced apical strain after apical myocardial infarction. (From Collier et al, A test in contest: Myocardial strain measured by speckle-tracking echocardiography. *J Am Coll Cardiol* 2017;69:1043–56)

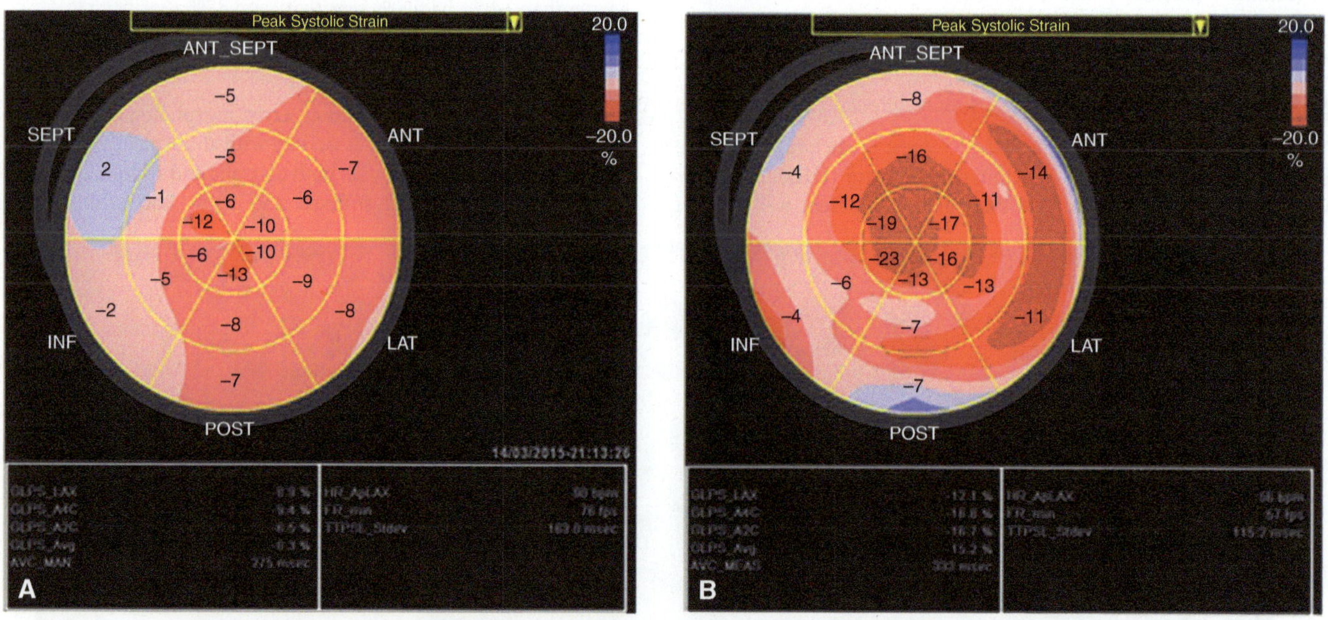

Fig. 10.17 Examples of the longitudinal strain bull's eye plot in patients with hypertrophic cardiomyopathy (HCM). (A) HCM patient with asymmetric hypertrophy. (B) HCM patient with concentric hypertrophy. (Courtesy of Specklepedia.com and Liu, D., et al., Effect of Combined Systolic and Diastolic Functional Parameter Assessment for Differentiation of Cardiac Amyloidosis From Other Causes of Concentric Left Ventricular Hypertrophy. Circulation: Cardiovascular Imaging, 2013. 6(6): p. 1066–1072.)

progression toward congestive heart failure. Furthermore, different MF deposition patterns can help in differentiating the etiology of heart failure. For example, the hallmark of ischemic scar is macroscopic substitutive fibrosis, while diffuse interstitial and/or perivascular fibrosis is generally seen in nonischemic cardiomyopathies and valvular heart diseases (reactive fibrosis). Early diagnosis of subclinical stages of cardiac remodeling and fibrosis is of importance. Harmonic phase (HARP) analysis of tagged MRI images and T1 mapping to quantify extracellular expansion and volume are currently the most widely used methods.[42]

The evaluation of LV deformation by 2-D STE allows better assessment of the subtle early changes of myocardial contractile behavior and remodeling due to MF compared to LV EF, which is not as sensitive until the disease becomes more advanced. Patients with MF detected on cardiac MRI show more impaired LV GLS as compared with patients without, despite preserved LV EF. In a study of 101 consecutive Fabry patients, MF was associated with lower longitudinal strain in the fibrotic wall segments as confirmed by late enhancement in MRI.[43] In another recent study of 36 patients with severe aortic stenosis and preserved EF, reduced regional and global LV myocardial strain, correlated with fibrosis determined by biopsy, shows an inverse relationship between strain and fibrosis burden.[44]

CLINICAL UTILITY OF DEFORMATION INDICES

Diagnosis of HFpEF

Despite its frequency, diagnosis of HFpEF remains a riddle. As of yet, it remains mostly a diagnosis of exclusion. For this and other reasons, the pharmacologic treatment of HFpEF remains difficult, with no randomized controlled trials having shown improved survivals except in a small series of transthyretin (TTR) amyloidosis, even though many drugs have been linked to functional benefit. Therefore new imaging techniques and technology are warranted for better and early diagnosis.

STE early diastolic strain rate is an excellent modality for evaluation of diastolic function. It reflects the myocardial lengthening rate and untwisting rate, which are tightly coupled to restoring forces and diastolic suction. However, as of yet strain rate has not been able to replace TDI e′ due to its greater signal noise and lower reproducibility.

GLS is a very promising method to identify patients with systolic dysfunction that has not resulted in reduced EF. A recent study comparing longitudinal and circumferential global strain in 301 patients with symptomatic HFpEF and diastolic dysfunction to controls free from cardiovascular disease and hypertensive patients with diastolic dysfunction but no heart failure found lower longitudinal and circumferential strain in HFpEF patients compared to the other groups.[45]

In patients with HFpEF, impaired diastolic filling may be affected by spatial heterogeneity and temporal dyssynchrony of function. In a study where artificial intelligence (machine learning) was used to analyze the spatiotemporal characteristics of measured velocity, strain, and strain rate traces in 100 subjects imaged at rest and during semisupine bicycle exercise, temporal and spatial variations in regional myocardial function and functional reserve were identified in patients with HFpEF.[46] To date the application of strain imaging in HFpEF is still lacking in clinical practice, but in the future it is likely to become a useful tool when evaluating patients with unexplained heart failure symptoms.[47]

Prognosis

Prognosis in cardiac disease is closely related to systolic function. An increasing number of studies have suggested that GLS is superior to EF as a measure of LV function and as a predictor of mortality and cardiac events. Among patients with HFpEF enrolled in the Treatment of Preserved Cardiac Function Heart Failure with an Aldosterone Antagonist (TOPCAT) trial, LV longitudinal strain was worse when compared to controls without heart failure matched for demographics and comorbidities, and was associated with a higher risk of the composite end point of heart failure hospitalization, cardiovascular death, or aborted sudden death. Furthermore, after adjusting for clinical and conventional echocardiographic factors and measures, lower GLS was associated with cardiovascular death and heart failure hospitalization risk alone.[48] In another study where GCS was obtained in 201 patients hospitalized for acute heart failure, lower GCS was an independent prognosticator of cardiac events in heart failure regardless of age, LV EF, and E/e′, and has greater prognostic power than GLS or LV EF.[49] Other studies have reported that reduced GLS is a powerful and independent predictor for vascular events such as stroke, MI, and new onset of atrial fibrillation in the general population.[50] Lower GLS also demonstrated prognostic value for adverse outcomes in patients with valvular heart disease, including asymptomatic degenerative mitral regurgitation, and in patients with severe aortic stenosis undergoing aortic valve replacement.[51,52]

In a study of 546 patients, GLS proved to be a superior predictor of all-cause mortality when compared with LV EF and myocardial wall motion score index in patients with CAD.[53]

Furthermore, a drop in longitudinal strain measurements can detect early systolic LV impairment in patients undergoing chemotherapy, and as per American Society of Echocardiography guidelines, a drop in GLS greater than 15% from baseline in patients undergoing chemotherapy is associated with cardiac events and dysfunction.[54] In a large group of obstructive hypertrophic cardiomyopathy patients with preserved LV EF, abnormal LV GLS is independently associated with higher cardiac events, whereas myectomy is associated with improved outcomes.[55]

FUTURE DIRECTIONS

Potential future improvement in speckle tracking echocardiography will be focused on shorter analysis time and improved tracking and border recognition with the application of greater automation and machine learning protocols, which may lead to more widespread adoption of the technique. Furthermore, ongoing development of 3-D strain may overcome limitations caused by out-of-plane speckle motion and should improve diagnostic potential from the technology.

KEY POINTS

- Myocardial velocities can be obtained from multiple locations of the myocardium using tissue Doppler imaging. TDI velocities are affected not only by regional LV mechanical events but also by global translation and rotation of the heart.
- Strain is a unitless measurement of deformational/geometry change of the myocardium and is often expressed as a percentage. Thus changes in LV geometry during LV systole relate primarily to radial (short axis), longitudinal (long axis), circumferential, and torsional strain.
- Speckle tracking echocardiography is based on B mode gray scale tracking of 2-D speckles. 2-D speckle tracking–derived strain is angle-independent and provides mechanical analysis of the whole thickness of myocardium seen in one echocardiographic view.

- Modern STE techniques can measure LV rotation and twist by quantifying apical and basal twist rotation followed by the calculation of LV torsion from short axis projections.
- GLS, GCS, GRS, and strain rates can be applied in the evaluation of HFpEF, interstitial fibrosis, myocardial ischemia, and cardiomyopathies. They also proved to be important indices in the prognosis of cardiac disease.

REVIEW QUESTIONS

1. Which of the following combinations of views may be used to obtain all global longitudinal, radial, and circumferential strain?
   a. Basal, midventricular, and apical short axis views
   b. Parasternal long and midventricular short axis views
   c. Apical four-chamber and two-chamber views
   d. Apical four-chamber, two-chamber, and long axis views
2. Compared to TDI-derived strain, speckle tracking–derived strain:
   a. is less angle dependent.
   b. provides higher temporal resolution.
   c. is less affected by translational motion.
   d. requires fundamental imaging.
3. Which of the following represents global longitudinal strain?
   a. The sum of the basal, mid-, and apical segments strain values
   b. The average of the basal, mid-, and apical segments strain values
   c. The average of the three apical views percentage change in length from base to base around the extent of the LV wall
   d. The average difference between basal and apical strain values

REFERENCES

1. Klein AL, Hatle LK, Burstow DJ, et al. Doppler characterization of left ventricular diastolic function in cardiac amyloidosis. *J Am Coll Cardiol.* 1989;13(5):1017–1026.
2. Rihal CS, Nishimura RA, Hatle LK, Bailey KR, Tajik AJ. Systolic and diastolic dysfunction in patients with clinical diagnosis of dilated cardiomyopathy. Relation to symptoms and prognosis. *Circulation.* 1994;90(6):2772–2779.
3. Redfield MM, Jacobsen SJ, Burnett JC Jr, Mahoney DW, Bailey KR, Rodeheffer RJ. Burden of systolic and diastolic ventricular dysfunction in the community: appreciating the scope of the heart failure epidemic. *JAMA.* 2003;289(2):194–202.
4. Støylen A. *Strain Rate Imaging of the Left Ventricle by Ultrasound. Feasibility, Clinical Validation and Physiological Aspects.* Trondheim, Norway: Norwegian University of Science and Technology; 2001.
5. Collier P, Phelan D, Klein A. A test in context: myocardial strain measured by speckle-tracking echocardiography. *J Am Coll Cardiol.* 2017;69(8):1043–1056.
6. Potter E, Marwick TH. Assessment of left ventricular function by echocardiography: the case for routinely adding global longitudinal strain to ejection fraction. *JACC. Cardiovasc Imag.* 2018;11(2 Part 1):260–274.
7. Mirea O, Duchenne J, Voigt J. Recent advances in echocardiography: strain and strain rate imaging [version 1; referees: 3 approved]. *F1000Research.* 2016;5(787):000.
8. Opdahl A, Helle-Valle T, Skulstad H, Smiseth OA. Strain, strain rate, torsion, and twist: echocardiographic evaluation. *Curr Cardiol Rep.* 2015;17(3):568.
9. Rüssel IK, Götte MJ, Bronzwaer JG, Knaapen P, Paulus WJ, van Rossum A. Left ventricular torsion: an expanding role in the analysis of myocardial dysfunction. *JACC. Cardiovasc Imag.* 2009;2(5):648–655.
10. Helle-Valle T, Crosby J, Edvardsen T, et al. New noninvasive method for assessment of left ventricular rotation. *Circulation.* 2005;112(20):3149–3156.
11. Kaku K, Takeuchi M, Tsang W, et al. Age-related normal range of left ventricular strain and torsion using three-dimensional speckle-tracking echocardiography. *J Am Soc Echocardiogr.* 2014;27(1):55–64.
12. Salvo GD, Pergola V, Fadel B, Bulbul ZA, Caso P. Strain echocardiography and myocardial mechanics: from basics to clinical applications. *J Cardiovasc Echogr.* 2015;25(1):1–8.
13. Sengupta PP, Tajik AJ, Chandrasekaran K, Khandheria BK. Twist mechanics of the left ventricle: principles and application. *JACC. Cardiovasc Imag.* 2008;1(3):366–376.
14. Sallin EA. Fiber orientation and ejection fraction in the human left ventricle. *Biophys J.* 1969;9(7):954–964.
15. Abduch MCD, Alencar AM, Mathias W Jr, Vieira ML. Cardiac mechanics evaluated by speckle tracking echocardiography. *Arquivos Brasileiros De Cardiologia.* 2014;102(4):403–412.
16. Notomi Y, Lysyansky P, Setser RM, et al. Measurement of ventricular torsion by two-dimensional ultrasound speckle tracking imaging. *J Am Coll Cardiol.* 2005;45(12):2034–2041.
17. Sengupta PP, Tondato F, Khandheria BK, Belohlavek M, Jahangir A. Electromechanical activation sequence in normal heart. *Heart Fail Clin.* 2008;4(3):303–314.
18. Ingels NB JR, Hansen DE, Daughters GT, Stinson EB, Alderman EL, Miller DC. Relation between longitudinal, circumferential, and oblique shortening and torsional deformation in the left ventricle of the transplanted human heart. *Circ Res.* 1989;64(5):915–927.
19. Khan SG, Klettas D, Kapetanakis S, Monaghan MJ. Clinical utility of speckle-tracking echocardiography in cardiac resynchronisation therapy. *Echo Res Prac.* 2016;3(1):R1–R11.
20. Seo Y, Ishizu T, Kawamura R, et al. Three-dimensional propagation imaging of left ventricular activation by speckle-tracking echocardiography to predict responses to cardiac resynchronization therapy. *J Am Soc Echocardiogr.* 2015;28(5):606–614.
21. Nesser HJ. Wall motion tracking and activation imaging—latest developments and applications for patients with heart failure. *Eur Cardiol.* 2012;8(1):51–55.
22. Nguyen JS, Lakkis NM, Bobek J, Goswami R, Dokainish H. Systolic and diastolic myocardial mechanics in patients with cardiac disease and preserved ejection fraction: impact of left ventricular filling pressure. *J Am Soc Echocardiogr.* 2010;23(12):1273–1280.
23. Kosmala W, Plaksej R, Strotmann JM, et al. Progression of left ventricular functional abnormalities in hypertensive patients with heart failure: an ultrasonic two-dimensional speckle tracking study. *J Am Soc Echocardiogr.* 2008;21(12):1309–1317.
24. Hasselberg NE, Haugaa KH, Sarvari SI, et al. Left ventricular global longitudinal strain is associated with exercise capacity in failing hearts with preserved and reduced ejection fraction. *Eur Heart J Cardiovasc Imag.* 2015;16(2):217–224.
25. Singh A, Addetia K, Maffessanti F, Mor-Avi V, Lang RM. LA strain for categorization of LV diastolic dysfunction. *JACC. Cardiovasc Imag.* 2017;10(7):735–743.
26. Kawasaki M, Tanaka R, Ono K, et al. A novel ultrasound predictor of pulmonary capillary wedge pressure assessed by the combination of left atrial volume and function: a speckle tracking echocardiography study. *J Cardiol.* 2015;66(3):253–262.
27. Jugdutt BI. Aging-related changes in cardiac extracellular matrix: implications for heart failure in older patients. *J Cardiol Curr Res.* 2015;3(3):00101.
28. Vizir VA, Sadomov AS, Nasonenko OV, Age-related changes in myocardial deformation and arterial stiffness in hypertensive males. *Zaporozhye Medical Journal.* 2016;6(99):21–24.10.14739/2310-1210.2016.6.85487.
29. Gehlen H, Bildheim LM. Speckle-tracking analysis of myocardial deformation in correlation to age in healthy horses. *J Vet Sci.* 2018;19(5):676–682.

30. de Lucia C, Wallner M, Eaton DM, Zhao H, Houser SR, Koch WJ. Echocardiographic strain analysis for the early detection of left ventricular systolic/diastolic dysfunction and dyssynchrony in a mouse model of physiological aging. *J Gerontol. Series A, Biol Sci Med Sci.* 2018;74:455–461.
31. Cacciapuoti F, Paoli VD, Scognamiglio A, Caturano M, Cacciapuoti F. Left atrial longitudinal speckle tracking echocardiography in healthy aging heart. *J Cardiovasc Echogr.* 2015;25(2):40–45.
32. Serri K, Reant P, Lafitte M, et al. Global and regional myocardial function quantification by two-dimensional strain: application in hypertrophic cardiomyopathy. *J Am Coll Cardiol.* 2006;47(6):1175–1181.
33. Saito M, Okayama H, Yoshii T, et al. Clinical significance of global two-dimensional strain as a surrogate parameter of myocardial fibrosis and cardiac events in patients with hypertrophic cardiomyopathy. *Eur Heart J Cardiovasc Imag.* 2012;13(7):617–623.
34. Phelan D, Collier P, Thavendiranathan P, et al. Relative apical sparing of longitudinal strain using two-dimensional speckle-tracking echocardiography is both sensitive and specific for the diagnosis of cardiac amyloidosis. *Heart.* 2012;98:1442–1448.
35. Liu D, Hu K, Niemann M, et al. Effect of combined systolic and diastolic functional parameter assessment for differentiation of cardiac amyloidosis from other causes of concentric left ventricular hypertrophy. *Circ. Cardiovasc Imag.* 2013;6(6):1066–1072.
36. Pislaru C, Belohlavek M, Bae RY, Abraham TP, Greenleaf JF, Seward JB. Regional asynchrony during acute myocardial ischemia quantified by ultrasound strain rate imaging. *J Am Coll Cardiol.* 2001;37(4):1141–1148.
37. Biering-Sorensen T, Biering-Sørensen T, Hoffmann S, et al. Myocardial strain analysis by 2-dimensional speckle tracking echocardiography improves diagnostics of coronary artery stenosis in stable angina pectoris. *Circ. Cardiovasc Imag.* 2014;7(1):58–65.
38. Choi JO, Cho SW, Song YB, et al. Longitudinal 2D strain at rest predicts the presence of left main and three vessel coronary artery disease in patients without regional wall motion abnormality. *Eur J Echocardiogr.* 2009;10(5):695–701.
39. Dahlslett T, Karlsen S, Grenne B, et al. Early assessment of strain echocardiography can accurately exclude significant coronary artery stenosis in suspected non-ST-segment elevation acute coronary syndrome. *J Am Soc Echocardiogr.* 2014;27(5):512–519.
40. Gjesdal O, Hopp E, Vartdal T, et al. Global longitudinal strain measured by two-dimensional speckle tracking echocardiography is closely related to myocardial infarct size in chronic ischaemic heart disease. *Clin Sci (London, England).* 2007;113(6):287–296.
41. Grenne B, Eek C, Sjøli B, et al. Acute coronary occlusion in non-ST-elevation acute coronary syndrome: outcome and early identification by strain echocardiography. *Heart (British Cardiac Society).* 2010;96(19):1550–1556.
42. Donekal S, Venkatesh BA, Liu YC, et al. Interstitial fibrosis, left ventricular remodeling, and myocardial mechanical behavior in a population-based multiethnic cohort. *Circ. Cardiovasc Imag.* 2014;7(2):292–302.
43. Krämer J, Niemann M, Liu D, et al. Two-dimensional speckle tracking as a non-invasive tool for identification of myocardial fibrosis in Fabry disease. *Eur Heart J.* 2013;34(21):1587–1596.
44. Fabiani I, Scatena C, Mazzanti CM, et al. Micro-RNA-21 (biomarker) and global longitudinal strain (functional marker) in detection of myocardial fibrotic burden in severe aortic valve stenosis: a pilot study. *J Trans Med.* 2016;14(1):248.
45. Kraigher-Krainer E, Shah AM, Gupta DK, et al. Impaired systolic function by strain imaging in heart failure with preserved ejection fraction. *J Am Coll Cardiol.* 2014;63(5):447–456.
46. Tabassian M, Sunderji I, Erdei T, et al. Diagnosis of heart failure with preserved ejection fraction: machine learning of spatiotemporal variations in left ventricular deformation. *J Am Soc Echocardiogr.* 2018;31(12):1272–1284. e9.
47. Smiseth OA, Torp H, Opdahl A, Haugaa KH, Urheim S. Myocardial strain imaging: how useful is it in clinical decision making? *Eur Heart J.* 2016;37(15):1196–1207.
48. Shah AM, Claggett B, Sweitzer NK, et al. Prognostic importance of impaired systolic function in heart failure with preserved ejection fraction and the impact of spironolactone. *Circulation.* 2015;132(5):402–414.
49. Cho GY, Marwick TH, Kim HS, Kim MK, Hong KS, Oh DJ. Global 2-dimensional strain as a new prognosticator in patients with heart failure. *J Am Coll Cardiol.* 2009;54(7):618–624.
50. Russo C, Jin Z, Elkind MS, et al. Prevalence and prognostic value of subclinical left ventricular systolic dysfunction by global longitudinal strain in a community-based cohort. *Eur J Heart Fail.* 2014;16(12):1301–1309.
51. Lancellotti P, Cosyns B, Zacharakis D, et al. Importance of left ventricular longitudinal function and functional reserve in patients with degenerative mitral regurgitation: assessment by two-dimensional speckle tracking. *J Am Soc Echocardiogr.* 2008;21(12):1331–1336.
52. Dahl JS, Videbæk L, Poulsen MK, Rudbæk TR, Pellikka PA, Møller JE. Global strain in severe aortic valve stenosis: relation to clinical outcome after aortic valve replacement. *Circ. Cardiovasc Imag.* 2012;5(5):613–620.
53. Stanton T, Leano R, Marwick TH. Prediction of all-cause mortality from global longitudinal speckle strain: comparison with ejection fraction and wall motion scoring. *Circ. Cardiovasc Imag.* 2009;2(5):356–364.
54. Plana JC, Galderisi M, Barac A, et al. Expert consensus for multimodality imaging evaluation of adult patients during and after cancer therapy: a report from the American Society of Echocardiography and the European Association of Cardiovascular Imaging. *J Am Soc Echocardiogr.* 2014;27(9):911–939.
55. Tower-Rader A, Betancor J, Popovic ZB, et al. Incremental prognostic utility of left ventricular global longitudinal strain in hypertrophic obstructive cardiomyopathy patients and preserved left ventricular ejection fraction. *J Am Heart Assoc.* 2017;6(10):e006514.

11

Color M-mode Doppler

Leonardo Rodriguez and Marie Stugaard

OUTLINE

INTRODUCTION

Pulsed-wave Doppler velocities of mitral inflow are the most commonly used indices of diastolic function. Their application is nevertheless limited by their load dependency. Flow propagation (Vp) using color M mode Doppler has been proposed as a complementary technique to evaluate left ventricular (LV) relaxation.

Color M mode Doppler echocardiography provides a spatiotemporal map of blood distribution within the heart, with a typical temporal resolution of 5 msec, a spatial resolution of 300 microns, and a velocity resolution of 3 cm/sec. By aligning the cursor parallel to the streamlines of flow we can observe the propagation of flow from the mitral valve to the apex (Fig. 11.1). Assessment of diastolic flow propagation has offered novel information about LV filling dynamics and has been applied in a variety of clinical conditions. Since the initial description of Jacobs[1] and later Brun,[2] computer simulation,[3] in vitro modeling,[4] animal,[5,6] and clinical studies[2,5–8] have improved our understanding of the determinants of Vp but also have shown the complexity of this index. The Vp appears to be relatively independent of loading conditions and therefore may overcome one of the main limitations of Doppler-based techniques.[2,5,7,9]

In this chapter we will review the current understanding of how flow propagates from the base to apex of the left ventricle, its major determinants, how to properly obtain a color M mode (CMM) tracing, and clinical situations where this technique may be applied. We will also describe its application in the calculation of intraventricular pressure gradients.

Case Study

A 53-year-old female patient presents with shortness of breath putting on shoes and climbing one flight of stairs. She reports a fullness in the epigastric area. There is no lower extremity edema. Normal coronaries.

Echo shows dilated left atrium, mild respiratory variation, but septal bounce. This color M-mode was obtained showing rapid flow propagation from base to apex (Fig. 11.2).

BACKGROUND

It is now well recognized that in early diastole there are small but significant intraventricular mitral-to-apex pressure gradients that are generated.[10,11] These intraventricular pressure gradients (IVPG) are related to elastic recoil[12–14] and represent one of the driving forces of the blood entering the left ventricle (ventricular suction). As a result, when the mitral valve opens, a column of blood accelerates from the atrium toward the ventricular apex. In normal ventricles, flow propagates very rapidly (Fig. 11.3A) while in dilated, poorly contracted ventricles it occurs rather slowly[2] (see Fig. 11.3B).

Mitral inflow flow propagation displayed by CMM has a complex pattern. The earliest CMM velocities often occur during isovolumic relaxation. After the mitral valve opens there is a rapid initial component (phase I) often followed by a slower component (phase II). Finally the last component in late diastole is associated with atrial contraction (see Fig. 11.1).

Computer and in vitro modeling have helped to understand the complex phenomenon of flow propagation. During phase I, blood moves almost simultaneously in the whole left ventricle behaving as an incompressible fluid column (columnar flow).[3,4] Phase II is a flow wave thought to be caused by propagation of a ring vortex formed at the ventricular base.[3,4,15,16] Advances in imaging techniques have expanded our understanding of vortex formation and propagation (Figs. 11.4 and 11.5).[17,18] It has been suggested that vortex formation may contribute to increased efficiency of LV filling.[17,19] The formation of a vortex is affected by the size and eccentricity of the mitral orifice[4] as well as the geometry and size of the left ventricle.[20] In small, tubular ventricles there is predominant columnar flow with no space from the mitral leaflets to the ventricular wall for vortex formation. In dilated ventricles with decreased ratio of mitral valve orifice to ventricular diameter there would be predominant vortex formation and propagation[4] (see Fig. 11.4). In dilated cardiomyopathy vortices move flow toward the LV outflow tract in diastole with little loss in energy and without significant increase in pressure. By in vitro modeling, the ratio of flow velocity to vortex propagation is around 2:1.[4]

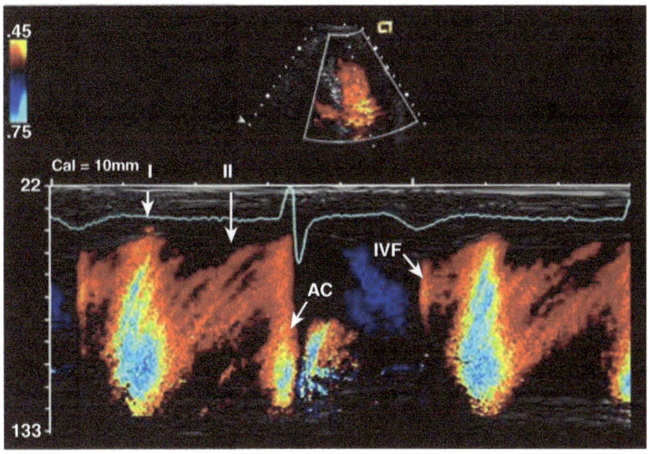

Fig. 11.1 Color M-mode of mitral inflow obtained from the apical window. Several components can be appreciated from this tracing. Phase I is faster, followed by the slower phase II (vortex) component. A short flow *(IVF)* during isovolumetric relaxation is also seen as well as late flow during atrial contraction *(AC)*.

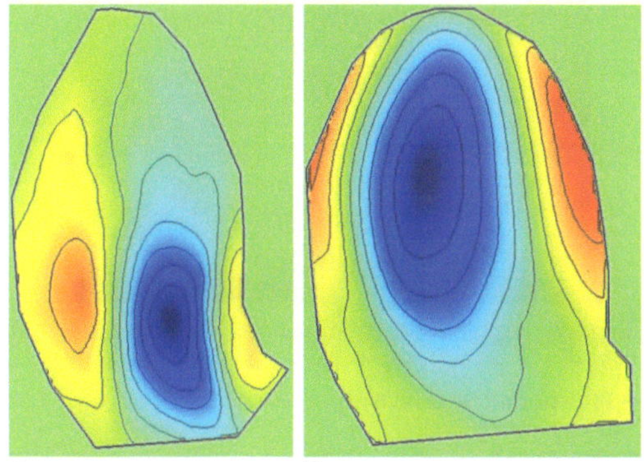

Fig. 11.4 Streamlines and color map of the vorticity field showing vortex formation in a normal subject (A) and in a patient with dilated cardiomyopathy (B). Note a larger vortex displaced to the apex in the patient with dilated cardiomyopathy. (From Mele D, Smarrazzo V, Pedrizzety G, Capasso F, Pepe M, Severino S, et al, Intradiac flow analysis: Techniques and potential clinical applications. *J Am Soc Echocardiogr.* 2019;3:319–332.)

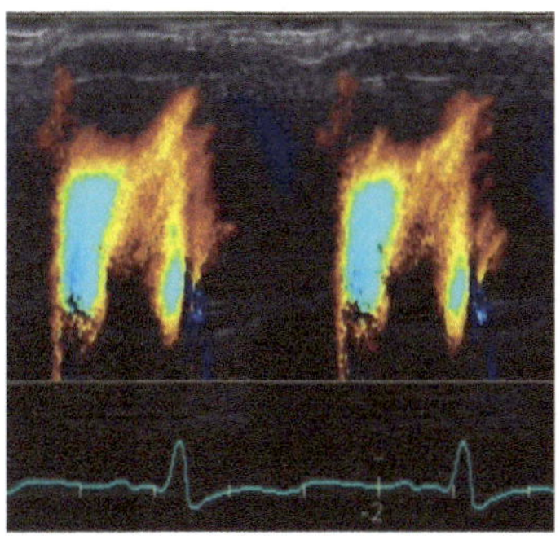

Fig. 11.2 This color M-mode was obtained showing rapid flow propagation from base to apex.

Obtaining and Measuring Flow Propagation

CMM flow propagation is usually measured from the apical four-chamber view. The M mode cursor is carefully aligned with direction of flow, maximizing the distance from mitral tips to apex. At least 4 cm of CMM depth should be obtained and displayed at 100 cm/sec sweep speed. In the initial description by Brun,[2] CMM flow propagation was measured as the slope of color-noncolor interface. The use of the slope of the color-noncolor interface is limited by its interference with isovolumic flow. Since then, several other methods have been proposed, and this constitutes one of the main limitations of this technique and makes it difficult to compare studies among different authors. The slope of the first aliasing velocity has also been used by several authors, setting the aliasing velocity at a percentage (40–70%) of the maximal inflow velocity[5,21] (see Fig. 11.3). An aliasing velocity of 40% of the peak E wave velocity appears to be more reproducible and better reflect the velocity of propagation.[21] There is no consensus guidelines whether phase I or phase II should be measured. Garcia et al.[22] proposed the use of phase II when present.

Stugaard et al. used a computer algorithm to detect the maximal velocities along the center of the flow propagation wave and measured the time delay between the velocity at mitral tips and apex.[8] This method is attractive for it appears to be more objective, but it is not widely available. An automated way to measure the slope of Vp has been described.[23]

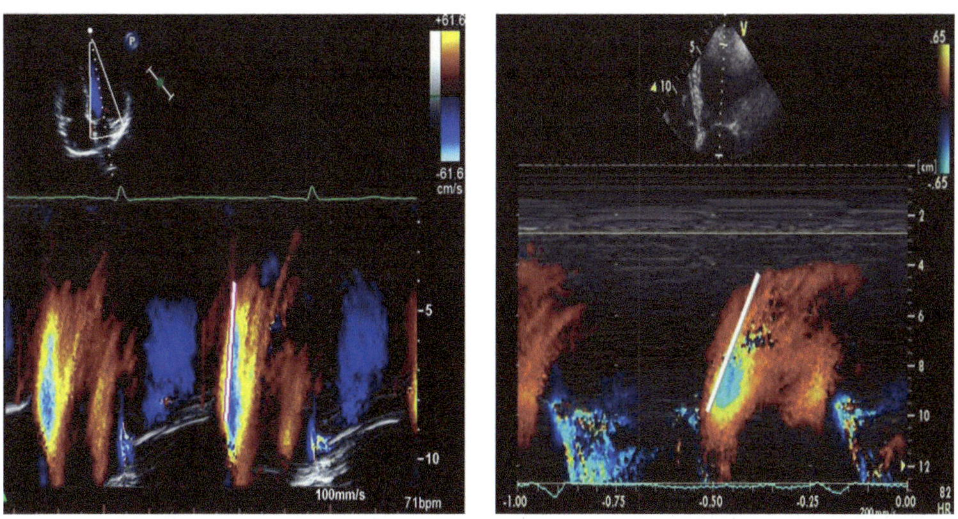

Fig. 11.3 Example of a young normal individual (A) and a patient with delayed relaxation (B). Note the difference in color M mode (CMM) Vp slope between the two.

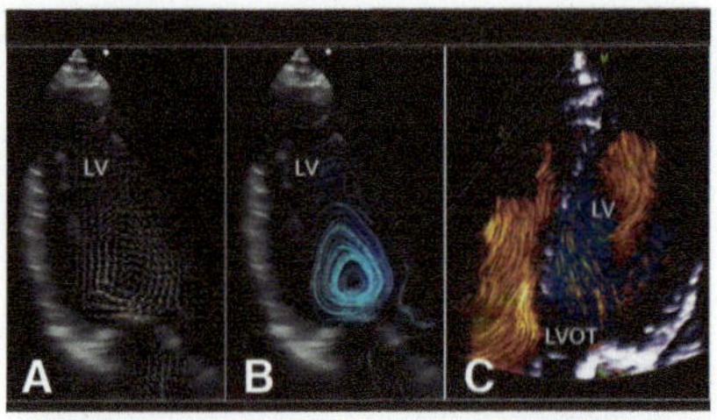

Fig. 11.5 Echocardiographic techniques for vortex visualization. (From Mele D, Smarrazzo V, Pedrizzetti G, et al. Intracardiac flow analysis: techniques and potential clinical applications. *J Am Soc Echocardiogr.* 2019;32:319–332.)

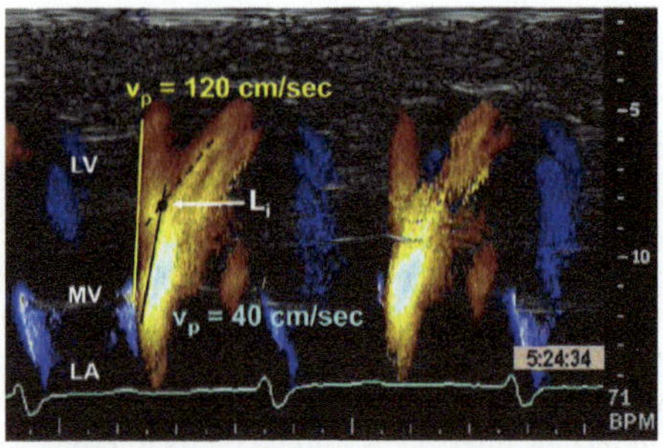

Fig. 11.6 Flow velocity propagation and deceleration point. L1 is the distance between annulus and deceleration point. (From Thomas JD. Flow propagation analysis computer or eyeball? *JACC Cardiovasc Imag.* 2011;4:47–49.)

Normal values of Vp depend on the methodology used. The slope of first aliasing (40%–50% of peak E velocity) values less than 45 cm/sec are considered abnormal. The interobserver variability of Vp measurements has been reported to be around 12%[24] but can be as high as 20%.[15]

More recently Stewart et al.[25] proposed a semiautomated method taking into account the change of the slope of the curvilinear isovelocity contours. Using statistical point-change analysis, the authors defined the deceleration point. Thus the contour was divided at the deceleration point into the initial propagation and the terminal propagation. Finally a new parameter, the strength of early filling (Vs), was calculated as the product of the distance from the position of the mitral annulus to the deceleration point and the initial Vp (Fig. 11.6). The authors showed that in a validation study of 160 patients, Vs was more accurate than Vp to assess diastolic dysfunction (as defined by reduced diastolic intraventricular pressure gradient, elevated pulmonary capillary wedge pressure (PCWP), or elevated B-type natriuretic peptide). In diastolic dysfunction, the initial velocity was slower and the deceleration point occurred closer to the mitral annulus than with normal filling. Although promising to better describe flow propagation properties, further studies are needed in other laboratories to test the feasibility and usefulness of this method.

Late (A Wave) CMM Flow Propagation

Most of the studies have focused on the propagation of early mitral inflow. There are limited data about the importance and clinical significance of the propagation of flow during atrial contraction (Vpa). One study that includes 75 healthy adult subjects age 18 to 79 years revealed a large range of values of Vpa from 26 to 179 cm/sec.[26] Vpa was mainly dependent on age, gender, and LV mass.

There is a fundamental difference between the early and late flow propagation. During early propagation blood is pulled into the ventricle, while during late propagation it is pushed (atrial contraction). A ratio of early to late flow propagation has been reported in patients with pseudonormal filling pattern,[27] although the advantage of this over early Vp alone or E/Vp is unclear. Further studies are required to explore the importance and clinical significance of late diastolic flow propagation.

CMM Intraventricular Pressure Gradients

Given the complexity of CMM inflow pattern and the variability of measurements of flow propagation, a more objective analysis of LV filling is desirable.

It is well known that the presence of regional pressure differences in the left ventricle is related to LV relaxation and suction. Ling et al.[10] demonstrated in a canine model the presence of regional diastolic IVPG between the base and apex of the left ventricle. These gradients resulted in the active filling of the left ventricle. Courtois et al.[11,28] validated these findings and later demonstrated reduction in IVPG during myocardial ischemia in an animal model. These IVPG relate to elastic recoil and apical untwisting.[29] Greenberg and Thomas[30] used the Euler equation to calculate local pressure gradients:

$$\frac{\partial p}{\partial s} = -\rho\left[\frac{\partial v}{\partial t} + v\frac{\partial v}{\partial s}\right]$$

where p, s, t, and v are pressure, distance, time, and velocity, respectively. Integrating the Euler equation from the LV base to apex IVPG can be estimated

$$\Delta P_{IV}(t) = \int_{base}^{apex} \frac{\partial p}{\partial s} ds$$

where $\Delta P_{IV}(t)$ represents IVPG.[31]

This methodology has been reproduced by others[32] and opens the possibility of evaluating diastole in a more fundamental way by measuring one of the driving forces of early filling.

Pathophysiology

In abnormal ventricles, when intraventricular pressure gradients are blunted[28] or even reversed, the initial, faster phase is then lost. Vortex formation predominates over columnar flow, decreasing the initial slowing of the progression of flow toward the apex. Factors that can affect the formation of intraventricular pressure gradients include regional wall motion abnormalities, increased end-systolic volume, and dyssynchrony of relaxation.[15] The magnitude of pressure gradient formation also depends on ventricular size. In small ventricles intraventricular gradient formation is enhanced. Vortex formation and propagation require that the ventricular diameter exceed the mitral diameter.[4]

CMM DOPPLER AND DIASTOLIC FUNCTION

Human and animal studies have shown that Vp of early transmitral flow correlates well with the time constant of isovolumic relaxation (tau).[2,5,6,33] This correlation is maintained under a variety of loading and inotropic[5] conditions and also in children.[34] The strength of the correlation varies according to the technique used to measure Vp, with r values ranging from 0.5 to 0.9.[5,6,33,34] The Vp is also related to -dP/dt and minimal LV diastolic pressure.[33] The Vp appears to be a more complex parameter than a simple index of ventricular relaxation.[35,36] The Vp is influenced not only by the rate of LV relaxation but also by ventricular geometry,[37] the ratio between mitral orifice size and LV cavity size, and dyssynchrony of relaxation.[4,36,38]

Because Vp correlates well with tau, which is preload independent, CMM flow propagation has been proposed as a load-insensitive method of assessing LV relaxation.[5,7] Although most clinical studies have found that Vp is relatively load independent, there is still some controversy particularly in patients with normal systolic function and hypertrophy.[36,39–42] In these groups of patients LV geometry may play a predominant role. There are also reports that in patients with congestive heart failure Vp may decrease after medical treatment and is correlated with changes in PCWP.[43]

CLINICAL RELEVANCE

Pseudonormal Filling Pattern

In patients with elevated left atrial pressure (LAP), the mitral inflow Doppler pattern can be indistinguishable from those with normal diastolic function. This important limitation of pulsed Doppler of the mitral inflow has led to search for other techniques. One of the early applications of CMM was to differentiate normal from pseudonormal filling pattern.

In patients with pseudonormal mitral filling pattern the CMM will show slow flow propagation.[33,44]

Estimation of LV Filling Pressures

The main determinants of Doppler peak E wave velocity (E) are LA pressure and relaxation. By using 1/Vp as a surrogate for relaxation, it is in theory possible to estimate LAP. Substituting Vp α 1/tau in E α LAP/tau to yield E α LAP × Vp and then rearranged LAP α E/Vp.

This method has been investigated in patients under several conditions, including in sinus rhythm[22] and atrial fibrillation.[45] Garcia et al. studied 45 patients and found a robust correlation of E/Vp with PCWP (r = 0.80) with a regression equation:

$$PCWP = 5.27 \times (E/Vp) + 4.6$$

The limitations of this method to calculate a numerical value for LAP lie in the difficulty in measuring a reliable and reproducible slope of the CMM. As an example, the same group published the relation of PCWP and Vp in normal subjects. The regression equation in this group was:

$$PCWP = 25.6 \times Vp - 26.1 (r = 0.81)$$

Adding isovolumic relaxation time to the calculation appears to improve the correlation with PCWP. Gonzalez-Vilchez and Ares[46] modified the Weiss equation to derive:

$$PCWP = (0.9 \times SBP) \times e^{-IVRT \times Vp}$$

Using this equation they found improved correlation compared to E/Vp ratio alone (r: 0.80 vs. 0.55).[46]

Another approach is to use the ratio of E/Vp to identify patients with normal versus elevated PCWP. An E/Vp of more than 1.4 or 1.5 appears to have high sensitivity and reasonable specificity to identify patients with PCWP greater than 15 mmHg in patients in sinus rhythm or even in atrial fibrillation.[45] Other authors[46] have used a ratio of 2.5 to predict elevated PCWP, once again reflecting variability in measuring the slope of Vp.

Use of CMM in Clinical Settings

Abnormalities in Vp have been described in ischemic heart disease,[6,8,44,47,48] before cardiac resynchronization,[49] constrictive pericarditis,[50] and in dilated,[1,27] hypertrophic,[51] and restrictive cardiomyopathies.[52,53] In all clinical conditions with abnormal relaxation the velocity of propagation is diminished. In patients with isolated constrictive physiology where the intrinsic properties of the myocardium are normal, and the left ventricle has small end-systolic volume, Vp is normal or even augmented despite elevated filling pressures.[50]

The prognostic value of Vp has been investigated in patients after their initial myocardial infarction (MI). Patients with pseudonormal pattern defined by normal E/A ratio and slow Vp had an adverse prognosis.[44] The same authors found that an E/Vp greater than 1.5 was a strong predictor of in-hospital heart failure in patients with acute MI (Fig. 11.7).[54]

The Vp has been studied in patients with congestive heart failure. The E/Vp ratio has a modest correlation with brain natriuretic peptide (BNP) levels.[55] In patients with hypertensive heart disease and normal function who present with dyspnea to the emergency room, E/Vp has a sensitivity of 73.7%, specificity of 75%, and accuracy of 74.3% for diagnosis of heart failure for the optimal cutoff of 1.5.[56] Others have found that an E/Vp of 1.8 has a sensitivity of 83% and specificity of 86% to predict pulmonary congestion in patients with normal or low ejection fraction (EF) and correlated with LV end-diastolic pressure

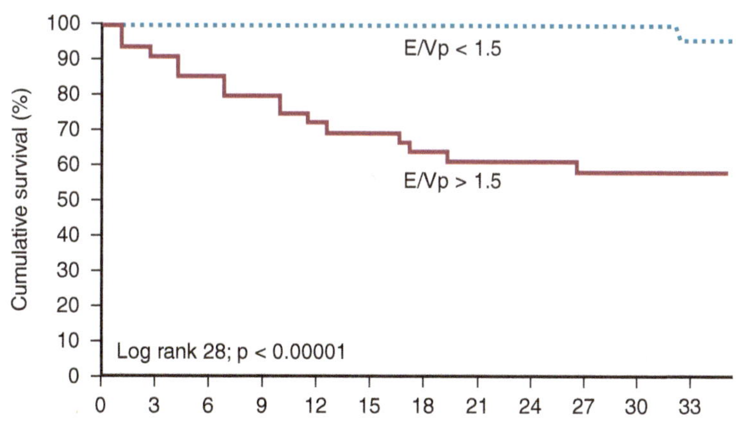

Fig. 11.7 Kaplan-Meier curves showing the effect of the ratio of peak E wave velocity and flow propagation velocity (E/Vp) on cardiac survival in patients after first myocardial infarction. (From Moller JE, Sondergaard E, Seward JB, Appleton CP, Egstrup K. Ratio of left ventricular peak E-wave velocity to flow propagation velocity assessed by color M-mode Doppler echocardiography in first myocardial infarction: prognostic and clinical implications. *J Am Coll Cardiol.* 2000;35:363–370.)

(r = 0.73).[57] As mentioned previously, in patients with heart failure, Vp may show some dependency on loading conditions,[43,58] and Vp can be lower after heart failure treatment. This may limit the application of Vp for assessing therapy in patients with congestive heart failure. In this situation E/Vp appears to be still useful as E decreases more than Vp, and therefore the ratio diminishes in the direction of hemodynamic improvement. In patients with systolic heart failure E/Vp greater than 2.7 independently predicts the composite end point of death, transplantation, or hospitalization.[58]

In a study by Ohara et al.,[59] Vp was tested to detect diastolic dysfunction in the clinical setting of 90 patients undergoing dobutamine stress echocardiography (DSE), with coronary angiography as the reference method. Vp increased significantly in the non–coronary artery disease (non-CAD) group at peak dobutamine infusion (from 56 ± 19 cm/sec to 66 ± 25 cm/sec), but not in the CAD group. Receiver operating characteristic analysis showed that sensitivity of DSE and reliability to exclude CAD was improved using peak Vp. The calculation of IVPG using CMM has yielded important information in patients with hypertrophic cardiomyopathy and has been used as a tool to study basic physiologic changes of aging[31] and exercise.[29,31,60] Rovner et al.[60] found that exercise capacity and VO_2 max have a tight relationship with changes in IVPG with exercise. Notably the basal IVPG was not related to exercise capacity. IVPGs are influenced by tau and preload.[31] Ohara et al. further extended these observations and reported that in patients with diastolic dysfunction and preserved EF, there is reduced adrenergic augmentation of IVPG from mid-LV to apex during dobutamine echo, indicating less apical suction.[61]

Normal aging impairs the relationship between IVPGs and preload, probably through age-dependent decline in relaxation, and is independent of changes in ventricular compliance.[31] More recently, a close relation between IVPGs and velocity of apical untwisting has been shown at rest and with exercise.[29] The increase in IVPGs during exercise appears to be an essential mechanism to augment stroke volume during this condition.

The precise relationship between CMM-derived IVPGs and Vp has not been well characterized yet. This relationship is probably complex involving not only the absolute pressure difference but also the temporal and spatial location of local pressure gradients. In an animal model of ischemia, time delay of Vp from base to apex correlated closely with IVPGs (r = 0.94).[62]

Limitations of CMM Indices

The main limitation of Vp is the high variability in measuring the slope of CMM. There is no agreement in how to measure it and, even if we agree in how to do it, the color display is often complex, bifurcated, and curvilinear. In some patients prominent isovolumic flow interferes with measurement of the slope.

Normal or increased Vp in patients in whom we expect delayed relaxation has been described,[40] a condition named by some authors as pseudonormalization of Vp.[15] This appears to be limited to small, hypertrophic ventricles with small end-systolic volumes.

VECTOR FLOW MAPPING

Vector flow mapping (VFM) is a novel echocardiographic method based on the continuity equation applied to color Doppler and speckle tracking velocities. VFM estimates flow velocity vectors accurately. Thereby vortex formation and characteristics of vorticity can be evaluated.

This technique has allowed visualization of vortex location and morphology and other parameters such as vortex strength and vortex pulsation correlation.[20,63] Vortex formation time has been described as an index of early LV diastolic filling.[19,64]

VFM also allows computation of the amount of energy dissipated by viscous friction, in addition to wall shear stress. These parameters have been applied in different conditions (congenital heart disease, valve disease, hypertrophic cardiomyopathy, diabetes mellitus, renal disease, cardiac resynchronization therapy) as measures of cardiac function and severity of disease from the aspect of cardiac load.[65–68]

Furthermore, by applying the divergence operation of the Navier-Stokes equation to velocity fields obtained by VFM, ultrasonic relative pressure imaging (RPI) has been developed. This method calculates pressure differences noninvasively and visualizes relative pressure distribution in color codes within cardiac chambers. RPI provides a promising method to quantify regional LV flow dynamics from the aspect of intraventricular pressures.

Finally, advances in VFM visualization make this an increasingly appealing technique.

FUTURE DIRECTIONS

The recent guidelines for evaluation of diastolic function/dysfunction do not include CMM Vp in the initial algorithm, and in most laboratories CMM is not routinely acquired.

The application of this technique remains hampered by the lack of consistent quantification. Without the incorporation of quantitative analysis by the manufacturers of echo machines it is unlikely that this technology will further evolve.

The clinical role of more complex flow visualization techniques, such as vortex imaging and vector flow mapping, remains to be established but appears promising. In the same manner as color M mode, incorporation of these techniques with automatic analysis within commercial packages and machines will be necessary to validate their role in clinical cardiology.

KEY POINTS

- Color M-mode allows visualization of velocity of early ventricular filling.
- Intraventricular pressure gradients can be derived from the information contained in CMM.
- There are differences in the CMM slope between normal individuals and patients with delayed relaxation and abnormal LV filling.

REVIEW QUESTIONS

1. What is the main determinant of flow propagation velocity (Vp)?
   a. Left ventricular relaxation
   b. Left ventricular geometry
   c. Minimum dP/dt
   d. Minimal left ventricular diastolic pressure
   e. All the above
2. What is the hemodynamic mechanism of Vp?
   a. Formation of a ring vortex
   b. Motion of an incompressible fluid column

c. Convective forces
d. All the above

3. What is the normal value of Vp?
 a. Above 45 cm/sec
 b. Above 30 cm/sec
 c. Depends on the method used
 d. None of the above

4. In what condition is Vp not reliable?
 a. Severe concentric LV hypertrophy
 b. Constrictive pericarditis
 c. Restrictive cardiomyopathy
 d. LV systolic dysfunction

REFERENCES

1. Jacobs LE, Kotler MN, Parry WR. Flow patterns in dilated cardiomyopathy: a pulsed-wave and color flow Doppler study. *J Am Soc Echocardiogr.* 1990;3:294–302.
2. Brun P, Tribouilloy C, Duval AM, et al. Left ventricular flow propagation during early filling is related to wall relaxation: a color M-mode Doppler analysis. *J Am Coll Cardiol.* 1992;20: 420–432.
3. Vierendeels JA, Dick E, Verdonck PR. Hydrodynamics of color M-mode Doppler flow wave propagation velocity V(p): a computer study. *J Am Soc Echocardiogr.* 2002;15:219–224.
4. Steen T, Steen S. Filling of a model left ventricle studied by colour M mode Doppler. *Cardiovasc Res.* 1994;28:1821–1827.
5. Garcia MJ, Smedira NG, Greenberg NL, et al. Color M-mode Doppler flow propagation velocity is a preload insensitive index of left ventricular relaxation: animal and human validation. *J Am Coll Cardiol.* 2000;35:201–208.
6. Stugaard M, Smiseth OA, Risoe C, Ihlen H. Intraventricular early diastolic velocity profile during acute myocardial ischemia: a color M-mode Doppler echocardiographic study. *J Am Soc Echocardiogr.* 1995;8:270–279.
7. Garcia MJ, Palac RT, Malenka DJ, Terrell P, Plehn JF. Color M-mode Doppler flow propagation velocity is a relatively preload-independent index of left ventricular filling. *J Am Soc Echocardiogr.* 1999;12:129–137.
8. Stugaard M, Brodahl U, Torp H, Ihlen H. Abnormalities of left ventricular filling in patients with coronary artery disease: assessment by colour M-mode Doppler technique. *Eur Heart J.* 1994;15:318–327.
9. Abali G, Tokgozoglu L, Ozcebe OI, Aytemir K, Nazli N. Which Doppler parameters are load independent? A study in normal volunteers after blood donation. *J Am Soc Echocardiogr.* 2005;18:1260–1265.
10. Ling D, Rankin JS, Edwards II CH, McHale PA, Anderson RW. Regional diastolic mechanics of the left ventricle in the conscious dog. *Am J Physiol.* 1979;236:H323–H330.
11. Courtois M, Kovacs Jr SJ, Ludbrook PA. Transmitral pressure-flow velocity relation. Importance of regional pressure gradients in the left ventricle during diastole. *Circulation.* 1988;78:661–671.
12. Nikolic SD, Feneley MP, Pajaro OE, Rankin JS, Yellin EL. Origin of regional pressure gradients in the left ventricle during early diastole. *Am J Physiol.* 1995;268:H550–H557.
13. Suga H, Goto Y, Igarashi Y, Yamada O, Nozawa T, Yasumura Y. Ventricular suction under zero source pressure for filling. *Am J Physiol.* 1986;251: H47–H55.
14. Ingels Jr NB, Daughters GT, Nikolic SD, et al. Left ventricular diastolic suction with zero left atrial pressure in open-chest dogs. *Am J Physiol.* 1996;270:H1217–H1224.
15. De Boeck BW, Oh JK, Vandervoort PM, Vierendeels JA, van der Aa RP, Cramer MJ. Colour M-mode velocity propagation: a glance at intra-ventricular pressure gradients and early diastolic ventricular performance. *Eur J Heart Fail.* 2005;7:19–28.
16. Nakamura M, Wada S, Mikami T, Kitabatake A, Karino T. Computational study on the evolution of an intraventricular vortical flow during early diastole for the interpretation of color M-mode Doppler echocardiograms. *Biomech Model Mechanobiol.* 2003;2:59–72.
17. Martinez-Legazpi P, Bermejo J, Benito Y, et al. Contribution of the diastolic vortex ring to left ventricular filling. *J Am Soc Echocardiogr.* 2014;64:1711–1721.
18. Sengupta PP, Narula J, Chandrashekhar Y. The dynamic vortex of a beating heart: wring out the old and ring in the new! *J Am Soc Echocardiogr.* 2014;64:1722–1724.
19. Gharib M, Rambod E, Kheradvar A, Sahn DJ, Dabiri JO. Optimal vortex formation as an index of cardiac health. *Proc Natl Acad Sci USA.* 2006;103:6305–6308.
20. Mele D, Smarrazzo V, Pedrizzetti G, et al. Intracardiac flow analysis: techniques and potential clinical applications. *J Am Soc Echocardiogr.* 2019;32:319–332.
21. Seo Y, Ishimitsu T, Ishizu T, et al. Assessment of propagation velocity by contrast echocardiography for standardization of color Doppler propagation velocity measurements. *J Am Soc Echocardiogr.* 2004;17:1266–1274.
22. Garcia MJ, Ares MA, Asher C, Rodriguez L, Vandervoort P, Thomas JD. An index of early left ventricular filling that combined with pulsed Doppler peak E velocity may estimate capillary wedge pressure. *J Am Coll Cardiol.* 1997;29:448–454.
23. Greenberg NL, Firstenberg MS, Cardon LA, et al. Automated assessment of noninvasive filling pressure using color Doppler M-mode echocardiography. *Comput Cardiol.* 2001;28:601–604.
24. Khan S, Bess RL, Rosman HS, Nordstrom CK, Cohen GI, Gardin JM. Which echocardiographic Doppler left ventricular diastolic function measurements are most feasible in the clinical echocardiographic laboratory? *Am J Cardiol.* 2004;94:1099–1101.
25. Stewart KC, Kumar R, Charonko JJ, Ohara T, Vlachos PP, Little WC. Evaluation of LV diastolic function from color M-mode echocardiography. *JACC Cardiovasc Imag.* 2011;4:37–46.
26. Vanhercke D, Claessens T, Pardaens S, et al. Assessment of variables affecting late left ventricular flow propagation velocity. *Acta Cardiol.* 2012;67:391–397.
27. Patrianakos AP, Parthenakis FI, Mavrakis HE, Zacharis EA, Vardas PE. Late left ventricular color M-mode Doppler in the assessment of diastolic dysfunction in patients with dilated cardiomyopathy. *J Am Soc Echocardiogr.* 2005;18:979.
28. Courtois M, Kovacs SJ, Ludbrook PA. Physiological early diastolic intraventricular pressure gradient is lost during acute myocardial ischemia. *Circulation.* 1990;81:1688–1696.
29. Notomi YM-M, Oryszak SJ, Shiota T, et al. Enhanced ventricular untwisting during exercise: A mechanistic manifestation of elastic recoil described by Doppler tissue imaging. *Circulation.* 2006;113(21):2524–2533.
30. Greenberg NL, Vandervoort PM, Firstenberg MS, Garcia MJ, Thomas JD. Estimation of diastolic intraventricular pressure gradients by Doppler M-mode echocardiography. *Am J Physiol Heart Circ Physiol.* 2001;280:H2507–H2515.
31. Popovic ZB, Prasad A, Garcia MJ, et al. Relationship among diastolic intraventricular pressure gradients, relaxation, and preload: impact of age and fitness. *Am J Physiol Heart Circ Physiol.* 2006;290:H1454–H1459.
32. Bermejo J, Antoranz JC, Yotti R, Moreno M, Garcia-Fernandez MA. Spatio-temporal mapping of intracardiac pressure gradients. A solution to Euler's equation from digital postprocessing of color Doppler M-mode echocardiograms. *Ultrasound Med Biol.* 2001;27:621–630.
33. Takatsuji H, Mikami T, Urasawa K, et al. A new approach for evaluation of left ventricular diastolic function: spatial and temporal analysis of left ventricular filling flow propagation by color M-mode Doppler echocardiography. *J Am Coll Cardiol.* 1996;27:365–371.
34. Border WL, Michelfelder EC, Glascock BJ, et al. RH, et al. Color M-mode and Doppler tissue evaluation of diastolic function in children: simultaneous correlation with invasive indices. *J Am Soc Echocardiogr.* 2003;16:988–994.
35. Stoylen A, Skjelvan G, Skjaerpe T. Flow propagation velocity is not a simple index of diastolic function in early filling. A comparative study of early diastolic strain rate and strain rate propagation, flow and flow propagation in normal and reduced diastolic function. *Cardiovasc Ultrasound.* 2003;1:3.

36. Barbier P, Grimaldi A, Alimento M, Berna G, Guazzi MD. Echocardiographic determinants of mitral early flow propagation velocity. *Am J Cardiol.* 2002;90:613–619.
37. Baccani B, Domenichini F, Pedrizzetti G, Tonti G. Fluid dynamics of the left ventricular filling in dilated cardiomyopathy. *J Biomech.* 2002;35: 665–671.
38. Smiseth OA, Thompson CR. Atrioventricular filling dynamics, diastolic function and dysfunction. *Heart Fail Rev.* 2000;5:291–299.
39. Ie EH, Vletter WB, ten Cate FJ, et al. Preload dependence of new Doppler techniques limits their utility for left ventricular diastolic function assessment in hemodialysis patients. *J Am Soc Nephrol.* 2003;14:1858–1862.
40. Alegret JM, Borras X, Carreras F, Duran I, Pons-Llado G. Restrictive left ventricular filling and preserved ventricular function: A limitation in the noninvasive estimation of pulmonary wedge pressure by Doppler echocardiography. *J Am Soc Echocardiogr.* 2002;15:334–338.
41. Hsiao SH, Huang WC, Lee TY, Sy CL, Lin SK, Liu CP. Preload and flow propagation velocity: Insight into patients with uremia and different left ventricular systolic function. *J Am Soc Echocardiogr.* 2005;18:1254–1259.
42. Hsiao SH, Huang WC, Sy CL, Lin SK, Lee TY, Liu CP. Doppler tissue imaging and color M-mode flow propagation velocity: are they really preload independent? *J Am Soc Echocardiogr.* 2005;18:1277–1284.
43. Seo Y, Ishimitsu T, Ishizu T, et al. Preload-dependent variation of the propagation velocity in patients with congestive heart failure. *J Am Soc Echocardiogr.* 2004;17:432–438.
44. Moller JE, Sondergaard E, Poulsen SH, Egstrup K. Pseudonormal and restrictive filling patterns predict left ventricular dilation and cardiac death after a first myocardial infarction: a serial color M-mode Doppler echocardiographic study. *J Am Coll Cardiol.* 2000;36:1841–1846.
45. Nagueh SF, Kopelen HA, Quinones MA. Assessment of left ventricular filling pressures by Doppler in the presence of atrial fibrillation. *Circulation.* 1996;94:2138–2145.
46. Gonzalez-Vilchez F, Ares M, Ayuela J, Alonso L. Combined use of pulsed and color M-mode Doppler echocardiography for the estimation of pulmonary capillary wedge pressure: an empirical approach based on an analytical relation. *J Am Coll Cardiol.* 1999;34:515–523.
47. De Sutter J, De Mey S, De Backer J, et al. Diastolic dysfunction, infarct size, and exercise capacity in remote myocardial infarction: a combined approach of mitral E-wave deceleration time and color M-mode flow propagation velocity. *Am J Cardiol.* 2002;89:593–595.
48. Stugaard M, Smiseth OA, Risoe C, Ihlen H. Intraventricular early diastolic filling during acute myocardial ischemia, assessment by multigated color M-mode Doppler echocardiography. *Circulation.* 1993;88:2705–2713.
49. Waggoner AD, Faddis MN, Gleva MJ, et al. Cardiac resynchronization therapy acutely improves diastolic function. *J Am Soc Echocardiogr.* 2005;18:216–220.
50. Rajagopalan N, Garcia MJ, Rodriguez L, et al. Comparison of new Doppler echocardiographic methods to differentiate constrictive pericardial heart disease and restrictive cardiomyopathy. *Am J Cardiol.* 2001;87: 86–94.
51. Nishihara K, Mikami T, Takatsuji H, et al. Usefulness of early diastolic flow propagation velocity measured by color M-mode Doppler technique for the assessment of left ventricular diastolic function in patients with hypertrophic cardiomyopathy. *J Am Soc Echocardiogr.* 2000;13:801–808.
52. Palecek T, Linhart A, Lubanda JC, et al. Early diastolic mitral annular velocity and color M-mode flow propagation velocity in the evaluation of left ventricular diastolic function in patients with Fabry disease. *Heart Vessels.* 2006;21:13–19.
53. Salemi VM, Picard MH, Mady C. Assessment of diastolic function in endomyocardial fibrosis: value of flow propagation velocity. *Artif Organs.* 2004;28:343–346.
54. Moller JE, Sondergaard E, Seward JB, Appleton CP, Egstrup K. Ratio of left ventricular peak E-wave velocity to flow propagation velocity assessed by color M-mode Doppler echocardiography in first myocardial infarction: prognostic and clinical implications. *J Am Coll Cardiol.* 2000;35:363–370.
55. Troughton RW, Prior DL, Pereira JJ, et al. Plasma B-type natriuretic peptide levels in systolic heart failure: importance of left ventricular diastolic function and right ventricular systolic function. *J Am Coll Cardiol.* 2004;43:416–422.
56. Arques S, Roux E, Sbragia P, et al. Comparative accuracy of color M-mode and tissue Doppler echocardiography in the emergency diagnosis of congestive heart failure in chronic hypertensive patients with normal left ventricular ejection fraction. *Am J Cardiol.* 2005;96:1456–1459.
57. Schwammenthal E, Popescu BA, Popescu AC, et al. Association of left ventricular filling parameters assessed by pulsed wave Doppler and color M-mode Doppler echocardiography with left ventricular pathology, pulmonary congestion, and left ventricular end-diastolic pressure. *Am J Cardiol.* 2004;94:488–491.
58. Troughton RW, Prior DL, Frampton CM, et al. Usefulness of tissue Doppler and color M-mode indexes of left ventricular diastolic function in predicting outcomes in systolic left ventricular heart failure (from the adept study). *Am J Cardiol.* 2005;96:257–262.
59. Ohara T, Hashimoto Y, Suzuki M, Matsumura A, Isobe M. Early diastolic flow propagation velocity detects induced diastolic dysfunction during dobutamine stress echocardiography. *Echocardiography.* 2011;28:335–341.
60. Rovner A, Greenberg NL, Thomas JD, Garcia MJ. Relationship of diastolic intraventricular pressure gradients and aerobic capacity in patients with diastolic heart failure. *Am J Physiol Heart Circ Physiol.* 2005;289: H2081–H2088.
61. Ohara T, Niebel CL, Stewart KC, et al. Loss of adrenergic augmentation of diastolic intra-LV pressure difference in patients with diastolic dysfunction: evaluation by color M-mode echocardiography. *JACC Cardiovasc Imaging.* 2012;5:861–870.
62. Steine K, Stugaard M, Smiseth OA. Mechanisms of retarded apical filling in acute ischemic left ventricular failure. *Circulation.* 1999;99:2048–2054.
63. Rodriguez Munoz D, Moya Mur JL, Fernandez-Golfin C, et al. Left ventricular vortices as observed by vector flow mapping: main determinants and their relation to left ventricular filling. *Echocardiography.* 2015;32: 96–105.
64. Poh KK, Lee LC, Shen L, et al. Left ventricular fluid dynamics in heart failure: echocardiographic measurement and utilities of vortex formation time. *Eur Heart J Cardiovasc Imaging.* 2012;13:385–393.
65. Stugaard M, Koriyama H, Katsuki K, et al. Energy loss in the left ventricle obtained by vector flow mapping as a new quantitative measure of severity of aortic regurgitation: a combined experimental and clinical study. *Eur Heart J Cardiovasc Imaging.* 2015;16:723–730.
66. Ji L, Hu WZ, Yong YH, Wu HP, Zhou L, Xu D. Left ventricular energy loss and wall shear stress assessed by vector flow mapping in patients with hypertrophic cardiomyopathy. *Int J Cardiovas Imag.* 2018;34:1383–1391.
67. Li CM, Bai WJ, Liu YT, Tang H, Rao L. Dissipative energy loss within the left ventricle detected by vector flow mapping in diabetic patients with controlled and uncontrolled blood glucose levels. *Int J Cardiovasc Imaging.* 2017;33:1151–1158.
68. Stugaard M, Kamimukai T, Masuda K, Asanuma T, Nakatani S. Characterization of relative pressure profiles in the inflow tract of the normal and ischemic left ventricle. A study by new ultrasonic relative pressure imaging. *Eur Heart J.* 2017;38:892–1892.
69. Thomas JD. Flow propagation analysis computer or eyeball? *JACC Cardiovasc Imaging.* 2011;4:47–49.

12

Assessment of Left Atrial Size and Function

Katsuji Inoue and Satoshi Nakatani

OUTLINE

Case Study 1

A 68-year-old woman was transferred to the emergency room with paroxysmal nocturnal dyspnea. She had comorbidities with obesity, hypertension, and glucose intolerance and had been treated with calcium channel and angiotensin-II receptor blockers. On admission, her oxygen saturation was 90%, blood pressure 186/102 mmHg, and heart rate 102 bpm with regular rhythm. The point-of-care echocardiography revealed mildly reduced left ventricular (LV) systolic function with concentric hypertrophy, while LV ejection fraction was visually estimated to be 50%. The left atrium and inferior vena cava were dilated. Physical examination confirmed jugular venous dilatation and edema in bilateral lower extremities. Laboratory tests showed that estimated glomerular filtration rate was 36 mL/min/1.73 m^2 and B-type natriuretic peptide level was 360 pg/mL. Her symptoms and signs of heart failure were controlled by adding loop diuretics, whereas Doppler echocardiography showed that E wave velocity was 84 cm/sec, A wave velocity was 40 cm/sec, E/e′ 21, and left atrial volume index was 42 mL/m^2, indicating that LV filling pressure remained to be elevated.

This is a typical case with heart failure with preserved ejection fraction (HFpEF). Enlarged left atrial (LA) size is an important characteristic of HFpEF besides signs of impaired diastolic function. Because the number of patients with HFpEF is increasing, routine measurement of LA size is mandatory when scanning a patient with heart failure symptoms.

INTRODUCTION

The left atrium is the most posteriorly positioned among all cardiac chambers. The four pulmonary veins (right superior, right inferior, left superior, left inferior) enter from the posterior part of the left atrium. The left atrium also has a continuum of mitral leaflets in conjunction with the left ventricle. In front of the left atrium, the ascending aorta exists, and the tracheal bifurcation, the esophagus, the descending aorta, and the vertebra column coexist behind.[1] The walls of the left atrium consist of thin musculature with nonuniform features and include the left atrial (LA) appendage with pectinate muscles.[2] In one cardiac cycle, the LA dimension changes mainly at anteroposterior and superoinferior directions, producing the phasic LA volumetric changes. The left atrium has three functions (see Chapter 4), including reservoir, conduit, and booster pump, and can be a buffer chamber to modulate left ventricular (LV) filling. During ventricular systole, the left atrium actively relaxes and passively dilates through the descent of cardiac base. The LA reservoir capacity thus enables to sufficiently collect the pulmonary venous inflow and then functions as a conduit, allowing the passage of stored blood from the left atrium and the left ventricle. During LV late diastole, the left atrium acts as a booster pump. The LA booster function contributes to one-third of the LV filling and plays an important role in maintaining normal cardiac output through the Frank-Starling mechanism.[3]

The left atrium gradually enlarges due to a burden of elevated LV filling pressure and diastolic dysfunction.[4,5] Thus the LA size is widely recognized as a novel marker of cardiovascular risks in the general population and various cardiovascular diseases.[6,7] The LA function can be assessed using transthoracic echocardiography (TTE) from phasic changes of LA volumes, transmitral flow and mitral annular velocities, and atrial deformation indices.[8–10] The estimation of LA functional parameters in addition to LA size leads to a better understanding of LA mechanics as well as risk stratification of cardiovascular outcomes.

MEASUREMENT OF LEFT ATRIAL SIZE

Two-Dimensional Echocardiography

To measure the LA size, TTE is recommended by the American Society of Echocardiography.[11] Transesophageal echocardiography (TEE) should not be used for the measurement of the LA size because the entire left atrium frequently cannot be included within the image plane with TEE.

M Mode Echocardiography (Internal Linear Dimensions)

M mode echocardiography was the first TTE application used to assess LA size. The LA internal dimensions should be measured at LV end

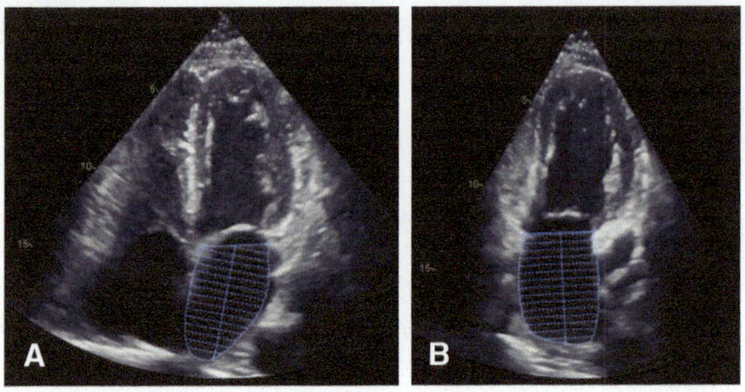

Fig. 12.1 Measurement of left atrial volume using the biplane disk summation algorithm. Apical four-chamber (A) and two-chamber (B) views are obtained when the left atrium maximally expands just before mitral valve opening.

systole when the LA chamber reaches its maximal dimension, from the parasternal long axis view perpendicular to the aortic root long axis. After the cursor is set at the level of the aortic sinuses, the anteroposterior diameter can be calculated by trailing the leading edge of the posterior aortic wall to the leading edge of the posterior LA wall.

B Mode Echocardiography (Two-Dimensional Guided Linear Dimensions, Area, Volume)

When the M mode cursor is not perpendicular to LA posterior wall, two-dimensional (2-D) guided linear measurement should be performed to measure LA anteroposterior diameter. Despite its lower temporal resolution, 2-D guidance provides the optimal orientation for obtaining the anteroposterior linear dimension of the left atrium. While the anteroposterior diameter is the most reproducible measurement, the left atrium also expands in the superoinferior direction through LV long axis shortening. Thus M mode or 2-D guided linear methods for determination of LA size underestimate LA volume due to geometric assumption. Consequently the inconsistencies are pronounced among patients with LA remodeling.[12]

Instead of linear dimensions, LA area can be planimetered from the apical views. The measurements of LA area overcome the inaccuracy of the M mode method because LA enlargement is not uniform. While recording images for the measurements of optimal LA area, care should be taken to avoid foreshortening of the left atrium.

LA volume can be used as a biomarker of the burden and chronicity of LV diastolic dysfunction. LA volume can be estimated using the biplane calculation of the LA area-length from apical four-chamber and two-chamber views.[13] The area-length method is based on the assumption of an ellipsoidal LA shape.[14] Accordingly, the biplane disk summation algorithm, similar to its application for measurements of LV volume, should be used for the standard of the LA volumetric assessment.[15] Mathematically, the measurements of the LA volume can be performed by adding the volumes of a series of elliptic cylinders of known height (h):

$$\text{Volume} = \pi/4(h)\sum(D_1)(D_2)$$

where D_1 and D_2 are orthogonal minor and major transverse axes of each cylinder (Fig. 12.1). When the left atrium maximally expands just before mitral valve opening, the LA volume should be measured on the optimal frame ensuring alignment along the true long axis of the left atrium. The tracings of LA endocardial border should exclude the area under mitral annular plane, the pulmonary veins, and the LA appendages. The upper normal indexed maximal LA volume of 34 mL/m^2 is recommended to use in a risk-based approach for determination of cutoffs between a normal and an enlarged left atrium.[11] The measurements of the LA volume using B mode echocardiography are still limited in accuracy due to the asymmetrical process of LA remodeling. 2-D echocardiographic methods significantly underestimate the LA volume compared with computed tomography (CT).[16]

Three-Dimensional Echocardiography

Three-dimensional (3-D) echocardiography is not based on geometric assumption, providing more accurate measurement of the LA volume and greater prognostic ability than a 2-D approach.[17] The 3-D technique enables to accurately display a maximized LA plane without LA foreshortening in the apical four-chamber and two-chamber views in which LA and LV axes do not lie in the same plane.[18,19] Despite these advantages, 3-D echocardiography has limitations to analyze the LA volume in a clinical practice because of low spatiotemporal resolution, lack of standardized methodology, and limited normative data compared with the 2-D method. Another limitation may be the time and training required to obtain accurate and reproducible 3-D volumetric data. A recent advance of automated cardiac chamber quantification technique allows simultaneous quantification of LA and LV volumes with a short acquisition time (Fig. 12.2).[20]

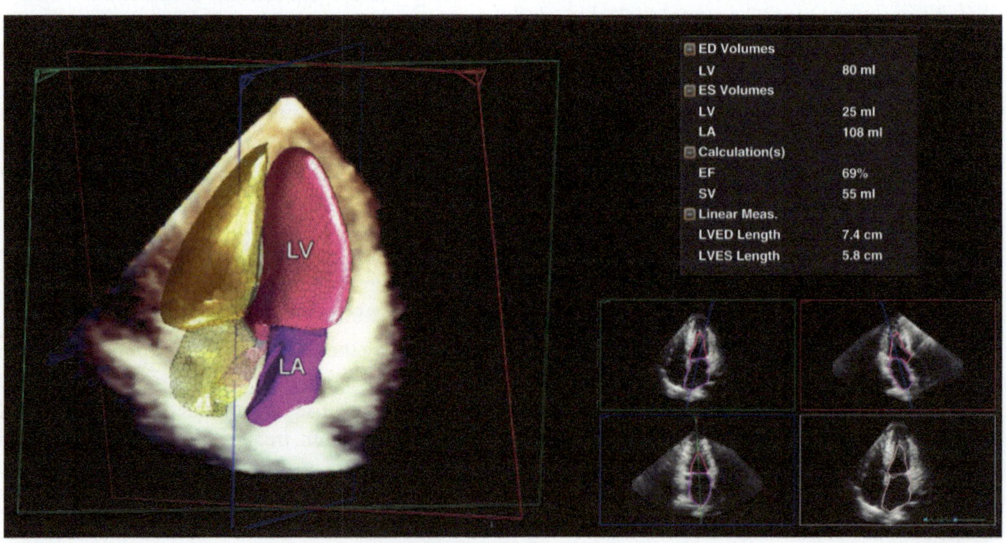

Fig. 12.2 Automated cardiac chamber quantification technique allows integration of volumetric left atrial *(LA)* and left ventricular *(LV)* measurements with 3-D echocardiography. (HeartModel, courtesy of Philips Healthcare.)

ASSESSMENT OF LEFT ATRIAL FUNCTION

The left atrium acts to modulate LV filling and performance through three functions: (1) booster (active contraction), (2) reservoir (active relaxation and passive dilatation), and (3) conduit (passive emptying).[7] The instantaneous changes in LA pressure and volume during a cardiac cycle can facilitate to understand the LA functions (Fig. 12.3). The LA pre-A volume (LAV_{pre-A}) can be measured at the beginning of the electrocardiogram (ECG) P wave when the left atrium is completely relaxed. The left atrium acts as a contractile chamber to produce an A wave in the LA pressure tracing, while the LA volume is minimized (LAV_{min}). The A wave is interrupted by the C wave, which is a transmitted wave by closure of the mitral valve. During LV isovolumic contraction, the left atrium intrinsically relaxes to enhance LA early filling. Thus the x descent, which is the first nadir of LA pressure, correlates with LA early filling, resulting in a rapid increase of LA volume. The change of slope in the upsloping curve of the LA volume indicates a transition between the LA early and late reservoir phases.[21] The late reservoir phase is determined by the LV long axis shortening of the cardiac base and LA chamber stiffness.[22] At the late reservoir phase, the pulmonary venous blood progressively flows into the left atrium, causing the V wave, while the LA volume is maximized (LAV_{max}). With mitral valve opening, the blood rapidly drains into the left ventricle, and the LA volume decreases (passive emptying), causing the y descent. During LV diastole, LA conduit function is mainly influenced by LV diastolic properties.

Volumetric Changes

2-D Echocardiography

The volumetric changes of the left atrium may be estimated from biplane disk summation algorithm with 2-D echocardiography. The LA volumes are measured at different time points as follows: (1) LAV_{pre-A}: LA volume preceding atrial contraction at the beginning of a P wave, (2) LAV_{min}: minimal LA volume just at the mitral valve closure, and (3) LAV_{max}: maximal LA volume just before the mitral valve opening (Fig. 12.4).[23] By using these volumes, the volumetric differences or fractions at active (contractile), passive (conduit), and total filling (reservoir) phases can be calculated (Fig. 12.5).

3-D Echocardiography

3-D echocardiography allows the automatic quantification of the LA volumetric changes with avoidance of geometric assumptions and foreshortened views.[24] The 3-D multibeat integration is limited to use in patients without irregular rhythm and significant respiratory motion. The real-time 3-D echocardiography can capture entire cardiac motion in a single cardiac beat, despite being of lower spatiotemporal resolution than that of the multibeat method.

Doppler Indices

Transmitral Inflow

Pulsed Doppler echocardiography usually reveals early (E) and late diastolic (A) waves.

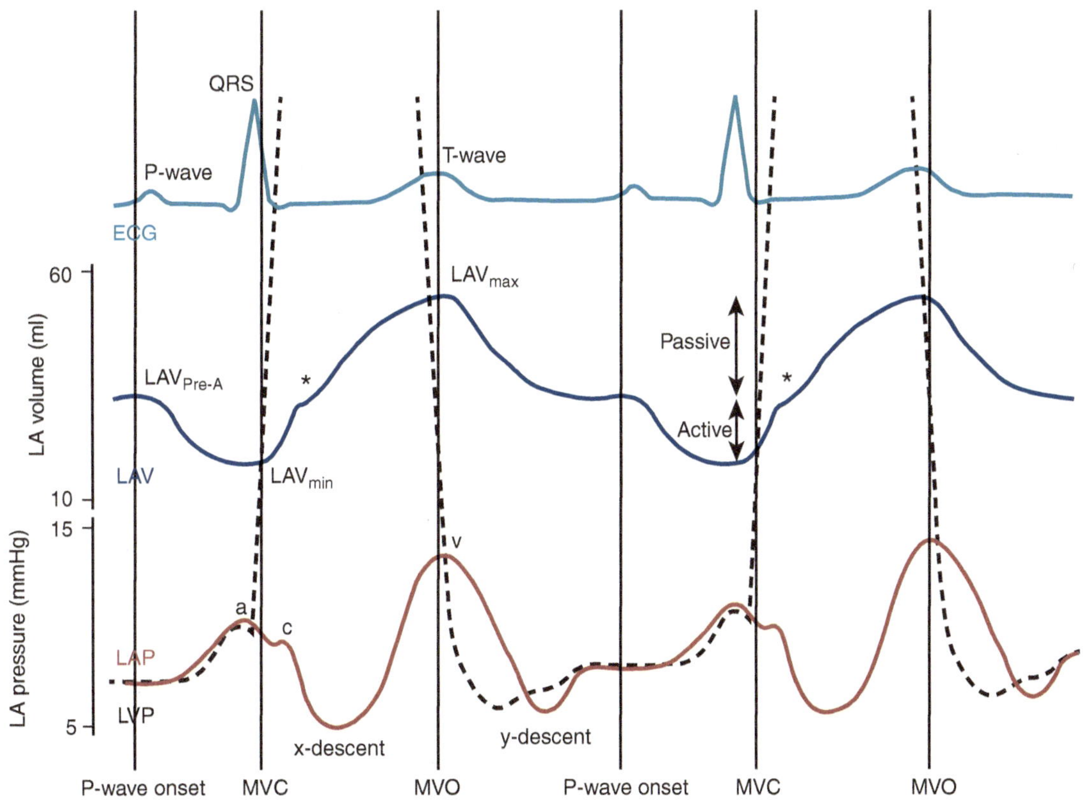

Fig. 12.3 Scheme of instantaneous changes in left atrial *(red line)* and left ventricular *(black dotted line)* pressures as well as left atrial volume *(blue line)* in two cardiac cycles. The asterisk indicates a transition between LA early and late filling during ventricular systole. *LAP,* Left atrial pressure; *LAV,* left atrial volume; *LAV_{max},* maximal LA volume; *LAV_{min},* minimal LA volume; *LAV_{Pre-A},* LA volume at the beginning of P wave; *LVP,* left ventricular pressure; *MVC,* mitral valve closure; *MVO,* mitral valve opening.

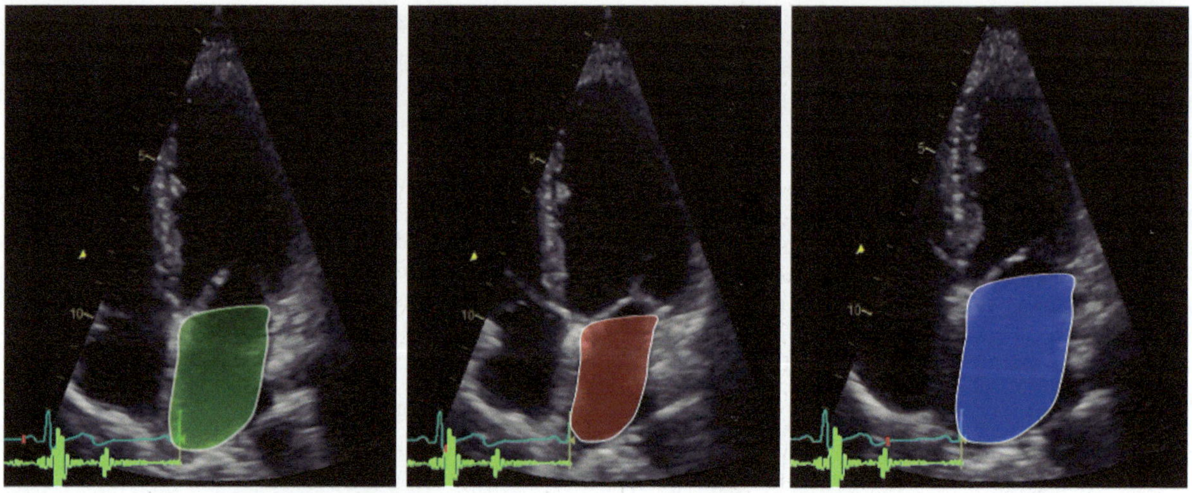

A B C

Fig. 12.4 Three different phases to measure left atrial (LA) volumes. (A) LA volume at the beginning of P wave ($LAV_{pre\text{-}A}$), (B) minimal LA volume just at the mitral valve closure (LAV_{min}), and (C) maximal LA volume just before the mitral valve opening (LAV_{max}).

LA active (booster) function
- LA active emptying volume: $LAV_{pre\text{-}A} - LAV_{min}$
- LA active emptying fraction: $(LAV_{pre\text{-}A} - LAV_{min}) / LAV_{pre\text{-}A}$

LA passive (conduit) function
- LA passive emptying volume: $LAV_{max} - LAV_{pre\text{-}A}$
- LA passive emptying fraction: $(LAV_{max} - LAV_{pre\text{-}A}) / LAV_{max}$
- Conduit volume: LV stroke volume $- (LAV_{max} - LAV_{min})$

LA total reservoir function
- LA total emptying volume: $LAV_{max} - LAV_{min}$
- LA total emptying fraction: $(LAV_{max} - LAV_{min}) / LAV_{max}$

Fig. 12.5 Calculations of left atrial (LA) volumetric differences or fractions at active (booster), passive (conduit), and total filling (reservoir) phases. *LAV_{max}*, Maximal LA volume; *LAV_{min}*, minimal LA volume; *$LAV_{Pre\text{-}A}$*, LA volume at the beginning of P wave; *LV*, left ventricular.

A pressure gradient between the left atrium and the left ventricle results in transmitral inflow during diastole. When LV filling pressure is abnormally elevated, the E wave velocity increases and the A wave velocity decreases, resulting in a pseudonormal inflow pattern (E/A >1). The decrease of the A wave in the pseudonormal pattern might reflect a lack of an increase in LA systolic (ejection) force.[25] Braunwald et al. first described the important contribution of the LA systolic force to maintain the stroke volume with a lower mean LA pressure in patients with LV dysfunction.[26]

Pulmonary Venous Flow

Pulmonary venous flow can be obtained from the apical four-chamber view with pulse wave Doppler, when the sample volume is placed 1 to 2 cm into the right (or left) upper pulmonary veins. The pulmonary venous flow consists of two forward flows during ventricular systole and early diastole with a reversed flow during atrial systole.[27] TEE allows obtaining a complete pulmonary venous flow compared with the transthoracic approach.

Tissue Doppler

Pulse wave tissue Doppler echocardiography is widely used to assess LV early diastolic function with peak early diastolic tissue velocity (e′) at mitral annular level. The following peak negative velocity during atrial systole (a′) has a potential to estimate LA contractility.[28] In addition, the time difference from the P wave onset to the peak a′ velocity is known as an echocardiographic index of atrial electromechanical coupling.[29]

Transesophageal Echocardiography (Left Atrial Appendage)

TEE enables us to characterize the structure and function of the LA appendage (LAA). Partially, the LAA is a source to produce LA contraction and distensibility.[30] When LAA immobility and blood stasis are ensured, thrombus formation responsible for stroke frequently occurs within the LA appendage.[31] The LAA is a remnant of the primordial left atrium. The LAA shape is variable and categorized as four types: cactus, chicken wing, windsock, and cauliflower. The chicken wing morphology has lesser embolic event than the non–chicken wing categories.[32] 3-D TEE is applicable to classify these four types of the LAA morphology.[33]

The LAA flow can be detected by pulse wave Doppler method during TTE examinations.[34] In patients with atrial fibrillation (AFib), the active LAA flow is observed with a sawtooth appearance, despite insufficient flow velocity of the transmitral A wave. Because there are variations of the LAA flow from relatively preserved contraction to atrial standstill, the lower LAA flow velocities are associated with the higher risk of stroke in these patients.

Deformation Indices

Myocardial deformation (strain) can be measured by tissue Doppler imaging or speckle tracking echocardiography. Tissue Doppler imaging may be used to derive strain, but its accuracy is limited by angle dependency. In contrast, speckle tracking echocardiography utilizes natural acoustic markers (speckles) in grey scale images within myocardial tissue, which can be tracked in any direction. Despite the reduced width of the left atrial wall, speckle tracking allows the diagnostician to estimate percentage of LA circumferential change in cavity circumference, which is concordant with average LA longitudinal strain.[35] This method enables quantification of the three components of LA function from apical four-chamber and two-chamber views. The strain analysis from apical long axis view is problematic because the ascending aorta is difficult to separate from the LA wall.

There are two approaches to estimate the LA function depending on the reference points to define an initial length of the left atrium: (1)

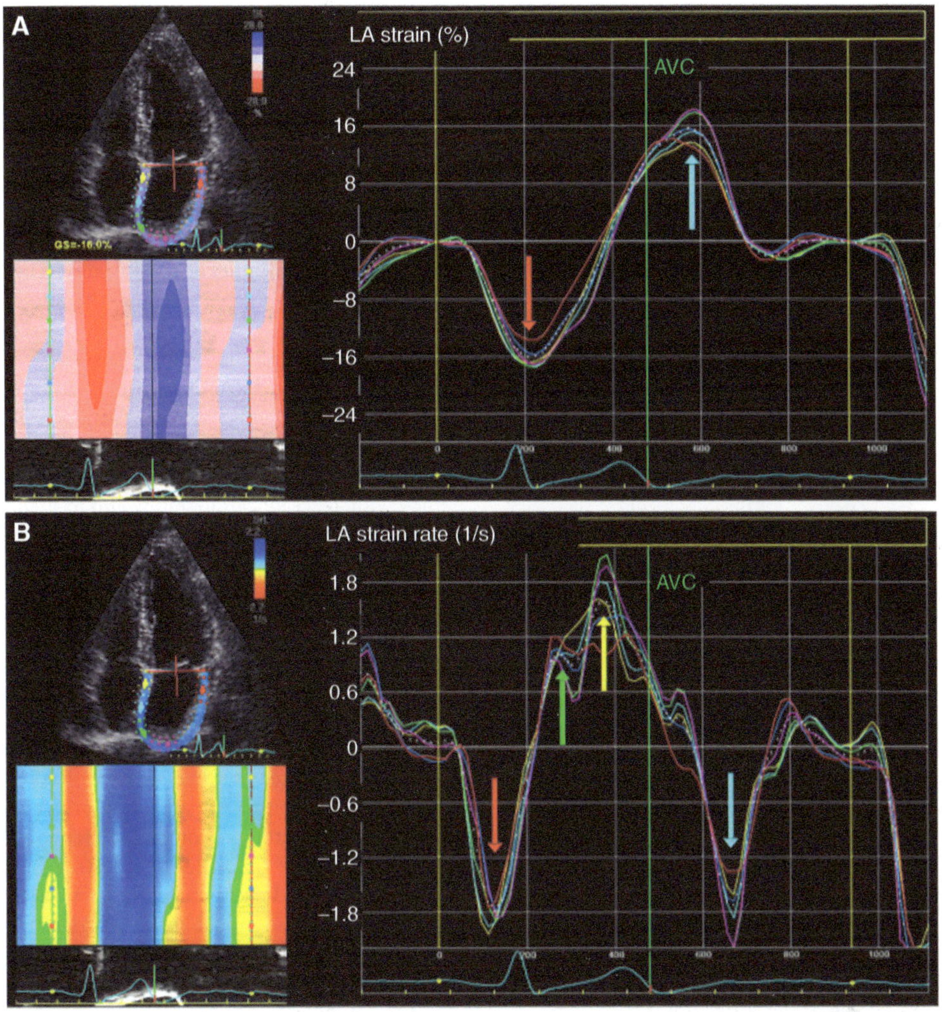

Fig. 12.6 Representative curves of left atrial (LA) strain and strain rate with speckle tracking echocardiography in a control subject (P-P gating method). (A) LA strain consists of an initial negative peak *(red arrow)* corresponding to LA contraction and a positive peak *(pale arrow)* corresponding to LA conduit function. The sum of the absolute values of the two peaks corresponds to LA total reservoir function. (B) LA strain rate curve consists of a first negative peak *(red arrow)* corresponding to LA contraction, an initial positive peak *(green arrow)* to LA relaxation, followed by a second positive peak *(yellow arrow)* to left ventricular (LV) systolic shortening, and a second negative peak *(pale arrow)* to early diastolic LV filling. *AVC,* Aortic valve closure.

P-P gating (starting on the P wave), and (2) R-R gating (starting on the QRS complex).[36] When the P-P gating is used, the morphology of the LA strain shows a sinusoidal waveform with a first negative wave corresponding to LA contraction and a following positive wave to LA reservoir function. Fig. 12.6 demonstrates the representative curves of the LA strain and strain rate using the P-P gating.[37,38] When the R-R gating is used, the LA strain curve has two positive peaks corresponding to LA reservoir and booster functions. The R-R gating enables estimation of the LA strain even in patients with AFib. Fig. 12.7 shows the different methods of LA strain measurements using P-P gating and R-R gating. Recently, the European Association of Cardiovascular Imaging/American Society of Echocardiography/Industry Task Force states that ventricular end diastole (R-R gating) is recommended as the time reference to define the zero baseline for LA strain curves. LA strain values obtained with either zero baseline approach can be converted into the other, if the respective LA strain during contraction phase is available.[39] When ECG trigger is used as time reference, it may be misleading to define ventricular end diastole in patients with bundle branch block. The Task Force recommends that both ventricular end diastole and onset of atrial contraction be defined according to the mitral valve inflow profile. In an LA strain curve with typical morphology, the curve itself could guide the correct measurement points.

Estimation of Pressure-Volume and Pressure-Strain Loops

The instantaneous acquisitions of the LA pressure and volume produce the LA pressure-volume loop (Fig. 12.8). The loop shows a characteristic figure-8 configuration, which consists of the A loop and V loop.[40] The A loop represents active contraction and relaxation, and the V loop represents passive dilatation and emptying. By using the V loop, the LA chamber stiffness can be estimated from the ascending limb of the V loop during LA passive dilatation. The sum of the areas of the A and V loops has been proposed as an index of the LA work.[22] Speckle tracking echocardiography or real-time 3-D echocardiography has potential to evaluate the LA pressure-volume as well as pressure-strain relationships.[21,41]

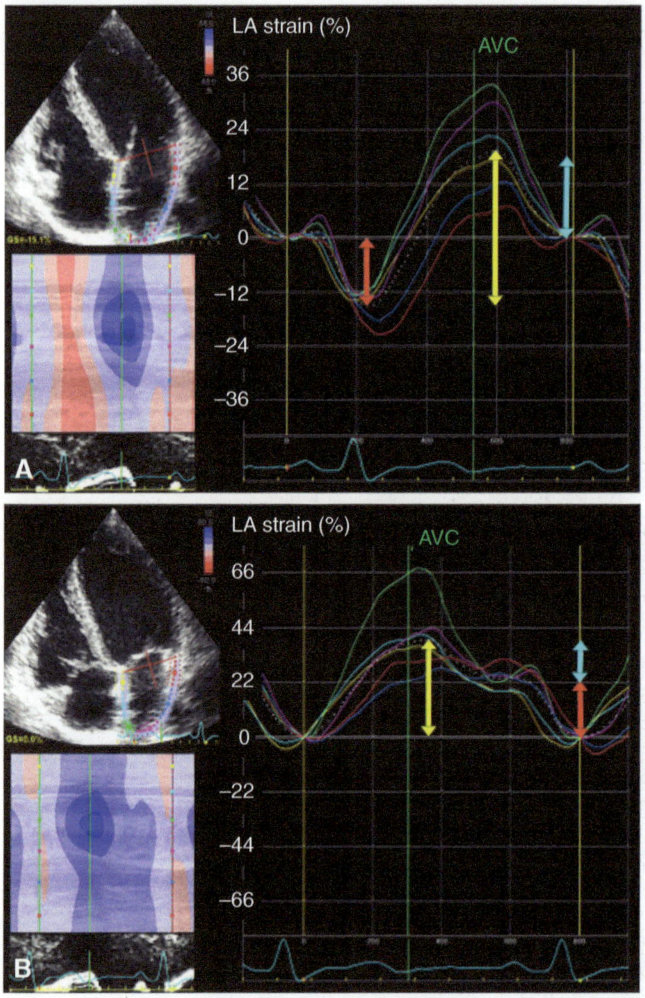

Fig. 12.7 Representatives curves of left atrial *(LA)* strain using the P-P gating method (A) and the R-R gating method (B) with speckle tracking echocardiography. The closed red, yellow and pale arrows indicate left atrial *(LA)* booster, reservoir, and conduit strain, respectively. AVC, aortic valve closure.

RISK STRATIFICATION AND PROGNOSTIC PREDICTION WITH LEFT ATRIAL SIZE AND FUNCTION

LA Enlargement

Epidemiologic studies have established that patients with HFpEF are increasing over time.[42,43] In the I-PRESERVE echocardiographic substudy, LA size and LV mass were independently associated with an increased risk of morbidity and mortality.[44] The indexed LAV_{max} greater than 34 mL/m^2 is a key structural alteration found in patients with HFpEF.[45] This cutoff value has been adopted by the American Society of Echocardiography and European Association of Cardiovascular Imaging guideline document on evaluation of LV diastolic function (see Chapter 19).[46] Alternatively, the indexed LAV_{min}, which includes LA contractile capacity, has an ability to identify LV diastolic dysfunction rather than the indexed LAV_{max} in a community-based cohort study with 2-D echocardiography and to predict prognosis in patients with various cardiovascular risks with 3-D echocardiography.[47,48]

LA Dysfunction

LA Booster Pump Dysfunction

LA booster pump function contributes to maintaining stroke volume. Its failure is often associated with a transition from asymptomatic state to overt heart failure. A loss of LA transport in AFib predisposes to life-threatening complications such as heart failure and stroke. Previous studies reported that in patients with AFib, LA contractile factors, including a′ velocity, LAA velocities, or LA booster strain, improved after successful cardioversion or catheter ablation when sinus rhythm was restored.[29,49,50] Fig. 12.9 demonstrates a patient with persistent AFib who received successful catheter ablation. Although transmitral A wave was reduced probably due to atrial stunning just after the ablative therapy, the A wave velocity was markedly increased at 1 year after the procedure, indicating the recovery of LA booster function.

The LA booster function is enhanced during increased afterload, which is one of the key triggers for the onset of acute (flash) pulmonary edema. During an acute increase of blood pressure, the left atrium immediately reacts to the hemodynamic overload by enhancing LA contraction and relaxation. In an experimental study where LA

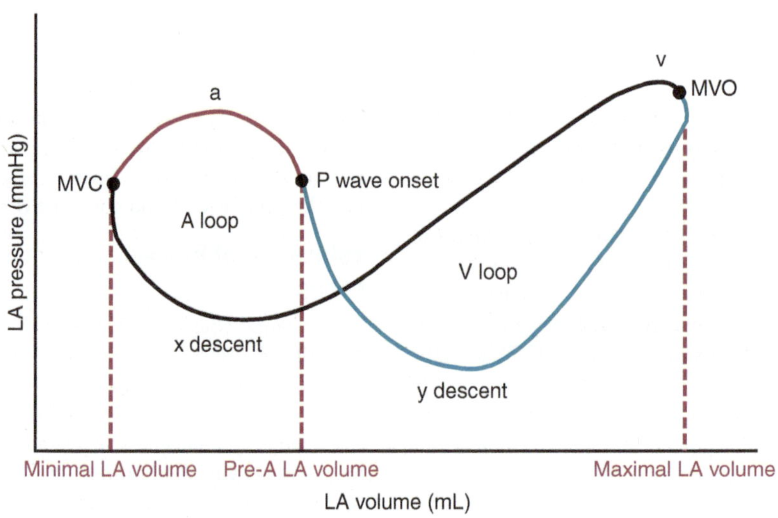

Fig. 12.8 Scheme of left atrial (*LA*) pressure and volume loop. LA pressure-volume relationship typically represents a figure-8 pattern. The A loop corresponds to active contraction and relaxation (counterclockwise rotation), and the V loop to passive filling and emptying (clockwise rotation). The area inside of each loop represents LA external work. *MVC,* Mitral valve closure; *MVO,* mitral valve opening.

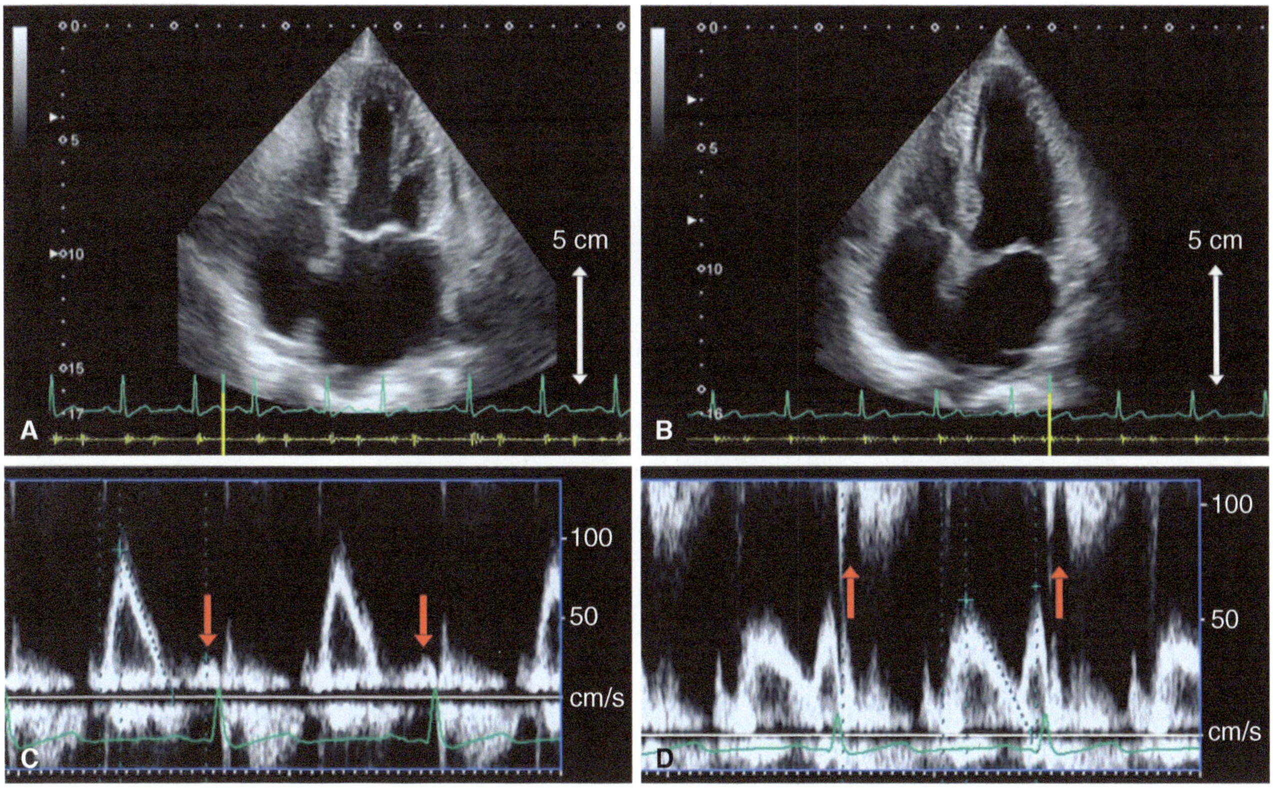

Fig. 12.9 A representative case of persistent atrial fibrillation undergoing catheter ablation. (A) Apical four-chamber image just after the procedure. Maximal left atrial (LA) volume index was estimated as 56.2 mL/m². (B) Apical four-chamber view at 1 year after the procedure. Maximal LA volume index was decreased as 24.8 mL/m². (C) Transmitral flow just after the procedure. The E wave and A wave *(downward red arrow)* velocities were 93 cm/sec and 25 cm/sec, respectively. (D) Transmitral flow at 1 year after the procedure. The E wave and A wave *(upward red arrow)* velocities were 59 cm/sec and 65 cm/sec, respectively. The catheter ablation was effective to reduce LA volume and to augment LA booster function in this patient.

pressure-strain loop was recorded, during acute afterload increase, the A loop area, which corresponds to LA contraction and relaxation, immediately increased to maintain stroke volume, whereas the V loop area remained unchanged.[21] The augmentation of LA contractility to an increased afterload was impaired in patients with hypertensive heart disease or HFpEF.[51] The lower strain values of LA active contraction and relaxation assessed by speckle tracking echocardiography are associated with higher incidence of AFib and heart failure hospitalization in patients with hypertrophic cardiomyopathy.[37] Fig. 12.10 shows the distinct strain patterns of LA active function in two representative cases of hypertrophic cardiomyopathy with or without heart failure hospitalization.

LA Reservoir Dysfunction

The assessments of LA reservoir function are helpful for the prediction of the burden of LV diastolic dysfunction and future cardiovascular risks. The LA total emptying fraction has been reported as an independent predictor for new onset AFib or flutter in elderly patients.[52] In the general population, the LA total emptying fraction is superior to LAV_{max} for the identification of individuals at an increased risk of adverse outcomes.[6] The decreased LA reservoir strain with speckle tracking echocardiography is a powerful clinical and prognostic factor in patients with HFpEF, above and beyond LA size.[53]

Impaired LV longitudinal function, LV hypertrophy, and concentric geometry are characteristic in patients with HFpEF. In these, it appears that compensatory circumferential shortening preserves LV ejection fraction.[54] According to a recent meta-analysis, LV global longitudinal strain appears to have superior prognostic value for predicting major adverse cardiac events beyond LV ejection fraction.[55] Because the LA reservoir function is closely affected by LV longitudinal function, the LA reservoir strain could be an important surrogate of LA-LV interaction that determines LA stiffness.

LA Stiffness

Suga et al., by using a circulatory analog model, reported that cardiac output increases in response to increases in the atrial compliance.[56] When the left atrium is fully relaxed, it is ideal to estimate the degrees of LA stiffening. The LA stiffness constant has been rigorously modeled with an exponential fitting of the ascending limb of the V loop from the LA pressure-area curve.[57] Alternatively, Melenovsky et al. simplified this concept to estimate the LA stiffness index by connecting maximal and minimal pressure-volume points in heart failure patients undergoing right heart catheterization and echocardiography, demonstrating that HFpEF is characterized by increased LA stiffness.[58] Alternatively, the LA stiffness index may be estimated noninvasively using the E/e′ ratio as a surrogate of LA pressure in conjunction with LA reservoir strain.[59] Although the LA pressure-strain loop could be utilized to identify the LA stiffening during catheterization, it remains to be cumbersome to apply in a clinical setting.[60] Fig. 12.11 demonstrates different LA behavior in two patients with hypertrophic cardiomyopathy and cardiac amyloidosis. As compared with a patient with hypertrophic cardiomyopathy, the blunted volumetric changes of the left atrium in a patient with cardiac amyloidosis may indicate the LA chamber stiffening is due to amyloid deposition in the left atrium. A vigilant screening for restrictive LA motion might help diagnose cardiac amyloid patients.

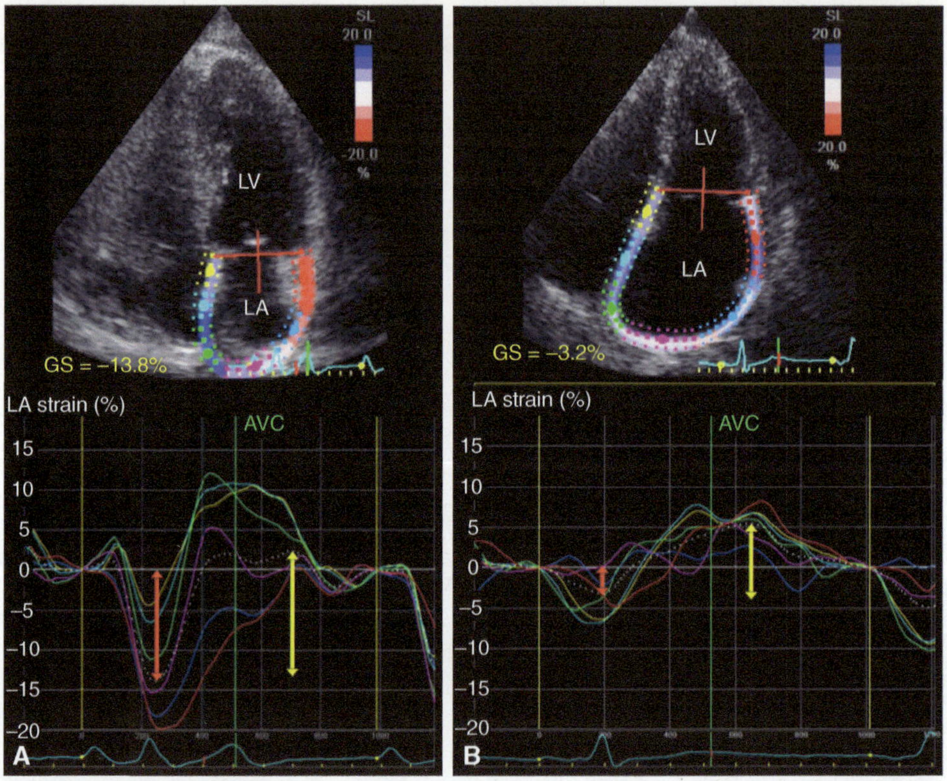

Fig. 12.10 **Two representative cases of hypertrophic cardiomyopathy: one free from cardiac events (A) and the other requiring repeated heart failure hospitalization (B).** The LA reservoir strain *(closed yellow arrow)*, especially at late reservoir phase, was decreased in both cases. The LA booster strain *(closed red arrow)* was severely decreased concomitantly with LA enlargement in a patient with refractory heart failure. *AVC*, aortic valve closure; *LA*, left atrial; *LV*, left ventricular.

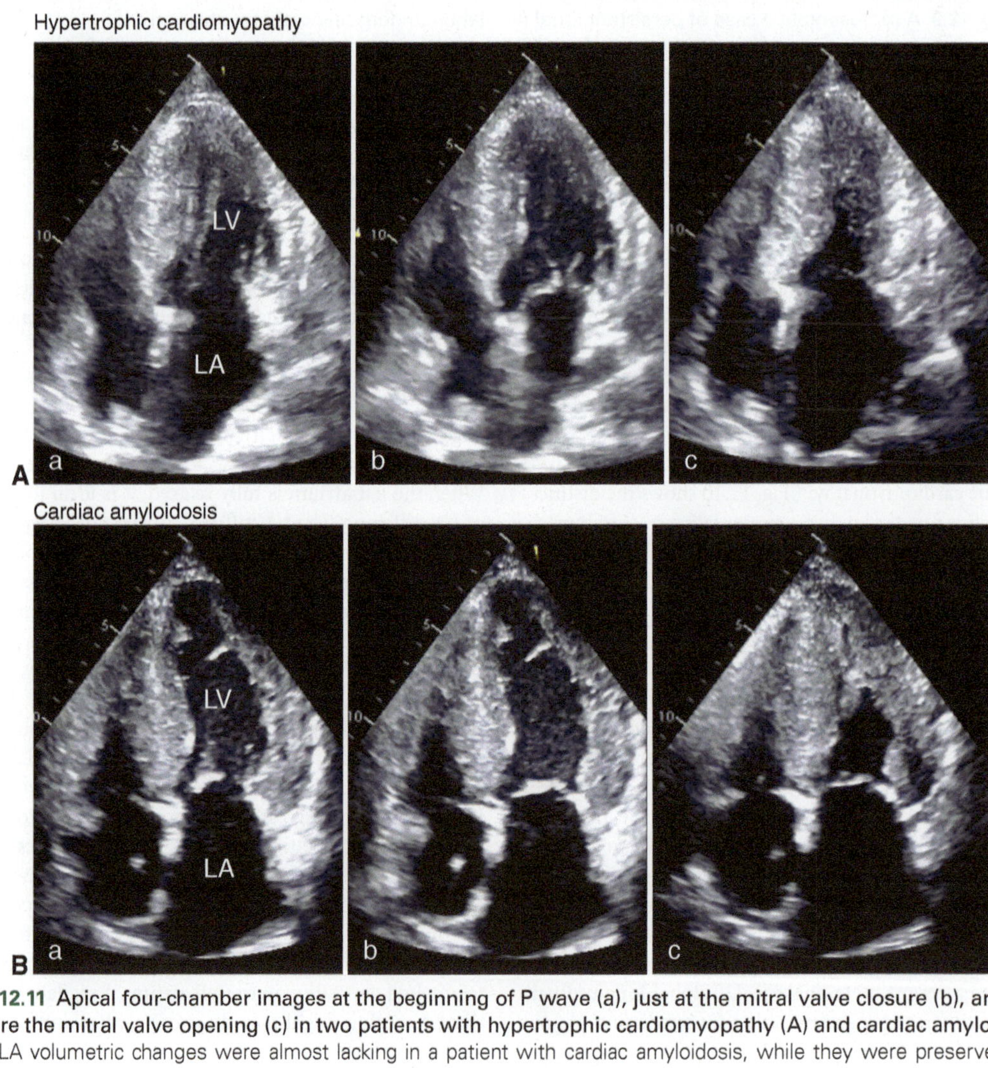

Fig. 12.11 **Apical four-chamber images at the beginning of P wave (a), just at the mitral valve closure (b), and just before the mitral valve opening (c) in two patients with hypertrophic cardiomyopathy (A) and cardiac amyloidosis (B).** LA volumetric changes were almost lacking in a patient with cardiac amyloidosis, while they were preserved in a patient with hypertrophic cardiomyopathy. *LA*, Left atrial; *LV*, left ventricular.

FUTURE DIRECTIONS

Because the assessment of LA size provides important prognostic information, practical approaches for the measurement of LA size with echocardiography are necessary for a routine clinical use. Observers should recognize some critical limitations of 2-D echocardiography, including that LA images are easily obtained to be foreshortened from apical windows, and the measurement is based on geometric assumption. 3-D echocardiography could resolve these issues according to the advances in technology. Recently fusion of echocardiography with CT or magnetic resonance imaging (MRI), by providing anatomic information and tissue characterization, has been developed to evaluate LA size and function. Among them, real-time fusion imaging of 2-D echocardiography with CT for the use of anatomic guidance could be easy to implement.

The assessments of LA function add incremental prognostic value to LA size quantification. Automatic endocardial border detection of the left atrium based on 3-D or speckle tracking echocardiography could produce the volumetric curves of the left atrium, computing several prognostic values of LA maximal or minimal volume as well as LA total or active emptying fraction. The speckle tracking–based method could also estimate LA booster, reservoir, and conduit strains for better understanding of LA mechanics. Especially LA reservoir strain has the largest evidence supporting its prognostic utility. Due to the exponential LA pressure-volume relationship, LA deformation at reservoir phase could decrease when LV filling pressure is high.[35] LA reservoir strain may be a candidate for estimating LV filling pressure and grading LV diastolic function. The clinical utilities of LA strain measurements need to be evaluated by further studies of a large cohort of healthy individuals and patients with various cardiovascular diseases.

The left atrium is seated around the ascending aorta, the left ventricle, and the right atrium. Accordingly, the understandings of the LA mechanics should be advanced in the viewpoints of unknown interactions between the left atrium and these vital structures in addition to intrinsic LA function.

KEY POINTS

- LA size is recognized as a novel marker of cardiovascular risks in the general population and various cardiovascular diseases.
- A main pathologic alteration in patients with HFpEF is characterized as LV diastolic dysfunction, leading to elevated LV filling pressure and LA enlargement.
- The biplane disk summation algorithm should be used as the standard method of 2-D echocardiography for the LA volumetric assessment. 3-D echocardiography allows quantifying LA volumes without geometric assumption.
- The left atrium acts to modulate LV filling and performance through three functions of booster, reservoir, and conduit.
- LA volumetric parameters include (1) LA volume preceding atrial contraction at the beginning of a P wave ($LAV_{pre\text{-}A}$), (2) minimal LA volume just at the mitral valve closure (LAV_{min}), and (3) maximal LA volume just before the mitral valve opening (LAV_{max}).
- Transmitral and pulmonary venous flows, mitral annular velocities, and deformation indices can be utilized to estimate LA function.
- TEE is useful to characterize the structure and function of LA appendage.
- The LA pressure-volume curve shows a characteristic figure-8 configuration, which consists of the A and V loops. The A loop represents active contraction and relaxation, and the V loop represents passive dilatation and emptying.
- Patients with limited LA booster and reservoir function or advanced LA stiffness have an increased risk of adverse outcomes.
- The understanding of LA mechanics should be advanced in the viewpoints of unknown interactions between the left atrium and neighboring vital structures in addition to intrinsic LA function.

Case Study 2 (Video 12.1)

A 74-year-old man was admitted to the hospital because of worsening exertional dyspnea. Chest x-ray findings showed mild cardiomegaly. A 12-lead ECG confirmed sinus rhythm, poor R progression in leads V1 to V3, and nonspecific intraventricular conduction delay. Echocardiography was performed to diagnose whether his symptoms were related to cardiac or noncardiac disorder.

REVIEW QUESTIONS

1. Video 12.1 shows a cine loop from an apical four-chamber view. Choose the appropriate echocardiographic findings.
   a. Eccentric left ventricular hypertrophy
   b. Reduced left ventricular ejection fraction
   c. Relative preservation of apical function rather than basal or midventricular function
   d. Lack of left atrial expansion
   e. Increased wall thickness in right ventricle
2. Fig. 12.12 shows transmitral inflow velocities. Choose an appropriate transmitral flow pattern in terms of left ventricular diastolic function.
   a. Normal mitral inflow pattern
   b. Grade 1 diastolic dysfunction
   c. Grade 2 diastolic dysfunction
   d. Grade 3 diastolic dysfunction
   e. Undetermined mitral inflow pattern
3. Fig. 12.13 shows mitral annular velocity at the septal corner. Choose the appropriate interpretation of mitral annular velocity.
   a. Because s′ velocity is preserved, left ventricular systolic function is normal.
   b. Because s′ velocity is reduced, left ventricular systolic function is abnormal.
   c. Because e′ velocity is preserved, left ventricular diastolic function is normal.
   d. Because e′ velocity is reduced, left ventricular diastolic function is abnormal.
   e. Because a′ velocity is preserved, left atrial function is normal.
4. Fig. 12.14 demonstrates two strain curves of left atrium (A) and left ventricle (B). Choose the appropriate explanations of the strain curves. The white dotted curve corresponds to global longitudinal strain.
   a. Left atrial strain is analyzed using the P-P gating method.
   b. Left ventricular strain is analyzed using the R-R gating method.
   c. Left atrial booster strain is preserved.
   d. Left atrial reservoir strain is reduced.
   e. Left ventricular apical sparing is observed.

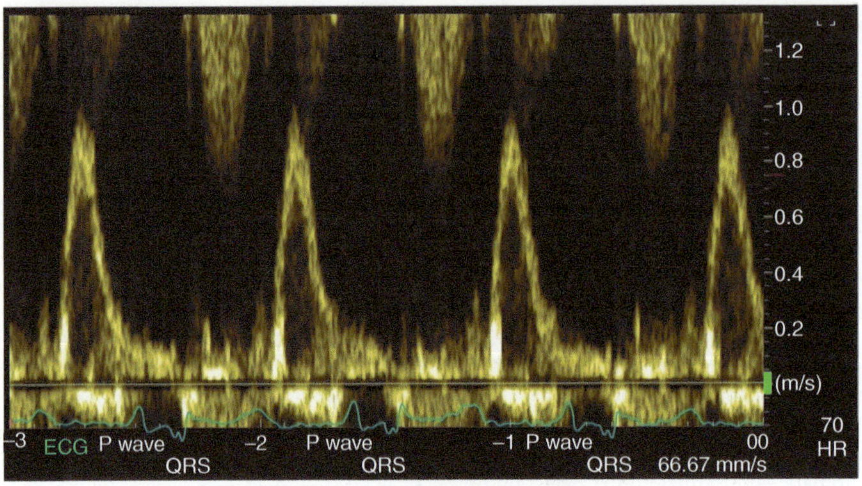

Fig. 12.12 A still frame from a video.

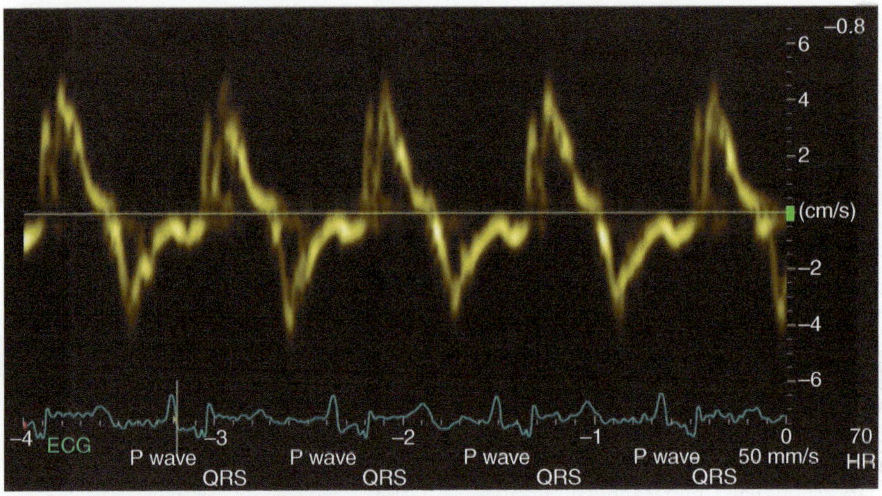

Fig. 12.13 A still frame from a video.

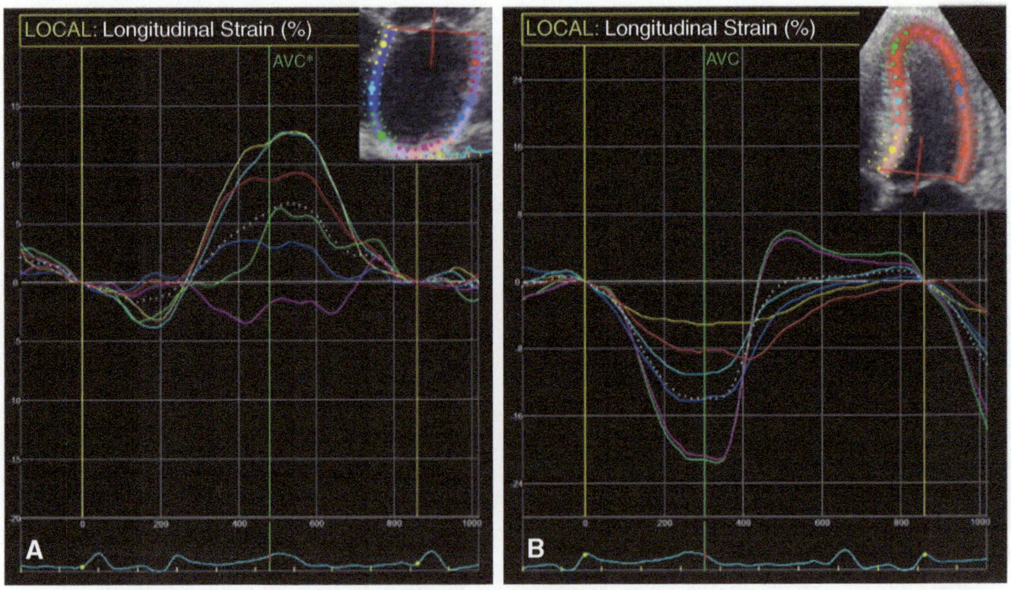

Fig. 12.14 A still frame from a video.

REFERENCES

1. Ho SY, Cabrera JA, Sanchez-Quintana D. Left atrial anatomy revisited. *Circ Arrhythm Electrophysiol.* 2012;5:220–228.
2. Al-Saady NM, Obel OA, Camm AJ. Left atrial appendage: structure, function, and role in thromboembolism. *Heart.* 1999;82:547–554.
3. Spencer KT, Mor-Avi V, Gorcsan III J, et al. Effects of aging on left atrial reservoir, conduit, and booster pump function: a multi-institution acoustic quantification study. *Heart.* 2001;85:272–277.
4. Tsang TS, Barnes ME, Gersh BJ, Bailey KR, Seward JB. Left atrial volume as a morphophysiologic expression of left ventricular diastolic dysfunction and relation to cardiovascular risk burden. *Am J Cardiol.* 2002;90: 1284–1289.
5. Simek CL, Feldman MD, Haber HL, Wu CC, Jayaweera AR, Kaul S. Relationship between left ventricular wall thickness and left atrial size: comparison with other measures of diastolic function. *J Am Soc Echocardiogr.* 1995;8:37–47.
6. Gupta S, Matulevicius SA, Ayers CR, et al. Left atrial structure and function and clinical outcomes in the general population. *Eur Heart J.* 2013;34:278–285.
7. Hoit BD. Left atrial size and function: role in prognosis. *J Am Coll Cardiol.* 2014;63:493–505.
8. Prioli A, Marino P, Lanzoni L, Zardini P. Increasing degrees of left ventricular filling impairment modulate left atrial function in humans. *Am J Cardiol.* 1998;82:756–761.
9. Khankirawatana B, Khankirawatana S, Peterson B, Mahrous H, Porter TR. Peak atrial systolic mitral annular velocity by Doppler tissue reliably predicts left atrial systolic function. *J Am Soc Echocardiogr.* 2004;17:353–360.
10. Singh A, Addetia K, Maffessanti F, Mor-Avi V, Lang RM. LA strain for categorization of LV diastolic dysfunction. *JACC Cardiovasc Imag.* 2017;10:735–743.
11. Lang RM, Badano LP, Mor-Avi V, et al. Recommendations for cardiac chamber quantification by echocardiography in adults: an update from the American Society of Echocardiography and the European Association of Cardiovascular Imaging. *J Am Soc Echocardiogr.* 2015;28:1–39. e14.
12. Lester SJ, Ryan EW, Schiller NB, Foster E. Best method in clinical practice and in research studies to determine left atrial size. *Am J Cardiol.* 1999;84:829–832.
13. Pritchett AM, Jacobsen SJ, Mahoney DW, Rodeheffer RJ, Bailey KR, Redfield MM. Left atrial volume as an index of left atrial size: a population-based study. *J Am Coll Cardiol.* 2003;41:1036–1043.
14. Faustino A, Providência R, Barra S, et al. Which method of left atrium size quantification is the most accurate to recognize thromboembolic risk in patients with non-valvular atrial fibrillation? *Cardiovasc Ultrasound.* 2014;12:28.
15. Lang RM, Bierig M, Devereux RB, et al. Recommendations for chamber quantification: a report from the American Society of Echocardiography's Guidelines and Standards Committee and the Chamber Quantification Writing Group, developed in conjunction with the European Association of Echocardiography, a branch of the European Society of Cardiology. *J Am Soc Echocardiogr.* 2005;18:1440–1463.
16. Miyasaka Y, Tsujimoto S, Maeba H, et al. Left atrial volume by real-time three-dimensional echocardiography: validation by 64-slice multidetector computed tomography. *J Am Soc Echocardiogr.* 2011;24:680–686.
17. Caselli S, Canali E, Foschi ML, et al. Long-term prognostic significance of three-dimensional echocardiographic parameters of the left ventricle and left atrium. *Eur J Echocardiogr.* 2010;11:250–256.
18. Badano LP, Miglioranza MH, Mihăilă S, et al. Left atrial volumes and function by three-dimensional echocardiography: reference values, accuracy, reproducibility, and comparison with two-dimensional echocardiographic measurements. *Circ Cardiovasc Imag.* 2016;9:e004229.
19. Medvedofsky D, Mor-Avi V, Byku I, et al. Three-dimensional echocardiographic automated quantification of left heart chamber volumes using an adaptive analytics algorithm: feasibility and impact of image quality in nonselected patients. *J Am Soc Echocardiogr.* 2017;30:879–885.
20. Tsang W, Salgo IS, Medvedofsky D, et al. Transthoracic 3D echocardiographic left heart chamber quantification using an automated adaptive analytics algorithm. *JACC Cardiovasc Imag.* 2016;9:769–782.
21. Inoue K, Asanuma T, Masuda K, Sakurai D, Higaki J, Nakatani S. Compensatory increase of left atrial external work to left ventricular dysfunction caused by afterload increase. *Am J Physiol Heart Circ Physiol.* 2015;308:H904–H912.
22. Barbier P, Solomon SB, Schiller NB, Glantz SA. Left atrial relaxation and left ventricular systolic function determine left atrial reservoir function. *Circulation.* 1999;100:427–436.
23. Blume GG, Mcleod CJ, Barnes ME, et al. Left atrial function: physiology, assessment, and clinical implications. *Eur J Echocardiogr.* 2011;12:421–430.
24. Anwar AM, Geleijnse ML, Soliman OI, Nemes A, ten Cate FJ. Left atrial Frank-Starling law assessed by real-time, three-dimensional echocardiographic left atrial volume changes. *Heart.* 2007;93:1393–1397.
25. Manning WJ, Silverman DI, Katz SE, Douglas PS. Atrial ejection force: a noninvasive assessment of atrial systolic function. *J Am Coll Cardiol.* 1993;22:221–225.
26. Braunwald E, Frahm CJ. Studies on Starling's law of the heart IV. Observations on the hemodynamic functions of the left atrium in man. *Circulation.* 1961;24:633–642.
27. Tabata T, Thomas JD, Klein AL. Pulmonary venous flow by Doppler echocardiography: revisited 12 years later. *J Am Coll Cardiol.* 2003;41:1243–1250.
28. Khankirawatana B, Khankirawatana S, Peterson B, Mahrous H, Porter TR. Peak atrial systolic mitral annular velocity by Doppler tissue reliably predicts left atrial systolic function. *J Am Soc Echocardiogr.* 2004;17:353–360.
29. Fujii A, Inoue K, Nagai T, et al. Clinical utility of atrial electromechanical conduction time measured with speckle tracking echocardiography after catheter ablation in patients with atrial fibrillation: a validation study with electroanatomical mapping. *Echocardiography.* 2016;33:1317–1325.
30. Hoit BD, Shao Y, McMannis K, Gabel M, Walsh RA. Determination of left atrial volume using sonomicrometry: a cast validation study. *Am J Physiol.* 1993;264:H1011–H1016.
31. Beigel R, Wunderlich NC, Ho SY, Arsanjani R, Siegel RJ. The left atrial appendage: anatomy, function, and noninvasive evaluation. *JACC Cardiovasc Imag.* 2014;7:1251–1265.
32. Di Biase L, Santangeli P, Anselmino M, et al. Does the left atrial appendage morphology correlate with the risk of stroke in patients with atrial fibrillation? Results from a multicenter study. *J Am Coll Cardiol.* 2012;60:531–538.
33. Sommer M, Roehrich A, Boenner F, et al. Value of 3D TEE for LAA morphology. *JACC Cardiovasc Imag.* 2015;8:1107–1110.
34. Agmon Y, Khandheria BK, Gentile F, Seward JB. Echocardiographic assessment of the left atrial appendage. *J Am Coll Cardiol.* 1999;34:1867–1877.
35. Smiseth OA, Torp H, Opdahl A, Haugaa KH, Urheim S. Myocardial strain imaging: how useful is it in clinical decision making? *Eur Heart J.* 2016;37:1196–1207.
36. Pathan F, D'Elia N, Nolan MT, Marwick TH, Negishi K. Normal ranges of left atrial strain by speckle-tracking echocardiography: a systematic review and meta-analysis. *J Am Soc Echocardiogr.* 2017;30:59–70.e8.
37. Fujimoto K, Inoue K, Saito M, et al. Incremental value of left atrial active function measured by speckle tracking echocardiography in patients with hypertrophic cardiomyopathy. *Echocardiography.* 2018;35:1138–1148.
38. Vianna-Pinton R, Moreno CA, Baxter CM, Lee KS, Tsang TS, Appleton CP. Two-dimensional speckle-tracking echocardiography of the left atrium: feasibility and regional contraction and relaxation differences in normal subjects. *J Am Soc Echocardiogr.* 2009;22:299–305.
39. Badano LP, Kolias TJ, Muraru D, et al. Standardization of left atrial, right ventricular, and right atrial deformation imaging using two-dimensional speckle tracking echocardiography: a consensus document of the EACVI/ASE/Industry Task Force to standardize deformation imaging. *Eur Heart J Cardiovasc Imag.* 2018;19:591–600.
40. Stefanadis C, Dernellis J, Toutouzas P. A clinical appraisal of left atrial function. *Eur Heart J.* 2001;22:22–36.
41. Bauer F, Jones M, Qin JX, et al. Quantitative analysis of left atrial function during left ventricular ischemia with and without left atrial ischemia: a real-time 3-dimensional echocardiographic study. *J Am Soc Echocardiogr.* 2005;18:795–801.

42. Lam CSP, Voors AA, de Boer RA, Solomon SD, van Veldhuisen DJ. Heart failure with preserved ejection fraction: from mechanisms to therapies. *Eur Heart J.* 2018;39:2780–2792.
43. Redfield MM. Heart failure with preserved ejection fraction. *N Engl J Med.* 2016;375:1868–1877.
44. Melenovsky V, Hwang SJ, Redfield MM, Zakeri R, Lin G, Borlaug BA. Left atrial remodeling and function in advanced heart failure with preserved or reduced ejection fraction. *Circ Heart Fail.* 2015;8:295–303.
45. Paulus WJ, Tschöpe C, Sanderson JE, et al. How to diagnose diastolic heart failure: a consensus statement on the diagnosis of heart failure with normal left ventricular ejection fraction by the Heart Failure and Echocardiography Associations of the European Society of Cardiology. *Eur Heart J.* 2007;28:2539–2550.
46. Nagueh SF, Smiseth OA, Appleton CP, et al. Recommendations for the evaluation of left ventricular diastolic function by echocardiography: an update from the American Society of Echocardiography and the European Association of Cardiovascular Imaging. *J Am Soc Echocardiogr.* 2016;29:277–314.
47. Russo C, Jin Z, Homma S, et al. Left atrial minimum volume and reservoir function as correlates of left ventricular diastolic function: impact of left ventricular systolic function. *Heart.* 2012;98:813–820.
48. Wu VC, Takeuchi M, Kuwaki H, et al. Prognostic value of LA volumes assessed by transthoracic 3D echocardiography: comparison with 2D echocardiography. *JACC Cardiovasc Imag.* 2013;6:1025–1035.
49. Sanders P, Morton JB, Kistler PM, et al. Reversal of atrial mechanical dysfunction after cardioversion of atrial fibrillation: implications for the mechanisms of tachycardia-mediated atrial cardiomyopathy. *Circulation.* 2003;108:1976–1984.
50. Thomas L, Boyd A, Thomas SP, Schiller NB, Ross DL. Atrial structural remodelling and restoration of atrial contraction after linear ablation for atrial fibrillation. *Eur Heart J.* 2003;24:1942–1951.
51. Melenovsky V, Borlaug BA, Rosen B, et al. Cardiovascular features of heart failure with preserved ejection fraction versus nonfailing hypertensive left ventricular hypertrophy in the urban Baltimore community: the role of atrial remodeling/dysfunction. *J Am Coll Cardiol.* 2007;49:198–207.
52. Abhayaratna WP, Fatema K, Barnes ME, et al. Left atrial reservoir function as a potent marker for first atrial fibrillation or flutter in persons > or = 65 years of age. *Am J Cardiol.* 2008;101:1626–1629.
53. Freed BH, Daruwalla V, Cheng JY, et al. Prognostic utility and clinical significance of cardiac mechanics in heart failure with preserved ejection fraction: importance of left atrial strain. *Circ Cardiovasc Imag.* 2016;9:e003754.
54. Stokke TM, Hasselberg NE, Smedsrud MK, et al. Geometry as a confounder when assessing ventricular systolic function: comparison between ejection fraction and strain. *J Am Coll Cardiol.* 2017;70:942–954.
55. Kalam K, Otahal P, Marwick TH. Prognostic implications of global LV dysfunction: a systematic review and meta-analysis of global longitudinal strain and ejection fraction. *Heart.* 2014;100:1673–1680.
56. Suga H. Importance of atrial compliance in cardiac performance. *Circ Res.* 1974;35:39–43.
57. Stefanadis C, Dernellis J, Stratos C, et al. Assessment of left atrial pressure-area relation in humans by means of retrograde left atrial catheterization and echocardiographic automatic boundary detection: effects of dobutamine. *J Am Coll Cardiol.* 1998;31:426–436.
58. Melenovsky V, Hwang SJ, Redfield MM, Zakeri R, Lin G, Borlaug BA. Left atrial remodeling and function in advanced heart failure with preserved or reduced ejection fraction. *Circ Heart Fail.* 2015;8:295–303.
59. Kurt M, Wang J, Torre-Amione G, Nagueh SF. Left atrial function in diastolic heart failure. *Circ Cardiovasc Imag.* 2009;2:10–15.
60. Inoue K, Iio C, Kawakami H, et al. Prominent v wave as a result of left atrial stiffening. *J Echocardiogr.* 2018;16:47–48. [2]

13

Evaluation of Intracardiac Filling Pressures

Miguel A. Quinones

OUTLINE

Case Study

A 69-year-old woman presents with a 2-month history of dyspnea that has progressed to a NYHA Class III, occurring with minimal exertion. Fig. 13.1 shows a four-chamber view at end systole and a continuous wave (CW) Doppler recording of tricuspid regurgitation (TR) enhanced by saline contrast. Fig. 13.2 shows a pulse wave (PW) Doppler recording of the transmitral velocity (MV) and tissue Doppler recording of lateral and septal annulus velocities. Would you say that the filling pressures are normal, elevated, or indeterminate? The answer to the question will become clear as we proceed with a comprehensive discussion of how to assess left ventricular (LV) filling pressures.

DEFINITION OF FILLING PRESSURES

The term *left ventricular filling pressure* (LVFP) refers to the LV pressures during diastole. They are illustrated in Fig. 13.3 and include LV minimal pressure, pre-A wave pressure, and LV end-diastolic pressure (LVEDP). In the absence of mitral inflow obstruction, mean left atrial pressure (LAP) and mean pulmonary capillary wedge pressure (PCWP) are surrogates of LVFP.

LV minimal pressure occurs very early in diastole and is greatly influenced by the relaxation properties of the left ventricle.[1] As relaxation worsens, LV minimal pressure rises. To have an accurate measurement of this pressure, the recording must be made with a high-fidelity micromanometer catheter, and for this reason, this measurement is rarely used clinically.

In the presence of sinus rhythm, LVEDP occurs after atrial contraction. It is influenced by the strength and effectiveness of the LA contraction (i.e., the amount of volume entering with the atrial kick), and the end-diastolic stiffness of the LV. With an effective atrial contraction, patients with diastolic dysfunction can maintain a normal mean LA pressure despite having an elevated LVEDP (see Fig. 13.3).

The pre-A pressure reflects the diastolic pressure in the LV during the passive phase of filling and is within a few mmHg of the mean LAP or PCWP.[2] These are the pressures responsible for passive pulmonary congestion. Therefore when evaluating patients with dyspnea, the noninvasive estimation of these pressures is of greater importance than the estimation of LVEDP. Consequently, most of the discussion in this chapter will focus on ways to estimate mean LAP or PCWP. Because the pre-A LV pressure relates closely to mean LAP, this pressure should be reported when one is performing a left heart catheterization. This is discussed in greater detail in Chapter 8.

MECHANISMS OF DIASTOLIC PRESSURE ELEVATION

The role of the left ventricle during diastole is to provide an adequate inflow of volume (i.e., preload) to generate the stroke volume and cardiac output necessary to support body functions at rest and during a wide range of physical activies and heart rates, and to accomplish this while maintaining low filling pressures. The mechanisms responsible for normal diastolic function and the abnormalities that result in elevations of filling pressures are discussed in detail in Chapter 2; Chapters 4 and 5 discuss the determinants of diastolic flow and role of LA function, respectively. In simplified terms, early LV filling depends on a rapid and complete relaxation of the ventricle, which is an active, energy-consuming process, while filling during mid- to late diastole depends greatly on the passive elastic properties of the ventricle (i.e., stiffness) and the effectiveness of atrial contraction.

Impaired LV relaxation has been shown to be present in the vast majority of patients with conditions leading to or associated with diastolic heart failure or heart failure with preserved ejection fraction (HFpEF).[3–7] These conditions are also associated with increased diastolic stiffness so that both factors become instrumental in the

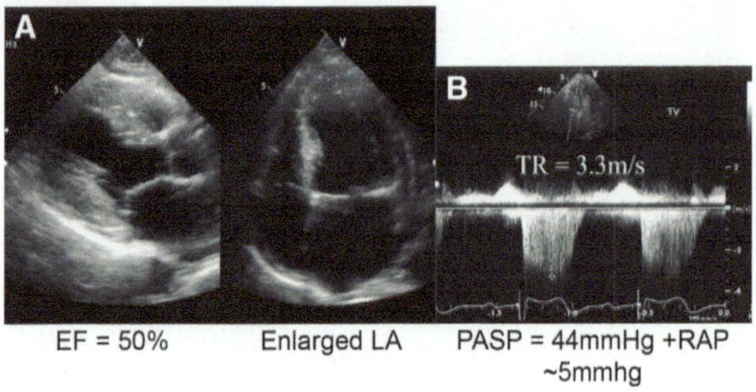

Fig. 13.1 Case study: (A) Parasternal and apical four-chamber view taken at end systole in Case Study 1. (B) Tricuspid regurgitant velocity enhanced by saline contrast from Case Study 1. *EF*, LV ejection fraction; *LA*, left atrium; *PASP*, pulmonary artery systolic pressure; *RAP*, right atrial pressure. See text for details.

elevation of filling pressures either at rest or with exercise. As a rule, it can be stated that when diastolic function is normal (i.e., normal relaxation and stiffness), heart failure is highly unlikely to occur. Mean LAP may be elevated in normally relaxing hearts with pericardial constriction, obstruction to mitral inflow, or a rapid and severe increase in preload such as with acute aortic or mitral regurgitation.

If we accept the premise that patients with HFpEF have abnormalities of LV relaxation and stiffness (i.e., diastolic dysfunction), we can derive an algorithm for the estimation of LVFP by echocardiography/Doppler (two-dimensional [2-D]/Doppler) that is based on first determining if they have diastolic dysfunction with impaired relaxation and then looking for findings indicative of elevated LVFP. This chapter will review the algorithm currently recommended by the American Society of Echocardiography (ASE) that integrates findings

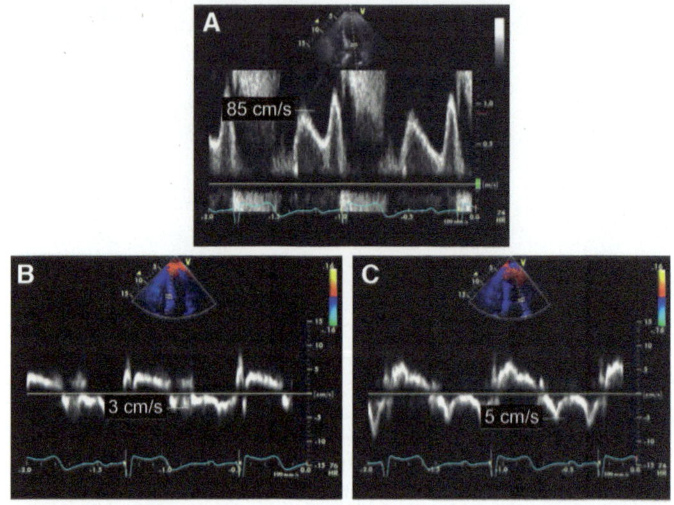

Fig. 13.2 Case Study: PW Doppler recording of transmitral velocity (A), tissue Doppler recording of septal (B), and lateral (C) taken from Case Study 1. See text for details. *IVRT*, Isovolumic relaxation time; *LVFP*, left ventricular filling pressure.

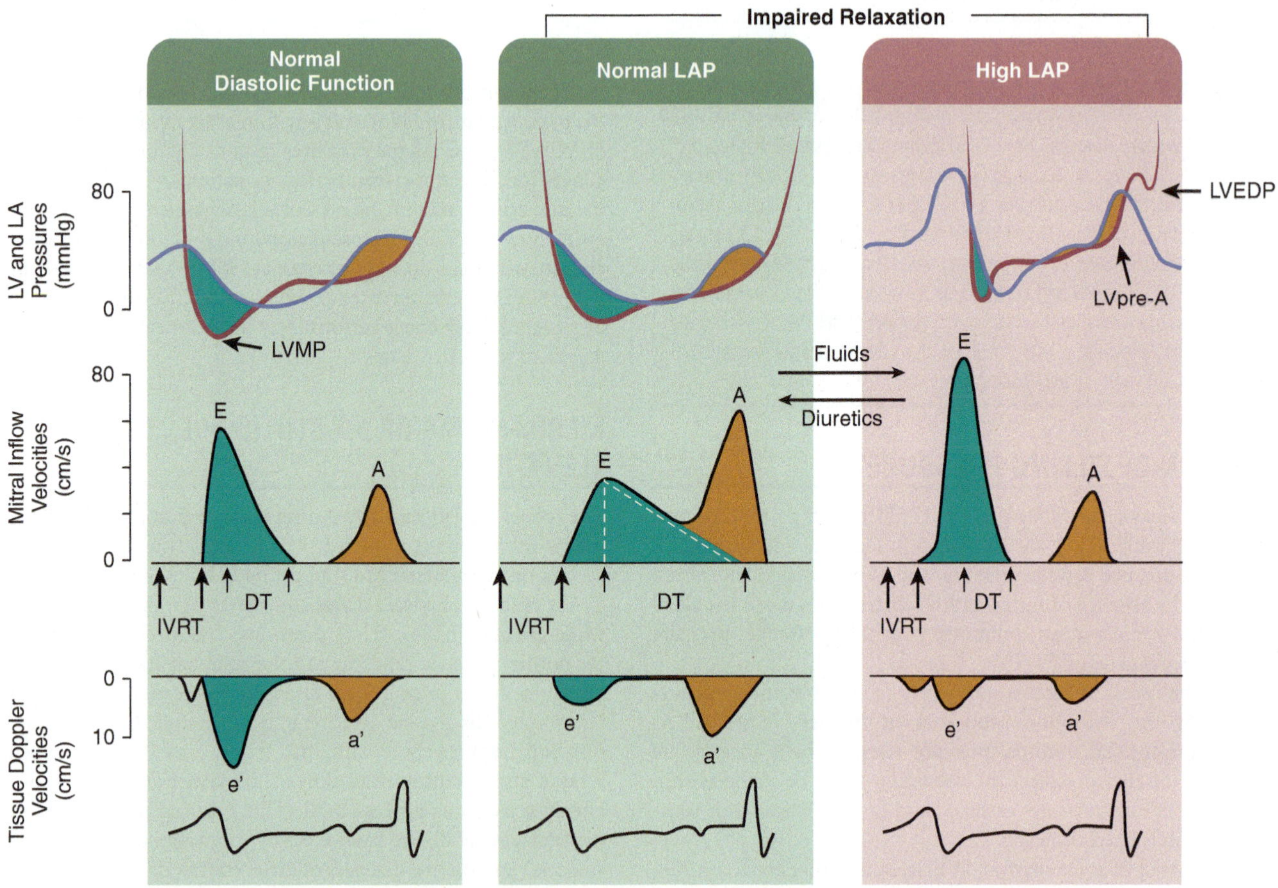

Fig. 13.3 Diagrammatic illustrations of LV and LA pressures, transmitral velocity, and tissue Doppler velocity from the lateral annulus in a normal heart and in grade I *(middle panel)* and grade III *(right panel)* diastolic dysfunction. Reproduced by permission from the American Society of Echocardiography. See text for explanations. *DT*, Deceleration time; *IVRT*, isovolumic relaxation time; *LVEDP*, LV end-diastolic pressure; *LVMP*, LV minimal pressure; *LVpre-A*, LV pre-A pressure. ASE: https://asecho-prod.force.com/CPBase__item?id=a2l4A000001tJb3QAE.

derived from 2-D, PW and CW Doppler, and tissue Doppler recordings.[8] We will also present an approach to managing indeterminate findings and evaluating challenging clinical scenarios. A limited discussion of new developments and recommendations on how to create a clinically meaningful diastolic function report will be presented.

EVALUATING LV RELAXATION

LV relaxation is an active process; consequently conditions affecting the myocardium such as pathologic hypertrophy, ischemia or infarction, excessive afterload, and any form of cardiomyopathy will result in impaired relaxation. Therefore one may have a high index of suspicion for the presence of impaired relaxation in patients with known coronary artery disease (CAD) and in those with chronic systemic hypertension (HTN).[8] In addition, relaxation gradually declines with age so that with very advanced aging (≥80 years) the decline may be significant enough to impair diastolic filling (see Chapter 2).[9,10]

Several 2-D findings are highly indicative of diastolic dysfunction; these include reduced EF, concentric left ventricular hypertrophy (LVH) not caused by athletic training, and regional wall motion abnormalities (Fig. 13.4). In addition, LA enlargement is a sensitive marker of impaired relaxation,[11–13] given that patients with diastolic dysfunction often have transient increases in LAP that serve as a stimulus for LA dilation. However, this finding is less specific as it can be seen with high cardiac output states, athletic hearts, primary mitral regurgitation (MR), and atrial fibrillation (AFib)/flutter. Eccentric LVH occurring with athletic training or with the early stages of chronic mitral or aortic regurgitations is usually not associated with diastolic dysfunction.

A detail discussion of the relation of PW and tissue Doppler velocities, and color flow Doppler recordings to diastolic filling dynamics and filling pressures, can be found in Chapters 9, 10, and 11. Doppler measurements suggestive of impaired relaxation include reduced transmitral E/A ratio (<0.8), prolonged isovolumic relaxation time (IVRT >90 msec), reduced flow propagation velocity (Vp) by color Doppler, and reduced early mitral annular velocity (e′) by tissue Doppler (lateral e′ <10 cm/sec; septal e′ <7 cm/sec). As it has been discussed in previous chapters, these measurements are imperfect markers of relaxation, and many are influenced by loading conditions. In addition, Vp may remain normal in patients with small end-systolic volumes despite having impaired relaxation and is therefore less valuable in HFpEF.[14,15] For this reason, the ASE guidelines recommend the use of multiple 2-D/Doppler findings in patients who lack clear-cut evidence by 2-D of impaired relaxation (Fig. 13.5; also see Fig. 13.4). These are usually the ones with preserved EF and without regional wall motion abnormalities or pathologic LVH.

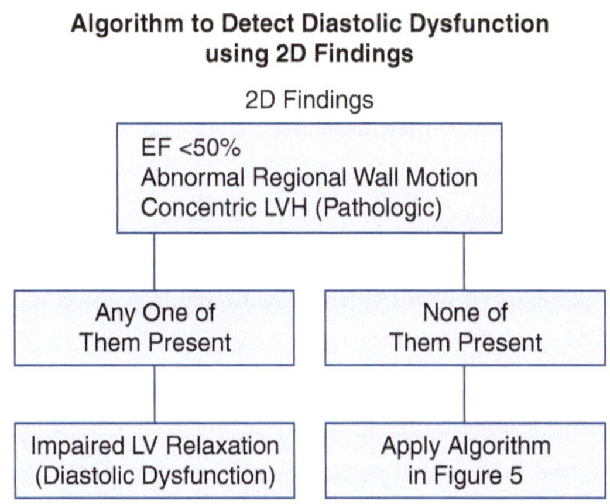

Fig. 13.4 Algorithm to assess LV relaxation using 2-D findings.

As can be seen in Fig. 13.5, the proposed ASE algorithm for detecting diastolic dysfunction incorporates four parameters: septal and lateral e′ as an index of relaxation, average E/e′ ratio (E/ average of septal and lateral e′) as an index of LAP, peak velocity of TR as surrogate for pulmonary artery systolic pressure [PASP]), and LA volume. Patients with three or more normal values are classified as having normal relaxation, while those with three or more abnormal values are diagnosed with diastolic dysfunction. Patients with only two normal/abnormal parameters are classified as indeterminate in recognition that it may not always be possible to correctly assess diastolic function. This new algorithm was proposed to reduce the number of false positive diagnoses of diastolic dysfunction created by using only a reduced e′. However, by doing this, the algorithm can miss patients with impaired relaxation. A good example of such is a 72-year-old woman with chronic HTN (a clinical setting that often results in impaired relaxation), normal EF without concentric LVH or LA enlargement, a TR velocity of 2.7 m/sec, an average E/e′ of 10, and a lateral e′ of 5 cm/sec. The patient will be classified by the new algorithm as normal (i.e., 3/4 negative and 1 positive), although it is possible that she could have early diastolic dysfunction. Likewise, a patient with dyspnea who has an average E/e′ greater than 14 and LA enlargement with a normal right ventricular systolic pressure (RVSP) and low-normal e′, although classified as indeterminate, is likely to have diastolic dysfunction with elevated LVFP and may warrant application of the algorithm for estimating LVFP (see upcoming discussion). We have found that applying these concepts in routine clinical practice allows an assessment of diastolic function in over 90% of patients examined. The algorithm is limited in the presence of sinus tachycardia, marked bradycardia, or AFib.

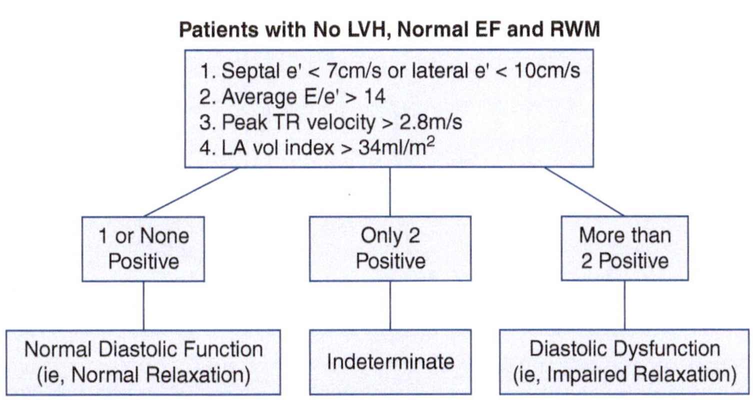

Fig. 13.5 Algorithm recommended by the ASE guidelines for detection of diastolic dysfunction in patients without positive 2-D findings.

ESTIMATING FILLING PRESSURES IN SINUS RHYTHM

Patients with HFpEF may have normal or elevated LVFP at rest depending on the severity of the relaxation abnormality, degree of chamber stiffness of the ventricle, loading conditions, and effectiveness of atrial contraction. Their diastolic pressure-volume (P-V) relation is typically shifted to the left in contrast to the marked shift to the right seen in patients with heart failure with reduced ejection fraction (HFrEF) (Fig. 13.6). Thus it is not uncommon to see patients with impaired relaxation that are compensated with normal mean LAP, even though they might have elevated LVEDP. However, many of these patients experience an increase in LV diastolic pressure with exercise or excessive fluid intake (shifting from point A to B or C in Fig. 13.6),[16] and as such are at risk for developing clinical heart failure. Likewise, with appropriate therapy, their P-V relation can shift from point B or C back to point A (see Fig. 13.6).

Once we have determined that a patient is likely to have diastolic dysfunction, the estimation of filling pressures is made by integrating several echo/Doppler findings given that no single parameter is perfect for estimating filling pressures. In the past, several equations were proposed in the literature to derive mean PCWP.[13,17–22] Many of them incorporated multiple Doppler and 2-D measurements, and some utilized the E/e′ ratio alone or combined with other measurements. They all performed better in patients with depressed LV function and were less accurate in those with normal EF. Rather than trying to make a precise estimate of LAP or PCWP, the current ASE guidelines recommend combining Doppler findings with LA volume to classify diastolic dysfunction into three grades: grade I, which is generally associated with normal mean LAP (<15 mmHg); grade II, which is generally associated with a mild to moderate elevation (15–25 mmHg); and grade III, which is generally associated with marked elevation of mean LAP (>25 mmHg). The primary Doppler findings include the transmitral E velocity and E/A ratio, average E/e′ ratio, and peak TR velocity; other measurements such as deceleration time of the E velocity (DT), IVRT, and pulmonary vein velocity measurements can be used in selected situations (see upcoming discussion).

Transmitral Velocity

The transmitral velocity is driven by two major factors: mitral valve orifice area and flow. Both of these combined result in a given instantaneous transvalvular pressure gradient and velocity (see Fig. 13.3).[23,24] During early diastole, and with normal mitral valve orifice area, active relaxation and LAP are the principal determinants of flow and transvalvular gradients. With normal relaxation, the LV pressure decay during isovolumic relaxation occurs rapidly (thus a shorter time constant of relaxation [tau]), and early ventricular suction is enhanced. This results in a higher E velocity, an E/A ratio greater than 1, and a shorter DT and IVRT; the opposite occurs with impaired relaxation: less suction, lower E velocity, E/A ratio less than 1, and longer DT and IVRT. Increasing LA pressure (and LV-LA crossover pressure) also results in shortening of IVRT, higher LA-LV transmitral gradient, higher E velocity, E/A ratio greater than 0.8, and shorter DT (see Fig. 13.3);[25,2627] the pattern observed resembles that of normal diastolic function and thus was referred to as pseudonormal (currently classified as grade II diastolic dysfunction). The opposite occurs with lower LAP. At the extremes, an E/A ratio of 0.8 or less with an E of 50 cm/sec or less, in a patient with impaired relaxation, usually implies a mean PCWP less than 15 mmHg;

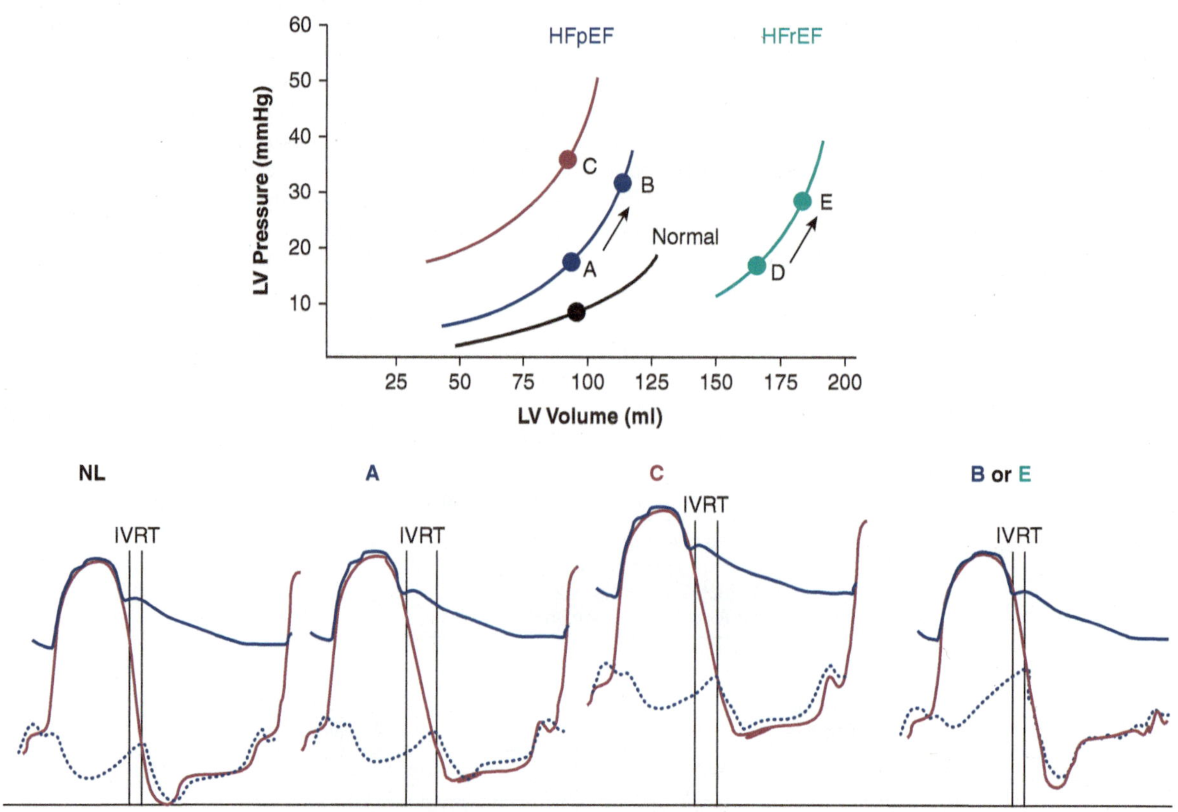

Fig. 13.6 The upper panel shows a diagrammatic illustration of diastolic LV pressure-volume curves in a normal heart, a dilated LV with heart failure, and two stages of diastolic dysfunction with preserved EF. The lower panel shows a diagrammatic illustration of LV, central aortic and LA pressures in a normal heart, and the different stages of heart failure shown in the upper panel. See text for explanation.

likewise, an E/A ratio above 2 with a short DT less than 150 msec is highly predictive of a high mean PCWP (see Fig. 13.3).

In the era prior to the use of annular velocities by tissue Doppler, the response of the transmitral velocity to the Valsalva maneuver was used to distinguish a grade II pseudonormal pattern from normal relaxation (see Chapter 9).[28] The maneuver acutely reduces venous return to the left atrium, which in a normal heart leads to a lowering of both E and A velocities. By contrast, patients with a pseudonormal pattern respond to Valsalva by changing to a grade I diastolic dysfunction pattern (i.e., E/A ratio <0.8). With the advent of annular velocities, the need for performing a Valsalva maneuver has been greatly diminished though at times it can be useful (see upcoming discussion).

Annular Velocities and E/e′

Mitral annular e′ has been shown to be an index of LV relaxation. Consequently, E/e′ corrects the E velocity for the influence of relaxation and has been shown to relate directly with mean PCWP; an E/e′ greater than 14 is predictive of a mean LAP of 15 mmHg or more, while a ratio less than 8 is often predictive of a mean PCWP below 15 mmHg.[13,21–23] As with the other diastolic indices, E/e′ relates better with mean PCWP in patients with depressed EF.[14,21,23] The annular a′ velocity reflects the longitudinal expansion of the LV during atrial contraction. Reduction of a′ has been associated with increased LV end-diastolic stiffness and reduced survival in patients with HFrEF.[29] This measurement has been of lesser value in HFpEF. Because e′ is a regional index, the ASE guidelines recommend averaging the septal and lateral e′ values to have a closer assessment of global LV relaxation.

Pulmonary Vein Velocities

Pulmonary vein velocities are useful in estimating the LVEDP. During atrial contraction with an elevated LVEDP, LV pressure may rise over LA pressure (see Fig. 13.3) producing a reverse gradient that shortens the duration of the transmitral A velocity (AMV) relative to the pulmonary vein retrograde A velocity (APV) (Fig. 13.7). The interval APV-AMV has been found to relate directly with LVEDP; whenever APV-AMV exceeds 20 msec, LVEDP is likely to be higher than 20 mmHg (see Chapter 9).[30] This finding is fairly reliable as long as the PR interval is within a normal range (i.e., neither too short nor too long).

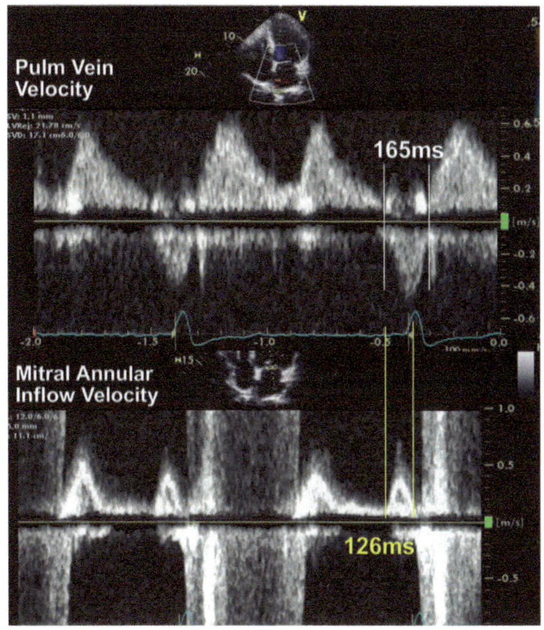

Fig. 13.7 Pulmonary vein velocity and mitral annular inflow velocity recorded in a patient with elevated LVEDP. Note the longer duration of the retrograde pulmonary A wave relative to the mitral antegrade A wave.

The value of pulmonary vein velocities in estimating mean LAP is limited. With an elevated V wave as seen in patients with grade III (and sometimes with grade II) diastolic dysfunction, systolic antegrade flow velocity (S) in the pulmonary vein is diminished, while diastolic flow velocity (D) is augmented (S/D ratio <1) (Fig. 13.8). However, these changes are often accompanied by increasing E/A and E/e′ ratios so that the contribution of the pulmonary veins is diminished. Furthermore, in patients with normal EF, S/D often remains above 1 despite elevated LVFP.[23,31,32]

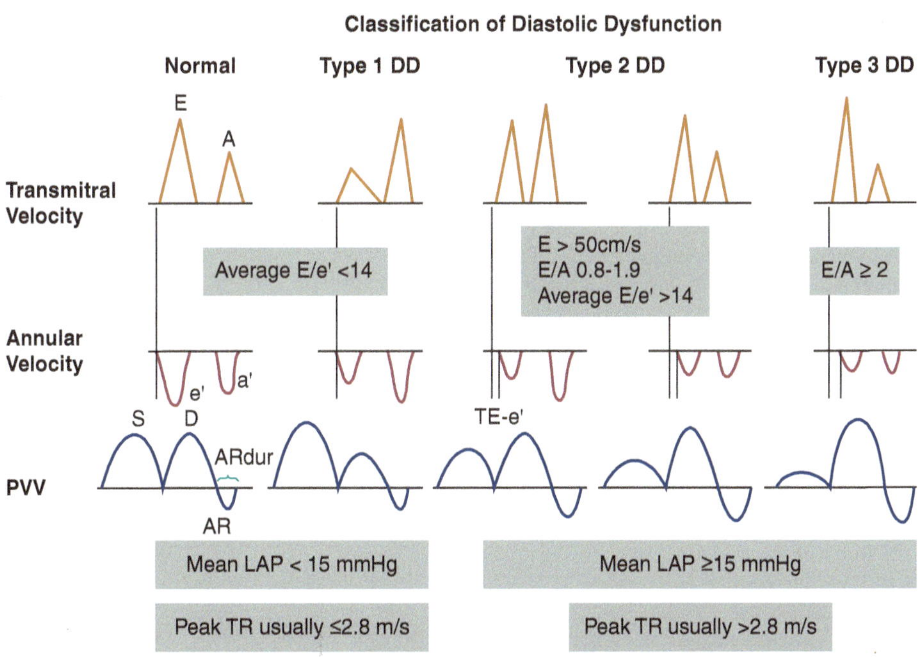

Fig. 13.8 Diagrammatic illustration of the transmitral velocity, annular tissue Doppler velocity, and pulmonary vein velocity (PVV) in a normal heart and the three grades of diastolic dysfunction (DD).

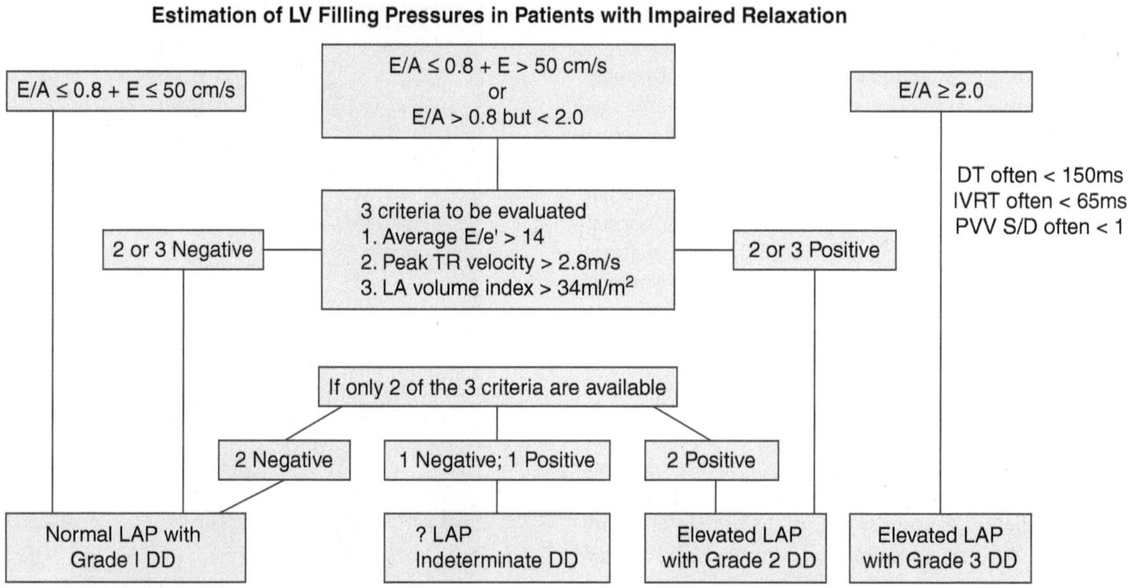

Fig. 13.9 Algorithm recommended by the ASE guidelines for the estimation of LV filling pressures in patients with impaired relaxation.

Peak TR Velocity

Peak TR velocity provides an estimate of the instantaneous pressure gradient between right ventricle (RV) and right atrium (RA). A peak velocity of 2.9 m/sec is converted with the $4V^2$ equation into a pressure gradient of 34 mmHg. In the absence of RV outflow obstruction, peak systolic pulmonary artery pressure (PASP) is 34 plus mean RA pressure. Therefore most patients with a peak TR velocity greater than 2.8 m/sec will have an elevated PASP above 37 mmHg. It has been shown that in patients with impaired LV relaxation, in the absence of increased pulmonary vascular resistance, a peak TR velocity greater than 2.8 m is predictive of an elevated mean PCWP, particularly if accompanied by LA enlargement.[33,34]

Applying an Algorithm to Estimate LVFP

In patients with depressed EF, grading diastolic dysfunction and detection of elevated LVFP can often be established using the E/A ratio and pulmonary vein S/D. E/e′ and peak TR velocity may corroborate the E/A ratio and pulmonary veins and are helpful in cases where E/A is between 0.8 and 1.5. However, in patients with normal EF (and thus with HFpEF), the evaluation is more challenging, and the ASE algorithm recommends integration of multiple findings, the concept being that the more findings that predict normal or elevated LVFP, the more likely that the prediction is accurate. The algorithm also recognizes that there are times when it may not be possible to make an accurate estimation of LVFP.

The algorithm usually applied to patients with myocardial pathology and evidence of impaired relaxation starts with the E/A ratio followed by adding average E/e′, peak TR velocity, and LA volume, as needed (Fig. 13.9). An E of 50 cm/sec or less with an E/A of 0.8 or less is predictive of a grade I diastolic dysfunction with normal LAP. Likewise, an E/A of 2 or more is predictive of grade III diastolic dysfunction with a high LAP. The challenge is deciphering the in-between findings (i.e., when E/A is <0.8 with an E velocity >50 cm/sec or when E/A is between 0.9 and 1.9). In these cases, the algorithm recommends incorporating the following three parameters:

- Average E/e′ >14
- TR peak velocity >2.8 m/sec
- LA volume index >34 mL/m^2

If two of the three parameters are absent, LAP is estimated to be normal. If two of the three parameters are present, mean LAP is elevated (grade II diastolic dysfunction). If only one of the three parameters is present, the estimation becomes indeterminate. At times, this may occur because no TR velocity was recorded, and in these cases, the use of saline contrast can be of great value in resolving the estimation. Keep in mind that the cutoff value of 2.8 m/sec for peak TR velocity is meant to predict a PASP greater than 37 mmHg. However, there are times when PASP will be elevated with a peak TR less than 2.8 if the RA pressure is elevated. Sometimes other measurements—such as DT, IVRT, pulmonary vein S/D or APV-AMV, and more recently global longitudinal strain (GLS) and LA strain can help in establishing a more precise determination of the LVFP, particularly in patients with indeterminate findings and in those with challenging conditions such as AFib and mitral annular calcification (MAC) (see upcoming discussion).

The ASE algorithm was recently validated in a prospective investigation carried out by Andersen and associates in five international centers (three in North America, one in Norway, and one in South Korea).[35] The study enrolled 450 patients undergoing 2-D/Doppler examination and invasive hemodynamics as part of routine clinical evaluation (mean PCWP measured in 293; pre-A LV diastolic pressure in 157). LVEF was 50% or more in 54% of the patients, and LVFP by catheterization was elevated in 58%. Although no single echo/Doppler parameter performed well enough to be used alone, applying the ASE algorithm distinguished between normal and elevated LVFP in 87% patients (84% in patients with EF ≥ 50%). Accuracy was highest in patients with EF less than 50% (91%) and in those with CAD (93%), and lowest in patients with chronic kidney disease (79%) and pulmonary parenchymal or vascular disease (81%).

Let us now apply the ASE algorithm to the case presented at the beginning of the chapter. The patient has an EF of 50% with a dilated LA (volume index, 46 mL/m^2) and a peak TR velocity of 3.3 m/sec (see Fig. 13.1). In addition, she has a septal e′ of 3 cm/sec, a lateral e′ of 5 cm/sec, and an average E/e′ of 21 (see Fig. 13.2). With an E velocity of 85 cm/sec and an E/A of 0.8, the collective findings are indicative of grade II diastolic dysfunction (impaired relaxation with elevated LVFP), predictive of a mean PCWP between 16 and 25 mmHg.

Incorporating Other Parameters

There are times when other parameters of diastolic function (such as IVRT ≤65 msec, DT ≤150 msec, pulmonary vein S/D <1, and

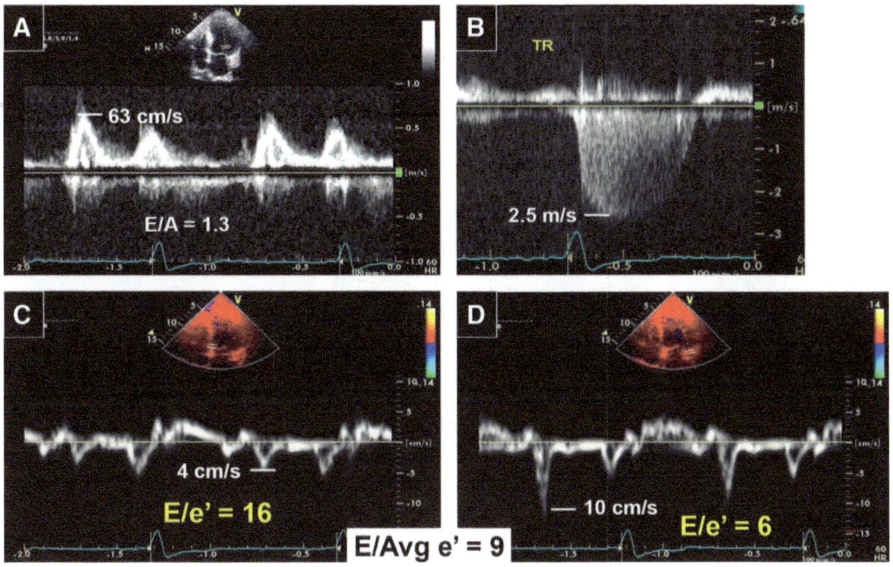

Fig. 13.10 Case study: Transmitral velocity (A), tricuspid regurgitant velocity by CW Doppler (B), tissue Doppler velocity at the septal (C), and lateral (D) annulus in the same patient shown in Fig. 13.8. See text for details.

APV-AMV >20 msec or response of E/A to Valsalva) can help resolve an indeterminate grade of diastolic dysfunction. A common situation is when some of the measurements proposed by the ASE algorithm are not available or their values are in a borderline or gray zone. For instance, a hypertensive patient with class 2 dyspnea and concentric LVH has an E/A of 1.2, absent TR velocity, LA volume index right at 34 mL/m^2, and an average E/e′ of 14. These findings could be classified either as normal LAP or as indeterminate. In such a patient, a pulmonary vein S/D less than 1, a short IVRT, and/or a positive response to Valsalva can change the estimate from indeterminate to elevated LVFP.

Fig. 13.10 illustrates another example where using other measurements provided greater insight into the patient's diastolic function. The patient was a 67-year-old man with known CAD. The 2-D examination showed an EF of 50% with akinesis of the distal anterior/septal segments and apex; LA volume index was 38 mL/m^2. The transmitral velocity had an E velocity of 67 cm/sec with an E/A of 1.3. Peak TR velocity was 2.5 m/sec indicative of normal PASP. While lateral e′ was normal (10 cm/sec), septal e′ was much reduced (4 cm/sec), a finding commonly seen in patients with CAD reflecting the impact of regional wall motion on annular velocities. Septal E/e′ is 16, lateral E/e is 6, and average E/e′ is 9. Are filling pressures normal or elevated? The patient clearly has impaired relaxation demonstrated by the resting wall motion abnormalities. With two of three negative ASE criteria, the algorithm predicts a normal mean LAP. The pulmonary vein velocity tracing shown in Fig. 13.7 was taken from this patient. While the S/D ratio is near 1, APV-AMR is greater than 20 msec, which is consistent with an elevated LVEDP. Integration of these findings allowed the report to state, "Impaired relaxation with normal mean LAP and elevated LVEDP."

EVALUATION IN CHALLENGING CASES

AFib and Other Rhythm Disorders

AFib presents multiple challenges to the evaluation of diastolic function and estimation of LVFP. The transmitral and annular velocities lack an atrial component, and the beat-by-beat variation in R-R interval results in beat-to-beat variation in E and e′ as well as in DT and IVRT. Thus measurements must be averaged over several cardiac cycles or, alternatively, made in three to five cycles with cycle lengths within 10% to 20% of the average heart rate. Furthermore, LA enlargement frequently occurs regardless of filling pressures.

There is a frequent association between AFib and diastolic dysfunction. Diastolic dysfunction causes LA dilation, which can result in AFib[36–38]; likewise, AFib is frequently seen in patients with heart failure, regardless of the EF. Many patients with AFib have advanced age, concentric LVH, reduced EF below 50%, and/or abnormal regional wall motion, all of which are clues for diastolic dysfunction/impaired relaxation. In the setting of impaired relaxation, the following Doppler findings can be combined to estimate LVFP[39–44]:

- IVRT <65 msec
- DT of transmitral velocity (DT*mv*) ≤160 msec
- DT of pulmonary venous diastolic velocity (DT*pv*) <220 msec
- Septal E/e′ >11
- Peak TR >2.8 m/sec
- Peak acceleration rate of mitral E velocity (PkE*acc*) ≥1900 cm/sec

Peak acceleration rate, although accurate in detecting elevated LAP, is difficult to measure in routine clinical practice. Because beat-to-beat variability in e′ is more prominent in the lateral mitral annular corner, it is preferable to use the septal E/e′. As with sinus rhythm, these parameters are more accurate in patients with EF less than 45%. In clinical practice, we have found that peak TR greater than 2.8 m/sec, septal E/e′ greater than 11, and IVRT less than 65 msec are the best parameters to combine in patients with preserved EF. Of the three, peak TR above 2.8 has significant weight given that with a normal EF and stroke volume, PASP exceeds 37 mmHg in most patients with elevated LAP. When all three are positive, likelihood of an elevated LAP is very high and vice versa (Fig. 13.11). Accuracy of the estimation diminishes in the absence of TR, even if IVRT and E/septal e′ are positive. In these instances, a positive DT*mv*, DT*pv*, and/or PkE*acc* may enhance the estimation of an elevated LAP.

There are insufficient validated studies to propose a practical algorithm to estimate LVFP in patients with advanced degrees of atrioventricular (AV) block, paced rhythms, or junctional rhythms. The suggestions recommended for AFib may be used, recognizing that the accuracy of estimates is diminished. Once again, an IVRT less than 65 msec, septal E/e′ above 11, and peak TR greater than 2.8 m/s may be the most reliable ones to combine.

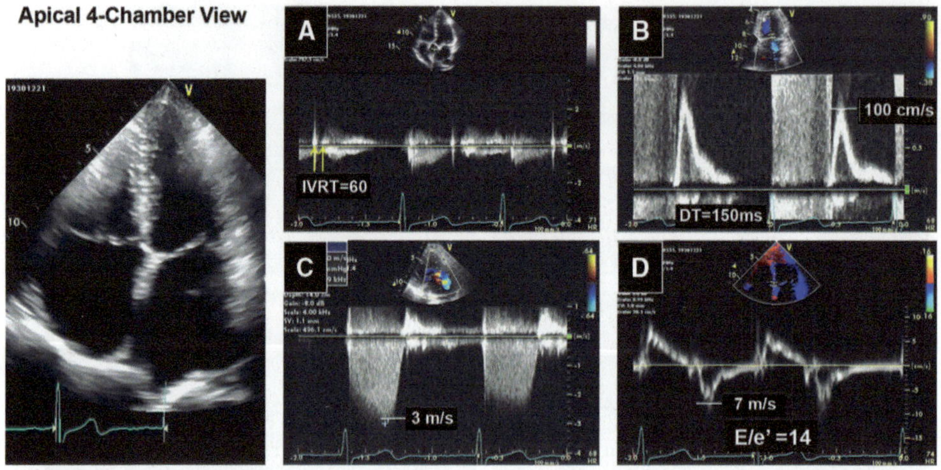

Fig. 13.11 Apical four-chamber view recorded at end systole in a patient with atrial fibrillation and elevated mean PCWP. Recordings of aortic and mitral inflow velocities with (A) CW Doppler, (B) transmitral velocity, (C) TR velocity, and (D) septal annular velocity are shown. The isovolumic relaxation time (IVRT) is measured as the time interval between end of aortic flow and onset of mitral inflow (A, *arrows*). Note the short IVRT (60 msec), short deceleration time (DT, 150 msec), elevated TR velocity (3 m/sec), and increased E/septal e′ (14). See text for details.

Mitral Annular Calcification

MAC has long been considered an obstacle to the evaluation of diastolic function and estimation of LVFP for two primary reasons: (1) concern that e′ recorded in the proximity of the calcified annulus does not reflect myocardial relaxation accurately, and (2) the presence of variable degrees of mitral inflow obstruction due to reduction in mitral valve area may alter the relation of E/A with LAP and invalidates E/e′ as an index of LVFP.

The recent ASE guidelines did not provide any recommendations for estimating LVFP in patients with MAC. However, recently Abudiab and associates combined E/A with IVRT to predict whether mean PCWP was normal or greater than 15 mmHg.[45] An E/A greater than 1.8 was 100% predictive of elevated LVFP, while an E/A less than 0.8 was 92% predictive of normal LVFP. In patients with E/A between 0.8 and 1.8, an IVRT less than 80 msec was 90% predictive of elevated LVFP, while a longer IVRT was 64% predictive of normal pressures. Overall the algorithm was 85% sensitive and 95% specific for elevated LVFP with positive and negative predictive values of 97% and 78%, respectively ($n = 71$). These encouraging results will need to be validated in a larger and diverse population.

High Cardiac Output

Patients with HFpEF can have a high cardiac output, particularly when associated with arteriovenous fistulas for dialysis and/or chronic anemia. These patients often have LA enlargement as a result of the high output, thus limiting the diagnostic value of LA volume measurements. When E/A is 2.0 or higher, average E/e′ is above 14, and peak TR velocity is above 2.8 m/sec, an elevated LVFP is predicted with high specificity; however, sensitivity may be lower.[35] A particularly challenging group includes those with chronic anemia or liver cirrhosis and EF above 65%; except for LA enlargement, their hearts appear normal by 2-D and often have an E/A above 2 and average E/e′ below 14. In these cases, a positive Valsalva maneuver and a peak TR greater than 2.8 may be the only clues that LVFP is elevated. Even then, the margin of error is greater in these patients. When in doubt, it is appropriate to recommend invasive hemodynamic evaluation, particularly when the patient presents with dyspnea.

Mitral Regurgitation

Primary valvular MR may occur in patients with normal LV and no diastolic dysfunction. However, the large regurgitant volume seen with moderate or severe MR will increase E velocity and E/A, shorten IVRT, reduce the pulmonary vein S/D ratio, and preserve e′, particularly at the lateral annular corner. The ASE guidelines recommend abstaining from evaluating diastolic function in these patients. From a clinical decision-making point of view, the estimation of PASP is more relevant than the evaluation of diastolic function.

In contrast to primary MR, patients with functional or ischemic MR have myocardial disease; as such, they have diastolic dysfunction. Although E velocity and E/A ratio may be increased by the regurgitant volume, studies have shown that the application of the ASE algorithm as a rule works well in the estimation of LVFP, particularly when a TR velocity is available.[46,47]

NEWER DEVELOPMENTS

TE-e′ Time Interval

The time interval between the onset of mitral E velocity and annular velocity e′ (TE-e′) is an index of LV relaxation that relates directly with the time constant of relaxation (tau). It can be combined with IVRT to estimate LV filling pressures.[48] With elevated LAP, mitral inflow starts before the onset of e′. Consequently, IVRT shortens while TE-e′ remains prolonged (see Fig. 13.8). IVTR/TE-e′ is therefore an index that corrects the effect of relaxation on IVRT. IVRT/TE-e′ has been found to have an inverse curvilinear relation with mean PCWP. A ratio less than 2 had a sensitivity of 91% and a specificity of 89% in detecting PCWP above 15 mmHg.[48] An important advantage of this parameter is that it can be applied to patients with mitral valve disease (either stenosis or regurgitation).[49] The main limitation of IVRT/TE-e′ is the inability to measure TE-e′ directly given that most ultrasound instruments cannot record tissue Doppler and PW Doppler simultaneously. Consequently this interval must be derived indirectly by measuring the time from the peak of the R wave to onset of E, and from peak R to e′ at the four corners of the mitral annulus. TE-e′ is derived as follows: (average R-e′)–(R-E). Applying this method in routine clinical practice requires meticulous attention to recording and measurement techniques to reduce variability and maintain the reproducibility of the method. If properly learned, IVRT/TE-e′ can be helpful in determining LVFP when the ASE algorithm results in an indeterminate grading.

Strain by Speckle Tracking

Measurement of longitudinal strain and strain rate with speckle tracking provides insight into myocardial performance during systole and diastole. Measurements made during isovolumic relaxation relate well with tau and, when combined with the mitral E velocity, have provided estimates of LVFP.[50–52] Although results are encouraging, technical challenges and variability between measurements made by different software and ultrasound systems limit the application of this method in routine clinical practice.

LA Strain

Speckle tracking can be applied to the left atrium to obtain measurements of LA strain. An inverse relation has been observed between peak longitudinal LA strain and LVFP.[53,54] Although promising, there are still technical challenges in obtaining an accurate measurement, particularly in patients with significant LA enlargement or when the entire chamber is not completely imaged. At this time, LA strain remains as a research tool used to better understand LA function and atrioventricular interactions.

PREPARING A CLINICALLY MEANINGFUL REPORT

Assessment of diastolic function and estimation of LVFP provides important information to the clinician and often alters further diagnostic and therapeutic decisions. For this reason, every comprehensive echocardiography/Doppler report should include a comment regarding diastolic function. The ASE guidelines recommend that the report include a statement regarding the relaxation properties of the LV and another regarding resting filling pressures. If an accurate evaluation is not possible for technical or functional reasons (as with marked tachycardia), it should be stated. A reasonable statement to make is, "Evaluation of diastolic function is not possible due to ___."

Although many equations have been proposed to estimate LVFP, none are accurate enough to precisely derive mean PCWP. Thus current guidelines recommend general statements, such as normal relaxation and LVFP (i.e., normal function), impaired relaxation with normal LVFP (grade I diastolic dysfunction), impaired relaxation with elevated LVFP (grade II diastolic dysfunction), and impaired relaxation with restrictive LV filling and a mean PCWP of 25 mmHg or greater (grade III diastolic dysfunction). As discussed earlier, there are times when one can assess relaxation but cannot give an estimate of LVFP. A case example would be a hypertensive patient with concentric LVH and enlarged left atrium (highly predictive of impaired relaxation) but with sinus tachycardia that impedes accurate measurement of E and e′, and no TR recorded. In such cases, a reasonable statement to make is, "Impaired LV relaxation; unable to estimate LV filling pressure." Likewise, there are times when relaxation is indeterminate, but the other findings are predictive of normal LVFP. A case example would be a 78-year-old woman with normal LV and LA size, average e′ of 6 cm/sec, and an average E/e′ of 9. The average e′ of 6 cm/sec could be due to her age but we cannot completely exclude impairment in relaxation, thus it is better not to make a categorical statement on relaxation. Nevertheless, the remaining findings are highly predictive of normal LVFP; therefore a reasonable statement to make is, "Indeterminate LV relaxation with normal LV filling pressures."

FUTURE DIRECTIONS

LV diastolic pressures are not static but dynamic. Patients with HFpEF may have normal resting filling pressures, but these can increase with volume loading or exercise. Documentation of increasing LVFP with exercise not only helps in establishing a diagnosis of HFpEF, but can help in following a response to therapy. Consequently there are times when recommending a diastolic stress test is appropriate. The most common scenario is in a patient with grade I diastolic dysfunction, who presents with exercise dyspnea. The diastolic stress test is discussed in detail in Chapter 18.

The most accurate assessment of intracardiac and pulmonary hemodynamics is provided by invasive measurements, and there are times when the 2-D/Doppler report should recommend a right heart catheterization (invasive hemodynamics assessment is discussed in Chapter 8). The most common is when clinical findings are suggestive of HFpEF, and the 2-D/Doppler evaluation results in an indeterminate grading of filling pressures. In these cases, a statement such as the following is appropriate: "Recommend invasive hemodynamic evaluation to better determine resting filling pressures." A less common scenario is when findings are indicative of a grade II or III diastolic dysfunction and the estimated PASP is greater than 64 mmHg. These patients have severe pulmonary HTN, which might be all secondary to marked elevation of mean PCWP. However, they might also have wedge-driven, reactive pulmonary HTN, whereby the pulmonary pressures are elevated out of proportion to the increased PCWP.[55] The diagnosis is made by demonstrating an elevated PCWP and a PA diastolic-to-mean PCWP gradient of 7 mmHg or above. Wedge-driven, reactive pulmonary HTN occurs in ~12% of patients with HFpEF. It is very difficult to treat and is associated with a poor prognosis.[55] In these cases, the following statements are suggested: "The mark elevation of PASP noted in this patient may be in part due to reactive, wedge-driven pulmonary HTN. Recommend invasive hemodynamic evaluation to determine if this condition is present given that it is associated with a worse prognosis."

KEY POINTS

- The term *left ventricular filling pressure* is most frequently interpreted as synonymous with mean LAP or PCWP. However, it can also be used in reference to the LV pre-A pressure or LVEDP.
- LV diastolic dysfunction (impaired relaxation with varying degrees of increased stiffness) is a universal finding in patients with HFpEF.
- Impaired relaxation can be inferred by several clinical scenarios (ischemic heart disease, cardiomyopathies, hypertension, advanced age) and 2-D findings (impaired global and/or regional systolic function, concentric LVH, dilated LA).
- Use of a combination of 2-D, Doppler, and tissue Doppler findings provides more accurate assessment of filling pressures than any parameter used by itself.
- A diastolic stress test should be considered in patients with exercise-induced dyspnea and grade I diastolic dysfunction.
- Invasive hemodynamic evaluation should be recommended in patients with NYHA Class III to IV dyspnea who are suspected of having HFpEF, but in whom the echo/Doppler findings are inconclusive.

REVIEW QUESTIONS

1. Which measurement of diastolic LV pressures approximates best the mean LA pressure?
   a. LVEDP
   b. LV pre-A pressure
   c. LV minimal pressure
   d. LV pressure at the time of mitral valve opening
2. Which of the following measurements is not indicative of elevated filling pressures in a patient with myocardial pathology?
   a. E/A ratio >2
   b. Average E/e′ >14
   c. Ratio of systolic antegrade flow velocity (S) to diastolic flow velocity (D) in the pulmonary vein <1
   d. Peak mitral E velocity <50 cm/sec
3. In the absence of RV outflow obstruction, a peak TR velocity greater than 2.8 m/sec can be used as a criterion to estimate an elevated mean LAP
   a. as long as the average E/e′ is greater than 14 and/or LA is dilated, and there is no evidence of increased vascular resistance.
   b. as long as the estimated mean RA pressure is 10 mmHg or higher.
   c. at all times.
   d. as long as the transmitral E/A ratio is greater than 2.
4. In the presence of atrial fibrillation
   a. LV filling pressures cannot be estimated.
   b. a dilated LA is very predictive of an elevated mean LAP.
   c. estimation of elevated mean LAP using an IVRT less than 65 msec or transmitral DT less than 160 msec accompanied by increased septal E/e′ greater than 11 and/or peak TR velocity greater than 2.8 m/sec is more accurate in patients with EF below 45%.
   d. can be estimated using the same algorithm recommended for patients in sinus rhythm.
5. The presence of mitral regurgitation
   a. precludes the estimation of LV filling pressures with the ASE algorithm.
   b. precludes the evaluation of diastolic function when the MR is of a primary valvular etiology and moderate or greater in severity.
   c. does not affect the estimation of mean LAP with the ASE algorithm.
   d. indicates only a peak TR velocity above 2.8 m/sec can be used as an index of an elevated LAP.

REFERENCES

1. Nagueh SF, Sun H, Kopelen HA, Middleton KJ, Khoury DS. Hemodynamic determinants of the mitral annulus diastolic velocities by tissue Doppler. *J Am Coll Cardiol.* 2001;37:278–285.
2. Rahimtoola SH, Loeb HS, Ehsani A, et al. Relationship of pulmonary artery to left ventricular diastolic pressures in acute myocardial infarction. *Circulation.* 1972;46:283–290.
3. Habib GB, Zoghbi WA. Doppler assessment of right ventricular filling dynamics in systemic hypertension: comparison with left ventricular filling. *Am Heart J.* 1992;124:1313–1320.
4. Wachtell K, Bella JN, Rokkedal J, et al. Change in diastolic left ventricular filling after one year of antihypertensive treatment: the Losartan Intervention for Endpoint Reduction in Hypertension (LIFE) Study. *Circulation.* 2002;105:1071–1076.
5. Nishimura RA, Appleton CP, Redfield MM, Ilstrup DM, Holmes DR, Tajik AJ. Noninvasive Doppler echocardiographic evaluation of left ventricular filling pressures in patients with cardiomyopathies: a simultaneous Doppler echocardiographic and cardiac catheterization study. *J Am Coll Cardiol.* 1996;28:1226–1233.
6. Quiñones MA,. Doppler assessment of left ventricular diastolic function. Navin C, ed. *Doppler Echocardiography* 2nd ed. Philadelphia, PA: Lea & Febiger; 1992:197–215.
7. Sartori MP, Quiñones MA, Kuo LC. Relation of Doppler-derived left ventricular filling parameters to age and radius/thickness ratio in normal and pathologic states. *Am J Cardiol.* 1987;59:1179–1182.
8. Nagueh SF, Smiseth OA, Appleton CP, et al. Recommendations for the evaluation of left ventricular diastolic function by echocardiography: an update from the American Society of Echocardiography and the European Association of Cardiovascular Imaging. *J Am Soc Echocardiogr.* 2016;29:277–314.
9. Caballero L, Kou S, Dulgheru R, et al. Echocardiographic reference ranges for normal cardiac Doppler data: results from the NORRE Study. *Eur Heart J Cardiovasc Imag.* 2015;16:1031–1041.
10. Leibowitz D, Stessman-Lande I, Jacobs JM, et al. Cardiac structure and function as predictors of mortality in persons 85 years of age. *Am J Cardiol.* 2012;109:901–905.
11. Basnight MA, Gonzalez MS, Kershenovich SC, Appleton CP. Pulmonary venous flow velocity: relation to hemodynamics, mitral flow velocity and left atrial volume, and ejection fraction. *J Am Soc Echocardiogr.* 1991;4:547–558.
12. Appleton CP, Galloway JM, Gonzalez MS, Gaballa M, Basnight MA. Estimation of left ventricular filling pressures using two-dimensional and Doppler echocardiography in adult patients with cardiac disease. Additional value of analyzing left atrial size, left atrial ejection fraction and the difference in duration of pulmonary venous and mitral flow velocity at atrial contraction. *J Am Coll Cardiol.* 1993;22:1972–1982.
13. Dokainish H, Nguyen JS, Sengupta R, et al. Do additional echocardiographic variables increase the accuracy of E/e' for predicting left ventricular filling pressure in normal ejection fraction? An echocardiographic and invasive hemodynamic study. *J Am Soc Echocardiogr.* 2010;23:156–161.
14. Rivas-Gotz C, Manolios M, Thohan V, Nagueh SF. Impact of left ventricular ejection fraction on estimation of left ventricular filling pressures using tissue Doppler and flow propagation velocity. *Am J Cardiol.* 2003;91:780–784.
15. Wang J, Khoury DS, Yue Y, Torre-Amione G, Nagueh SF. Left ventricular untwisting rate by speckle tracking echocardiography. *Circulation.* 2007;116:2580–2586.
16. Zile MR, Baicu CF, Gaasch WH. Diastolic heart failure—abnormalities in active relaxation and passive stiffness of the left ventricle. *N Engl J Med.* 2004;350:1953–1959.
17. Appleton CP, Galloway JM, Gonzalez MS, Gaballa M, Basnight MA. Estimation of left ventricular filling pressures using two-dimensional and Doppler echocardiography in adult patients with cardiac disease. Additional value of analyzing left atrial size, left atrial ejection fraction and the difference in duration of pulmonary venous and mitral flow velocity at atrial contraction. *J Am Coll Cardiol.* 1993;22:1972–1982.
18. Nagueh SF, Kopelen HA, Zoghbi WA. Feasibility and accuracy of Doppler echocardiographic estimation of pulmonary artery occlusive pressure in the intensive care unit. *Am J Cardiol.* 1995;75:1256–1262.
19. Vanoverschelde JL, Robert AR, Gerbaux A, Michel X, Hanet C, Wijns W. Noninvasive estimation of pulmonary arterial wedge pressure with Doppler transmitral flow velocity pattern in patients with known heart disease. *Am J Cardiol.* 1995;75:383–389.
20. Pozzoli M, Capomolla S, Pinna G, Cobelli F, Tavazzi L. Doppler echocardiography reliably predicts pulmonary artery wedge pressure in patients with chronic heart failure with and without mitral regurgitation. *J Am Coll Cardiol.* 1996;27:883–893.
21. Nagueh SF, Middleton KJ, Kopelen HA, Zoghbi WA, Quiñones MA. Doppler tissue imaging: a noninvasive technique for evaluation of left ventricular relaxation and estimation of filling pressures. *J Am Coll Cardiol.* 1997;30:1527–1535.

22. Ommen SR, Nishimura RA, Appleton CP, et al. Clinical utility of Doppler echocardiography and tissue Doppler imaging in the estimation of left ventricular filling pressures: a comparative simultaneous Doppler-catheterization study. *Circulation.* 2000;102:1788–1794.
23. Nagueh SF, Lakkis NM, Middleton KJ, Spencer WH III, Zoghbi WA, Quiñones MA. Doppler estimation of left ventricular filling pressures in patients with hypertrophic cardiomyopathy. *Circulation.* 1999;99:254–261.
24. Ishida Y, Meisner JS, Tsujioka K, et al. Left ventricular filling dynamics: influence of left ventricular relaxation and left atrial pressure. *Circulation.* 1986;74:187–196.
25. Nishimura RA, Tajik AJ. Evaluation of diastolic filling of left ventricle in health and disease: Doppler echocardiography is the clinician's Rosetta Stone. *J Am Coll Cardiol.* 1997;30:8–18.
26. Choong CY, Abascal VM, Thomas JD, Guerrero JL, McGlew S, Weyman AE. Combined influence of ventricular loading and relaxation on the transmitral flow velocity profile in dogs measured by Doppler echocardiography. *Circulation.* 1988;78:672–683.
27. Little WC, Ohno M, Kitzman DW, Thomas JD, Cheng CP. Determination of left ventricular chamber stiffness from the time for deceleration of early left ventricular filling. *Circulation.* 1995;92:1933–1939.
28. Schwammenthal E, Popescu BA, Popescu AC, et al. Noninvasive assessment of left ventricular end-diastolic pressure by the response of the transmitral A-wave velocity to a standardized Valsalva maneuver. *Am J Cardiol.* 2000;86:169–174.
29. Yamamoto T, Oki T, Yamada H, et al. Prognostic value of the atrial systolic mitral annular motion velocity in patients with left ventricular systolic dysfunction. *J Am Soc Echocardiogr.* 2003;16:333–339.
30. Rossvoll O, Hatle LK. Pulmonary venous flow velocities recorded by transthoracic Doppler ultrasound: relation to left ventricular diastolic pressures. *J Am Coll Cardiol.* 1993;21:1687–1696.
31. Nishimura R, Appleton C, Redfield M, Ilstrup D, Holmes D, Tajik A. Noninvasive Doppler echocardiographic evaluation of left ventricular filling pressures in patients with cardiomyopathies: a simultaneous Doppler echocardiographic and cardiac catheterization study. *J Am Coll Cardiol.* 1996;28:1226–1233.
32. Yamamoto K, Nishimura RA, Chaliki HP, Appleton CP, Holmes DR Jr, Redfield MM. Determination of left ventricular filling pressure by Doppler echocardiography in patients with coronary artery disease: critical role of left ventricular systolic function. *J Am Coll Cardiol.* 1997;30:1819–1826.
33. Bouchard JL, Aurigemma GP, Hill JC, Ennis CA, Tighe DA. Usefulness of the pulmonary arterial systolic pressure to predict pulmonary arterial wedge pressure in patients with normal left ventricular systolic function. *Am J Cardiol.* 2008;101:1673–1676.
34. Dokainish H, Nguyen J, Sengupta R, et al. New, simple echocardiographic indexes for the estimation of filling pressure in patients with cardiac disease and preserved left ventricular ejection fraction. *Echocardiography.* 2010;27:946–953.
35. Andersen OS, Smiseth OA, Dokainish H, et al. Estimating left ventricular filling pressure by echocardiography. *J Am Coll Cardiol.* 2017;69:1937–1948.
36. Tsang TS, Gersh BJ, Appleton CP, Tajik AJ, et al. Left ventricular diastolic dysfunction as a predictor of the first diagnosed nonvalvular atrial fibrillation in 840 elderly men and women. *J Am Coll Cardiol.* 2002;40:1636–1644.
37. Vasan RS, Larson MG, Levy D, Galderisi M, Wolf PA, Benjamin EJ. Doppler trans-mitral flow indexes and risk of atrial fibrillation (the Framingham Heart Study). *Am J Cardiol.* 2003;91:1079–1083.
38. Jons C, Joergensen RM, Hassager C, et al. Diastolic dysfunction predicts new-onset atrial fibrillation and cardiovascular events in patients with acute myocardial infarction and depressed left ventricular systolic function: a CARISMA sub-study. *Eur J Echocardiogr.* 2010;7:602–607.
39. Nagueh SF, Kopelen HA, Quiñones MA. Doppler estimation of left ventricular filling pressure in atrial fibrillation. *Circulation.* 1996;94:2138–2145.
40. Temporelli PL, Scapellato F, Corrà U, Eleuteri E, Imparato A, Giannuzzi P. Estimation of pulmonary wedge pressure by transmitral Doppler in patients with chronic heart failure and atrial fibrillation. *Am J Cardiol.* 1999;83:724–727.
41. Chirillo F, Brunazzi MC, Barbiero M, et al. Estimating mean pulmonary wedge pressure in patients with chronic atrial fibrillation from transthoracic Doppler indexes of mitral and pulmonary venous flow velocity. *J Am Coll Cardiol.* 1997;30:19–26.
42. Kusunose K, Yamada H, Nishio S, et al. Clinical utility of single-beat E/e′ obtained by simultaneous recording of flow and tissue Doppler velocities in atrial fibrillation with preserved systolic function. *J Am Coll Cardiol Imag.* 2009;2:1147–1156.
43. Wada Y, Murata K, Tanaka T, et al. Simultaneous Doppler tracing of transmitral inflow and mitral annular velocity as an estimate of elevated left ventricular filling pressure in patients with atrial fibrillation. *Circ J.* 2012;76:675–681.
44. Li C, Zhang J, Zhou C, Huang L, Tang H, Rao L. Will simultaneous measurement of E/e' index facilitate the non-invasive assessment of left ventricular filling pressure in patients with non-valvular atrial fibrillation? *Eur J Echocardiogr.* 2010;11:296–301.
45. Abudiab MM, Chebrolu LH, Schutt RC, Nagueh SF, Zoghbi WA. Doppler echocardiography for the estimation of LV filling pressure in patients with mitral annular calcification. *JACC Cardiovasc Imag.* 2017;10:1411–1420.
46. Bruch C, Stypmann J, Gradaus R, Breithardt G, Wichter T. Usefulness of tissue Doppler imaging for estimation of filling pressures in patients with primary or secondary pure mitral regurgitation. *Am J Cardiol.* 2004;93:324–328.
47. Bruch C, Klem I, Breithardt G, Wichter T, Gradaus R. Diagnostic usefulness and prognostic implications of the mitral E/e' ratio in patients with heart failure and severe secondary mitral regurgitation. *Am J Cardiol.* 2007;100:860–865.
48. Rivas-Gotz C, Khoury DS, Manolios M, Rao L, Kopelen HA, Nagueh SF. Time interval between onset of mitral inflow and onset of early diastolic velocity by tissue Doppler: a novel index of left ventricular relaxation: experimental studies and clinical application. *J Am Coll Cardiol.* 2003;42:1463–1470.
49. Diwan A, McCulloch M, Lawrie GM, Reardon MJ, Nagueh SF. Doppler estimation of left ventricular filling pressures in patients with mitral valve disease. *Circulation.* 2005;111:3281–3289.
50. Wang J, Khoury DS, Thohan V, Torre-Amione G, Nagueh SF. Global diastolic strain rate for the assessment of left ventricular relaxation and filling pressures. *Circulation.* 2007;115:1376–1383.
51. Dokainish H, Sengupta R, Pillai M, Bobek J, Lakkis N. Usefulness of new diastolic strain and strain rate indexes for the estimation of left ventricular filling pressure. *Am J Cardiol.* 2008;101:1504–1509.
52. Kimura K, Takenaka K, Ebihara A, et al. Speckle tracking global strain rate E/e' predicts LV filling pressure more accurately than traditional tissue Doppler E/e'. *Echocardiography.* 2012;29:404–410.
53. Wakami K, Ohte N, Asada K, et al. Correlation between left ventricular end-diastolic pressure and peak left atrial wall strain during left ventricular systole. *J Am Soc Echocardiogr.* 2009;22:847–851.
54. Singh A, Addetia K, Maffessanti F, Mor-Avi V, Lang RM. LA Strain for categorization of LV diastolic dysfunction. *JACC Cardiovasc Imag.* 2017;10:735–743.
55. Gerges M, Gerges C, Pistritto AM, et al. Pulmonary hypertension in heart failure. Epidemiology, right ventricular function, and survival. *Am J Respir Crit Care Med.* 2015;192:1234–1246.

14

Evaluation of Right Ventricular Diastolic Function

Dimitrios Maragiannis and Sherif F. Nagueh

OUTLINE

Case Study

A 63-year-old man presented with acute onset of shortness of breath. Body surface area (BSA) is 2.04 m^2 with body mass at 199 lb. An echocardiogram was obtained as a stat test. Blood pressure (BP) was 105/65 mmHg, with heart rate at 95 bpm. Parasternal views show normal left ventricular (LV) size and function. In all of the required views, the right ventricle (RV) is enlarged and its systolic function is severely depressed with markedly reduced fractional area change. RV tissue Doppler (TD) shows reduced systolic velocities at RV basal and midsegments as noted in the apical four-chamber view. While tricuspid regurgitation (TR) jet is incomplete, peak velocity is at least 3.5 m/sec, and septal motion in the parasternal short axis view is consistent with RV pressure overload. TD shows markedly reduced segmental e′ velocity but increased a′ velocity (average 12.8 cm/sec), thus e′/a′ ratio markedly is less than 0.5. Inferior vena cava (IVC) is dilated without a decrease in its diameter with sniffing consistent with elevated mean right atrial (RA) pressure. The acute event was due to pulmonary embolism, and the echocardiographic images show a large thrombus (2 × 4 cm) prolapsing across the tricuspid valve and across patent foramen ovale into the left atrium.

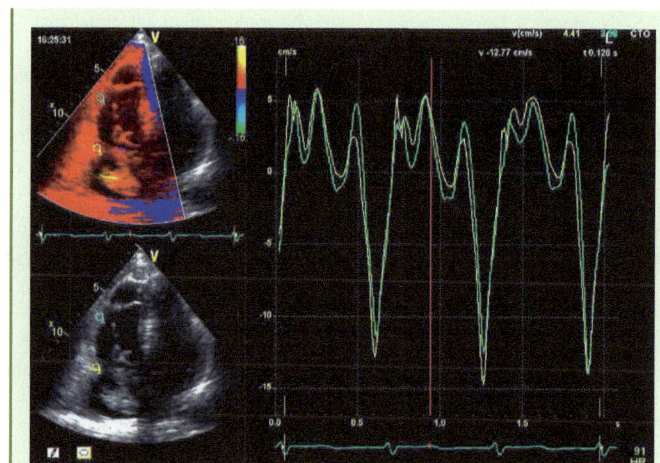

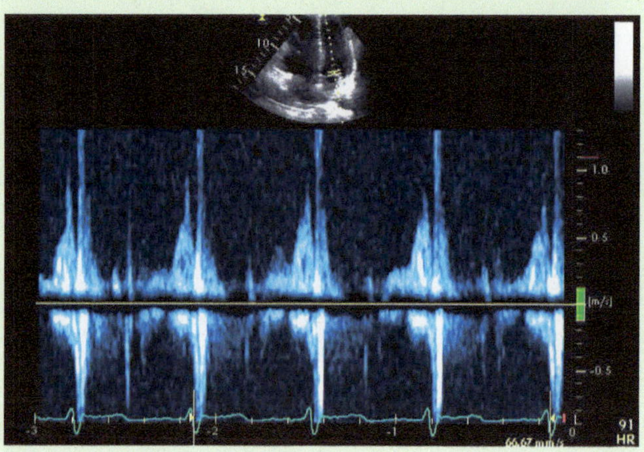

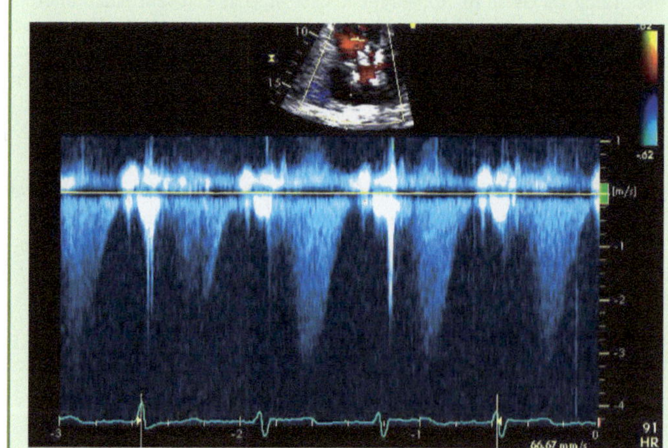

INTRODUCTION

Echocardiography plays an important role in the evaluation of RV function. Importantly, noninvasive indices of RV diastolic function are associated with worse outcomes in patients with pulmonary hypertension (HTN) and chronic heart failure.[1,2] There are several diseases associated with RV diastolic dysfunction, including group I pulmonary HTN, congenital heart disease, pulmonary embolism, right ventricular ischemia or infarction, and cardiomyopathies. Echocardiographic assessment of RV diastolic function relies on several two-dimensional (2-D) and Doppler variables (Box 14.1). This chapter reviews the noninvasive indices of RV diastolic function, including their correlation with RV filling pressures.

INVASIVE ASSESSMENT OF RV DIASTOLIC FUNCTION

The right ventricle ejects blood into the low-pressure and high-compliance pulmonary circulation. In healthy subjects, the right ventricle has brief isovolumic contraction and relaxation periods. RV filling during early diastole occurs as RV relaxation leads to a positive pressure gradient between the right atrium and the right ventricle. RV filling depends on active relaxation, chamber stiffness, and transtricuspid pressure gradient. Active relaxation is among the important determinants of RV diastolic function and is dependent on calcium reuptake by the sarcoplasmic reticulum, intrinsic contractility, uniformity of relaxation, and the load-dependent properties of relaxation. Load-dependent parameters of RV function can be evaluated invasively.[3,4] Insights into impaired RV relaxation can be appreciated using high-fidelity pressure catheters to measure peak rate of RV pressure decline (−dP/dt) and the time constant of pressure decay during isovolumic relaxation (tau [τ]). Abnormal RV relaxation occurs in patients with coronary artery disease with RV involvement,[5] pulmonary HTN,[4] hypertrophic cardiomyopathy,[6] and heart failure with preserved ejection fraction (HFpEF).[7]

BOX 14.1 Echocardiographic Indices for Assessment of Right Ventricular (RV) Diastolic Function and Estimation of Mean Right Atrial (RA) Pressure

1. RA volumes (maximum, minimum, and emptying volume)
2. Right atrial strain (reservoir, conduit, and pump-related strain)
3. Inferior vena cava maximum diameter and diameter change with inspiration
4. Tricuspid inflow early (E), late (A) diastolic velocities, E/A ratio, and deceleration time of E velocity
5. Hepatic vein flow velocities (systolic, diastolic, and atrial reversal)
6. Tricuspid annulus velocities by tissue Doppler: early (e′) and late (a′) diastolic velocities
7. Tricuspid E/e′ ratio
8. Tricuspid e′/a′ ratio
9. Isovolumic relaxation time (time between end of systolic velocity and beginning of e′ velocity)
10. RV early and late diastolic strain rates
11. Deceleration time of pulmonary regurgitation signal
12. Forward diastolic flow into RV outflow tract with restrictive right ventricle
13. Rate of decline of RV pressure (–dP/dt) from tricuspid regurgitation signal by continuous wave Doppler

During late diastole, RV stiffness and RA contraction are the important determinants of RV filling. RV chamber stiffness is dependent on myocardial stiffness, RV volume and mass, ventricular interdependence, and pericardial and pleural constraints. There is a curvilinear relationship between RV diastolic volume and pressure. RV chamber stiffness can be characterized by the end-diastolic pressure-volume relationship.[3,8] RV stiffness constant (beta [β]) is measured using high-fidelity conductance catheters.[9] Increased RV stiffness contributes to the increased RV filling pressure in patients with HFpEF.[7] In patients with pulmonary HTN, preserved RA booster pump function is associated with lower likelihood of progression to heart failure.[10]

Throughout diastole, tissue mechanics, fluid dynamics, and intracavitary vorticity provide insight into diastolic function. Animal studies using three-dimensional (3-D) real-time echocardiography have revealed the formation of vortices during early diastolic RV filling, which is impaired with chamber dilatation.[11] Recently, using four-dimensional flow cardiac magnetic resonance imaging (MRI), a correlation of vorticity with echocardiographic indices of RV diastolic function was shown in patients with pulmonary HTN.[12]

RIGHT ATRIAL SIZE

RA size is related to RV systolic and diastolic function. Accordingly, RA enlargement is a predictor of adverse outcomes in patients with pulmonary arterial HTN and chronic heart failure.[2,13–15] Traditionally, evaluation of RA size includes measurement of RA diameters (minor and major) and RA area using 2-D imaging in the apical four-chamber view (Fig. 14.1). The upper limits of normal are 4.4 cm and 5.3 cm,

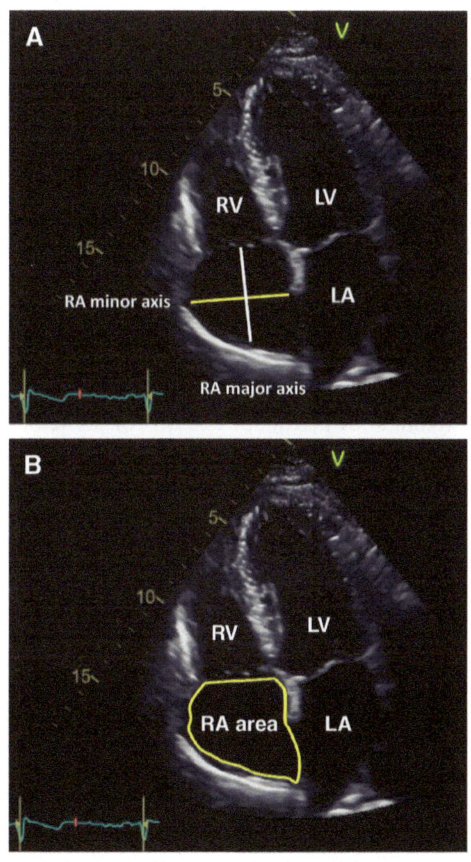

Fig. 14.1 (A) RA linear dimensions: RA minor axis at the midatrial level is the distance between the medial and lateral right atrial walls *(yellow)* and the major axis corresponds to the right atrial long axis (superior inferior axis in *white*). (B) RA area measured in a healthy individual.

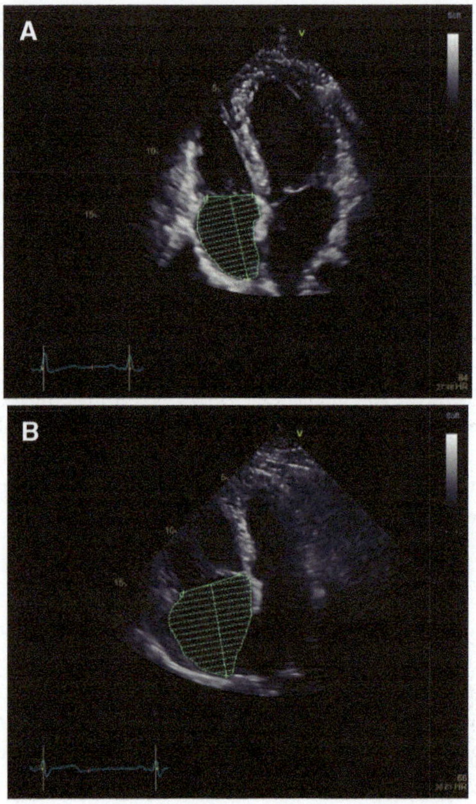

Fig. 14.2 (A) Normal 2-D–derived right atrial end-systolic volume (31 mL) from a healthy individual. (B) Severely enlarged right atrium (98 mL) from a 48-year-old male with ostium secundum atrial septal defect and pulmonary hypertension. Notice the presence of enlarged right ventricle end-systolic area also.

respectively, for RA minor axis and major axis dimensions. For RA area, the upper limit of normal is 18 cm^2.[16] Similar to the relation between the left atrium and the left ventricle, RA volume is usually increased in patients with RV diastolic dysfunction. It is reasonable to consider RA volumes when drawing conclusions about RA pressure in patients with equivocal findings with other signals. RA maximum volume is measured at the end of RV systole before tricuspid valve opening, whereas RA minimum volume is measured at end diastole after RA contraction. Similar to the left atrium, RA emptying fraction can be computed as the difference between RA maximum and minimum volumes/RA maximum volume. For RA volume measurements, RA volume can be obtained using single-plane area length or disk summation techniques in a dedicated apical four-chamber view[17] (Fig. 14.2), and normal reference ranges have been published.[18,19]

In patients with increased mean RA pressure, RA maximum and minimum volumes are increased, whereas RA emptying fraction is decreased.[20] While statistically significant, the correlation of RA volumes with RA pressure is weak and is affected by RA stiffness and contractility. In addition, RA volumes may be increased for reasons other than diastolic dysfunction, such as hyperdynamic state, athletic training, atrial fibrillation, and tricuspid valve disorders.

More recently, it has been recognized that 2-D echocardiography underestimates true RA volumes as measured by cardiac MRI. Nowadays, 3-D echocardiography can be utilized in daily clinical laboratory practice (Fig. 14.3). 3-D RA volumes by transthoracic echocardiography (TTE) have a stronger correlation with RA volumes by cardiac MRI, as well as lower bias than 2-D RA volumes versus cardiac MRI.[21] Real-time RA volumes by 3-D echocardiography have satisfactory reproducibility.[22] While promising, only few studies have

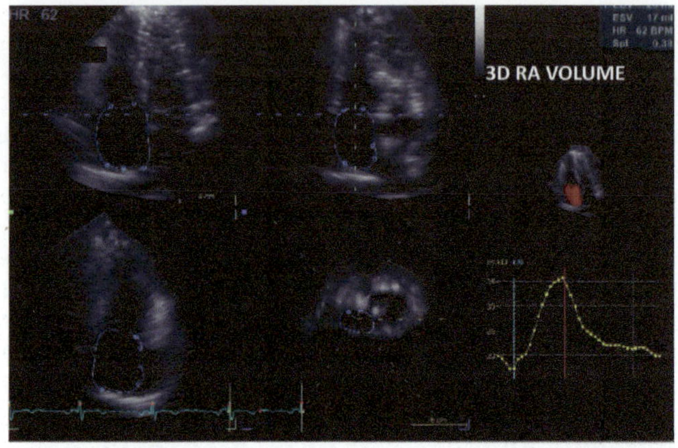

Fig. 14.3 3-D echocardiographic evaluation of right atrial (RA) volume. To the left, three orthogonal views of the maximal RA volume are shown. To the right, changes in RA volume over the cardiac cycle against the time are presented.

reported on the normal reference ranges for 3-D RA volumes.[18,22–23] More importantly using 3-D echocardiography, investigators reported that in patients with acutely decompensated heart failure, 3-D RA maximum volume index, in conjunction with IVC parameters, has a high accuracy in the detection of elevated RA pressure.[24]

RIGHT ATRIAL FUNCTION

The RA serves as a reservoir during systole, as a conduit during early diastole, and as a pump during late diastole. RA volume changes and phasic function can be quantified using maximum, minimum, and pre-A RA volumes as recorded by 2-D and 3-D echocardiography.[18] RA ejection fraction provides assessment of RA systolic function and can be obtained as the difference between RA pre-A volume and RA minimum volume divided by RA pre-A volume. While RA ejection fraction is an index of RA systolic function, RA emptying fraction is an index of RA reservoir function. Reduced right atrial emptying fraction is associated with increased risk of death in patients with pulmonary arterial HTN.[25]

In addition to 2-D–derived RA volumes, RA myocardial mechanics can be evaluated using speckle tracking (Fig. 14.4). There are emerging data on normal values for RA longitudinal strain as well as phasic 3-D

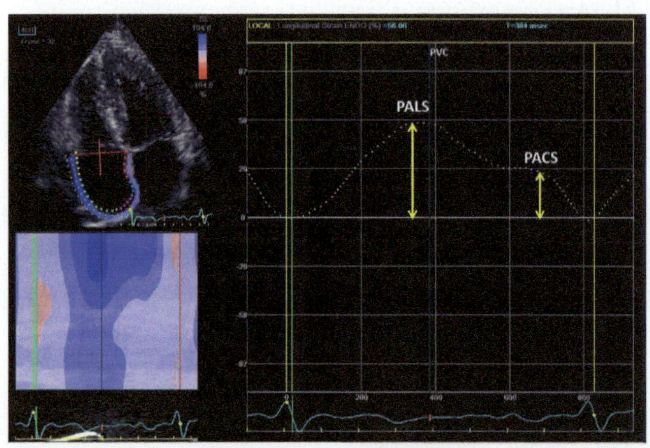

Fig. 14.4 Right atrial (RA) strain by speckle tracking from a healthy individual. Average RA longitudinal strain throughout the cardiac cycle is shown. RA peak systolic strain is a measure of RA reservoir function *(PALS)*. End-diastolic RA strain *(PACS)* is a measure of RA systolic function. The difference between both corresponds to RA conduit function.

RA volumes and ejection fraction in healthy individuals.[18] RA longitudinal systolic strain and early diastolic longitudinal strain rate, representing RA reservoir and conduit functions, respectively, are reduced in patients with pulmonary arterial HTN when compared to controls.[26] Likewise, abnormal RA strain has been reported in patients with right ventricular infarction and inferior wall myocardial infarction when compared with patients with inferior wall myocardial infarction but without RV involvement.[27] In addition, investigators have shown that reduced RA strain is predictive of abnormal hemodynamics and adverse clinical outcomes in patients with pulmonary arterial HTN.[28] It remains to be seen whether RA strain can add to the noninvasive assessment of RV filling pressures.

RV MORPHOLOGY: SIZE AND WALL THICKNESS

The right ventricle has a complex geometry. Current guidelines recommend the use of multiple acoustic windows to assess RV size with 2-D echocardiography.[17] The RV-focused apical four-chamber view is needed to determine RV end-diastolic area, end-systolic area, and fractional area change. Notwithstanding, the left parasternal long and short axis views, the left parasternal RV inflow view, and subcostal views can also be used to gain insight into RV size. An RV end-diastolic diameter greater than 41 mm at the base and greater than 35 mm at the midlevel in the RV-focused view denotes RV enlargement.[17]

3-D echocardiography overcomes the limitations of 2-D imaging. 3-D echocardiography has been compared with cardiac MRI. A good correlation is observed between 3-D echocardiographic and cardiac MRI volumes; values obtained by 3-D echocardiography tend to be smaller.[29] RV end-diastolic volumes of 87 mL/m^2 in men and 74 mL/m^2 in women, and RV end-systolic volumes of 44 mL/m^2 for men and 36 mL/m^2 for women, have been recommended as the upper limits of the corresponding normal ranges.[17] Normative ranges for RV size based on age, body size, and gender have been published.[30] Importantly, investigators have shown that the use of contrast enhancement to assess RV size improves reproducibility and accuracy.[31] More recently, investigators evaluated 3-D echocardiographic values for RV regional curvature indices from 3-D endocardial surfaces in a large group of individuals with a normal right ventricle.[32] They depicted some age-related differences in the RV shape, which may be due to increased chamber stiffness. These newly described indices could be of value in the evaluation of RV diastolic function. In addition, RV free wall thickness greater than 5 mm is consistent with RV hypertrophy, which is also associated with diastolic dysfunction. RV free wall thickness can be measured using either M mode or 2-D imaging in the subcostal view.[17]

RV SYSTOLIC FUNCTION PARAMETERS

A comprehensive evaluation of RV diastolic function should incorporate the evaluation of the RV systolic function, as systolic and diastolic functions are closely related. Patients with reduced RV systolic performance have diastolic dysfunction. Multiple variables defining regional and global RV function have been applied to assess RV systolic function. Tricuspid annular plane systolic excursion (TAPSE) using M mode echocardiography reflects RV function along the RV long axis. TAPSE less than 17 mm is associated with RV systolic dysfunction.[17] Tissue Doppler tricuspid systolic lateral annular velocity (s′) is another measure of RV longitudinal function.[17] RV index of myocardial performance is a measure of global RV function (Tei index). In addition, 2-D RV fractional area change (FAC) obtained by echocardiography correlates significantly with RV ejection fraction by cardiac MRI,[33] and RV FAC below 35% denotes

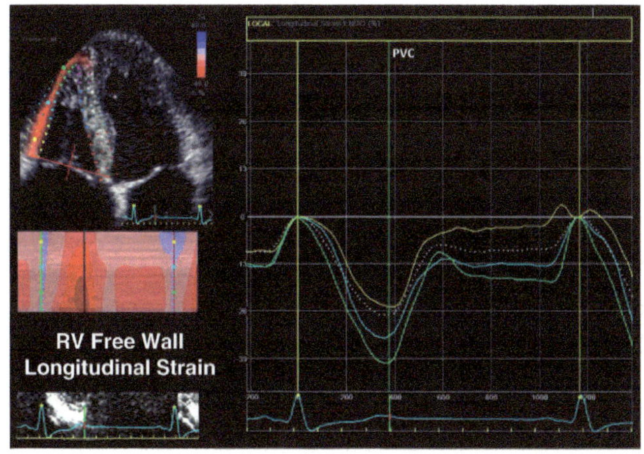

Fig. 14.5 Normal RV free wall longitudinal strain from a healthy 37-year-old man assessed in RV focused four-chamber view with 2-D speckle tracking echocardiography. The dotted white line corresponds to average global RV longitudinal strain.

impaired RV systolic function. Quantitative evaluation of RV function using 3-D volumetric imaging has been explored in several recent studies. 3-D ejection fraction has demonstrated its superiority over the 2-D method when compared with cardiac MRI as the gold standard. Specifically, 3-D RV ejection fraction less than 45% is consistent with depressed RV systolic function.[17] RV longitudinal strain (RVLS) and strain rate using tissue Doppler imaging or speckle tracking techniques can be measured in the RV focused apical four-chamber view (Fig. 14.5). RVLS provides important information on regional tissue mechanics.[34] A global longitudinal RV free wall strain greater than -20% is considered abnormally depressed.[17]

Doppler hemodynamic estimate of RV dP/dt is feasible in patients with satisfactory tricuspid regurgitation signal by continuous wave Doppler. RV-RA peak systolic pressure gradient can be calculated from the TR signal by continuous wave Doppler and applying the modified Bernoulli equation. The rate of rise and fall in TR jet velocity parallels the corresponding events in RV pressure, assuming minimal fluctuations of RA pressure over the time period when the change in RV systolic or diastolic pressure is measured. In one study, a strong correlation was observed between the invasive measurement and the noninvasive estimate of peak negative dP/dt.[35] For clinical application, one depends more on the shape of the signal (slow rise of the velocity from baseline) than the actual measurement.

NONINVASIVE ESTIMATION OF MEAN RIGHT ATRIAL PRESSURE

Inferior Vena Cava Diameter and Respiratory Collapse

IVC dimensions can be measured in the subcostal view with the patient lying supine at 1 to 2 cm from the RA-IVC junction at end expiration.[17] IVC diameter and the magnitude of inspiratory collapse have been traditionally used to estimate RA pressure noninvasively. Ideally, imaging the IVC should be made during spontaneous respiration and during a sniff test, and the diameter should be measured perpendicular to the IVC long axis. In particular, IVC expiratory and inspiratory diameters as well as percent collapse (Table 14.1) were reported to have significant relations with RA pressure in patients with spontaneous respiration.[20,36-38] Current ASE guidelines recommend that an IVC diameter less than 2.1 cm that collapses more than 50% with a sniff suggests normal RA pressure

TABLE 14.1 Estimation of Mean Right Atrial Pressure Based on Inferior Vena Cava Diameter Change With Inspiration (Collapse) and Hepatic Venous Flow

Mean Right Atrial Pressure	Inferior Vena Cava Collapse	Hepatic Vein Velocities
0–5 mmHg	≥50%	Systolic > Diastolic velocity
6–10 mmHg	≥50%	Systolic = Diastolic velocity
11–15 mmHg	<50%	Systolic < Diastolic velocity
16–20 mmHg	<50%	Forward flow only during diastole

(range, 0–5 mmHg). The presence of an IVC diameter greater than 2.1 cm that collapses below 50% with a sniff suggests elevated RA pressure (range, 10–20 mmHg).[17] Fig. 14.6 shows two examples for IVC diameter measurements and its change with inspiration. Of note, various echocardiographic indices of RA pressure can be used when IVC parameters lead to indeterminate conclusions about RA pressure.

There are several limitations to using IVC size and percent inspiratory collapse as surrogates of mean RA pressure. Variation of the IVC diameter in different positions has been reported, with underestimation of the IVC diameter in the left lateral position.[39] Likewise, IVC can be dilated in young healthy athletes,[40] which if not recognized can result in erroneous conclusions about RA pressure. Mechanical ventilation limits the accuracy of IVC diameter and collapse in predicting mean RA pressure. Specifically, in patients on mechanical ventilation, IVC percent collapse is not a reliable index of mean RA pressure,[20,41] whereas IVC diameter at end expiration has a significant but modest correlation with RA pressure ($r = 0.58$). An IVC diameter less than 12 mm appears highly accurate in identifying patients with an RA pressure less than 10 mmHg, whereas a diameter greater than 12 mm has no predictive value in this patient population.[41]

In addition, it is possible to image the left hepatic vein from the same window. In one study, the transverse diameter of this vein at end-expiratory apnea was shown to relate significantly to mean RA pressure in a group of 32 patients presenting with acute myocardial infarction.[42] Assessment of the left hepatic vein diameter could be helpful in patients where the IVC is not well visualized. However, there is a paucity of data on the clinical application of this approach in patients on mechanical ventilation.

Hepatic Vein Flow

A comprehensive interpretation of RV diastolic function should include the analysis of the Doppler patterns of the hepatic vein flow. The flow pattern in the hepatic veins is in part determined by RA pressure during the cardiac cycle. In addition, RA relaxation, RA compliance, tricuspid annular systolic descent, tricuspid valve disease, RV systolic and diastolic functions, and pericardial compliance can alter the flow pattern. Normally, hepatic vein flow exhibits variations during respiration.[43] In healthy subjects, pulse wave Doppler interrogation of the hepatic veins reveals a prominent forward flow during systole (S wave), a brief retrograde flow follows in late ventricular systole, an antegrade flow in diastole (D wave), and a small retrograde flow due to RA contraction occurs in late diastole (Ar wave).[44] The hepatic vein flow patterns have a direct association with right heart hemodynamics. During early to mid-systole, the S wave (forward systolic flow into RA from hepatic vein) occurs due to the fall

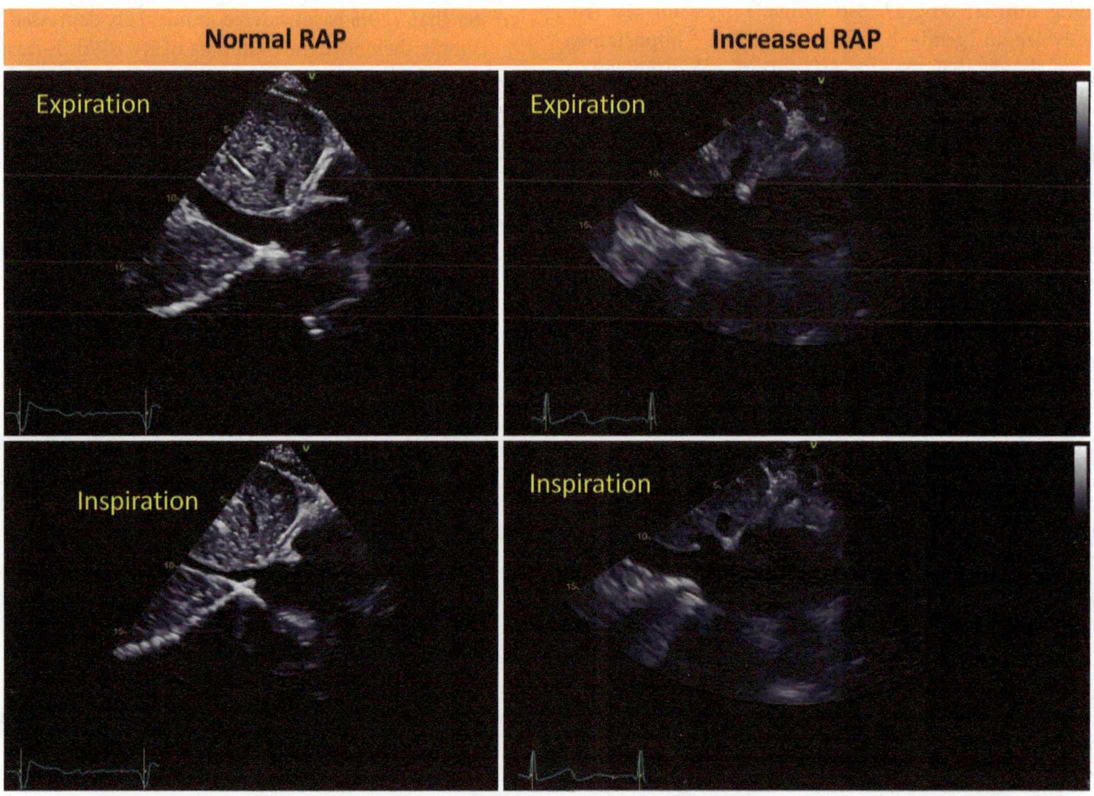

Fig. 14.6 Examples of inferior vena cava (IVC) diameter changes with inspiration from a patient with normal right atrial pressure *(RAP) (left panel)* and another with increased RAP *(right panel)*. In the left panel there is complete collapse of the IVC with inspiration, whereas in the right panel the IVC is dilated with less than 50% change in its diameter with inspiration.

of the RA pressure following RA relaxation and tricuspid annulus apical displacement. The late systolic wave is related to the transient rise in RA pressure just before the opening of the tricuspid valve. In diastole, the D wave corresponds to the fall of the RA pressure during RV filling as RA empties. The Ar wave follows atrial contraction and the late rise in RA pressure at end diastole. In older patients in sinus rhythm and in the presence of a normal RA pressure, predominant flow occurs in systole. Examples of hepatic vein flow are shown in Figs. 14.7, 14.8, 14.9, and 14.10.

Pulse wave Doppler imaging of the hepatic veins should include recordings of five to seven consecutive cardiac cycles or signals acquired at end-expiratory apnea.[45] The sample volume (3–4 mm) should be positioned 1 to 2 cm into the hepatic veins, close to their entrance into the IVC. Concomitant imaging of the hepatic veins with recording of the respiratory changes may unmask and support diagnosis in various disease states.[46] Quantitative measurements include the peak velocity, the duration, and the time velocity integral (TVI) of velocity at each of the cardiac phases described earlier, as well as the proportion of forward flow during systole and diastole, using either peak velocity or TVI measurements to derive the ratio.

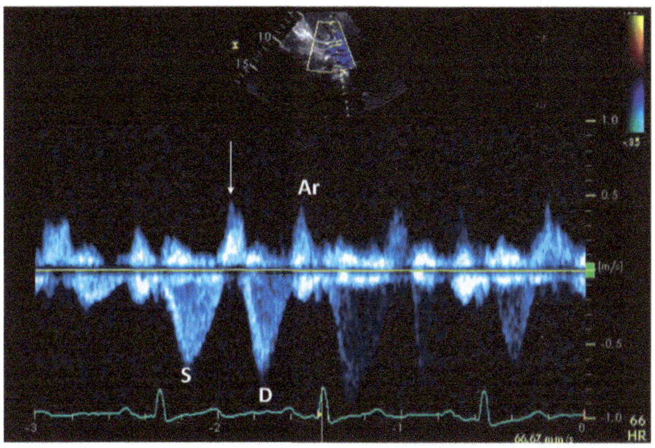

Fig. 14.7 Hepatic vein flow shows flow during systole *(S)*, during diastole *(D)*, and with atrial contraction *(Ar)*. Flow during systole, and most of diastole, is from hepatic veins to the right atrium and shown as velocities below the baseline (as flow is away from the transducer in the subcostal position). During atrial contraction, flow is from the right atrium toward the hepatic veins and the transducer in the subcostal position and thus appears above the baseline. The white arrow points to end-systolic flow into the hepatic vein from the right atrium related to C wave rise in right atrial pressure.

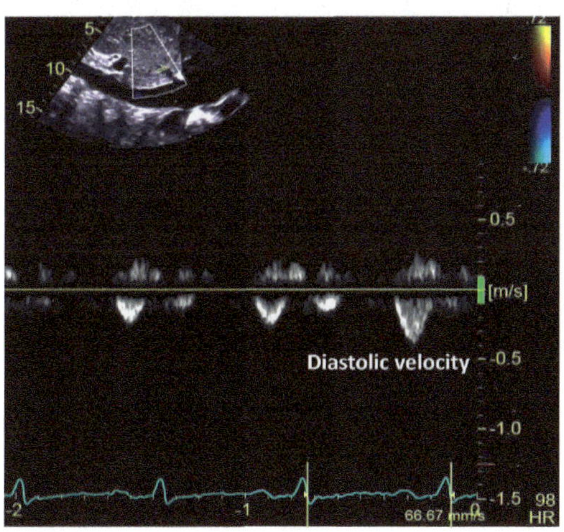

Fig. 14.8 Hepatic vein flow from a patient with markedly elevated right atrial pressure. Forward flow is present only during diastole.

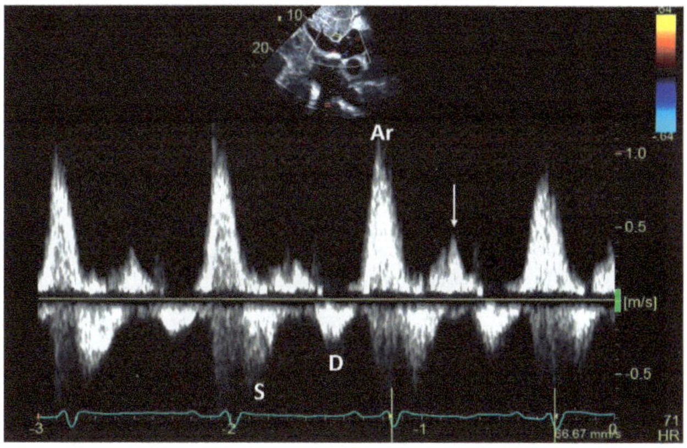

Fig. 14.9 Hepatic vein flow from a patient with markedly elevated right ventricular end-diastolic pressure. Notice the presence of a giant Ar end-diastolic velocity. This velocity corresponds clinically to the giant A wave seen in jugular venous pressure when examining the neck veins in these patients. S refers to forward systolic flow, D refers to forward diastolic flow, and the white arrow points to end-systolic reversal, which can be seen in normal hearts but is more prominent in patients with restrictive right ventricular filling.

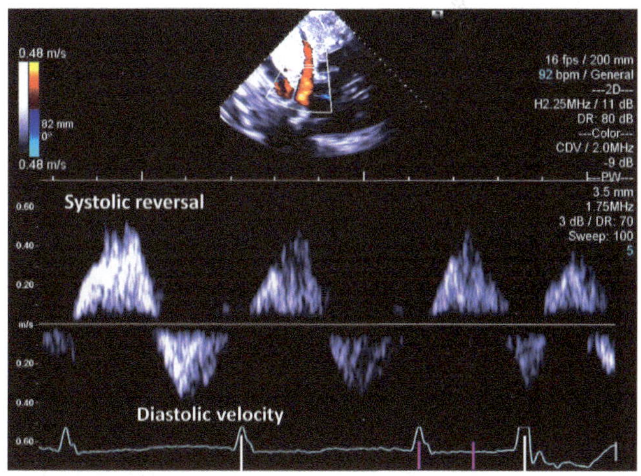

Fig. 14.10 Hepatic vein flow from a patient with severe tricuspid regurgitation. Forward flow occurs during diastole but there is flow from the right atrium to the hepatic vein during systole due to severe tricuspid regurgitation (systolic reversal).

Diastolic flow predominance in the hepatic veins in patients with cardiac disease usually reflects elevated RA pressure. With increased RA systolic pressure, the pressure gradient between the hepatic veins and the right atrium decreases, and correspondingly forward systolic flow decreases.[20] The hepatic venous systolic filling fraction (systolic flow/total antegrade flow), derived from either TVIs or maximal velocities, has been successfully applied to estimate mean RA pressure noninvasively. A systolic filling fraction less than 55% correlates with an RA pressure more than 8 mmHg[20] in patients with a variety of diseases, including those on mechanical ventilation. Likewise, in patients with restrictive physiology, prominent inspiratory or expiratory reversals are seen in the hepatic veins and correspond to elevated RA pressure.[47] Ar duration is of particular interest, as it has been shown to relate to mean RA and to late diastolic RV pressures.[20,48] The previous inferences about RA pressure based on hepatic vein flow should not be applied to patients in nonsinus rhythms, patients with

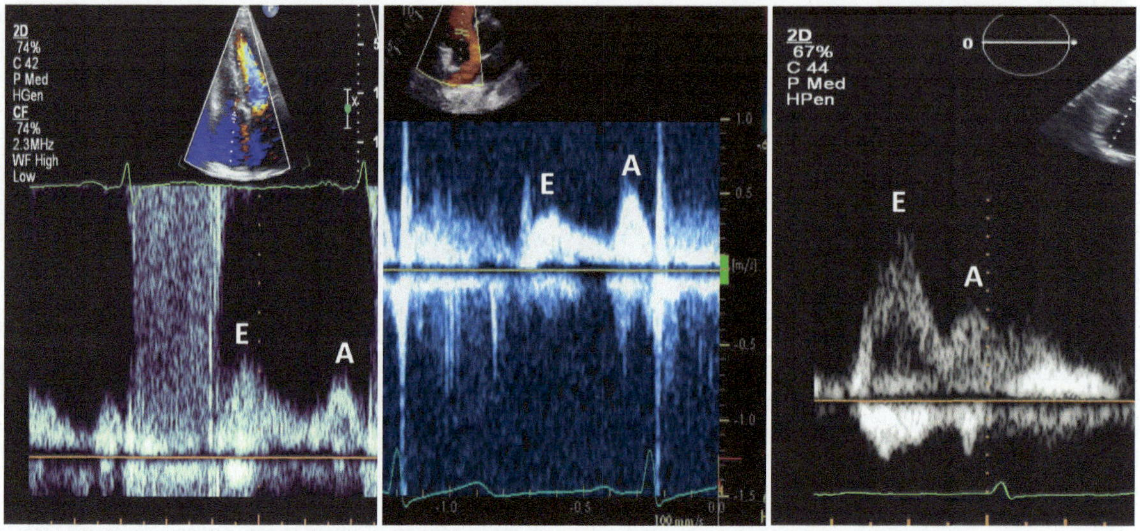

Fig. 14.11 Examples of tricuspid inflow from a normal subject *(left)*, a patient with impaired relaxation pattern *(middle)*, and a patient with restrictive filling pattern *(right)*.

heart transplant, tricuspid valve disease (significant stenosis or regurgitation and prosthetic valves), or pericardial compression syndromes. Hepatic venous flow can help differentiate pericardial constriction from restrictive cardiomyopathy.[49] Table 14.1 shows a practical summary for estimating mean RA pressure using IVC collapse index and hepatic venous flow.

Tricuspid Inflow

The principles of evaluation of RV diastolic function using transtricuspid flow with pulse wave Doppler is similar to the use of the transmitral inflow recording to assess LV diastolic function. Diastolic blood flow through the tricuspid valve has an early filling velocity (E) and a late active filling velocity (A) due to RA contraction. Acquisition of tricuspid inflow at the level of tricuspid leaflets tips and at the valve annulus is obtained by positioning a sample volume of 1 mm to 2 mm with pulse wave Doppler at these locations, paying attention to correct alignment with the direction of blood flow.[50] Angulation between the ultrasound beam and the direction of blood flow will lead to underestimation of peak velocity. Appropriate filter and gain adjustments are usually needed to obtain a clear signal. Doppler recordings are best obtained at end expiration to avoid respiratory variation. Alternatively, the average of five to seven consecutive cardiac cycles can be performed.[51] Doppler variables as the peak early (E) and late (A) diastolic velocity, deceleration time (DT) of E velocity, and duration of A velocity can be measured (Fig. 14.11). All measurements except for the A duration are obtained from the Doppler recordings at the level of the valve tips. Tricuspid A velocity duration is measured from the recordings acquired at the level of the tricuspid annulus. Additionally, RA contribution to RV filling (atrial filling fraction [AFF]) and E/A ratio can be calculated. Early diastolic RV filling velocity and filling rate as well as E/A ratio are reduced with normal aging, which should be considered when drawing conclusions about RV diastolic function using tricuspid inflow velocities.[51–53] In the presence of RV disease, tricuspid E/A ratio less than 0.8 suggests impaired RV relaxation, whereas an E/A ratio greater than 2.1 along with DT less than 120 msec are consistent with restrictive filling.[16] As RA pressure increases, E/A ratio increases and DT shortens. However, the individual response is highly variable and dependent on the interplay between many hemodynamic parameters, such that the E/A ratio has a significant positive relation with mean RA pressure but with a wide scatter. Nevertheless, in patients with RV systolic dysfunction, a short DT is usually associated with increased RV filling pressures.[20] In addition, diastolic TR, when present in the absence of atrioventricular (AV) block, indicates the presence of increased RV stiffness and increased RV filling pressures.[47]

Tissue Doppler Imaging

Tricuspid Annulus Velocities

Pulsed tissue Doppler imaging is applied to acquire tricuspid annular velocities during systole and diastole. Diastolic tissue Doppler signals include an early diastolic (e′) velocity and a late diastolic (a′) velocity (Fig. 14.12). Tricuspid annular velocity is recorded from the apical four-chamber view by positioning the pulse wave Doppler sample volume (4–5 mm) at the RV free wall at the tricuspid annulus level, paying attention to proper alignment with the plane of RV longitudinal motion.

In healthy adults, e′ velocity decreases with aging,[54] and e′ velocity is dependent on RV relaxation, but preload also affects e′ velocity in

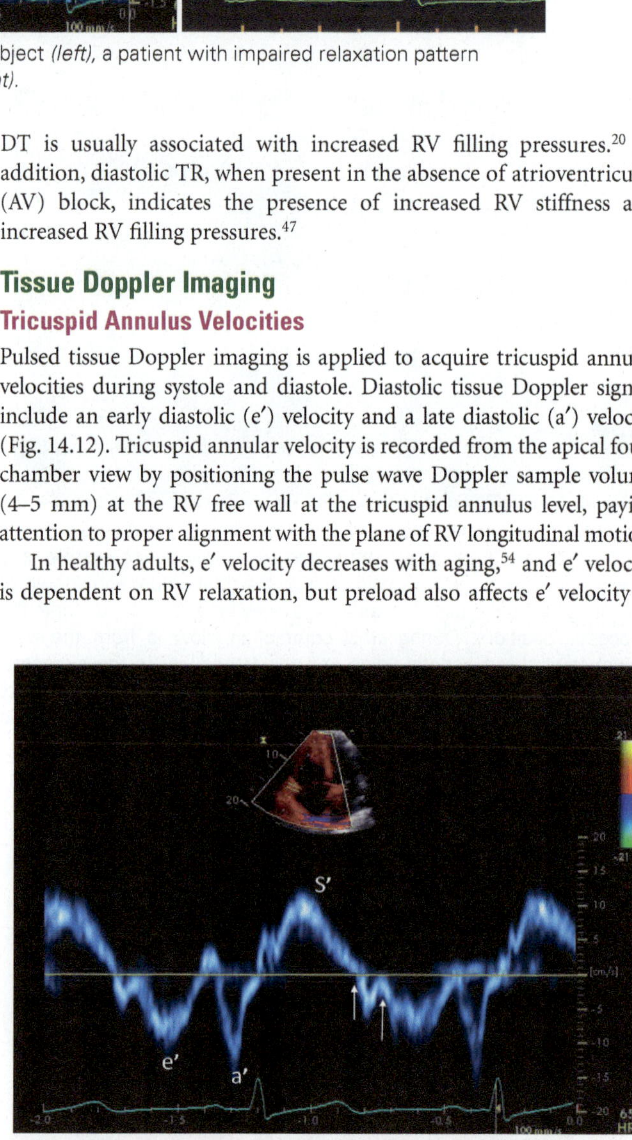

Fig. 14.12 Tissue Doppler recordings of tricuspid annulus. S′ refers to systolic velocity related to annulus descent toward the apex. The early (e′) and late (a′) diastolic velocities occur in early and late diastole, respectively, with the atrial velocity related to right atrium systolic function. White arrows show the time interval between end systole and beginning of early diastolic velocity. This time interval corresponds to the isovolumic relaxation time.

normal ventricles.[55] Notwithstanding, in patients with abnormal RV function, the existing studies support the conclusion that tricuspid annulus e′ velocity is not significantly affected by preload given the presence of an inverse correlation between e′ velocity and mean RA pressure in cardiac patients.[56] Therefore, in patients with RV dysfunction, a tricuspid E/A ratio of 0.8 to 2 with an E/e′ ratio greater than 6 is consistent with pseudonormal RV filling due to elevated RA pressure.

Tricuspid E/e′ Ratio

Peak tricuspid E velocity is directly related to RA pressure as well as RV relaxation. Likewise, tricuspid annulus e′ velocity is directly related to RV relaxation (the better the relaxation, the higher the e′ velocity) and is not strongly influenced by RA pressure in patients with RV dysfunction. Thus tricuspid E/e′ ratio is directly related to RA pressure and can be used to estimate RA pressure in patients with cardiac disease. Tricuspid e′/a′ ratio appears unaffected with preload reduction.[55] The hemodynamic correlates of tricuspid E/e′ ratio were examined in animal models[57] and in human studies.[56,58] A ratio greater than 6 is usually associated with mean RA pressure above 10 mmHg,[56] and can be applied in patients on mechanical ventilation. In cardiac transplant recipients a ratio greater than 8 had a sensitivity of 78% and a specificity of 85% for RA pressure of at least 10 mmHg.[58] In patients following cardiac surgery, weaker correlations were reported.[59]

In addition to the tricuspid E/e′ ratio, the time interval between the end of tricuspid annular systolic velocity and the onset of e′ velocity (see Fig. 14.12) has been evaluated as an index of RA pressure. A time interval less than 59 msec has a sensitivity of 80% and a specificity of 88% in identifying patients with RA pressure greater than 8 mmHg.[60]

Forward Flow Into the Pulmonary Artery and Pulmonary Regurgitation Signal by Continuous Wave Doppler as Indices of RV Diastolic Function

Restrictive filling of the right ventricle occurs in the setting of elevated RA and RV diastolic pressures. The net effect of a stiff right ventricle in conjunction with a vigorous RA contraction is the generation of an early ejection of flow into the main pulmonary artery during late diastole. The manifestation of end-diastolic forward flow into the pulmonary artery detected by Doppler echocardiography has been recognized as a sign of a noncompliant right ventricle (Fig. 14.13).

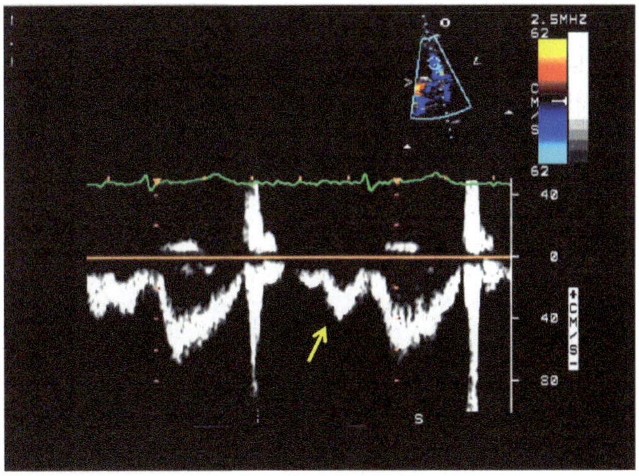

Fig. 14.13 Flow through the right ventricular outflow tract is shown. End-diastolic forward flow *(yellow arrow)* with pulse wave Doppler is present, consistent with elevated right ventricular end-diastolic pressure.

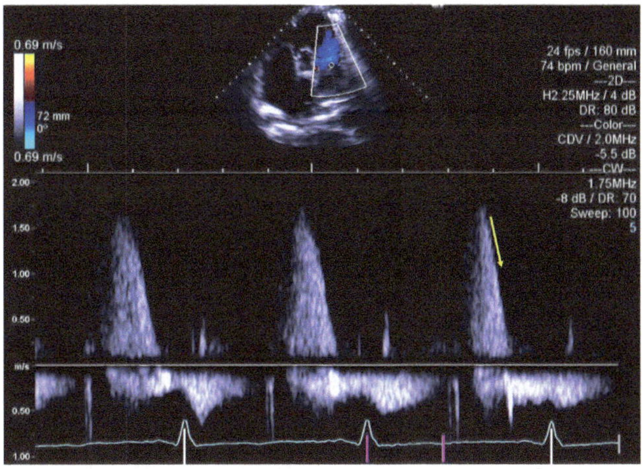

Fig. 14.14 Pulmonary regurgitation signal by continuous wave Doppler from a patient with right ventricular diastolic dysfunction and elevated right ventricular end-diastolic pressure. Notice the steep deceleration of the pulmonary regurgitation velocity *(yellow arrow)*.

This phenomenon occurs when RV diastolic pressure exceeds PA diastolic pressure. The presence of end-diastolic forward flow into the pulmonary artery is not specific for restrictive RV physiology, and other mechanisms may be linked to its occurrence.[61,62] Pulmonary artery end-diastolic forward flow can sometimes occur in patients with severe pulmonary regurgitation (PR) who have reduced pulmonary artery diastolic pressure but higher right ventricular late diastolic pressure.

Analysis of the PR signal by continuous wave Doppler yields important insights into RV compliance. In the absence of significant PR, a steep deceleration slope or a short pressure half-time of the PR jet by continuous wave Doppler indicates abnormally increased RV stiffness. Patients with increased RV stiffness exhibit a steep rise in RV diastolic pressure leading to rapid equalization of the pressure gradient between the pulmonary artery and the right ventricle and therefore a short pressure half-time (Fig. 14.14).

Doppler echocardiography, identifying distinctive flow features from the pulmonary regurgitation signal, has been applied to evaluate RV involvement in patients with inferior wall acute myocardial infarction. In one study, which used right heart catheterization, a pressure half-time of PR >/= 150 msec was the best predictor of RV infarction.[63] In addition, the same investigators reported that this parameter was the only predictor of overall in-hospital clinical events in the same patient population.[64]

In addition to evaluating RV diastolic function, PR signal by continuous wave Doppler can be applied to estimate mean PA pressure and PA diastolic pressure. Mean pulmonary artery pressure and pulmonary artery diastolic pressure can be estimated using the modified Bernoulli equation by using the sum of mean RA pressure and four times the peak PR velocity squared or end-diastolic PR velocity squared, respectively.[65] Discrepancies between invasive measurements and noninvasive estimation can occur if RV end-diastolic pressure is significantly higher than mean RA pressure or with erroneous noninvasive estimation of RA pressure.

FUTURE DIRECTIONS

Evaluation of RV function is important clinically. 2-D echocardiography and Doppler techniques provide complementary methods for evaluation of RV diastolic function and prediction of mean RA pressure. These include size and function of the RV and the RA, IVC diameter and its change with respiration, RV myocardial velocities, tricuspid inflow, and hepatic venous flow patterns. The availability of 3-D technology has undoubtedly improved quantification of RV volumes and systolic function. Whether 3-D technology will further improve the evaluation of RV diastolic function remains to be determined, as it is possible to obtain rates of RV filling and RA volumetric changes based on 3-D volumes.

Myocardial diastolic strain rate with speckle tracking can provide additional information about RV diastolic function, though incremental role of diastolic strain rate is yet to be determined. It is possible that early diastolic strain rate may help in the earlier diagnosis of RV diastolic dysfunction in cardiomyopathy disorders, as in patients with arrhythmogenic cardiomyopathy, where conventional echocardiography may not be diagnostic of RV disease. Vortex formation plays a key role in the interaction between cardiac tissue and intraventricular flow. Changes in intraventricular fluid dynamics may reflect impaired diastolic function. Analysis of vortices in the right ventricle may detect abnormalities before alterations in tissue mechanics occur. However, further development is needed to accurately characterize and quantify vortices in the right ventricle. RV systolic and diastolic dyssynchrony affect RV diastolic function, and this extends to the impact of different sites of RV pacing on RV performance. Additional work is needed in this area to explore the potential of the noninvasive assessment of these variables and their clinical relevance. Finally, it is potentially informative to look at tracking RV systolic and diastolic functions in response to medical and surgical therapies as a guide to patient-tailored treatment.

KEY POINTS

- In patients with increased RA pressure, RA maximum and minimum volumes are increased while RA emptying fraction is reduced.
- RA reservoir strain and conduit strain are reduced in patients with pulmonary arterial HTN and are predictive of adverse clinical outcomes.
- RV systolic function can be assessed using RV fractional area change (normal >35%), TPASE (normal >17 mm), global longitudinal RV free wall strain (normal >20%), and RV ejection fraction by 3-D echocardiography (normal >45%).
- It is possible to estimate mean RA pressure based on IVC maximum diameter and its change with inspiration. An IVC diameter greater than 2.1 cm with less than 50% collapse with sniffing are consistent with markedly elevated RA pressure.
- In older subjects, reduced systolic to diastolic velocity ratio in hepatic vein flow is consistent with elevated mean RA pressure.
- Tricuspid E/e′ ratio greater than 6 is usually associated with mean RA pressure above 10 mmHg and can be applied in patients on mechanical ventilation.
- The presence of end-diastolic forward flow into the pulmonary artery detected by Doppler echocardiography is a sign of a noncompliant right ventricle, in the absence of severe pulmonary regurgitation.
- In the absence of significant pulmonary regurgitation, a steep deceleration, A short pressure half-time of the PR jet by continuous wave Doppler indicates abnormally increased RV stiffness.

REVIEW QUESTIONS

1. A 30-year-old female patient with primary pulmonary hypertension is referred for evaluation of RV systolic function. Which of these measurements is indicative of abnormally reduced RV systolic function?
   a. RV fractional area change at 38%
   b. TAPSE at 21 mm
   c. RV free wall strain at −25%
   d. Tricuspid annulus systolic velocity by tissue Doppler at 12 cm/sec
   e. RV ejection fraction by 3-D echocardiography at 40%
2. A 65-year-old male patient with primary pulmonary hypertension is referred for evaluation of mean RA pressure. Which of these measurements is indicative of abnormally elevated mean RA pressure?
   a. IVC maximum diameter at 1.5 cm at end expiration and 0.5 cm with sniffing
   b. Hepatic vein systolic velocity at 65 cm/sec and diastolic velocity at 34 cm/sec
   c. RA maximum volume index of 25 mL/m^2
   d. Tricuspid E/e′ ratio at 8
   e. Peak tricuspid regurgitation velocity at 3.6 m/sec
3. Pulmonary regurgitation can be acquired by continuous wave Doppler. Assuming a complete jet has been recorded, which of these statements is correct?
   a. Peak velocity can be used to estimate PA systolic pressure.
   b. End-diastolic velocity can be directly used to estimate mean PA pressure.
   c. PR pressure half-time at 200 msec is consistent with RV involvement in patients with inferior wall myocardial infarction.
   d. PR pressure half-time at 130 msec predicts worse outcome in patients with inferior wall myocardial infarction and RV involvement.
   e. PR end-diastolic velocity of 2.5 m/sec is consistent with elevated RA pressure.

REFERENCES

1. Tei C, Dujardin KS, Hodge DO, et al. Doppler echocardiographic index for assessment of global right ventricular function. *J Am Soc Echocardiogr.* 1996;9(6):838–847.
2. Sallach JA, Tang WH, Borowski AG, et al. Right atrial volume index in chronic systolic heart failure and prognosis. *JACC Cardiovasc Imag.* 2009;2(5):527–534.
3. Leeuwenburgh BP, Steendijk P, Helbing WA, Baan J. Indexes of diastolic RV function: load dependence and changes after chronic RV pressure overload in lambs. *Am J Physiol Heart Circ Physiol.* 2002;282:H1350–H1358.
4. Stein PD, Sabbah HN, Mazilli M, Anbe DT. Effect of chronic pressure overload on the maximal rate of pressure fall of the right ventricle. *Chest.* 1980;78:10–15.
5. Darsinos JT, Evagelou AM, Rassidakis AN. Rate of pressure fall in right ventricle during isovolumic relaxation. *Angiology.* 1974;25: 520–526.
6. Maeda M, Yamakado T, Nakano T. Right ventricular diastolic function in patients with hypertrophic cardiomyopathy—an invasive study. *Jpn Circ J.* 1999;63:681–687.
7. Rommel KP, von Roeder M, Oberueck C, et al. Load-independent systolic and diastolic right ventricular function in heart failure with preserved

ejection fraction as assessed by resting and handgrip exercise pressure-volume loops. *Circ Heart Fail.* 2018;11(2):e004121.

8. Pasipoularides A, Shu M, Shah A, Silvestry S, Glower DD. Right ventricular diastolic function in canine models of pressure overload, volume overload, and ischemia. *Am J Physiol Heart Circ Physiol.* 2002;283: H2140–H2150.
9. Burkhoff D, Mirsky I, Suga H. Assessment of systolic and diastolic ventricular properties via pressure-volume analysis: a guide for clinical, translational, and basic researchers. *Am J Physiol Heart Circ Physiol.* 2005;289:H501–H512. doi: 10.1152/ajpheart.00138.2005.
10. Gaynor SL, Maniar HS, Bloch JB, Steendijk P, Moon MR. Right atrial and ventricular adaptation to chronic right ventricular pressure overload. *Circulation.* 2005;112:I212–I218.
11. Pasipoularides A, Shu M, Shah A, Womack MS, Glower DD. Diastolic right ventricular filling vortex in normal and volume overload states. *Am J Physiol Heart Circ Physiol.* 2003;284:H1064–H1072.
12. Fenster BE, Browning J, Schroeder JD, Schafer M, Podgorski CA, Smyser J, et al. Vorticity is a marker of right ventricular diastolic dysfunction. *Am J Physiol Heart Circ Physiol.* 2015;309(6):H1087–H1093.
13. Raymond RJ, Hinderliter AL, Willis PW, et al. Echocardiographic predictors of adverse outcomes in primary pulmonary hypertension. *J Am Coll Cardiol.* 2002;39(7):1214–1219.
14. Cioffi G, de Simone G, Mureddu G, Tarantini L, Stefenelli C. Right atrial size and function in patients with pulmonary hypertension associated with disorders of respiratory system or hypoxemia. *Eur J Echocardiogr.* 2007;8(5):322–331.
15. Grapsa J, Gibbs JS, Cabrita IZ, et al. The association of clinical outcome with right atrial and ventricular remodeling in patients with pulmonary arterial hypertension: study with real-time three-dimensional echocardiography. *Eur Heart J Cardiovasc Imag.* 2012;13(8):666–672.
16. Rudski LG, Lai WW, Afilalo J, et al. Guidelines for the echocardiographic assessment of the right heart in adults: a report from the American Society of Echocardiography endorsed by the European Association of Echocardiography, a registered branch of the European Society of Cardiology, and the Canadian Society of Echocardiography. *J Am Soc Echocardiogr.* 2010;23(7):685–713.
17. Lang RM, Badano LP, Mor-Avi V, et al. Recommendations for cardiac chamber quantification by echocardiography in adults: an update from the American Society of Echocardiography and the European Association of Cardiovascular Imaging. *J Am Soc Echocardiogr.* 2015;28(1):1–39.
18. Peluso D, Badano LP, Muraru D, et al. Right atrial size and function assessed with three-dimensional and speckle-tracking echocardiography in 200 healthy volunteers. *Eur Heart J Cardiovasc Imag.* 2013;14:1106–1114.
19. Kou S, Caballero L, Dulgheru R, et al. Echocardiographic reference ranges for normal cardiac chamber size: results from the NORRE study. *Eur Heart J Cardiovasc Imag.* 2014;15:680–690.
20. Nagueh SF, Kopelen HA, Zoghbi WA. Relation of mean right atrial pressure to echocardiographic and Doppler parameters of right atrial and right ventricular function. *Circulation.* 1996;93:1160–1169.
21. Keller AM, Gopal AS, King DL. Left and right atrial volume by freehand three-dimensional echocardiography: in vivo validation using magnetic resonance imaging. *Eur J Echocardiogr. 2000*;1(1):55–65.
22. Aune E, Baekkevar M, Roislien J, Rodevand O, Otterstad JE. Normal reference ranges for left and right atrial volume indexes and ejection fractions obtained with real-time three-dimensional echocardiography. *Eur J Echocardiogr.* 2009;10(6):738–744.
23. Quraini D, Pandian NG, Patel AR. Three-dimensional echocardiographic analysis of right atrial volume in normal and abnormal hearts: comparison of biplane and multiplane methods. *Echocardiography.* 2012;29:608–613.
24. Patel AR, Alsheikh-Ali AA, Mukherjee J, et al. 3D echocardiography to evaluate right atrial pressure in acutely decompensated heart failure correlation with invasive hemodynamics. *JACC Cardiovasc Imag.* 2011;4(9):938–945.
25. Brunner NW, Haddad F, Kobayashi Y, et al. Prognostic utility of right atrial emptying fractions in pulmonary arterial hypertension. *Pulm Circ.* 2015;5(3):473–480.
26. Querejeta Roca G, Campbell P, Claggett B, Solomon SD, Shah AM. Right atrial function in pulmonary arterial hypertension. *Circ Cardiovas Imag.* 2015;8(11):e003521.
27. Nourian S, Hosseinsabet A, Jalali A, Mohseni-Badalabadi R. Evaluation of right atrial function by two-dimensional speckle-tracking echocardiography in patients with right ventricular myocardial infarction. *Int J Cardiovasc Imag.* 2017;33(1):47–56.
28. Bhave NM, Visovatti SH, Kulick B, Kolias TJ, McLaughlin VV. Right atrial strain is predictive of clinical outcomes and invasive hemodynamic data in group 1 pulmonary arterial hypertension. *Int J Cardiovasc Imag.* 2017;33(6):847–855.
29. Shimada YJ, Shiota M, Siegel RJ, Shiota T. Accuracy of right ventricular volumes and function determined by three-dimensional echocardiography in comparison with magnetic resonance imaging: a meta-analysis study. *J Am Soc Echocardiogr.* 2010;23:943–953.
30. Maffessanti F, Muraru D, Esposito R, et al. Age-, body size-, and sex-specific reference values for right ventricular volumes and ejection fraction by three-dimensional echocardiography: a multicenter echocardiographic study in 507 healthy volunteers. *Circ Cardiovasc Imag.* 2013;6: 700–710.
31. Medvedofsky D, Mor-Avi V, Kruse E, et al. Quantification of right ventricular size and function from contrast-enhanced three-dimensional echocardiographic images. *J Am Soc Echocardiogr.* 2017;30(12): 1193–1202.
32. Addetia K, Maffessanti F, Muraru D, Singh A, Surkova E, Mor-Avi V. Morphologic analysis of the normal right ventricle using three-dimensional echocardiography-derived curvature indices. *J Am Soc Echocardiogr.* 2018;31(5):614–623.
33. Anavekar NS, Gerson D, Skali H, Kwong RY, Yucel EK, Solomon SD. Two-dimensional assessment of right ventricular function: an echocardiographic-MRI correlative study. *Echocardiography.* 2007;24(5): 452–456.
34. Mor-Avi V, Lang RM, Badano LP, et al. Current and evolving echocardiographic techniques for the quantitative evaluation of cardiac mechanics: ASE/EAE consensus statement on methodology and indications endorsed by the Japanese Society of Echocardiography. *J Am Soc Echocardiogr.* 2011;24(3):277–313.
35. Imanishi T, Nakatani S, Yamada S, et al. Validation of continuous wave Doppler–determined right ventricular peak positive and negative dP/dt: effect of right atrial pressure on measurement. *J Am Coll Cardiol.* 1994;23:1638–1643.
36. Simonson JS, Schiller NB. Sonospirometry: a non-invasive method for estimation of mean right atrial pressure based on two dimensional echocardiographic measurements of the inferior vena cava during measured inspiration. *J Am Coll Cardiol.* 1988;11:557–564.
37. Kircher BJ, Himelman RB, Schiller NB. Non-invasive estimation of right atrial pressure from the inspiratory collapse of the inferior vena cava. *Am J Cardiol.* 1990;66:493–496.
38. Brennan JM, Blair JE, Goonewardena S, et al. Reappraisal of the use of inferior vena cava for estimating right atrial pressure. *J Am Soc Echocardiogr.* 2007;20:857–861.
39. Nakao S, Come PC, McKay RG, Ransil BJ. Effects of positional changes on inferior vena caval size and dynamics and correlations with right-sided cardiac pressure. *Am J Cardiol.* 1987;59:125–132.
40. Goldhammer E, Mesnick N, Abinader EG, Sagiv M. Dilated inferior vena cava: a common echocardiographic finding in highly trained elite athletes. *J Am Soc Echocardiogr.* 1999;12:988–993.
41. Jue J, Chung W, Schiller NB. Does inferior vena caval size predict right atrial pressure in mechanically ventilated patients? *J Am Soc Echocardiogr.* 1992;5:613–619.
42. Luca L, Mario P, Giansiro B, Maurizio F, Antonio M, Carlo M. Non-invasive estimation of mean right atrial pressure utilizing the 2-D echo transverse diameter of the left hepatic vein. *Int J Cardiac Imag.* 1992;8:191–195.
43. Fadel BM, Alkalbani A, Husain A, Dahdouh Z, Di Salvo G. Respiratory hemodynamics in the hepatic veins–normal pattern. *Echocardiography.* 2015;32:585–588.

44. Appleton CP, Hatle LK, Popp RL. Superior vena cava and hepatic vein Doppler echocardiography in healthy adults. *J Am Coll Cardiol.* 1987;10:1032–1039.
45. Pinto FJ, Wranne B, St Goar FG, Schnittger I, Popp RL. Hepatic venous flow assessed by transesophageal echocardiography. *J Am Coll Cardiol.* 1991;17:1493–1498.
46. Fadel BM, Alkalbani A, Husain A, Dahdouh Z, Di Salvo G. Respiratory hemodynamics in the hepatic veins—abnormal patterns. *Echocardiography.* 2015;32(4):705–710.
47. Appleton CP, Hatle LK, Popp RL. Demonstration of restrictive ventricular physiology by Doppler echocardiography. *J Am Coll Cardiol.* 1988;11: 757–768.
48. Ommen SR, Nishimura RA, Hurrell DG, Klarich KW. Assessment of right atrial pressure with 2-dimensional and Doppler echocardiography: a simultaneous catheterization and echocardiographic study. *Mayo Clin Proc.* 2000;75:24–29.
49. Oh JK, Hatle LK, Seward JB, et al. Diagnostic role of Doppler echocardiography in constrictive pericarditis. *J Am Coll Cardiol.* 1994;23:154–162.
50. Appleton CP, Jensen JL, Hatle LK, Oh JK. Doppler evaluation of left and right ventricular diastolic function: a technical guide for obtaining optimal flow velocity recordings. *J Am Soc Echocardiogr.* 1997;10:271–292.
51. Zoghbi WA, Habib JB, Quiñones MA. Doppler assessment of right ventricular filling in a normal population: comparison with left ventricular filling dynamics. *Circulation.* 1990;82:1316–1324.
52. Berman G, Reicheck N, Brownson D, Douglas PS. Effects of sample volume location, imaging view, heart rate and age on tricuspid velocimetry in normal subjects. *Am J Cardiol.* 1990;65:1026–1030.
53. Innelli P, Esposito R, Olibet M, Nistri S, Galderisi M. The impact of ageing on right ventricular longitudinal function in healthy subjects: a pulsed tissue Doppler study. *J Am Soc Echocardiogr.* 2009;10(4):491–498.
54. Chia EM, Hsieh CH, Boyd A, et al. Effects of age and gender on right ventricular systolic and diastolic function using two-dimensional speckle-tracking strain. *J Am Soc Echocardiogr.* 2014;27(10):1079–1086.
55. Pela G, Regolisti G, Coghi P, et al. Effects of the reduction of preload on left and right ventricular myocardial velocities analyzed by Doppler tissue echocardiography in healthy subjects. *J Am Soc Echocardiogr.* 2004;5:262–271.
56. Nageh MF, Kopelen HA, Zoghbi WA, Quiñones MA, Nagueh SF. Estimation of mean right atrial pressure using tissue Doppler imaging. *Am J Cardiol.* 1999;84:1448–1451.
57. Boissiere J, Gautier M, Machet MC, Hanton G, Bonnet P, Eder V. Doppler tissue imaging in assessment of pulmonary hypertension-induced right ventricle dysfunction. *Am J Physiol Heart Circ Physiol.* 2005;289: H2450–H2455.
58. Sundereswaran L, Nagueh SF, Vardan S, et al. Estimation of left and right ventricular filling pressures after heart transplantation by tissue Doppler imaging. *Am J Cardiol.* 1998;82:352–357.
59. Sade LE, Gulmez O, Eroglu S, Sezgin A, Muderrisoglu H. Noninvasive estimation of right ventricular filling pressure by ratio of early tricuspid inflow to annular diastolic velocity in patients with and without recent cardiac surgery. *J Am Soc Echocardiogr.* 2007;20:982–988.
60. Abbas A, Lester S, Moreno FC, Srivathsan K, Fortuin D, Appleton C. Noninvasive assessment of right atrial pressure using Doppler tissue imaging. *J Am Soc Echocardiogr.* 2004;17:1155–1160.
61. Mori Y, Murakami T, Inoue N, Kaneko S, Nakashima Y, Koide M. Is the presence of end-diastolic forward flow specific for restrictive right ventricular physiology in repaired tetralogy of Fallot? *Int J Cardiol.* 2017;240:187–193.
62. Kutty S, Valente AM, White MT, et al. Usefulness of pulmonary arterial end-diastolic forward flow late after tetralogy of Fallot repair to predict a "restrictive" right ventricle. *Am J Cardiol.* 2018;121(11):1380–1386.
63. Cohen A, Guyon P, Chauvel C, et al. Relations between Doppler tracings of pulmonary regurgitation and invasive hemodynamics in acute right ventricular infarction complicating inferior wall left ventricular infarction. *Am J Cardiol.* 1995;75:425–430.
64. Cohen A, Logeart D, Costagliola D, et al. Usefulness of pulmonary regurgitation Doppler tracings in predicting in-hospital and long-term outcome in patients with inferior wall acute myocardial infarction. *Am J Cardiol.* 1998;81:276–281.
65. Masuyama T, Kodama K, Kitabatake A, Sato H, Nanto S, Inoue M. Continuous-wave Doppler echocardiographic detection of pulmonary regurgitation and its application to noninvasive estimation of pulmonary artery pressure. *Circulation.* 1986;74:484–492.

15

Evaluation of Diastolic Function by Cardiac Magnetic Resonance Imaging

Laura Young and Deborah Kwon

OUTLINE

Case Study

A 62-year-old male was admitted to the hospital with progressive dyspnea on exertion and presyncope. His workup in the emergency room included a troponin T, which was found to be mildly elevated. Further evaluation thus far has included an unrevealing coronary angiogram. Transthoracic echocardiogram (TTE) showed normal left ventricular ejection fraction (LV EF) of 65% with moderate LV hypertrophy and a moderate pericardial effusion. Infiltrative heart disease is suspected. Diastolic function is uninterpretable due to fusion of the E and A waves. His electrocardiogram (ECG) demonstrates sinus rhythm with low voltage. The admitting team is considering magnetic resonance imaging (MRI) to evaluate for infiltrative heart disease and asks for your opinion as to whether this will be useful (Figs. 15.1 and 15.2).

INTRODUCTION

In the past few decades, cardiac MRI has become an integral tool for the diagnosis and management of cardiovascular disease. Cardiac MRI offers excellent spatial and temporal resolution that allows for anatomic and functional assessment in a noninvasive manner. It is widely viewed as the gold standard for measurement of cardiac chamber volume in terms of precision and reproducibility.[1–3] Cardiac MRI provides the most comprehensive phenotypic assessment of cardiac disease by providing quantitative assessment of ventricular size/function, myocardial perfusion, myocardial fibrosis, tissue characterization, and flow quantification. While TTE remains the first-line diagnostic tool for cardiac imaging and diastolic assessment, imaging quality can be suboptimal if there are limited acoustic windows, which is common in patients with increased body habitus. Because of the ability for cardiac MRI to provide comprehensive quantitative assessment, it has emerged as an important tool for the evaluation of cardiac disease resulting in abnormal diastolic function.

PHYSICS OF MRI

Cardiac MRI relies on the inherent feature of hydrogen nuclei known as nuclear spin, in which the hydrogen proton produces a small positive electric charge that allows it to spin at a rapid rate and to ultimately produce a small but measurable magnetic field. Cardiac MRI capitalizes on the fact that hydrogen atoms are extremely abundant in the human body and produce these small magnetic fields randomly oriented throughout the human body. Therefore, when the protons are placed in an MRI scanner, they will accordingly align or repel against the MRI scanner's strong magnetic field. This alignment can be disturbed by applying additional small radiofrequency pulses that stimulate the protons to enter into a more excited state. When the hydrogen protons subsequently relax and return to their original state, a

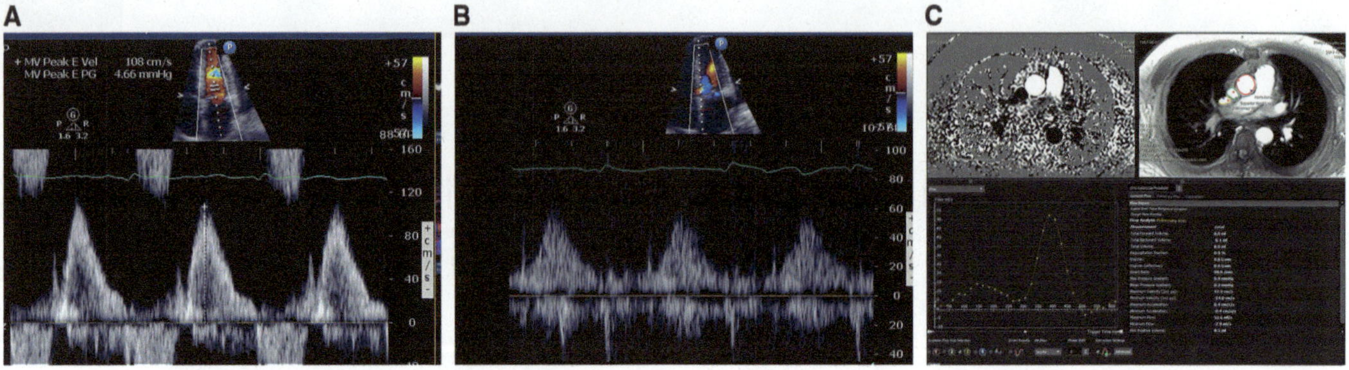

Fig. 15.1 Case study: (A) Transmitral inflow assessment. (B) Pulmonary venous flow assessment by echo. (C) Pulmonary flow by cardiac MRI.

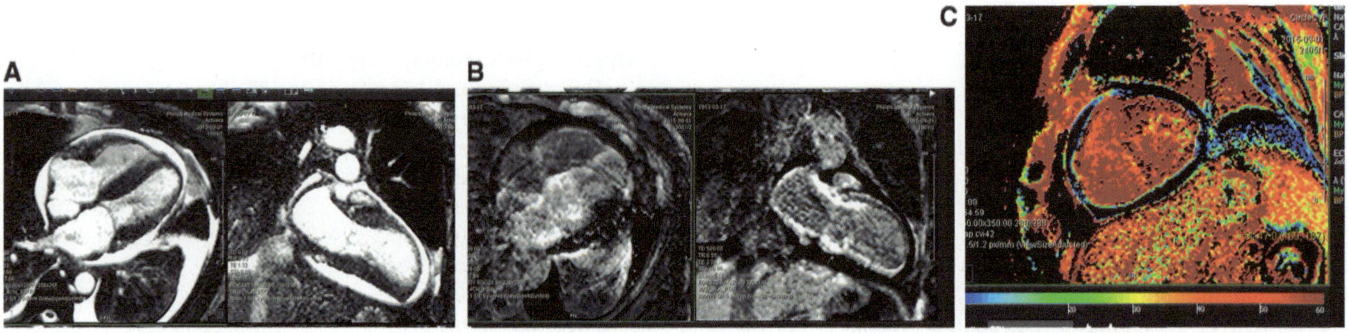

Fig. 15.2 Case study: (A) Steady-state free precession (SSFP) imaging demonstrating diffuse thickening of the ventricular walls, interatrial septum, and left atrial wall as well as a moderate pericardial effusion. (B) Late gadolinium enhancement imaging demonstrating diffuse enhancement of the right and left ventricular walls, interatrial septum, and left atrial wall. (C) Diffuse increase in extracellular volume quantification with T1 mapping; electrochemical capacitance voltage (ECV) is 61%.

radiofrequency signal will be emitted, which can be measured and used to produce a clinical image.

BASIC IMAGING SEQUENCES

Various MRI images can be obtained by using different gradient coils and radiofrequency pulses in specified sequences. The characteristics of these imaging sequences result in different signal characteristics of the hydrogen protons. The imaging sequences can be used in combination to specifically evaluate various properties of the cardiac structures, including tissue characterization, flow quantification, contractility, and diastolic function. The most common imaging sequences and those that are helpful for evaluating diastolic function are outlined in the following sections.

Spin Echo Technique—Black Blood Imaging

Black blood imaging sequences provide morphologic images of the heart in still frames. In these sequences, flowing blood moves quickly and thereby will not be consistently exposed to the radiofrequency pulses. This results in a signal void that appears black on final imaging (Fig. 15.3). Conversely, because the myocardium and great vessels that remain within the imaging plane are exposed to the sequence of radiofrequency pulses, they yield high contrast signals that allow for accurate morphologic assessment. Spin echo sequences can be processed to emphasize different relaxation properties of the protons, which are known as T1-weighted or T2-weighted images. Black blood imaging is not used specifically in the assessment of diastolic function. However, their excellent tissue contrast and anatomic detail allow for careful assessment of morphology, which provide essential context for assessing the underlying etiology of diastolic dysfunction.

Gradient Echo Technique

These pulse sequences are considerably faster than dark blood imaging and therefore can interpret the signal coming from flowing blood so that it appears white (see Fig. 15.3). Gradient echo (GRE) sequences will result in cine images that can be used to assess cardiac function and valvular flow. The biggest advantage of GRE sequences is that they allow for accurate and reproducible measurements of ventricular volumes without any need for geometric assumptions.

GRE sequencing can be used to derive time-volume LV filling curves for assessment of diastolic function but is notably a time-consuming process due to the significant number of images needed to be obtained for processing (on average, 200–300 images). The peak filling rate (PFR) is defined as the maximum change in LV volume per second during the rapid filling phase of ventricular diastole and can be identified as the highest positive slope on the volume curve. Time to PFR is the time between end systole and the point at which PFR occurs. Both of these parameters will typically be prolonged in patients with diastolic dysfunction (see Chapter 16).[4,5]

PHASE VELOCITY OR PHASE CONTRAST IMAGING

The term *phase* in cardiac MRI refers to the manner in which protons rotate about a particular axis. As hydrogen nuclei move through a magnetic field, they will shift their phase in proportion to their velocity. This allows for the direct measurement of blood flow velocity by

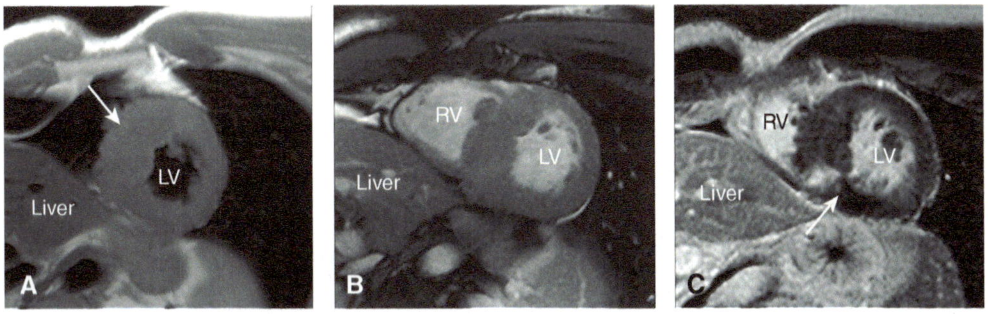

Fig. 15.3 Hypertrophic obstructive cardiomyopathy. (A) Short axis spin echo image. Moving blood is black, whereas myocardium and fat have intermediate and high signal intensities, respectively. Note the prominent interventricular septum *(arrow)*. The right ventricle is not well seen on this image. (B) Gradient echo (GRE) still frame image at the same level. Blood is bright *(white)* on this image. (C) Delayed enhancement (DE) MRI image at the same level. Note the area of hyperenhanced *(bright)* myocardium in the inferoseptal wall *(arrow)* near the right ventricular (RV) insertion point, which represents scarred or fibrotic tissue. *LV,* Left ventricle.

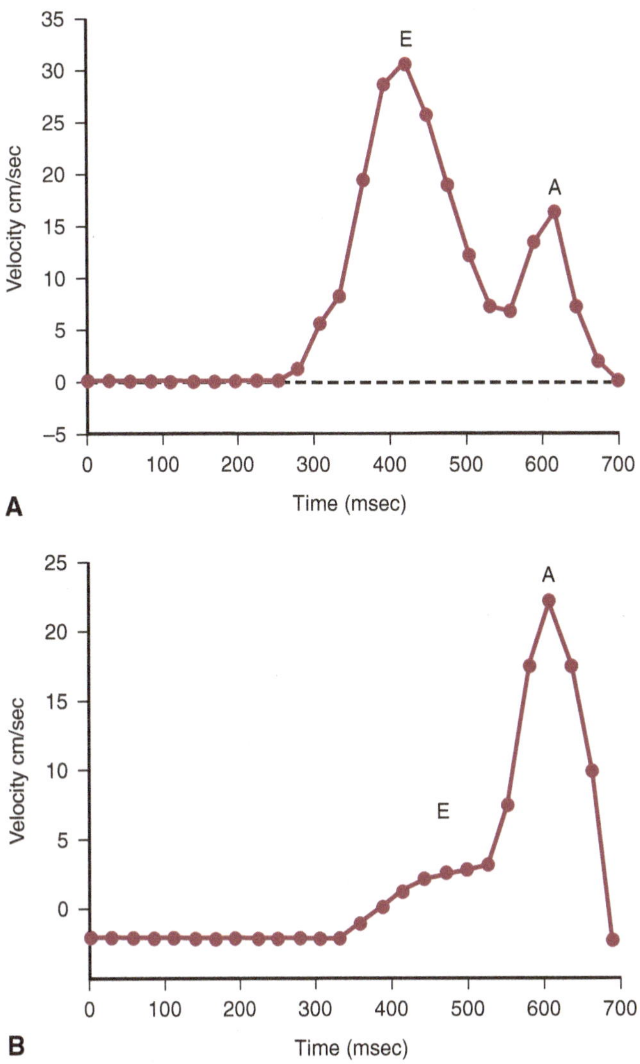

Fig. 15.4 (A) Mitral inflow pattern using phase contrast MRI in a 24-year-old healthy subject, depicting normal E/A ratio. (B) Severe myocardial relaxation disturbance leading to reversal of the E/A ratio. The early filling velocities are strongly decreased (E), whereas the late-filling velocities are increased (A). (From Bogaert J. Cardiac function. In Bogaert J et al, eds. *Clinical Cardiac MRI*. New York, NY: Springer-Verlag; 2005:99–141.)

phase contrast cardiac MRI, whereby an imaging plane perpendicular to the path of interest is selected to ultimately create a velocity encoded cine image. This technique will then provide data for the measurement of transvalvular velocities and gradients, regurgitant volumes, and shunt flow calculation (Qp/Qs).

Transmitral flow (TMF) serves to directly quantify the filling gradient between the left atrium and the left ventricle. Numerous studies have shown sufficient correlation between cardiac MRI and TTE for measurement of flow velocities[6–8] (Fig. 15.4). As with TTE, there are limitations to the use of TMF such as in patients with tachycardia or irregular rhythms, where interpretation will be difficult due to fusion or absence of the conventional filling pattern waves. It may also be more difficult to interpret TMF filling patterns in the more elderly population, in which there is an expected, age-related reduction in E wave velocity that is thought to be most often related to systemic hypertension resulting in slow LV relaxation rate.[9] This may be deceiving in that a normal filling pattern in patients over 60 years of age may indeed represent a pseudonormal filling pattern.

Pulmonary venous flow can be measured using phase contrast cardiac MRI (Fig. 15.5) and can help differentiate between normal TMF and pseudonormalization. In such cases, a normal TMF pattern (where E > A) may actually be pseudonormalization. In patients with pseudonormal TMF, the duration of the pulmonary A wave will be longer than that of the mitral A wave.[10–12] The main advantage of cardiac MRI is that pulmonary venous flow (PVF) can be measured in virtually all cardiac MRI cases as opposed to only 68% of TTE cases due to improved image quality with cardiac MRI.[7]

Phase velocity cardiac MRI can be used to assess longitudinal myocardial velocities; these are comparable to those obtained by tissue Doppler imaging on TTE, although they are only validated in small sample sizes as of yet.[6] Midwall longitudinal fractional shortening has been shown to correlate with LV diastolic function and can also be reliably and easily measured by cardiac MRI.[13]

MYOCARDIAL STRAIN

Myocardial strain can be assessed by myocardial tagging, which is unique to cardiac MRI and essentially allows for visualization of myocardial deformation during contraction by use of magnetic labels with a rectangular or radial grid (Fig. 15.6). Tagging of these grids can be obtained every 20 msec, allowing for high temporal resolution. Myocardial tagging may allow for earlier recognition of subclinical diastolic dysfunction, as demonstrated by Edvarsen et al. in a study of 218

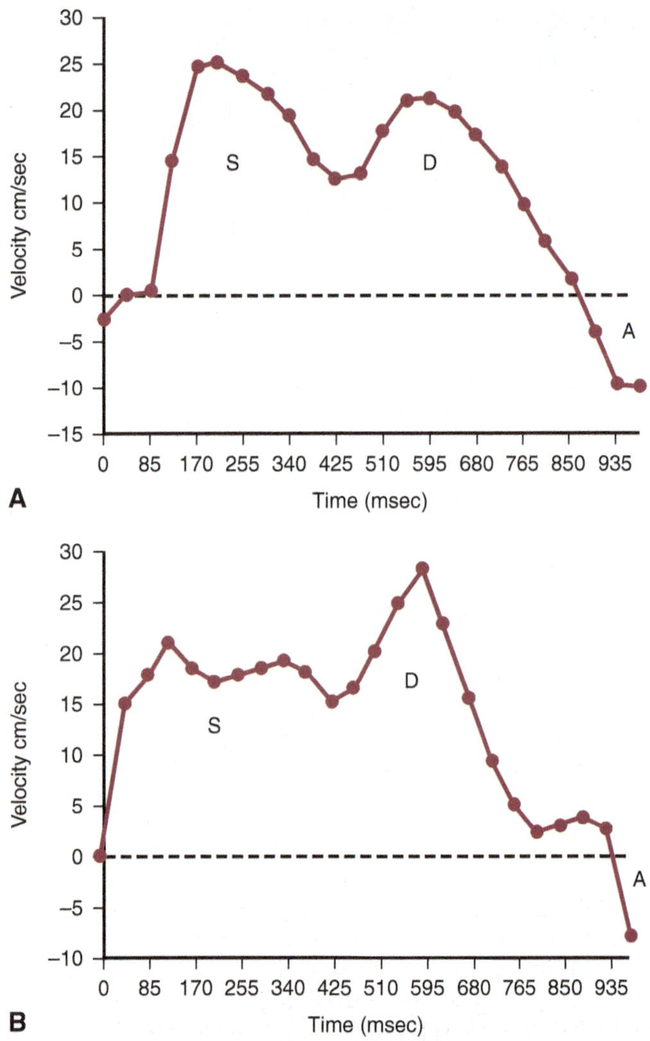

Fig. 15.5 Pulmonary venous flow assessment by echocardiography and cardiac MRI. (A) Transmitral inflow assessment by echocardiography. (B) Pulmonary venous flow assessment by echo. (C) Pulmonary flow by phase contrast cardiac MRI.

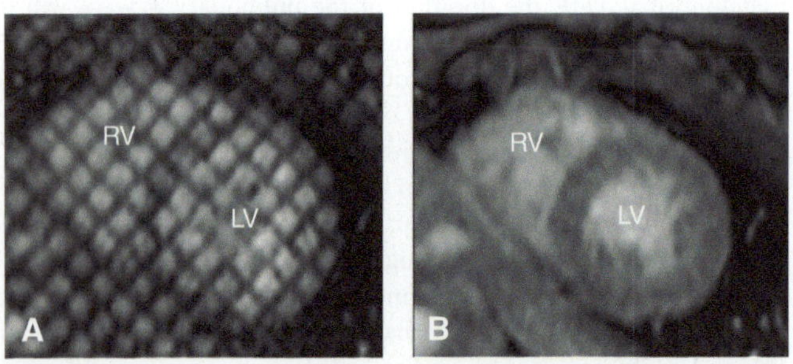

Fig. 15.6 Myocardial tagging in a healthy individual demonstrating normal patterns of myocardial deformation between end diastole (A) and end systole (B).

asymptomatic patients with LV hypertrophy (LVH) who were found to have regional diastolic dysfunction despite no clinical cardiovascular disease or LV dysfunction.[14] Several other methods for measuring myocardial strain have emerged recently, including strain-encoded imaging (SENC), phase velocity mapping, and deformation encoding with stimulated echoes (DENSE), and feature tracking with cine steady-state free precession (SSFP) imaging. Recently, left atrial (LA) function and strain have been recognized as important predictors of cardiovascular morbidity and mortality in patients with diastolic dysfunction.[15–17] Myocardial tracking can also be applied to the left atrium as well for quantification of LA function.[18,19] Early recognition may allow for aggressive risk factor modification and management to prevent progression of disease, although this has not been well established in clinical practice as of yet.

MAGNETIC RESONANCE SPECTROSCOPY

Magnetic resonance spectroscopy utilizes ^{31}P signals as opposed to H^1. This thereby allows for definition of regional adenosine triphosphate (ATP) and phosphocreatine (PCr) contents, which can be indirectly suggestive of energy status and viability of the myocardium.[20–22] Diastolic function is an active, energy-dependent process and therefore changes in PCr and ATP levels can be quantified by ^{31}P–cardiac MRI; altered high-energy phosphate metabolism has been associated with diastolic dysfunction.[23] Currently[19] the clinical utility of ^{31}P–cardiac MRI is limited by the low intrinsic signal-to-noise ratio of ^{31}P in humans, thereby making its acquisition technically demanding. Recent data using 7T cardiac MRI allowed for more precise quantification of the spectra when compared to conventional 3T, which may be useful in future practice.[24]

LATE GADOLINIUM ENHANCEMENT

Intravenous gadolinium-chelated contrast agents can be used to detect areas of fibrosis, often defined as late gadolinium enhancement (LGE), as the prolonged washout of the contrast correlates with a reduction in functional capillary density in the irreversibly injured myocardium. Myocardial fibrosis has a well-established role in the development and progression of both systolic and diastolic heart failure. LGE typically represents areas with replacement fibrosis or myocardial infarction, and the pattern of LGE can be useful in regard to identifying the underlying myocardial pathology (Fig. 15.7). Recent studies have indeed shown a correlation between LGE suggestive of fibrosis and diastolic dysfunction in various cardiovascular disease states.[25–27] The clinical significance of LGE in patients with diastolic dysfunction is yet to be determined, although hypertrophic cardiomyopathy (HCM) patients with LGE have worse outcomes than counterparts without LGE.[28–30]

QUANTITATIVE T1 MAPPING AND EXTRACELLULAR VOLUME MEASUREMENTS

Deposition of myocardial collagen results in diffuse myocardial fibrosis or myocyte replacement/replacement fibrosis.[31] Diffuse myocardial fibrosis can negatively impact diastolic filling and systolic function of the left ventricle. Recently there have been numerous studies demonstrating the utility and accuracy of quantifying myocardial fibrosis with T1 mapping and extracellular measurements in patients with heart failure with preserved ejection fraction (HFpEF), hypertensive heart disease, valvular heart disease, HCM, amyloidosis, and Fabry disease[32–38] (Fig. 15.8).

T1 times and extracellular volume measurements have been shown to correlate with diastolic dysfunction.[37,39,40]

DIFFUSION TENSOR IMAGING

Cardiac myocytes are organized into sheetlets, which are laminar microstructures that reorganize during cardiac systole from longitudinal to radial planes and thereby are thought to significantly contribute to LV wall thickening.[41,42] Although well established within

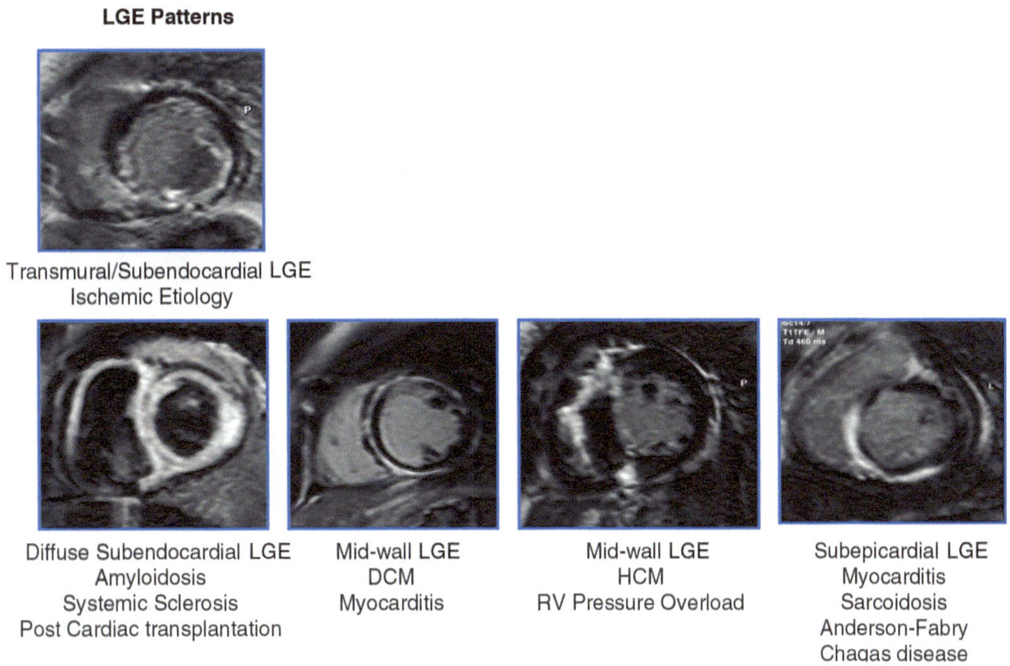

Fig. 15.7 Late Gadolinium Enhancement (LGE) patterns seen in common clinical conditions. If hyperenhancement is present, the endocardium should be involved in patients with ischemic disease. Isolated midwall, epicardial, or global hyperenhancement strongly suggests a nonischemic etiology

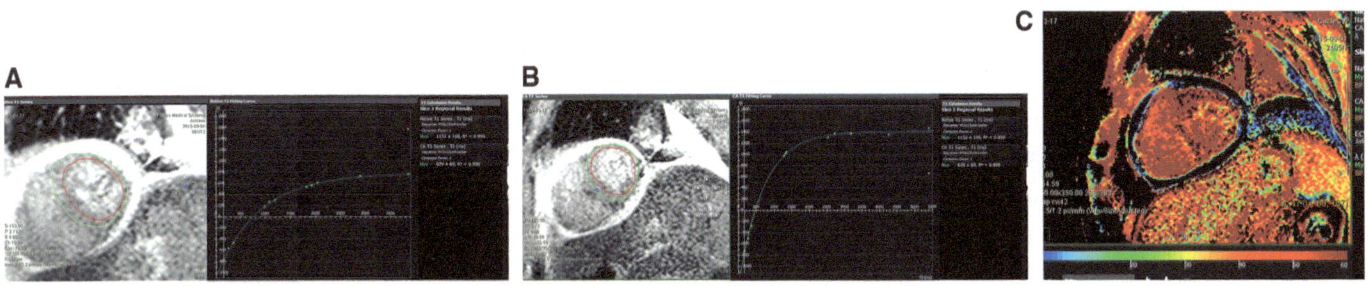

Fig. 15.8 Quantification of diffuse fibrosis using T1 mapping with cardiac MRI. (A) Precontrast T1 mapping images; (B) postcontrast T1 mapping images; (C) extracellular volume quantification.

the neuroimaging realm, cardiac diffusion tensor imaging (DTI) is a relatively new technique that allows for in vivo functional assessment of anisotropy and orientation of the sheetlets. Patients with HCM or ischemic heart disease may have altered tissue integrity that can be identified by DT-MRI.[43,44] (Fig. 15.9).

MR ELASTOGRAPHY

MR elastography is a technique that can measure myocardial shear wave amplitudes (SWA). The development of this technique was based on the principle that myocardial relaxation is related to decreases in the shear modulus, which is determined by the combination of active relaxation and passive stiffness. As such, shear modulus should serve as a marker for diastolic function. Recent data have shown that patients with diastolic dysfunction have significant reductions of SWA within the left ventricle[45–47] (Fig. 15.10).

FOUR-DIMENSIONAL FLOW

Four-dimensional (4-D) cardiac MRI is a specialized phase contrast cardiac MRI technique that allows for a more comprehensive evaluation of volumetric flow by enabling multidirectional and multidimensional image acquisition. Intracavitary LV blood flow kinetic energy, a marker of myocardial workload, can be semiautomatically quantified by 4-D cardiac MRI. A recent study demonstrated that kinetic energy parameters derived from 4-D cardiac MRI did indeed correlate with diastolic dysfunction but moreover demonstrated increased correlation with age.[48] Further studies are necessary to determine the clinical relevance of these findings (Fig. 15.11).

CLINICAL CORRELATION

Left Atrial Morphology and Function

Left atrial size and volume remain integral measurements in the evaluation of diastolic dysfunction and can be accurately performed in a reproducible manner with cardiac MRI. As previously discussed, LA pressure is directly affected by LV filling pressure during diastole. Increased LA pressure will result in LA dilation, which thereby serves as a marker of elevated LV filling pressures in patients with chronic diastolic dysfunction. LA enlargement is known to be a poor prognostic factor and thus serves as an important clinical tool in managing patients with diastolic dysfunction.[49–51]

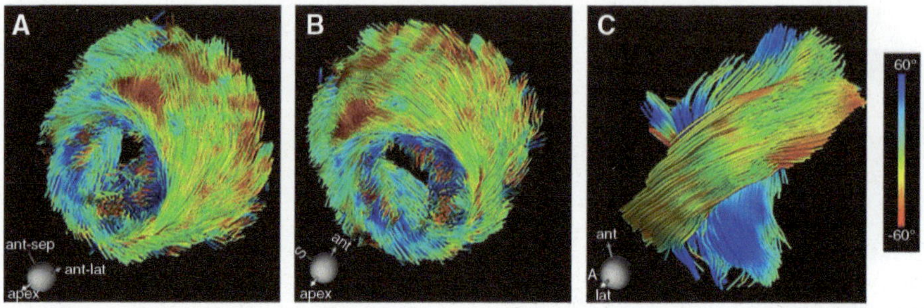

Fig. 15.9 High-resolution diffusion tensor imaging (DTI) tractography of the human heart in vivo. The images are of a healthy human volunteer imaged with the velocity-compensated pulse gradient spin echo (PGSE) sequence. (A, B) Coherent tracts with the correct orientation can be resolved in all regions of the myocardium. (Dispersion of hydroxyapatite [HA] over the papillary muscles and trabeculations of the left ventricle is a normal finding.) (C) Magnified view of fibers crossing a region of interest (ROI) in the midlateral wall of the left ventricle reveals the characteristic crossing pattern of myofibers in the subendocardium and subepicardium. *A,* Apex; *S,* septum. The higher signal-to-noise ratio (SNR) of the PGSE sequence enabled a resolution of $2 \times 2 \times 4$ mm^3 to be achieved, three times better than the resolution obtained with the stimulated echo (STE) approach. (From Mekkaoui C, Reese TG, Jackowski MP, et al. Diffusion MRI in the heart. *NMR Biomed.* 2017;30(3):e3426.)

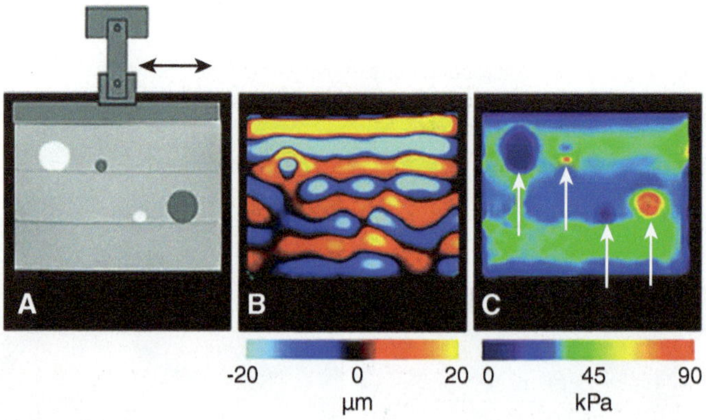

Fig. 15.10 Steps involved in magnetic resonance elastography (MRE). (A) A mechanical driver is used to introduce shear waves in the sample with soft *(bright)* and stiff *(dark)* inclusions. Shear waves are encoded into the phase image (B) obtained using an MRE sequence. Waves in the stiffer areas have longer wavelengths. An inversion algorithm is utilized to compute the stiffness map (C) using the phase image. (Khan S, Fakhouri F, Majeed W, et al. Cardiovascular magnetic resonance elastography: a review. *NMR Biomed.* 2018;31(10):e3853. doi:10.1002/nbm.3853.)

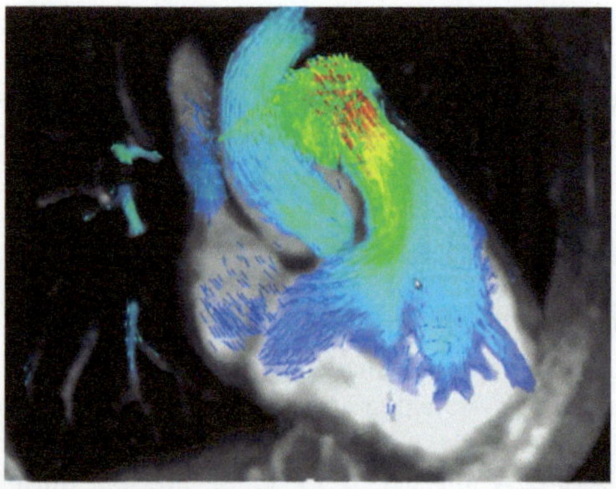

Fig. 15.11 4-D flow through the pulmonary artery.

Measurement of LA size and volume with cardiac MRI uses the same techniques as with TTE or computed tomography (CT) imaging, including the gold standard technique of Simpson's volumetric method or, alternatively, biplane area-length volumetry versus four-chamber planimetry.[52] It is important to note that cardiac MRI is considered the gold standard for quantifying LA volume and function, and can be an important tool in identifying the effects of diastolic dysfunction on the left atrium.[53–55] LA function can be quantified by various parameters, including left atrial strain; total left atrial emptying fraction (LAEF) [$100 \times$ (LAVmax – LAVmin)/LAVmax]; passive LAEF [$100 \times$ (LAVmax – LAVpre-a)/LAVmax]; and the active LAEF [$100 \times$ (LAVpre-A – LAVmin)/LAVpre-A]. Because several studies have demonstrated the prognostic importance of identifying abnormal LA size and function,[55–58] careful attention and dedicated assessment of the left atrium is an important part of evaluating diastolic function and the presence of cardiovascular disease (Fig. 15.12).

LV MASS

Increased LV mass has been independently associated with diastolic dysfunction and therefore is an important parameter in the evaluation of diastolic dysfunction.[59,60] This can be easily calculated using cine short axis views of the left ventricle to define the myocardial contours. Myocardial contouring is usually performed manually to determine LV volume, which is multiplied by myocardial density to yield the LV mass.

HYPERTROPHIC CARDIOMYOPATHY

Cardiac MRI has taken a much more prominent role in the diagnosis and management of patients with HCM, which is characterized as inappropriate myocardial hypertrophy without an alternative cause. It allows for differentiation of different forms of HCM, determination of obstructive versus nonobstructive disease, and prognostication. In addition, a significant proportion of patients with HCM can present with LV outflow obstruction in the absence of significant LVH. These patients typically have abnormal papillary muscle or mitral valve morphology, which are best identified by cardiac MRI.[61]

In patients with thickened myocardium, diastolic dysfunction is thought to be one of the initial and most prominent pathophysiologic mechanisms of clinical disease, manifesting as diastolic heart failure. These patients will often have a globally preserved or increased ejection fraction, but regional assessment with myocardial tagging via cardiac MRI has shown regional reduction in systolic wall thickening in hypertrophied areas.[62–64]

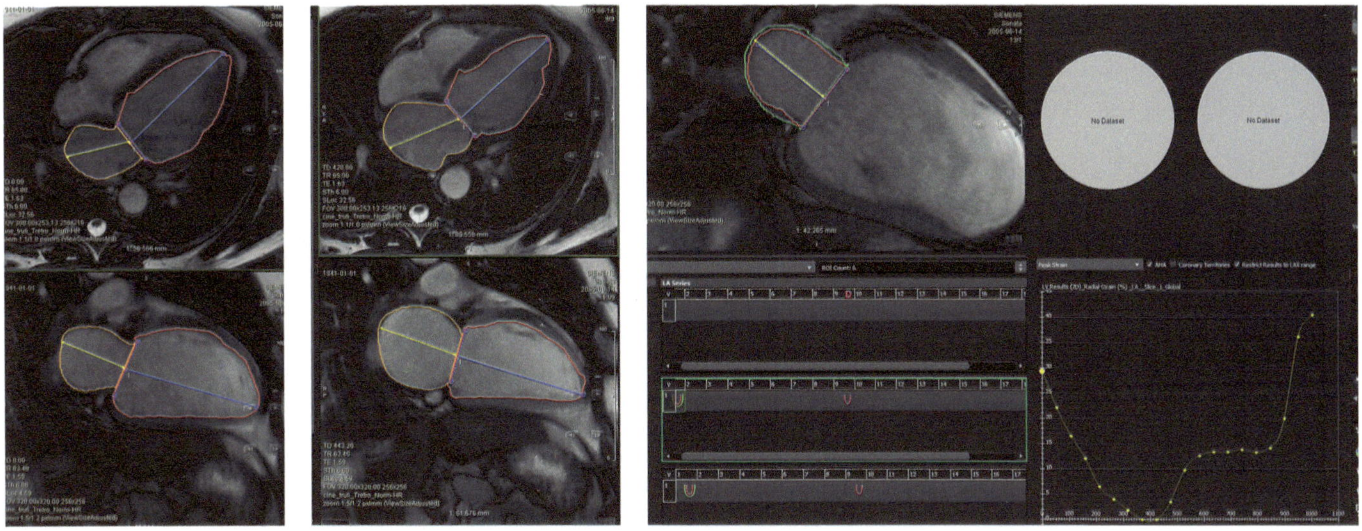

Fig. 15.12 Left atrial function and strain analysis. (A) Left atrial systole; (B) atrial diastole; (C) left atrial strain analysis.

Approximately 80% of HCM patients will have some degree of abnormal delayed enhancement when gadolinium is administered during cardiac MRI, even in those who are asymptomatic.[65,66] LGE usually is present in areas with hypertrophied myocardium and is typically seen in a patchy pattern with multiple foci predominating in the middle third of the ventricular wall and often notable near the insertion points of the RV free walls onto the interventricular septum. The clinical implication of deformation encoding (DE) in HCM patients has been established in numerous retrospective studies, whereby DE has been shown to portend an increased risk of sudden cardiac death or aborted sudden cardiac death.[28–30,67] Determining the severity of diastolic dysfunction in patients with HCM is challenging, particularly with cardiac MRI.

Recently myocardial elastography was shown to correlate with myocardial stiffness in patients with HCM and may become a clinically useful tool for quantifying diastolic function. The authors demonstrated significant positive correlation between myocardial stiffness by myocardial elastography and early diastolic peak/early diastolic mitral annular velocity, $r = 0.783$; early diastolic peak/transmitral flow propagation velocity, $r = 0.616$; LA volume index, $r = 0.623$; and with fibrosis markers in cardiac magnetic resonance (late gadolinium enhancement, $r = 0.804$; myocardial T1 precontrast, $r = 0.711$).[68]

However, currently quantifying the degree of diastolic function in patients with HCM remains challenging with the clinically available MRI protocols. Morphologic assessment of the extent of LVH and myocardial fibrosis are likely the most useful clinical correlates with the degree of diastolic dysfunction.[25,69]

Hypertension and Aortic Stenosis

Patients with uncontrolled hypertension or significant aortic stenosis develop organized LVH related to chronic LV pressure overload. While sarcomere organization is eccentric in patients with HCM, patients with hypertension and aortic stenosis develop new sarcomeres in parallel in an attempt to normalize wall tension, which results in concentric hypertrophy. This process can also alter the passive elastic properties and myocardial stiffness, resulting in diastolic dysfunction. Altered LV filling can be assessed using GRE sequences to identify early patterns of diastolic dysfunction such as prolonged time to PFR and an early filling percentage. These abnormalities in filling will be evident before changes in the transmitral flow pattern.[70] Reduced LA contractile function as calculated by cardiac MRI has been shown to be a poor prognostic factor in terms of cardiovascular risk in hypertensive patients, even in those without overt diastolic dysfunction.[71] In advanced hypertensive heart disease, the classic changes in TMF filling patterns will be evidence on phase contrast cardiac MRI, similar to that seen on TTE.[72]

^{31}P-MR spectroscopy can also reveal early changes with a reduced PCr/ATP ratio despite no evidence of LVH.[23] The clinical significance of this finding has not yet been established.

Myocardial tagging in these patients will often yield a prolonged LV untwisting time and, perhaps more clinically tangible, a reduction in regional strain in asymptomatic patients with LVH.[14,73]

Coronary Artery Disease

Diastolic dysfunction is often the earliest sign of myocardial ischemia and as such may often be underappreciated in patients with ischemic heart disease. Certainly, prior to the advent of cardiac MRI, it was an essentially unrecognized entity of patients with coronary artery disease (CAD). Diastolic filling patterns within this cohort will often be complex, related to the regional heterogeneity of myocardial function in ischemic, scarred, stunned, or hibernating areas. These regional changes in diastolic function can be accurately assessed using three-dimensional (3-D) tagging with cardiac MRI, which will typically reveal reduced regional strain most notable in the infarcted regions and delayed, prolonged, and nonuniform LV untwisting in infarcted or hibernating areas of myocardium.[74–77] This has been demonstrated in animal models as well, where normal untwisting was restored after reperfusion.[74]

Phase contrast imaging can also be used to assess for diastolic function in patients with established ischemic heart disease, wherein TMF patterns will be typical of other patients with diastolic dysfunction.[8]

Constrictive Pericarditis

Cardiac MRI provides excellent evaluation of the pericardium due to its excellent tissue characterization, multiplanar imaging, and superior contrast resolution. Cardiac MRI can provide a comprehensive assessment for patients with suspected pericardial disease, including T1-weighted and T2-weighted spin echo, GRE, and tagged cine

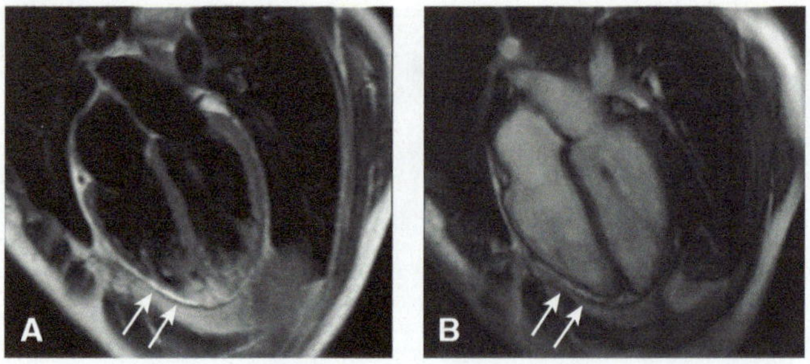

Fig. 15.13 Normal pericardium in a healthy individual, four-chamber view. (A) The pericardium appears as a thin band of low signal intensity *(black)* on a spin echo image. (B) The pericardium appears as a band of intermediate signal intensity *(grey)* on a gradient echo (GRE) image.

sequences to assess cardiac function and morphology, pericardial thickening and tethering, and presence of interventricular dependence. Normal pericardial thickness is typically 2 mm and best seen on T1/T2-weighted spin echo images, where the pericardium is seen as a thin rim of tissue between the mediastinal and epicardial fat. A pericardial thickness of 5 to 6 mm has a relatively high specificity for constrictive pericarditis.[78,79] Pericardial calcification or fibrosis will have low signal intensity and therefore appear black on spin echo images (Fig. 15.13). Because pericardial calcification is difficult to identify and distinguish from noncalcified thickened pericardium with cardiac MRI, CT imaging is the recommended imaging modality to identify and quantify the extent of pericardial calcification.

T2-weighted fat-suppressed spin echo and delayed enhancement imaging techniques can be used to assess for pericardial inflammation and edema in cases of suspected acute pericarditis (Fig. 15.14). Tissue characterization of the pericardium is of great clinical importance in determining the optimal treatment strategy for patients with constrictive pericarditis. Delayed hyperenhancement of the pericardium distinguished underlying acute pericarditis as the etiology of constrictive physiology versus chronic pericarditis, two entities that are managed differently.[80]

Cine tagged images can be used to evaluate for tethering or adhesion of the parietal pericardium to the visceral pericardium (Fig. 15.15). Conical deformity of the ventricles, diastolic tethering or restraint of any of the cardiac chambers, and a prominent diastolic bounce can also be seen on cine imaging due to the rapid and then abrupt cessation of filling during diastole, which are classic cardiac MRI findings in the setting of constrictive pericarditis. This respirophasic, interventricular-dependent filling can be identified on free-breathing cine sequences.[81]

Free-breathing cine GRE sequences are used for evaluation of interventricular dependence, whereby the interventricular septum will shift toward the left ventricle during inspiration and toward the right ventricle during expiration due to limited ability to expand in constrictive pericarditis (Fig. 15.16). This technique notably relies on patient cooperation for following instructions regarding adequate inspiratory effort. Similar to echocardiography, respirophasic flow across

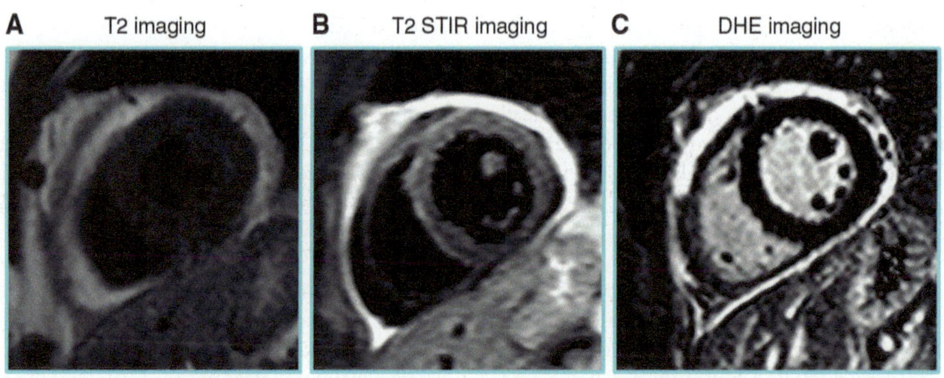

Fig. 15.14 Acute pericarditis. (A) Black blood T2 spin echo imaging demonstrating significant pericardial thickening. (B) T2 fat suppressed spin echo imaging demonstrates severe acute edema of the pericardium. (C) Late gadolinium enhancement imaging demonstrates severe inflammation of the pericardium.

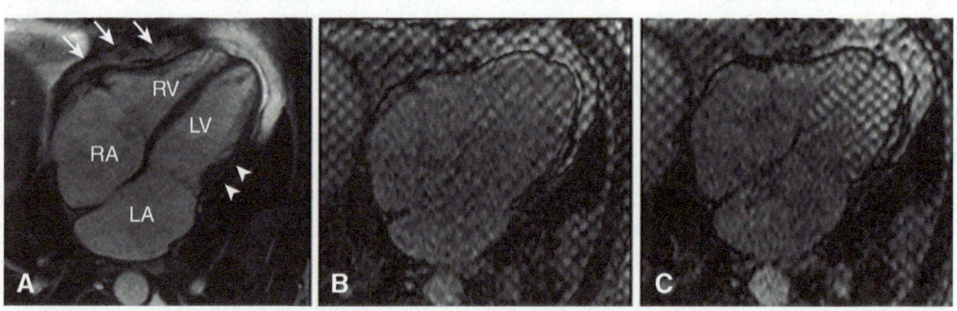

Fig. 15.15 Characteristic cardiac MRI findings in a patient with constrictive pericarditis. (A) Four-chamber gradient echo (GRE) image depicting the common tubular-shaped deformity of the ventricles and atrial dilatation. Note the thickened fibrous pericardium over the right ventricular free wall *(arrows)* and the darker area of calcified pericardium over the lateral wall of the left ventricle *(arrowheads)*. (B, C) Diastolic and systolic still frame from cine tagged four-chamber images shows the characteristic tethering of the pericardium to the epicardial surface during diastole. *LA,* Left atrium; *LV,* left ventrical; *RA,* right atrium; *RV,* right ventricle.

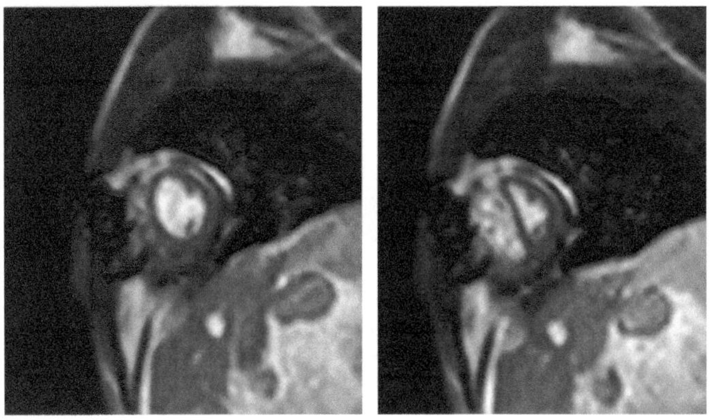

Fig. 15.16 Free-breathing cine sequence demonstrating septal flattening during inspiration in a patient with constrictive pericarditis. There is significant septal flattening during inspiration.

the mitral valve can also be assessed by real-time phase contrast imaging in spontaneously breathing patients. In a small study, respiratory variation greater than 25% across the mitral was highly sensitive and specific for identifying constrictive pericarditis.[82]

Restrictive Cardiomyopathy

By definition, all patients with restrictive cardiomyopathy will have evidence of diastolic dysfunction and restrictive filling patterns on all imaging modalities. This will be demonstrated on cardiac MRI cine tagged images, phase contrast cardiac MRI, LV filling curves, and ^{31}P-MR spectroscopy. Cardiac MRI can provide additional diagnostic utility in patients with restrictive cardiomyopathy by helping to establish the underlying etiology based on a pattern of functional and morphologic characteristics.

Cardiac Amyloidosis

Over 25 unique amyloidogenic proteins have been identified, but the frequency and severity of cardiac involvement can vary significantly among genotypes. Cardiac involvement can carry a significant prognostic and management impact and should therefore be identified as early as possible. LGE on cardiac MRI can identify early cardiac involvement of amyloidosis as demonstrated in one study where 47% of patients with known systemic amyloidosis were found to have cardiac involvement by cardiac MRI despite normal wall thickness on TTE.[83] However, typically there is diffuse deposition of the amyloid proteins throughout the cardiac structures, which can result in significant increase in thickness of the myocardium, atrial walls, interatrial septum, and occasionally valvular apparatus.

Patients with amyloidosis will typically demonstrate a diffuse pattern of LGE in a noncoronary distribution that is usually limited to subendocardial involvement[84] (Fig. 15.17). Additionally, native T1 measurements and electrochemical capacitance voltage (ECV) measurements can identify cardiac amyloidosis at earlier stages (Fig. 15.18) and provide powerful prognostic risk stratification in patients with both transthyretin amyloidosis and primary amyloidosis.[85,86]

Diastolic dysfunction results with increasing cardiac amyloid deposition, and Maceira et al. demonstrated a significant correlation with postcontrast T1 relaxation times and diastolic function (r = 0.42, p = 0.025).[84]

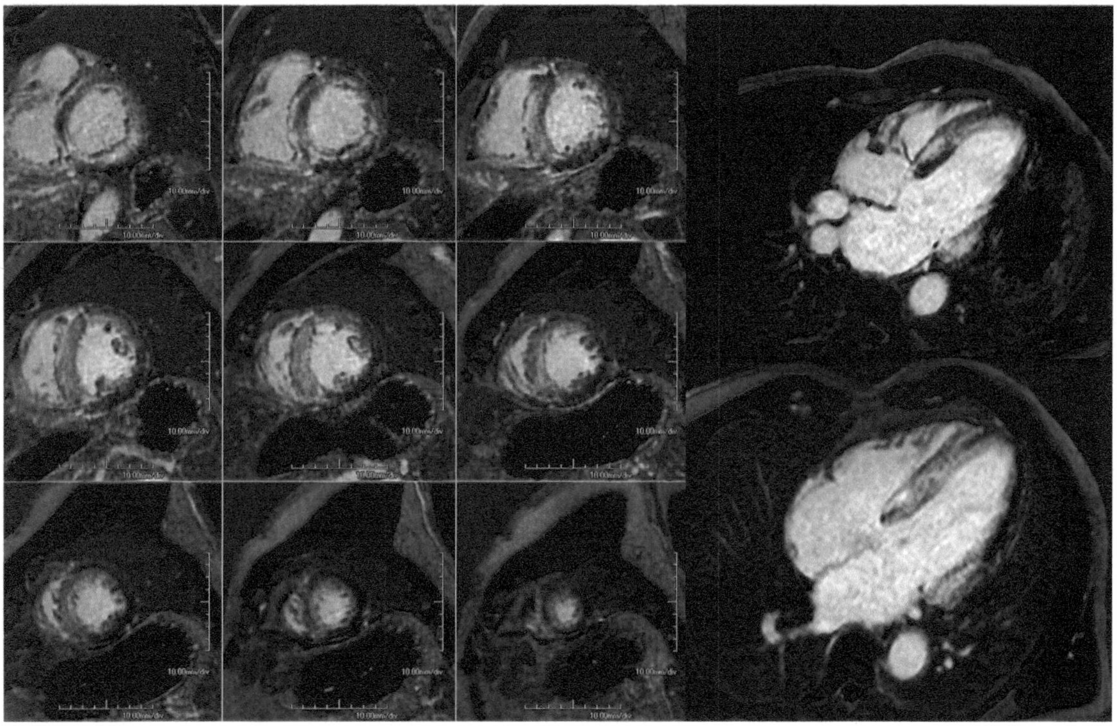

Fig. 15.17 A 64-year-old asymptomatic male with increased left ventricular wall thickness. Late gadolinium enhancement demonstrates diffuse gadolinium enhancement in a pattern suspicious for amyloidosis. The patient underwent endomyocardial biopsy and was found to have transthyretin (TTR) amyloidosis. (From Stegman BM, Kwon D, Rodriguez ER, et al. Left ventricular hypertrophy in a runner: things are not always what they seem. *Circulation* 2014;130(7):590–592. doi:10.1161/CIRCULATIONAHA.114.009362.)

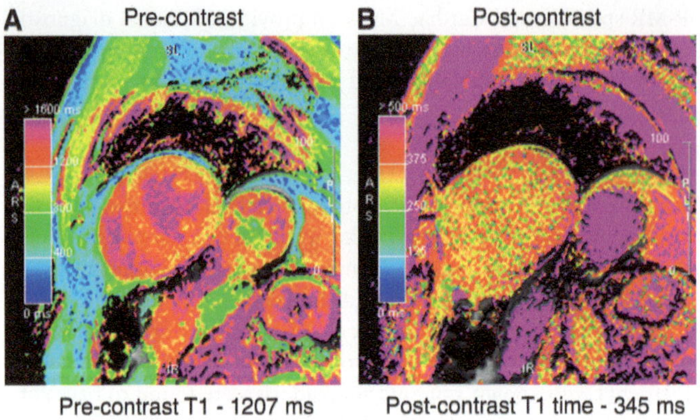

Fig. 15.18 Precontrast and postcontrast T1 mapping of the myocardium demonstrates markedly abnormal T1 times and expanded extracellular volume. (From Stegman BM, Kwon D, Rodriguez ER, et al. Left ventricular hypertrophy in a runner: things are not always what they seem. *Circulation* 2014;130(7):590–592. doi:10.1161/CIRCULATIONAHA.114.009362.)

Sarcoidosis

Approximately 5% of patients with systemic sarcoidosis are found to have clinically active cardiac involvement, while a further 20% of patients have evidence of cardiac involvement on autopsy.[87,88]

Cardiac MRI can help to identify active myocardial inflammation in patients with concern for clinically active disease. This will manifest as focal enhancements on T2-weighted spin echo images due to associated inflammation. Patchy LGE can be seen on delayed enhancement imaging in correlation with areas of caseating granulomas, which will thus be in a pattern of noncoronary distribution[89] (Fig. 15.19). LGE has been associated with an increased risk of adverse cardiac events, including death, within cardiac sarcoidosis patients.[90] In cases of chronic cardiac sarcoidosis, ventricular wall thinning and aneurysms may be more prominent features and most commonly involve the basal anteroseptal wall.

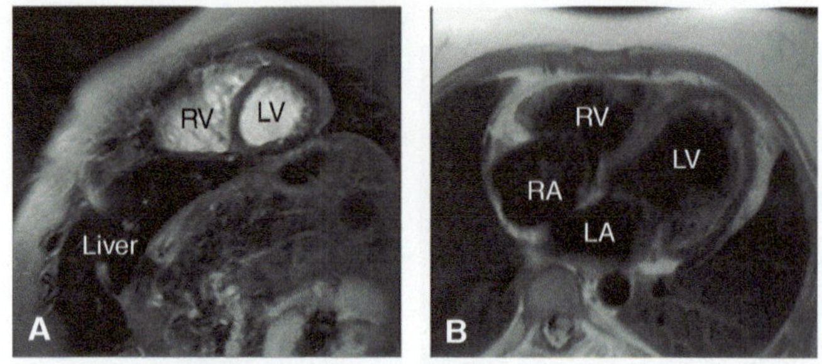

Fig. 15.20 Secondary hemochromatosis in a patient with iron overload due to recurrent blood transfusions for hereditary anemia. (A) Short axis gradient echo (GRE) image demonstrates the characteristic low signal over the liver due to accumulation of iron particles. (B) Axial T2-weighted spin echo image demonstrates the abnormally low signal intensity of the myocardium due to iron accumulation within myocardial tissue.

Hemochromatosis

Patients with myocardial iron overload are generally asymptomatic until advanced stages where global systolic dysfunction becomes the primary pathophysiologic mechanism. Cardiac MRI findings of hemochromatosis are generally less specific than for other restrictive cardiomyopathies. Restrictive diastolic filling is typically seen when there is cardiac involvement, and it typically precedes the development of systolic dysfunction.[91,92] In early stages, cardiac imaging will often demonstrate a dilated cardiomyopathy with increased LV wall thickness and LV end-diastolic volume, which will be evident on GRE sequences. The myocardium will appear dark on T2-weighted spin echo images as a result of loss of signal intensity due to iron accumulation (Fig. 15.20).

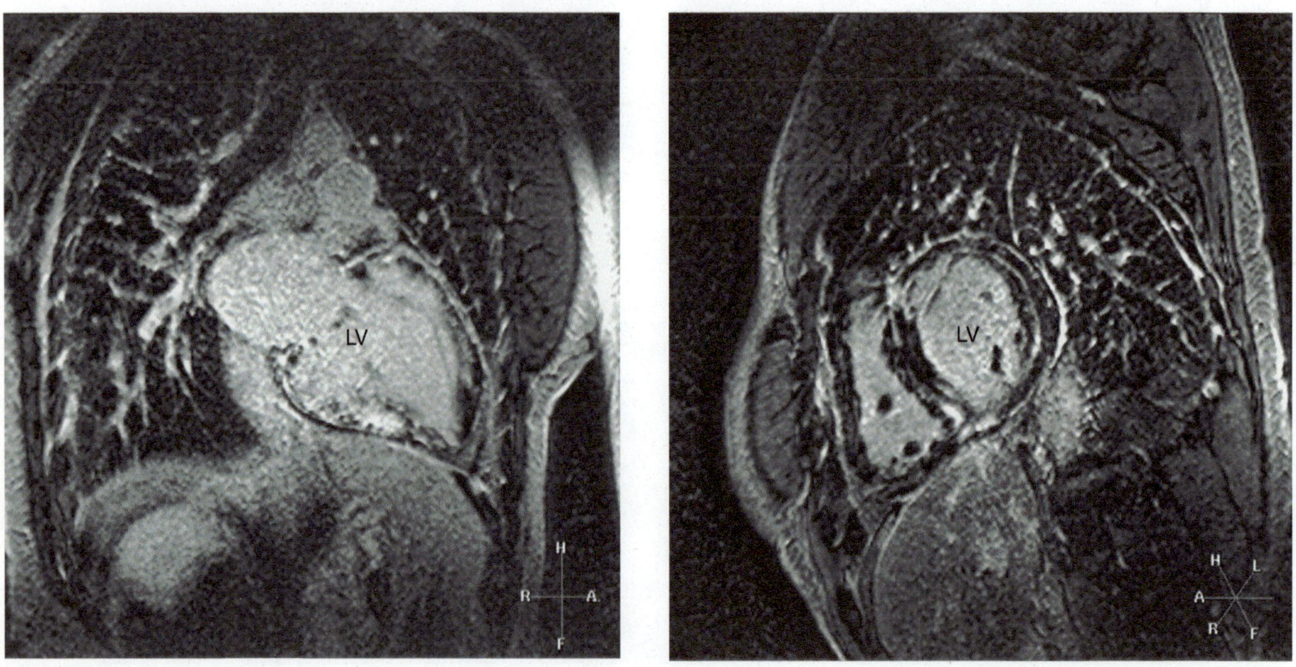

A

B

Fig. 15.19 Two-chamber (A) and midventricular short axis (B) late gadolinium enhancement images of a patient with cardiac sarcoidosis. Note the typical patchy pattern of hyperenhancement that occurs in a noncoronary distribution. Cine gradient echo (GRE) images *(not shown)* demonstrated reduced systolic function with regional wall motion abnormalities.

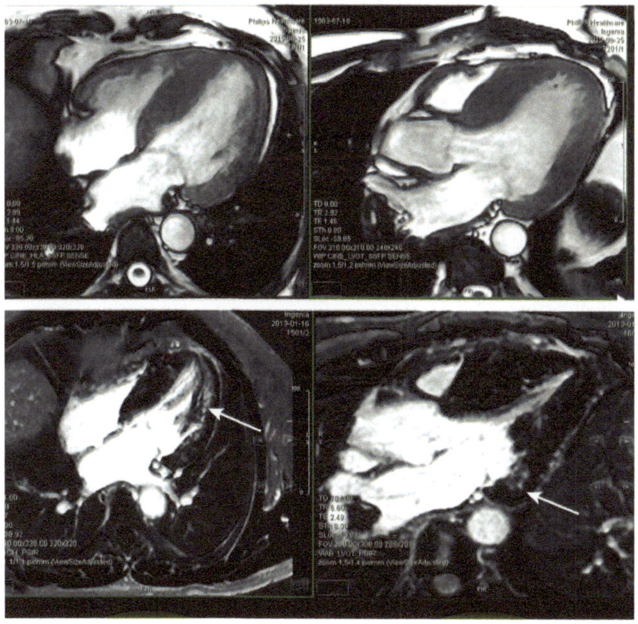

Fig. 15.21 A 27-year-old male with Fabry disease. (A) Steady-state free precession (SSFP) imaging demonstrating diffuse increased left ventricular thickness. (B) Late gadolinium enhancement demonstrating characteristic pattern of enhancement in the lateral wall *(arrows)*.

Fabry Disease

Fabry disease is an X-linked inherited disorder that is characterized by α-galactosidase A deficiency, a lysosomal enzyme, which leads to intracellular glycosphingolipid deposition in tissues, including the myocardium. LVH is a common manifestation of Fabry disease and can be difficult to differentiate from alternative etiologies of HCM, with significant implications for treatment options.

Fabry disease may result in prolonged T2 relaxation compared to those with HCM.[93] Concentric thickening will be evident on black blood imaging and inferolateral basal or midmyocardial fibrosis with subendocardial sparing on LGE[94] (Fig. 15.21). Finally, noncontrast T1 mapping can be significantly reduced in patients with Fabry disease when compared to both healthy controls and those with concentric hypertrophy, and this finding can be particularly useful in identifying the presence of Fabry disease.[95]

Friedreich Ataxia

Friedreich ataxia (FA) is an autosomal recessive mitochondrial disorder caused by deoxyribonucleic acid (DNA) triplet repeats of frataxin gene, which results in deficiency of the inner mitochondrial protein frataxin, leading to mitochondrial iron accumulation. Associated cardiomyopathy is the primary cause of mortality in patients with FA and is usually a result of end-stage heart failure or fatal arrhythmias.[96,97] FA results in HCM, often with preserved systolic function but impaired diastology.[98] LV mass in FA patients has been shown to directly correlate with GAA repeat number and age of disease onset.[99] Cardiac MRI may demonstrate myocardial fibrosis on LGE, although specific patterns of LGE distribution have not been established to differentiate FA from other hypertrophic cardiomyopathies.[100]

Glycogen Storage Disorders

Glycogen storage disorders (GSDs) are a broad classification of those diseases due to some degree of impairment of the metabolism or synthesis of glycogen. Cardiac involvement is common related to pathologic glycogen accumulation within the myocardium. Characteristic findings include significant LVH and areas of late gadolinium enhancement (Fig. 15.22).

LIMITATIONS AND CONTRAINDICATIONS OF CARDIAC MRI

Despite the expanding indications for cardiac MRI, it is important to recognize the limitations and contraindications for this imaging. While pacemakers and defibrillators previously were absolute contraindications, MRI conditional devices are now frequently being implanted. It is important to recognize that while it is safe to perform cardiac MRI in patients with these devices, the image quality and the artifact that arises from the device generator can result in significant image degradation and can significantly limit accurate or complete cardiac evaluation by cardiac MRI. Nonferromagnetic metallic devices include mechanical heart valves and sternal wires, which are safe to image although again may produce significant image artifact.

The ability for patients to follow instructions and hold their breath for 10 to 15 seconds is of critical importance to image quality. Furthermore, patients with claustrophobia may have difficulty tolerating the imaging procedure as they must reside within a small and confined space for 30 to 60 minutes. Moderate sedation can be used for patients with significant claustrophobia, but such sedation can alter the patient's ability to follow instruction and perform adequate breath holds. Arrhythmia will limit accuracy as well due to associated difficulty gating images postprocessing and inability to assess velocity or flow quantification by phase contrast cardiac MRI. Finally, patients should be carefully screened in regard to their renal function. Due to the risk of nephrogenic sclerosing fibrosis, patients with glomerular filtration rate (GFR) less than 30 should not be given gadolinium contrast agents; a decreased gadolinium dose should be given to patients with GFR between 30 and 60. Therefore it is important to carefully review the patient's clinical context and to determine if adequate imaging can be obtained safely.

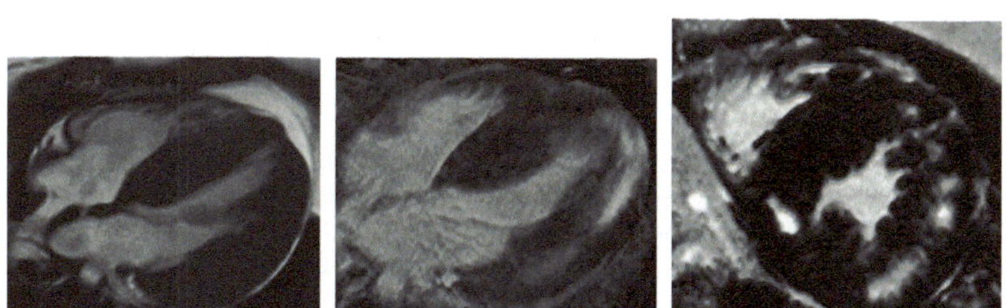

Fig. 15.22 A 19-year-old female with Danon disease. Severe concentric left ventricular hypertrophy (LVMi = 204 gm/m²; basal anteroseptum = 3.0 cm), with relative apical sparing. Severe late gadolinium enhancement in a midmyocardial distribution affecting distal anterior, apical and distal inferior wall segments, basal-to-distal lateral wall and inferoseptal wall segments, and the right ventricular insertion points, compatible with interstitial fibrosis.

FUTURE DIRECTIONS

There have been significant advancements in the role of cardiac MRI for the diagnosis of diastolic dysfunction over the past decades, with further techniques under development for clinical use. The field is continually expanding, and technology is constantly advancing. Further studies are needed to determine if MR elastography, diffusion tensor imaging, and 4-D flow will demonstrate incremental improvement in diagnostic abilities that will impact clinical management.

KEY POINTS

- Cardiac MRI offers excellent spatial and temporal resolution and can be used as an alternative modality to echo in the assessment of LV diastolic function.
- Gradient echo sequencing allows for calculation of the peak filling rate (PFR) and time to PFR, both of which will typically be prolonged in diastolic dysfunction.
- Phase contrast imaging can be used to measure transvalvular velocities and gradients. Transmitral flow and pulmonary venous flow can be useful in the identification of patients with diastolic dysfunction.
- Late gadolinium enhancement is a well-established marker of interstitial fibrosis and scarring, which plays a significant role in both systolic and diastolic dysfunctions. The pattern of myocardial LGE can be useful in identifying the underlying pathology.
- The use of cardiac MRI is contraindicated in patients with internal devices or implants that are ferromagnetic.

REVIEW QUESTIONS

The role of artificial intelligence for reproducible and quantitative reconstruction and advanced computation in interpretation and measurements of diastology is also an exciting prospect of this field but yet to be fully established.

1. Which of the following is an absolute contraindication for the patient in the chapter-opening case study to get a cardiac MRI?
   a. Coronary stents
   b. Permanent pacemaker
   c. Cochlear implant
   d. Mechanical heart valve
2. The case study patient's transmitral and pulmonary venous flow patterns are shown in Fig. 15.23. Which of the following statements is true?
   a. Both filling patterns are normal.
   b. The transmitral flow pattern is abnormal, and the pulmonary venous flow pattern is normal.
   c. The transmitral flow pattern is uninterpretable due to fused E and A waves, but the pulmonary venous flow pattern is abnormal suggestive of diastolic dysfunction.
   d. It is impossible to establish whether these patterns are normal with this information alone.

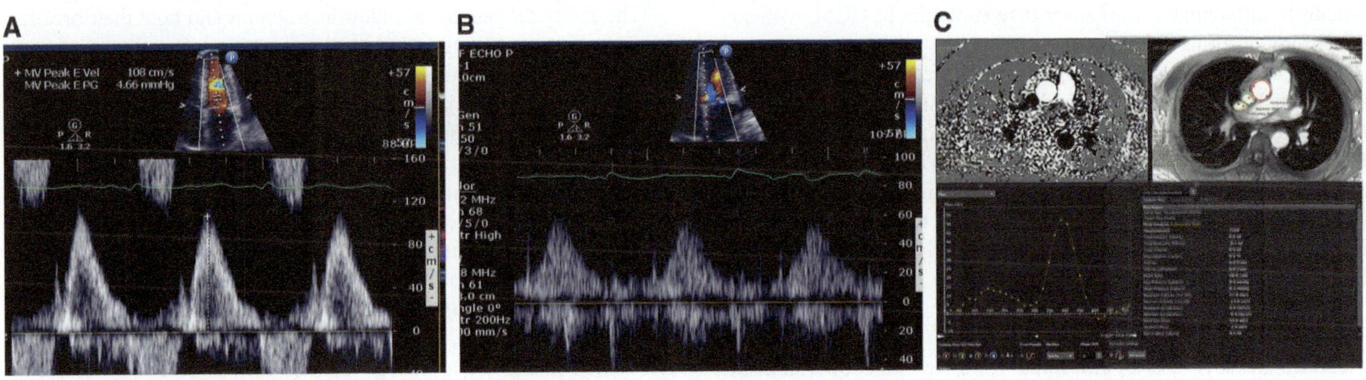

3. Intravenous gadolinium is given and the accompanying images are obtained (images showing patchy LGE). These findings are most suggestive of which diagnosis?
   a. Cardiac sarcoidosis
   b. Cardiac amyloidosis
   c. Ischemic cardiomyopathy
   d. Hypertrophic cardiomyopathy

REFERENCES

1. Grothues F, Smith GC, Moon JC, et al. Comparison of interstudy reproducibility of cardiovascular magnetic resonance with two-dimensional echocardiography in normal subjects and in patients with heart failure or left ventricular hypertrophy. *Am J Cardiol.* 2002;90(1):29–34.
2. Maceira AM, Prasad SK, Khan M, et al. Normalized left ventricular systolic and diastolic function by steady state free precession cardiovascular magnetic resonance. *J Cardiovasc Magn Reson.* 2006;8(3): 417–426.
3. Maceira AM, Cosin-Sales J, Roughton M, et al. Reference left atrial dimensions and volumes by steady state free precession cardiovascular magnetic resonance. *J Cardiovasc Magn Reson.* 2010;12:65.
4. Suzuki J, Caputo GR, Masui T, et al. Assessment of right ventricular diastolic and systolic function in patients with dilated cardiomyopathy using cine magnetic resonance imaging. *Am Heart J.* 1991;122(4 Pt 1):1035–1040.
5. Fujita N, Hartiala J, O'Sullivan M, et al. Assessment of left ventricular diastolic function in dilated cardiomyopathy with cine magnetic resonance imaging: effect of an angiotensin converting enzyme inhibitor, benazepril. *Am Heart J.* 1993;125(1):171–178.

6. Paelinck BP, de Roos A, Bax JJ, et al. Feasibility of tissue magnetic resonance imaging: a pilot study in comparison with tissue Doppler imaging and invasive measurement. *J Am Coll Cardiol.* 2005;45(7):1109–1116.
7. Rathi VK, Doyle M, Yamrozik J, et al. Routine evaluation of left ventricular diastolic function by cardiovascular magnetic resonance: a practical approach. *J Cardiovasc Magn Reson.* 2008;10:36.
8. Karwatowski SP, Brecker SJ, Yang GZ, et al. Mitral valve flow measured with cine MR velocity mapping in patients with ischemic heart disease: comparison with Doppler echocardiography. *J Magn Reson Imaging.* 1995;5(1):89–92.
9. Peverill RE, Chou B, Donelan L, et al. Possible mechanisms underlying aging-related changes in early diastolic filling and long axis motion-left ventricular length and blood pressure. *PLoS One.* 2016;11(6):e0158302.
10. Klein AL, Abdalla I, Murray RD, et al. Age independence of the difference in duration of pulmonary venous atrial reversal flow and transmitral A-wave flow in normal subjects. *J Am Soc Echocardiogr.* 1998;11(5):458–465.
11. Malkowski MJ, Guo R, Gray PG, et al. Is the pulmonary venous-transmitral A-wave duration difference altered by age and hypertension?. *Am J Cardiol.* 1995;76(10):722–724.
12. Rossvoll O, Hatle LK. Pulmonary venous flow velocities recorded by transthoracic Doppler ultrasound: relation to left ventricular diastolic pressures. *J Am Coll Cardiol.* 1993;(7):1687–1696.
13. Dusch MN, Thadani SR, Dhillon GS, et al. Diastolic function assessed by cardiac MRI using longitudinal left ventricular fractional shortening. *Clin Imaging.* 2014;38(5):666–668.
14. Edvardsen T, Rosen BD, Pan L, et al. Regional diastolic dysfunction in individuals with left ventricular hypertrophy measured by tagged magnetic resonance imaging--the Multi-Ethnic Study of Atherosclerosis (MESA). *Am Heart J.* 2006;151(1):109–114.
15. Posina K, McLaughlin J, Rhee P, et al. Relationship of phasic left atrial volume and emptying function to left ventricular filling pressure: a cardiovascular magnetic resonance study. *J Cardiovasc Magn Reson.* 2013;15:99.
16. Candan O, Ozdemir N, Aung SM, et al. Left atrial longitudinal strain parameters predict postoperative persistent atrial fibrillation following mitral valve surgery: a speckle tracking echocardiography study. *Echocardiography.* 2013;30(9): 1061–1068.
17. Hoit BD. Left atrial size and function: role in prognosis. *J Am Coll Cardiol.* 2014;63(6):493–505.
18. Kowallick JT, Kutty S, Edelmann F, et al. Quantification of left atrial strain and strain rate using cardiovascular magnetic resonance myocardial feature tracking: a feasibility study. *J Cardiovasc Magn Reson.* 2014;16:60.
19. Zareian M, Ciuffo L, Habibi M, et al. Left atrial structure and functional quantitation using cardiovascular magnetic resonance and multimodality tissue tracking: validation and reproducibility assessment. *J Cardiovasc Magn Reson.* 2015;17:52.
20. Friedrich J, Apstein CS, Ingwall JS. ^{31}P nuclear magnetic resonance spectroscopic imaging of regions of remodeled myocardium in the infarcted rat heart. *Circulation.* 1995;92(12):3527–3538.
21. Holloway CJ, Suttie J, Dass S, et al. Clinical cardiac magnetic resonance spectroscopy. *Prog Cardiovasc Dis.* 2011;54(3):320–327.
22. Bottomley PA, Wu KC, Gerstenblith G, et al. Reduced myocardial creatine kinase flux in human myocardial infarction: an in vivo phosphorus magnetic resonance spectroscopy study. *Circulation.* 2009;119(14):1918–1924.
23. Lamb HJ, Beyerbacht HP, van der Laarse A, et al. Diastolic dysfunction in hypertensive heart disease is associated with altered myocardial metabolism. *Circulation.* 1999;99(17):2261–2267.
24. Rodgers CT, Clarke WT, Snyder C, et al. Human cardiac 31P magnetic resonance spectroscopy at 7 Tesla. *Magn Reson Med.* 2014;72(2):304–315.
25. Motoyasu M, Kurita T, Onishi K, et al. Correlation between late gadolinium enhancement and diastolic function in hypertrophic cardiomyopathy assessed by magnetic resonance imaging. *Circ J.* 2008;72(3):378–383.
26. Moreo A, Ambrosio G, De Chiara B, et al. Influence of myocardial fibrosis on left ventricular diastolic function: noninvasive assessment by cardiac magnetic resonance and echo. *Circ Cardiovasc Imaging.* 2009;2(6): 437–443.
27. Nanjo S, Yoshikawa K, Harada M, et al. Correlation between left ventricular diastolic function and ejection fraction in dilated cardiomyopathy using magnetic resonance imaging with late gadolinium enhancement. *Circ J.* 2009;73(10):1939–1944.
28. Nojiri A, Hongo K, Kawai M, et al. Scoring of late gadolinium enhancement in cardiac magnetic resonance imaging can predict cardiac events in patients with hypertrophic cardiomyopathy. *J Cardiol.* 2011;58(3):253–260.
29. Weng Z, Yao J, Chan RH, et al. Prognostic value of LGE-CMR in HCM: a meta-analysis. *JACC Cardiovasc Imaging.* 2016;9(12):1392–1402.
30. Green JJ, Berger JS, Kramer CM, et al. Prognostic value of late gadolinium enhancement in clinical outcomes for hypertrophic cardiomyopathy. *JACC Cardiovasc Imaging.* 2012;5(4):370–377.
31. Mewton N, Liu CY, Croisille P, et al. Assessment of myocardial fibrosis with cardiovascular magnetic resonance. *J Am Coll Cardiol.* 2011;57(8):891–903.
32. Borbely A, van der Velden J, Papp Z, et al. Cardiomyocyte stiffness in diastolic heart failure. *Circulation.* 2005;111(6):774–781.
33. Zile MR, Baicu CF, Ikonomidis JS, et al. Myocardial stiffness in patients with heart failure and a preserved ejection fraction: contributions of collagen and titin. *Circulation.* 2015;131(14):1247–1259.
34. Aoki T, Fukumoto Y, Sugimura K, et al. Prognostic impact of myocardial interstitial fibrosis in non-ischemic heart failure. Comparison between preserved and reduced ejection fraction heart failure. *Circ J.* 2011;75(11):2605–2613.
35. Broadbent DA, Biglands JD, Larghat A, et al. Myocardial blood flow at rest and stress measured with dynamic contrast-enhanced MRI: comparison of a distributed parameter model with a Fermi function model. *Magn Reson Med.* 2013;70(6):1591–1597.
36. Flett AS, Hayward MP, Ashworth MT, et al. Equilibrium contrast cardiovascular magnetic resonance for the measurement of diffuse myocardial fibrosis: preliminary validation in humans. *Circulation.* 2010;122(2):138–144.
37. Iles L, Pfluger H, Phrommintikul A, et al. Evaluation of diffuse myocardial fibrosis in heart failure with cardiac magnetic resonance contrast-enhanced T1 mapping. *J Am Coll Cardiol.* 2008;52(19):1574–1580.
38. Sado DM, Flett AS, Banypersad SM, et al. Cardiovascular magnetic resonance measurement of myocardial extracellular volume in health and disease. *Heart.* 2012;98(19):1436–1441.
39. Mascherbauer J, Marzluf BA, Tufaro C, et al. Cardiac magnetic resonance postcontrast T1 time is associated with outcome in patients with heart failure and preserved ejection fraction. *Circ Cardiovasc Imaging.* 2013;6(6):1056–1065.
40. Su MY, Lin LY, Tseng YH, et al. CMR-verified diffuse myocardial fibrosis is associated with diastolic dysfunction in HFpEF. *JACC Cardiovasc Imaging.* 2014;7(10):991–997.
41. LeGrice IJ, Smaill BH, Chai LZ, et al. Laminar structure of the heart: ventricular myocyte arrangement and connective tissue architecture in the dog. *Am J Physiol.* 1995;269(2 Pt 2):H571–H582.
42. Hales PW, Schneider JE, Burton RA, et al. Histo-anatomical structure of the living isolated rat heart in two contraction states assessed by diffusion tensor MRI. *Prog Biophys Mol Biol.* 2012;110(2–3):319–330.
43. Wu MT, Tseng WY, Su MY, et al. Diffusion tensor magnetic resonance imaging mapping the fiber architecture remodeling in human myocardium after infarction: correlation with viability and wall motion. *Circulation.* 2006;114(10):1036–1045.
44. McGill LA, Ismail TF, Nielles-Vallespin S, et al. Reproducibility of in-vivo diffusion tensor cardiovascular magnetic resonance in hypertrophic cardiomyopathy. *J Cardiovasc Magn Reson.* 2012;14:86.
45. Elgeti T, Knebel F, Hattasch R, et al. Shear-wave amplitudes measured with cardiac MR elastography for diagnosis of diastolic dysfunction. *Radiology.* 2014;271(3):681–687.
46. Pernot M, Couade M, Mateo P, et al. Real-time assessment of myocardial contractility using shear wave imaging. *J Am Coll Cardiol.* 2011;58(1):65–72.
47. Kolipaka A, Araoz PA, McGee KP, et al. Magnetic resonance elastography as a method for the assessment of effective myocardial stiffness throughout the cardiac cycle. *Magn Reson Med.* 2010;64(3):862–870.
48. Crandon S, Westenberg JJM, Swoboda PP, et al. Impact of age and diastolic function on novel. 4D flow CMR biomarkers of left ventricular blood flow kinetic energy. *Sci Rep.* 2018;8(1):14436.
49. Abhayaratna WP, Seward JB, Appleton CP, et al. Left atrial size: physiologic determinants and clinical applications. *J Am Coll Cardiol.* 2006;47(12):2357–2363.

50. Tsang TS, Abhayaratna WP, Barnes ME, et al. Prediction of cardiovascular outcomes with left atrial size: is volume superior to area or diameter? *J Am Coll Cardiol.* 2006;7;47(5):1018–1023.
51. Pritchett AM, Jacobsen SJ, Mahoney DW, et al. Left atrial volume as an index of left atrial size: a population-based study. *J Am Coll Cardiol.* 2003;41(6):1036–1043.
52. Tops LF, van der Wall EE, Schalij MJ, et al. Multi-modality imaging to assess left atrial size, anatomy and function. *Heart.* 2007;93(11):1461–1470.
53. Whitlock M, Garg A, Gelow J, et al. Comparison of left and right atrial volume by echocardiography versus cardiac magnetic resonance imaging using the area-length method. *Am J Cardiol.* 2010;106(9):1345–1350.
54. Madueme PC, Mazur W, Hor KN, et al. Comparison of area-length method by echocardiography versus full-volume quantification by cardiac magnetic resonance imaging for the assessment of left atrial volumes in children, adolescents, and young adults. *Pediatr Cardiol.* 2014;35(4):645–651.
55. Hof IE, Velthuis BK, Van Driel VJ, et al. Left atrial volume and function assessment by magnetic resonance imaging. *J Cardiovasc Electrophysiol.* 2010;21(11):1247–1250.
56. Habibi M, Venkatesh BA, Lima JA. Feature tracking cardiac magnetic resonance imaging in the assessment of left atrial function. *J Am Coll Cardiol.* 2014;63(22):2434–2435.
57. Imai M, Ambale Venkatesh B, Samiei S, et al. Multi-ethnic study of atherosclerosis: association between left atrial function using tissue tracking from cine MR imaging and myocardial fibrosis. *Radiology.* 2014;273(3):703–713.
58. Markman TM, Habibi M, Venkatesh BA, et al. Association of left atrial structure and function and incident cardiovascular disease in patients with diabetes mellitus: results from multi-ethnic study of atherosclerosis (MESA). *Eur Heart J Cardiovasc Imaging.* 2017;18(10):1138–1144.
59. Lim YH, Lee JU, Kim KS, et al. Association between inappropriateness of left ventricular mass and left ventricular diastolic dysfunction: a study using the tissue Doppler parameter, e/e'. *Korean Circ J.* 2009;39(4):138–144.
60. de Simone G, Kitzman DW, Palmieri V, et al. Association of inappropriate left ventricular mass with systolic and diastolic dysfunction: the HyperGEN study. *Am J Hypertens.* 2004;17(9):828–833.
61. Patel P, Dhillon A, Popovic ZB, et al. Left ventricular outflow tract obstruction in hypertrophic cardiomyopathy patients without severe septal hypertrophy: implications of mitral valve and papillary muscle abnormalities assessed using cardiac magnetic resonance and echocardiography. *Circ Cardiovasc Imaging.* 2015;8(7):e003132.
62. Arrive L, Assayag P, Russ G, et al. MRI and cine MRI of asymmetric septal hypertrophic cardiomyopathy. *J Comput Assist Tomogr.* 1994;18(3):376–382.
63. van Dockum WG, Kuijer JP, Gotte MJ, et al. Septal ablation in hypertrophic obstructive cardiomyopathy improves systolic myocardial function in the lateral (free) wall: a follow-up study using CMR tissue tagging and 3D strain analysis. *Eur Heart J.* 2006;27(23):2833–2839.
64. Soler R, Rodriguez E, Monserrat L, et al. Magnetic resonance imaging of delayed enhancement in hypertrophic cardiomyopathy: relationship with left ventricular perfusion and contractile function. *J Comput Assist Tomogr.* 2006;30(3):412–420.
65. Moon JC, McKenna WJ, McCrohon JA, et al. Toward clinical risk assessment in hypertrophic cardiomyopathy with gadolinium cardiovascular magnetic resonance. *J Am Coll Cardiol.* 2003;41(9):1561–1567.
66. Choudhury L, Mahrholdt H, Wagner A, et al. Myocardial scarring in asymptomatic or mildly symptomatic patients with hypertrophic cardiomyopathy. *J Am Coll Cardiol.* 2002;40(12):2156–2164.
67. He D, Ye M, Zhang L, et al. Prognostic significance of late gadolinium enhancement on cardiac magnetic resonance in patients with hypertrophic cardiomyopathy. *Heart Lung.* 2018;47(2):122–126.
68. Villemain O, Correia M, Mousseaux E, et al. Myocardial stiffness evaluation using noninvasive shear wave imaging in healthy and hypertrophic cardiomyopathic adults. *JACC Cardiovasc Imaging.* 2018;00.
69. Finocchiaro G, Haddad F, Pavlovic A, et al. How does morphology impact on diastolic function in hypertrophic cardiomyopathy? A single centre experience. *BMJ Open.* 2014;4(6):e004814.
70. Hartiala JJ, Foster E, Fujita N, et al. Evaluation of left atrial contribution to left ventricular filling in aortic stenosis by velocity-encoded cine MRI. *Am Heart J.* 1994;127(3): 593–600.
71. Kaminski M, Steel K, Jerosch-Herold M, et al. Strong cardiovascular prognostic implication of quantitative left atrial contractile function assessed by cardiac magnetic resonance imaging in patients with chronic hypertension. *J Cardiovasc Magn Reson.* 2011;13:42.
72. Kudelka AM, Turner DA, Liebson PR, et al. Comparison of cine magnetic resonance imaging and Doppler echocardiography for evaluation of left ventricular diastolic function. *Am J Cardiol.* 1997;80(3):384–386.
73. Nagel E, Stuber M, Burkhard B, et al. Cardiac rotation and relaxation in patients with aortic valve stenosis. *Eur Heart J.* 2000;21(7):582–589.
74. Kroeker CA, Tyberg JV, Beyar R. Effects of ischemia on left ventricular apex rotation. An experimental study in anesthetized dogs. *Circulation.* 1995;92(12):3539–3548.
75. Garot J, Pascal O, Diebold B, et al. Alterations of systolic left ventricular twist after acute myocardial infarction. *Am J Physiol Heart Circ Physiol.* 2002;282(1):H357–H362.
76. Nagel E, Stuber M, Lakatos M, et al. Cardiac rotation and relaxation after anterolateral myocardial infarction. *Coron Artery Dis.* 2000;11(3):261–267.
77. Bogaert J, Bosmans H, Maes A, et al. Remote myocardial dysfunction after acute anterior myocardial infarction: impact of left ventricular shape on regional function: a magnetic resonance myocardial tagging study. *J Am Coll Cardiol.* 2000;35(6):1525–1534.
78. Maisch B, Seferovic PM, Ristic AD, et al. Guidelines on the diagnosis and management of pericardial diseases executive summary; the task force on the diagnosis and management of pericardial diseases of the European society of cardiology. *Eur Heart J.* 2004;25(7):587–610.
79. Soulen RL, Stark DD, Higgins CB. Magnetic resonance imaging of constrictive pericardial disease. *Am J Cardiol.* 1985;55(4):480–484.
80. Feng D, Glockner J, Kim K, et al. Cardiac magnetic resonance imaging pericardial late gadolinium enhancement and elevated inflammatory markers can predict the reversibility of constrictive pericarditis after anti-inflammatory medical therapy: a pilot study. *Circulation.* 2011;124(17): 1830–1837.
81. Francone M, Dymarkowski S, Kalantzi M, et al. Assessment of ventricular coupling with real-time cine MRI and its value to differentiate constrictive pericarditis from restrictive cardiomyopathy. *Eur Radiol.* 2006;16(4):944–951.
82. Thavendiranathan P, Verhaert D, Walls MC, et al. Simultaneous right and left heart real-time, free-breathing CMR flow quantification identifies constrictive physiology. *JACC Cardiovasc Imag.* 2012;5(1):15–24.
83. Syed IS, Glockner JF, Feng D, et al. Role of cardiac magnetic resonance imaging in the detection of cardiac amyloidosis. *JACC Cardiovasc Imag.* 2010;3(2):155–164.
84. Maceira AM, Joshi J, Prasad SK, et al. Cardiovascular magnetic resonance in cardiac amyloidosis. *Circulation.* 2005;111(2):186–193.
85. Fontana M, Pica S, Reant P, et al. Prognostic value of late gadolinium enhancement cardiovascular magnetic resonance in cardiac amyloidosis. *Circulation.* 2015;132(16):1570–1579.
86. Martinez-Naharro A, Treibel TA, Abdel-Gadir A, et al. Magnetic resonance in transthyretin cardiac amyloidosis. *J Am Coll Cardiol.* 2017;70(4):466–477.
87. Iwai K, Tachibana T, Takemura T, et al. Pathological studies on sarcoidosis autopsy. I. Epidemiological features of 320 cases in Japan. *Acta Pathol Jpn.* 1993;43(7–8):372–376.
88. Perry A, Vuitch F. Causes of death in patients with sarcoidosis. A morphologic study of 38 autopsies with clinicopathologic correlations. *Arch Pathol Lab Med.* 1995;119(2):167–172.
89. Ichinose A, Otani H, Oikawa M, et al. MRI of cardiac sarcoidosis: basal and subepicardial localization of myocardial lesions and their effect on left ventricular function. *AJR Am J Roentgenol.* 2008;191(3):862–869.
90. Greulich S, Deluigi CC, Gloekler S, et al. CMR imaging predicts death and other adverse events in suspected cardiac sarcoidosis. *JACC Cardiovasc Imag.* 2013;6(4):501–511.
91. Benson LP, Olivieri N, Rose V, et al. Left ventricular function in young adults with thalassemia. *Circulation.* 1989;80:274.
92. Liu SJ, Collins A, Olivieri N. Is there a predictable relationship between ventricular function and myocardial iron levels in patients with hemochromatosis. *Circulation.* 1993;88:183.
93. Imbriaco M, Spinelli L, Cuocolo A, et al. MRI characterization of myocardial tissue in patients with Fabry's disease. *AJR Am J Roentgenol.* 2007;188(3):850–853.

94. Deva DP, Hanneman K, Li Q, et al. Cardiovascular magnetic resonance demonstration of the spectrum of morphological phenotypes and patterns of myocardial scarring in Anderson-Fabry disease. *J Cardiovasc Magn Reson.* 2016;18:14.
95. Thompson RB, Chow K, Khan A, et al. T(1) mapping with cardiovascular MRI is highly sensitive for Fabry disease independent of hypertrophy and sex. *Circ Cardiovasc Imag.* 2013;6(5):637–645.
96. Bourke T, Keane D. Friedreich's ataxia: a review from a cardiology perspective. *Ir J Med Sci.* 2011;180(4):799–805.
97. Tsou AY, Paulsen EK, Lagedrost SJ, et al. Mortality in Friedreich ataxia. *J Neurol Sci.* 2011;307(1–2):46–49.
98. Dutka DP, Donnelly JE, Palka P, et al. Echocardiographic characterization of cardiomyopathy in Friedreich's ataxia with tissue Doppler echocardiographically derived myocardial velocity gradients. *Circulation.* 2000;102(11):1276–1282.
99. Rajagopalan B, Francis JM, Cooke F, et al. Analysis of the factors influencing the cardiac phenotype in Friedreich's ataxia. *Mov Disord.* 2010;25(7):846–852.
100. Mehta N, Chacko P, Jin J, et al. Serum versus imaging biomarkers in Friedreich ataxia to indicate left ventricular remodeling and outcomes. *Tex Heart Inst J.* 2016;43(4):305–310.

16

Evaluation of Diastolic Function by Radionuclide Techniques

Aldo L. Schenone, Wael A. Jaber, and Manuel D. Cerqueira

OUTLINE

Case Study

A 73-year-old man with a history of longstanding hypertension, diabetes mellitus, paroxysmal atrial fibrillation, and coronary artery disease (CAD) presents with progressive shortness of breath and exertional fatigue. Physical examination is notable for prominent apical impulse and a blood pressure of 140/90 mmHg. A transthoracic echocardiogram reported normal systolic function and concentric hypertrophy without significant valvular disease or regional wall motion abnormalities. An ischemic workup performed with a single-photon emission computed tomography (SPECT) stress test revealed ejection fractions of 0.67 at rest and 0.68 at stress without perfusion defects. However, the resting time-activity curve (TAC) showed a profoundly abnormal filling pattern (Fig. 16.1A), with a peak filling rate of 1.67 end-diastolic volume per second (EDV/sec) and a delayed time to maximal rate of 305 msec. Upon comparison to a SPECT perfusion study 1 year prior (see Fig. 16.1B), there is evidence of interval development of diastolic dysfunction with shifting of the diastolic curve to the left from a normal diastolic curve despite preserved systolic function.

Based on age and presence of concentric hypertrophy with interval development of diastolic dysfunction in the absence of ischemia on a radionuclide myocardial perfusion study, amyloid was considered in the differential diagnosis. A technetium (^{99m}Tc) pyrophosphate scan was performed with results consistent with transthyretin (TTR) cardiac amyloidosis (see Fig. 16.1C). Although the evaluation of diastolic function during perfusion studies is seldom conducted in clinical practice, this case illustrates the potential incremental benefit of such evaluation in selected patients undergoing ischemic evaluation with myocardial perfusion studies.

INTRODUCTION

The use of radioactive tracers in nuclear cardiology has been instrumental in the evaluation of patients with known or suspected cardiac disease. The majority of applications have been in the assessment of myocardial perfusion. These tracers can also be used to assess systolic and diastolic ventricular function in the following ways: injected as a bolus and tracked during first pass through the vascular system, attached to red blood cells and measured once in equilibrium within the vascular space, or as myocardial perfusion tracers that define the endocardial borders of the left ventricle.[1]

Historically equilibrium radionuclide angiocardiography (ERNA) and first-pass radionuclide angiography (FPRNA) were commonly used techniques for the evaluation of systolic and diastolic function both at rest and following exercise. The advantages of these modalities included absolute quantitation, high accuracy and reproducibility, and measurements based on true three-dimensional (3-D) measurements that were free of geometric assumptions. However, these techniques were time consuming, technically challenging, and not practical in most clinical settings. Optimal performance was achieved using single-headed, small field-of-view gamma cameras that are not currently widely available. The use of dual-headed, large field-of-view systems does not allow optimal, consistent isolation of the left ventricle. Thus they fell in disfavor and were overshadowed by the practicality and lack of radiation exposure of echocardiography in spite of an increase in interobserver variability and lower accuracy.[2]

Many of the concepts and methods developed for diastolic function analysis with ERNA and FPRNA may be adjunctively applied to electrocardiogram (ECG)–gated radionuclide myocardial perfusion

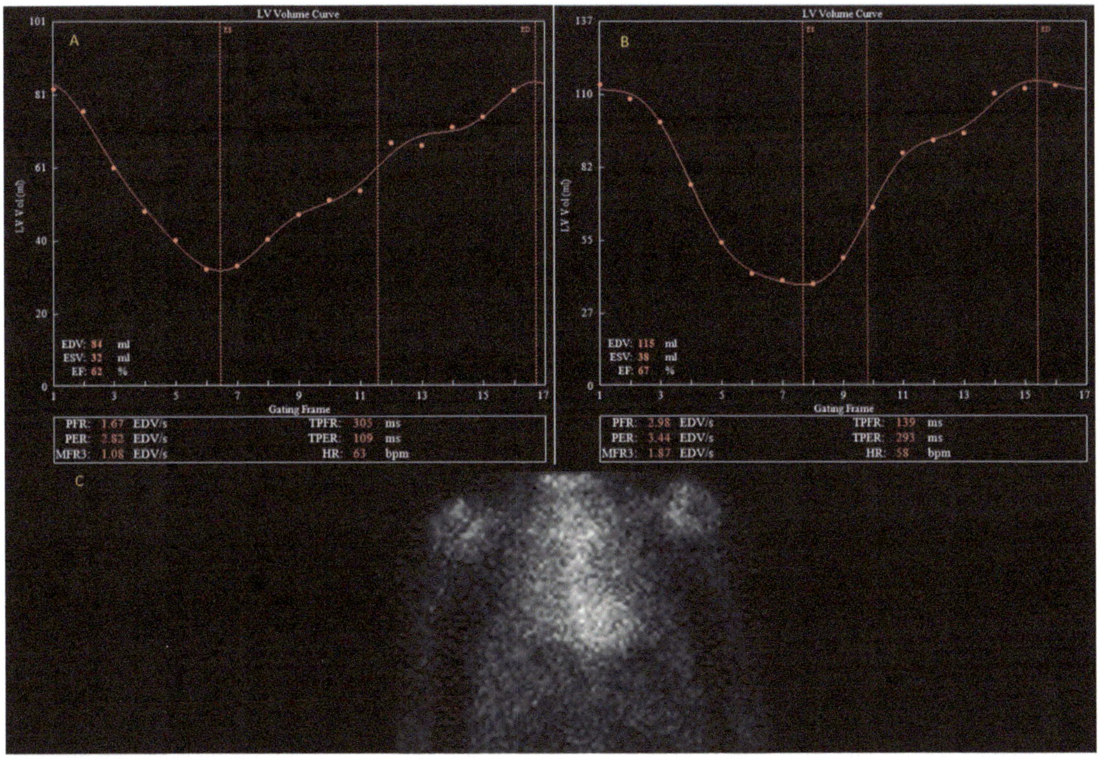

Fig. 16.1 (A) Resting time-activity curve (TAC) obtained on single-photon emission computed tomography (SPECT) perfusion study revealing a marked reduction in the peak filling rate (PFR) of 1.67 end-diastolic volume (EDV)/sec with a delayed time to maximal rate (TPFR) of 305 msec. (B) Resting TAC from a previous SPECT perfusion study 1 year prior exhibiting normal diastolic filling parameter with PFR of 2.98 EDV/sec and TPFR of 139 msec. (C) Technetium (^{99m}Tc) pyrophosphate scan revealing a cardiac silhouette with an elevated tracer retention exhibiting heart to contralateral chest (H/CL) ratio above 1.5 consistent with the diagnosis of transthyretin (TTR) cardiac amyloidosis.

imaging studies performed with SPECT or positron emission tomography (PET) tracers in the current era.[3,4] These may provide incremental and useful clinical data to the assessment of perfusion and systolic function. In some circumstances, diastolic dysfunction may even identify preclinical abnormalities in the absence of alterations of systolic function.[5–7]

This chapter will describe the concepts and methods of ERNA, FPRNA, and ECG-gated perfusion imaging to obtain diastolic information. It will also describe clinically useful diastolic findings obtained with these techniques resulting from abnormalities of the myocardium and ischemia.

BASIC PRINCIPLES OF RADIONUCLIDE ASSESSMENT OF DIASTOLIC FUNCTION

The radionuclide assessment of systolic and diastolic left ventricular (LV) function requires the generation of a curve plotting the changes in radioactivity over time, which is proportional to changes in LV volume over time (Fig. 16.2). From this time-activity curve, the first derivative is obtained, which measures the rate of volume change over time expressed in EDV/sec.[8]

The left side of the TAC prior to end systole (ES in Fig. 16.2) provides information on the systolic function of the ventricle, including peak emptying rate and time to peak emptying rate. For ventricles with muscle damage or infiltration, or ischemia, the rate of emptying is decreased with prolongation of the time when the peak emptying rate is achieved. Diastole is represented to the right of end systole in Fig. 16.2 and is a much more complicated process, which consists of four distinct phases: isovolumic relaxation, early diastolic filling, diastasis, and atrial systole.[7]

Isovolumic relaxation starts at end systole, is an energy-dependent process, and has a short duration (usually <50 msec). Early diastolic filling is the next phase. The rate of volume change over time during this phase is used to calculate (1) the most rapid ventricular filling, namely peak filling rate (PFR), and (2) the time elapsed until the occurrence of such PFR, called time to peak filling rate (TPFR) (Box 16.1). The PFR is normalized to EDV/sec and is greater than 2.5 under

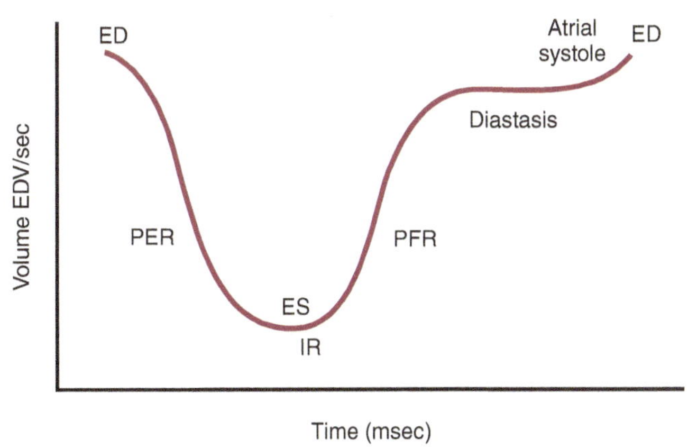

Fig. 16.2 The relationship between LV volume over time and the derived systolic and diastolic parameters. *ED,* End diastole; *EDV,* end-diastolic volume; *ES,* end systole; *IR,* isovolumic relaxation; *PER,* peak ejection rate; *PFR,* peak filling rate.

BOX 16.1 Important Radionuclide Parameters of Diastolic Function and Normal Values

1. Peak filling rate (PFR) (>2.5 end-diastolic volume/sec)
2. Time to peak filling rate (TPFR) (<180 msec)
3. Filling fraction (>69% during rapid filling)
4. A/E ratio <1:4

normal conditions. PFR is a very sensitive marker of diastolic function; however, it has been shown to be rapid in young and healthy hearts but declines in the elderly, even in the absence of pathology.[9,10] This parameter also varies with gender, heart rate, and left ventricular ejection fraction (LVEF). In contrast, TPFR is a more consistent measure of diastolic function less affected by these factors.[11] In normal ventricles, TPFR is less than 180 msec. In addition, there have also been attempts to look at the percent of EDV accumulated during the rapid filling phase as an indicator of disease. Generally, more than 69% of the EDV should be accumulated during the rapid filling portion; otherwise the presence of diastolic dysfunction is suggested.[7]

Following the rapid filling phase, diastasis ensues with minimal changes in volume. This phase is well appreciated only at lower heart rates and is followed by a distinct atrial phase. The PFR both during the early filling phase and atrial kick phase has been shown to correspond to the mitral inflow E and A waves of Doppler echocardiography. Thus they can be used to calculate an E/A ratio similar to that obtained by echocardiography. For nuclear techniques, an A/E ratio of less than 1:4 is normal, which increases with age. At faster heart rates, the duration of diastasis decreases and the rapid ventricular filling and atrial systolic portions of the TAC merge, making it difficult to calculate ratios and assess the relative contribution of the two phases.

Fig. 16.3 is a schematic representation of a normal TAC compared to a TAC in the presence of diastolic dysfunction (shown as the dashed line). With decreased relaxation, the rate of filling, expressed as EDV/sec, decreases and the TPFR is delayed and shifted to the left. Definitive abnormal threshold in the American population includes PFR less than 1.7 EDV/sec and TPFR greater than 208 msec.[11] Under such circumstances, the contribution of atrial systole may be increased and the E/A ratio shifted to a greater reliance on atrial filling. It is important to

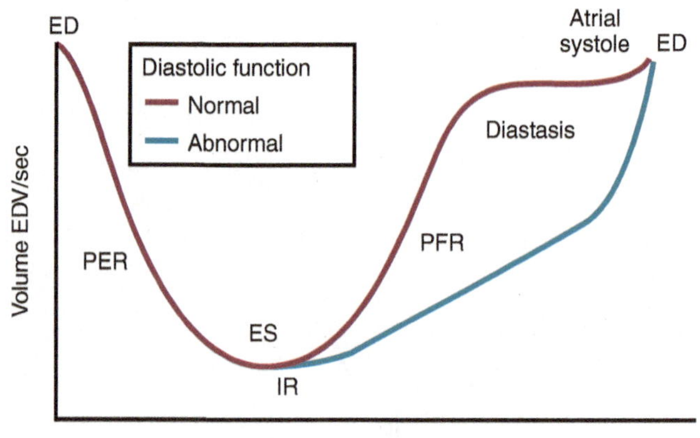

Fig. 16.3 Schematic of normal and abnormal diastolic function time-activity curves. The blue line shows that PFR has a flatter slope and is shifted to the right, indicating a delay in filling in comparison with the normal curve. *ED,* End diastole; *EDV,* end-diastolic volume; *ES,* end systole; *IR,* isovolumic relaxation; *PER,* peak ejection rate; *PFR,* peak filling rate.

recognize that patient factors such as age, heart rate, systolic function (EF), end-diastolic volume, adrenergic state, and medications as well as the methods of acquisition and processing can alter these parameters even in the absence of pathology.[2] Given the influence of these factors on the derived diastolic values, it is easy to see that single or even multiple variables may not accurately identify the presence or absence of pathology in a given individual.

DATA ACQUISITION AND ANALYSIS OF DIASTOLIC FUNCTION BY RADIONUCLIDE TECHNIQUES

Equilibrium Radionuclide Angiocardiography

Important variables for performing diastolic function analysis using ERNA are listed in Box 16.2.[12] ^{99m}Tc pertechnetate is attached to the patient's own red blood cells using one of three possible labeling methods, which vary in the time to perform labeling, expense, and labeling efficiency.[1] Acquisition is conducted once the radionuclide attached to red blood cells has achieved equilibrium within the vascular space. Planar and SPECT methods of acquisition are available, but nearly all studies were and are being performed using planar techniques. Finally, the diastolic assessment can be conducted at rest and/or following stress with exercise (upright or supine bicycle) or a pharmacologic agent (dobutamine).[12]

The patient is positioned in the supine or right lateral position for comfort, and a left anterior oblique (LAO) projection is obtained as the preferred one for diastolic assessment. This allows the best separation of the right and left ventricles for independent and accurate measurement of radioactivity within each chamber as a surrogate of volume.[12,13] An example of a typical LAO view is shown in Fig. 16.4. The labeled red blood cells circulate in the vascular space, and the patient's ECG signal is used to set the timing for acquisition of each heart beat at individual time points, which may vary from 10 to 150 msec depending on heart rate and the preset parameters. Information for each time point for each beat (usually >400 beats are acquired) is summed so that the final TAC is an average rather than information from a single beat or a small number of beats, as is provided by other modalities. For this reason, this technique may be more representative of overall function than are other methods due to the large number of beats averaged.[12,13]

BOX 16.2 Equilibrium Radionuclide Angiocardiography (ERNA): Methods of Acquisition for Diastolic Function Analysis

1. 20–30 millicuries ^{99m}Tc labeled red blood cells
2. Labeling methods
   a. In vivo: fastest and least expensive but lowest binding efficiency
   b. Modified in vivo/in vitro: compromise with good labeling efficiency
   c. In vitro: longest time and expense but best labeling efficiency
3. Planar or single photon emission computed tomography (SPECT)
4. Positioning: best septal separation, left anterior oblique (LAO)
5. Arrhythmia rejection: ±10% of mean R-R interval and drop postpremature beat
6. Temporal resolution: <50 msec or 16 to 32 frames/cycle
7. Acquisition
   a. Frame mode: simplest and least data intensive
   b. List mode: optimal but adds considerable processing time and data storage
   c. Forward-backward with buffered beat: compromise

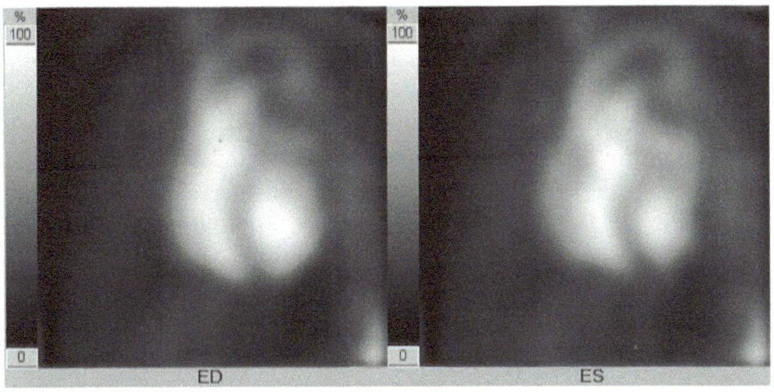

Fig. 16.4 Left anterior oblique planar equilibrium radionuclide angiocardiogram at end diastole *(ED)* and end systole *(ES)* in a patient with normal systolic and diastolic function. The time-activity curves for analysis are obtained from sequential definition of the edges of the left ventricle.

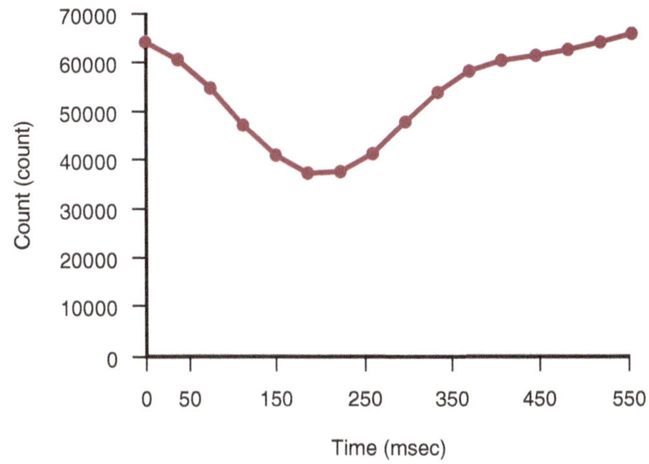

Fig. 16.5 A 16-time interval frame mode time-activity curve from the study in Fig. 16.4. The individual time points and triangles and the fitted curve are shown. All the fine diastolic detail shown in the schematics for Figs. 16.2 and 16.3 can be seen in this curve, even though the 16 time intervals provide less temporal sampling than a 24-frame or 32-frame study.

An adequate temporal sampling of the radioactivity within the left ventricle is crucial to capture the minor or subtle alterations in diastolic filling. To achieve a temporal resolution less than 50 msec usually requires 16 to 32 frames per heart cycle. Therefore the use of 32 frames for each R-R interval is favored when analyzing diastolic function, especially at slow heart rates to appropriately sample all phases and phase transitions of diastole.[12] Fig. 16.5 shows a 16-frame study, which can be contrasted to a study with 32 frame intervals shown in Fig. 16.6. The higher temporal resolution obtained with 32 frame intervals results in the acquisition of even more detail during the diastolic filling period.

Unlike systolic function analysis, diastolic parameters are markedly affected by changes in heart rate and arrhythmias during acquisition and processing. To avoid filling inconsistencies due to heart rate variability and arrhythmias from such a large number of beats, the R-R interval is sampled prior to acquisition and the parameters set up to reject individual beats that vary by ±10% of the mean R-R. Since the beat following a rejected beat has a longer filling period and will add variability to the measurements due to differences in EDV and EF, it is also rejected.[12]

There are three computer methods used to acquire ERNA studies: frame, list, and buffered beat acquisition.[12] Frame mode is the simplest method. It samples the R-R interval prior to acquisition, determines the number of time frames for each beat, and puts data into the appropriate time frame in real time for each beat using the set parameters until a new ECG gating signal identifies the beginning of a new contraction. Once a beat has been added to the particular time bin it cannot be removed. If there is an early beat, a new ECG trigger resets the acquisition so that the time bins toward the end of the heart cycle will have fewer beats contributing counts. The TAC generated from this method of acquisition suffers from count drop-off in the terminal frame(s) due to heart rate variability. Although these TACs with terminal count drop-offs provide accurate EF measurements, as the TPFR and smallest ventricular volume tend to stay constant regardless of heart rate and contractility state, they cannot be analyzed for diastolic parameters using harmonic analysis. Despite the disadvantages of the frame mode, this method is universally used for assessment of systolic function because of its simplicity and the small storage size of the retained data.[12]

List mode acquisition is considered the most accurate method. It retains the spatial distribution of the radiotracer for every millisecond of acquisition, along with the ECG trigger signal, so the data set can be reformatted after completion of acquisition into any timing interval and use the appropriate arrhythmia rejection during postprocessing. It provides maximal flexibility relative to heart rate variability but unfortunately at the expense of prolonged processing time and massive data

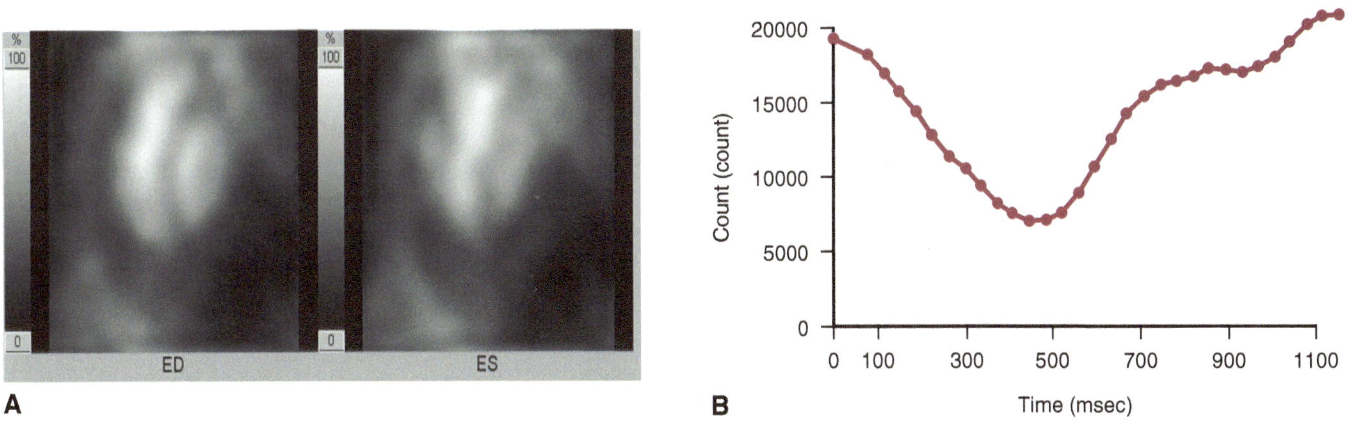

A B

Fig. 16.6 An equilibrium radionuclide angiocardiogram shown in representative end diastole and end systole for (A) the actual study and with (B) the 32-time frame-derived curve. With 32 frames, finer detail can be seen for all four phases of diastole.

storage. This technique was used exclusively for all studies performed by the group at the US National Institutes of Health (NIH).[12,14]

A hybrid method, the buffered beat approach, is an attempt to provide realistic flexibility for heart rate variability while keeping data size to a manageable limit. It uses a temporary memory buffer to examine each beat and the ECG gating signal with regard to the set baseline parameters and makes an instant decision to keep or reject the beat. An additional feature of this method is a forward-backward curve generation technique to avoid discontinuities or count drop-off in the last several frames, which precludes harmonic analysis of the TAC.[12]

Finally, the processed images are filtered to reduce statistical noise, the edges of the left ventricle are defined using manual or automated edge detection software, and background subtraction is performed. The radioactive counts within these boundaries is proportional to the total volume in the ventricle and are used to produce a TAC. A TAC from a frame mode of 16 time intervals acquired from a clinical study is shown in Fig. 16.5. All the fine detail shown schematically in Fig. 16.2 is retained in this curve, which does not have any drop-off in counts in the terminal frames that may be seen in the presence of even minor sinus arrhythmias but is much more pronounced in the presence of atrial or ventricular arrhythmias.[12]

First-Pass Radionuclide Angiography

First-pass techniques for assessment of diastolic function require administration of a compact intravenous (IV) bolus of radioactivity and use of a very high temporal resolution and high count rate camera system to follow the radioactivity as it traverses the right and left ventricles rather than after achieving equilibrium in the vascular space as with ERNA. Serial gated images at 25 to 50 msec of temporal resolution are acquired, and the resultant TACs allow systolic and diastolic function analysis of the right and left ventricles at rest or following exercise or pharmacologic stress. This technique often requires multicrystal camera systems to capture enough counts in the limited acquisition time of 8 to 10 beats during first pass. Such systems are no longer commercially produced. Newer cadmium-zinc-telluride (CZT) camera systems provide high sensitivity and spatial resolution and may potentially be used for FPRNA. The basic requirements for performing studies are shown in Box 16.3 and will be discussed in the following section.[15]

Any ^{99m}Tc radiolabeled compound can be used for bolus administration. When assessment is to be made at rest and following stress on one day, an agent that is cleared by the kidneys (^{99m}Tc dimethyl sulfoxide [DMSO] or diethylenetriaminepentaacetic acid [DTPA]) can be given first, followed by an agent that is cleared by the liver (^{99m}Tc sulfur colloid) or a heart perfusion tracer (^{99m}Tc tetrofosmin or sestamibi), so that there is no interference during the second study from the initial dose. The total dose administered can be lower when a multicrystal camera is used, but with a single crystal camera that is not capable of high count rates, 25 to 30 millicuries (mCi) are required. The total dose must be given as a tight IV bolus over 2 or 3 seconds, which requires at least an 18-gauge IV in the antecubital fossa or the external jugular. If such venous access is not available, the study should not be attempted.[15]

Anterior images are acquired with the patient supine or upright with the chest directly on the camera head. Exercise is best performed on a bicycle, which allows the chest to be relatively stationary and the images free of motion artifacts. Studies have been acquired during treadmill exercise, but this requires placement of external radioactive markers that can be used to correct for motion. Since only 8 to 10 beats can be used to analyze right ventricular (RV) or LV function without having bolus overlap in the chambers, heart rate variability or arrhythmias will further limit the number of beats that can be processed and will result in sampling bias or overlap of tracer activity in more than one chamber. These sampling limitations may result in poor study quality and limit the conclusions that can be reached.[15]

BOX 16.3 Basics of First Pass Radionuclide Angiography (FPRNA): Methods of Acquisition for Diastolic Function Analysis

1. Radiopharmaceutical
   a. 10 to 30 millicuries of ^{99m}Tc sulfur colloid, diethylene triamine pentaacetic acid
   b. Bolus injection of ^{99m}Tc sestamibi or tetrofosmin in conjunction with perfusion, given rapidly in small volume
   c. Total dose injected adjusted for count rate capabilities of camera
2. Injection site
   a. Antecubital vein or external jugular with minimum of 18-gauge IV cannula
3. Camera types
   a. Multicrystal preferred due to high count rates
   b. Single crystal must be capable of 150,000 counts/sec
4. Temporal resolution: usually 25 msec
5. Acquire images in anterior position

ECG-Gated Perfusion Imaging Studies

Current ECG-gated myocardial perfusion techniques (SPECT and PET) offer the ability to adjunctively assess diastolic function using the concepts and methods from ERNA.[3] For the assessment of diastolic function, ECG-gated perfusion studies use perfusion tracers (T1-201, ^{99m}Tc tetrofosmin or sestamibi, Rb-82) rather than Tc-tagged red blood cells utilized in ERNA, but similar methods of processing are utilized with these two radionuclide techniques. Unlike ERNA and FPRNA that identify temporal changes in radioactivity to assess ventricular function, ECG-gated perfusion studies track the ventricular endocardial borders using perfusion tracers, which allows both the evaluation of ventricular volumes and the assessment of systolic and diastolic function. To correctly perform diastolic function analysis from gated perfusion images, there are limitations to overcome. These include the low temporal resolution, failure to perform optimal arrhythmia rejection, and poor edge detection due to the low information density contained in the perfusion data. Despite these limitations there are several groups that have shown the feasibility of such an approach.[5,13,16–18] Diastolic assessment using 32-frame gated SPECT correlated closely to evaluation obtained with ERNA studies.[4] Although these systems are capable of generating values for diastolic function indices, these are not routinely used in clinical practice as the major interest is in perfusion and systolic function.

Unlike ERNA and FPRNA, in which the injected radioactivity remains in the intravascular space, ^{99m}Tc perfusion agents are cleared by the liver and empty into the gastrointestinal tract. Typically 20 mCi of ^{99m}Tc pertechnetate are injected and remain in the vascular space, whereas with the perfusion tracers 15 to 30 mCi are administered with only a small percentage taken up by the myocardium. This means that a smaller percentage of the injected dose is in the myocardium when imaging is performed and that the counts are low, mandating that the time intervals for each beat be relatively long to achieve adequate information density in each frame. Increasing the imaging time will improve total counts but decrease quality, as patients are likely to move. Most studies are acquired for 8 to 16 frames; however, acquisition at 8 frames might lack sufficient temporal resolution to adequately separate out and analyze the various components of diastole with low heart rates (125 msec/frame at a heart rate of 60 bpm). Conversely, an

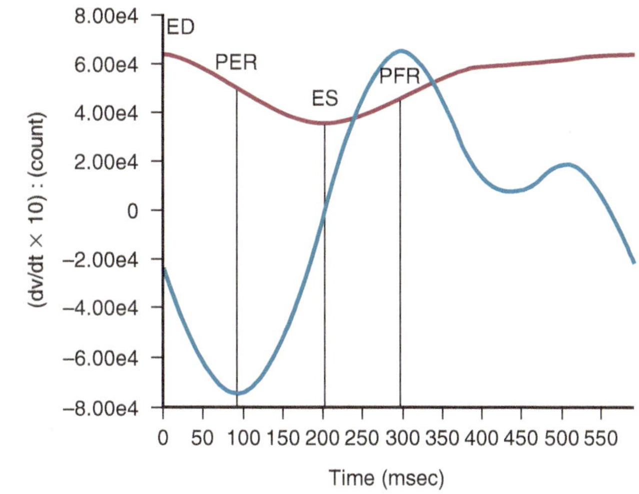

FITTING RESULTS

Item	Value
EDC (count)	64162
ESC (count)	36386
TES (msec)	202
TPE (msec)	92
PER(/SV) (%/sec)	718.8
TPE/T (%)	15.5
1/3EF(/SV) (%)	31.7
1/3ER(/SV) (%/sec)	471.4
TPF (msec)	94
PFR(/SV) (%/sec)	637.2
TPF/TF (%)	24.0
1/3FF(/SV) (%)	59.8
1/3FR(/SV) (%/sec)	460.2
1/2FF(/SV) (%)	11.2

Fig. 16.7 The graph shows the third harmonic fitted curve superimposed by the first derivative curve with the peak ejection rate and peak filling rate. To the right is the printout of all the variables that can be derived from the data. *ED,* End diastole; *ES,* end systole; *PER,* peak ejection rate; *PFR,* peak filling rate.

acquisition of 16 frames is optimal as it provides an improved temporal resolution of 63 msec at the cost of half the counts, yet adequate edge definition can still be performed.[5]

The other problem that requires resolution is getting a TAC without terminal frame count dropout. Currently, arrhythmia rejection for ECG-gated perfusion studies uses ±50% of the mean R-R interval to avoid compromising the perfusion study, which would either drop beats and lower total counts or prolong the acquisition time to achieve adequate counts. Some of the newer camera/workstation systems allow multiple acquisition windows so that arrhythmia rejection can be performed on one set of data while a separate window can be used for the perfusion data without arrhythmia rejection. Additional time is not added to the acquisition. If arrhythmias are present or there is a poor ECG signal due to bad skin contact or muscle interference, the ECG-gated data set will still be compromised, and quality control needs to be performed.[12]

The final hurdle is getting appropriate edge definition from the available algorithms to accurately track the endocardial borders of the ventricle. Existing software packages have been shown to handle the lower counts in 16-frame acquisition.[5] Definition of the mitral valve plane at the base of the heart is also difficult, as the transition from the left atrium, which has little uptake, to the myocardium in the area of the valves and membranous septum is difficult to identify. Failure to clearly delineate this separation will result in error in the volume of the cavity and the resultant TAC.

Data Analysis in the Evaluation of Diastolic Function by Radionuclides Techniques

Once the TAC has been generated there are two general methods of diastolic function analysis: digital filtering and mathematical curve fitting.[14] With digital filtering or harmonic analysis, three to five harmonics are applied to smooth noise in the TAC, and the first derivative is taken to define the point at which the greatest change in volume is present; this change and the time at which it occurs represents the PFR and TPFR. An example is shown in Fig. 16.7. An absolute requirement for harmonic analysis is that the EDV from the TAC start and end at the same volume point. Fig. 16.8 shows an example of count drop-off due to arrhythmias in a study acquired by frame mode. In the presence of count drop-off, error is introduced into the derived values from harmonic analysis. Discontinuity occurs in the terminal frames with

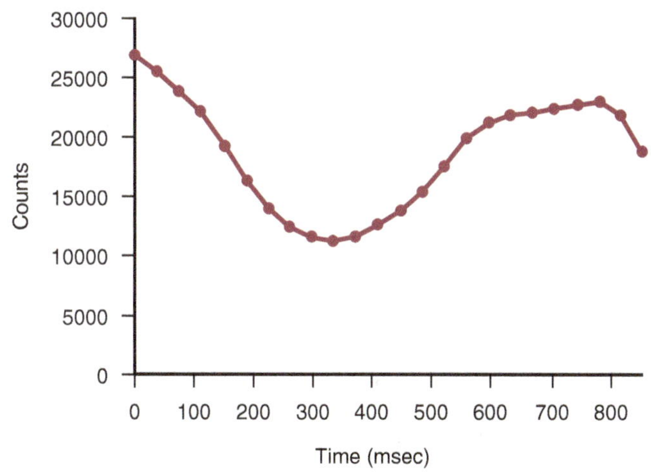

Fig. 16.8 Time-activity curve from a 32-frame study showing terminal frame drop-off in the last two frames due to an arrhythmia.

frame mode acquisition, and for this reason list or buffered beat acquisition with forward and backward reconstruction of the TAC is required to use harmonic methods of analysis. Diastolic function values derived using a mathematical curve fitting technique generally take the available data and apply a third-order polynomial equation to derive PFR and TPFR from the slope changes in the TAC. This method is less susceptible to discontinuities in the TAC.[12]

Currently most software packages on nuclear cardiology workstations are capable of generating diastolic function values from any TAC. A typical printout of results is shown in the right-hand panel of Fig. 16.7. Careful attention must be given to the accuracy of the ECG-gating mechanism, the presence or absence of count drop-off in the terminal frames, information density, and temporal resolution before applying these results to clinical practice.

CLINICAL RELEVANCE

Radionuclide methods for diastolic function analysis have been performed predominantly on a research basis and are not used on a day-to-day basis in general clinical cardiology practice. This is due in part to the lack of appropriate equipment, difficulty in accurately performing

BOX 16.4 Clinical Patient Populations Evaluated Using Radionuclide Diastolic Function Analysis

1. Coronary artery disease (CAD)
2. Heart failure with preserved ejection fraction (HFpEF) and microvascular dysfunction
3. Hypertrophic cardiomyopathy (HCM)
4. Hypertension
5. Aging
6. Cardio-oncology
7. Constrictive pericarditis and restrictive cardiomyopathy

the measurements, and variability in the measurements due to factors other than cardiac pathology. Even with these limitations this technique can be useful in certain disease states and clinical scenarios, especially in those with heart failure with preserved ejection fraction (HFpEF), as listed in Box 16.4. These will be discussed in detail.

Coronary Artery Disease

The utility of radionuclide techniques in the diagnosis of CAD predominantly relies on the measurement of myocardial perfusion or changes in systolic function at baseline and following stress. Nevertheless the analysis of diastolic function in conjunction with these other measures enhances the diagnostic accuracy for the detection of CAD.[8,19] The induction of LV ischemia halts the myosin-actin complex dissociation after a contraction. This impairs myocardial relaxation with a decreased PFR and an increased TPFR. Such diastolic dysfunction is a much earlier sign of myocardial ischemia than systolic dysfunction.[19] These are usually measurements of global changes, but regional analysis can also be performed in an attempt to increase sensitivity by measuring the small changes that may not be detected by a global filling value or time.[20]

A very high percentage (80%–90%) of patients with documented CAD have abnormal diastolic function at rest detected by ERNA, even in those with normal resting LV EF, no resting regional wall motion abnormalities, and no Q waves.[21] Thus these diastolic findings in CAD are independent of LV systolic function or previous myocardial infarction. In addition, patients with CAD tend to have lower PFR overall and a lower PFR in the first third of diastole during exertion. These diastolic abnormalities are more sensitive for detection of disease than the exertional wall motion abnormalities or abnormal EF response to exercise.[19] Finally, the presence of impaired LV filling and regional asynchrony predict a greater degree of exercise-induced ischemia, suggesting a greater extent of jeopardized myocardium.[22,23]

Once a diagnosis of CAD has been made, diastolic function analysis has also been used to document the response to treatment. In this regard, it has been reported that previously abnormal diastolic function resolves following target vessel revascularization.[24] This could be used to confirm successful revascularization but also to guide an optimal titration of medical therapy in patients with CAD.

Although the efficacy of diastolic function analysis for CAD diagnosis and monitoring was documented on ERNA and FPRNA studies, similar information can be derived from 16-frame ECG-gated perfusion studies. Thus, the addition of diastology may provide ancillary information beyond perfusion that may have a role in the management of patients with known or suspected CAD.

HFpEF and Microvascular Dysfunction

Patients with clinical symptoms of congestive heart failure generally have abnormal systolic function, but as many as 30% to 50% of these patients may have normal ejection fraction. The HFpEF population encompasses a heterogeneous group of patients ranging from those with infiltrative cardiomyopathies (amyloidosis, sarcoidosis), hypertrophic cardiomyopathy (HCM), hypertensive heart disease, ischemic heart disease, to idiopathic HFpEF.[25] Thus the pathophysiology behind idiopathic HFpEF is complex and poorly understood, yet diastolic dysfunction with elevated filling pressures is well recognized as a key player among other factors.[26–28]

Radionuclide techniques, including myocardial perfusion studies, identify diastolic abnormalities in a proportion of patients with HFpEF even after excluding obstructive CAD. At least 38% of patients with the diagnosis of HFpEF present with a reduction in PFR below 2.5 EDV/sec, while an additional 24% had probable diastolic dysfunction with values of 2.5 to 3 EDV/sec.[27] The quantification of cardiac volumes during radionuclide studies can also help identify those with small LV cavities that could contribute to the pathophysiology behind HFpEF.[25] Moreover, the identification of profound diastolic dysfunction in the absence of ischemia can trigger, in the right clinical context, the evaluation of secondary causes of diastolic dysfunction such as amyloidosis or other infiltrative cardiomyopathies as illustrated in the case presented earlier.

The conduction of myocardial perfusion assessment with PET can also provide information about the coexistence of diastolic dysfunction and reduced coronary flow reserved (CFR). CFR is a novel marker of large-vessel and small-vessel ischemia calculated as the ratio of hyperemic to rest myocardial blood flow (MBF). The accuracy of myocardial blood flow and CFR with PET has been validated in animal and human studies with well-established reproducibility.[29] Similar to diastolic assessment, MBF is derived from a TAC generated from the activity of perfusion tracers in the blood pool and myocardial tissue. The rate of myocardial uptake provides the estimate of MBF in mL/min/g.[29] In the absence of obstructive epicardial CAD, a depressed CFR (<2) is used as a marker of coronary microvascular dysfunction (CMD). New evidence has demonstrated that coronary CMD is independently associated with diastolic dysfunction in patients with HFpEF.[30,31] The underlying mechanism behind diastolic dysfunction with CMD resembles that of obstructive CAD with blunting of myocardial perfusion causing diffuse myocardial ischemia.[29,30] This novel concept is supported by prior studies, which demonstrated that diabetic patients without obstructive CAD tend to have lower PFR than their nondiabetic counterparts.[32] This impairment in diastolic function responds at least in part to microvascular dysfunction in the diabetic population known to have coronary endothelial dysfunction.[29,33] It might also explain the presence of HFpEF in those with cardiovascular risk factors such as hypertension, hyperlipidemia, and obesity.[33] This well-defined phenotype of very low CFR without obstructive CAD has been reported to be more prevalent in patients with HFpEF as well as other subsets, including women, atrial fibrillation, metabolic syndrome, and cardio-oncology complications.[29] Finally, the coexistence of diastolic dysfunction and CMD provides prognostic information as this combination has been found to be independently associated with an increased risk of major cardiovascular events, including heart failure hospitalization.[31]

The adjunctive assessment of diastolic function during ECG-gated perfusion studies may provide useful diagnostic and prognostic information in patients with or at risk of HFpEF, especially when evaluated in combination with a CFR during a perfusion study with PET. It is important to recognize that radionuclide studies lack specificity and thus provide less useful information than that provided by echocardiography. Thus, the evaluation of diastolic function with radionuclides techniques should be seen as an added benefit during the evaluation of myocardial ischemia and not as the reason to order a radionuclide study.

Hypertrophic Cardiomyopathy

Patients with HCM have been extensively evaluated in terms of diagnosis and management using radionuclide techniques because of the interest and expertise of National Heart, Lung and Blood Institute (NHLBI) investigators.[34–38] The major abnormalities in HCM patients include prolonged isovolumic relaxation caused by myocardial ischemia and intracellular calcium overloading, as well as delayed rapid ventricular filling and a greater dependence on the atrial contribution to filling. In addition to documenting these abnormalities, radionuclide techniques have been used to monitor the effects of treatment. The calcium blockers verapamil and nifedipine have been shown to improve LV relaxation and filling with IV administration and with long-term oral administration. In addition to improving hemodynamic parameters there are clinical improvements in exercise tolerance and heart failure symptoms.[34,35] It was shown that the early and late improvement in symptoms with verapamil was related to the extent of improvement in diastolic filling. These findings also explain why HCM patients can go into severe heart failure when they are not in sinus rhythm and lose atrial contraction, which makes a larger than normal contribution to ventricular filling in these abnormal ventricles.

At this stage of our understanding of the etiology and management of HCM, it is accepted that diastolic dysfunction is present, and there is no need to document its existence with radionuclide studies beyond the results available from echocardiography.

Hypertension

In the presence of hypertension there are alterations in diastolic function independent of alterations in systolic function or the presence of CAD that can be measured by radionuclide methods.[39,40] Resting diastolic function can detect early changes in myocardial function in patients with essential hypertension predicting abnormal response during stress such as drop in ejection fraction. These changes are not directly related to previously identified modifiers of diastolic parameters such as age, heart rate, and the extent and severity of hypertension. Conversely, these abnormalities are directly related to myocardial mass.[39] These studies suggest that diastolic function analysis may be used for preclinical detection of myocardial dysfunction in patients with hypertension. Moreover, serial assessment could document the improvement in diastolic function with medical therapy in hypertensive patients.[41]

Aging

There are age-related changes in ventricular relaxation and filling that are independent of the increasing prevalence of hypertension, CAD, increased LV mass, and altered response to catecholamines, and they suggest that there are primary effects of aging on diastolic function.[10,42,43] It has been documented by many methods that with increasing age there is a decrease in PFR and TPFR and an increase in the atrial component of diastole. The etiology of these changes is multifactorial but may be reversed in part through exercise training and with the use of calcium blockers.[10,42] It is also possible that fibrosis or protein deposition within the myocardium may mediate the abnormalities.[44] Documentation of these abnormalities is most useful when diastolic radionuclide parameters are being used to diagnose ischemia. Thus adjusting for age is critical in order not to confuse age-related changes with the presence of CAD.

Cardio-Oncology

Advances in cancer treatment have unequivocally led to improvements in overall survival in this patient population. In a number of patients, the development of cardiotoxicity from cancer treatments offsets this benefit with an increase in cardiovascular morbidity and mortality. The use of noninvasive imaging modalities pioneered with radionuclide angiography has allowed the prompt detection of cardiotoxicity earlier in the disease process avoiding or minimizing the irreversible consequences.[45,46]

Although serial LV EF assessment has been the gold standard measurement in cardio-oncology,[47] some have proposed that diastolic dysfunction could be an earlier and more sensitive marker of cardiotoxicity.[48–50] However, studies evaluating the cardiotoxic effect of anthracyclines and trastuzumab reported that diastolic dysfunction (lower PFR and longer TPFR) does not uniformly precede but rather parallels reduction in LV EF.[51,52] Diastolic dysfunction assessment using radionuclide technique provides enhanced sensitivity for identifying early cardiotoxicity from cancer treatment, but whether its identification adds to the standard of care prediction of heart failure remains unknown.[48]

Constrictive Pericarditis and Restrictive Cardiomyopathy

Constrictive pericarditis and restrictive cardiomyopathy often have near identical clinical presentation and share similar hemodynamic profile. The differentiation of one condition from the other is often challenging. Clinicians must use every tool at hand to solve this diagnostic dilemma when present, to provide the appropriate treatment to patients.

Scarce data suggest that the evaluation of LV filling using nuclear studies might help in the differentiation between constrictive pericarditis and restrictive cardiomyopathy. Small studies have postulated that filling fraction might be useful in differentiating constrictive pericarditis and restrictive cardiomyopathy. The former exhibits a high filling fraction with 85% of LV filling occurring early followed by an abrupt halt in late diastole due to a noncompliant pericardium. Conversely, the latter presents with a lower filling fraction with 45% of early filling due to a more uniform delay in ventricular filling through the whole diastole. This is contrasted to an average filling fraction of 65% in normal controls.[53–55] Subsequent analyses of the TAC in these two conditions demonstrate that constrictive pericarditis presents with an asymmetric curve due to a diastolic limb that is steeper than the systolic limb. Meanwhile, restrictive cardiomyopathy exhibits an asymmetry TAC at the expense of a less steep diastolic limb compared to the systolic limb. Therefore higher PFR and a shorter TPFR are seen with constrictive pericarditis compared to restrictive cardiomyopathy. Finally, the Fourier ratio (PFR/peak LV emptying rate) that accounts for changes in heart and contractility is another index that could discriminate between those two conditions. It is higher (>1) in constrictive pericarditis compared to restrictive cardiomyopathy (~1) and normal controls (<1). Interestingly, findings associated with constrictive pericarditis seems to revert after pericardiectomy.[54]

Although current practice relies on echocardiography, cardiac magnetic resonance, and invasive hemodynamic to differentiate between constrictive pericarditis and restrictive cardiomyopathy, the adjunctive analysis of diastolic function on ECG-gated perfusion studies performed for different reasons can offer helpful insight on diastolic function that could aid in the resolution of the constriction-restriction dilemma.

LIMITATIONS

Despite the extensive literature on the use of radionuclide methods for analysis of diastolic function, the clinical utility of these techniques is limited.[2] Measurements are difficult to perform using the standard methods of acquisition and processing in clinical practice, and efforts to achieve greater accuracy and reproducibility are time consuming, computer intensive, and not practical in most clinical settings. Even with the easier acquisition with myocardial perfusion studies, techniques such as echocardiography and cardiovascular magnetic resonance provide similar information on diastolic function and much more information on heart valves, wall thickness, LV mass, chamber pressures, flow dynamics, and the integrity of the pericardium. This additional information makes these techniques much more valuable for patient evaluation and management. Finally, the value of measuring relaxation rates and time intervals is questionable, as there might be a poor correlation between these parameters and the LV end-diastolic pressure and overall time constant of relaxation.[2]

FUTURE DIRECTIONS

Given the widespread use of ECG-gated perfusion studies, the ability to assess diastolic function from these perfusion studies would allow the screening of diastolic dysfunction in a larger patient population during the assessment for obstructive CAD. In addition, new software packages with enhanced digital storage capabilities could streamline the use of radionuclide techniques in the assessments of diastolic function in clinical practice and perhaps impulse the renaissance of these techniques for selected cases. The assessment of diastolic dysfunction along with CFR with PET could be of potential investigational interest in patients with microvascular dysfunction with or at risk for HFpEF. Similarly, the accuracy and reproducibility of radionuclide techniques in the evaluation of diastolic function can be used to determine if these parameters can be used in predicting systolic dysfunction in patients receiving cancer treatments.

KEY POINTS

- The radionuclide assessment of systolic and diastolic LV function requires the generation of a curve plotting the changes in radioactivity over time, which is proportional to changes in LV volume over time.
- To achieve an optimal temporal resolution (<50 msec) 16 to 32 frames per heart cycle are usually required.
- The accuracy of the ECG-gated mechanism, the presence or absence of count drop-off in the terminal frames, information density, and temporal resolution must be quality reviewed before applying results to clinical practice.
- The principles and concepts of diastolic function assessment by radionuclide techniques can be adjunctively applied to ECG-gated perfusion studies.
- A reduced peak filling rate, a longer time to peak filling rate, and an increased ratio between early and late filling are the most important radionuclide metrics suggesting diastolic dysfunction.
- The assessment of diastolic function during ECG-gated myocardial perfusion study enhances the sensitivity of the test in detecting myocardial ischemia.
- Radionuclide studies are rarely performed for the sole assessment of diastolic function in current practice, yet if conducted for other reasons they may identify preclinical cardiac abnormalities or assess response to treatment in patients with hypertensive heart disease, chemotherapy cardiotoxicity, or even microvascular dysfunction.

REVIEW QUESTIONS

1. With regard to data acquisition for evaluation of diastolic function with radionuclides techniques, which of the following statements is true?
   a. Arrhythmias during data acquisition have no impact on the quality of data acquisition.
   b. Diastolic function can be evaluated with equilibrium radionuclide angiography (ERNA) and first-pass radionuclide angiography (FPRNA) but not with ECG-gated myocardial perfusion studies.
   c. Optimal temporal resolution is obtained with acquisition of eight frames per cycle.
   d. Diastolic function is assessed by analyzing volume changes and rate of changes during diastole derived from a curve plotting the changes in radioactivity over time.
2. With regard to data analysis during evaluation of diastolic function with radionuclides techniques, which of the following statements is true?
   a. The most important metrics of diastolic function are obtained during atrial systole.
   b. The peak filling rate and time to peak filling rate are the most important metrics utilized during the evaluation of diastolic function.
   c. Diastolic dysfunction is suggested when peak filling time is greater than 2.5 EDV/sec and/or time to peak filling time is less than 180 msec.
   d. Radionuclides techniques have a high specificity in the detection of diastolic dysfunction.
3. With regard to the clinical utility of diastolic evaluation with radionuclides techniques, which of the following statements is true?
   a. The impairment in diastolic function seen in patients with hypertensive heart disease is solely and directly related to the severity of hypertension.
   b. Radionuclide techniques can detect diastolic dysfunction in more than 80% of patients carrying the diagnosis of HFpEF.
   c. The adjunctive evaluation of diastolic function during an ischemic evaluation with myocardial perfusion studies is of no utility in the evaluation of a patient with cardiorespiratory symptoms.
   d. The assessment of diastolic function with radionuclides techniques may allow the preclinical identification of cardiac abnormalities in patients with hypertensive heart disease, chemotherapy-induced cardiotoxicity, or microvascular dysfunction.

REFERENCES

1. Cerqueira M. *Nuclear Cardiology*. Boston, MA: Blackwell Scientific; 1994.
2. Arrighi JA, Soufer R. Left ventricular diastolic function: physiology, methods of assessment, and clinical significance. *J Nucl Cardiol.* 1995;2:525–543.
3. Nagamachi S, Wakamatsu H, Fujita S, et al. Assessment of diastolic function using 16-frame 201Tl gated myocardial perfusion SPECT: a comparative study of QGS2 and pFAST2. *Ann Nucl Med.* 2008;22(2):115–122. doi:10.1007/s12149-007-0091-2.
4. Kumita SI, Cho K, Nakajo H, et al. Assessment of left ventricular diastolic function with electrocardiography-gated myocardial perfusion SPECT:

comparison with multigated equilibrium radionuclide angiography. *J Nucl Cardiol.* 2001;8(5):568–574. doi:10.1067/mnc.2001.116853.
5. Akincioglu C, Berman D, Nishina H, et al. Assessment of diastolic function using 16-frame 99mTc-sestamibi gated myocardial perfusion SPECT: normal values. *J Nucl Med Tech.* 2005;46:1102–1108.
6. Germano G, Kiat H, Kavanagh PB, et al. Automatic quantification of ejection fraction from gated myocardial perfusion SPECT. *J Nucl Med Tech.* 1995;36(11):2138–2147.
7. Mitra D, Basu U. Equilibrium radionuclide angiocardiography: its usefulness in current practice and potential future applications. *World J Radiol.* 2012;4(10):421. doi:10.4329/wjr.v4.i10.421.
8. Bonow R. Radionuclide angiographic evaluation of left ventricular diastolic function. *Circulation.* 1991;84:I208–I2015.
9. Johannessen KA, Cerqueira M, Veith RC, Stratton JR. The relation between radionuclide angiography and Doppler echocardiography during contractile changes with infusions of epinephrine. *Int J Cardiol.* 1991;33(1):149–157. doi:10.1016/0167-5273(91)90163-J.
10. Levy WC, Cerqueira MD, Abrass IB, Schwartz RS, Stratton JR. Endurance exercise training augments diastolic filling at rest and during exercise in healthy young and older men. *Circulation.* 1993;88(1):116–126. doi:10.1161/01.CIR.88.1.116.
11. Matsuo S, Nakajima K, Kinuya S. Clinical use of nuclear cardiology in the assessment of heart failure. *World J Cardiol.* 2010;2(10):344–356. doi:10.4330/wjc.v2.i10.344.
12. Corbett JR, Akinboboye OO, Bacharach SL, et al. Equilibrium radionuclide angiocardiography. *J Nucl Cardiol.* 2006;13(6):e56–e79. doi:10.1016/j.nuclcard.2006.08.007.
13. Higuchi T, Taki J, Nakajima K, et al. Left ventricular ejection and filling rate measurement based on the automatic edge detection method of ECG-gated blood pool single-photon emission tomography. *Ann Nucl Med.* 2004;18(6):507–511. doi:10.1007/BF02984568.
14. Bacharach SL, Green MV, Borer JS. Instrumentation and data processing in cardiovascular nuclear medicine: evaluation of ventricular function. *Semin Nucl Med.* 1979;9(4):257–274. doi:10.1016/S0001-2998(79)80013-6.
15. Friedman JD, Berman DS, Borges-Neto S, et al. First-pass radionuclide angiography. *J Nucl Cardiol.* 2006;13(6):e42–e55. doi:10.1016/j.nuclcard.2006.08.006.
16. Kikkawa M, Nakamura T, Sakamoto K, et al. Assessment of left ventricular diastolic function from quantitative electrocardiographic-gated 99mTc-tetrofosmin myocardial SPET. *Eur J Nucl Med.* 2001;28(5):593–601. doi:10.1007/s002590100487.
17. Higuchi T, Nakajima K, Taki J, Kinuya S, Bunko H, Tonami N. Assessment of left ventricular systolic and diastolic function based on the edge detection method with myocardial ECG-gated SPET. *Eur J Nucl Med.* 2001;28(10):1512–1516. doi:10.1007/s002590100619.
18. Sakamoto K, Nakamura T, Zen K, et al. Identification of exercise-induced left ventricular systolic and diastolic dysfunction using gated SPECT in patients with coronary artery disease. *J Nucl Cardiol.* 2004;11(2):152–158. doi:10.1016/j.nuclcard.2003.12.007.
19. Reduto L, Wickemeyer W, Young J, et al. Left ventricular diastolic performance at rest and during exercise in patients with coronary artery disease: assessment with first-pass radionuclide angiography. *Circulation.* 1981;63:1228–1237.
20. Bonow RO, Vitale DF, Bacharach SL, Frederick TM, Kent KM, Green MV. Asynchronous left ventricular regional function and impaired global diastolic filling in patients with coronary artery disease: reversal after coronary angioplasty. *Circulation.* 1985;71(2):297–307. doi:10.1161/01.CIR.71.2.297.
21. Bonow R, Bacharach S, Green M, et al. Impaired left ventricular diastolic filling in patients with coronary artery disease: assessment with radionuclide angiography. *Circulation.* 1981;64:315–323.
22. Perrone-Filardi P, Bacharach SL, Dilsizian V, Bonow RO. Effects of regional systolic asynchrony on left ventricular global diastolic function in patients with coronary artery disease. *J Am Coll Cardiol.* 1992;19(4):739–744. doi:10.1016/0735-1097(92)90511-K.
23. Perrone-Filardi P, Bacharach SL, Dilsizian V, Bonow RO. Impaired left ventricular filling and regional diastolic asynchrony at rest in coronary artery disease and relation to exercise-induced myocardial ischemia. *Am J Cardiol.* 1991;67(5):356–360. doi:10.1016/0002-9149(91)90041-I.
24. Bonow RO, Kent KM, Rosing DR, et al. Improved left ventricular diastolic filling in patients with coronary artery disease after percutaneous transluminal coronary angioplasty. *Circulation.* 1982;66:1159–1167. doi:10.1161/01.CIR.66.6.1159.
25. Gupta DK, Solomon SD. Imaging in heart failure with preserved ejection fraction. *Heart Fail Clin.* 2014;10:419–434. doi:10.1016/j.hfc.2014.04.004.
26. Redfield MM. Heart failure with preserved ejection fraction. *N Engl J Med.* 2016;375(19):1868–1877. doi:10.1056/NEJMcp1511175.
27. Soufer R, Wohlgelernter D, Vita NA, et al. Intact systolic left ventricular function in clinical congestive heart failure. *Am J Cardiol.* 1985;55(8):1032–1036.
28. Watanabe J, Levine MJ, Bellotto F, Johnson RG, Grossman W. Effects of coronary venous pressure on left ventricular diastolic distensibility. *Circ Res.* 1990;67(4):923–932.
29. Taqueti VR, Di Carli MF. Clinical significance of noninvasive coronary flow reserve assessment in patients with ischemic heart disease. *Curr Opin Cardiol.* 2016;31(6):662–669. doi:10.1097/HCO.0000000000000339.
30. Giamouzis G, Schelbert EB, Butler J. Growing Evidence Linking Microvascular Dysfunction With Heart Failure With Preserved Ejection Fraction. *J Am Heart Assoc.* 2016;5(2): :e003259. Published 2016 Feb 23. doi:10.1161/JAHA.116.003259.
31. Taqueti VR, Solomon SD, Shah AM, et al. Coronary microvascular dysfunction and future risk of heart failure with preserved ejection fraction. *Eur Heart J.* 2018;39(10):840–849. doi:10.1093/eurheartj/ehx721.
32. Korkmaz A, Caliskan B, Erdem F. Evaluation of diastolic function in patients with normal perfusion and type 2 diabetes mellitus with gated single-photon emission computed tomography. *World J Nucl Med.* 2017;16(3):206–211.
33. Bairey Merz CN, Pepine CJ, Walsh MN, Fleg JL. Ischemia and no obstructive coronary artery disease (INOCA). *Circulation.* 2017;135:1075–1092. doi:10.1161/CIRCULATIONAHA.116.024534.
34. Bonow RO, Dilsizian V, Rosing DR, Maron BJ, Bacharach SL, Green MV. Verapamil-induced improvement in left ventricular diastolic filling and increased exercise tolerance in patients with hypertrophic cardiomyopathy: short- and long-term effects. *Circulation.* 1985;72(4):853–864. doi:10.1161/01.CIR.72.4.853.
35. Bonow RO, Rosing DR, Bacharach SL, et al. Effects of verapamil on left ventricular systolic function and diastolic filling in patients with hypertrophic cardiomyopathy. *Circulation.* 1981;64(4):787–796. doi:10.1161/01.CIR.64.4.787.
36. Bonow RO, Vitale DF, Maron BJ, Bacharach SL, Frederick TM, Green MV. Regional left ventricular asynchrony and impaired global left ventricular filling in hypertrophic cardiomyopathy: effect of verapamil. *J Am Coll Cardiol.* 1987;9(5):1108–1116.
37. Cannon RO, Rosing DR, Maron BJ, et al. Myocardial ischemia in patients with hypertrophic cardiomyopathy: contribution of inadequate vasodilator reserve and elevated left ventricular filling pressures. *Circulation.* 1985;71:234–243.
38. Marian AJ, Braunwald E. Hypertrophic cardiomyopathy: genetics, pathogenesis, clinical manifestations, diagnosis, and therapy. *Circ Res.* 2017;121(7):749–770. doi:10.1161/CIRCRESAHA.117.311059.
39. Cuocolo A, Sax FL, Brush JE, Maron BJ, Bacharach SL, Bonow RO. Left ventricular hypertrophy and impaired diastolic filling in essential hypertension. Diastolic mechanisms for systolic dysfunction during exercise. *Circulation.* 1990;81(3):978–986. doi:10.1161/01.CIR.81.3.978.
40. Inouye I, Massie B, Loge D, et al. Abnormal left ventricular filling: an early finding in mild to moderate systemic hypertension. *Am J Cardiol.* 1984;53(1):120–126. doi:10.1016/0002-9149(84)90695-7.
41. Brush JE Jr, Udelson JE, Bacharach SL, et al. Comparative effects of verapamil and nitroprusside on left ventricular function in patients with hypertension. *J Am Coll Cardiol.* 1989;14(2):515–522. doi:10.1016/0735-1097(89)90210-6.
42. Arrighi JA, Dilsizian V, Perrone-Filardi P, Diodati JG, Bacharach SL, Bonow RO. Improvement of the age-related impairment in left ventricular diastolic filling with verapamil in the normal human heart. *Circulation.* 1994;90(1):213–219. doi:10.1161/01.CIR.90.1.213.

43. Bonow RO, Vitale DF, Bacharach SL, Maron BJ, Green MV. Effects of aging on asynchronous left ventricular regional function and global ventricular filling in normal human subjects. *J Am Coll Cardiol.* 1988;11(1):50–58. doi:10.1016/0735-1097(88)90166-0.
44. Topol EJ, Traill TA, Fortuin NJ. Hypertensive hypertrophic cardiomyopathy of the elderly. *N Engl J Med.* 1985;312(5):277–283. doi:10.1056/NEJM198501313120504.
45. Alexander J, Dainiak N, Berger HJ, et al. Serial assessment of doxorubicin cardiotoxicity with quantitative radionuclide angiocardiography. *N Engl J Med.* 1979;300(6):278–283. doi:10.1056/NEJM197902083000603.
46. Schwartz RG, McKenzie WB, Alexander J, et al. Congestive heart failure and left ventricular dysfunction complicating doxorubicin therapy. Seven-year experience using serial radionuclide angiocardiography. *Am J Med.* 1987;82(6):1109–1118. doi:10.1016/0002-9343(87)90212-9.
47. Russell RR, Alexander J, Jain D, et al. The role and clinical effectiveness of multimodality imaging in the management of cardiac complications of cancer and cancer therapy. *J Nucl Cardiol.* 2016;23(4):856–884. doi:10.1007/s12350-016-0538-8.
48. Schwartz RG, Venci N. Can serial changes of diastolic dysfunction signal incremental risk of chemotherapy-induced heart failure missed by the timing of declining LV ejection fraction? *J Nucl Cardiol.* 2016;23(4):833–836. doi:10.1007/s12350-015-0194-4.
49. Serrano JM, González I, Del Castillo S, et al. Diastolic dysfunction following anthracycline-based chemotherapy in breast cancer patients: incidence and predictors. *Oncologist.* 2015;20(8):864–872. doi:10.1634/theoncologist.2014-0500.
50. Boyd A, Stoodley P, Richards D, et al. Anthracyclines induce early changes in left ventricular systolic and diastolic function: a single centre study. *PLoS One.* 2017;12(4):e0175544. doi:10.1371/journal.pone.0175544.
51. Cottin Y, Touzery C, Coudert B, et al. Impairment of diastolic function during short-term anthracycline chemotherapy. *Brit Heart J.* 1995;73(1):61–64.
52. Reuvekamp EJ, Bulten BF, Nieuwenhuis AA, et al. Does diastolic dysfunction precede systolic dysfunction in trastuzumab-induced cardiotoxicity? Assessment with multigated radionuclide angiography (MUGA). *J Nucl Cardiol.* 2016;23(4):824–832. doi:10.1007/s12350-015-0164-x.
53. Tyberg TI, Goodyer AVN, Hurst VW, Alexander J, Langou RA. Left ventricular filling in differentiating restrictive amyloid cardiomyopathy and constrictive pericarditis. *Am J Cardiol.* 1981;47:791–796. doi:10.1016/0002-9149(81)90175-2.
54. Gerson M, Colthar M, Fowler N. Differentiation of constrictive pericarditis and restrictive cardiomyopathy by radionuclide ventriculography. *Am Heart J.* 1989;118(1):114–120.
55. Aroney CN, Ruddy TD, Dighero H, Fifer MA, Boucher CA, Palacios IF. Differentiation of restrictive cardiomyopathy from pericardial constriction: assessment of diastolic function by radionuclide angiography. *J Am Coll Cardiol.* 1989;13:1007–1014. doi:10.1016/0735-1097(89)90252-0.

17

Diastolic Echocardiographic Examination

Bonita A. Anderson and Darryl J. Burstow

OUTLINE

Case Study 1

A 68-year-old female presents with Class II heart failure. Her echocardiogram (see figure) showed normal left ventricular (LV) systolic function with the LV ejection fraction (EF) estimated at 67% by the Simpson's biplane method (A). There was no significant valvular heart disease. Diastolic function parameters include the transmitral inflow profile (B), septal and lateral mitral annular velocities (C), the peak tricuspid regurgitant (TR) velocity (D), and the indexed left atrial (LA) volume (E). See Box 17.1 for the interpretation of diastolic function pertaining to this case study.

BOX 17.1 Interpretation of Diastolic Function in Case Study 1 Using Key Parameters

As the patient has a normal LVEF of 67%, interpretation of diastolic function begins with Algorithm A (Fig. 17.1). The average E/e′ ratio is above 14; both the septal and lateral e′ velocities are below the cutoff values of 7 cm/sec and 10 cm/sec, respectively; the peak TR velocity is greater than 2.8 m/sec; and the indexed LA volume exceeds 34 mL/m^2. As four of four parameters are positive, diastolic dysfunction is present. To determine the left ventricular filling pressure (LVFP) and grade of diastolic dysfunction, algorithm B is applied. This begins by considering the transmitral inflow profile. As the E/A ratio is between 0.8 and 2.0, to determine the grade of LV diastolic function, an additional three parameters are considered: the average E/e′ ratio, the peak TR velocity, and the indexed LA volume. All three of these parameters are positive; hence there is grade II diastolic dysfunction with an elevated LAP. See text for further details.

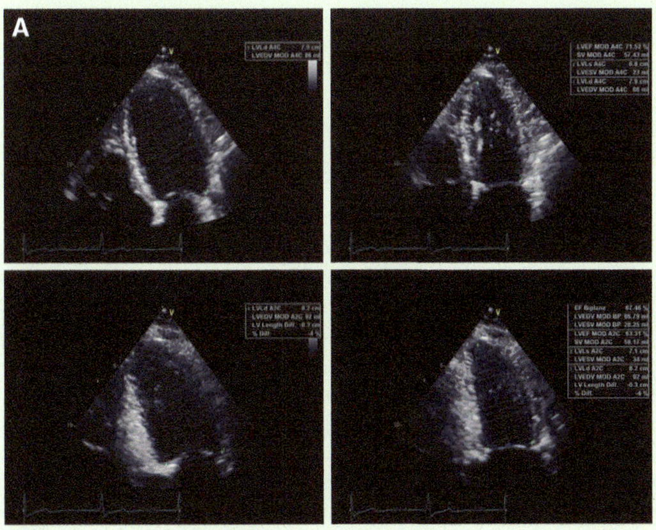

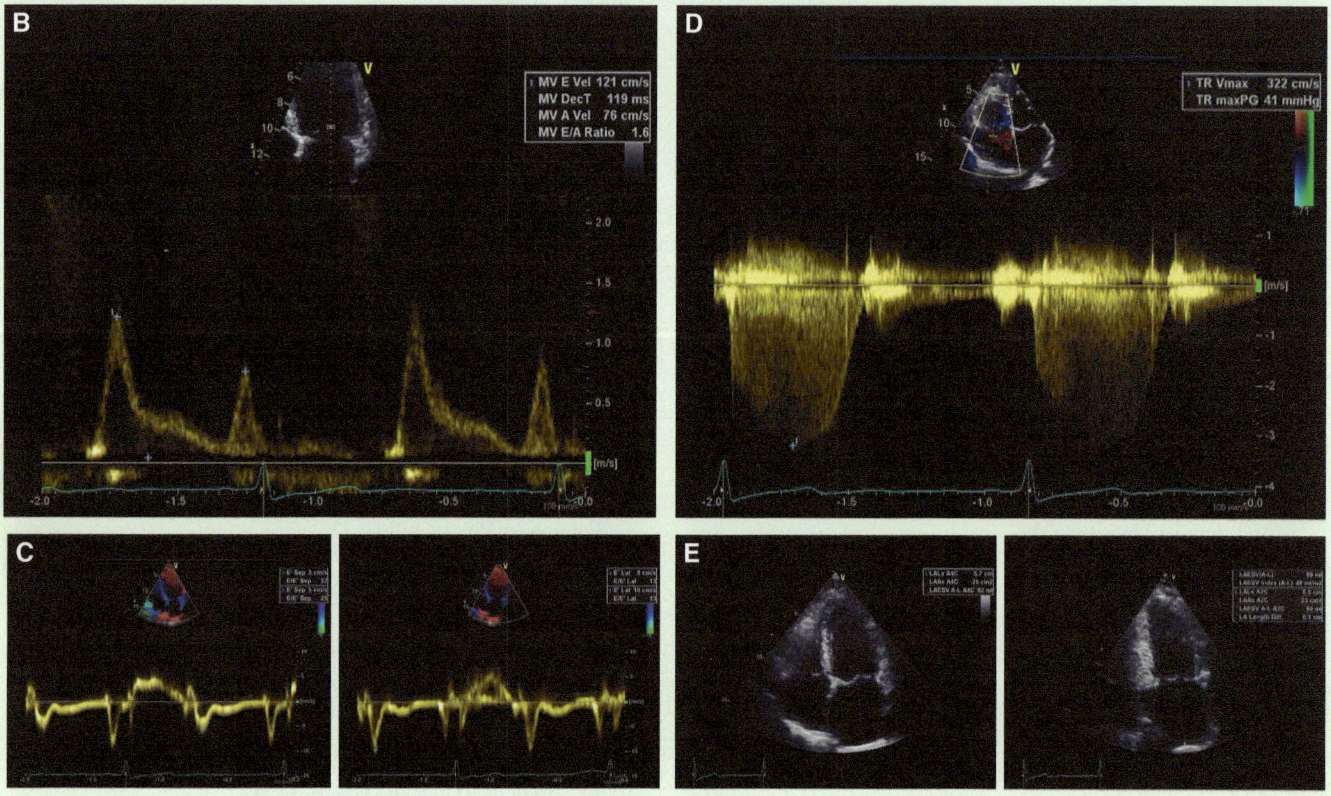

(A) The biplane LV ejection fraction (EF) derived from the end-diastolic and end-systolic volumes from the apical four-chamber *(top)* and apical two-chamber *(bottom)* views is 67%. (B) From the transmitral inflow trace the peak early diastolic (E) velocity is 121 cm/sec, the peak velocity with atrial contraction (A) velocity is 76 cm/sec with an E/A ratio of 1.6. (C) The peak e′ velocity acquired at the septal *(left)* and lateral *(right)* mitral annulus is 5 cm/sec and 9 cm/sec, respectively. The average E/e′ ratio is 17. (D) The peak tricuspid regurgitant velocity (TR) is 322 cm/sec (or 3.2 m/sec). (E) The biplane left atrial (LA) volume, indexed to the body surface area, is 48 mL/m^2.

INTRODUCTION

In 2016 the American Society of Echocardiography (ASE) along with the European Association of Cardiovascular Imaging (EACVI) produced an updated document for the assessment of LV diastolic function.[1] The primary goal of this update is to simplify the approach to the assessment of LV diastolic function and thus increase the utility of the guidelines in daily clinical practice by applying the most useful, reproducible, and feasible two-dimensional (2-D) and Doppler measurements for the estimation of LV filling pressures (LVFP) and the grading of LV diastolic dysfunction. Importantly, there is no single diastolic parameter, with perhaps the exception of the E/A ratio in depressed LVEF, that is reliable enough to determine the presence or grading of LV diastolic function. For this reason, an integrated approach, considering multiple parameters, in addition to the clinical data and patient's age, is required to identify the presence of LV diastolic dysfunction and to provide a reliable estimation of LVFP.

Based on the 2016 ASE/EACVI recommendations, four key parameters have been proposed for the evaluation LV diastolic function: transmitral inflow profile, mitral annular velocities, peak tricuspid regurgitant (TR) velocity, and indexed LA volume. Complementary measurements can also be used for the assessment of LV diastolic function when key variables are inconclusive. The justification for the use of each of these indices is briefly described in the chapter. This is followed by a detailed description of the echocardiographic technique for acquiring, optimizing, and measuring each parameter.

KEY ECHOCARDIOGRAPHIC PARAMETERS

LV diastolic dysfunction is characterized by abnormal myocardial mechanics resulting initially in the development of impaired LV relaxation, followed by increased chamber stiffness and an associated progressive rise in LVFP as the severity or grade of diastolic dysfunction worsens. Therefore useful parameters for the assessment of diastolic function will be able to detect impaired LV relaxation and/or elevated LVFP. However, as there is no single variable that can be used to establish the grade of LV diastolic function with high accuracy, a multiparameter approach is required whereby multiple variables are considered. Algorithms (Fig. 17.1), with concordance between two or more parameters in an individual patient, can then be applied to determine the presence (see Fig. 17.1A) and grading (see Fig. 17.1B) of diastolic dysfunction.

Transmitral Inflow

The transmitral inflow profile consists of an early diastolic (E) and atrial contraction (A) velocities (Fig. 17.2). The ratio between these two peak velocities (E/A ratio) has a satisfactory correlation with LVFP in patients with established or recognized LV diastolic dysfunction. This means that when there is known diastolic dysfunction, the transmitral E/A ratio alone can often be used to accurately estimate LVFP. For example, a decreased E/A ratio (≤ 0.8) due to a low E velocity (≤ 50 cm/sec) and increased filling at atrial contraction (A velocity), along with prolongation of the deceleration time (DT), is consistent

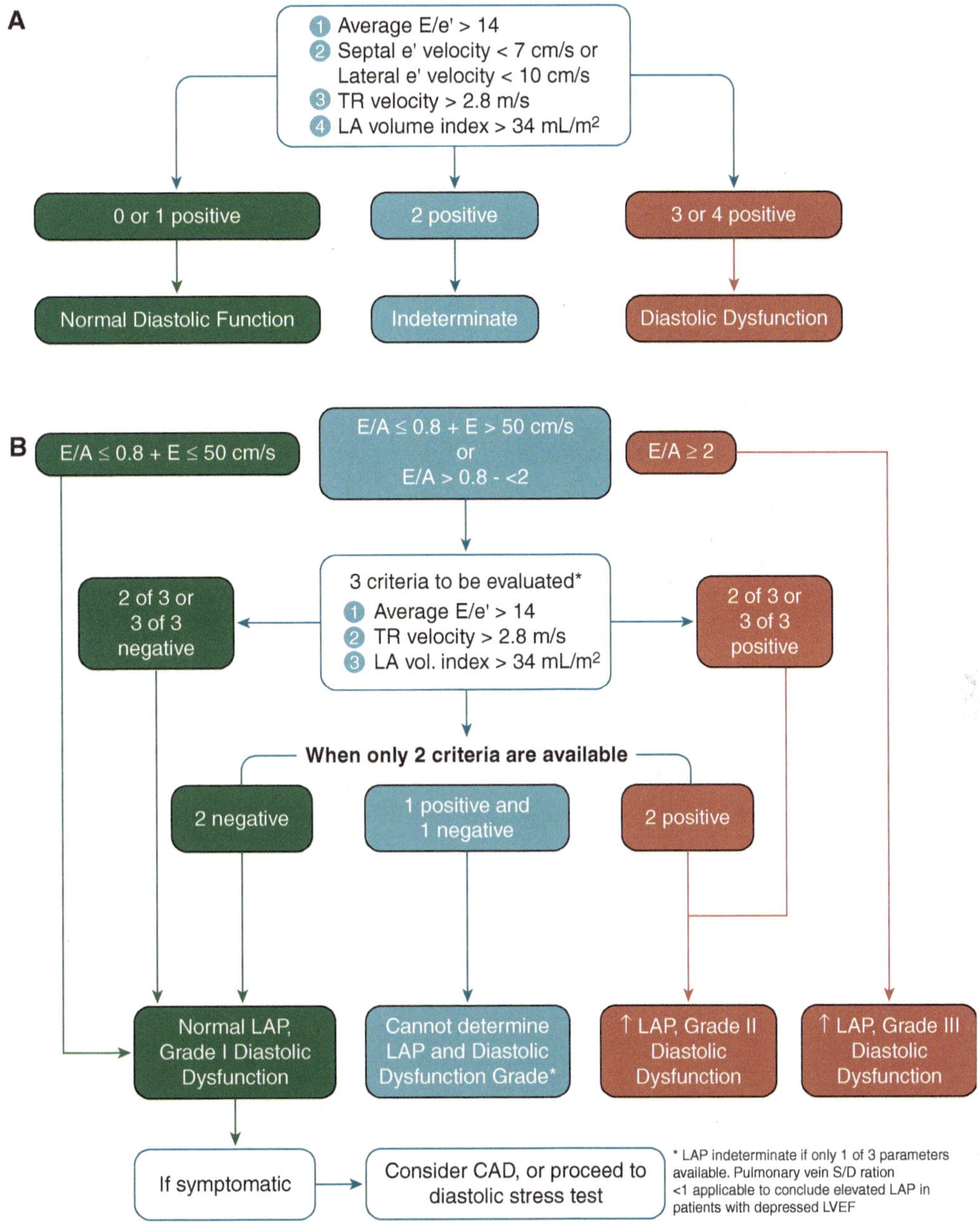

Fig. 17.1 (A) Algorithm for diagnosis of left ventricular (LV) diastolic dysfunction in subjects with a normal LV ejection fraction (EF). (B) Algorithm for estimation of LV filling pressures and grading LV diastolic function in patients with depressed LVEFs, patients with normal LVEF and diastolic dysfunction (DD), or patients with normal LVEF and myocardial disease, after consideration of clinical and other 2-D data. (Adapted from Nagueh SF, Smiseth OA, Appleton CP, Byrd III BF, Dokainish H, Edvardsen T, et al. Recommendations for the evaluation of left ventricular diastolic function by echocardiography: an update from the American Society of Echocardiography and the European Association of Cardiovascular Imaging. *J Am Soc Echocardiogr.* 2016;29(4):277–314.)

with impaired relaxation and normal LVFP; while a markedly increased E/A ratio (≥2.0), with a high E velocity and a low A velocity, along with a short DT, is consistent with advanced diastolic dysfunction and a marked elevation in LVFP.[2]

One of the limitations of using the transmitral inflow profile alone for assessing LVFP relates to the competing effects of impaired relaxation and rising LVFP. That is, in the setting of impaired relaxation in conjunction with a moderate reduction in LV compliance and a moderate increase in LA pressure (LAP), the decreased E/A ratio and prolonged DT that are typical of impaired relaxation will normalize to create a pseudonormal transmitral inflow profile.[2] For this transmitral inflow pattern, additional parameters are still required to accurately estimate LV filling pressures. Furthermore, the normal values for transmitral indices are age dependent.[3] As such, age should be taken into account when evaluating the significance of transmitral Doppler filling patterns.[1] The normal values for various age groups are listed in Table 17.1.

Mitral Annular Velocities

The peak mitral annular e′ velocity acquired with tissue Doppler imaging (TDI) reflects LV relaxation in early diastole.[4] In particular, the

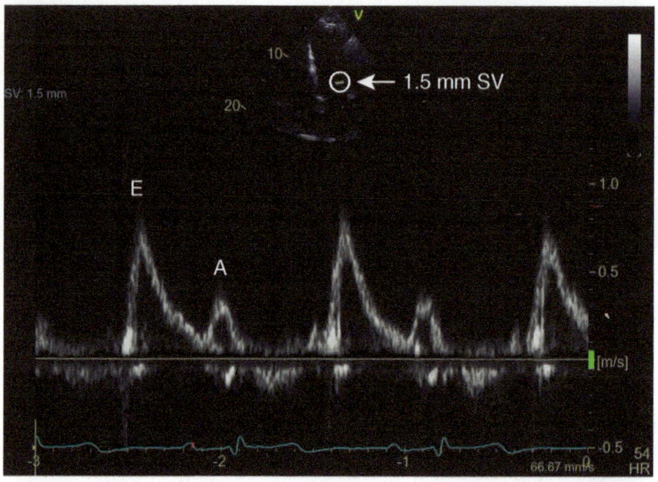

Fig. 17.2 Transmitral inflow is recorded from an apical four-chamber view with a pulsed-wave Doppler with a sample volume (SV) between 1–3 mm in size placed at the tips of the mitral valve and aligned parallel with LV inflow. The normal profile displays two prominent velocity peaks above the zero baseline: The peak early diastolic *(E)* occurs after the T wave of the electrocardiogram (ECG), and the peak atrial contraction *(A)* occurs just after the P wave of the ECG.

peak e′ velocity is inversely related to the time constant of isovolumic relaxation (tau [τ]); thus when there is prolongation of LV relaxation (a longer τ), there is a lower e′ velocity.[5] Importantly, the e′ velocity is relatively load independent and since in most patients impaired relaxation is present across all grades of diastolic dysfunction, a reduction in the e′ velocity is also present across all stages of diastolic dysfunction. However, as for the transmitral inflow velocities, the normal values for the e′ velocity are age dependent.[3] In addition, normal values for the e′ velocity is dependent on the sampled location (septal vs. lateral annulus). Therefore age as well as sampled location should be considered when evaluating these velocities.[1] The normal e′ values for various age groups and sample locations are listed in Table 17.1.

Another application of the e′ velocity is in the calculation of the E/e′ ratio. As stated, the transmitral inflow profile is load dependent, while the e′ velocity is relatively load independent. Hence the E/e′ ratio predominately adjusts for the influence of LV relaxation on the transmitral inflow profile. For example, in the individual with normal LAP, both the transmitral E and e′ velocities are normal; therefore the E/e′ ratio will be low. With impaired relaxation plus an elevated preload (LAP), the E velocity is normal or increased but the e′ velocity will be reduced; therefore the E/e′ ratio will be increased. Numerous studies have shown that there is a strong relationship between the E/e′ ratio, with the e′ acquired at either the septal or lateral annulus, and the LVFP.[6–10] In particular, an E/e′ ratio (averaged at the septal and lateral annulus) greater than 14 is rarely seen in normal individuals of any age (see Table 17.1).[3]

Tricuspid Regurgitant Velocity

In the absence of pulmonary stenosis or right ventricular outflow tract (RVOT) obstruction, the peak TR velocity combined with right atrial pressure (RAP) can be used to estimate the pulmonary artery systolic pressure (PASP). In the absence of pulmonary vascular disease, an elevated PASP is seen as a marker of elevated LVFP.[1] In this instance, it is assumed that the increased PASP is due to left heart disease (or

TABLE 17.1 Normal Transmitral Inflow, Mitral Annular e′ and E/e′ Ratios for Age

	Age (yrs)			
Measurement	**20–40**	**40–60**	**≥60**	**All**
Transmitral Inflow				
Peak E (cm/sec)	0.82 ± 0.16 (0.53–1.22)	0.75 ± 0.17 (0.46–1.13)	0.70 ± 0.16 (0.39–1.03)	0.76 ± 0.17 (0.46–1.12)
Peak A (cm/sec)	0.50 + 0.13 (0.30–0.87)	0.62 ± 0.15 (0.37–0.97)	0.74 ± 0.16 (0.40–1.04)	0.60 ± 0.17 (0.35–0.98)
DT (msec)	178.2 ± 43.1 (105.2–269.0)	187.6 ± 45.5 (114.6–288.1)	208.9 ± 62.7 (114.0–385.9)	188.0 ± 49.4 (112.8–296.4)
E/A ratio	1.71 ± 0.52 (0.89–3.18)	1.24 ± 0.39 (0.71–2.27)	0.98 ± 0.29 (0.53–1.80)	1.37 ± 0.51 (0.64–2.74)
Mitral Annular e′ Velocities				
Septal e′ (cm/sec)	12.1 ± 2.5 (8.0–17.0)	9.8 ± 2.6 (5.0–16.0)	7.6 ± 2.3 3.0–13.0	10.3 ± 3.0 (5.0–17.0)
Lateral e′ (cm/sec)	16.4 ± 3.4 (10.0–23.0)	12.5 ± 3.0 (6.0–18.0)	9.6 ± 2.8 (4.0–17.0)	13.5 ± 4.0 (6.0–22.0)
E/e′ Ratio				
Septal E/e′	6.9 ± 1.6 (4.4–10.6)	8.1 ± 2.3 (4.3–13.2)	9.7 ± 2.8 (5.0–16.9)	7.9 ± 2.4 (6.1–9.2)
Lateral E/e′	5.1 ± 1.3 (3.1–8.5)	6.3 ± 2.2 (3.7–12.0)	7.8 ± 2.2 (4.2–12.8)	6.1 ± 2.1 (4.6–7.3)
Average septal and lateral E/e′	5.8 ± 1.3 (3.6–9.1)	7.0 ± 2.1 (4.2–11.5)	8.5 ± 2.2 (4.6–13.5)	6.8 ± 2.1 (5.4–7.9)

DT, Deceleration time.

Data are expressed as mean ± 1 standard deviation (95% confidence interval).

From Caballero L, Kou S, Dulgheru R, Gonjilashvili N, Athanassopoulos GD, Barone D, et al. Echocardiographic reference ranges for normal cardiac Doppler data: results from the NORRE Study. *Eur Heart J Cardiovasc Imaging.* 2015;16(9):1031–1041.

postcapillary pulmonary hypertension) where there is an elevation in the LAP, which leads to increased back pressure to the lungs and a subsequent increase in PASP. A peak TR velocity value of 2.8 m/sec or less is generally considered normal.[11] Hence a peak TR velocity value greater than 2.8 m/sec, in the absence of pulmonary vascular disease, indicates elevated LVFP.[1]

Indexed LA Volume

The LA size is considered a morphophysiologic expression of LV diastolic dysfunction and increased LVFP.[12] For instance, a dilated LA suggests a chronic elevation in LAP. It has been found that an indexed LA volume of 34 mL/m^2 distinguished the presence of elevated LVFP (defined by a septal E/e′ >15) with 86% sensitivity and 66% specificity.[13] Thus an indexed LAV greater than 34 mL/m^2 may indicate an increased LAP secondary to chronically increased LVFP.

COMPLEMENTARY ECHOCARDIOGRAPHIC PARAMETERS

Complementary or supplementary measurements such as an abnormal Valsalva maneuver on the mitral inflow profile, an increased, pulmonary venous flow atrial reversal velocity, or the presence of an L wave in the mitral inflow (see upcoming discussion) can also be used for the assessment of LV diastolic function when key variables are inconclusive or when the presence or grading of LV diastolic dysfunction is deemed indeterminate. These complementary parameters indicate either the presence of underlying impaired LV relaxation and/or provide additional evidence of elevated LVFP.

LV Wall Thickness and Mass

Hypertensive heart disease is the most common abnormality leading to diastolic heart failure.[12] As increased LV wall thickness and mass are common findings associated with hypertensive heart disease, the mere presence of increased LV wall thickness and mass are clues to the presence of abnormal myocardial structure and thus underlying LV diastolic dysfunction. For instance, when there is a marked increase in LV wall thickness and LV mass, an impaired relaxation pattern is expected on the transmitral inflow profile. The absence of an impaired relaxation pattern suggests a decrease in LV compliance and an increased LAP.

Pulmonary Venous Inflow

The normal pulmonary venous profile is characterized by three distinct waveforms: (1) systolic forward flow (S velocity), (2) diastolic forward flow (D velocity), and (3) atrial flow reversal during atrial systole (Ar velocity) (see Fig. 17.8 later in the chapter). In approximately one-third of normal individuals, the S waveform may be biphasic consisting of an S1 velocity and an S2 velocity.[14]

Pulmonary venous waveforms are influenced by LA contraction, relaxation, and pressure as well as by LV compliance and filling pressures.[12] The pulmonary venous S velocity is closely related to the LAP. The pulmonary venous D velocity is influenced by changes in LV filling and compliance, and essentially parallels the transmitral E velocity. The magnitude and duration of the Ar waveform is influenced by LV late diastolic pressures, atrial preload, and LA contractility. In particular, increased LAP decreases the pulmonary venous-to-LA pressure gradient in systole and increases the pulmonary vein–LA pressure gradient during diastole; this results in a decreased peak S velocity, an increased peak D velocity, and a subsequent decrease in the S/D ratio.[15] Generally a decreased S/D ratio less than 1 in adult patients with a depressed LVEF is indicative of increased LAP.[1]

The pulmonary venous flow profile can also be used to identify patients with an elevated LV end-diastolic pressure (LVEDP). When the LVEDP is increased, there is an earlier than normal crossover of pressures between the LA and the LV, which effectively shortens the transmitral A wave duration. As a result, the pulmonary venous Ar duration is longer than the transmitral A duration since the transmitral A duration is shortened by the elevated LVEDP. Difference between the pulmonary vein Ar and the transmitral A durations has shown a strong correlation with the LVEDP[16–18] with a difference of 30 msec or more providing a good indicator for an elevated LVEDP above 15 mmHg.[1,12,16]

Isovolumic Relaxation Time

The isovolumic relaxation time (IVRT) is the time interval between aortic valve closure and mitral valve opening. When LV relaxation is impaired, the fall in LV pressure is slow so that the normal crossover between the LA and LV pressures is delayed, which also delays the opening of the mitral valve and prolongs the IVRT. However, as for the transmitral inflow profile, the IVRT is both load dependent and age dependent (Table 17.2). Importantly, despite the presence of impaired relaxation, increased LAP normalizes the IVRT; with a further elevation in the LAP, the IVRT shortens. Hence the use of the IVRT in isolation has limited accuracy in the assessment of LV diastolic function. However, when combined with other key variables, the IVRT may be useful in assessing LV diastolic function in patients with heart failure and reduced LVEF, coexistent mitral valve disease, mitral annular calcification, or atrial fibrillation.[1,19–22]

Color M-mode Propagation Velocity

Similar to transmitral inflow, LV intracavitary filling is comprised of two waveforms: an early diastolic wave and an atrial contraction wave (see Fig. 17.10 later in the chapter). Using color M-mode (CMM), these waveforms can be mapped as blood flows from the mitral annulus toward the LV apex. The flow propagation velocity (Vp) is a measurement of the velocity at which flow propagates within the LV during early diastole. The Vp is indirectly related to the time constant of relaxation (τ) such that the longer it takes for the ventricle to relax, the slower the Vp.[23,24]

The E/Vp ratio has been found to correlate with the LVFP.[25–28] Like the E/e′ ratio, the E/Vp unmasks the influence of LV relaxation on the transmitral inflow profile. For example, in the individual with normal LAP, both the transmitral E velocity and Vp are normal; therefore the

TABLE 17.2 Normal Isovolumic Relaxation Time (IVRT) for Age

	Age Group (yrs)			
Measurement	**16–20**	**21–40**	**41–60**	**> 60**
IVRT (msec)	50 ± 9 (32–68)	67 ± 8 (51–83)	74 ± 7 (60–88)	87 ± 7 (73–101)

Data are expressed as mean ± 1 standard deviation (95% confidence interval).
From Klein AL, Burstow DJ, Tajik AJ, Zachariah PK, Bailey KR, Seward JB. Effects of age on left ventricular dimensions and filling dynamics in 117 normal persons. *Mayo Clin Proc.* 1994;69:212–224.

E/Vp ratio will be low. With impaired relaxation plus an elevated preload (LAP), the E velocity is normal or increased but the Vp is slow; therefore the E/Vp ratio will be increased. However, the Vp can fall into the normal range in patients with normal LV cavity size and ejection fraction, despite the presence of impaired relaxation; hence the E/Vp ratio may not accurately predict LVFP in these patients.[29]

A more detailed description of the role of CMM propagation velocity in the assessment of LV diastolic function is discussed in Chapter 11.

LV and LA Strain

LV global longitudinal strain (GLS) is a measure of longitudinal deformation of the LV during systole, and abnormally low values indicate impaired global longitudinal function. A reduction in GLS can precede the development of overt systolic dysfunction as measured by traditional methods such as LVEF.[30] Thus abnormal LV GLS identifies patients with abnormal myocardial mechanics and therefore suggests the presence of diastolic dysfunction, but as a single parameter it has not been found to be an accurate predictor of LVFP.

LV global diastolic strain rate (GDSR) in the isovolumic relaxation period and in early diastole has demonstrated good correlation with the time constant of relaxation (τ). Reduced values suggest the presence of impaired relaxation. When combined with the transmitral E velocity, GDSR has been shown to correlate with LVFP.[31]

LA strain is an emerging parameter used for the assessment of LA function. Peak LA strain has been shown to be abnormal in patients with systolic and diastolic heart failure.[32] In patients with preserved LVEF, peak LA strain values have demonstrated a stepwise decline with increasing grades of diastolic dysfunction[33] and thus may allow more accurate categorization of diastolic dysfunction severity.

LV and LA strain, although not part of the current diagnostic algorithms for diastolic function assessment, are promising parameters and await ongoing validation in larger clinical studies. A more detailed description of the application of strain imaging in the assessment of LV diastolic function is discussed in Chapter 10 and 12.

ACQUISITION AND MEASUREMENT OF KEY ECHOCARDIOGRAPHIC VARIABLES

The methodology for acquiring the four key parameters utilized for the evaluation LV diastolic function described in this section is based on ASE recommendations.[1,12,37] Table 17.3 provides a summary of the technical aspects for the acquisition, optimization, and measurement of each parameter. All measurements should be averaged over at least two cardiac cycles for patients in sinus rhythm and three to five cardiac cycles for patients in atrial fibrillation. For the LA volume, measurement from one representative beat is acceptable in the clinical setting. Furthermore, a number of potential pitfalls may lead to measurement error and sonographers, and reporting physicians need to be mindful of these and understand how these errors can be avoided and/or overcome (Table 17.4).

Transmitral Inflow

Transmitral inflow is interrogated from the apical four-chamber view using pulsed-wave (PW) Doppler with the Doppler beam aligned parallel with inflow and the sample volume positioned centrally at the tips of the open mitral valve leaflets. When there is sinus rhythm, the transmitral velocity profile consists of early diastolic (E) and atrial contraction (A) velocities appearing above the zero baseline (see examples in Case Study 1 and 2, and in Fig. 17.2). The trace is optimized by using a small sample volume size (1–3 mm) and by ensuring that there is parallel alignment with LV inflow. Color Doppler and off-axis imaging may be used to optimize the alignment. Off-axis imaging is especially important in the dilated LV where transmitral inflow is directed progressively more posterolaterally. The sweep speed (50–100 mm/sec), filters, Doppler gain, baseline, and velocity scale are adjusted to display an optimal trace (see Table 17.3).

Routine measurements performed include the peak E velocity, the peak A velocity, the E/A ratio, the DT, and the A wave duration (Fig. 17.3). DT is measured from the peak E wave velocity, along the deceleration slope, to the zero baseline. The A duration is measured from the beginning of the A wave to the end of the A wave. When there are prominent flow eddies at the end of the A wave, moving the sample volume a few millimeters closer to the mitral annulus may better define the end of the A wave and improve measurement accuracy. There are several potential pitfalls that may lead to measurement error (see Table 17.4) (Fig. 17.4).

Mitral Annular Velocities

Mitral annular signals are acquired from the apical four-chamber view at the septal and lateral annulus using TDI with the Doppler beam aligned parallel with myocardial motion and the sample volume positioned at the fibrous mitral annulus. When there is sinus rhythm, the annular profile is characterized by three distinct waveforms: (1) an apically directed systolic myocardial velocity (s′) above the zero baseline, (2) an early diastolic atrially directed myocardial velocity (e′) below the zero baseline, and (3) a late diastolic atrially directed myocardial velocity (a′) below the zero baseline (see examples in Case Study 1 and 2) (Fig. 17.5). In addition to these three distinct velocities, less prominent velocity spikes may be seen between the s′ and e′ waves during the isovolumic relaxation period and between the a′ and s′ waves during the isovolumic contraction period. These velocity spikes are often biphasic appearing above and below the zero baseline. The trace is optimized by using a large sample volume size (5–10 mm) to ensure sampling of the annular excursion over systole and diastole. Off-axis imaging may be required to improve this alignment, especially when interrogating the lateral mitral annulus. As myocardial velocities are much slower, and amplitudes are much higher than conventional PW Doppler, when performing TDI the filters are set to detect low velocities (<20 cm/sec) and high amplitudes (>40 dB). Most current ultrasound systems have TDI presets, which should be selected to ensure the proper display of velocity scale and filter settings. The sweep speed, Doppler gain, and baseline are adjusted to display optimal signals (see Table 17.3).

For LV diastolic function assessment, the peak e′ velocity is measured at the septal and lateral annulus. The E/e′ can be calculated from the septal and lateral e′ velocities. The averaged E/e′ is calculated from the averaged septal E/e′ and lateral E/e′ ratios. While some laboratories only acquire septal or lateral velocities, recording of the TDI profiles at both annuli is encouraged. This is especially useful in aiding the diagnosis of constrictive pericarditis (CP) (Box 17.2). The most pitfalls leading to measurement error relate to nonparallel alignment and sample volume placement (see Table 17.4).

Tricuspid Regurgitant Velocity

The peak TR velocity is measured via continuous wave (CW) Doppler ensuring parallel alignment with the TR jet (see examples in Case Study 1 and 2). The peak TR velocity should be averaged over the respiratory cycle or measured at end expiration. The trace is optimized by ensuring that there is parallel alignment between the Doppler beam and the TR jet. Off-axis imaging is often required to improve alignment. The sweep speed, filters, Doppler gain, baseline, and velocity scale are adjusted to display the TR velocities, including forward flow, over multiple cardiac cycles (see Table 17.3). The compression and/or reject should also be optimized to enhance the peak TR velocity.

TABLE 17.3 Technical Aspects for Left Ventricular Diastology Parameters

Parameter	Acquisition	Optimization	Measurements Performed
Key Diastology Parameters			
Transmitral inflow	Apical four-chamber PW Doppler 1–3mm SV placed between MV leaflet tips Color Doppler and/or off-axis imaging may be used to aid alignment with inflow	Parallel alignment with inflow Sweep speed 100 mm/sec Low wall filters enabling a clear depiction of the onset and cessation of flow Low signal gain with minimal background speckling Velocity scale and baseline set to display full spectrum	Peak E velocity Peak A velocity E/A ratio DT A duration
Mitral annular velocities	Apical four-chamber TDI 5–10mm SV placed at septal and lateral mitral annulus	TDI preset (low velocity, high amplitude settings) Parallel alignment with myocardial motion Sweep speed 50–100 mm/sec (display two complete cardiac cycles) Low signal gain with minimal background speckling Velocity scale and baseline set to display full spectrum	Septal e′ velocity Lateral e′ velocity
TR velocity	Any view where parallel alignment with TR jet is achieved CW Doppler	Parallel alignment with TR jet Sweep speed 50–75 mm/sec (display a full respiratory cycle) Low signal gain with minimal background speckling Velocity scale and baseline set to display full spectrum (including forward flow signal) Decrease compression or increase reject to minimize spectral broadening	Peak TR velocity
LA volume	Apical four-chamber and two-chamber views End systole (one to two frames prior to opening of the MV) LA area traced at blood-tissue interfaces LA length measured from the center of the mitral annulus to the center of the LA superior wall	Open up and elongate LA (without concern for the LV) Optimize 2-D gains and TGC to ensure blood pool is echo free Adjust the field of view to see the entire LA and/or utilize the zoom function Utilize other available 2-D controls to optimize image Ensure differences between LA lengths is <5 mm	Apical four-chamber LA area and LA length Apical two-chamber LA area and LA length Biplane LA volume is indexed to the BSA
Complementary Diastology Parameters			
LV wall thickness and mass	Parasternal LAX 2-D or M-mode End diastole Perpendicular to LAX of LV Just distal to MV leaflet tips Calipers placed at blood-tissue interfaces	Ensure the 2-D image is on-axis For M-mode, ensure the cursor is aligned perpendicular to the LV LAX and just distal to MV leaflet tips Optimize 2-D/M-mode gains and TGC to ensure blood pool is echo free Adjust the field of view to see the entire LV Utilize other available 2-D controls to optimize image	IVS thickness LV internal dimension Posterior LV wall thickness
PV inflow	Apical four-chamber or five-chamber view PW Doppler 3–5mm SV placed 1 cm into PV Color Doppler especially useful in aiding alignment with inflow	Parallel alignment with inflow Sweep speed 100 mm/sec Low wall filters enabling a clear depiction of the onset and cessation of flow Low signal gain with minimal background speckling Velocity scale and baseline set to display full spectrum Low PRF	Peak S velocity Peak D velocity S/D ratio Ar velocity Ar duration
IVRT	Apical five-chamber or apical LAX view PW Doppler (3–5 mm SV) or CW Doppler Color Doppler useful in identifying region of inflow/outflow	Sweep speed 100 mm/sec Low wall filters enabling a clear depiction of the onset and cessation of flow Velocity scale and baseline set to display full spectrum	IVRT (time interval between aortic valve closure and mitral valve opening)
Color M-mode Vp	Apical four-chamber view Color Doppler of LV inflow M-mode cursor placed within the center of LV inflow color jet Decrease color velocity scale to 30–50 cm/sec or shift color baseline upwards (forward velocity scale to 30–50 cm/sec) so central highest velocity jet is blue	Avoid apical foreshortening Color box adjusted to cover LV cavity and mitral annulus Color gain to just below background speckling Image depth decreased to include the entire LV and a small portion of LA M-mode sweep speed 100–200 mm/sec Color velocity scale adjusted as opposite to enhance demarcation of the Vp slope on M-mode trace	Vp (slope of first aliased velocity during early filling from the level of the mitral annulus to 4 cm into the LV cavity)

(Continued)

TABLE 17.3 Technical Aspects for Left Ventricular Diastology Parameters (*Cont.*)

Parameter	Acquisition	Optimization	Measurements Performed
LV strain	Apical LAX view Apical four-chamber view Apical two-chamber view Acquire three-beat loops at end expiration	Ensure apical images are on-axis Optimize for best endocardial definition Narrow sector width and use a shallow image depth (ensure LV epicardial border within imaging sector) Ensure high frame rates between ~50 and 90 fps	Segmental systolic strain and global longitudinal strain (see Chapter 10)
LA strain	Apical four-chamber view Apical two-chamber view Acquire three-beat loops at end expiration	Ensure non-foreshortened images of the LA Optimize for best endocardial definition Narrow sector width and use a shallow image depth Ensure high frame rates between ~50 and 90 fps	Peak reservoir, conduit and contractile strain (see Chapter 12)

BSA, Body surface area; *CW,* continuous wave; *DT,* deceleration time; *IVRT,* isovolumic relaxation time; *IVS,* interventricular septum; *LA,* left atrial; *LAX,* long axis; *LV,* left ventricular; *MV,* mitral valve; *PRF,* pulse repetition frequency; *PV,* pulmonary venous; *PW,* pulsed-wave; *RV,* right ventricular; *SV,* sample volume; *TDI,* tissue Doppler imaging; *TGC,* time gain compensation; *TR,* tricuspid regurgitant; *TV,* tricuspid valve; *Vp,* velocity propagation.

TABLE 17.4 Common Errors for Left Ventricular Diastology Parameters

Parameter	Common Errors	How to Avoid/Overcome
Key Diastology Parameters		
Transmitral inflow	Nonparallel alignment with inflow (poor quality trace, underestimation of velocities)	Use off-axis imaging to improve alignment Use color Doppler to identify inflow direction
	Sample volume too far into LV or too close to annulus (underestimation of velocities)	Zoom on the MV to assist with SV placement
	SV too large (spectral broadening)	Ensure SV size is between 1 and 3 mm
	Not measuring along modal velocity (overestimation of velocities and DT)	Reduce Doppler signals, decrease compression or increase reject to minimal spectral broadening Measure at the center of the most solid edge of the signal
	A duration due to flow eddies at end of A wave (overestimation A duration)	Move the SV toward the mitral annulus (only measure A duration at this level)
	E/A fusion (DT and A duration not accurate)	Do not measure the DT or A duration
Mitral annular velocities	Nonparallel alignment with myocardial motion (poor quality trace, underestimation of velocities)	Use off-axis imaging to improve alignment
	SV too low into the basal LV segments (blunting of velocities)	Zoom on the MV to assist with SV placement
	Measurement of the isovolumic relaxation (IVR) spike instead of the e′ velocity	Look at the ECG for timing, IVR spike occurs on the T wave while the e′ velocity occurs after the T wave
TR velocity	Nonparallel alignment with the TR (underestimation of peak TR velocity)	Use off-axis imaging to improve alignment Use color Doppler to identify inflow direction Attempt a reversed apical four-chamber view to improve alignment
	Measuring beard rather than chin of the signal (overestimation of peak TR velocity)	Decrease compression or increase reject to eliminate beard
LA volume	Foreshortening of the LA (overestimation of LA volume)	Attempt imaging from a lower intercostal space
	>5 mm difference in LA lengths between apical four-chamber and two-chamber views (overestimation or underestimation of LA volume)	Usually results due to foreshortening of the apical two-chamber; see previous comment
	LA length not measured to center of LA superior wall (underestimation of LA length)	Measure the longest length of the LA from the center of the mitral anulus to the center of the superior LA wall
	Poor tracing of LA area (overestimation or underestimation of LA volume)	Optimize 2-D image first ensuring that the LA is opened up and that 2-D gains/TCG are appropriately adjusted Trace at the blood-tissue interface If 2-D images are suboptimal, do not attempt
Complementary Diastology Parameters		
LV wall thickness and mass	Off-axis images (inaccurate measurements)	Reposition patient steeper, move the transducer to a higher intercostal space, and/or ask patient to breath out and hold
	M-mode cursor not aligned perpendicular to LAX of LV or off-axis image (inaccurate measurements)	See earlier discussion
	2-D measurements not perpendicular to LV LAX (inaccurate measurements)	Measurements should be performed perpendicular to the theoretical LAX of the LV
	M-mode cursor too far into LV cavity (underestimation LVID)	Ensure cursor is placed just distal to the MV leaflet tips during diastole
	Measured too far into LV cavity (underestimation LVID)	Measure just distal to the MV leaflet tips at end diastole
	Anterior caliper for IVS too anterior (overestimation IVS thickness)	Be aware of TV apparatus or RV trabeculations; exclude these from the measurement

TABLE 17.4 Common Errors for Left Ventricular Diastology Parameters (*Cont.*)

Parameter	Common Errors	How to Avoid/Overcome
PV inflow	SV placed too high at LA-PV junction or within LA; SV not in center of vein—signal contaminate by wall motion (poor trace quality and inaccurate measurements)	Ensure that the SV is placed at least 1 cm into the center of PV Use color Doppler to identify PV inflow while angling/tilting the transducer
	End caliper for Ar duration placed too early (underestimation of Ar duration)	End of the AR velocity coincides with the onset of the next S velocity
	Wall filters set too high (inaccurate Ar measurements)	Low wall filters are required to clearly see the onset and cessation of venous flow; especially when measuring the Ar duration
	High PRF (superimposition of PV and transmitral inflow leading to overestimation of peak S and D velocities)	Decrease velocity scale to remove second SV May need to move baseline down for S and D velocity measurements and then move up for Ar measurements
IVRT	Poor aortic closing clicks (inaccurate measurements)	Attempt alternative views and slight transducer manipulations to improve signal Use a larger SV size for PW Doppler attempts
	Difficulty in identifying onset of transmitral inflow (inaccurate measurements)	As earlier Increase wall filters to minimize flow contamination at zero baseline
Color M-mode Vp	Incorrect M-mode cursor alignment (inaccurate measurements)	Ensure M-mode cursor is aligned with color aliasing of LV inflow

CW, Continuous wave; *DT*, deceleration time; *DTI*, Doppler tissue imaging; *IVRT*, isovolumic relaxation time; *IVS*, interventricular septum; *LA*, left atrial; *LAX*, long axis; *LV*, left ventricular; *LVID*, left ventricular internal dimension; *MV*, mitral valve; *PV*, pulmonary venous; *PW*, pulsed-wave; *RV*, right ventricular; *SV*, sample volume; *TR*, tricuspid regurgitant; *TV*, tricuspid valve; *Vp*, velocity propagation.

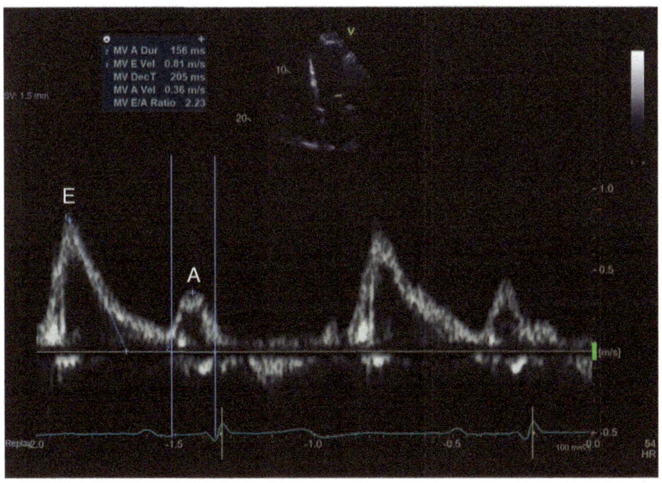

Fig. 17.3 Transmitral inflow measurements include the peak E velocity (MV E Vel), the deceleration time (MV DecT), the peak A velocity (MV A Vel), and the A duration (MV A Dur). The E/A ratio is derived from the peak E and peak A velocities.

The most common measurement errors relate to underestimation of the peak TR velocity due to nonparallel alignment of the Doppler beam with the TR jet and overestimation of the TR velocity caused by intrinsic spectral broadening and/or nonlaminar flow (see Table 17.4). Frequently the TR signal may include a chin, which represents the maximal spectral Doppler signal intensity, and a beard, which is the less intense and more poorly defined envelope with a higher velocity contour (Fig. 17.6). In this instance, the chin rather than the beard should be measured to avoid overestimation of the peak TR velocity.[39] The use of an ultrasound enhancing agent (contrast) may also be employed to enhance trivial or suboptimal TR Doppler signals.[40,41]

Indexed LA Volume

The LA volume can be measured via the area-length method or the method of discs. Measurements are performed at end systole from the apical four-chamber and apical two-chamber views. The image is optimized to ensure that the LA is not foreshortened. This can be achieved by tilting and/or angling the transducer and/or by sliding to a lower intercostal space. 2-D images are optimized in the standard manner by considering adjustable 2-D image controls such as the transducer frequency, field of view, focus, 2-D gain, and time-gain compensation (TGC).

The LA area is traced at the blood-tissue interface from annulus to annulus, excluding the mitral valve funnel, LA appendage, and pulmonary inlets. The LA length is measured from the center of the mitral annulus to the center of the superior wall of the left atrium (see examples in Case Study 1 and 2). The difference in LA lengths between the apical four-chamber and apical two-chamber views should be less than 5 mm. The LA volume is then divided by the body surface area to calculate the indexed LA volume. The most common measurement errors for the LA volume, as well as how these errors can be overcome or avoided, are listed in Table 17.4.

ACQUISITION AND MEASUREMENT OF COMPLEMENTARY ECHOCARDIOGRAPHIC PARAMETERS

The measurement techniques for acquiring complementary parameters described in the chapter are based on ASE recommendations.[1,12,34] As for the key parameters, all measurements should be averaged over at least two cardiac cycles for patients in sinus rhythm and three to five cardiac cycles for patients in atrial fibrillation. For the left ventricle, measurements from one representative beat is acceptable in the clinical setting. Table 17.3 provides a summary of the technical aspects for the acquisition, optimization, and measurement of each parameter. Table 17.4 lists the potential pitfalls that may lead to measurement error and how these errors can be avoided and/or overcome.

LV Wall Thickness and LV Mass

LV wall thickness includes the measurement of the interventricular septum (IVS) and posterior LV wall. LV mass by linear measurements is calculated from the thickness of the IVS and posterior LV wall and from the LV internal dimension (LVID). Measurements are performed from a 2-D image or M-mode trace acquired from the parasternal long axis view. Measurements are performed at end diastole, perpendicular

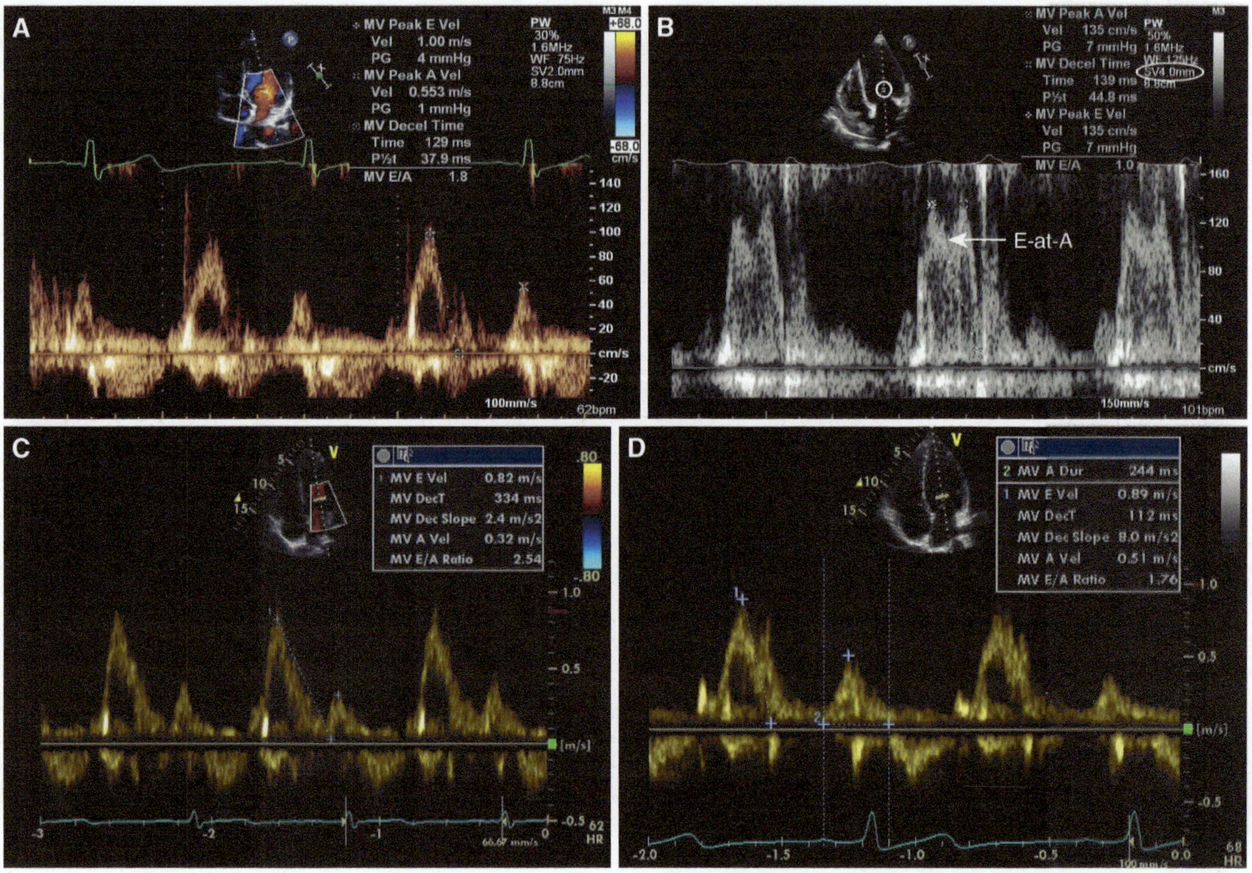

Fig. 17.4 Examples of transmitral measurement errors. (A) This trace shows poor alignment between the Doppler beam and LV inflow *(see image above the Doppler trace)*. As a result there is a poor-quality transmitral inflow signal, and measurement accuracy is compromised. (B) This trace was acquired with a sample volume size of 4 mm; this has resulted in marked spectral broadening. In addition, there is tachycardia (heart rate is 101 bpm). As a result, there is E/A fusion and the deceleration time (DT) cannot be accurately measured. Furthermore, when the E velocity at the onset of the A velocity ("E-at-A") is greater than 20 cm/sec, the A velocity is higher than it would be at slower heart rates, so the E/A ratio is not accurate. (C) The DT is overestimated as the measurement is not performed at the modal velocity. (D) The A duration is significantly overestimated with the right caliper placed well beyond the mitral valve closing click. When there are prominent flow eddies at the end of the A wave as in this example, the sample volume should be moved a few millimeters toward the mitral annulus.

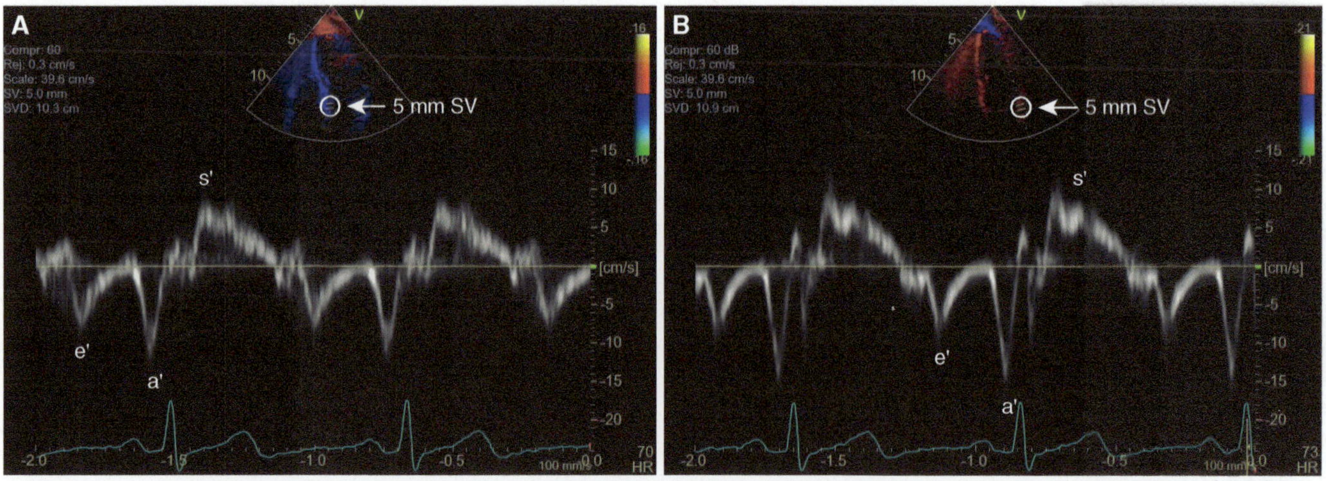

Fig. 17.5 Mitral annular velocities are recorded via tissue Doppler imaging (TDI) from an apical four-chamber view with a 5–10mm sample volume (SV) placed at the septal (A) and lateral (B) fibrous mitral annulus, aligned parallel with myocardial motion. The normal profile displays three prominent velocity peaks. The early diastolic myocardial velocity (e′) occurs after the T wave of the electrocardiogram (ECG) and appears below the zero baseline. The late diastolic myocardial velocity (a′) occurs just after the P wave of the ECG and appears below the zero baseline. The systolic myocardial velocity (s′) coincides with the T wave of the ECG and appears above the zero baseline.

BOX 17.2 Annulus Reversus in Constrictive Pericarditis

In the normal individual, the lateral e′ velocity is slightly higher than the septal e′ velocity. In patients with constrictive pericarditis, the reverse occurs; that is, the septal e′ velocity is higher than the lateral e′ velocity. This phenomenon is referred to as annulus reversus and is thought to occur due to tethering of the lateral annulus to the adjacent fibrotic and scarred pericardium.[38]

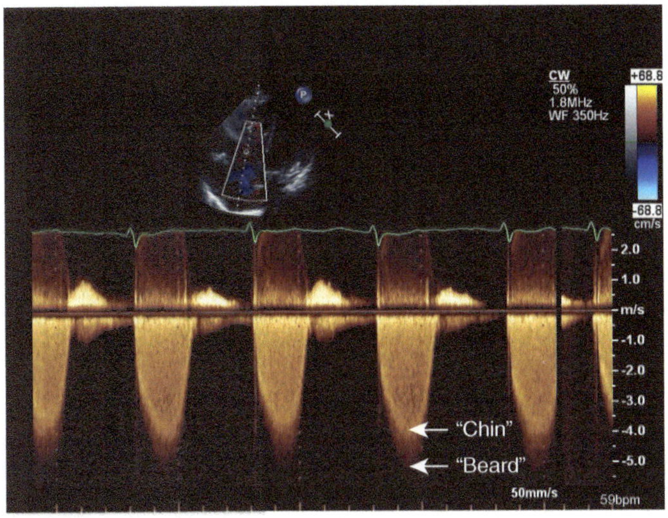

Fig. 17.6 This tricuspid regurgitant continuous wave *(CW)* Doppler traces shows the chin and the beard. When measuring the peak tricuspid regurgitation (TR) velocity, the chin rather than the beard should be measured to avoid overestimation of the peak TR velocity.

to the long axis of the LV and just distal to the mitral valve leaflet tips, and at the blood-tissue interfaces (Fig. 17.7). 2-D images and M-mode traces are optimized in the standard manner by considering adjustable image controls such as the transducer frequency, field of view, focus, gain, and TGC. The sweep speed for the M-mode trace is set to display at least two complete cardiac cycles (between 50 and 100 mm/sec).

Pulmonary Venous Inflow

Pulmonary venous inflow is interrogated from the apical four-chamber or apical five-chamber view using PW Doppler with the Doppler beam aligned parallel with inflow and with a sample volume (3–5 mm) positioned approximately 1 cm into the pulmonary vein (Fig. 17.8, left). When there is sinus rhythm, the pulmonary venous profile consists of three waveforms: systolic forward flow (S) velocity (above the zero baseline), diastolic forward flow (D) velocity (above the zero baseline), and atrial flow reversal (Ar) velocity (below the zero baseline). The trace is optimized by ensuring that there is parallel alignment with LV inflow. Color Doppler is especially useful in identifying and aligning pulmonary venous flow. The sweep speed (between 50 and 100 mm/sec), filters, Doppler gain, baseline, and velocity scale are adjusted to display an optimal trace (see Table 17.3).

Routine measurements performed include the peak S velocity, the peak D velocity, the S/D ratio, the peak Ar velocity, and the Ar wave duration (see Fig. 17.8, right). The Ar duration is measured from the beginning of the Ar wave to the end of the Ar wave or from the end of the D wave to the onset of the next S wave. When the pulmonary venous S signal appears biphasic (S1 and S2 components are distinctly separated), for the purposes of measuring the pulmonary venous S/D ratio, the peak of S2 is measured as this component is more reflective of LA pressure as well as LA and LV compliance.

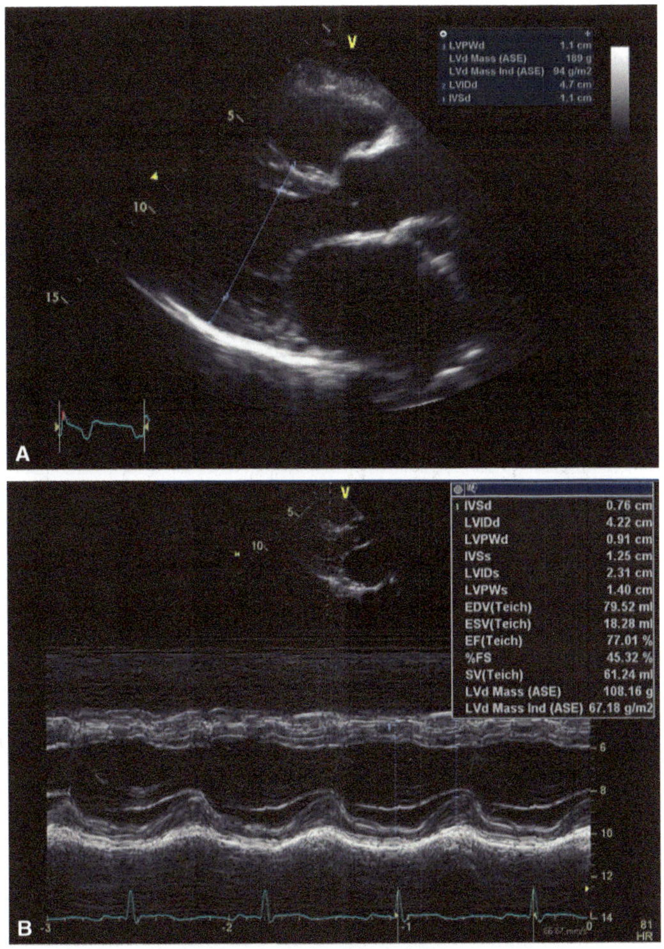

Fig. 17.7 (A) From a 2-D parasternal long axis view image, the interventricular septum *(IVSd)*, the LV cavity *(LVIDd)*, and the posterior wall *(LVPWd)* are measured perpendicular to the long axis of the LV and just distal to the mitral leaflet tips. Measurements are performed at the blood-tissue interfaces at end diastole. (B) Via M-mode, the interventricular septum *(IVSd)*, the LV cavity *(LVIDd)*, and the posterior LV wall *(LVPWd)* are measured from the parasternal long axis view with the M-mode cursor aligned perpendicular to the long axis of the LV and just distal to the mitral leaflet tips. Measurements are performed at the blood-tissue interfaces at end diastole.

Isovolumic Relaxation Time

The IVRT is obtained from the apical five-chamber or apical long axis view by aligning the Doppler beam between LV inflow and LV outflow. PW Doppler (3–5mm sample volume) or CW Doppler can be used to acquire this signal. Color Doppler is useful in aiding the alignment of the Doppler beam between the two flow regions. The IVRT is optimally displayed when the closing click of the aortic valve is depicted both above and below the zero baseline. Delineation of this closing click is important as it coincides with the cessation of systolic blood flow and the end of systole. The IVRT is measured as the time interval between aortic valve closure and mitral valve opening (Fig. 17.9).

Color M-mode Propagation Velocity

The Vp is measured by CMM from the apical four-chamber view with the color Doppler box covering the region of LV inflow, including the mitral annulus. The image is further optimized by decreasing the image depth or zooming to include the entire LV and a small portion of the LA. The color gain is adjusted to just below speckling, and the color velocity scale is decreased so that the central highest velocity jet is blue.

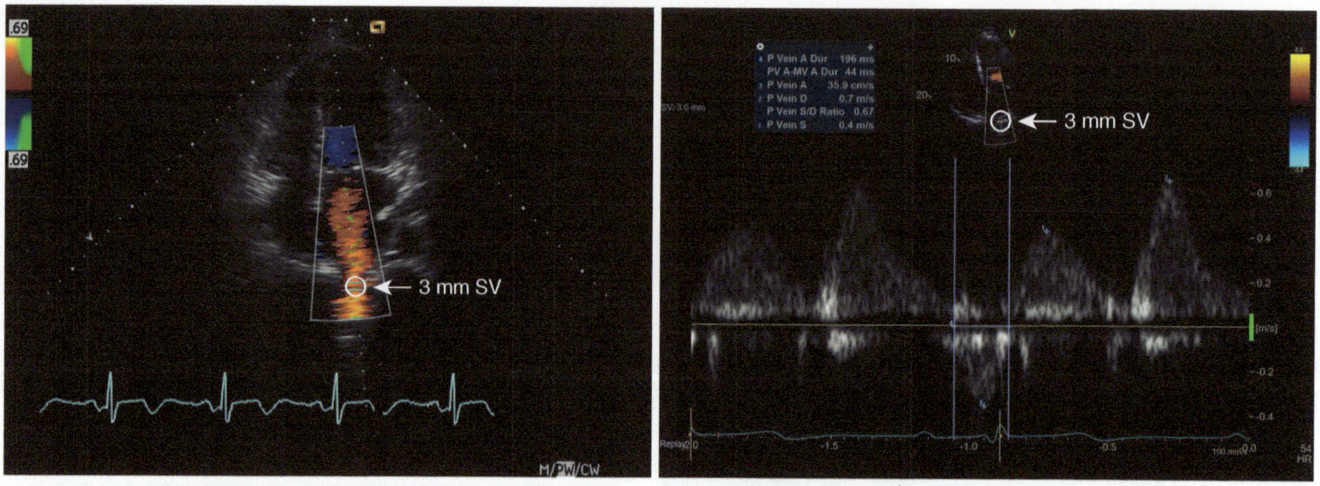

Fig. 17.8 Pulmonary venous inflow is recorded from an apical four-chamber or apical five-chamber view with a 3–5-mm pulsed-wave (PW) Doppler sample volume (SV) placed 1 cm into the pulmonary vein, aligned parallel with inflow *(left)*. The normal profile displays prominent systolic *(S)* and the diastolic *(D)* velocities above the zero baseline and a smaller atrial reversal *(Ar)* velocity below the zero baseline. The peak velocities of the S (P Vein S), D (P Vein D), S/D ratio (P Vein S/d), and Ar (P Vein A) are measured along with the Ar duration (P Vein A Dur) *(right)*.

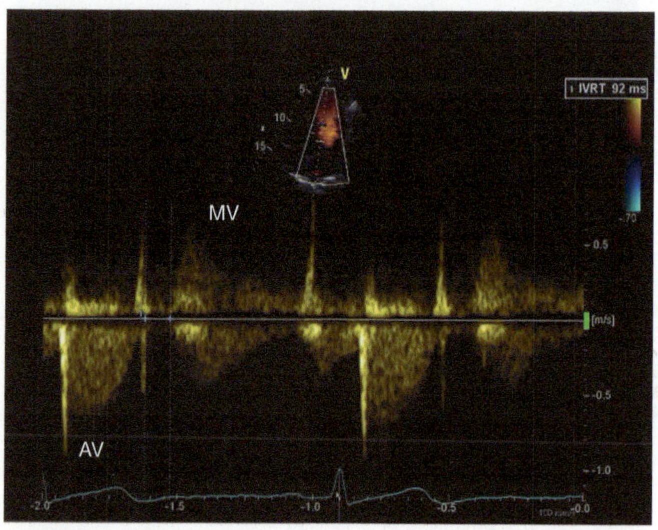

Fig. 17.9 Measurement of the isovolumic relaxation time *(IVRT)* is performed via continuous wave (CW) Doppler with the Doppler beam aligned to intercept flow between LV inflow *(MV)* and LV outflow *(AV)*. The IVRT is measured as the time interval between aortic valve closure and mitral valve opening.

The M-mode cursor is placed through the center of the LV inflow blood column from the mitral valve to the LV apex (Fig. 17.10, left). The Vp slope is measured along the first aliased velocity, during early diastole, from the level of the mitral annulus to a distance of at least 4 cm into the LV cavity (see Fig. 17.10, right). Shifting the Doppler baseline and/or adjusting the Nyquist limit to a value below the pulsed Doppler peak E velocity helps in demarcating the edge of the first aliasing velocity, where the slope of Vp is measured. A more detailed description of the Vp in the assessment of LV diastolic function is discussed in Chapter 11.

LV and LA Strain

LV and LA strain are derived using 2-D speckle tracking software. 2-D image optimization is crucial to ensure adequate speckle tracking[42,43]; hence appropriate time must be spent optimizing 2-D images prior to storing for later analysis. The focus (if available) should be positioned at an intermediate depth to optimize the 2-D image, and sector depth and width should be narrowed to include as little as possible outside the region of interest, thus increasing the frame rate. The recommended frame for rate analysis is between 40 and 80 frames per second. On-axis images are then acquired on a three-beat loop at end expiration and with a stable ECG recording. For LA strain, using the apical four-chamber, the LA endocardial border is traced from the border of the mitral annulus up to the opposite mitral annulus side, extrapolating across the pulmonary veins, and/or LA appendage orifices. The apical two-chamber view can also be analysed to obtain a biplane calculation of the LA strain.[33] There are two distinct options with respect to which reference frame should be set to zero LA strain.[34] That is, the timing of initial zero reference point may be at either the onset of the P-wave (P-P gating) or QRS complex (R-R gating).[35,36] For the purposes of diastolic assessment, R-R gating is recommended. For LV strain, images are acquired from the apical long axis, apical four-chamber, and apical two-chamber views. The endocardial border is traced and the width of the region of interest is adjusted to exclude the pericardium.[42] GLS for the LV can be displayed in a quad format or as a bull's eye plot (Fig. 17.11). Importantly, there is a significant learning curve associated with LV strain analysis,[44] and therefore the same may be expected for the LA strain analysis. As previously mentioned in this chapter, the application of LV and LA strain for LV diastolic function assessment is still in the investigative stage. Furthermore, there is currently a lack of dedicated tracking algorithms for LA strain assessment. Assessment of LA strain is also compromised due to the thinness of the LA wall and dropout of the interatrial septum. A more detailed description of strain imaging in the assessment of LV diastolic function is discussed in Chapter 10 and 12.

RESPIRATORY MONITORING AND SPECIAL MANEUVERS

Constrictive pericarditis is a treatable cause of diastolic heart failure, hence recognition of this disorder is crucial (see Chapter 26). This condition can be identified based on characteristic echocardiographic findings, which include exaggerated respiratory variation in chamber dimensions and Doppler diastolic filling profiles.[45] The precise timing

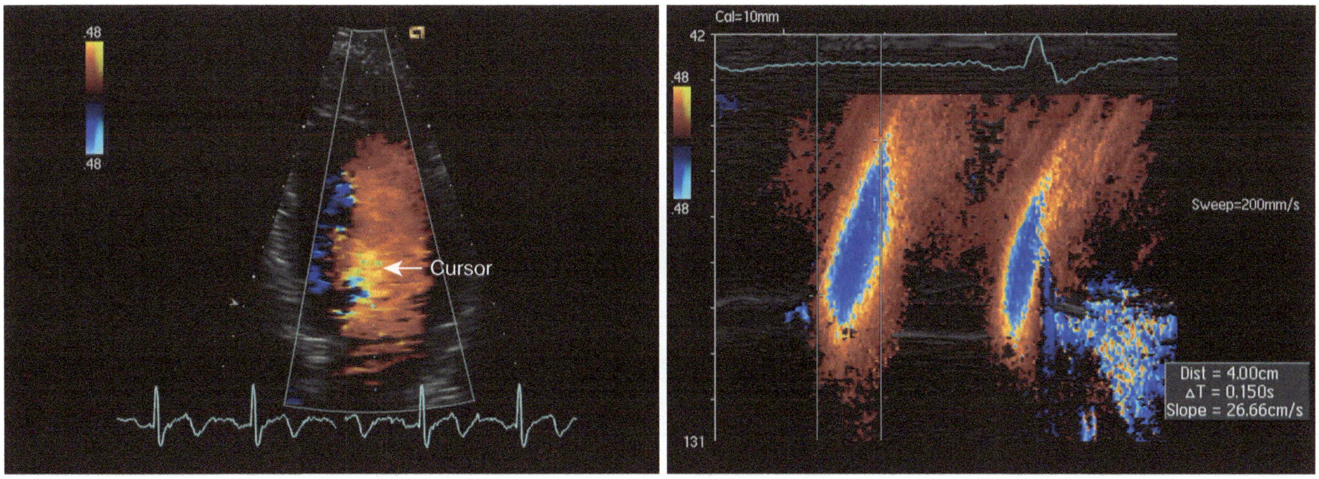

Fig. 17.10 Measurement of the Vp is performed from the color M-mode trace of transmitral inflow acquired from the apical four-chamber view. The M-mode cursor is positioned through the center of the LV inflow blood column *(left)*. The Vp is then measured along the early diastolic slope of the first aliased velocity *(red-blue interface)* from the level of the mitral annulus to 4 cm into the LV cavity *(right)*.

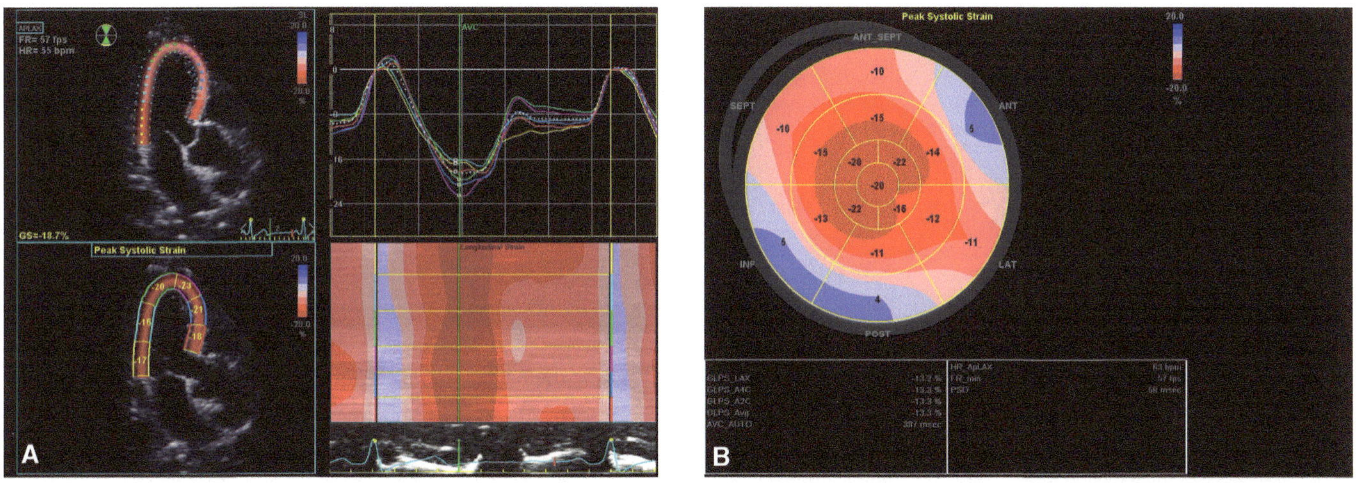

Fig. 17.11 (A) LV global longitudinal strain (GLS) can be displayed in a quad format for each apical view. This includes a color-encoded region of interest or parametric preview *(top left)*, segmental strain curves *(top right)*, a peak segmental strain map *(bottom left)*, and a curved anatomic color M-mode trace *(bottom right)*. For each of these images, six LV segments are displayed, and each segment is easily recognized based on a color coding for each. In this apical long axis view, the basal inferolateral wall is yellow, the midinferolateral wall is blue, the inferior apex is green, the anterior apex is pink, the midanterior septum is dark blue, and the basal anterior septum is red. (B) LV GLS is more commonly shown as a bull's eye plot. On this plot, 17 segments of the LV are displayed along with the peak systolic strain for that segment. An average of all 17 segments of the LV is then combined into one single number to provide the GLS. As GLS represents systolic shortening, the strain values are negative. Normal strain is identified as red (values at ≥−20%). When strain values are less negative than −20%, segments are color coded brighter shades of red and pink. When strain values become positive, representing lengthening rather than shortening, segments are color coded various shades of blue.

of this respirophasic variation can be documented by using a respirometer.

Load-altering maneuvers may also be incorporated into the examination to assist in the diagnosis of CP as well as for the interpretation of LV diastolic function and LVFP. In CP, the characteristic respiratory variations in left heart filling may be absent when there is a marked elevation in LAP. Unmasking of these respiratory variations may be achieved by positional preload reducing maneuvers.[46] For diastology, as previously mentioned, several parameters are preload dependent. For example, an increase in LAP may normalize the transmitral inflow profile despite the presence of an underlying relaxation abnormality. Thus, by reducing preload, the normalizing effect of increased LAP is removed, and the underlying relaxation abnormality can be unmasked.[46,47] The Valsalva maneuver is the most commonly used preload-reducing technique to reduce preload. Preload augmentation by passive leg raise might also be useful as an alternative to diastolic stress testing in patients who have a lower diastolic functional reserve and lower exercise capacity.[48,49] In constrictive pericarditis, the sitting-up position can be used as well to lower preload.

Respiratory Monitoring

Respiratory monitoring can be achieved using a nasal thermistor (in the past) or by using the physiologic respiratory control linked to the ECG on the ultrasound machine. The nasal thermistor detects breathing from temperature changes in the nose. The tip of the nasal thermistor is placed inside the patient's nose, but not touching the nasal wall; the patient is required to breathe through the nose. The

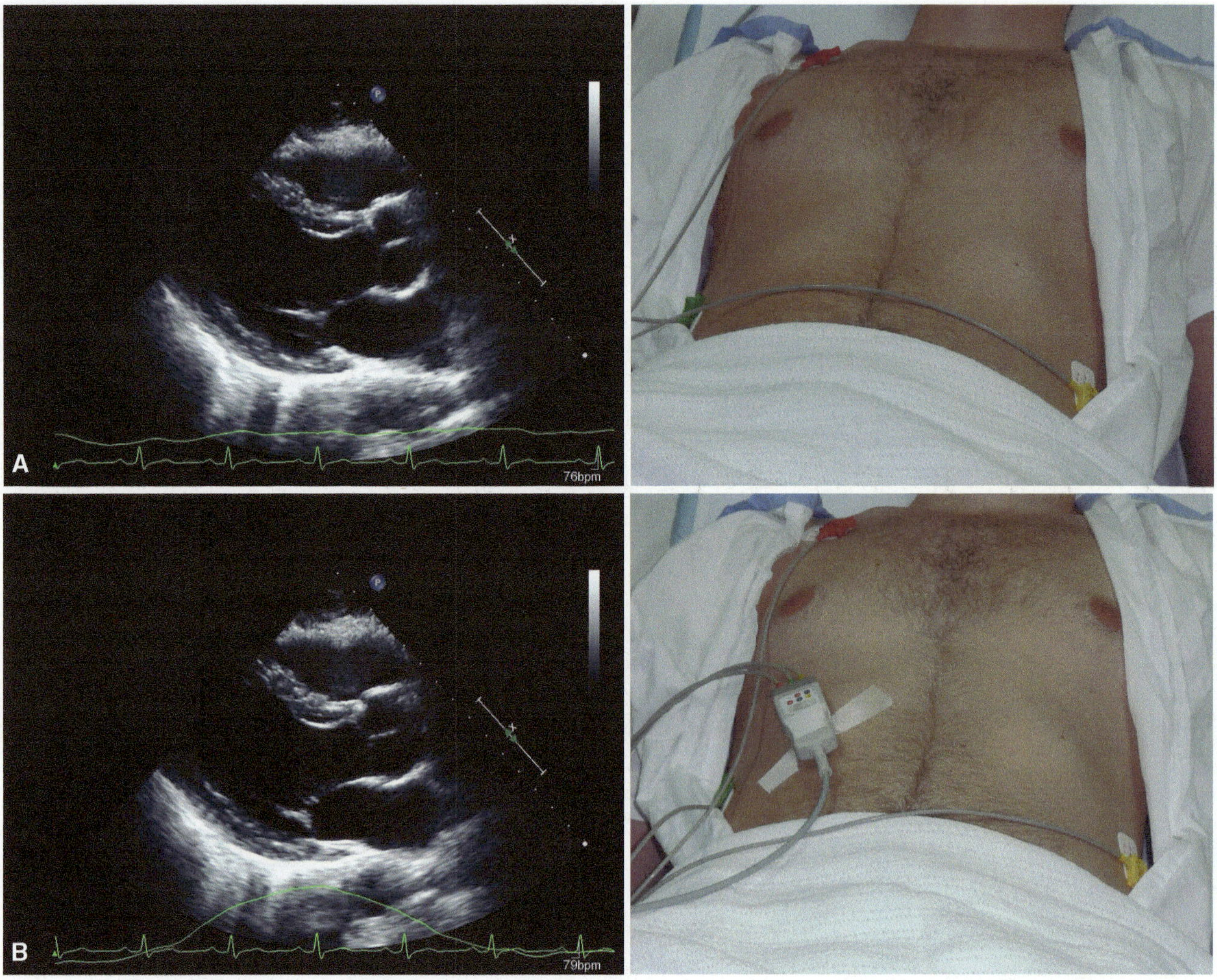

Fig. 17.12 Respiration via the electrocardiogram (ECG) is based on detecting the motion of the diaphragm through the ECG cables and/or the cable box. (A) On the echocardiographic image, the superimposed respiratory tracing is poor and displays no obvious inspiratory or expiratory variation. The photo to the right shows the ECG cables, which are not flat against the chest; the cable box is also well away from the patient. (B) On the echocardiographic image, the respiratory tracing is much improved with a clear upward deflection representing inspiration and a downward deflection representing expiration. The photo to the right shows that the ECG cables are flush against the chest wall with the ECG cable box securely taped onto the lower chest wall. This enables better detection of the motion of the diaphragm during respiration.

respiration trace is displayed approximately 30 sec after the system detects a steady breathing rate.

Via the ECG, respiration is detected as diaphragmatic movement through the ECG cables. For an optimal respiratory recording, the ECG cables (leads) and the cable box should be placed flush against the chest wall (Fig. 17.12).

The respirometer trace is typically displayed such that an upward deflection represents inspiration and a downward deflection represents expiration. When documenting respiratory variation, the sweep speed is slowed to display at least two to three complete respiratory cycles. The use of a respirometer is recommended when there is an apparent greater than normal respiratory variation in transmitral inflow velocities and to determine the precise timing of the respirophasic variation in the spectral Doppler signals. Typically, in CP and other pericardial diseases, the respiratory variation seen in Doppler diastolic filling profiles is maximal on the onset of the first beat of inspiration and expiration, underscoring the importance of the precise documentation of the phase of respiration.[50]

A respirometer is also useful in observing the respirophasic variation of the inferior vena cava (IVC). For example, a dilated IVC without any inspiratory collapse suggests a markedly increased RAP of greater than 15 mmHg.[37]

Valsalva Maneuver

The Valsalva maneuver is achieved by straining against a closed airway for 10 to 15 sec following a deep inspiration. The aim of this maneuver is to elevate intrathoracic pressure to about 40 mmHg.[47,51] Analogies that may help the patient to understand what is required include, "Hold your nose and try to pop your ears as you would do on an airplane," "Pretend that you have a belt around your tummy and try to bust this," and "Place your thumb in your mouth and try to blow it up as though it is a balloon." During the strain phase of the Valsalva maneuver, intrathoracic pressure exceeds the pressure in the great veins resulting in a positive intrathoracic pressure, which leads to decreased venous return to the heart and thus a decreased preload.

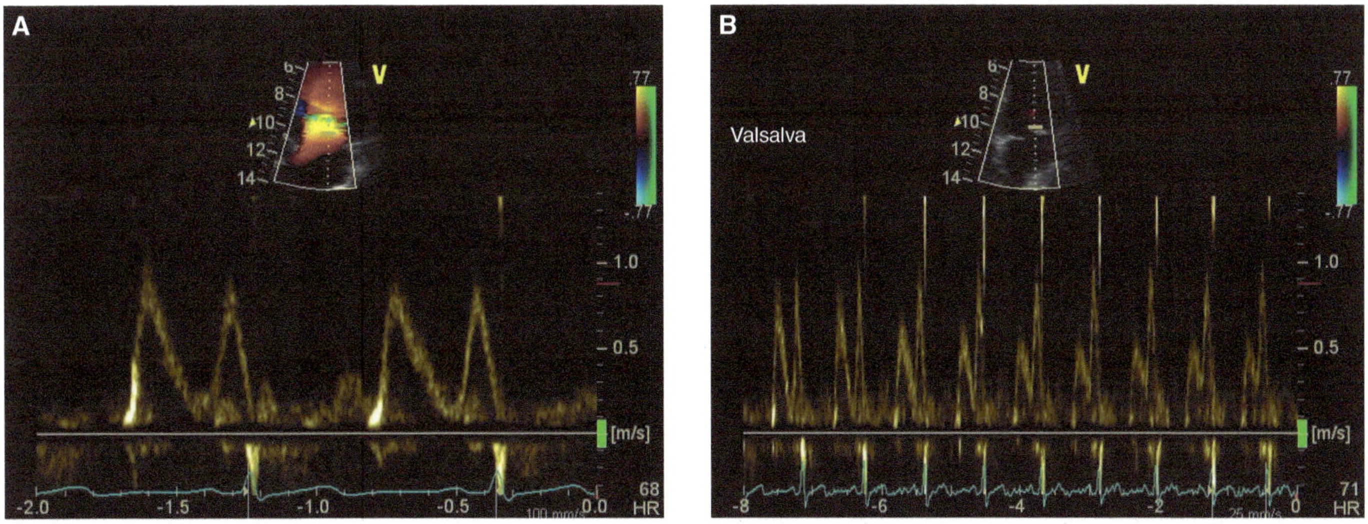

Fig. 17.13 A 67-year-old man, with normal LV size and systolic function and moderately dilated left atrium. (A) Transmitral inflow pattern appears normal at rest. (B) During Valsalva maneuver the E/A ratio decreased from 1.0 to 0.7 and peak A velocity increased from 90 to 97 cm/sec, unmasking the impaired relaxation pattern.

This maneuver is usually performed while interrogating transmitral inflow. An adequate Valsalva attempt is a 10% reduction in the peak transmitral E velocity from the baseline value.[52] Technical challenges in performing this maneuver include having the patient generate a sufficient increase in intrathoracic pressure for at least 10 sec while the sonographer maintains an image with the sample volume correctly positioned between the mitral leaflet tips.

The effect of decreased preload on a normal transmitral trace is a comparable reduction in both the E and A velocities with the resultant E/A ratio remaining essentially unchanged, while in patients with elevated LVFP there is a decrease in the E/A ratio of 50% or more.[53] Therefore, when there is a pseudonormal transmitral inflow profile, preload reduction unmasks the underlying impaired relaxation pattern (Fig. 17.13). Hence the Valsalva maneuver may be useful in distinguishing normal LV filling from pseudonormal filling.

The Valsalva maneuver may also be useful in differentiating reversible restrictive filling from an irreversible restrictive filling.[1,12] When there is reversible restrictive filling, preload reduction will result in a reversal of this filling profile to either a pseudonormal filling profile or even to an impaired relaxation filling profile. When there is irreversible restrictive filling, the transmitral inflow profile remains unchanged.

Postural Maneuvers

Postural changes that result in preload reduction include a head-up tilt or changing the patient position from a supine to a standing or sitting position. A decrease in preload occurs by causing blood to pool in the venous beds of the legs, which decreases venous return. These maneuvers may be attempted when patients cannot perform an effective Valsalva or in patients with suspected CP when specific observation of respirophasic changes, due to preload reduction, are required.

Diastolic reserve refers to the ability of LVFP to remain normal during exercise. In patients with a lower diastolic reserve, LVFP increases abnormally with exercise due in part to an increase in preload. One of the primary roles of diastolic stress testing is to determine if LVFP increases abnormally with exertion (see Chapter 18). However, not all patients are able to exercise. Preload augmentation by passive leg raise is a nonexercise alternative that can be used in patients with a lower exercise capacity and may be able to identify an abnormal increase in LVFP when the preload in increased.[49,54] Passive leg raise is performed by passively elevating the patient's legs using a hinged examination table to an angle of 60 degrees for 3 minutes. Doppler echocardiographic parameters such as transmitral inflow, e′ velocities at the septal and lateral annulus, and the peak TR velocity are remeasured in the leg-raised state.

DIASTOLIC STRESS TESTING

Diastolic stress echocardiography is indicated when resting echocardiographic findings do not explain the patient's symptoms, when there is subclinical diastolic dysfunction, or when findings are equivocal. For example, in some patients with exertional dyspnea, symptoms develop secondary to an abnormal increase in LVFP upon exertion, which occurs to maintain adequate LV filling and subsequent stroke volume. However, at rest the patient's LVFP may be normal, and thus the cause of the patient's symptoms may be missed. To determine if LVFP increases abnormally with exertion, a diastolic stress echocardiogram can be performed.

In normal individuals with normal myocardial relaxation, increasing the heart rate with stress leads to a proportional increase in both the E and e′ velocities, so the E/e′ ratio remains unchanged or may even be reduced.[55] However, in patients with elevated LVFP during exercise, the e′ does not augment with exercise; hence the E/e′ ratio increases.[56,57] An increase in the PASP with exercise has also been shown to parallel increases in the LVFP.[58] The most appropriate patient population for diastolic exercise testing is the group that exhibits grade I diastolic dysfunction, which indicates impaired myocardial relaxation and normal LAP at rest.[1]

The recommended method for diastolic exercise testing is supine bicycle, as this more easily allows Doppler interrogation during exercise.[1,49] During the supine bicycle test, 2-D images, transmitral inflow velocities, mitral annular TDI velocities, and peak TR velocity are acquired at baseline, during each stage of exercise (including peak exercise), and in recovery.[1] A total of 5 to 10 cardiac cycles should be acquired with the transmitral E and TDI e′ signals recorded at heart rates between 100 and 110 bpm when the E and A and e′ and a′ waves are not yet fused.[49]

Preload augmentation (as previously mentioned in this chapter) and treadmill exercise are alternative methods that can be used.

Although treadmill exercise does not allow the acquisition of Doppler signals during exercise, it should be remembered that the E velocity remains increased for several minutes after the termination of exercise while the e′ velocity remains reduced at baseline, exercise, and recovery.[12,59] Therefore measurements of the E and e′ velocities can be acquired following treadmill exercise in the recovery stage, after 2-D images have been obtained for wall motion analysis, and after acquisition of the peak TR velocity.

A more detailed description of stress testing in the assessment of LV diastolic function is provided in Chapter 18.

RIGHT VENTRICULAR DIASTOLIC FUNCTION

In the presence of CP, suspected primary abnormality of RV myocardium, or unexplained right heart failure, assessment of RV diastolic parameters is required. RV diastolic function is evaluated by considering multiple parameters such as transtricuspid inflow, TDI of the lateral tricuspid valve annulus, hepatic venous flow, superior vena cava (SVC) flow, as well as assessment of the IVC size and collapsibility. The tricuspid E/e′ ratio, hepatic venous inflow, and the IVC can be used in the estimation of RAP.[60]

The methodology for acquiring these parameters described in the chapter and summarized in Table 17.5 is based on ASE recommendations.[1,12,37] As many of the velocities in right heart Doppler profiles vary with respiration, signals should be averaged over a full respiratory cycle or measured at end-expiratory apnea. The exception to this includes the assessment of the IVC and in cases of suspected CP where precise timing of the respirophasic variation is required for the diagnosis. Images and traces are optimized in a similar manner as described for the LV diastolic function assessment earlier. A more detailed discussion on RV diastolic function can be found in Chapter 14.

Tricuspid Inflow

Transtricuspid inflow may be interrogated from any view where parallel alignment between tricuspid inflow and the Doppler beam can be achieved. Most commonly this is from the apical four-chamber view. Using PW Doppler, a sample volume (1–3 mm) is positioned

TABLE 17.5 Technical Aspects for Right Ventricular Diastology Parameters

Parameter	Acquisition	Optimization	Measurements Performed
Key Diastology Parameters			
Transtricuspid inflow	Apical four-chamber (or other view where parallel alignment with RV inflow is achieved) PW Doppler 1–3mm SV placed between TV leaflet tips Color Doppler and/or off-axis imaging may be used to aid alignment with inflow	Parallel alignment with inflow Sweep speed 50–100 mm/sec[a] Low wall filters enabling a clear depiction of the onset and cessation of flow Low signal gain with minimal background speckling Velocity scale and baseline set to display full spectrum	Peak E velocity Peak A velocity E/A ratio +/- DT
Tricuspid annular velocities	Apical four-chamber TDI 5–10 mm SV placed at lateral tricuspid annulus or within basal RV myocardium	TDI preset (low velocity, high amplitude settings) Parallel alignment with myocardial motion Sweep speed 50–100 mm/sec (display two complete cardiac cycles) Low signal gain with minimal background speckling Velocity scale and baseline set to display full spectrum	Lateral e′ velocity +/- rIVRT
Hepatic venosus inflow	Subcostal SAX PW Doppler 3–5 mm SV placed 1–2 cm into HV from its junction with IVC	Parallel alignment with inflow Sweep speed 50–100 mm/sec[a] Low wall filters enabling a clear depiction of the onset and cessation of flow Low signal gain with minimal background speckling Velocity scale and baseline set to display full spectrum	Observation and/or measurement of peak S and D velocities or TVIs
SVC	Right supraclavicular fossa	Parallel alignment with inflow Sweep speed 50–100 mm/sec[a] Low wall filters enabling a clear depiction of the onset and cessation of flow Low signal gain with minimal background speckling Velocity scale and baseline set to display full spectrum	Observation of peak S and D velocities over respiratory cycle
IVC	Subcostal SAX	Open up long axis of IVC Optimize 2-D gains and TGC to ensure blood pool is echo free Adjust the field of view and/or utilize the zoom function for IVC Utilize other available 2-D controls to optimize image	Observation and/or measurement of IVC maximum and minimal dimensions over respiratory cycle

DT, Deceleration time; *HV*, hepatic venous; *IVC*, inferior vena cava; *PW*, pulsed-wave; *rIVRT*, regional isovolumic relaxation time; *RV*, right ventricular; *SAX*, short axis; *SV*, sample volume; *SVC*, superior vena cava; *TDI*, tissue Doppler imaging; *TGC*, time gain compensation; *TV*, tricuspid valve; *TVI*, time velocity integrals.

[a]Use slower sweep speed to display two complete respiratory cycles when the aim is to display precise timing of the respirophasic variation such as in the case of confirmed or suspected constrictive pericarditis.

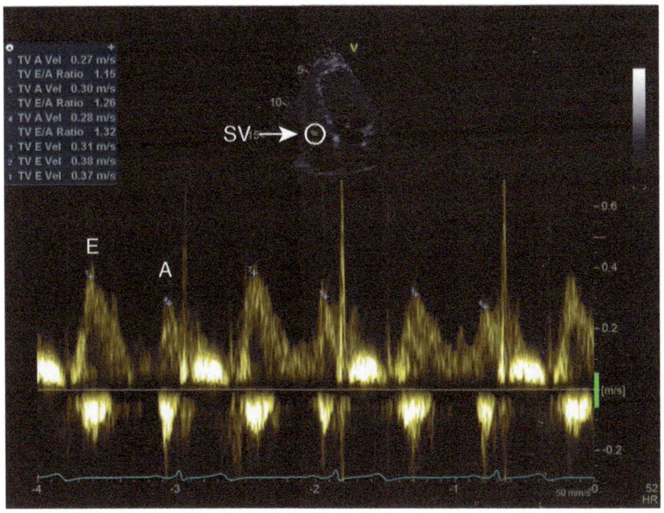

Fig. 17.14 Transtricuspid inflow may be recorded from an apical four-chamber view with a 1–3mm pulsed-wave (PW) Doppler sample volume (SV) placed at the tips of the tricuspid valve, aligned parallel with RV inflow. The normal profile displays two prominent velocity peaks above the zero baseline: The peak early diastolic *(E)* occurs after the T wave of the electrocardiogram (ECG), and the peak atrial contraction *(A)* occurs just after the P wave of the ECG. Transtricuspid inflow measurements include the peak E velocity (TV E Vel) and the peak A velocity (TV A Vel); the E/A ratio is derived from these two velocities. The deceleration time can also be measured from the peak E velocity, along the deceleration slope, to the zero baseline.

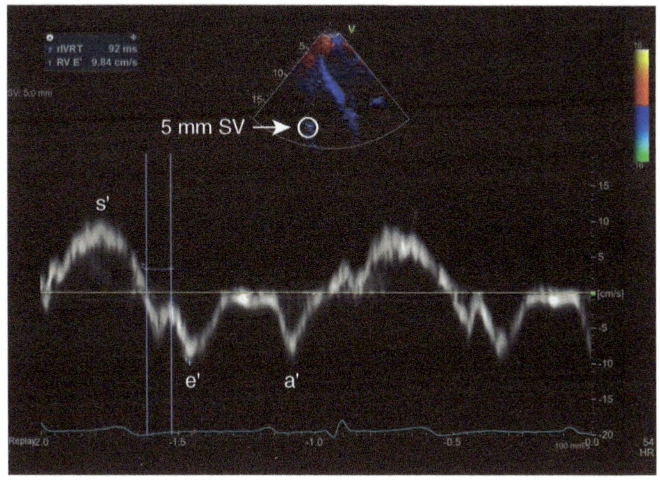

Fig. 17.15 Tricuspid annular velocities are recorded via tissue Doppler imaging (TDI) from an apical four-chamber view with a 5–10 mm sample volume (SV) placed at the lateral tricuspid annulus, aligned parallel with myocardial motion. The early diastolic myocardial velocity *(e')* occurs after the T wave of the electrocardiogram (ECG) and appears below the zero baseline. The late diastolic myocardial velocity *(a')* occurs just after the P wave of the ECG and appears below the zero baseline. The systolic myocardial velocity *(s')* coincides with the T wave of the ECG and appears above the zero baseline. In addition to the measurement of the peak e′ velocity, the regional isovolumic relaxation time (rIVRT) can be measured from the end of s′ velocity to onset of e′.

centrally at the tips of the open tricuspid valve leaflets. As for transmitral inflow, when there is sinus rhythm the transtricuspid velocity profile consists of early diastolic (E) and atrial contraction (A) velocities appearing above the zero baseline (Fig. 17.14). Normal transtricuspid inflow values vary slightly with respiration, with a slight increase in both E and A velocities upon inspiration. Routine measurements performed include the peak E velocity, the peak A velocity, the E/A ratio, and the DT. One of the primary limitations of acquiring optimal traces is the frequent inability to align the Doppler beam with tricuspid inflow.

Tricuspid Annular Velocities

Tricuspid annular signals are acquired from the apical four-chamber view at the lateral tricuspid annulus using the TDI preset. The Doppler beam is aligned parallel with myocardial motion and a sample volume (5–10 mm) is positioned at either the lateral tricuspid annulus or within the basal RV myocardium. As for mitral annular signals, when there is sinus rhythm the annular profile is characterized by three distinct waveforms representing a systolic myocardial velocity (s′) above the zero baseline, an early diastolic myocardial velocity (e′) below the zero baseline, and a late diastolic myocardial velocity (a′) below the zero baseline (Fig. 17.15). For RV diastolic function assessment, the peak e′ velocity is measured to calculate the tricuspid E/e′ ratio. The regional IVRT (rIVRT) can also be measured from this trace to provide an estimation of RAP.[61] The rIVRT is measured from the end of s′ velocity to the onset of the next e′ (see Fig. 17.15).

Hepatic Venous Inflow

Hepatic venous (HV) inflow is interrogated from the subcostal short axis view using PW Doppler with the Doppler beam aligned parallel with inflow and with a sample volume (3–5 mm) positioned approximately 1 to 2 cm into the HV proximal to its junction with the IVC (Fig. 17.16, left). The normal inflow profile consists of four waveforms: systolic forward flow (S) velocity (below the zero baseline), diastolic forward flow (D) velocity (below the zero baseline), atrial flow reversal (Ar) velocity (above the zero baseline), and ventricular (end-systolic) flow reversal (Vr) velocity (above the zero baseline) (see Fig. 17.16, right). The trace is optimized by ensuring that there is parallel alignment with HV inflow. Color Doppler is especially useful in identifying and aligning HV flow. Peak velocities vary with respiration; with inspiration there is a slight increase in both S and D velocities, while with expiration there is a slight increase in the Ar and Vr velocities. One of the primary limitations of acquiring optimal HV traces relates to the horizontal movement of the HV during respiration, hence maintaining the sample volume within the HV is difficult.

Measurements of HV inflow are not routinely performed. However, measurement of the peak S velocity or time velocity integral (TVI) and the peak D velocity or TVI can be performed to estimate the systolic filling fraction (SSF), which can then be used in the estimation of RAP.[57,58] SSF is calculated as the S velocity (or TVI) divided by the sum of the S velocity (or TVI) and the D velocity (or TVI).

Superior Vena Cava Inflow

SVC inflow is interrogated from the right supraclavicular fossa using PW Doppler with a sample volume (3–5 mm) positioned approximately 5 to 7 cm into the SVC (Fig. 17.17, left). Identification of the SVC may be aided using color Doppler imaging by identifying the appearance of blue laminar flow down the vessel and away from the transducer. The normal SVC profile consists of three waveforms: systolic forward flow (S) velocity (below the zero baseline), diastolic forward flow (D) velocity (below the zero baseline), and atrial flow reversal (Ar) velocity (above the zero baseline) (see Fig. 17.17, right). Infrequently a fourth waveform representing ventricular (end-systolic) reversal is seen. As for HV flow, the SVC flow profile also shows respiratory changes. Therefore in the normal SVC

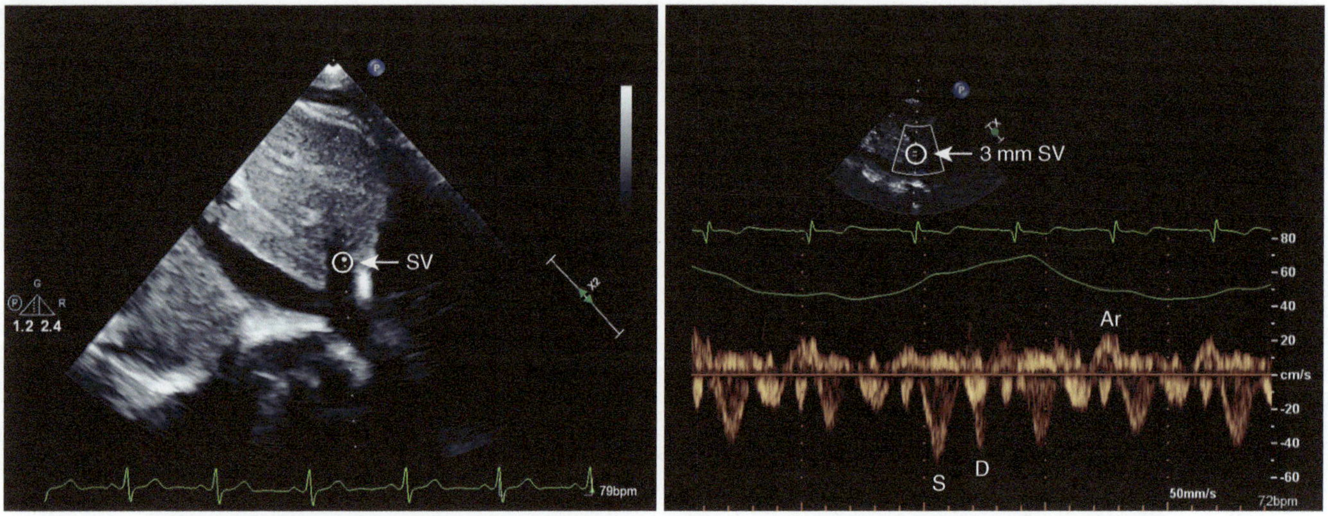

Fig. 17.16 Hepatic venous (HV) inflow is recorded from the subcostal short axis view with a 3–5mm pulsed-wave (PW) Doppler sample volume (SV) placed 1 to 2 cm into the HV *(left)*. The normal profile displays prominent systolic *(S)* and the diastolic *(D)* velocities below the zero baseline and a smaller atrial reversal *(Ar)* velocity above the zero baseline *(right)*. A small ventricular flow reversal (Vr) may also be seen above the zero baseline but is often difficult to differentiate from other low velocity flow close to the zero baseline. Normal respiratory variation shows a slight increase in both S and D velocities with inspiration and a slight increase in the Ar velocity with expiration.

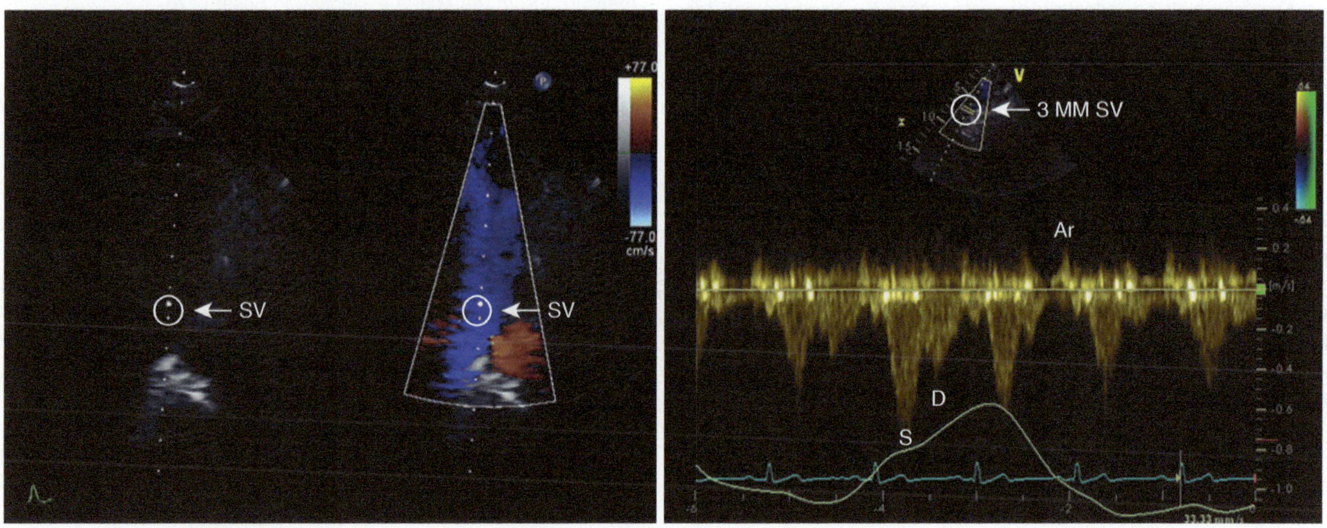

Fig. 17.17 Superior vena cava (SVC) inflow is recorded from the right supraclavicular view with a 3–5mm pulsed-wave (PW) Doppler sample volume (SV) placed 5 to 7 cm into the SVC *(left)*. The normal profile displays prominent systolic *(S)* and diastolic *(D)* velocities below the zero baseline and a smaller atrial reversal *(Ar)* velocity above the zero baseline *(right)*. Normal respiratory variation shows a slight increase in both S and D velocities with inspiration and a slight increase in the Ar velocity with expiration.

profile there is a slight increase in forward flow velocities during inspiration, while during expiration there is a slight increase in the Ar velocity. Measurements of SVC inflow are not routinely performed. However, evaluation of the SVC flow profile is useful when considering the presence or absence of hemodynamic effects caused by pericardial diseases such as CP.[51] In these instances, observation of respirophasic variation is important, hence use of a respirometer is recommended with the sweep speed slowed to display at least two complete respiratory cycles. An increase in HV Ar velocity with a simultaneous reduction in forward flow velocities on expiration are important findings for confirming the diagnosis of CP[45].

Inferior Vena Cava

As previously mentioned in this chapter, the IVC can be used in the estimation of RAP. The long axis of the IVC is imaged from the subcostal short axis view with the patient in a supine position. The maximum and minimum IVC diameters are measured using the inner edge–to–inner edge technique, perpendicular to the long axis of the IVC and just proximal to the junction of IVC with hepatic veins or about 1 to 2 cm proximal to the IVC-RA junction. IVC measurements may be performed via 2-D linear measurements (Fig. 17.18) or by M-mode, providing the M-mode cursor can be aligned perpendicular to the IVC (Fig. 17.19). When right-sided filling pressures are increased,

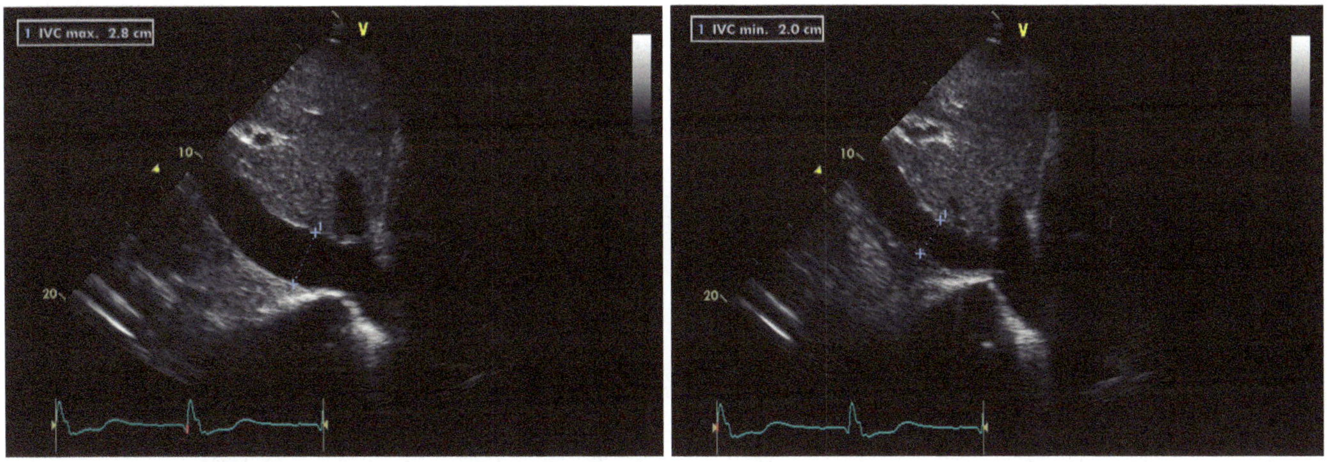

Fig. 17.18 Via 2-D echocardiography, the maximum *(left)* and minimum *(right)* dimensions of the inferior vena cava (IVC) are measured from the subcostal view, perpendicular to the IVC long axis, and about 1 to 2 cm proximal to the IVC-RA junction. The measurement technique is inner edge to inner edge.

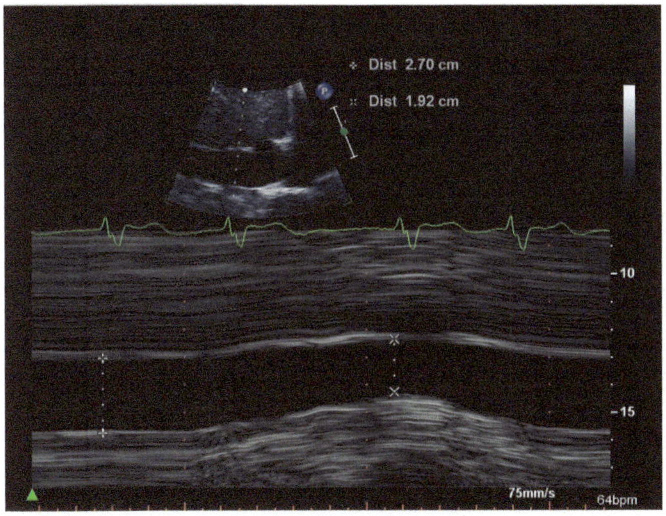

Fig. 17.19 Via M-mode, the maximum and minimum dimensions of the inferior vena cava (IVC) are measured from the subcostal view, with the M-mode cursor aligned perpendicular to the IVC long axis and about 1 to 2 cm proximal to the IVC-RA junction. The measurement technique is inner edge to inner edge.

the normal inspiratory collapse of the IVC is diminished or absent (IVC plethora). Dilatation or distension of the IVC and/or dilatation of the hepatic veins may also ensue. Therefore the maximum dimension and the degree of collapse of the IVC during respiration are useful indicators of RAP. Occasionally only a minimal change in the inspiratory diameter of the IVC may be observed due to variations in the force of inspiratory effort or the inability of some patients to inspire deeply due to severe breathlessness. In these patients, a sniff maneuver may be required to differentiate patients with a normal RAP from those with a genuinely increased RAP.[60]

FUTURE DIRECTIONS

Successful interpretation of diastolic examinations depends on study quality, consistency, and reliability. Dedicated and lifelong learning is essential to master the acquisition of a complete and accurate study. Online tutorials, simulation training, and interactive feedback in real time should continue to be developed and offered to cardiac sonographers in practice. The use of artificial intelligence may facilitate consistency in measurements and the preliminary interpretation of diastology studies.

KEY POINTS

- An integrated approach, considering multiple parameters, in addition to the clinical data and patient age, is required to identify the presence of LV diastolic dysfunction and to provide a reliable estimation of LVFP.
- The four key diastology parameters include the transmitral inflow profile, mitral annular velocities, the peak TR velocity, and the indexed LA volume.
- Algorithms, with concordance between two or more parameters in an individual patient, can be applied to determine the presence and grading of diastolic dysfunction.
- Complementary parameters can be used when key variables are inconclusive, when the presence or grading of diastolic dysfunction is deemed indeterminate, or to further support interpretation. Additional parameters include LV thickness and mass, pulmonary venous inflow, IVRT, and color M-mode propagation velocity.
- Emerging parameters such as GDSR and LA strain are promising and may further aid in the interpretation of diastolic function. GLS is useful in detecting subclinical LV dysfunction.
- Careful attention to the technique of acquisition and measurement of parameters, as well as an awareness of potential pitfalls, is required to ensure accurate, consistent, and reproducible measurements.
- Respiratory monitoring and special maneuvers to alter loading conditions can be incorporated into the examination to provide respiratory cycle timing information, to aid in the diagnosis of CP, and to enhance the interpretation of LV diastolic function and LVFP.
- Assessment of RV diastolic parameters is important in the presence of right heart failure or confirmed or suspected CP.

Case Study 2

A 46-year-old male presents with progressive shortness of breath on exertion and presyncope. Echocardiographic images provided for this case include video clips of the LV acquired from the parasternal long (Video 17.1) and short axis (Video 17.2) views, and the apical four-chamber (Video 17.3), apical two-chamber (Video 17.4), and apical long axis (Video 17.5) views. Other images (see figure) include the transmitral inflow profile (A), septal and lateral mitral annular velocities (B), pulmonary venous trace (C), TR trace (D), transmitral inflow profile with Valsalva (E), and the indexed LA volume (F). The strain GLS bull's eye plot is also provided (G).

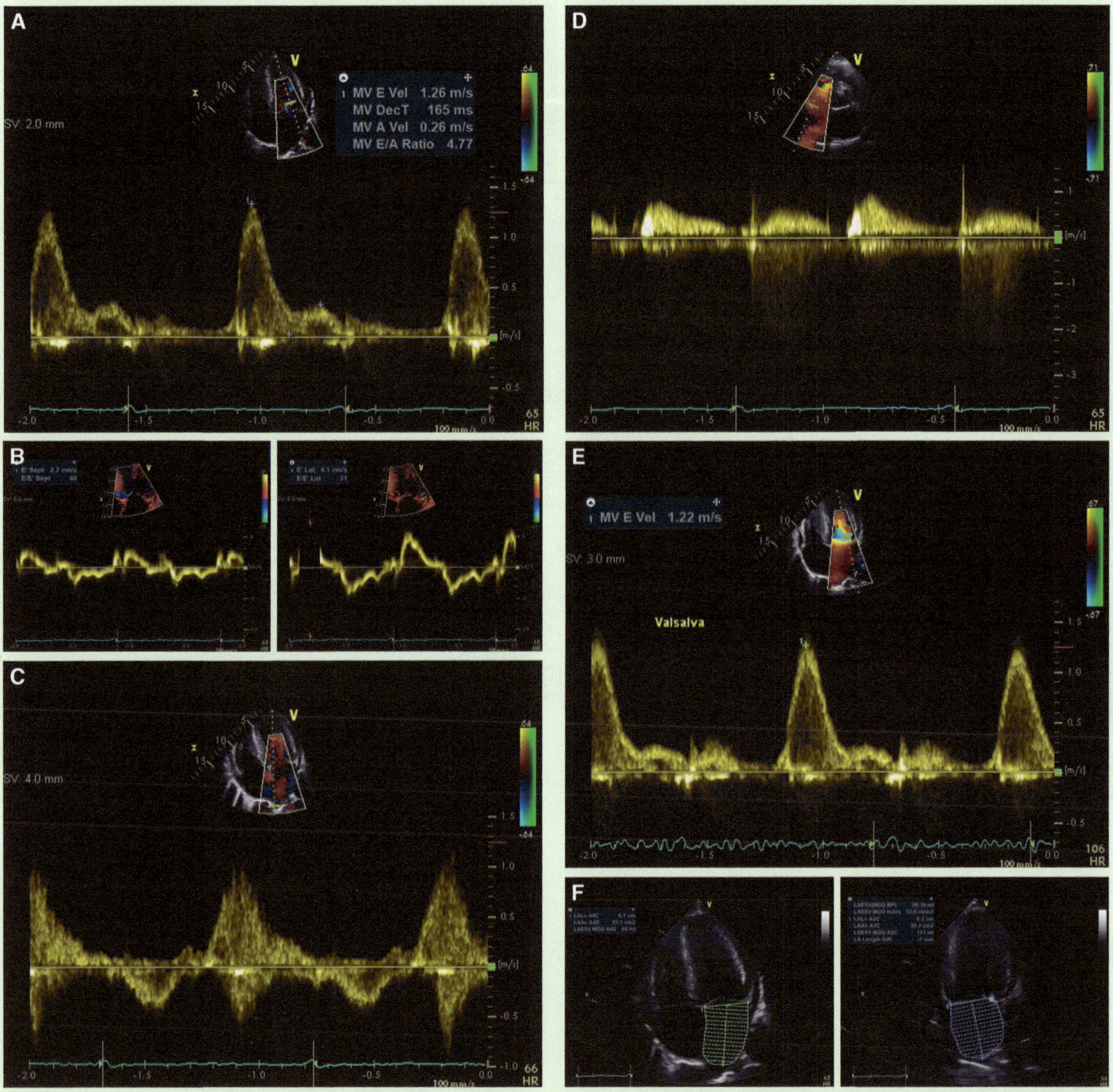

(A) From the transmitral inflow trace the peak early diastolic (E) velocity is 1.26 m/sec, the peak velocity with atrial contraction (A) velocity is 0.26 m/sec with an E/A ratio of 4.8. (B) The peak e′ velocity acquired at the septal *(left)* and lateral *(right)* mitral annulus is 2.7 cm/sec and 4.1 cm/sec, respectively. The average E/e′ ratio is 37. (C) The pulmonary venous signal is acquired unmeasured. (D) The tricuspid regurgitant signal cannot be accurately measured as the signal is weak and the envelope is incomplete. (E) The peak E velocity on the transmitral inflow trace with a Valsalva attempt is measured at 1.22 m/sec. (F) The biplane left atrial (LA) volume, indexed to the body surface area, is 53 mL/m^2.

Case Study 2 (*Cont.*)

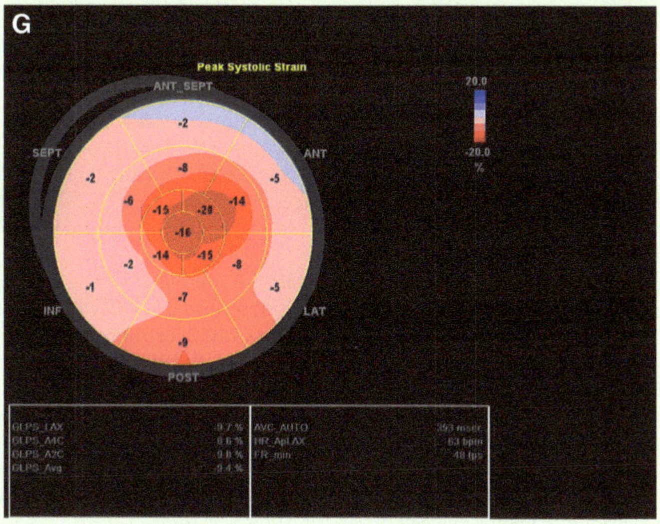

(G) Global longitudinal strain (GLS) is −9.4%.

REVIEW QUESTIONS

Note: Review questions pertain to Case Study 2.

1. Based on the images provided for this case, LV diastology is graded as
   a. indeterminate.
   b. Grade I.
   c. Grade II.
   d. Grade III.
2. Based on the grade of diastolic dysfunction, the Vp and IVRT if measured in this case would reveal
   a. both Vp and IVRT would be prolonged.
   b. both Vp and IVRT would be shortened.
   c. Vp would be prolonged and IVRT shortened.
   d. Vp would be shortened and IVRT prolonged.
3. The Valsalva maneuver was performed in this patient (see E in Case Study 2 figure). Which statement is true with respect to the finding in this case example?
   a. There is evidence of a reversible restrictive LV filling.
   b. There is no evidence of a reversible restrictive LV filling.
   c. This is a suboptimal Valsalva attempt.
   d. This attempt is unnecessary as grading has been already established.
4. Observe the pulmonary venous PW Doppler trace (see C in Case Study 2 figure). This trace is not truly reflective of pulmonary venous inflow because
   a. the velocity scale is set too high.
   b. the wall filter is set too low.
   c. the sample volume size is too big.
   d. the sample volume is not in the pulmonary vein.

REFERENCES

1. Nagueh SF, Smiseth OA, Appleton CP, et al. Recommendations for the evaluation of left ventricular diastolic function by echocardiography: an update from the American Society of Echocardiography and the European Association of Cardiovascular Imaging. *J Am Soc Echocardiogr.* 2016;29(4):277–314.
2. Nishimura RA, Tajik AJ. Evaluation of diastolic filling of left ventricle in health and disease: Doppler echocardiography is the clinician's Rosetta Stone. *J Am Coll Cardiol.* 1997;30(1):8–18.
3. Caballero L, Kou S, Dulgheru R, et al. Echocardiographic reference ranges for normal cardiac Doppler data: results from the NORRE Study. *Eur Heart J Cardiovasc Imag.* 2015;16(9):1031–1041.
4. Mitter SS, Shah SJ, Thomas JD. A test in context: E/A and E/e′ to assess diastolic dysfunction and LV filling pressure. *J Am Coll Cardiol.* 2017;69(11):1451–1464.
5. Sohn DW, Chai IH, Lee DJ, et al. Assessment of mitral annulus velocity by Doppler tissue imaging in the evaluation of left ventricular diastolic function. *J Am Coll Cardiol.* 1997;30(2):474–480.
6. Nagueh SF, Middleton KJ, Kopelen HA, Zoghbi WA, Quiñones MA. Doppler tissue imaging: a noninvasive technique for evaluation of left ventricular relaxation and estimation of filling pressures. *J Am Coll Cardiol.* 1997;30(6):1527–1533.
7. Ommen SR, Nishimura RA, Appleton CP, et al. Clinical utility of Doppler echocardiography and tissue Doppler imaging in the estimation of left ventricular filling pressures: a comparative simultaneous Doppler-catheterization study. *Circulation.* 2000;102(15): 1788–1794.
8. Rivas-Gotz C, Manolios M, Thohan V, Nagueh SF. Impact of left ventricular ejection fraction on estimation of left ventricular filling pressures using tissue Doppler and flow propagation velocity. *Am J Cardiol.* 2003;91(6): 780–784.
9. Kim YJ, Sohn DW. Mitral annulus velocity in the estimation of left ventricular filling pressure: prospective study in 200 patients. *J Am Soc Echocardiogr.* 2000;13(11):980–985.
10. Kasner M, Westermann D, Steendijk P, et al. Utility of Doppler echocardiography and tissue Doppler imaging in the estimation of diastolic function in heart failure with normal ejection fraction: a comparative Doppler-conductance catheterization study. *Circulation.* 2007;116(6):637–647.
11. Parasuraman S, Walker S, Loudon BL, et al. Assessment of pulmonary artery pressure by echocardiography—a comprehensive review. *Int J Cardiol Heart Vasc.* 2016;12:45–51.
12. Nagueh SF, Appleton CP, Gillebert TC, et al. Recommendations for the evaluation of left ventricular diastolic function by echocardiography. *J Am Soc Echocardiogr.* 2009;22(2):107–133.

13. Tsang TS, Barnes ME, Gersh BJ, Bailey KR, Seward JB. Left atrial volume as a morphophysiologic expression of left ventricular diastolic dysfunction and relation to cardiovascular risk burden. *Am J Cardiol.* 2002;90(12): 1284–1289.
14. Klein AL, Burstow DJ, Tajik AJ, Zachariah PK, Bailey KR, Seward JB. Effects of age on left ventricular dimensions and filling dynamics in 117 normal persons. *Mayo Clin Proc.* 1994;69(3):212–224.
15. Kuecherer HF, Muhiudeen IA, Kusumoto FM, et al. Estimation of mean left atrial pressure from transesophageal pulsed Doppler echocardiography of pulmonary venous flow. *Circulation.* 1990;82(4):1127–1139.
16. Appleton CP, Galloway JM, Gonzalez MS, Gaballa M, Basnight MA. Estimation of left ventricular filling pressures using two-dimensional and Doppler echocardiography in adult patients with cardiac disease. Additional value of analyzing left atrial size, left atrial ejection fraction and the difference in duration of pulmonary venous and mitral flow velocity at atrial contraction. J Am Coll Cardiol. 1993;22:1972–1982.
17. Yamamoto K, Nishimura RA, Chaliki HP, Appleton CP, Holmes DR Jr, Redfield MM. Determination of left ventricular filling pressure by Doppler echocardiography in patients with coronary artery disease: critical role of left ventricular systolic function. *J Am Coll Cardiol.* 1997;30:1819–1826.
18. Rossi A, Cicoira M, Golia G, Anselmi M, Zardini P. Mitral regurgitation and left ventricular diastolic dysfunction similarly affect mitral and pulmonary vein flow Doppler parameters: the advantage of end-diastolic markers. *J Am Soc Echocardiogr.* 2001;14:562–568.
19. Nagueh SF. Non-invasive assessment of left ventricular filling pressure. *Eur J Heart Fail.* 2018;20(1):38–48.
20. Diwan A, McCulloch M, Lawrie GM, Reardon MJ, Nagueh SF. Doppler estimation of left ventricular filling pressures in patients with mitral valve disease. *Circulation.* 2005;111:3281–3289.
21. Abudiab MM, Chebrolu LH, Schutt RC, Nagueh SF, Zoghbi WA. Doppler echocardiography for the estimation of LV filling pressure in patients with mitral annular calcification. *JACC Cardiovasc Imag.* 2017;10:1411–1420.
22. Nagueh SF, Kopelen HA, Quiñones MA. Assessment of left ventricular filling pressures by Doppler in the presence of atrial fibrillation. *Circulation.* 1996;94:2138–2145.
23. Garcia MJ, Ares MA, Asher C, Rodriguez L, Vandervoort P, Thomas JD. An index of early left ventricular filling that combined with pulsed Doppler peak E velocity may estimate capillary wedge pressure. *J Am Coll Cardiol.* 1997;29(2):448–454.
24. Garcia MJ, Smedira NG, Greenberg NL, et al. Color M-mode Doppler flow propagation velocity is a preload insensitive index of left ventricular relaxation: animal and human validation. *J Am Coll Cardiol.* 2000;35(1):201–208.
25. Gonzalez-Vilchez F, Ares M, Ayuela J, Alonso L. Combined use of pulsed and color M-mode Doppler echocardiography for the estimation of pulmonary capillary wedge pressure: an empirical approach based on an analytical relation. *J Am Coll Cardiol.* 1999;34(2):515–523.
26. González-Vilchez F, Ayuela J, Ares M, Mata NS, González AG, Durán RM. Comparison of Doppler echocardiography, color M-mode Doppler, and Doppler tissue imaging for the estimation of pulmonary capillary wedge pressure. *J Am Soc Echocardiogr.* 2002;15(10 Pt 2):1245–1250.
27. Dini FL, Ballo P, Badano L, et al. Validation of an echo-Doppler decision model to predict left ventricular filling pressure in patients with heart failure independently of ejection fraction. *Eur J Echocardiogr.* 2010;11(8):703–710.
28. Nagueh SF, Bhatt R, Vivo RP, et al. Echocardiographic evaluation of hemodynamics in patients with decompensated systolic heart failure. *Circ Cardiovasc Imag.* 2011;4(3):220–227.
29. Rivas-Gotz C, Manolios M, Thohan V, Nagueh SF. Impact of left ventricular ejection fraction on estimation of left ventricular filling pressures using tissue Doppler and flow propagation velocity. *Am J Cardiol.* 2003;91:780–784.
30. Potter E and Marwick TH. Assessment of Left Ventricular Function by Echocardiography: The Case for Routinely Adding Global Longitudinal Strain to Ejection Fraction. JACC Cardiovasc Imaging. 2018 Feb;11(2 Pt 1):260–274.
31. Dokainish H, Sengupta R, Pillai M, Bobek J, Lakkis N. Usefulness of new diastolic strain and strain rate indexes for the estimation of left ventricular filling pressure. *Am J Cardiol.* 2008;101:1504–1509.
32. Melenovsky V, Hwang SJ, Redfield MM, Zakeri R, Lin G, Borlaug BA. Left atrial remodeling and function in advanced heart failure with preserved or reduced ejection fraction. *Circ Heart Fail.* 2015;8:295–303.
33. Singh A, Addetia K, Maffessanti F, Mor-Avi V, Lang RM. LA Strain for categorization of LV diastolic dysfunction. *J Am Coll Cardiol Imag.* 2017;10: 735–743.
34. Badano LP, Kolias TJ, Muraru D, et al. Standardization of left atrial, right ventricular, and right atrial deformation imaging using two-dimensional speckle tracking echocardiography: a consensus document of the EACVI/ASE/Industry Task Force to standardize deformation imaging [published correction appears in Eur Heart J Cardiovasc Imaging. 2018 Jul 1;19(7):830-833]. *Eur Heart J Cardiovasc Imaging.* 2018;19(6):591–600.
35. Thomas L, Marwick TH, Popescu BA, Donal E, Badano LP. Left Atrial Structure and Function, and Left Ventricular Diastolic Dysfunction: JACC State-of-the-Art Review. *J Am Coll Cardiol.* 2019;73(15):1961–1977.
36. Haji K, Wong C, Wright L, Ramkumar S, Marwick TH. Left Atrial Strain Performance and its Application in Clinical Practice. *JACC Cardiovasc Imaging.* 2019;12(6):1093–1101.
37. Lang RM, Badano LP, Mor-Avi V, et al. Recommendations for cardiac chamber quantification by echocardiography in adults: an update from the American Society of Echocardiography and the European Association of Cardiovascular Imaging. *J Am Soc Echocardiogr.* 2015;28(1):1–39.
38. Reuss CS, Wilansky SM, Lester SJ, et al. Using mitral 'annulus reversus' to diagnose constrictive pericarditis. *Eur J Echocardiogr.* 2009;10(3):372–375.
39. Kyranis SJ, Latona J, Platts D, et al. Improving the echocardiographic assessment of pulmonary pressure using the tricuspid regurgitant signal-The "chin" vs the "beard." *Echocardiography.* 2018;35:1085–1096.
40. Platts DG, Vaishnav M, Burstow DJ, Hamilton-Craig C, Chan J, Sedgwick JF, Scalia GM. Contrast microsphere enhancement of the tricuspid regurgitant spectral Doppler signal - Is it still necessary with contemporary scanners?. *Int J Cardiol Heart Vasc.* 2017 Dec;17:1–10.
41. Porter TR, Mulvagh SL, Abdelmoneim SS, Becher H, Belcik JT, Bierig M, et al. Clinical Applications of Ultrasonic Enhancing Agents in Echocardiography: 2018 American Society of Echocardiography Guidelines Update. *J Am Soc Echocardiogr.* 2018 Mar;31(3):241–274.
42. Negishi K, Negishi T, Kurosawa K, et al. Practical guidance in echocardiographic assessment of global longitudinal strain. *JACC Cardiovasc Imag.* 2015;8(4):489–492.
43. Collier P, Phelan D, Klein A. A test in context: myocardial strain measured by speckle-tracking echocardiography. *J Am Coll Cardiol.* 2017;69(8):1043–1056.
44. Chan J, Shiino K, Obonyo NG, et al. Left ventricular global strain analysis by two-dimensional speckle-tracking echocardiography: the learning curve. *J Am Soc Echocardiogr.* 2017;30(11):1081–1090.
45. Sun JP, Abdalla IA, Yang XS, et al. Respiratory variation of mitral and pulmonary venous Doppler flow velocities in constrictive pericarditis before and after pericardiectomy. *J Am Soc Echocardiogr.* 2001;14(11):1119–1126.
46. Oh JK, Tajik AJ, Appleton CP, Hatle LK, Nishimura RA, Seward JB. Preload reduction to unmask the characteristic Doppler features of constrictive pericarditis. A new observation. *Circulation.* 1997;95(4):796–799.
47. Mottram PM, Marwick TH. Assessment of diastolic function: what the general cardiologist needs to know. *Heart.* 2005;91:681–695.
48. Ginghina C, Beladan CC, Iancu M, Calin A, Popescu BA. Respiratory maneuvers in echocardiography: a review of clinical applications. *Cardiovasc Ultrasoun.* 2009;7:42. doi: 10.1186/1476-7120-7-42.
49. Lancellotti P, Pellikka PA, Budts W, et al. The clinical use of stress echocardiography in non-ischaemic heart disease: recommendations from the European Association of Cardiovascular Imaging and the American Society of Echocardiography. *J Am Soc Echocardiogr.* 2017;30(2):101–138.
50. Klein AL, Abbara S, Agler DA, et al. American Society of Echocardiography clinical recommendations for multimodality cardiovascular imaging of patients with pericardial disease: endorsed by the Society for Cardiovascular Magnetic Resonance and Society of Cardiovascular Computed Tomography. *J Am Soc Echocardiogr.* 2013;26(9):965–1012. e15.
51. Pstras L, Thomaseth K, Waniewski J, Balzani I, Bellavere F. The Valsalva manoeuvre: physiology and clinical examples. *Acta Physiologica (Oxford).* 2016;217(2):103–119.
52. Dumesnil JG, Gaudreault G, Honos GN, Kingma JG Jr. Use of Valsalva maneuver to unmask left ventricular diastolic function abnormalities by Doppler echocardiography in patients with coronary artery disease or systemic hypertension. *Am J Cardiol.* 1991;68(5):515–519.

53. Hurrell DG, Nishimura RA, Ilstrup DM, Appleton CP. Utility of preload alteration in assessment of left ventricular filling pressure by Doppler echocardiography: a simultaneous catheterization and Doppler echocardiographic study. *J Am Coll Cardiol.* 1997;30:459–467.
54. Choi EY, Shim CY, Kim SA, et al. Passive leg-raise is helpful to identify impaired diastolic functional reserve during exercise in patients with abnormal myocardial relaxation. *J Am Soc Echocardiogr.* 2010;23(5):523–530.
55. Ha JW, Lulic F, Bailey KR, et al. Effects of treadmill exercise on mitral inflow and annular velocities in healthy adults. *Am J Cardiol.* 2003;91(1):114–115.
56. Burgess MI, Jenkins C, Sharman JE, Marwick TH. Diastolic stress echocardiography: hemodynamic validation and clinical significance of estimation of ventricular filling pressure with exercise. *J Am Coll Cardiol.* 2006;47(9): 1891–1900.
57. Ha JW, Oh JK, Pellikka PA, et al. Diastolic stress echocardiography: a novel noninvasive diagnostic test for diastolic dysfunction using supine bicycle exercise Doppler echocardiography. *J Am Soc Echocardiogr.* 2005;18(1):63–68.
58. Borlaug BA, Nishimura RA, Sorajja P, Lam CS, Redfield MM. Exercise hemodynamics enhance diagnosis of early heart failure with preserved ejection fraction. *Circ Heart Fail.* 2010;3(5):588–595.
59. Ha JW, Choi EY, Choi D, et al. Time course of recovery of left ventricular filling pressure after exercise in healthy subjects. *Circ J.* 2008;72(2):186–188.
60. Beigel R, Cercek B, Luo H, Siegel RJ. Noninvasive evaluation of right atrial pressure. *J Am Soc Echocardiogr.* 2013;26(9):1033–1042.
61. Abbas A, Lester S, Moreno FC, Srivathsan K, Fortuin D, Appleton C. Noninvasive assessment of right atrial pressure using Doppler tissue imaging. *J Am Soc Echocardiogr.* 2004;17(11):1155–1160.
62. Nagueh SF, Kopelen HA, Zoghbi WA. Relation of mean right atrial pressure to echocardiographic and Doppler parameters of right atrial and right ventricular function. *Circulation.* 1996;93(6):1160–1169.
63. Ommen SR, Nishimura RA, Hurrell DG, Klarich KW. Assessment of right atrial pressure with 2-dimensional and Doppler echocardiography: a simultaneous catheterization and echocardiographic study. *Mayo Clin Proc.* 2000;75(1):24–29.

18

Diastology Stress Test

Jong-Won Ha

OUTLINE

Case Study

A 71-year-old man presents with exertional dyspnea progressing over several months. He has known diabetes mellitus and hypertension, both well controlled on medications. Chest x-ray and electrocardiogram (ECG) are unremarkable. His resting transthoracic echocardiogram shows normal-size cardiac chambers and left ventricular (LV) ejection fraction of 70%. Mitral inflow shows reduced early (E) to late (A) diastolic filling ratio and prolonged deceleration time of E velocity, suggesting impaired relaxation. E/e′ ratio of 12 suggests normal LV filling pressure at rest. No other valvular or pericardial abnormalities are observed. Diastolic stress echocardiography (SE) is performed with supine bicycle exercise, and exercise is stopped at 50 W due to severe dyspnea. During exercise there is significant increase in mitral E velocity with shortened deceleration time, but minimal change in mitral annular e′ velocity suggests elevated LV filling pressure with exercise (Fig. 18.1).

EPIDEMIOLOGY

Exertional dyspnea is one of the most common presenting symptoms in our routine practice. The mechanisms responsible for dyspnea may vary significantly. Although cardiac or pulmonary diseases are major causes of pathologic dyspnea, other systemic conditions such as anemia, obesity, neuromuscular diseases, and metabolic acidosis should be suspected as possible causes. By accurately identifying the correct etiology of dyspnea in a patient, the appropriate treatment can be implemented. Cardiac causes of dyspnea include right, left, or biventricular heart failure with systolic dysfunction, coronary artery disease, hypertensive heart disease, cardiomyopathy, valvular dysfunction, pericardial disease, arrhythmia, congenital heart disease, and pulmonary arteriovenous malformations. Regardless of ejection fraction, demonstration of an elevated LV filling pressure is the most important hemodynamic parameter when a cardiac etiology is suspected. Frequently, exertional dyspnea cannot be explained by the variables of LV systolic and diastolic functions at rest. Therefore, for patients who report severe exertional symptoms, it may be desirable to measure the hemodynamic response to exercise to ensure that these symptoms are due to LV dysfunction.

Heart failure is the most common hospital discharge diagnosis in patients 65 years or older and is a major cardiovascular disorder that is still increasing. It has become increasingly evident that LV diastolic function has a major role in producing signs and symptoms in patients presenting with heart failure.[1–4] Primary diastolic dysfunction is the cause of up to 50% of cases of heart failure, and it is also a determinant of prognosis. Impaired myocardial relaxation, manifested echocardiographically as reduced early to late (E/A) ratio or prolonged deceleration time of E velocity, is the most common finding in LV diastolic dysfunction, and it is recognized as an early manifestation in the spectrum of diastolic abnormalities. However, because of its ubiquity, this abnormality is often recognized as an incidental finding. Many elderly subjects and patients with hypertension or LV hypertrophy have Doppler echocardiographic evidence of impaired diastolic function but do not have any symptoms of heart failure at rest. More commonly, symptoms of diastolic dysfunction occur only during exertion when filling pressures are normal at rest and increase only with exertion. Therefore exercise could unmask diastolic abnormalities not evident under resting conditions. Despite this, the majority of measures used to characterize the severity of heart failure and prognosis are obtained at rest.

PATHOPHYSIOLOGY

Abnormalities of ventricular relaxation and filling contribute to heart failure because these result in an abnormally high ventricular diastolic pressure in relation to diastolic volume. The most important factors that determine the relation between pressure and volume during ventricular diastole are the rate and extent of myocardial relaxation and the generation of restoring forces, both of which are important determinants of early diastolic filling. The passive pressure-volume relationship (PVR) of the ventricle determines mid- to late diastolic filling after the relaxation is complete.[5–8]

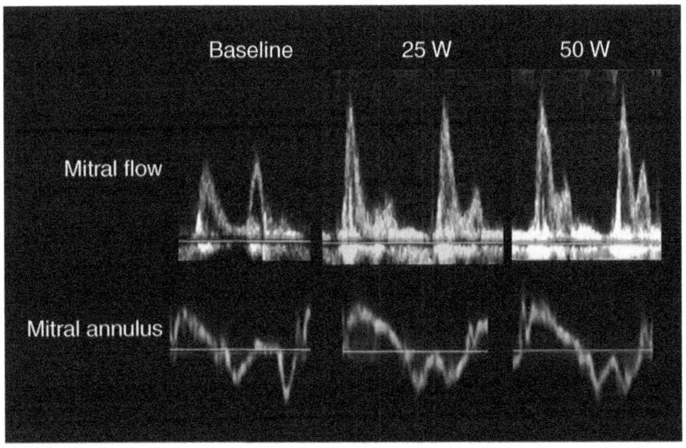

Fig. 18.1 Case study: Pulsed-wave Doppler recordings obtained at baseline and during diastolic bicycle stress test at 25 and 50 Watts (W) loads.

Myocardial Relaxation

The normal cardiac contraction/relaxation cycle requires a precise, transient rise and fall of intracellular calcium ions (see Chapter 2). The sarcoplasmic reticulum (SR) has a central role in orchestrating the movement of calcium during each contraction and relaxation.[9,10] Contraction of cardiac muscle is initiated by the cellular action potential that causes the opening of L-type sarcolemmal calcium channels, through which calcium ions enter the cytosol. Influx of calcium ions through L-type channels results in the release of large amounts of calcium ions from the adjacent SR through ryanodine receptor channels, a process termed calcium-induced calcium release. These calcium ions bind to troponin C, which ultimately disinhibits the interaction of actin and myosin with resultant cross-bridge formation.[5,6] Myocardial relaxation is accomplished primarily by removal of calcium ions from troponin C by an enzyme located in SR, called SR calcium ATPase or $SERCA_2$ and the sarcolemmal sodium-calcium (Na-Ca) exchanger. In humans, approximately 75% of calcium ions are removed by $SERCA_2$ and 25% by the Na-Ca exchanger.[11] The activity of $SERCA_2$ is modulated by phospholamban, another SR protein located near $SERCA_2$. By virtue of phosphorylation by protein kinase A and other kinases, phospholamban enhances the calcium ion uptake by $SERCA_2$.[12] Failure of normal mechanisms of reuptake and extrude calcium ions released during contraction can result in the slowing of relaxation or an inability to return cytosolic calcium concentration to normal diastolic levels. The latter causes diastolic calcium overload and incomplete relaxation with excessive diastolic tension or stiffening.[13–15] In an experimental model of senescence, it has been demonstrated that the decrease in SR Ca^{2+} uptake during relaxation is associated with a decrease in the content and activity of $SERCA_2$.[16] More recently, $SERCA_2$ protein levels were found to be significantly decreased in senescent human myocardium.[17] This decrease in $SERCA_2$ levels was associated with impaired myocardial function at baseline, and further deterioration occurred during hypoxic conditions.[17] Thus decrease in $SERCA_2$ content and an associated decrease in SR Ca^{2+} uptake has been suggested to play a major role in the diastolic dysfunction. The vulnerability of calcium reuptake is a contributing factor for abnormal LV relaxation early in cardiac disease states despite normal systolic function.

Myocardial relaxation is also modulated by external factors. Endocardial and vascular endothelial modulators have been proposed as important factors for the physiology of myocardial relaxation.[5,18] Vascular endothelium also appears to play an important role in these responses. In an experimental papillary muscle preparation, Brutsaert et al. found that denudation of the endocardium resulted in an earlier and rapid relaxation in conjunction with a very modest reduction of developed force.[5] Although effects are less clear in normal hearts, angiotensin II has been shown to slow myocardial relaxation in hypertrophied hearts.[18] Other locally released substances that may influence myocardial relaxation include endothelin-1, natriuretic peptides, prostaglandins, and adenyl purines. The physiologic and pathophysiologic significance of these modulators of relaxation remains to be elucidated.

Interestingly, the relevance of caffeine for facilitating diastolic dysfunction in the intact heart was demonstrated in the experimental canine model of demand ischemia.[19] It was also suggested that caffeine affected myocardial relaxation favorably without altering contractility.[20]

Restoring Forces

Restoring forces are generated when the ventricle contracts to an end-systolic volume (ESV) less than its equilibrium volume (Vo), the volume in the fully relaxed state when transmural pressure is zero, thereby storing energy by compressing the elastic elements in the myocardium.[7,18] The physical properties of the normal ventricular chamber allow potential energy to be stored during systole in the form of a lower ventricular pressure. This potential energy is converted to kinetic energy in the form of elastic recoil, with the resultant suction of blood from the left atrium into the ventricle early during diastole.[21] Other factors, especially complex shape changes during systole, may also play a role in causing suction during subsequent diastole.[22] During systole, the left ventricle demonstrates a counterclockwise twist extending from apex to base, and in early diastole the left ventricle untwists clockwise releasing the stored energy and creating a suction force not unlike the release of a compressed spring. Suction is most important under conditions of stress, when contractility is high and ESV is small, and filling must be enhanced such as during exercise. Conversely, when contractility is impaired, ESV is larger and suction is reduced or lost as a mechanism of filling.[23]

The Passive Pressure-Volume Relation of the Ventricle

The Laplace law provides the relationship between pressure and chamber geometry when a stress is applied to the ventricle. In the simplest case of a sphere, the Laplace law states that pressure is proportional to the radius of the chamber divided by its wall thickness. Thus a chamber with thicker walls requires a larger distending pressure to achieve a given volume. The intrinsic stiffness of the tissue in the ventricular wall is the other key determinant of the distending force required to passively fill the chamber. At low filling pressures, the elastic properties are most responsible for wall stiffness.[24] At higher distending pressures, the myocardial connective tissue matrix assumes a key role. The intrinsic passive stiffness of any tissue, including the myocardium, can be quantified as the change in stress required to produce a given change in stretch (or strain). Biologic tissues have a curvilinear passive stress-strain relationship. The amount of blood contained in the vessels in the wall is also a determinant of the stiffness of the myocardial tissue, contributing to the pressure-volume relationship.[25] As a result, a greater distending pressure is required to fill the chamber when the myocardial blood volume increases. The PVR of the passive ventricle is curvilinear, paralleling the passive stress-strain relationship. At any point on this curve, the ratio of change in pressure to change in volume represents the operating chamber stiffness; its inverse is operating compliance. Like the stress-strain relationship, the PVR can be converted into a linear relationship by the plotting of operating chamber stiffness versus pressure (Fig. 18.2). The slope of this relation is the chamber-stiffness constant. The parietal pericardium and right ventricle form external constraints

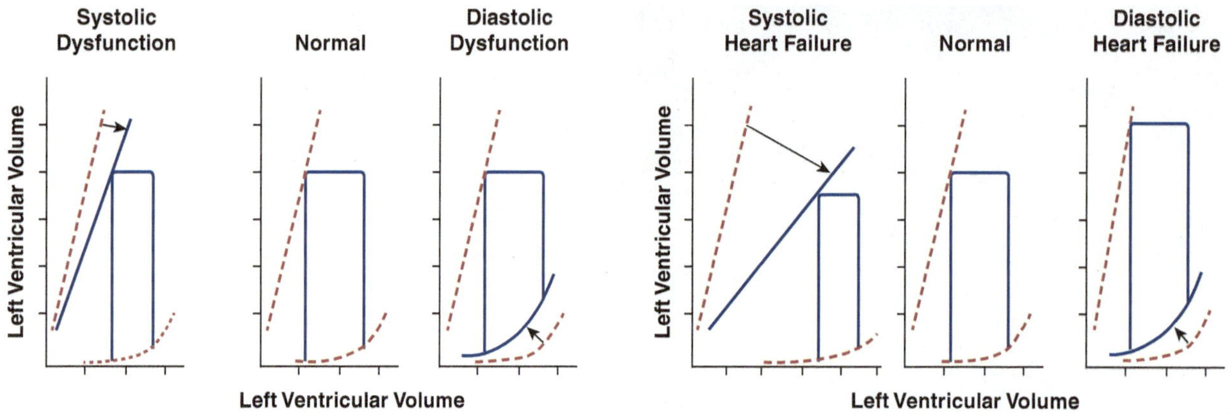

Fig. 18.2 Diagram of left ventricular pressure-volume loops in systolic dysfunction, normal and diastolic dysfunction (left panel) and in systolic heart failure, normal, and diastolic heart failure (right panel). (Adapted from Zile MR, et al. Diastolic heart failure: definitions and terminology. *Prog Cardiovasc Dis.* 2005;47:3017–3013.)

to filling that influence the PVR as well. The parietal pericardium has a very compliant PVR at low volumes but then makes a sharp transition to a very steep relationship. Increases in right ventricular (RV) diastolic volume and pressure influence the LV PVR similarly, albeit more modestly, because the RV changes are transmitted to the left ventricle via the ventricular septum. This phenomenon is termed diastolic ventricular interaction and is based on the fact that total cardiac volume within the pericardial sac remains constant, hence overfilling of the right ventricle will result in reduced filling of the left ventricle, and vice versa. This is most dramatically manifested in constrictive pericarditis. The ventricular and pericardial effects on the LV PVR are often linked.

During exercise there is less time for diastolic filling of the left ventricle because tachycardia decreases the duration of diastole. To maintain or augment the stroke volume, myocardial relaxation should be faster and LV suction should be exaggerated. There can be a spectrum of alterations in diastolic function during exercise. Therefore exercise could unmask diastolic abnormalities not evident under rest conditions.

DIAGNOSTIC EVALUATION

Invasive Diastology Stress Test

LV diastolic pressure is the main parameter that characterizes LV filling properties. The term LV filling pressures can refer to mean pulmonary capillary wedge pressure (PCWP), mean left atrial (LA) pressure (LAP), LV pre-A pressure, mean LV diastolic pressure, and LV end-diastolic pressure (LVEDP).[26,27] In the early stages of diastolic dysfunction, LVEDP is the only abnormally elevated pressure, while mean PCWP and LAP remain normal. With tachycardia and/or increased LV afterload, mean PCWP and LAP increase, which provides the basis for the diastolic stress testing. Catheterization is performed while subjects are doing an exercise on a variable-load bicycle ergometer specially mounted at the catheterization table in a supine position. Changes of PCWP, an indirect estimate of LV diastolic pressures, during exercise can be assessed by right heart catheterization through the right internal jugular vein. A study examined hemodynamic responses to exercise measured invasively in consecutive patients with preserved LV ejection fraction who were referred for catheterization to evaluate the cause of exertional dyspnea. Despite normal resting PCWP, more than half of the patients had an abnormal increase in PCWP during exercise, with symptoms of exercise intolerance. The increase in PCWP during peak exercise was greater in heart failure with preserved ejection fraction (HFpEF) than in noncardiac dyspnea.[28] Alternately, LV diastolic pressures at rest and during exercise can be obtained by introducing a pigtail catheter into the left ventricle from a radial arterial access site. By this approach, LV systolic pressure, minimal LV pressure, LVEDP, and mean LV diastolic pressure can be measured. Previous studies utilizing an invasive measurement of LV pressure demonstrate that augmenting LV suction is important to produce the early diastolic mitral valve gradient for more rapid mitral valve flow in early diastole, particularly during exercise, which shortens the diastolic period.[29,30] Thus a decrease in minimal LV pressure reflecting the augmented LV suction during exercise is crucial to maintain early LV diastolic filling without an increase in LAP.

A normal heart can increase transmitral flow during exercise with little or no increase in LAP by lowering minimum LV diastolic pressure. In the failing heart, however, there was no fall in minimum LV diastolic pressure with exercise, and an increase in transmitral gradient and mitral flow was achieved by elevation of LAP (Fig. 18.3). Possibly a similar mechanism explains elevated LAP during exercise in patients with heart failure. Representative cases of LV pressure curves at rest and at maximal exercise from two individuals show minimal LV pressure at rest was −2 mmHg, and it decreased up to −5 mmHg during maximal exercise in patient A, whereas minimal LV pressure at rest was 7 mmHg, and it increased up to 16 mmHg in patient B (Fig. 18.4). Although cardiac catheterization remains the gold standard and provides several important hemodynamic parameters, it is not practical to submit many patients presenting with dyspnea and suspicion of heart failure to invasive studies. A simultaneous echocardiographic-catheterization study prospectively conducted at rest and during exercise in subjects with invasively proven HFpEF and participants with dyspnea but no identifiable cardiac pathology has demonstrated that exercise E/e′ data improve sensitivity and negative predictive value; thus these results reinforce the value of exercise testing using invasive and noninvasive hemodynamic assessments to definitively confirm or refute the diagnosis of HFpEF.[31]

Noninvasive Diastology Stress Test (Diastolic Stress Echocardiography)

Diastolic stress echocardiography (SE) generally refers to the use of exercise Doppler echocardiography to detect impaired LV diastolic functional reserve and the resulting increase in LV filling pressures.[27,32,33] It is valuable particularly in patients with suspected HFpEF and borderline diastolic abnormalities at rest.[34] Early studies showed that diastolic SE is technically feasible for demonstrating the change in

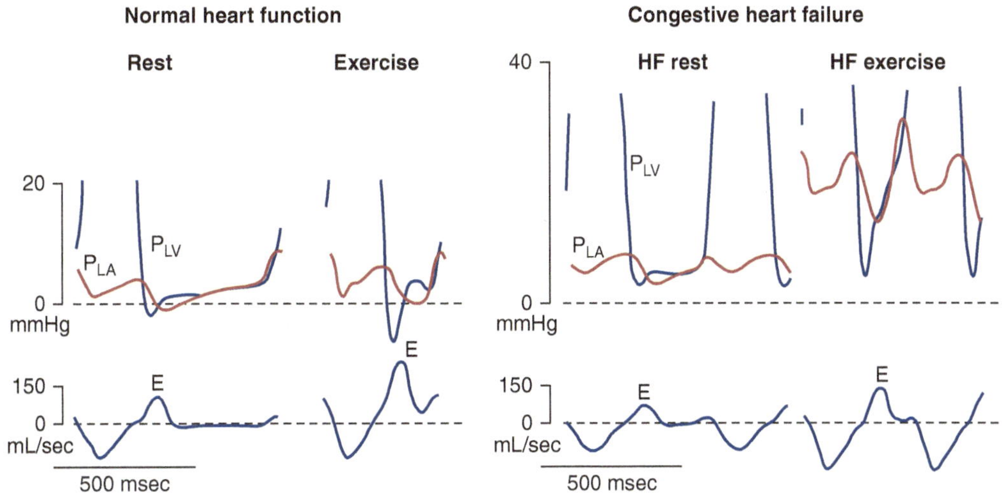

Fig. 18.3 Invasive diastrology stress test in the failing heart. (Adapted from Smiseth OA. Need for better diastolic stress test: twistin' time is here? *Eur Heart J Cardiovasc Imag.* 2018;19:20–22.)

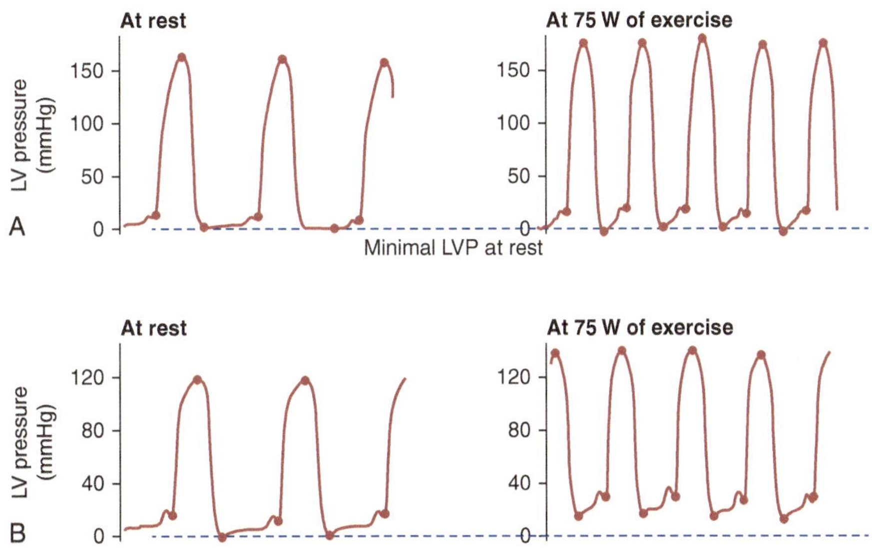

Fig. 18.4 Representative cases of LV pressure curves at rest and at maximal exercise from two individuals.

E/e′ (i.e., filling pressure) with exercise, and that the hemodynamic consequences of an exercise-induced increase in LV filling pressure can be demonstrated noninvasively with this technique. This test potentially can be an excellent way to distinguish between cardiac and noncardiac dyspnea in patients with multiple coexisting conditions that can cause exertional dyspnea.[35]

How to Perform a Diastolic Stress Echocardiogram

Supine bicycle ergometry is the recommended modality for diastolic SE, as it allows the acquisition of Doppler recordings throughout the test. Treadmill exercise SE is an alternative, as diastolic abnormalities may persist even after cessation of exercise. Preload augmentation by passive leg raise might also represent a nonexercise alternative in patients who cannot exercise since it provides additional information identifying patients with exercise-induced LV filling pressure elevation and lower exercise capacity.[34] Mitral E, A, E/A (1–2-mm sample volume pulse wave [PW] Doppler placed at the tip of the mitral valve), e′ (2–5-mm sample volume PW tissue Doppler, septal, and/or lateral mitral annulus with a Nyquist limit at 15–20 cm/sec with adjustment of gain and filter), E/e′, and systolic pulmonary artery pressure (SPAP) should be recorded at baseline, at low-level exercise, and during the recovery period. E and e′ are usually recorded at 100 to 110 bpm, when E and A waves are not yet fused. Postexercise assessment during the recovery period can be performed, especially when there has been a premature tachycardia even with a low level of exercise.[19] Recordings are obtained using the apical four-chamber view, and a total of 5 to 10 cardiac cycles should be acquired. During passive leg raise, in which the patient's legs are passively elevated for 3 minutes,[36] similar Doppler echocardiographic parameters are recorded. In supine bicycle exercise, the workload starts at 25 W and increases in increments of 25 W every 3 minutes. It is needed to record mitral inflow by pulsed Doppler echocardiography at the level of mitral tips, mitral annular velocities by spectral Doppler echocardiography, and tricuspid regurgitation jet by continuous wave Doppler at baseline, during exercise, and recovery period after the termination of exercise.

Diastolic stress echo data acquired before and after a symptom-limited supine bicycle exercise SE performed in a subject with impaired relaxation at rest is shown in Fig. 18.5. During exercise, there is an

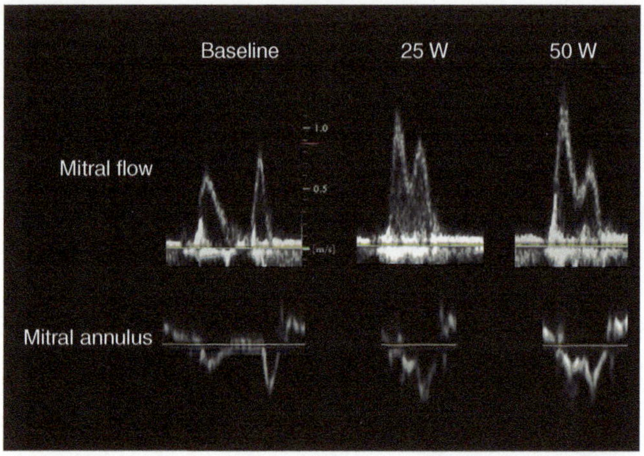

Fig. 18.5 Diastolic stress echo data acquired before and after a symptom-limited supine bicycle exercise stress echocardiography performed in a subject with impaired relaxation at rest.

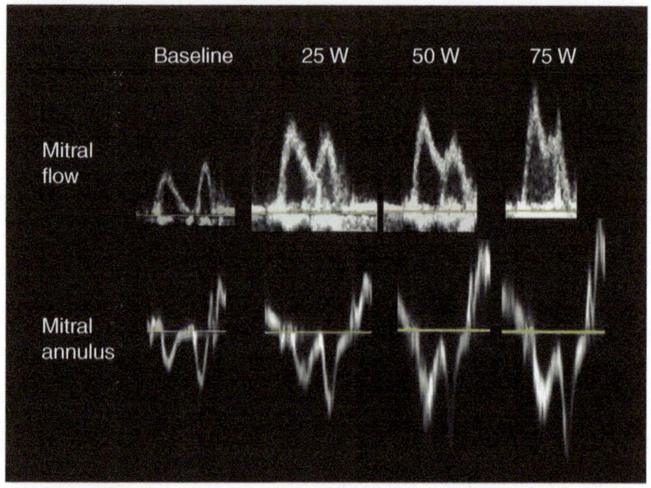

Fig. 18.6 Diastolic stress echo data acquired before and after a symptom-limited supine bicycle exercise performed in another subject with impaired relaxation at rest.

increase in mitral E velocity but minimal change in e′ with exercise, suggestive of elevated LV filling pressures with exercise. It is not yet known whether impaired relaxation leads invariably to elevated LV filling pressure during exercise. Diastolic stress echo data acquired before and after a symptom-limited supine bicycle exercise performed in another subject with impaired relaxation at rest is shown in Fig. 18.6. During exercise there is a concordant rise in both mitral E velocity and mitral annular e′ velocity with exercise, without an overall change in the mitral E/e′ ratio. These findings further underscore the fact that, in patients with a similar grade of diastolic dysfunction at rest, there can be a spectrum of alterations in diastolic function during exercise.

How to Interpret a Diastolic Stress Echocardiogram

Diastolic SE is definitively normal if the septal E/e′ is less than 10 at rest and with exercise, and the peak tricuspid regurgitation (TR) velocity is less than 2.8 m/sec at rest and with stress. A study is definitively abnormal when the septal E/e′ ratio is above 15, peak TR velocity is above 2.8 m/sec with exercise, and septal e′ velocity is below 8 cm/sec at baseline.[26,27,34,37] Systolic pulmonary artery pressure measurement with exercise has been found to be helpful in aiding the assessment of diastolic filling pressure with exercise.[27,28] It has been shown that the upper normal SPAP is less than 35 mmHg at rest and less than 43 mmHg at exercise (Fig. 18.7). Exercise E/septal e′ greater than 13, lower amplitude of changes in diastolic longitudinal velocities, and induced pulmonary hypertension (PH) (SPAP ≥50 mmHg) are markers of adverse outcomes.

Detection of Early Myocardial Disease and the Concept of Diastolic Reserve

The increase of e′ during exercise, a marker of longitudinal functional reserve, can be used as a parameter for the evaluation of LV diastolic reserve during exercise. Longitudinal diastolic functional reserve can be calculated as follows: $\Delta e' \, [1 - (1/e'_{base})]$, where $\Delta e'$ is the change of e′ from baseline to 25 or 50 W of exercise, and e'_{base} is early diastolic mitral annular velocity at rest.[38] LV diastolic reserve has been reported to be reduced in various diseases that are associated with diastolic dysfunction, including hypertrophic cardiomyopathy, diabetes mellitus, and a subtype

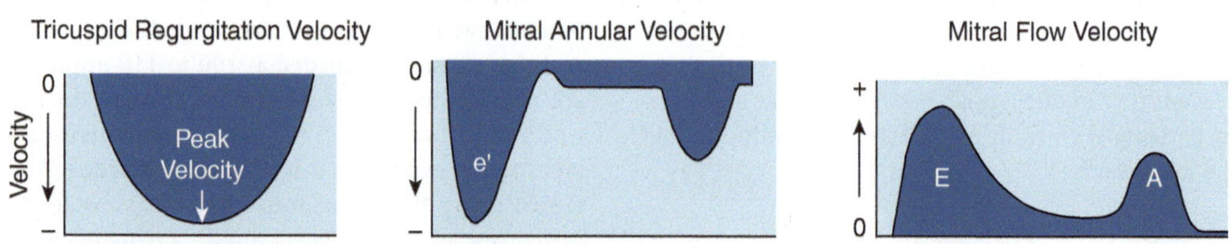

Parameter	Cutoff value
E/e'	>15
Peak TR velocity	>2.8 m/sec
E' at rest	<8 cm/sec

Fig. 18.7 Parameters used to define abnormal diastolic function during stress testing.

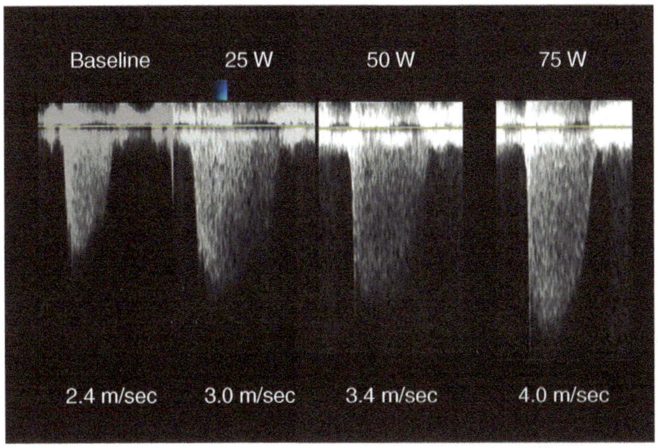

Fig. 18.8 Diastolic stress echo data acquired before and after a symptom-limited supine bicycle exercise in an individual with exertional dyspnea.

of hypertension.[38–40] It has been shown that exercise E/e′ and diastolic reserve are both associated with exercise capacity, but E/e′ has greater specificity for elevated filling pressure and is more closely associated with the expected parameters of diastolic dysfunction. However, high sensitivity of diastolic reserve makes it a better test for screening for exercise-induced diastolic dysfunction.[41]

Exercise-Induced LV Filling Pressure Elevation and Exercise-Induced Pulmonary Hypertension

Exercise-induced PH is common in subjects with reduced as well as preserved LV ejection fraction,[42] and it is considered an important cause of exertional dyspnea and exercise intolerance.[42,43] Fig. 18.8 shows the diastolic stress echo data acquired before and after a symptom-limited supine bicycle exercise in an individual with exertional dyspnea. The patient showed an increase in TR velocity during exercise, suggesting exercise-induced PH (see Fig. 18.8). A previous study has shown that subjects with exercise-induced PH associated with an increase in E/e′ have significantly worse outcomes, whereas no significant difference of clinical outcomes was found among subjects with exercise-induced PH without an increase in E/e′ and subjects without exercise-induced PH.[44] Thus exercise-induced PH when associated with an increase in LV filling pressure portends the worst clinical outcome. Therefore preventing or treating exercise-induced PH should be focused on improving LV diastolic properties and decreasing the LV filling pressure at rest and during exercise. Diastolic SE has a significant role in this regard since it can provide information regarding SPAP as well as LV filling pressure both at rest and during exercise.

In addition to limited LV functional reserve, patients with HFpEF had impaired RV reserve during exercise that is associated with high LV filling pressures and inadequate cardiac output responses. These findings underscore the importance of biventricular dysfunction in HFpEF and suggest that novel therapies targeting myocardial reserve in both the left and right heart may be effective in improving clinical status.[45]

Technical Challenges

One of the practical drawbacks of diastolic SE is technical difficulty obtaining adequate two-dimensional and Doppler echocardiographic parameters within a limited time, particularly during exercise. Fortunately patients with marked diastolic dysfunction revealed diagnostic changes even at mild or moderate exertion with a moderately increased heart rate. Despite this, a subset of patients develop premature tachycardia even at mild exertion, which makes a meaningful analysis difficult. In a previous report, the test was unsuccessful in 10% of enrolled patients because of tachycardia with low levels of exercise and exercise-induced atrial tachyarrhythmia.[32] It has been shown that diastolic dysfunction induced by exercise or ischemia persists well beyond recovery of myocardial ischemia or cessation of exercise.[46] In one study, 73 healthy subjects underwent supine bicycle exercise, and mitral inflow parameters and diastolic velocities of the mitral annulus were recorded at baseline and during recovery 2, 5, and 10 minutes after cessation of exercise. None of the patients had an E/e′ above 15 at rest, during exercise, and at the recovery phase, for up to 10 minutes after cessation of exercise.[47] Since the E/e′ was not elevated in healthy subjects, elevated E/e′ during recovery may be helpful to detect exercise-induced diastolic dysfunction in subjects with tachycardia even at low levels of exercise. If the evaluation of mitral flow and annular velocities during exercise is not optimal due to premature tachycardia, another way is to evaluate these parameters during the recovery period after cessation of exercise.

Diastolic Stress Testing in Recent Guidelines

Recent guidelines from the American Society of Echocardiography (ASE) and the European Association of Cardiovascular Imaging (EACVI) regarding the evaluation of LV diastolic function by echocardiography[26,27] and the clinical use of SE in nonischemic heart disease[34,37] included diastolic SE as a valuable tool for the evaluation of patients with unexplained dyspnea and subclinical LV diastolic dysfunction (see Chapter 19).

FUTURE DIRECTIONS

Most of the previous studies regarding diastolic SE excluded patients with significant coronary artery disease to avoid confounding effects from myocardial ischemia to diastolic dysfunction.[32,33,38,39] However, in reality, patients with significant coronary artery disease with or without myocardial ischemia represent an important subset of patients in whom the assessment of an exercise-induced increase in LV filling pressure would be critically important. Future studies would be warranted in patients with diastolic dysfunction and ischemic heart disease since the clinical value of diastolic SE has been established mostly in patients with preserved LV systolic function, without regional LV dysfunction, mitral valve disease, or atrial fibrillation.

Recently it has been shown that absence of a decrease in minimal LV pressure during exercise, a manifestation of impaired LV suction, was closely linked with impaired LV untwisting during exercise.[48] In patients with a normal LV ejection fraction, previously treated for coronary artery disease, a range of responses of minimum LV diastolic pressure, tau, and untwisting velocity was reported. Patients with a decrease in minimum LV diastolic pressure had a most marked increase in LV untwisting velocity with exercise (Fig. 18.9). Furthermore, e′ velocity during exercise was highest in patients with a decrease in minimum LV diastolic pressure (Fig. 18.10). These findings imply that dynamic changes in LV apical back rotation during exercise can be used as a noninvasive parameter of diastolic suction during exercise. More work would be needed to refine and standardize the methodology for measuring twisting deformation, but provided the technique is improved, untwisting velocity may become an important addition to the diastolic SE.[49]

The decades of investigation into the diastology stress test have provided us with many important insights into cardiovascular hemodynamics and have improved our delivery of care for patients with diastolic dysfunction and exertional dyspnea. With these efforts and the recommendations from the recent guidelines, it is quite evident that the integration of the diastology stress test into clinical practice will certainly enhance our understanding and better management to our patients.[50]

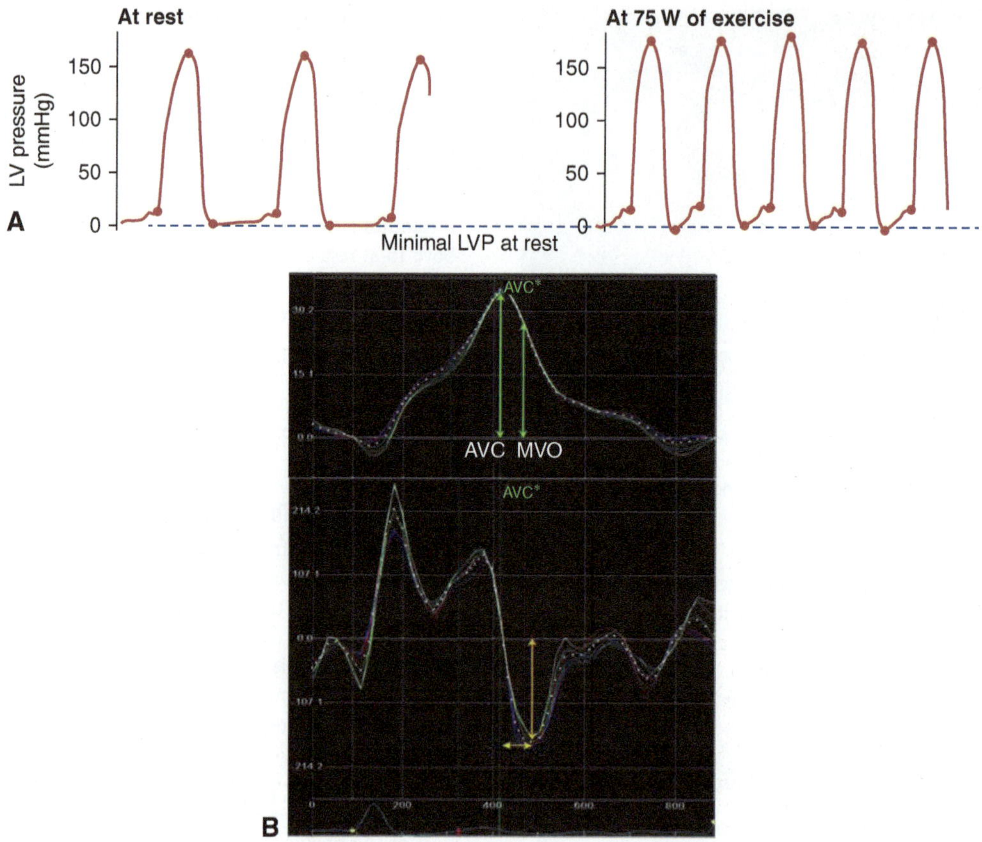

Fig. 18.9 Changes of minimal LV pressure and apical back rotation during exercise. Patients with decrease in minimum LV diastolic pressure during exercise had greater increase in LV untwisting velocity with exercise. From (Reference 48).

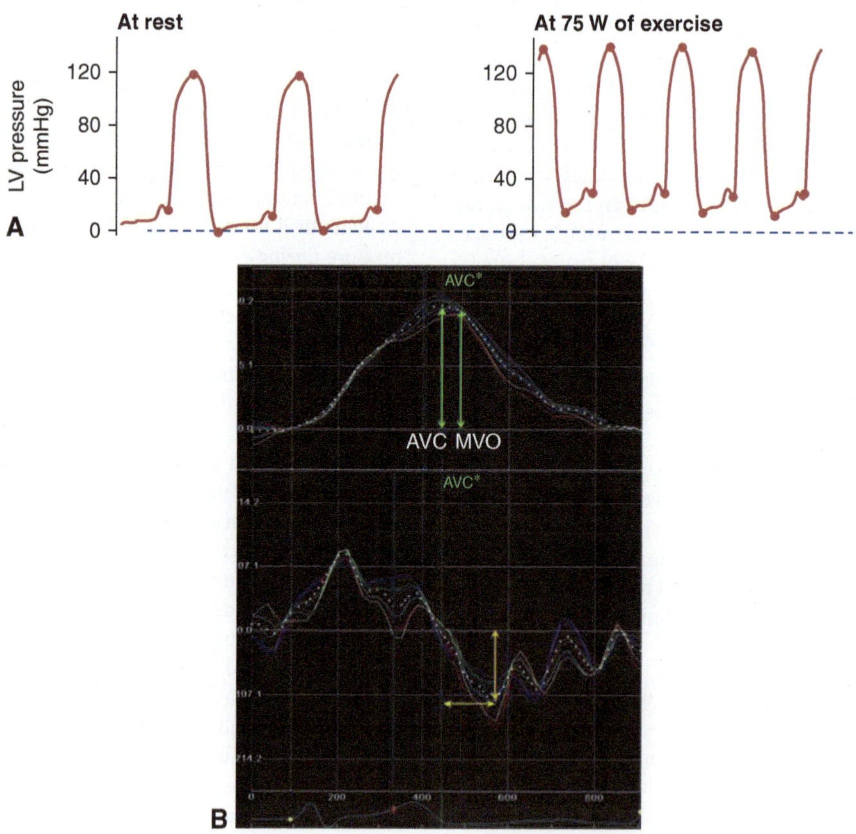

Fig. 18.10 Changes of minimal LV pressure and apical back rotation during exercise. Patients with increase in minimum LV diastolic pressure during exercise had less degree of increase in LV untwisting velocity with exercise. From: (reference 48).

KEY POINTS

- Despite similar resting diastolic parameters, exercise hemodynamic responses are different.
- Although presenting symptom of exertional dyspnea is similar, exercise hemodynamic responses are different.
- Diastolic stress echo not only can rule out exercise-induced increase in LV filling pressures in patients with exertional dyspnea but also can detect other causes of dyspnea.
- Exercise-induced PH is common, and prognosis is poor when it is associated with exercise-induced increase in E/e′.
- Unsuccessful test can occur in some patients because of premature tachycardia with low levels of exercise, but observation of LV filling pattern during recovery period is helpful since diastolic abnormalities usually persist even after cessation of exercise.

REVIEW QUESTIONS

1. To assess LV diastolic function with stress, which modality would be most appropriate?
   a. Dobutamine
   b. Pacing
   c. Exercise
2. Diastolic stress echocardiography is indicated when
   a. elevated LV filling pressures are at rest.
   b. normal hearts and diastolic function are at rest.
   c. subjects with exertional dyspnea and grade I diastolic dysfunction are at rest.
3. Diastolic stress echocardiography is considered abnormal if
   a. septal E/e′ is above 15 with exercise.
   b. peak tricuspid regurgitation velocity is greater than 2.8 m/sec with stress.
   c. septal e′ velocity is less than 8 cm/sec at baseline.
   d. all of these occur.

REFERENCES

1. Packer M. Abnormalities of diastolic function as a potential cause of exercise intolerance in chronic heart failure. *Circulation.* 1990;81:S78–S86.
2. Gaasch WH, Levine HJ, Quinones MA, Alexander JK. Left ventricular compliance: mechanisms and clinical implications. *Am J Cardiol.* 1976;38:645–653.
3. Grossman W, McLaurin L. Diastolic properties of the left ventricle. *Ann Intern Med.* 1976;84:316–326.
4. Grossman W, Barry WH. Diastolic pressure-volume relations in the diseased heart. *Fed Proc.* 1980;39:148–155.
5. Brutsaert DL, Meulemans AL, Sipido KR, Sys SU. Effects of damaging the endocardial surface on the mechanical performance of isolated cardiac muscle. *Circ Res.* 1988;62:358–366.
6. Weiss JL, Frederiksen JW, Weisfeldt ML. Hemodynamic determinants of the time-course of fall in canine left ventricular pressure. *J Clin Invest.* 1976;58:751–760.
7. Yellin EL, Hori M, Yoram C, Sonnenblick EH, Gabbay S, Frater RW. Left ventricular relaxation in the filling and nonfilling intact canine heart. *Am J Physiol.* 1993;250:H620–H629.
8. Gaasch WH. *Passive Elastic Properties of the Left Ventricle.* Philadelphia, PA: Lea & Febiger; 1994.
9. Wahr PA, Michele DE, Metzger JM. Parvalbumin gene transfer corrects diastolic dysfunction in diseased cardiac myocytes. *Proc Nat Acad Sci USA.* 1999;96:11982–11985.
10. Ebashi S. Excitation-contraction coupling and the mechanism of muscle contraction. *Ann Rev Physiol.* 1991;53:1–16.
11. Hasenfuss G. Calcium pump overexpession and myocardial function: implications for gene therapy of myocardial failure. *Circ Res.* 1998;83:966–968.
12. Koss KL, Kranias EG. Phospholamban: a prominent regulator of myocardial contractility. *Circ Res.* 1996;79:1059–1063.
13. Taffet GE, Michael LA, Tate CA. Exercise training improves lusitropy by isoproterenol in papillary muscles from aged rats. *J Appl Physiol.* 1996;81: 1488–1494.
14. Takagishi Y, Rothery S, Issberner J, Levi A, Severs NJ. Spatial distribution of dihydropyridine receptors in the plasma membrane of guinea pig cardiac myocytes investigated by correlative confocal microscopy and label-fracture electron microscopy. *J Electron Microsc.* 1997;46:165–170.
15. Tate CA, Helgason T, Hyek MF, et al. SERCA2a and mitochondrial cytochrome oxidase expression are increased in hearts of exercise-trained old rats. *Am J Physiol.* 1996;271:H68–H72.
16. Taffet GE, Pham TT, Bick DL, Entman ML, Pownall HJ, Bick RJ. The calcium uptake of the rat heart sarcoplasmic reticulum is altered by dietary lipid. *J Membr Biol.* 1993;131:35–42.
17. Cain BS, Meldrum DR, Joo KS, et al. Human SERCA2a levels correlate inversely with age in senescent human myocardium. *J Am Coll Cardiol.* 1998;32:458–467.
18. Shah AM, Grocott-Mason RM, Pepper CB, et al. The cardiac endothelium: cardioactive mediators. *Progr Cardiovas Dis.* 1996;39:239–262.
19. Paulus WJ, Serizawa T, Grossman W. Altered left ventricular diastolic properties during pacing-induced ischemia in dogs with coronary stenoses. Potentiation by caffeine. Circ Res. 1982;50:218–227.
20. Leite-Moreira AF, Correia-Pinto J, Gillebert TC. Load dependence of left ventricular contraction and relaxation. Effects of caffeine. *Basic Res Cardiol.* 1999;94:284–293.
21. Hori M, Yellin EL, Sonnenblick EH. Left ventricular diastolic suction as a mechanism of ventricular filling. *Jpn Circ J.* 1982;46:124–129.
22. Ingels NB Jr, Hansen DE, Daughters GT, Stinson EB, Alderman EL, Miller DC. Relation between longitudinal, circumferential, and oblique shortening and torsional deformation in the left ventricle of the transplanted heart. *Circ Res.* 1989;64:915–927.
23. Solomon SB, Nikolic SD, Glantz SA, Yellin EL. Left ventricular diastolic function of remodeled myocardium in dogs with pacing induced heart failure. *Am J Physiol.* 1998;274:H945–H954.
24. Bell SP, Fabian J, LeWinter MM. Effects of dobutamine on left ventricular restoring forces. *Am J Physiol.* 1998;275:H190–H194.
25. Apstein CS, Grossman W. Opposite initial effects of supply and demand ischemia on left ventricular diastolic compliance. The ischemia-diastolic paradox. *J Molecul Cell Cardiol.* 1987;19:119–128.
26. Nagueh SF, Smiseth OA, Appleton CP, et al. Recommendations for the evaluation of left ventricular diastolic function by echocardiography: an update from the American Society of Echocardiography and the European Association of Cardiovascular Imaging. *J Am Soc Echocardiogr.* 2016;29:277–314.
27. Nagueh SF, Smiseth OA, Appleton CP, et al. Recommendations for the evaluation of left ventricular diastolic function by echocardiography: an update from the American Society of Echocardiography and the European Association of Cardiovascular Imaging. *Eur Heart J Cardiovasc Imag.* 2016;17:1321–1360.
28. Borlaug BA, Nishimura RA, Sorajja P, Lam CS, Redfield MM. Exercise hemodynamics enhance diagnosis of early heart failure with preserved ejection fraction. *Circ Heart Fail.* 2010;3:588–595.
29. Cheng CP, Igarashi Y, Little WC. Mechanism of augmented rate of left ventricular filling during exercise. *Circ Res.* 1992;70:9–19.
30. Udelson JE, Bacharach SL, Cannon RO, Bonow RO. Minimum left ventricular pressure during beta-adrenergic stimulation in human subjects. Evidence for elastic recoil and diastolic "suction" in the normal heart. Circulation. 1990;82:1174–1182.

31. Obokata M, Kane GC, Reddy YN, Olson TP, Melenovsky V, Borlaug BA. Role of diastolic stress testing in the evaluation for heart failure with preserved ejection fraction: a simultaneous invasive-echocardiographic study. *Circulation.* 2017;135:825–838.
32. Ha JW, Oh JK, Pellikka PA, et al. Diastolic stress echocardiography: a novel noninvasive diagnostic test for diastolic dysfunction using supine bicycle exercise Doppler echocardiography. *J Am Soc Echocardiogr.* 2005;18:63–68.
33. Burgess MI, Jenkins C, Sharman JE, Marwick TH. Diastolic stress echocardiography: hemodynamic validation and clinical significance of estimation of ventricular filling pressure with exercise. *J Am Coll Cardiol.* 2006;47:1891–1900.
34. Lancellotti P, Pellikka PA, Budts W, et al. The clinical use of stress echocardiography in non-ischaemic heart disease: recommendations from the European Association of Cardiovascular Imaging and the American Society of Echocardiography. *Eur Heart J Cardiovasc Imag.* 2016;17:1191–1229.
35. Ha JW, Oh JK. Echocardiographic evaluation of chronic dyspnea. In: Bax JJ, Kramer CM, Marwick TH, Wijns W, eds. *Cardiovascular Imaging; A Handbook for Clinical Practice.* Malden: Blackwell Publishing 2005;164–174.
36. Choi EY, Shim CY, Kim SA, et al. Passive leg-raise is helpful to identify impaired diastolic functional reserve during exercise in patients with abnormal myocardial relaxation. *J Am Soc Echocardiogr.* 2010;23:523–530.
37. Lancellotti P, Pellikka PA, Budts W, et al. The clinical use of stress echocardiography in non-ischaemic heart disease: recommendations from the European Association of Cardiovascular Imaging and the American Society of Echocardiography. *J Am Soc Echocardiogr.* 2017;30:101–138.
38. Ha JW, Ahn JA, Kim JM, et al. Abnormal longitudinal myocardial functional reserve assessed by exercise tissue Doppler echocardiography in patients with hypertrophic cardiomyopathy. *J Am Soc Echocardiogr.* 2006;19:1314–1319.
39. Ha JW, Lee HC, Kang ES, et al. Abnormal left ventricular longitudinal functional reserve in patients with diabetes mellitus: implication for detecting subclinical myocardial dysfunction using exercise tissue Doppler echocardiography. *Heart.* 2007;93:1571–1576.
40. Choi EY, Ha JW, Yoon SJ, et al. Increased plasma aldosterone-to-renin ratio is associated with impaired left ventricular longitudinal functional reserve in patients with uncomplicated hypertension. *J Am Soc Echocardiogr.* 2008;21:251–256.
41. Gibby C, Wiktor DM, Burgess M, Kusunose K, Marwick TH. Quantitation of the diastolic stress test: filling pressure vs. diastolic reserve. *Eur Heart J Cardiovasc Imag.* 2013;14:223–227.
42. Ha JW, Choi D, Park S, et al. Determinants of exercise-induced pulmonary hypertension in patients with normal left ventricular ejection fraction. *Heart.* 2009;95:490–494.
43. Tolle JJ, Waxman AB, Van Horn T, Pappagianopoulos PP, Systrom DM. Exercise-induced pulmonary arterial hypertension. *Circulation.* 2008;118:2183–2189.
44. Shim CY, Kim SA, Choi D, et al. Clinical outcomes of exercise-induced pulmonary hypertension in subjects with preserved left ventricular ejection fraction: implication of an increase in left ventricular filling pressure during exercise. *Heart.* 2011;97:1417–1424.
45. Borlaug BA, Kane GC, Melenovsky V, Olson TP. Abnormal right ventricular-pulmonary artery coupling with exercise in heart failure with preserved ejection fraction. *Eur Heart J.* 2016;37:3293–3302.
46. Ishii K, Imai M, Suyama T, et al. Exercise-induced post-ischemic left ventricular delayed relaxation or diastolic stunning: is it a reliable marker in detecting coronary artery disease? *J Am Coll Cardiol.* 2009;53:698–705.
47. Ha JW, Choi EY, Choi D, et al. Time course of recovery of left ventricular filling pressure after exercise in healthy subjects. *Circ J.* 2008;72:186–188.
48. Hong SJ, Shim CY, Kim D, et al. Dynamic change in left ventricular apical back rotation: a marker of diastolic suction with exercise. *Eur Heart J Cardiovasc Imag.* 2008;19:12–19.
49. Smiseth OA. Need for better diastolic stress test: twistin' time is here? *Eur Heart J Cardiovasc Imag.* 2018;19:20–22.
50. Oh JK, Kane GC. Diastolic stress echocardiography: the time has come for its integration into clinical practice. *J Am Soc Echocardiogr.* 2014;27:1060–1063.

19

ASE/EACVI Diastolic Guidelines: Strength and Limitations

Otto A. Smiseth and Øyvind Senstad Andersen

OUTLINE

Case Study

A 56-year-old obese woman with exertional dyspnea was referred for evaluation of suspected heart failure with preserved ejection fraction (HFpEF). She had a past medical history of Crohn Crohn's disease, hypothyroidism, and asthma. She had been medically treated for hypertension for several years.

Over the last several years, she was hospitalized several times with pneumonia and exacerbations of asthma. Between these admissions, she was experiencing shortness of breath on moderate activity, which was attributed to the combination of moderate asthma and obesity. She was referred to echocardiography to determine if cardiac dysfunction contributed to her dyspnea.

Echocardiography revealed normal systolic function, with left ventricular (LV) ejection fraction (EF) of 54%. She had LV hypertrophy with septal wall thickness of 1.2 cm (Fig. 19.1). Peak mitral early diastolic flow velocity (E) was 73 cm/sec, mitral early diastolic flow velocity/atrial induced inflow velocity ratio (E/A) 0.9, and E deceleration time (DT) 222 msec (Fig. 19.2). Septal mitral annulus velocity (e′) was 6 and lateral e′ 7 cm/sec (Fig. 19.3). The presence of LV hypertrophy gives suspicion of diastolic dysfuncion.

By following algorithm B in the 2016 American Society of Echocardiography (ASE)/European Association of Cardiovascular Imaging (EACVI) guidelines (Fig. 19.4), she is in the intermediate group where the three additional criteria E/e′, left atrial (LA) volume, and peak tricuspid regurgitation (TR) velocity need to be considered. Although E/e′ is 10 (normal), LA volume is mildly increased to 37 mL/m^2, and TR velocity is increased to 3.0 m/sec (Fig. 19.5). Thus values are above cutoff for two of the three criteria, supporting that LV filling pressure is elevated. With regard to grading of diastolic dys function, she is classified as grade II diastolic dysfunction.

DEFINITION AND GRADING OF DIASTOLIC DYSFUNCTION

One important change from the ASE/EACVI 2009 to 2016 guidelines for evaluation of diastolic function is that the definition of diastolic dysfunction was changed. In the 2009 ASE/EACVI guidelines, diastolic dysfunction was defined according to Fig. 19.6 and included a scheme for grading of diastolic dysfunction as mild (grade I), moderate (grade II), and severe (grade III). In the 2009 ASE/EACVI guidelines, the idea was that grade I diastolic dysfunction (mitral E/A <0.8) represented mainly patients with normal LV filling pressure, grade II (E/A 0.8–1.5) mild to moderate elevation of LV filling pressure, and grade III (E/A >1.5) patients with more marked elevation of LV filling pressure. In addition to mitral E/A, other Doppler indices that are related to filling pressure were used as criteria for grading (see Fig. 19.6).

In the 2016 guidelines, diastolic dysfunction is defined according to the scheme in Fig. 19.7, which represents a simplification relative to the 2009 guidelines. There are four criteria in the 2016 definition of diastolic dysfunction, with cutoff values for three of these criteria being consistent with elevated LV filling pressure. Therefore, even for patients with mild diastolic dysfunction, elevated LV filling pressure is probably present in many if not most subjects. For patients with reduced EF, it is assumed that there is coexisting diastolic dysfunction. Therefore patients with reduced EF are not included in the scheme for diagnosis of diastolic dysfunction. This is also the case in patients where the presence of diastolic dysfuncion for other reasons is likely, for instance in patients with LV hypertrophy. One problem with the algorithm to define whether there is diastolic dysfunction in the 2016 ASE/EACVI guidelines is that with four parameters, many patients remain unclassified, as they have two positive and two negative parameters.

With regards to grading, the 2016 guidelines recommend as a first step to use the algorithm in Fig. 19.7 to determine if there is diastolic dysfunction. The second step is to determine the grade of dysfunction by using the algorithm in Fig. 19.4B. By definition, grade I refers to patients without elevated LV filling pressure and grades II and III to diastolic dysfunction with elevated LV filling pressure. Furthermore, grade III is differentiated from grade II by a restrictive mitral filling pattern.

After the publication of the 2016 ASE/EACVI guidelines, there was debate regarding the definition of diastolic dysfunction. Since the definition used in the 2016 guidelines is based mainly on markers of elevated LV filling pressure, this definition would favor more advanced

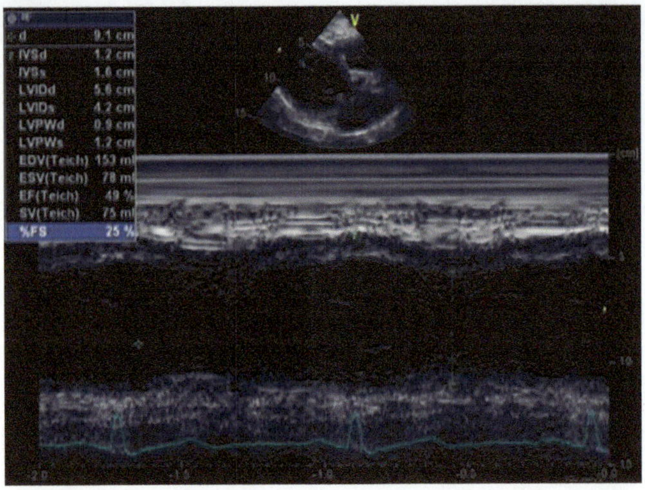

Fig. 19.1 M mode echocardiography revealed mild LV hypertrophy. This finding, often seen in patients with hypertension, is one of the key mechanisms of diastolic dysfunction.

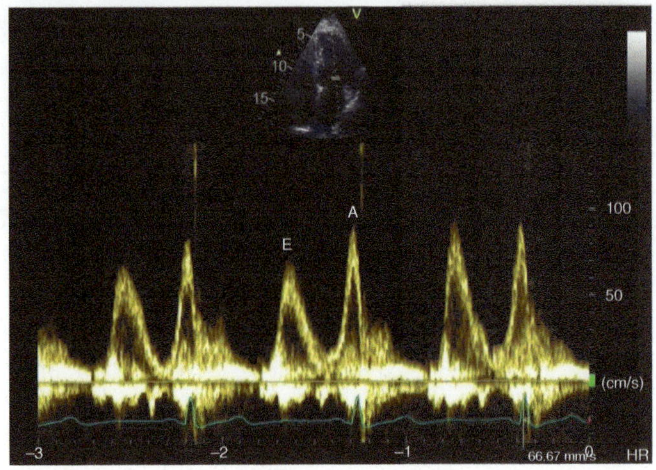

Fig. 19.2 **Mitral inflow velocities.** E velocity is 73 cm/sec and E/A 0.9.

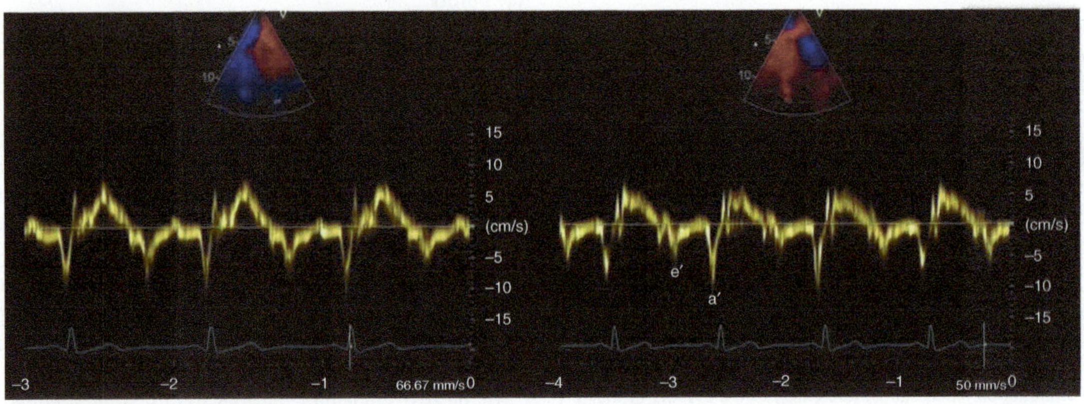

Fig. 19.3 Mitral annular velocity (e′) is reduced both in LV septum and in the lateral wall, 6 and 7 cm/sec, respectively.

diastolic dysfunction than the 2009 guidelines. Fig. 19.8 illustrates how this difference in diagnostic criteria alters the prevalence of diastolic dysfunction. In a study of 1000 apparently heart healthy individuals with a mean age of 62 years, Almeida et al. confirmed that the prevalence of diastolic dysfunction was much lower when using the 2016 guidelines than the 2009 recommendations.[1] Only 1% had diastolic dysfunction with the 2016 recommendations as compared to 38% when using the 2009 recommendations. This observation is consistent with the study of Huttin et al.[2]

Therefore, when applying the 2016 ASE/EACVI recommendations, the prevalence of diastolic dysfunction is much lower than with the 2009 recommendations, reflecting that the specificity is much higher, apparently at the cost of sensitivity. These differences do not necessarily imply limitations of the different versions of the ASE/EACVI guidelines but have a major impact on prevalence data.

Redfield et al. used a grading system somewhat similar to the 2009 version of the ASE/EACVI guidelines, showing in a cross-sectional survey that mild diastolic dysfunction was associated with increased mortality.[3] The prevalence of diastolic dysfunction was 28%, and of these 4.5% had clinical evidence of congestive heart failure.[3] This included 21% with mild diastolic dysfunction, defined as filling pattern of impaired LV relaxation. The latter group would not be identified by the ASE/EACVI 2016 recommendations, which are less suited to identify early stage diastolic dysfunction.

The validity and rationale for the grading scheme in the 2009 ASE/EACVI guidelines were challenged by a study that showed a relatively weak relationship between grades of diastolic dysfunction and LV filling pressure.[4] As shown by several studies, the criteria and cutoff values for diastolic dysfunction used in the 2016 version of the ASE/EACVI guidelines are relatively strong markers of elevated filling pressure.[5,6] The validity of relating grading based on the 2016 recommendations to filling pressure is supported by the study of Andersen et al., which showed that LV filling pressure differed significantly when comparing the three grades of diastolic dysfunction. It increased from 10 mmHg in grade I (interquartile range [IQR]: 7–12 mmHg) to 18 mmHg in grade II (IQR: 14–24 mmHg) and 24 mmHg in grade III (IQR: 19–30 mm Hg) (grade I vs. grade II: $p < 0.001$; grade I vs. grade III: $p < 0.001$; and grade II vs. grade III: $p < 0.006$ by the Dunn method).

Since elevated LV filling pressure is a compensatory mechanism, a diagnosis of diastolic dysfunction according to the 2016 guidelines will tend to reflect more advanced diastolic dysfunction. The utility of the relatively high specificity of the 2016 ASE/EACVI definition was demonstrated in a recent study, which showed that patients undergoing transcatheter aortic valve replacement (TAVR) had markedly increased cardiovascular risk when there was diastolic dysfunction.[7]

The issue of what is an optimal definition of diastolic dysfunction depends entirely on the purpose of the study. As shown in several

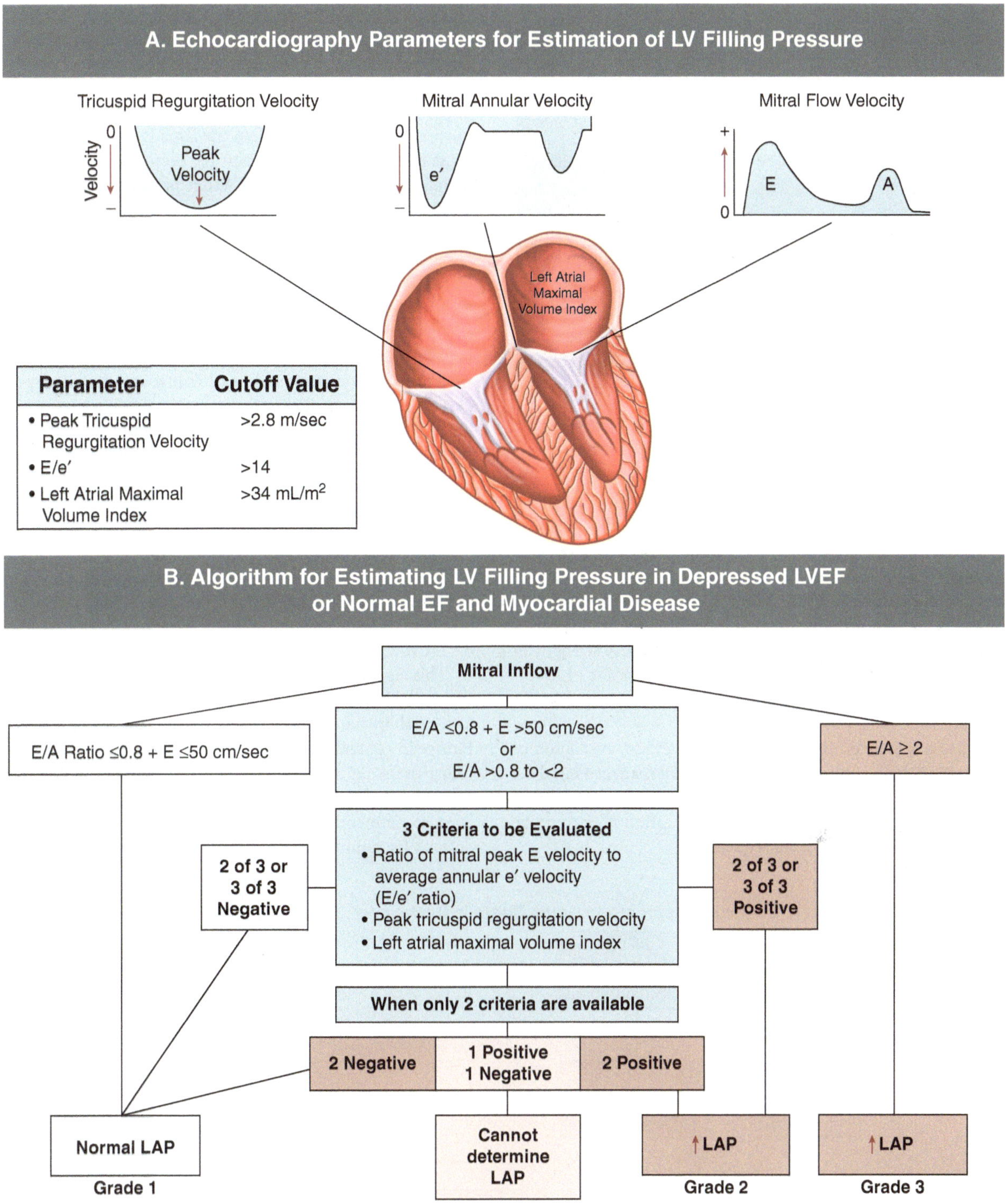

Fig. 19.4 Evaluation of LV filling pressure. (A) For evaluation of LV filling pressure, four echocardiographic parameters are used: E/A, E/e′, TR velocity, and LA volume indexed. Cutoff values for criteria used to decide if LV filling pressure is normal or not are indicated. (B) When E/A is 0.8 or less and E 50 cm/sec or less, LV filling pressure is assumed to be normal, and diastolic dysfunction grade I is assumed. When E/A is 2 or more, LV filling pressure is assumed to be elevated and diastolic dysfunction grade III is assumed. In the intermediate group, the three additional parameters are used. When the majority of these parameters are positive, LV filling pressure is assumed to be elevated. These patients are defined as having diastolic dysfunction grade II. When the majority of these parameters are negative, LV filling pressure is assumed to be normal, and grade I diastolic dysfunction is assumed. When one parameter is positive and one parameter is negative, LV filling pressure cannot be estimated. (Adapted from Andersen OS, Smiseth OA, Dokainish H, et al. Estimating left ventricular filling pressure by echocardiography. *J Am Coll Cardiol.* 2017;69:1937–1948.)

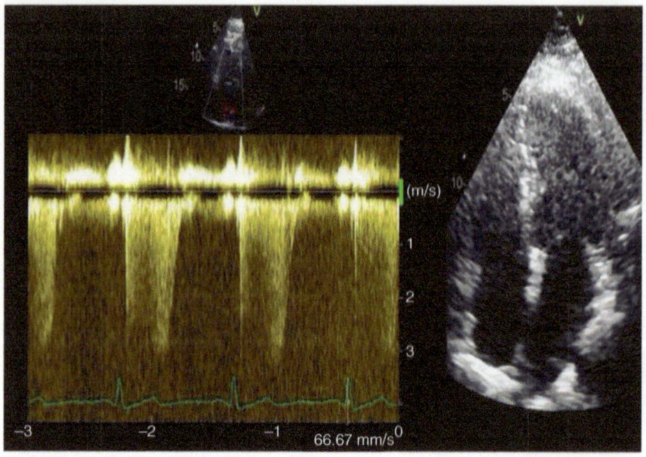

Fig. 19.5 LA volume is mildly increased to 37 mL/m^2, and TR velocity is increased to 3.0 m/sec.

studies, the demonstration of mild diastolic dysfunction provides important prognostic information, which may be lost when using the 2016 ASE/EACVI definition of diastolic dysfunction.[3,8,9] On the other hand, it is likely that the 2016 definition will help to identify patients with the highest risk; this may be important in clinical practice, as suggested by the study of TAVR patients.[7] The 2016 EACVI/ASE guidelines were written with the intent of increasing specificity, which explains the lower prevalence of diastolic dysfunction. A strength of the 2016 ASE/EACVI guidelines is that the parameters E/e′, LA volume, and systolic pulmonary artery pressure, which are used in the definition, are all relatively age independent.[10,11]

The next step is to determine in outcome studies how evaluation of diastolic function can be utilized to improve patient management. Due to the change in definition of diastolic dysfunction, it would be of particular interest to investigate whether identification of early stage diastolic dysfunction has clinical consequences.

DIAGNOSING HFpEF AND ESTIMATION OF LV FILLING PRESSURE

LV filling pressure refers to the pressure that fills the ventricle and is used differently depending on which pressure is available and what the purpose of the study is. When the issue is pulmonary congestion, the most relevant pressure is mean LA pressure, which may be approximated as pulmonary capillary wedge pressure (PCWP) and as LV pre-atrial contraction (pre-A) pressure.[12] When the issue is LV mechanical function, however, LV end-diastolic pressure (EDP) (ideally transmural end-diastolic pressure), which represents LV preload, is the preferred parameter of LV filling pressure. All these parameters are valid measures of LV filling pressure, although their relationships to Doppler parameters are slightly different. Fig. 19.9 illustrates how the different pressures are acquired.

Since early symptoms of heart failure are often nonspecific, an accurate noninvasive method to estimate LV filling pressure would be of great clinical value. The ASE/EACVI task force presented an algorithm for evaluating LV filling pressure (see Fig. 19.4). The algorithm suggested the use of four echocardiographic parameters to determine whether LV filling pressure was elevated:

1. The ratio between early mitral inflow velocity (E) and atrial-induced mitral inflow velocity (A) (E/A), and peak E velocity
2. The ratio between early mitral inflow velocity (E) and early mitral annular velocity (e′) (E/e′)
3. Peak TR velocity
4. LA volume indexed to body surface area (LAVI)

This algorithm was recently tested in two large multicenter studies, which used invasive filling pressure as the reference method.[5,6] Lancellotti et al. in the Euro-Filling study investigated 159 patients at nine European centers with simultaneous evaluation of echo estimates of filling pressures and invasive measurements of LVEDP.[6] Additionally, the ASE/EACVI recommendations from 2009 were compared to the 2016 recommendations. The study showed that the 2016 recommendations for noninvasive assessment of LV filling pressure were reliable

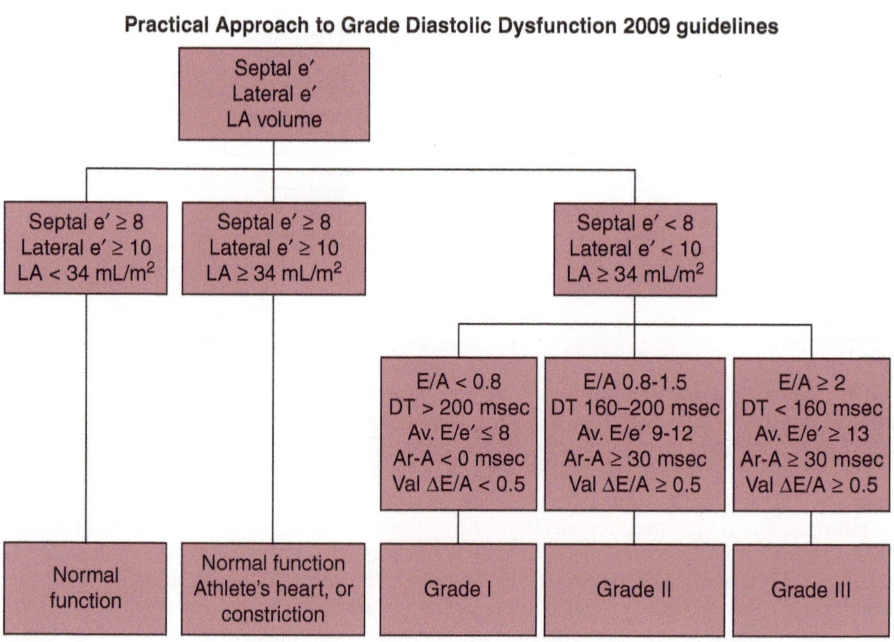

Fig. 19.6 Scheme for grading of LV diastolic dysfunction from 2009 guidelines. Ar, pulmonary venous atrial reversal wave *Av*, Average; DT, deceleration time *LA*, left atrial; *Val*, Valsalva. (Adapted from Nagueh SF, Appleton P, Gillebert TC. Recommendations for the evaluation of left ventricular diastolic function by echocardiography. *J Am Soc Echocardiogr.* 2009;22(2):107–133.)

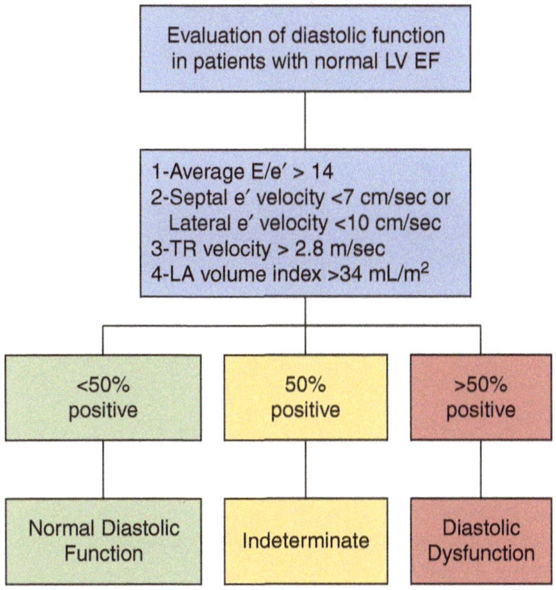

Fig. 19.7 Definition of diastolic dysfunction according to the 2016 ASE/EACVI guidelines. The scheme is intended for patients with normal ejection fraction. In HFrEF it is assumed that diastolic function is always impaired. For patients who are indeterminate, use additional criteria for diastolic dysfunction.

and clinically useful and, importantly, superior to the 2009 recommendations for estimating invasive LVEDP. In the other study, Andersen et al. included 450 patients in a multicenter trial with PCWP in 293 patients and LV pre-A pressure in 157 patients as references. The study demonstrated that the ASE/EACVI recommendations for echocardiographic assessment of LV filling pressure are readily available and can be performed with high feasibility and good accuracy. These two studies confirm that the new ASE/EACVI recommendations are clinically valuable and accurate and therefore very helpful in making a correct diagnosis of our patients. The algorithm for estimation of LV filling pressure may be applied in patients with normal LV EF and unexplained exertional dyspnea, and in patients with heart failure with reduced ejection fraction (HFrEF) when considering adjustment of diuretics or other medication.

The rationale behind the conclusion that LA pressure is normal when mitral E is less than 50 cm/sec combined with an E/A less than 0.8 is that a low E implies a small transmitral pressure gradient.[13,14] The combination with E/A less than 0.8 confirms that E is low also when compared with A. When E is tall and much higher than A, it implies a high transmitral gradient, which in turn implies high LA pressure. One exception is young healthy individuals who may have negative early diastolic pressure and therefore a high gradient and tall E with normal LA pressure.[15] For intermediate mitral filling patterns, the recommendation is to use E/e′, LA volume, and peak TR velocity in combination (see Fig. 19.4). The reason why elevated E/e′ is useful is because the combination of a high transmitral gradient (high E) on top of elevated minimum LV diastolic pressure (suggested by low e′) means high LA pressure.

An enlarged LA reflects the long-term effect of elevated LA pressure. High TR regurgitation velocity implies high pulmonary artery systolic pressure, which in the absence of either pulmonary disease or pulmonary vascular disease reflects elevated LV filling pressure.

When evaluating patients with potential HFpEF, one should always search to exclude diseases such as valve disease, coronary artery disease, pericardial disease, and right-sided heart disease before it is concluded that a patient suffers from HFpEF.

A limitation of this diagnostic algorithm is that patients with heart failure may have normal filling pressure at rest. However, when cardiac output increases with activity in these patients, it can only be done at the expense of elevated LV filling pressure. Therefore further development of a diastolic stress test is needed, in particular in patients with grade I diastolic dysfunction (see Chapter 18). In the 2016 ASE/EACVI guidelines, a diastolic stress test is recommended when resting echocardiography does not explain the symptoms of heart failure or dyspnea, especially with exertion. Fig. 19.10 shows how echocardiographic parameters change during activity as a reflection of elevated LV filling pressure.

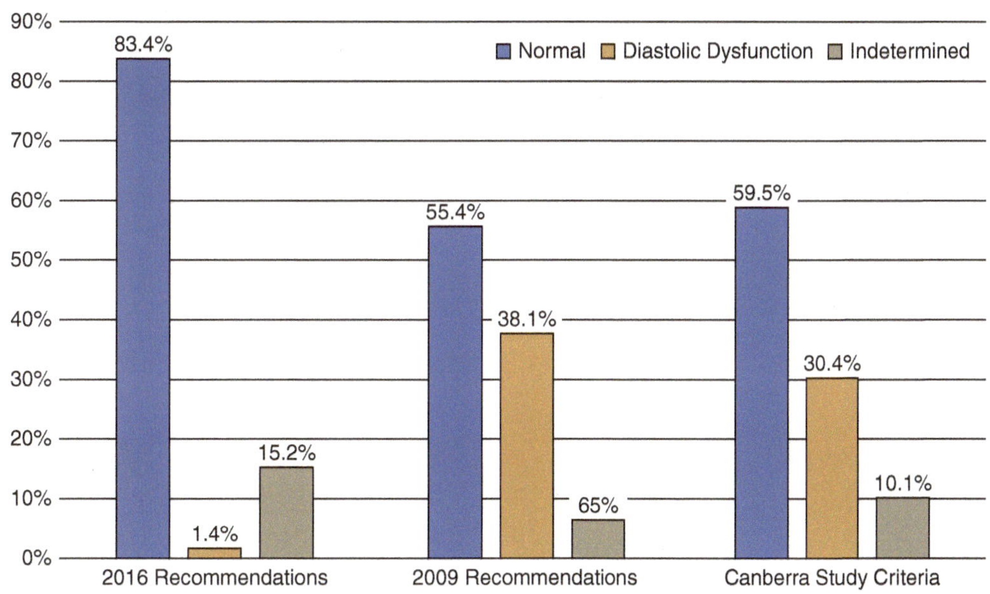

Fig. 19.8 Prevalence of diastolic dysfunction according to different diagnostic criteria in a population aged 45 years or more with no manifest cardiac disease. (Adapted from Almeida JG, Fontes-Carvalho R, Sampaio F, et al. Impact of the 2016 ASE/EACVI recommendations on the prevalence of diastolic dysfunction in the general population. *Eur Heart J Cardiovasc Imag.* 2008;19(4):380–386.)

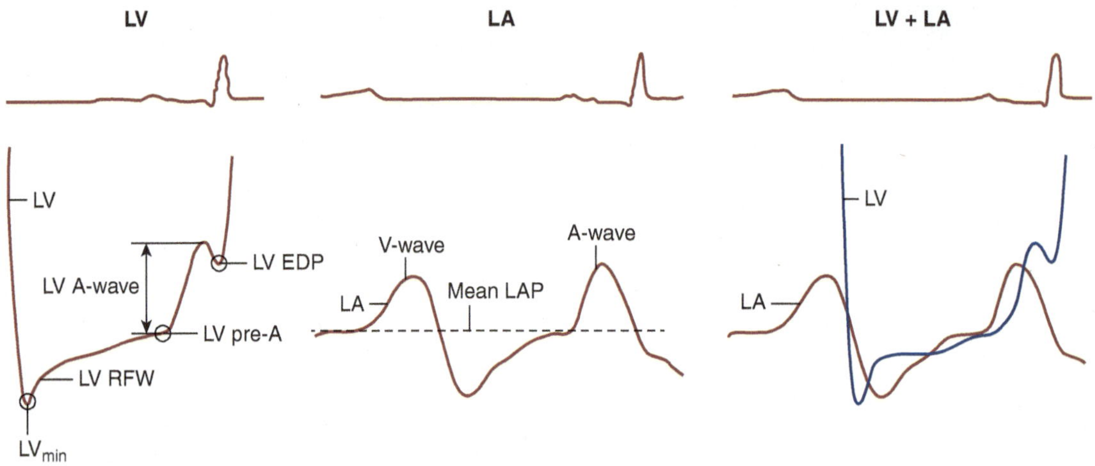

Fig. 19.9 *(Left)* LV diastolic pressures recording. Lines point to LV minimal pressure *(min)*, LV rapid filling wave *(RFW)*, LV pre-A pressure *(pre-A)*, A-wave rise with atrial contraction and end-diastolic pressure *(EDP)*. *(Middle)* LAP recording showing V- and A-waves. *(Right)* Simultaneous LV and LAP recording showing early and late transmitral pressure gradients. Notice that LA A-wave) pressure precedes the late diastolic rise *(LV A-wave)* in LV pressure.

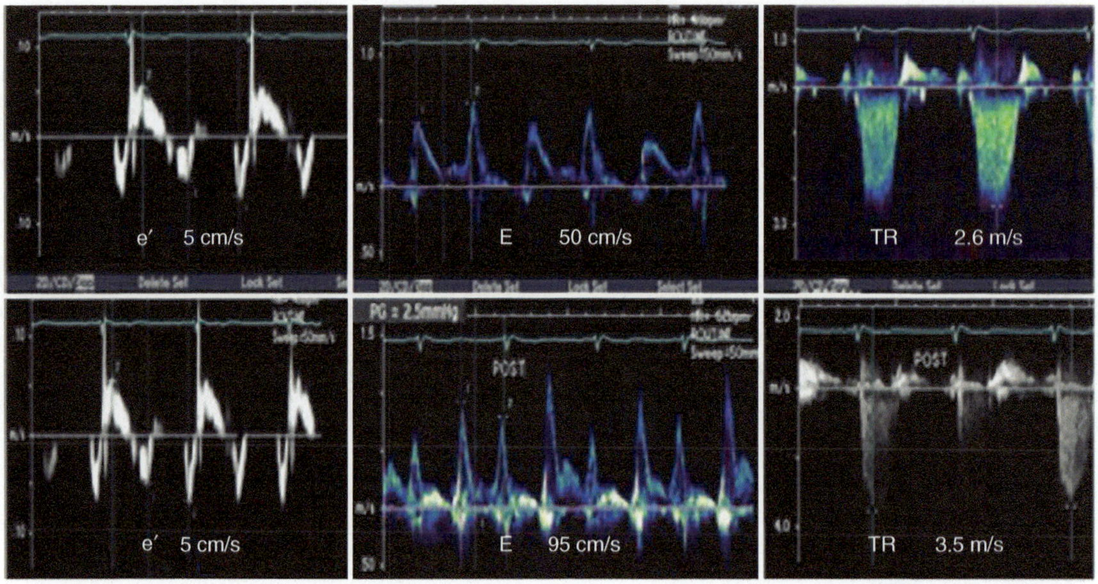

Fig. 19.10 Mitral septal annulus *(left)*, mitral inflow *(middle)*, and TR velocity *(right)* at rest *(top)* and immediately after treadmill exercise test *(bottom)*. At rest this is normal, with E/e′ of 10 and TR velocity 2.6 m/s. With exercise, e′ remains the same, whereas E velocity increased such that E/e′ increased to 19 along with an increase in TR velocity to 3.5 m/sec.

A common misinterpretation of the ASE/EACVI guidelines is that echocardiographic evaluation of filling pressure should start with a diagnostic algorithm to determine whether the patient has diastolic dysfunction. This is not needed when there is clinical suspicion of heart disease. Then one can go directly to the algorithm used to decide whether LV filling pressure is elevated (see Fig. 19.4). This can be illustrated by our chapter-opening case study, where the patient presented with LV hypertrophy and dyspnea, both indicative of underlying cardiac disease. In a similar way this algorithm can be used to assess filling pressure in patients with reduced LV EF. Fig. 19.11 provides a flow chart of how to evaluate LV diastolic function, suggested by Andersen et al. This flow chart demonstrates how a conclusion about diastolic function using the suggested algorithm can be reached in most patients, but also how further steps are sometimes needed to accurately diagnose patients. Of special notice, though many patients can be correctly classified as having normal or elevated LV filling pressure using a noninvasive approach, invasive measurement of PCWP, EDP, or pre-A pressure is still the gold standard to decide if heart failure is present.[16]

ADDITIONAL PARAMETERS TO BE USED IN THE EVALUATION OF DIASTOLIC FUNCTION

The combination of echocardiographic parameters suggested to decide whether LV filling pressure is elevated had an accuracy of 87% when investigated in a large multicenter trial.[5] This implies that a wrong conclusion about LV filling pressure was made in at least 1 in 10 patients. Therefore it is always important to interpret echocardiographic data on diastolic function in a clinical context. One should

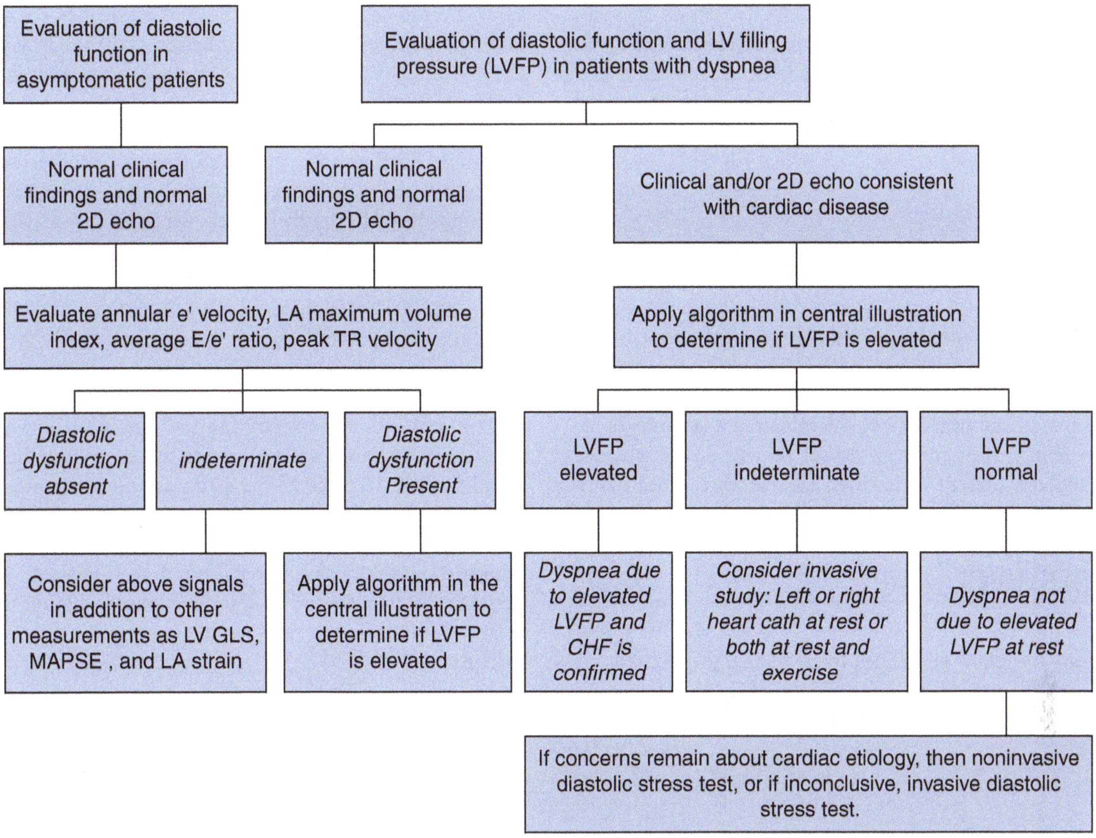

Fig. 19.11 Schematic illustration of how to evaluate LV diastolic function and filling pressure. The evaluation starts with clinical and 2D findings. Based on these findings, either the algorithm for evaluation of diastolic function *(left)* or the algorithm to estimate LV filling pressure *(right)* is used. When findings regarding diastolic function are indeterminate, other abnormalities that point to cardiac disease should be considered. If there is clinical suspicion of cardiac disease, and the algorithm used to decide if filling pressure is negative or indeterminate, cardiac catheterization with or without noninvasive or invasive diastolic stress testing should be applied to reach a conclusion about LV filling pressure. *CHF,* Congestive heart failure; *echo,* echocardiography; GLS, global longitudinal strain; LA, left atrial; *LVFP,* left ventricular filling pressure MAPSE, mitral annular plane systolic excursion.

always consider symptoms and clinical findings such as auscultation of lungs, jugular veins, and peripheral edema. Furthermore, pulmonary congestion on chest x-ray and elevated proBNP[17] provide strong support of elevated LV filling pressure.

Of note, the algorithm suggested in Fig. 19.4 should not be used when there is not clinical suspicion of heart failure.

Furthermore, novel echocardiographic parameters as LA reservoir strain and LV global longitudinal strain (GLS) have been shown to correlate well with LV filling pressure.[18,19] A reduction in LA reservoir strain is consistent with, but does not represent standalone evidence of elevated LV filling pressure. A reduction in LV GLS does not in itself indicate diastolic dysfunction, but it represents important evidence of LV disease as a mechanism of symptoms. As shown in Fig. 19.11, these parameters are of particular use when a conclusion about diastolic function cannot be made using the four parameters suggested for this purpose by the ASE/EACVI recommendations.

EVALUATION OF DIASTOLIC FUNCTION IN SPECIAL POPULATIONS

A substantial proportion of patients with diastolic dysfunction have comorbidities that complicate interpretation of the echocardiographic parameters normally used to evaluate whether diastolic dysfunction is present. Thus, the 2016 ASE/EACVI guidelines briefly describe how to evaluate diastolic function in patients with some of the most common comorbidities.

ATRIAL FIBRILLATION

It is challenging to assess diastolic function in patients with atrial fibrillation for various reasons. The left atrium is usually large, and there is no atrial contraction. Moreover, mitral inflow varies with different cardiac cycle lengths, and as there is no A wave, E/A cannot be calculated. Fortunately, studies have shown that E/e′ correlates well with PCWP in atrial fibrillation.[20] In this situation it would be best to obtain an average value from three to six consecutive cardiac cycles for E and e′ velocity. E/e′ of 11 or more is proposed as an indicator of elevated LV filling pressure. The lack of E velocity fluctuation or short E_{DT} (<160 m) also indicates increased filling pressure and/or a poor clinical outcome in atrial fibrillation.[21] Furthermore, TR velocity as the average of several beats can be used to estimate pulmonary artery systolic pressure.

MITRAL ANNULAR CALCIFICATION

Mitral annular calcification (MAC) is often seen in hypertensive heart disease and is associated with aortic stenosis, kidney disease, and coronary artery disease. The prevalence of MAC increases with increasing age. With severe MAC, the mitral orifice area will be decreased, resulting in increased diastolic transmitral velocity. Simultaneously, lateral and posterior e′ might be reduced due to restriction of the posterior mitral leaflet excursion. Thus in these patients, increased E/e′ does not necessarily imply diastolic dysfunction. A recent study showed that E/A ratio and isovolumic relaxation time (IVRT) could be useful in patients with severe MAC.[22]

HEART TRANSPLANTS

Evaluation of diastolic function in heart transplants is challenging, as several of the parameters used in normal individuals cannot be used in these patients. Due to the denervation of the donor heart, sinus tachycardia is common, resulting in a fusion of E/A. Thus E/A can often not be used, and E/e′ should be used with caution. The interaction between donor and recipient heart due to the midatrial anastomoses interfere with the ability of pulmonary venous flow to decide whether diastolic dysfunction is present.[23] However, TR velocity can be used to decide whether diastolic dysfunction is present.

FUTURE DIRECTIONS

The definition of diastolic dysfunction in the 2016 ASE/EACVI guidelines differs from the 2009 guidelines by reducing the number of parameters to be evaluated. In the 2009 guidelines, the algorithm used to define whether diastolic dysfunction was present was rather complex, including Valsalva maneuver, pulmonary venous flow, and E wave deceleration time. The definition of diastolic dysfunction in the 2016 ASE/EACVI guidelines was thus a simplification of the previous definition. Furthermore, the parameters used to decide whether diastolic dysfunction is present recommended in the 2016 ASE/EACVI guidelines could normally be obtained in all individuals.

The criteria for the diagnosis of diastolic dysfunction and classification as grade II diastolic dysfunction are more restrictive in the 2016 than in the 2009 version of the guidelines; they imply that individuals with early stage preclinical diastolic dysfunction may be lost. The 2016 guidelines have better specificity and may be better suited to identify high-risk patients.

The accuracy for identifying patients with elevated LV filling pressure is improved when applying the 2016 guidelines.[5,6] However, in at least 1 in 10 patients the estimate will be wrong, and therefore other signs of elevated filling pressure should always be part of the evaluation. LA reservoir strain and LV GLS are both promising echocardiographic parameters found to correlate with LV filling pressure.[18,19] Future studies should evaluate whether the addition of these parameters might increase diagnostic accuracy in heart failure patients.

KEY POINTS

Strengths

- Easier estimation of LV filling pressure: The simplified algorithm makes estimation of filling pressure easier. There are fewer parameters to be evaluated, and the parameters used in the algorithm are easily obtained in a majority of individuals referred to echocardiography.
- Validated in clinical trials: Two recent multicenter studies have confirmed the validity of the algorithm to estimate LV filling pressure. It was shown that echocardiographic evaluation of LV filling pressure significantly increased the diagnostic accuracy when compared to clinical evaluation alone.
- Algorithm for evaluation of diastolic function simplified: The algorithm to decide whether diastolic dysfunction is present has been simplified. Furthermore, specificity is increased, and studies have demonstrated that grading of diastolic function can be prognostically useful.

Limitations

- Which algorithm to use: It is difficult to know when to use algorithm A and B in combination and when algorithm B should be used as the first step.
- Many indeterminate patients: The use of four parameters in the initial algorithm to decide whether diastolic dysfunction is present renders many patients unclassified.
- Not a standalone method for estimation of LV filling pressure: At best there is 85% to 90% accuracy for estimation of LV filling pressure, which means that you are wrong in at least 1 in 10 patients. Therefore, in every patient you need additional diagnostic information.
- Supplementary indices to estimate LV filling pressure: Could have given more emphasis to alternative indices to use when the study is inconclusive regarding LV filling pressure. The following indices/parameters should be discussed in more detail. (Details regarding the data to support these indices will be discussed in other chapters.)
  - Pulmonary artery flow acceleration time as an alternative to TR jet[24]
  - LV GLS to confirm mild reduction in systolic function
  - LA reservoir strain as additional index of LV filling pressure
  - NT-proBNP as supplementary or alternative method to establish the diagnosis
  - LV hypertrophy may serve as a supportive finding
  - Chest x-ray to verify pulmonary congestion
  - Age adjustment of echocardiographic indices of diastolic function: There should be more guidance on how to age-adjust reference values for different parameters.
  - Ejection fraction to define systolic function: The validity of using LV EF to define systolic function should be discussed in more detail, as several studies have demonstrated how LV GLS is a more sensitive marker of systolic function.[25]

REVIEW QUESTIONS

1. A patient with dyspnea on exertion was evaluated with echocardiography. The patient had no cardiac history. LV ejection fraction and LV dimensions were normal. Septal e′ velocity was 6 cm/sec, mitral annular lateral velocity 7 cm/sec, mitral E wave 85 cm/sec, and E/e′ 13. LA volume index was 35 mL/m^2 and TR velocity 3.2 m/sec. How would you describe LV diastolic function?
   a. There is no diastolic dysfunction.
   b. Diastolic function is indeterminate.
   c. There is diastolic dysfunction.

2. LV filling pressure can be estimated by echocardiography using a combination of Doppler parameters and two-dimensional (2-D) echocardiography. A patient with a history of hypertensive heart disease presented with the following combination of echocardiographic parameters: E/A ratio 0.9, E velocity 65 cm/sec, LA volume index 38, E/e′ 12, and TR velocity 2.0 m/sec. Using these parameters, what would you say about LV filling pressure?
   a. LV filling pressure is elevated.
   b. LV filling pressure cannot be estimated in this patient.
   c. LV filling pressure is normal.
3. In atrial fibrillation, some of the parameters used to evaluate LV diastolic function and LV filling pressure cannot be used. Which of the following parameters can be used to evaluate LV filling pressure and diastolic function in patients with atrial fibrillation?
   a. E/e′
   b. LA volume
   c. E/A ratio
   d. TR velocity
4. The 2016 guidelines for evaluation of diastolic dysfunction differed from the 2009 guidelines by reducing the number of parameters used in the evaluation and by using a more restrictive definition of grade I diastolic dysfunction. In what way would you say that this changed diagnostic properties of the guidelines?
   a. Sensitivity was increased, specificity reduced.
   b. Specificity was increased, sensitivity reduced.
   c. The diagnostic properties were not changed.
5. A patient was presenting with dyspnea on exertion, suspicion of diastolic dysfunction, but normal echocardiography at rest. Which diagnostic tests could be used to reach a conclusion about diastolic function in this patient?
   a. Spirometry
   b. Coronary angiography
   c. Diastolic stress echocardiography

REFERENCES

1. Almeida JG, Fontes-Carvalho R, Sampaio F, Ribeiro J, Bettencourt P, Flachskampf FA, et al. Impact of the 2016 ASE/EACVI recommendations on the prevalence of diastolic dysfunction in the general population. *Eur Heart J Cardiovasc Imag.* 2018;19(4):380–386.
2. Huttin O, Fraser AG, Coiro S, Bozec E, Selton-Suty C, Lamiral Z, et al. Impact of changes in consensus diagnostic recommendations on the echocardiographic prevalence of diastolic dysfunction. *J Am Coll Cardiol.* 2007;69(25):3119–3121.
3. Redfield MM, Jacobsen SJ, Burnett JC Jr, Mahoney DW, Bailey KR, Rodeheffer RJ. Burden of systolic and diastolic ventricular dysfunction in the community: appreciating the scope of the heart failure epidemic. *JAMA.* 2003;289(2):194–202.
4. Grant AD, Negishi K, Negishi T, Collier P, Kapadia SR, Thomas JD, et al. Grading diastolic function by echocardiography: hemodynamic validation of existing guidelines. *Cardiovasc Ultrasound.* 2015;13:28.
5. Anderen OS, Smiseth OA, Dokainish H, Abudiab MM, Schutt RC, Kumar A, et al. Estimating left ventricular filling pressure by echocardiography. *J Am Coll Cardiol.* 2017;69:961–968.
6. Lancellotti P, Galderisi M, Edvardsen T, Donal E, Goliasch G, Cardim N, et al. Echo-Doppler estimation of left ventricular filling pressure: results of the multicentre EACVI Euro-Filling study. *Eur Heart J Cardiovasc Imag.* 2017;18(9):961–968.
7. Asami M, Lanz J, Stortecky S, Räber L, Franzone A, Heg D, et al. The impact of left ventricular diastolic dysfunction on clinical outcomes after transcatheter aortic valve replacement. *JACC Cardiovasc Interv.* 2018;11(6):593–601.
8. Kane GC, Karon BL, Mahoney DW, Redfield MM, Roger VL, Burnett JC Jr, et al. Progression of left ventricular diastolic dysfunction and risk of heart failure. *JAMA.* 2011;306(8):856–863.
9. AlJaroudi W, Alraies MC, Halley C, Rodriguez L, Grimm RA, Thomas JD, et al. Impact of progression of diastolic dysfunction on mortality in patients with normal ejection fraction. *Circulation.* 2012;125:782–788.
10. Caballero L, Kou S, Dulgheru R, Gonjilashvili N, Athanassopoulos GD, Barone D, et al. Echocardiographic reference ranges for normal cardiac Doppler data: results from the NORRE study. *Eur Heart J Cardiovasc Imag.* 2015;16(9):1031–1041.
11. Kou S, Caballero L, Dulgheru R, Voilliot D, De Sousa C, Kacharava G, et al. Echocardiographic reference ranges for normal cardiac chamber size: results from the NORRE study. *Eur Heart J Cardiovasc Imag.* 2014;15(6):680–690.
12. Rahimtoola SH, Loeb HS, Ehsani A, Sinno MZ, Chuquimia R, Lal R, et al. Relationship of pulmonary artery to left ventricular diastolic pressures in acute myocardial infarction. *Circulation.* 1972;46:283–290.
13. Edvardsen T, Smiseth OA. Evaluation of diastolic function by echocardiography: important progression, but issues to be resolved. *Eur Heart J Cardiovasc Imag.* 2018;19(4):387–388.
14. Smiseth OA. Evaluation of left ventricular diastolic function: state of the art after 35 years with Doppler assessment. *J Echocardiogr.* 2018;16(2):55–56.
15. Schirmer H, Lunde P, Rasmussen K. Mitral flow derived Doppler indices of left ventricular diastolic function in a general population—the Tromso study. *Eur Heart J.* 2000;21:1376–1386.
16. Paulus WJ, Tschöpe C, Sanderson JE, Rusconi C, Flachskampf FA, Rademakers FE, et al. How to diagnose diastolic heart failure: a consensus statement on the diagnosis of heart failure with normal left ventricular ejection fraction by the Heart Failure and Echocardiography Associations of the European Society of Cardiology. *Eur Heart J.* 2007;28:2539–2550.
17. Ponikowski P, Voors AA, Anker SD, Bueno H, Cleland JGF, Coats AJS, et al. 2016 ESC guidelines for the diagnosis and treatment of acute and chronic heart failure. *Eur Heart J.* 2016;37:2129–2200.
18. Camelli M, Lisi M, Mondillo S, Padeletti M, Ballo P, Tsioulpas C, et al. Left atrial longitudinal strain by speckle tracking echocardiography correlates well with left ventricular filling pressures in patients with heart failure. *Cardiovas Ultrasound.* 2010;8:14.
19. Wang J, Khoury DS, Thohan V, Torre-Amione G, Nagueh SF. Global diastolic strain rate for the assessment of left ventricular relaxation and filling pressures. *Circulation.* 2007;115:1376–1383.
20. Nagueh SF, Kopelen HA, Quiñones MA. Assessment of left ventricular filling pressures by Doppler in the presence of atrial fibrillation. *Circulation.* 1996;94:2138–2145.
21. Temporelli PL, Scapellato F, Corrà U, Eleuteri E, Imparato A, Giannuzzi P. Estimation of pulmonary wedge pressure by transmitral Doppler in patients with chronic heart failure and atrial fibrillation. *Am J Cardiol.* 1999;83:724–727.
22. Abudiab MM, Chebrolu LH, Schutt RC, Nagueh SF, Zoghbi WA. Doppler echocardiography for the estimation of LV filling pressure in patients with mitral annular calcification. *JACC Cardiovasc Imag.* 2017;10(12):1411-1420.
23. Dell'Aquila AM, Mastrobuoni S, Bastarrika G, Praschker BL, Aguero PA, Castano S, et al. Bicaval versus standard technique in orthotopic heart transplant: assessment of atrial performance at magnetic resonance and transthoracic echocardiography. *Interact Cardiovasc Thorac Surg.* 2012;14:457–462.
24. Tossavainen E, Söderberg S, Grönlund C, Gonzalez M, Henein MY, Lindqvist P. Pulmonary artery acceleration time in identifying pulmonary hypertension patients with raised pulmonary vascular resistance. *Eur Heart J Cardiovasc Imag.* 2013;14(9):890–897.
25. Stokke TM, Hasselberg NE, Smedsrud MK, Sarvari SI, Haugaa KH, Smiseth OA, et al. Geometry as a confounder when assessing ventricular systolic function. *J Am Coll Cardiol.* 2017;70:942–954.

20

Hypertension and Its Relation to Heart Failure With a Preserved Ejection Fraction

Lakshmi Nambiar and Martin M. LeWinter

OUTLINE

INTRODUCTION

Hypertension (HTN) is the single most important and widespread cardiovascular diagnosis in the developed world and, as such, an enormous public health problem.[1,2] With the recent change in guidelines reducing the systolic blood pressure (BP)–lowering target from 140 to 130 mmHg based on the landmark Systolic Blood Pressure Intervention Trial (SPRINT), it is now estimated that 46% of Americans should be considered to have treatable HTN.[3] HTN is both a major risk factor for other forms of cardiovascular disease (e.g., coronary artery disease [CAD] and stroke) and a direct cause and substrate of cardiovascular disease (e.g., concentric left ventricular [LV] hypertrophy [LVH] and remodeling and heart failure [HF]). Despite recognition of the importance of HTN, there remains uncertainty about what constitutes the appropriate threshold for treatment. The SPRINT study results showing that targeting a systolic BP of 120 mmHg rather than 140 mmHg improved long-term outcomes[3] begs the question, Should attempts be made to lower BP even further than 120 mmHg? In light of the SPRINT study, it is interesting to note that as recently as the 1960s there was some disagreement as to whether HTN should even be treated.

In view of the scope of the topic and the theme of this book, this chapter will focus on HTN and its relationship to concentric remodeling (CR), LV diastolic filling properties, and heart failure with a preserved LV ejection fraction (HFpEF). Of necessity, there are some weaknesses to this approach. First and most importantly, we largely disregard patients with a history of HTN without CR. Many of them undoubtedly have abnormal diastolic function, and a number clearly have HFpEF, but there are virtually no studies of ventricular or myocardial function or outcomes that have examined them as a distinct group. Second, many if not most patients with HTN and CR have comorbidities that contribute independently to CR and/or diastolic dysfunction. Thus we are usually not observing the effects of HTN in isolation. Third, many BP-lowering drugs have other properties (e.g., anti-inflammatory, antifibrotic) that contribute to their effects, so that HTN treatment typically involves more than simply lowering BP. Last, in considering HFpEF it is important to remember that not all patients have HTN, even after excluding specific diagnoses such as hypertrophic cardiomyopathy and amyloid heart disease. While small in number these patients have not been analyzed separately. The following case study serves as an introduction to the problem of HTN as it relates to these three main themes.

Case Study

A 58-year-old man is referred by his internist for evaluation of progressive dyspnea on exertion. He is sedentary, has longstanding HTN and obesity, and for many years has found that he becomes dyspneic going up more than one flight of stairs or carrying heavy bags of groceries. Over the last 6 to 8 months this complaint has been progressively worsening, such that he now becomes dyspneic walking on level ground at anything more than a normal pace for him. He is self-employed as a landscape architect and has had to cut down on his work because of his dyspnea. He also has obstructive sleep apnea (OSA), for which he is being treated with continuous positive airway pressure (CPAP). He sleeps on two pillows but denies paroxysmal nocturnal dyspnea or peripheral edema.

He denies chest discomfort, palpitations, dizziness, or syncope. His HTN has been somewhat difficult to control over the years, and despite various drugs his systolic BP routinely ranges from 150 to 160 mmHg. He has been told that he has "borderline-elevated blood sugar." He is a nonsmoker and does not consume significant amounts of alcohol.

His past medical history is significant only for gastroesophageal reflux disease manifest as occasional nonexertional epigastric burning relieved by a proton pump inhibitor, and osteoarthritis mainly affecting his knees.

His current medications include aspirin 81 mg daily, chlorthalidone 25 mg daily, metoprolol tartrate 50 mg twice daily, losartan 50 mg daily, furosemide 20 mg daily, atorvastatin 20 mg daily, and pantoprazole 40 mg daily.

On physical examination he appears in no acute distress and has central obesity. His BP is 155/95 mmHg (after sitting for 5 minutes), heart rate 75 bpm, and respiratory rate 14/min. He is 68 in. (150 cm) tall and weighs 235 lb (107 kg, BMI = 36). His chest is clear to auscultation, and his estimated jugular venous pressure is 7 cm. His carotid arterial pulses are normal. His cardiac point of maximal impulse cannot be palpated; S_1 and S_2 are normal, a fourth heart sound is present at the cardiac apex, and there are no murmurs. His abdomen is obese and nontender, and his extremities reveal 1+ bilateral pedal edema.

His laboratory data include a normal complete blood count (CBC), serum blood urea nitrogen (BUN) 26 mg/dL, creatinine 1.4 mg/dL, estimated glomerular filtration rate (GFR) 55 mL/min/1.73 m^2, and normal electrolytes with serum K+ 4.6 mEq/L. His fasting blood glucose is 105 mg/dl, and hemoglobin A1c is 6.3%. His total cholesterol is 210 mg/dL, low-density lipoprotein (LDL) 82 mg/dL, high-density lipoprotein (HDL) 38 mg/dL, and triglycerides 180 mg/dL. His N-terminal pro-brain natriuretic peptide (NT-proBNP) is 1050 pg/mL (normal <300).

His electrocardiogram (ECG) reveals normal sinus rhythm, borderline left axis deviation, and minor nonspecific ST-T abnormalities. A chest radiograph shows normal lung fields and pulmonary vascularity and a slightly enlarged cardiac silhouette.

An echocardiographic Doppler study reveals LV ejection fraction (EF) of 0.60 to 0.65, LV end-diastolic volume index 55 mL/m^2 (normal range 35–75), LV mass index 138 g/m^2 (normal range 49–115), left atrial (LA) volume index 39 mL/m^2 (normal <34), E/A ratio 0.9, and average E/e′ 13 (normal <10). An echocardiographic image illustrating this patient's concentric LVH is shown in Fig. 20.1.

His 6-minute walk test result is 340 m.

Following this initial evaluation and a discussion of diagnostic and treatment possibilities with the patient, spironolactone 25 mg daily is added to his regimen, and the dose of losartan is increased to 100 mg daily. In addition, a combined exercise-pharmacologic stress test with nuclear imaging is scheduled. Myocardial perfusion is subsequently reported as normal.

The patient returns in 2 weeks. He feels that his dyspnea may be mildly improved. He has not had any medication side effects. Repeat blood work obtained 4 days previous does not reveal any significant change in his renal function or electrolytes. His physical examination is unchanged except that his BP is now 128/80 mmHg. No further medication changes are made. A home exercise conditioning and weight-loss program is recommended to the patient as his insurance plan will not reimburse him for a formal cardiac rehabilitation program.

On return in 2 months, he has succeeded in losing 10 lb and he is taking a 2-mile daily walk, which takes about 1 hour to complete. He feels that his dyspnea is definitely improved, although still a significant problem. His BP is now 124/80 mmHg. On a repeat 6-minute walk test he walks 390 m.

This patient fulfils published diagnostic criteria for HFpEF, as delineated in Chapter 7.[4,5] Thus he has dyspnea on exertion in the absence of other medical conditions that can cause dyspnea (with the exception of obesity), concentric LVH with evidence of diastolic dysfunction, and a modestly elevated NT-proBNP. The results of the initial 6-minute walk test confirm that he has poor exercise tolerance. Although not routinely assessed as of yet, most such patients demonstrate abnormal elevations of LV filling pressures during upright bicycle exercise, further confirming the diagnosis of HF.[6]

This patient has the most common comorbidity associated with HFpEF: HTN,[4,5] which has not been optimally controlled. Like most patients with HFpEF he also has other comorbidities, including obesity, OSA, chronic kidney disease (CKD), and apparent insulin resistance.[5] HTN, especially if poorly controlled, is of course an important stimulus for concentric LVH. However, insulin resistance with associated hyperinsulinemia and most likely OSA are also contributory.[7,8] Thus the substrates for HFpEF and LVH overlap.

HTN and concentric LVH are associated with myocardial abnormalities that cause diastolic dysfunction,[9] specifically slowed actomyosin relaxation kinetics,[10] altered Na-Ca handling,[11,12] changes in titin phosphorylation and possibly isoforms,[13–15] and increased collagen content and crosslinking,[15,16] which are discussed in more detail later in the chapter. It is not known whether a history of HTN alone without CR or LVH is sufficient to cause any or all of these diverse myocardial abnormalities.

With respect to the management of HFpEF, there is an indication for stress testing in this patient as the incidence of coexistent CAD is high, he has multiple CAD risk factors, and his dyspnea on exertion could represent an angina equivalent.[17,18]

As discussed here and elsewhere in this book (see Chapter 35) no treatment has been clearly shown to favorably affect long-term outcomes in HFpEF. Therefore current guideline recommendations are general measures and include loop diuretics for volume overload, optimal BP control, treatment of comorbidities, and weight loss and exercise.[17,19] The patient in the case study has no overt evidence of volume overload other than the elevated NT-proBNP. Thus there is no clear indication for a loop diuretic for decongestion, but in light of his CKD and relatively resistant HTN, furosemide is appropriate as a component of BP control. Since his BP is poorly controlled, increasing his losartan dose is also entirely appropriate. Aldosterone blockers have unquestioned benefit in HF with reduced EF (HFrEF), but the situation is less clear in HFpEF. As discussed in more detail later in the chapter, the TOPCAT trial of spironolactone in HFpEF did not meet its primary end points, but there was a signal of possible benefit. Thus, while there is no definite proof of efficacy, there may be a role for spironolactone in patients who fit the TOPCAT entry criteria.[19] Like many patients with HFpEF, he is also receiving a beta blocker, which is typically prescribed for HTN and is one of the drug classes recommended for BP control as part of guideline-directed care of HFpEF.[17,19] However, as with other treatments there is once again no proof that beta blockers provide long-term benefit. Moreover, we and others have argued that beta blockers are not preferred for the treatment of HTN in general and may actually be harmful in patients with a normal LV EF.[20,21] Thus a case could be made for discontinuing metoprolol and substituting other BP-lowering drugs if necessary. Exercise conditioning programs (some including an explicit weight-loss component) have been shown in a number of relatively small studies to improve exercise capacity in HFpEF[22] and of course are also beneficial in treating most of the common comorbidities, including HTN.[23] While difficult to achieve, this is an important therapeutic recommendation for this patient.

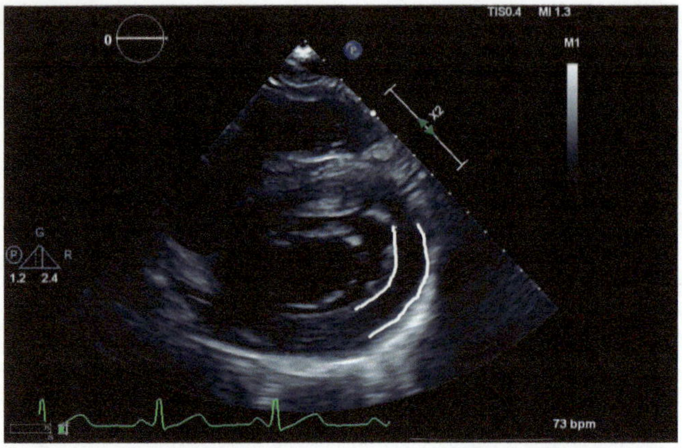

Fig. 20.1 Echocardiographic short axis LV end-diastolic image demonstrating an increased mass/volume ratio (i.e., concentric remodeling) *(endocardium and epicardium are highlighted).* In this case wall thickness is increased and LV diastolic volume is normal, indicating the presence of an increased mass and concentric hypertrophy. Some patients with concentric remodeling do not have overt hypertrophy but rather have normal wall thickness with a small diastolic volume.

EPIDEMIOLOGY OF HYPERTENSION IN HFpEF

The prevalence of a history of HTN in patients with HFpEF has been somewhat variable. An early registry of hospitalized patients[24] reported an incidence of 78%. In contrast, HTN was present in 96% of patients in the Mayo Clinic outpatient registry.[25] In CHARM-Preserved[26] HTN was present in ~65%, in the PEP trial[27] in 79%, and in SENIORS[28] in 77%. These three early randomized trials had EF inclusion cutoffs below 35% to 40%. In more recent large clinical trials, each of which required a LV EF of 45% or more, the prevalence of HTN has been consistently much higher. Thus in I-PRESERVE[29] it was 88%, in TOPCAT[30] 91%, and in the ongoing PARAGON trial[31] it is 96%. In view of the fact that a modern diagnosis of HFpEF requires a LV EF of 50% or more, it seems likely that the true incidence is more in line with the Mayo registry and the more recent clinical trials (i.e., >90%).

PATHOPHYSIOLOGY OF DIASTOLIC DYSFUNCTION IN HYPERTENSION AND HFpEF

Abnormalities of the relaxation and filling properties of the left ventricle are common in patients with asymptomatic HTN[32,33] and constitute a core component of the pathophysiology in patients with HFpEF.[29,34] Systemic HTN and other forms of pressure overload (PO) (e.g., aortic stenosis) cause an increase in LV mass/volume ratio, consisting of either an absolute increase in LV mass with a normal end-diastolic volume or an increase in mass/volume ratio without an absolute increase in mass.[33] These two variants are referred to as concentric remodeling.

As discussed, the great majority of patients with HFpEF have a history of HTN. In large clinical trials, greater than 50% have had CR,[26–28,30,35] although in the Mayo Clinic community registry only 42% had CR.[25] A small number of HFpEF patients have eccentric remodeling.[29] While HFpEF patients without CR appear to have abnormal LV diastolic properties,[25,29,34] understanding how or even if HTN contributes to diastolic dysfunction and the development of HFpEF in the absence of its signature cardiac end-organ effect is very difficult, and there are no reports focusing on myocardial determinants of diastolic dysfunction in such patients. In addition, while animal models of PO are useful in providing mechanistic insights, they frequently do not simulate human disease very well. This may be a particular problem with rodents because their underlying cardiovascular physiology is so different. Lastly, as noted earlier, despite the high prevalence of HTN in HFpEF patients it is important to keep in mind that other comorbidities may contribute to the development of CR and/or diastolic dysfunction (e.g., hyperinsulinemia and other effects associated with type 2 diabetes mellitus [T2DM]/insulin resistance, obesity, OSA, CAD, and normal aging).[7,8] It is impossible to know how much these comorbidities, as opposed to HTN per se, influence the development of CR. For these reasons we once again focus our discussion on diastolic function in patients with HTN and CR, understanding the difficulty of isolating the effects of HTN. When possible, we distinguish between patients with and without HFpEF and the effects of HTN versus comorbidities. In addition, we divide LV diastolic properties into the rate and completeness of active relaxation and passive, or fully relaxed, filling properties. A schematic representation of the time course of HTN and common comorbidities and their progression to concentric remodeling in relation to LV diastolic dysfunction and HFpEF is presented in Fig. 20.2.

Hypertension-Associated Concentric Remodeling and Diastolic Properties of the Intact Left Ventricle

All else being equal, based on Laplace's law, an increase in mass/volume ratio in and of itself reduces LV chamber distensibility (i.e., the LV passive pressure-volume relation [PVR] is shifted upward) with fully relaxed pressure higher at any volume. Rigorously defined, chamber compliance (the inverse of chamber stiffness) is the slope of the entire passive PVR, beginning at the LV equilibrium volume (Veq) (i.e., the volume at which the transmural pressure is zero). Since whether and

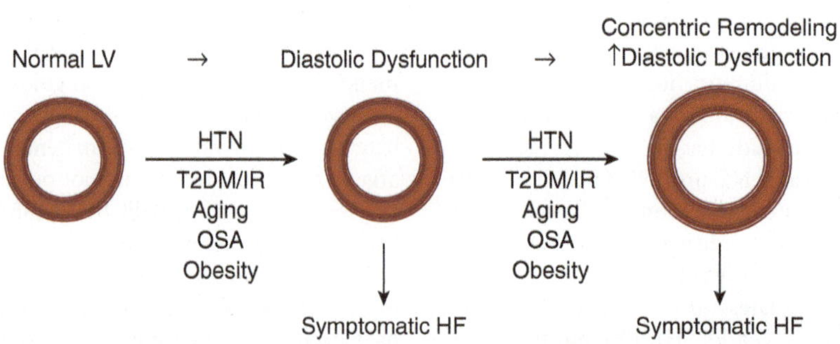

Fig. 20.2 Schematic representation of how hypertension (HTN) in conjunction with common comorbidities and aging causes diastolic dysfunction and progresses to concentric remodeling. Virtually all patients with HFpEF have evidence of diastolic dysfunction based on direct hemodynamic and/or echocardiographic Doppler assessment but not all have concentric remodeling when they present with heart failure (HF). Concentric remodeling is defined as an ↑ LV mass/volume ratio or ↑ relative wall thickness (wall thickness to radius ratio), whether or not an increased LV mass is present. *IR,* Insulin resistance; *OSA,* obstructive sleep apnea; *T2DM,* type 2 diabetes mellitus.

to what extent CR affects Veq is unknown, it cannot be stated with certainty that CR reduces chamber compliance, although it very likely does. CR also may impair LV twist-untwisting[36] and the closely related phenomenon of diastolic suction, an important mechanism that facilitates early diastolic filling. Suction results from conversion of potential energy stored during systole to kinetic energy during diastole.[37] Last, while not strictly speaking a result of CR, many patients with HTN have abnormally stiff systemic arteries,[38] which increases LV systolic pressure and total load, slowing LV relaxation. In addition, the velocity of arterial wave reflection is increased when arterial stiffness increases. Normally, reflected waves return to the LV near the time of aortic valve closure and facilitate relaxation. However, when they return to the LV earlier than normal, they add to total load and thus further slow relaxation.[39]

As discussed in the earlier case, diastolic dysfunction in patients with HFpEF, the great majority of whom have HTN, is exacerbated during exercise, as reported by Borlaug et al.[18] who have measured hemodynamics in patients during upright bicycle exercise (see Chapter 8). Thus patients with HFpEF typically demonstrate markedly abnormal elevations of the pulmonary capillary wedge pressure (PCWP) during exercise as well as impaired cardiac output responses, although once again it is impossible to isolate the effects of HTN-associated CR from those of other comorbidities. The mechanism of abnormal exercise hemodynamics is likely multifactorial and may include abnormalities at a myocardial level (e.g., abnormally elevated diastolic [Ca^{2+}]), at the whole organ level (e.g., increased vascular load), and subendocardial ischemia.[40]

Myocardial Determinants of LV Diastolic Properties in Hypertension-Associated Concentric Remodeling

The determinants of passive myocardial stiffness, and therefore passive chamber compliance, are collagen, whose content and crosslinking dictate stiffness of the extracellular matrix (ECM), and the giant myofilament spring protein titin, whose stiffness dictates cardiomyocyte passive tension.[15] The relative contribution of collagen versus titin to passive stiffness is sarcomere length dependent, with titin relatively more important at short and collagen more important at long sarcomere lengths.[41] There are important changes in both of these determinants in patients with HTN and CR that increase passive myocardial stiffness, keeping in mind once again that the aforementioned comorbidities coexist in many patients and may also modify collagen and titin. These passive stiffness changes appear to be much more prominent in patients with HTN and CR who have progressed to HFpEF (Fig. 20.3).

Based on postmortem studies, increased collagen content has been recognized for many years in patients with HTN and cardiac hypertrophy.[42,43] However, it is only rather recently that patients with HTN and CR with well-characterized clinical features and in vivo cardiac structure and function assessments based on modern techniques (mainly echocardiography-Doppler) have been studied. Thus using myocardial biopsies, recent studies have shown that collagen content is increased in patients with HFpEF.[15,16] In these studies, virtually all patients had a history of HTN and most had CR. Using strips dissected from myocardial biopsies obtained from patients undergoing coronary bypass surgery, we published the only report to date in which patients with HTN as an explicit study entry criterion and CR with and without HFpEF were analyzed and compared with control subjects.[15] We found that collagen content was increased only in HFpEF patients, although serum biomarkers suggested that alterations in the ECM were ongoing in HTN patients without HFpEF. Table 20.1 shows selected biomarkers in controls and HTN patients without HFpEF [(-)HFpEF] and with HFpEF [(+)HFpEF]. ST-2 is a proinflammatory biomarker, while MMP-7 and TIMP-1 reflect ECM remodeling. Note alterations in HTN(-) HFpEF patients and normalization of MMP-7 in HTN(+) HFpEF patients. We and others[15,16] have also documented increased collagen crosslinking in patients with HTN and HFpEF, which increases its stiffness. Surprisingly, coexistent T2DM did not appear to

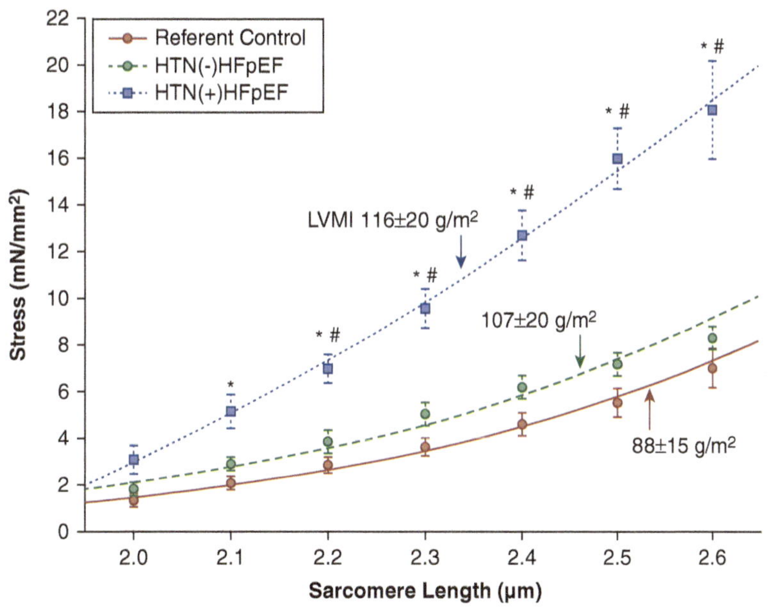

Fig. 20.3 Passive myocardial stiffness (stress vs sarcomere length) assessed in demembranated (skinned) strips dissected from LV epicardial biopsies obtained in the operating room in patients with HTN, concentric remodeling, and normal EF undergoing coronary bypass surgery. Patients were classified as HTN without HFpEF [(-)HFpEF)] or with HFpEF [(+)HFpEF] and compared with controls without HTN. There is a modest trend toward increased stiffness in HTN(-)HFpEF, but a marked increase in HTN(+)HFpEF (see text). LV mass index (LVMI) progressively increases from controls to HTN(-)HFpEF to HTN(+)HFpEF. Adapted from Zile MR, Baicu CF, Ikonomidis J. Myocardial Stiffness in Patients with Heart Failure and a Preserved Ejection Fraction: Contributions of Collagen and Titin. *Circulation.* 2015;131(14)1247–59.

TABLE 20.1 **Selected Biomarkers in Controls and HTN Patients Without HFpEF [(-)HFpEF] and with HFpEF [(+)HFpEF].**

		HYPERTENSION	
	Referent Control	**(-)HFpEF**	**(+)HFpEF**
CRP (mcg/mL)	2.4 ± 1.8	4.8 ± 2.9	4.2 ± 2.1
sST-2 (ng/mL)	25.6 ± 19.8	82.0 ± 35.7	105.5 ± 31.4
MMP-7 (pg/mL)	228 ± 132	468 ± 288	212 ± 210
TIMP-1 (ng/mL)	64 ± 27	101 ± 27	128 ± 34
NT-proBNP (pg/mL)	897 ± 629	1507 ± 976	2355 ± 1394

CRP, C-reactive protein; *HFpEF,* heart failure with preserved ejection fraction; *HTN,* hypertension; *MMP,* matrix metalloproteinase; *NT-proBNP,* N-terminal pro-brain natriuretic peptide; *sST-2,* soluble ST-2; *TIMP,* tissue inhibitor of MMPs.
From Zile MR, Baicu CF, Ikonomidis JS, Stroud RE, Nietert PJ, Bradshaw AD, et al. Myocardial stiffness in patients with heart failure and a preserved ejection fraction: contributions of collagen and titin. *Circulation* 2015;131(14):1247–1259.

have an additive effect on either collagen content or crosslinking.[15] Advanced glycation end-product (AGE) accumulation is a logical candidate to explain increased crosslinking as AGEs are known to accumulate and increase collagen crosslinking in the myocardium in experimental DM.[44] However, we found that ECM AGEs are barely detectable in myocardial biopsies from control patients and patients with HTN and HTN combined with T2DM.[9] Thus the mechanism of increased crosslinking is most likely something other than AGEs.

Alterations in titin, also based on studies using myocardial biopsies, have been implicated in patients with HFpEF[14] and with HTN and HFpEF with associated CR.[15] Titin stiffness can be modulated by isoform shifts, with smaller isoforms (N2B titin) being stiffer than larger isoforms (N2BA titin).[41] Increases in the stiffness of titin due to isoform switching (greater ratio of N2B:N2BA titin) have been somewhat inconsistent but are likely not of major importance. Changes in the phosphorylation state of titin can also modify its stiffness and appear to play a significant role in HFpEF. Titin has multiple phosphorylation sites. Protein kinases (PK) A and G phosphorylate identical sites, while other sites are phosphorylated by PKCα and several others.[42] Paulus et al.[14,45] reported reduced phosphorylation of PKG/A sites in association with reduced cardiomyocyte PKG activity and impaired nitric oxide (NO) availability, a change that increases titin stiffness and cardiomyocyte resting tension. Although most patients had HTN, they were not specifically selected for its presence. Paulus and Tschope have proposed that titin phosphorylation as well as other changes in diastolic function in HFpEF are related to an obesity-associated endothelial-based proinflammatory state.[46] We also reported a decrease in titin PKG/PKA site phosphorylation as well as increased phosphorylation of a PKC site[15]; the latter also increases titin stiffness. As with collagen, our study design allowed us to differentiate patients with HTN and CR with and without HFpEF; both types of phosphorylation changes were found in HFpEF patients but not in HTN patients without HFpEF, and here again coexistent T2DM did not have an additive effect. Changes in titin phosphorylation can result in rapid changes in titin and presumably myocardial stiffness (e.g., during exercise), and this could influence exercise responses in HFpEF.

Little is known about active relaxation at the myocardial level in HTN-associated CR and HFpEF. Our research group has focused on such patients, however, once again using strips obtained from intraoperative myocardial biopsies and the same paradigm comparing control subjects with patients with HTN and CR with and without HFpEF.[11,12] We have shown that such patients have abnormal Na^+-Ca^{2+} handling manifest as contraction-frequency dependent slowing and incomplete relaxation associated with elevated intracellular [Ca^{2+}]. The mechanism of this finding has been elusive to date but does not appear to be related to changes in the expression levels of Na^+-Ca^{2+} handling proteins or sarcolemmal Na^+ influx. Interestingly, in contrast to changes in passive filling properties, altered Na^+-Ca^{2+} handling is present in patients with HTN and CR whether or not they have HFpEF (Fig. 20.4).

We have also studied myofilament function, specifically actomyosin cross-bridge cycling kinetics, in skinned (demembranated) strips from patients with HTN and CR versus controls.[10] The number of patients in this study was too small to analyze those with HFpEF versus those without HFpEF, but we did exclude DM as a confounding factor. We found that cross-bridge detachment (relaxation) kinetics are slowed, which would contribute to slowed LV relaxation rate, and there was evidence of increased cross-bridge cycling at what are ordinarily relaxed levels of intracellular [Ca^{2+}], which would contribute to incomplete relaxation. Preliminary evidence suggests that hypophosphorylation of cardiac myosin-binding protein C and possibly troponin I underlies these findings.

A schematic representation of the various mechanisms acting on the left ventricle in patients with HTN that cause diastolic dysfunction at both the LV chamber and myocardial level is presented in Fig. 20.5.

In summary, in patients with HTN and CR, multiple mechanisms of diastolic dysfunction affecting both active relaxation and passive filling properties have been detected; some are present only when HFpEF is also present, while others do not require HFpEF. The effects of HTN on diastolic function in the absence of CR is uncertain. At present, the relative importance of these various mechanisms, the extent to which they vary between patients, and the importance of comorbidities are unknown

DIAGNOSTIC EVALUATION OF PATIENTS WITH HYPERTENSION AND HFpEF

As with any patient with HTN and HF, consideration should be given to secondary causes of HTN when appropriate, although these are quite unusual. It is also important to be sure that comorbidities, especially OSA, and unusual coexistent diagnoses such as hypertrophic cardiomyopathy are not missed. Details of diagnosing HFpEF and associated hemodynamic and imaging evaluations are provided in Part II. These are identical regardless if the patient has HTN.

Echocardiography-Doppler studies continue to be the most commonly used clinical modalities for assessment of diastolic function. Once again, we refer the reader to the detailed coverage of this topic in Part II. Briefly, as discussed earlier, the presence of CR in and of itself implies the presence of some component of diastolic dysfunction. Older mitral inflow Doppler indexes of diastolic function, which remain useful, include early peak filling rate (E velocity), E/A ratio, deceleration time of E velocity, and isovolumetric relaxation time (IVRT).

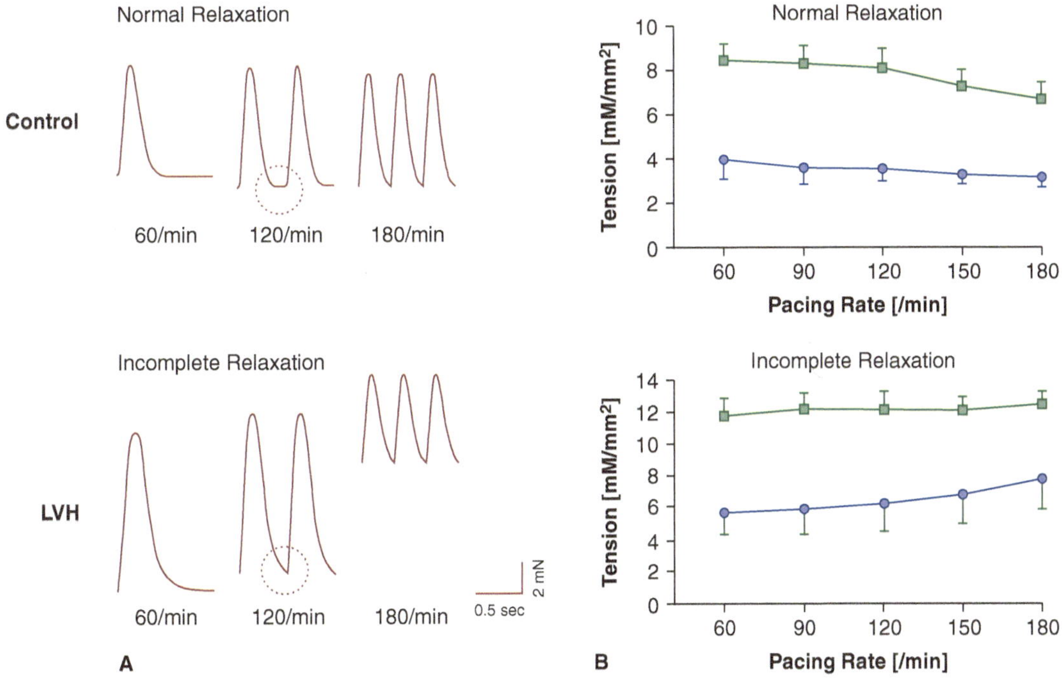

Fig. 20.4 Recordings of tension from excitable, isometrically contracting strips obtained from intraoperative epicardial biopsies from patients undergoing coronary bypass surgery. Controls are compared with patients with HTN and LV hypertrophy (LVH) at stimulation frequencies from 60 to 180/min. Note marked rise in diastolic tension due to incomplete relaxation as rate increases in strips from LVH patients. Adapted from Selby, D. E., Palmer, B. M., LeWinter, M. M., & Meyer, M. (2011). Tachycardia-induced diastolic dysfunction and resting tone in myocardium from patients with a normal ejection fraction. *Journal of the American College of Cardiology*, 58(2), 147–154.

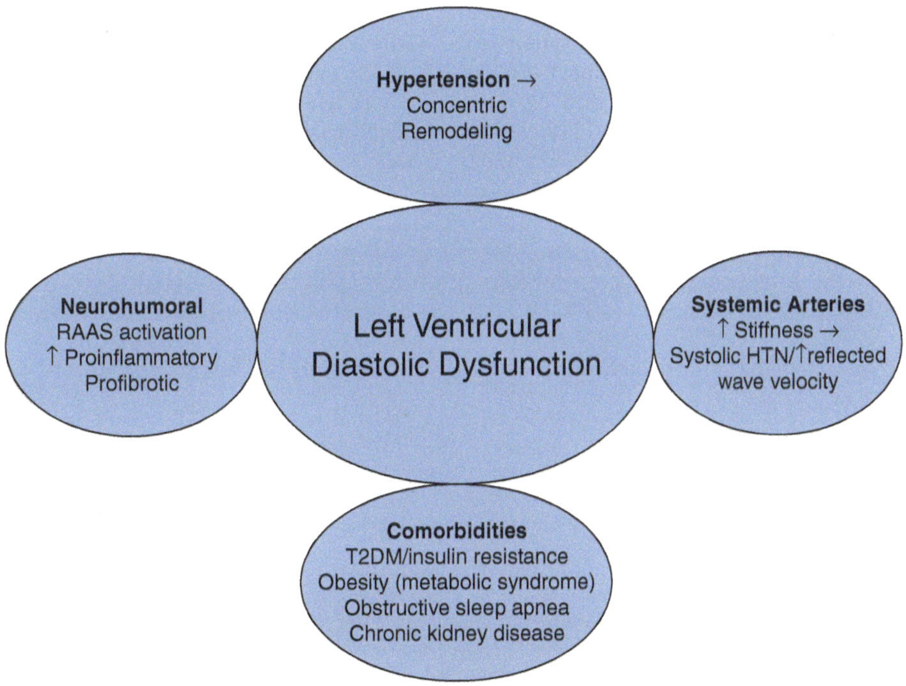

Fig. 20.5 Schematic representation of multiple factors that contribute to LV diastolic dysfunction in patients with hypertension and concentric remodeling, including neurohumoral activation, stiff systemic arteries, and common comorbidities. *RAAS*, Renin-angiotensin-aldosterone system; *T2DM*, type 2 diabetes mellitus.

In recent years combining mitral inflow with tissue Doppler measurements (E/e′ ratio) has gained favor because it correlates well with LV end-diastolic pressure. Increased LA dimension or volume is in many respects the most robust measure of abnormal diastolic function in the setting of a preserved EF as it is less susceptible to changes in loading conditions and has relatively low levels of noise. Longitudinal strain measurements have also found their way into clinical practice. A number of comparable diastolic function indexes can be derived from magnetic resonance imaging (MRI). Estimation of extracellular volume as a surrogate for collagen volume fraction is a particularly promising MRI approach.

HYPERTENSION TREATMENT: CURRENT STATUS IN RELATION TO HFpEF

In this section we focus on BP management in patients with HTN, with particular reference to prevention of HFpEF and its treatment in established HFpEF. There have been five modern randomized controlled trials (RCTs) in HFpEF of drugs that lower BP that were powered to detect changes in long-term outcomes, as summarized in Table 20.2.[26–28,30,35] Four of them tested commonly used BP-lowering drug classes. The fifth tested the mineralocorticoid antagonist spironolactone, which is usually used for resistant HTN. Each of these drugs of course has important, non-BP-lowering effects that might be efficacious in HFpEF. None of the trials met its primary end point. It is unclear if lack of benefit was due to the fact that some or all of these agents are simply ineffective or trial design was at fault. As an example of the latter, none of these RCTs met the modern EF cutoff of 50% required for the diagnosis of HFpEF, with the SENIORS trial classifying EFs as low as 35% as HFpEF. Interestingly, regression of CR was not observed in these trials but has been observed during the course of treatment for HTN in patients without HFpEF.[47]

As mentioned earlier, it is also important to note that a signal indicating possible benefit was detected in the TOPCAT trial of spironolactone. TOPCAT was an international trial in which sites from two of the contributing countries had markedly lower event rates than the rest of the sites, which effectively reduced the trial's power. With these sites eliminated from the analysis, there appeared to be a benefit. As a result, consideration of the use of spironolactone in HFpEF patients who meet the TOPCAT entry criteria has been encouraged,[48] especially since the drug improved quality of life.[48] With regard to ongoing trials, the results of the PARAGON trial of combined valsartan + sacubitril (Entresto),[31] which has been shown to have long-term benefit in HFrEF, are eagerly awaited.

Lacking evidence-based guidance from large HFpEF RCTs in regard to preferred BP-lowering strategies, it is very difficult to be dogmatic about treating HTN in HFpEF patients. Clinicians are dependent on published guidelines and expert opinion for treatment of HTN in general and in HFpEF patients in particular.[1,2,17,19] A detailed discussion of general HTN guidelines and their evidence base is beyond the scope of this chapter. For patients with T2DM and/or evidence of existing vascular disease (i.e., most HFpEF patients), interference with the renin-angiotensin system (RAS) with angiotensin-converting enzyme (ACE) inhibitors or angiotensin II receptor blockers (ARBs) has demonstrated long-term benefit in reducing cardiovascular and renal complications regardless of long-term effects on HFpEF per se, and current guidelines recommend their use for treating HTN in established HFpEF.[17,19] Beyond RAS inhibitors, management of HTN is empirical and should be guideline driven to the extent possible. The high incidence of resistant HTN, T2DM, and CKD in the HFpEF population often modifies HTN management, and multiple BP-lowering drugs are typically required. Thus, because of resistant HTN and comorbidities, spironolactone (in addition to its possible long-term benefit) and loop diuretics often have important roles. At the same time, CKD may limit use of renin-angiotensin-aldosterone system (RAAS) antagonists. Use of beta blockers in HFpEF has been mentioned in our illustrative case study. Current guidelines list beta blockers as having a Class IIA–C indication for treatment of HTN in HFpEF patients. However, it is our belief that the weight of evidence does not in fact support their use in the absence of some other indication (e.g., rate control in atrial fibrillation).[20,21] One negative effect of beta blockers that may be important in this regard is that while they reduce peripheral arterial BP they actually raise central arterial pressure.

Although nitrates are not commonly used to treat HTN, their use should also be avoided in established HFpEF because in the NEAT-HFpEF trial[50] isosorbide mononitrate failed to improve symptoms and exercise capacity and may have had deleterious effects.

TABLE 20.2 The Five Modern RCTs in HFpEF of Drugs That Lower BP Powered to Detect Changes in Long-Term Outcomes

	CHARM (candesartan)	SENIORS (nebivolol)	PEP-CHF (perindopril)	I-PRESERVE (irbesartan)	TOPCAT (spironolactone)
EF cutoff (%)	>40	>35	>40	>45	>45
Diastolic dysfunction required	No	No	Yes	Yes	Yes
Positive outcomes	↓ hospitalizations	Trend↓ mortality, hospitalizations	Trend↓ hospitalizations, symptoms at 2-year follow-up	None	Trend↓ CV death, hospitalizations

BP, Blood pressure; *CV*, cardiovascular; *EF*, ejection fraction; *HFpEF*, heart failure with preserved ejection fraction; *RCT*, randomized controlled trial.
Adapted from McMurray JJ, Ostergren J, Swedberg K, Granger CB, Held P, Michelson EL, et al. Effects of candesartan in patients with chronic heart failure and preserved left-ventricular ejection fraction: the CHARM-Preserved trial. *Lancet* 2003;362(9386):777–781; Cleland JG, Tendera M, Adamus J, Freemantle N, Polonski L, Taylor J. The perindopril in elderly people with chronic heart failure (PEP-CHF) study. *Eur Heart J.* 2006;27(19):2338–2345; van Veldhuisen DJ, Cohen-Solal A, Böhm M, Anker SD, Babalis D, Roughton M, et al. Beta-blockade with nebivolol in elderly heart failure patients with impaired and preserved left ventricular ejection fraction: data from SENIORS (Study of effects of nebivolol intervention on outcomes and rehospitalization in seniors with heart failure). *J Am Coll Cardiol.* 2009;53(23):2150–2158; Pitt B, Pfeffer MA, Assmann SF, Boineau R, Anand IS, Claggett B, et al. Spironolactone for heart failure with preserved ejection fraction. *N Engl J Med.* 2014;370(15):1383–1392; Massie BM, Carson PE, McMurray JJ, Komajda M, McKelvie R, Zile MR, et al. Irbesartan in patients with heart failure and preserved ejection fraction. *N Engl J Med.* 2008;359(23):2456–2467.

Prevention of HFpEF is clearly an important public health goal. A priori, it seems likely that effective treatment of HTN should contribute toward reduction of the subsequent development of HFpEF, and this is an extremely important research direction. To date no specific HTN treatment has been shown to accomplish this. However, no large HTN treatment trials have actually focused on development of HFpEF as an explicit end point. Thus there is no evidence to support the use of specific BP-lowering drugs in HFpEF prevention. At present we must rely once again on general HTN treatment guidelines[1,2] and hope that they achieve this goal. It is important to remember that chlorthalidone remains the general use BP-lowering drug with the strongest evidence for reduction in various long-term HTN complications, while RAAS inhibitors are again preferred agents in patients with T2DM/insulin resistance and/or overt vascular disease. Despite the current HTN guidelines[2] we believe that beta blockers should also be avoided for the general treatment of HTN in patients without other non-BP-lowering indications for their use.[20,21] Additional data to further clarify the use of beta blockers would be welcome.

Given the public health burden of HFpEF, prevention trials of HTN treatments focused on patients at elevated risk for HFpEF (e.g., those with metabolic syndrome) with echocardiography built into the design are worthy of consideration. In light of prior HFpEF RCT failures it may be that prevention will be easier to achieve than treatment of established HFpEF.

With respect to BP-lowering targets and HFpEF prevention, the landmark SPRINT trial may provide some clues or at least the basis for future research.[3] Briefly, SPRINT randomized HTN patients at elevated cardiovascular risk to a strategy of achieving a systolic BP of 120 mmHg or less versus achieving a BP of 140 mmHg or less. The protocol allowed the use of all approved BP-lowering agents and encouraged but did not mandate those with the strongest evidence for reduction in long-term HTN complications (e.g., chlorthalidone). The lower BP strategy was found to substantially reduce the risk of a composite end point of HTN complications, including acute decompensated HF. The SPRINT trial challenges our notion of what is meant by HTN. Based on its results roughly half of ostensibly healthy individuals may be considered to have treatable BP. Going forward, it may make more sense to simply define optimal BP goals rather than labeling patients as having HTN as a disease.

Of all the component end points in SPRINT, the decrease in incident HF was largest and statistically most significant. The results of SPRINT are still being incorporated into clinical practice. The fact that the lower BP strategy incurred a higher incidence of adverse effects will likely be a major issue with respect to how much influence the trial ultimately has. Nonetheless, the impressive reduction in incident HF suggests that the lower BP strategy may be effective in HFpEF prevention. However, several factors limit the applicability of SPRINT to HF prevention. The trial did not include a LV EF measurement, and therefore it is unknown whether the incidence of HFpEF was reduced. Moreover, the fact that the trial end point was acute decompensated HF excludes patients with HF who did not present in this fashion. The trial also specifically excluded patients with T2DM, eliminating a major component of the HFpEF population. Nonetheless, since SPRINT was a HTN trial, there is a strong likelihood that the occurrence of acute decompensated HFpEF was in fact reduced. Last, since the trial was largely agnostic with respect to BP-lowering agents, it does not provide guidance as to which agent(s) might be preferred for HF prevention. Thus, while SPRINT suggests that a lower BP target might prevent HFpEF in patients with HTN, this clearly remains to be proven. Moreover, the experience gained from SPRINT suggests that a somewhat smaller trial with HF as an end point, including EF measurement, could be adequately powered to assess BP-lowering targets in the prevention of HFpEF.

Recent HTN and HF guideline modifications[2,19] have incorporated the SPRINT results by recommending that the target for systolic BP lowering in general as well as in established HFpEF should be lowered from 140 mmHg and less to 130 mmHg and less. The selection of 130 mmHg instead of 120 mmHg SPRINT target recognizes both the higher incidence of adverse effects in the 120 mmHg target group in SPRINT as well as the fact that BPs in SPRINT were measured after 5 minutes in a quiet room, which is often not adhered to in routine practice.

FUTURE DIRECTIONS

As we have seen, optimal goals of BP management in HTN patients and whether there is a preferred BP-lowering regimen for prevention and treatment of HFpEF remain uncertain and constitute important knowledge gaps and goals for future research.

In view of the fact that patients with the complex of abnormalities constituting the metabolic syndrome (HTN, T2DM/insulin resistance, central obesity, elevated LDL cholesterol) constitute such a large proportion of the contemporary HFpEF population, it is important to mention the role of lifestyle modification, specifically weight loss and exercise. These are first-line treatments of HTN and are likely to receive greater emphasis in the future in prevention and treatment of HFpEF. Moreover, improvement in indexes of diastolic function, regression of LVH, and improved exercise tolerance have been reported after bariatric surgery.[51,52] Sustained, nonsurgical weight loss and exercise are difficult to achieve and maintain, but in small studies newer approaches have had improved success while ameliorating components of the metabolic syndrome,[23] improving exercise tolerance, and achieving LV mass regression and improved diastolic function in patients with established HFpEF.[22,53] There are no data in regard to prevention of HFpEF in such at-risk patients, but a priori it would seem likely that sustained weight loss and exercise would have a good chance of success. Moreover, there is ample evidence that HTN, insulin resistance, and even diastolic dysfunction and CR are detectable early in life in obese subjects.[54] Thus attempts to further develop and refine sustained weight loss and exercise programs, especially in young people, deserve additional future consideration in both the prevention and treatment of HFpEF. This might possibly be combined with pharmacologic approaches to weight loss (e.g., sodium glucose transporter-2 [SGLT-2] inhibitors), which result in both weight loss and modest BP reduction and strikingly reduce incident HF in patients with T2DM.[55]

In summary, in recent years much progress has been made in achieving a mechanistic understanding of how HTN affects the myocardium and the left ventricle, especially with reference to mechanisms of diastolic dysfunction and HFpEF. Recent years have also seen significant advances with respect to defining optimal BP goals and how to achieve them. These advances, along with an increasing emphasis on lifestyle modifications, especially in younger individuals, offer the promise of improved primary prevention of the adverse cardiovascular consequences of HTN, including HFpEF. Unfortunately, with the possible exception of spironolactone, attempts to treat established HFpEF with conventional BP-lowering drugs have been disappointing. While control of BP is undeniably important, it is notable that of the 22 currently active or planned HFpEF clinical trials,[56] only the PARAGON trial[31] is testing a BP-lowering drug (in combination with nephrolysin inhibition). Thus use of conventional BP-lowering drugs to impact the long-term prognosis of established HFpEF may be an idea whose time has passed.

KEY POINTS

- Hypertension is the most common underlying substrate for HFpEF.
- Hypertension causes concentric LV remodeling, which is present in a majority of HFpEF patients.
- Mechanisms of diastolic dysfunction reported in association with hypertension and concentric remodeling are multifactorial and include alterations in passive stiffness (collagen, titin), Na-Ca handling, and actomyosin cross-bridge dynamics.
- Various comorbidities that can also cause changes in the myocardium are common in HFpEF; therefore it is difficult to know to what extent diastolic dysfunction can be attributed to hypertension per se.
- Blood pressure management is a core component of the treatment of HFpEF.
- Because trials of BP-lowering drugs for HFpEF have been neutral, there is no evidence-based approach for preventing HFpEF in at-risk hypertensive patients or patients with established HFpEF.
- Published hypertension treatment guidelines should be followed in at-risk patients or patients with established HFpEF.
- In established HFpEF the guidelines emphasize use of RAAS blockade as well as chlorthalidone.
- The SPRINT trial has reset the target for systolic BP in general, and in HFpEF patients in particular, to 130 mmHg.
- In patients with metabolic syndrome, who make up a large portion of the HFpEF population, lifestyle modification (diet, exercise) should be an important part of the management of hypertension.

REVIEW QUESTIONS

1. Which of the following myocardial changes has been reported to contribute to diastolic dysfunction in hypertensive patients with HFpEF?
   a. Reduced activity of sarcoplasmic reticulum ATPase 2 (SERCA-2)
   b. Reduced phosphorylation of troponin I
   c. Decreased phosphorylation of PKA/PKG sites on titin
   c. Decreased extracellular matrix collagen
2. Which of the following is the most common comorbidity associated with HFpEF?
   a. Type 2 diabetes mellitus
   b. Obstructive sleep apnea
   c. Hypertension
   c. Chronic kidney disease
3. Guideline-recommended first-line BP-lowering agents in patients with HFpEF include which of the following?
   a. Hydralazine
   b. Isosorbide mononitrate
   c. Chlorthalidone
   c. Metoprolol tartrate

REFERENCES

1. Whelton PK, Carey RM, Aronow WS, Casey Jr DE, Collins KJ, Dennison Himmelfarb C, et al. 2017 ACC/AHA/AAPA/ABC/ACPM/AGS/APhA/ASH/ASPC/NMA/PCNA guideline for the prevention, detection, evaluation, and management of high blood pressure in adults: a report of the American College of Cardiology/American Heart Association Task Force on Clinical Practice Guidelines. *J Am Coll Cardiol.* 2018;71(19):e127–e248.
2. Reboussin DM, Allen NB, Griswold ME, Guallar E, Hong Y, Lackland DT, et al. Systematic review for the 2017 ACC/AHA/AAPA/ABC/ACPM/AGS/APhA/ASH/ASPC/NMA/PCNA guideline for the prevention, detection, evaluation, and management of high blood pressure in adults: a report of the American College of Cardiology/American Heart Association Task Force on Clinical Practice Guidelines. *J Am Coll Cardiol.* 2018;71(19):2176–2198.
3. SPRINT Research Group, Wright Jr JT, Williamson JD, Whelton PK, Snyder JK, Sink KM, et al. A randomized trial of intensive versus standard blood-pressure control. *N Engl J Med.* 2015;373(22):2103–2116.
4. Paulus WJ, Tschöpe C, Sanderson JE, Rusconi C, Flachskampf FA, Rademakers FE, et al. How to diagnose diastolic heart failure: a consensus statement on the diagnosis of heart failure with normal left ventricular ejection fraction by the Heart Failure and Echocardiography Associations of the European Society of Cardiology. *Eur Heart J.* 2007;28(20):2539–2550.
5. Lekavich CL, Barksdale DJ, Neelon V, Wu JR. Heart failure preserved ejection fraction (HFpEF): an integrated and strategic review. *Heart Fail Rev.* 2015;20(6):642–653.
6. Reddy YNV, Olson TP, Obokata M, Melenovsky V, Borlaug BA. Hemodynamic correlates and diagnostic role of cardiopulmonary exercise testing in heart failure with preserved ejection fraction. *JACC Heart Fail.* 2018;6(8):665–675.
7. Roca GQ, Shah AM. Sleep disordered breathing: hypertension and cardiac structure and function. *Curr Hypertens Rep.* 2015;17(12):91–100.
8. Jia G, DeMarco VG, Sowers JR. Insulin resistance and hyperinsulinaemia in diabetic cardiomyopathy. *Nat Rev Endocrinol.* 2016;12(3):144–153.
9. LeWinter MM, Meyer M. Mechanisms of diastolic dysfunction in heart failure with a preserved ejection fraction: if it's not one thing it's another. *Circ Heart Fail.* 2013;6(6):1112–1115.
10. Donaldson C, Palmer BM, Zile M, Maughan DW, Ikonomidis JS, Granzier H, et al. Myosin cross-bridge dynamics in patients with hypertension and concentric left ventricular remodeling. *Circ Heart Fail.* 2012;5(6):803–811.
11. Selby DE, Palmer BM, LeWinter MM, Meyer M. Tachycardia-induced diastolic dysfunction and resting tone in myocardium from patients with a normal ejection fraction. *J Am Coll Cardiol.* 2011;58(2):147–154.
12. Runte KE, Bell SP, Selby DE, Häußler TN, Ashikaga T, LeWinter MM, et al. Relaxation and the role of calcium in isolated contracting myocardium from patients with hypertensive heart disease and heart failure with preserved ejection fraction. *Circ Heart Fail.* 2017;10(8):e004311.
13. Borbély A, van der Velden J, Papp Z, Bronzwaer JG, Edes I, Stienen GJ, et al. Cardiomyocyte stiffness in diastolic heart failure. *Circulation.* 2005;111(6):774–781.
14. Obokata M, Reddy YNV, Melenovsky V, Kane GC, Olson TP, Jarolim P, et al. Myocardial injury and cardiac reserve in patients with heart failure and preserved ejection fraction. *J Am Coll Cardiol.* 2018;72(1):29–40.
15. Zile MR, Baicu CF, Ikonomidis JS, Stroud RE, Nietert PJ, Bradshaw AD, et al. Myocardial stiffness in patients with heart failure and a preserved ejection fraction: contributions of collagen and titin. *Circulation.* 2015;131(14):1247–1259.
16. Kasner M, Westermann D, Lopez B, Gaub R, Escher F, Kühl U, et al. Diastolic tissue Doppler indexes correlate with the degree of collagen expression and cross-linking in heart failure and normal ejection fraction. *J Am Coll Cardiol.* 2011;57(8):977–985.
17. Yancy CW, Jessup M, Bozkurt B, Butler J, Casey Jr DE, Drazner MH, et al. 2013 ACCF/AHA guideline for the management of heart failure: a report of the American College of Cardiology Foundation/American Heart Association Task Force on Practice Guidelines. *J Am Coll Cardiol.* 2013;62(16):e147–e239.

18. Hwang SJ, Melenovsky V, Borlaug BA. Implications of coronary artery disease in heart failure with preserved ejection fraction. *J Am Coll Cardiol.* 2014;63(25 Pt A):2817–2827.
19. Yancy CW, Jessup M, Bozkurt B, Butler J, Casey Jr DE, Colvin MM, et al. 2017 ACC/AHA/HFSA focused update of the 2013 ACCF/AHA guideline for the management of heart failure: a report of the American College of Cardiology/American Heart Association Task Force on Clinical Practice Guidelines and the Heart Failure Society of America. *J Am Coll Cardiol.* 2017;70(6):776–803.
20. Meyer M, Rambod M, LeWinter M. Pharmacological heart rate lowering in patients with a preserved ejection fraction-review of a failing concept. *Heart Fail Rev.* 2018;23(4):499–506.
21. Nambiar L, Meyer M. Beta-blockers in myocardial infarction and coronary artery disease with a preserved ejection fraction: recommendations, mechanisms, and concerns. *Coron Artery Dis.* 2-18;29(3):262-270.
22. Upadhya B, Haykowsky MJ, Kitzman DW. Therapy for heart failure with preserved ejection fraction: current status, unique challenges, and future directions. *Heart Fail Rev.* 2018;23:609–629.
23. Ades PA, Savage PD, Toth MJ, Harvey-Berino J, Schneider DJ, Bunn JY, et al. High-calorie-expenditure exercise: a new approach to cardiac rehabilitation for overweight coronary patients. *Circulation.* 2009;119(20):2671–2678.
24. Klapholz M, Maurer M, Lowe AM, Messineo F, Meisner JS, Mitchell J, et al. Hospitalization for heart failure in the presence of a normal left ventricular ejection fraction: results of the New York Heart Failure Registry. *J Am Coll Cardiol.* 2004;43(8):1432–1438.
25. Lam CS, Roger VL, Rodeheffer RJ, Bursi F, Borlaug BA, Ommen SR, et al. Cardiac structure and ventricular-vascular function in persons with heart failure and preserved ejection fraction from Olmsted County. *Minnesota. Circulation.* 2007;115(15):1982–1990.
26. McMurray JJ, Ostergren J, Swedberg K, Granger CB, Held P, Michelson EL, et al. Effects of candesartan in patients with chronic heart failure and preserved left-ventricular ejection fraction: the CHARM-Preserved trial. *Lancet.* 2003;362(9386):777–781.
27. Cleland JG, Tendera M, Adamus J, Freemantle N, Polonski L, Taylor J. The perindopril in elderly people with chronic heart failure (PEP-CHF) study. *Eur Heart J.* 2006;27(19):2338–2345.
28. van Veldhuisen DJ, Cohen-Solal A, Böhm M, Anker SD, Babalis D, Roughton M, et al. Beta-blockade with nebivolol in elderly heart failure patients with impaired and preserved left ventricular ejection fraction: data from SENIORS (Study of effects of nebivolol intervention on outcomes and rehospitalization in seniors with heart failure). *J Am Coll Cardiol.* 2009;53(23):2150–2158.
29. Zile MR, Gottdiener JS, Hetzel SJ, McMurray JJ, Komajda M, McKelvie R, et al. Prevalence and significance of alterations in cardiac structure and function in patients with heart failure and a preserved ejection fraction. *Circulation.* 2011;124(23):2491–2501.
30. Pitt B, Pfeffer MA, Assmann SF, Boineau R, Anand IS, Claggett B, et al. Spironolactone for heart failure with preserved ejection fraction. *N Engl J Med.* 2014;370(15):1383–1392.
31. Solomon SD, Rizkala AR, Gong J, Wang W, Anand IS, Ge J, et al. Angiotensin receptor neprilysin inhibition in heart failure with preserved ejection fraction: rationale and design of the PARAGON-HF Trial. *JACC Heart Fail.* 2017;5(7):471–482.
32. de Simone G, Greco R, Mureddu G, Romano C, Guida R, Celentano A, et al. Relation of left ventricular diastolic properties to systolic function in arterial hypertension. *Circulation.* 2000;101(2):152–157.
33. Messerli FH, Rimoldi SF, Bangalore S. The transition from hypertension to heart failure: contemporary update. *JACC Heart Fail.* 2017;5(8):543–551.
34. Zile MR, Baicu CF, Gaasch WH. Diastolic heart failure-abnormalities in active relaxation and passive stiffness of the left ventricle. *N Engl J Med.* 2004;350(19):1953–1959.
35. Massie BM, Carson PE, McMurray JJ, Komajda M, McKelvie R, Zile MR, et al. Irbesartan in patients with heart failure and preserved ejection fraction. *N Engl J Med.* 2008;359(23):2456–2467.
36. Takeuchi M, Borden WB, Nakai H, Nishikage T, Kokumai M, Nagakura T, et al. Reduced and delayed untwisting of the left ventricle in patients with hypertension and left ventricular hypertrophy: a study using two-dimensional speckle tracking imaging. *Eur Heart J.* 2007;28(22):2756–2762.
37. Bell SP, Fabian J, Watkins MW, LeWinter MM. Decrease in forces responsible for diastolic suction during acute coronary occlusion. *Circulation.* 1997;96:2348–2352.
38. Dumor K, Shoemaker-Moyle M, Nistala R, Whaley-Connell A. Arterial stiffness in hypertension: an update. *Curr Hypertens Rep.* 2018;20(8):72.
39. Zile MR, Gaasch WH. Mechanical loads and the isovolumic and filling indices of left ventricular relaxation. *Prog Cardiovasc Dis.* 1990;32(5):333–346.
40. Borbély A, Falcao-Pires I, van Heerebeek L, Hamdani N, Edes I, Gavina C, et al. Hypophosphorylation of the stiff N2B titin isoform raises cardiomyocyte resting tension in failing human myocardium. *Circ Res.* 2009;104(6):780–788.
41. LeWinter MM, Granzier HL. Cardiac titin and heart disease. *J Cardiovasc Pharmacol.* 2014;63(3):207–212.
42. Schwartzkopff B, Frenzel H, Dieckerhoff J, Betz P, Flasshove M, Schulte HD, et al. Morphometric investigation of human myocardium in arterial hypertension and valvular aortic stenosis. *Eur Heart J.* 1992;13(D):S17–S23.
43. Weber KT, Sun Y, Guarda E. Structural remodeling in hypertensive heart disease and the role of hormones. *Hypertension.* 1994;23(6 Pt 2):869–877.
44. Bodiga VL, Eda SR, Bodiga S. Advanced glycation end products: role in pathology of diabetic cardiomyopathy. *Heart Fail Rev.* 2014;19(1):49–63.
45. van Heerebeek L, Hamdani N, Falcão-Pires I, Leite-Moreira AF, Begieneman MP, Bronzwaer JG, et al. Low myocardial protein kinase G activity in heart failure with preserved ejection fraction. *Circulation.* 2012;126(7):830–839.
46. Paulus WJ, Tschope C. A novel paradigm for heart failure with preserved ejection fraction: comorbidities drive myocardial dysfunction and remodeling through coronary microvascular endothelial inflammation. *J Am Coll Cardiol.* 2013;62(4):263–271.
47. Lønnebakken MT, Izzo R, Mancusi C, Gerdts E, Losi MA, Canciello G, et al. Left ventricular hypertrophy regression during antihypertensive treatment in an outpatient clinic (the Campania Salute Network). *J Am Heart Assoc.* 2017;6(3):e004152.
48. Ferreira JP, Mentz RJ, Pizard A, Pitt B, Zannad F. Tailoring mineralocorticoid receptor antagonist therapy in heart failure patients: are we moving towards a personalized approach?. *Eur J Heart Fail.* 2017;19(8):974–986.
49. Lewis EF, Kim HY, Claggett B, Spertus J, Heitner JF, Assmann SF, et al. Impact of spironolactone on longitudinal changes in health-related quality of life in the treatment of preserved cardiac function heart failure with an aldosterone antagonist trial. *Circ Heart Fail.* 2016;9(3):e001937.
50. Redfield MM, Anstrom KJ, Levine JA, Koepp GA, Borlaug BA, Chen HH, et al. Isosorbide mononitrate in heart failure with preserved ejection fraction. *N Engl J Med.* 2015;373(24):2314–2324.
51. Owan T, Avelar E, Morley K, Jiji R, Hall N, Krezowski J, et al. Favorable changes in cardiac geometry and function following gastric bypass surgery: 2-year follow-up in the Utah obesity study. *J Am Coll Cardiol.* 2011;57(6):732–739.
52. Le Jemtel TH, Samson R, Jaiswal A, Lewine EB, Oparil S. Regression of left ventricular mass after bariatric surgery. *Curr Hypertens Rep.* 2017;19(9):68.
53. Kitzman DW, Brubaker PH, Morgan TM, Stewart KP, Little WC. Exercise training in older patients with heart failure and preserved ejection fraction. *Circ Heart Fail.* 2010;3(6):659–667.
54. Titmuss AT, Srinivasan S. Metabolic syndrome in children and adolescents: old concepts in a young population. *J Paediatr Child Health.* 2016;52(10):928–934.
55. Raz I, Cahn A. Heart failure: SGLT2 inhibitors and heart failure—clinical implications. *Nat Rev Cardiol.* 2016;13(4):185–186.
56. Parikh KS, Sharma K, Fiuzat M, Surks HK, George JT, Honarpour N, et al. Heart failure with preserved ejection fraction expert panel report: current controversies and implications for clinical trials. *JACC Heart Fail.* 2018;6(8):619–632.

21

Valve Disease

Ruxandra Beyer and Frank A. Flachskampf

OUTLINE

INTRODUCTION

Mild degrees of valvular heart disease are very prevalent in adult patients with heart failure symptoms. Given that these are often patients with hypertension, aortic valve sclerosis and mitral annular calcification, frequently accompanied by some degree of mitral regurgitation, are extremely common. They need to be taken into consideration when assessing such patients. On the other hand, severe left-sided valvular heart disease may also lead to the clinical syndrome of heart failure. Naturally, the hemodynamic consequences of severe valvular lesions (e.g., in aortic stenosis) take priority over the assessment of myocardial diastolic function for making clinical decisions. Nevertheless, it is helpful to review the impact of such lesions on diastolic left ventricular (LV) pressure levels and diastolic function, and their echocardiographic correlates, since following valve replacement many patients will have persisting symptoms caused by the long-term effect of LV remodeling leading to diastolic dysfunction.

EPIDEMIOLOGY OF VALVULAR HEART DISEASE

Valvular heart disease increases in prevalence with age. The most frequent valvular lesion requiring repair is aortic stenosis, followed by mitral regurgitation. Aortic stenosis is very prevalent (3%–5%) in the elderly population. Aortic regurgitation is considerably rarer, and severe mitral stenosis is almost exclusively rheumatic in origin and thus rare in developed countries. On the other hand, degenerative calcific mitral stenosis has become more frequent due to the aging of the general population, but mostly is hemodynamically mild. It does affect, however, parameters used in echocardiography to assess diastolic function, such as e′, and thus needs to be taken into account when interpreting such parameters.

Case Study 1

An 82-year-old man with aortic stenosis is admitted for repetitive transient loss of consciousness and progressive dyspnea. The patient is on insulin therapy for diabetes mellitus with vascular, neurologic, and renal complications. At admission, ankle edema and hepatomegaly are observed. Auscultation reveals a grade III-IV systolic ejection murmur and rales in the lungs. His BP is 110/80 mmHg and heart rate 65 bpm. His N-terminal pro-brain natriuretic peptide (NT-proBNP) is 985 pg/mL (normal: <125 pg/mL). Electrocardiogram (ECG) shows sinus rhythm, LV hypertrophy with discordant ST-T changes. An echocardiogram is performed, and selected images are shown (Figs. 21.1, 21.2, 21.3, 21.4, 21.5, 21.6, 21.7, and 21.8; Videos 21.1 and 21.2). Coronary angiography shows diffuse coronary disease without significant stenosis. The Euroscore II is 10.46%, and STS 5%. The patient will subsequently undergo percutaneous aortic valve implantation.

AORTIC STENOSIS

In aortic stenosis with preserved ejection fraction, LV concentric remodeling or hypertrophy leads to slowed myocardial relaxation in early diastole, low chamber compliance, and increased myocardial stiffness, especially at a higher age (see Case Study 1). These changes are at least partially reversible after aortic valve replacement.[1]

Additionally, long-standing aortic stenosis leads to myocardial interstitial fibrosis, and a considerable fraction of elderly patients with aortic stenosis also develop some degree of cardiac amyloidosis.[2] The latter is impossible to differentiate by echocardiography from concentric remodeling due the valvular stenosis, but can be characterized by cardiac magnetic resonance imaging (cardiac MRI) or nuclear imaging. Fibrosis and amyloidosis are known to impair LV diastolic function; thus their detection suggests indirectly possible diastolic dysfunction. Global longitudinal echocardiographic strain has been shown to correlate modestly with diffuse myocardial fibrosis in patients with aortic stenosis.[3]

On cardiac MRI, diffuse interstitial myocardial fibrosis leads to increased myocardial T1 values and increased extracellular volume estimates. Thus these parameters may be interpreted as markers of diastolic dysfunction, although the strength of the association between T1 values and histologic parameters of fibrosis, such as collagen volume fraction, is quite modest.[4] Furthermore, replacement fibrosis, or the presence of localized increases in extracellular space, may be visible as midwall late enhancement after gadolinium (cardiac MRI contrast)

Vmax 5.11 m/sec, gradients 104/69 mmHg

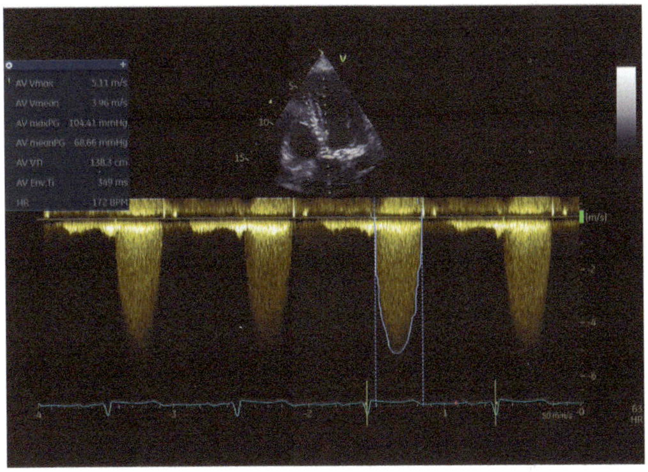

Fig. 21.1 Case 1: Continuous wave Doppler tracing of transaortic flow, showing severe aortic stenosis (Vmax 5.11 m/sec, gradients 104/69 mmHg).

E = 1.2 m/sec
E/A = 0.8

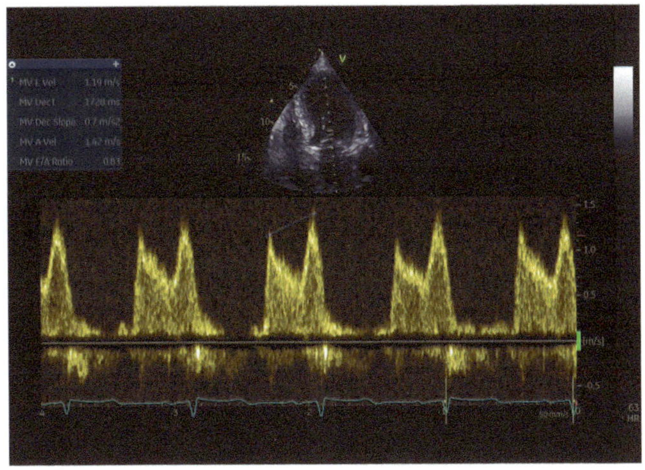

Fig. 21.3 Case 1: Pulsed-wave Doppler of transmitral inflow, showing E/A = 0.8 and Emax velocity of 1.2 m/sec.

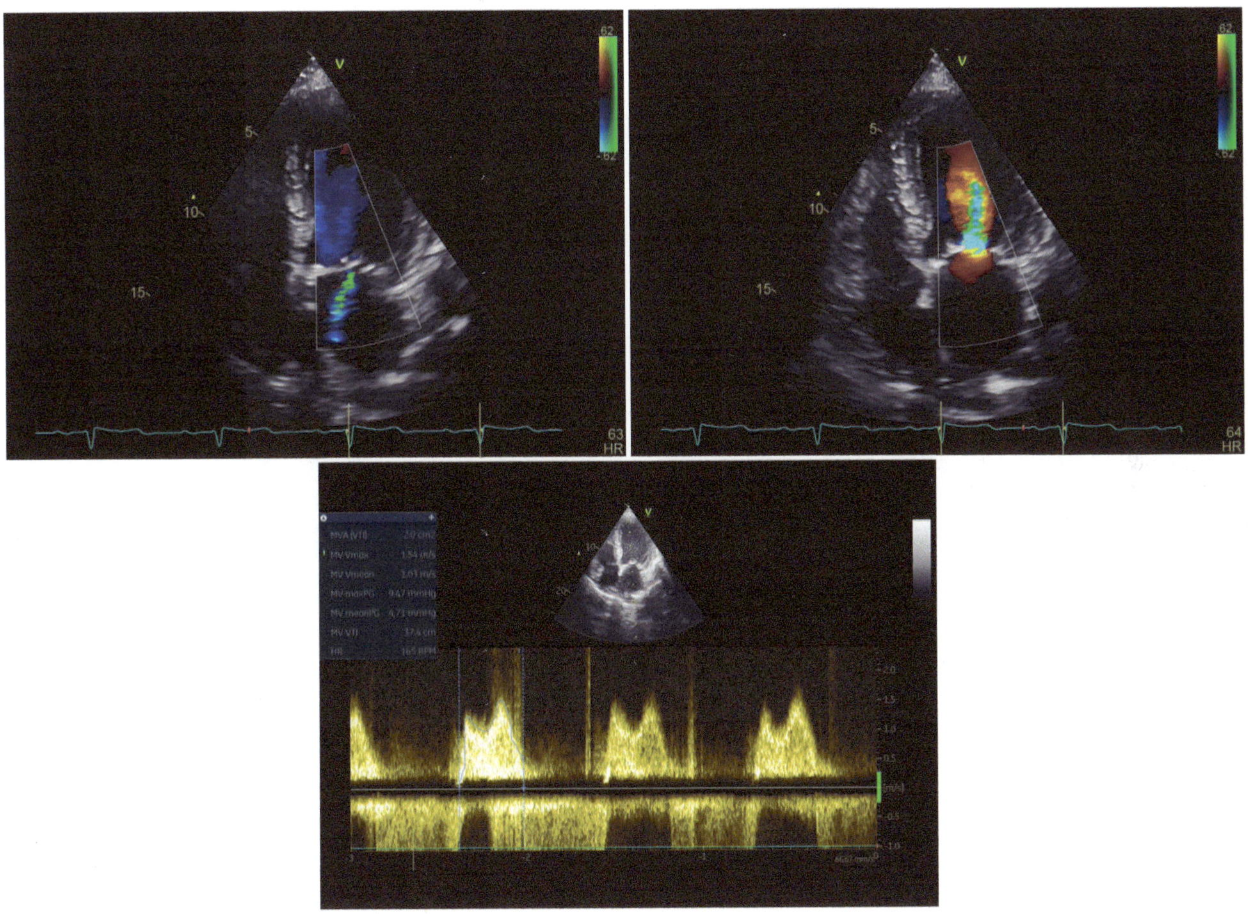

Mean transmitral gradient, 5 mmHg

Fig. 21.2 Case 1: Apical four-chamber color Doppler images in systole *(top left)* and diastole *(top right)*, together with continuous wave Doppler tracing of transmitral flow. Mild degenerative mitral stenosis and regurgitation are seen.

application. The importance of such findings in the individual patient, however, is unclear.

As in all forms of hypertrophy, longitudinal function and thus e′, as well as longitudinal strain parameters, such as global longitudinal strain (GLS), are reduced in aortic stenosis, while ejection fraction is preserved until late in the progression of the disease (see Case Study 1). Diastolic dysfunction is probably the prime cause of the chief symptom of aortic stenosis, dyspnea. Signs of diastolic dysfunction are therefore expected in the context of significant aortic stenosis and should not be construed as necessarily indicating an additional disease.

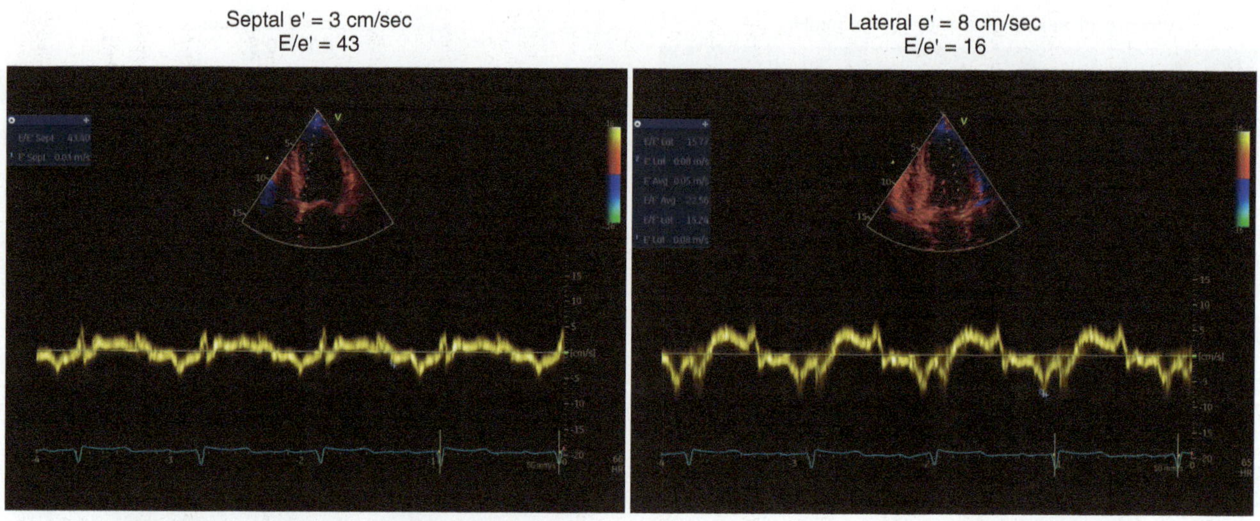

Fig. 21.4 Case 1: Septal *(left)* and lateral *(right)* tissue Doppler recordings from mitral annulus region, showing severely reduced septal e′ of 3 cm/sec and lateral 8 cm/sec. Corresponding E/e′ values are strongly elevated with 43 and 16, respectively.

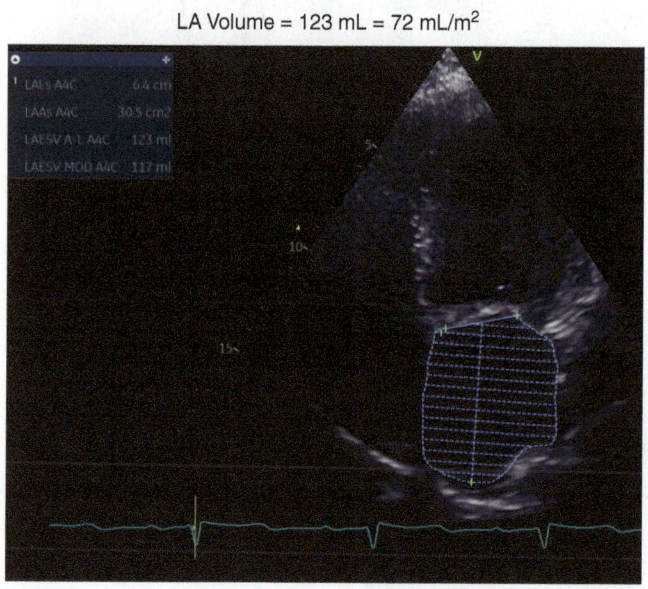

Fig. 21.5 Case 1: Calculation of left atrial volume from the apical four-chamber view at end systole (123 mL or 72 mL/m²).

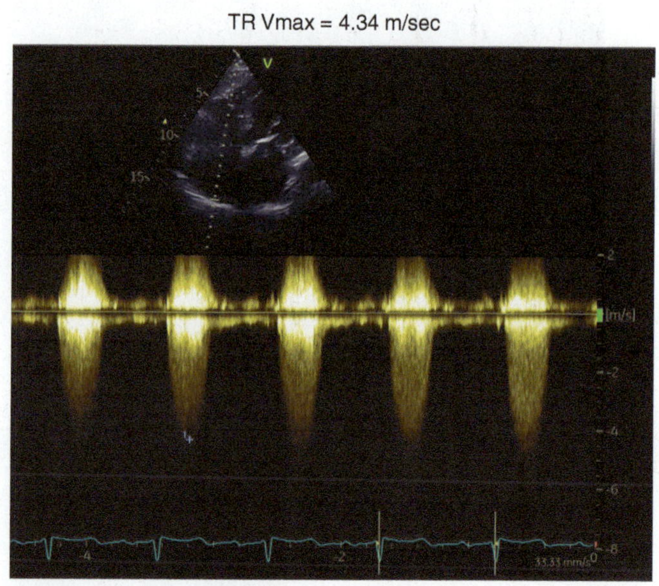

Fig. 21.6 Case 1: Continuous wave Doppler of tricuspid regurgitant velocity, with a maximal velocity of 4.34 m/sec.

However, concomitant hypertension, coronary artery disease, myocardial fibrosis, amyloidosis, and others may be present and contribute to diastolic functional impairment. Thus increased left atrial (LA) volume, low e′ and high E/e′, as well as right-sided pressure increase are frequent in moderate or severe aortic stenosis and indicate LV diastolic dysfunction with increased diastolic pressures. Note that low longitudinal strain is also frequently present in spite of preserved ejection fraction. Other imaging modalities such as cardiac MRI are generally unnecessary to assess diastolic function.

Diastolic LV function contains prognostic information in aortic stenosis. In 125 patients with severe aortic stenosis who were not operated for diverse reasons, E/e′ was the best echo predictor of 1-year survival, both in symptomatic and asymptomatic patients.[5] Recently, a retrospective study of 90 patients[6] undergoing transcatheter intervention for severe aortic stenosis reported that (1) preoperative grade of diastolic dysfunction was a strong predictor of postinterventional 1-year morbidity and mortality, and (2) diastolic dysfunction tended to improve after intervention, but improvement was not clearly related to prognosis (which might be due to study size and/or missing data). In the largest such study (n = 358), an effect of preoperative diastolic function grade on postinterventional mortality could not be shown; however, improvement in diastolic function after transcatheter intervention paralleled clinical improvement, and lack of improvement was associated with a worse prognosis.[7] After aortic valve replacement or intervention, regression of LV hypertrophy and improvement of systolic LV function (by ejection fraction, as well as by longitudinal strain) occur. There is regression of myocardial T1, likely paralleling decrease in myocardial fibrosis.[8] Diastolic function has been shown both invasively and noninvasively to improve over time. However, the degree of normalization varies. Patient-prosthesis mismatch is associated with persistent diastolic dysfunction and adverse prognosis.[9]

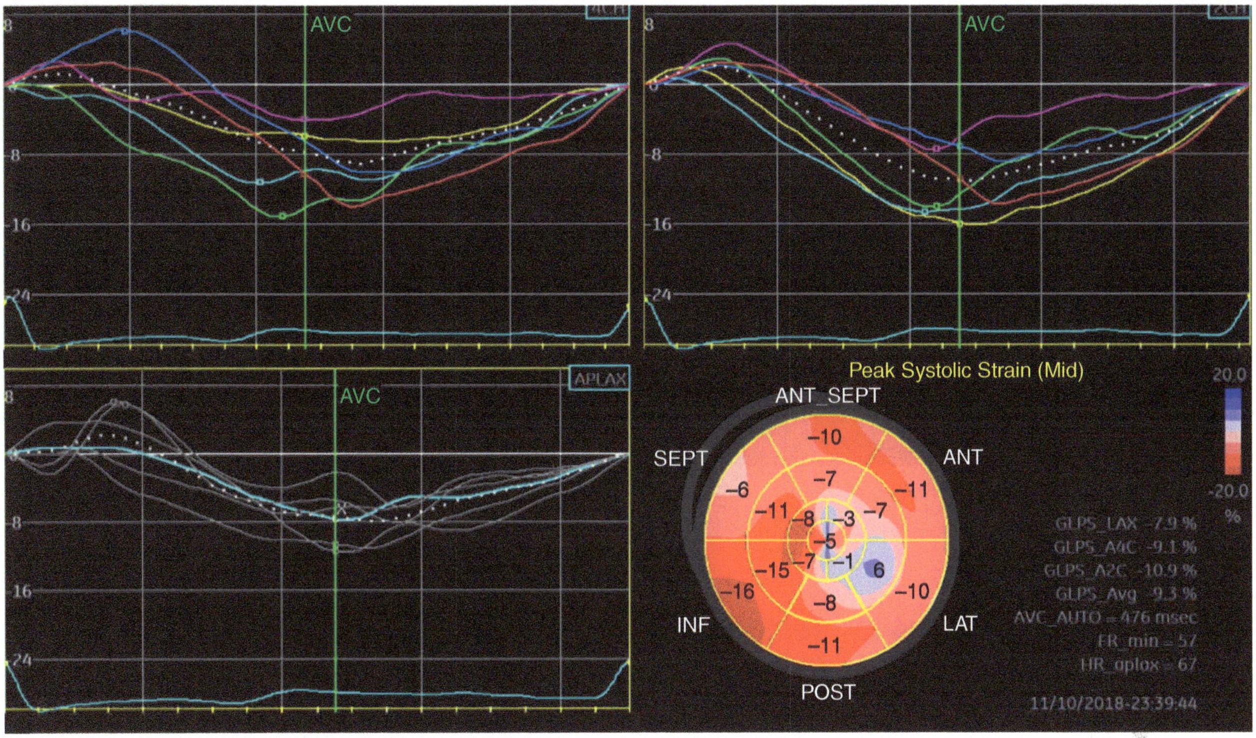

GLS – 9.3%

Fig. 21.7 Case 1: Regional curves and global bull's eye plot of longitudinal strain, with a global longitudinal peak systolic strain *(GLS)* of −9.3% (severely reduced).

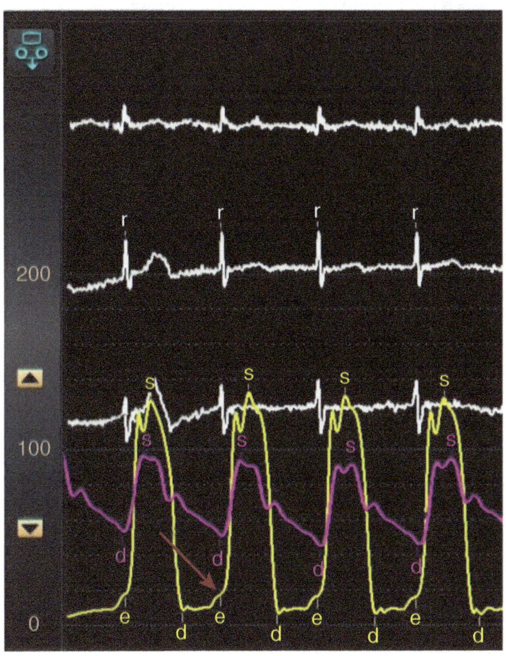

LVEDP 18 mmHg

Fig. 21.8 Case 1: Pressure tracings with superimposed aortic pressures in violet and left ventricular pressures in yellow. Red arrow shows left ventricular end-diastolic pressure *(LVEDP)* of 18 mmHg.

AORTIC REGURGITATION

In aortic regurgitation, the left ventricle in diastole fills through both the mitral and the aortic valve. Invasive studies have shown that LV remodeling in response to the volume load from severe aortic regurgitation leads to myocyte hypertrophy, slowed relaxation, increased chamber stiffness, and increased fibrosis on biopsy, which may partially regress after valve replacement.[10] Aortic regurgitation is therefore almost by definition associated with increased LV diastolic pressures, which may shorten E wave deceleration time. Current guidelines recommend applying the standard three criteria (LA size, E/e′, and right ventricular [RV] pressure) for diagnosis of diastolic dysfunction, but, similar to the situation in mitral regurgitation, it appears problematic to tease out noninvasively the effects of volume overload and genuine myocardial diastolic dysfunction. Acute aortic regurgitation may occur with infective endocarditis or aortic dissection involving the ascending aorta and is characterized by severe hemodynamic impairment, leading to excessively high diastolic pressures and acute pulmonary hypertension. Transmitral E wave deceleration is short (<150 msec), the A wave may be truncated or absent, and diastolic mitral regurgitation may be present.

Case Study 2

A 42-year-old woman was admitted to the hospital for new New York Heart Association (NYHA) III heart failure symptoms and a 4/6 systolic murmur best heard in the left axillary region. Her ECG showed sinus rhythm. NT-proBNP was 445 pg/mL (normal, <125 pg/mL). Transthoracic and transesophageal echocardiograms were performed, and selected images are shown (Figs. 21.9, 21.10, 21.11, 21.12, 21.13, and 21.14; Videos 21.3 and 21.4). As shown, the average E/e′ was elevated.[11] Likewise, pulmonary venous flow showed reduced systolic fraction, which could be due to mitral regurgitation, diastolic dysfunction, or both. The findings indicate diastolic pressure elevation (diastolic dysfunction grade II), but the absence of increased RV pressure suggests that diastolic dysfunction and the effect of mitral regurgitation on central pressures are modest (only slightly elevated E/A ratio). Catheterization revealed a LV end-diastolic pressure of 20 mmHg.

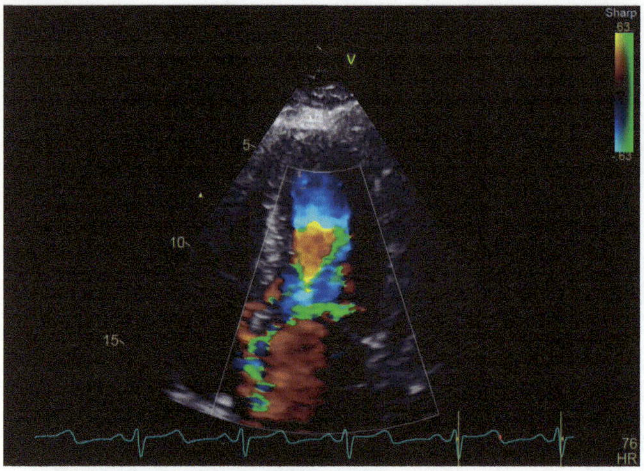

Fig. 21.9 Case 2: Apical four-chamber view. Color Doppler shows a large eccentric anteroseptal regurgitation jet. See also Video 12.3.

MITRAL REGURGITATION

Mild mitral regurgitation of nonischemic origin is nearly universally present in the elderly. Although no conclusive data exist on the long-term impact of mild mitral regurgitation, it is generally believed to have no physiologic consequences. Higher degrees of mitral regurgitation, however, clearly lead to LV and atrial enlargement to accommodate the additional regurgitant volume. In acute mitral regurgitation, the additional volume increases diastolic pressure in the left atrium and ventricle, as has been shown in animal experiments.[12] Over time, the chambers adapt by dilatation, and diastolic pressures fall, although generally, they remain somewhat elevated. Long term, degenerative or primary mitral regurgitation in patients causes a decrease in chamber stiffness, as long as ejection fraction is preserved.[13] Thus diastolic pressures in chronic mitral regurgitation may be only mildly or not at all elevated. However, severe acute mitral regurgitation is usually characterized by increased diastolic pressures (see Case Study 2, which shows a case of new-onset degenerative severe mitral regurgitation). The assessment by echocardiography is hampered by the fact that most signs

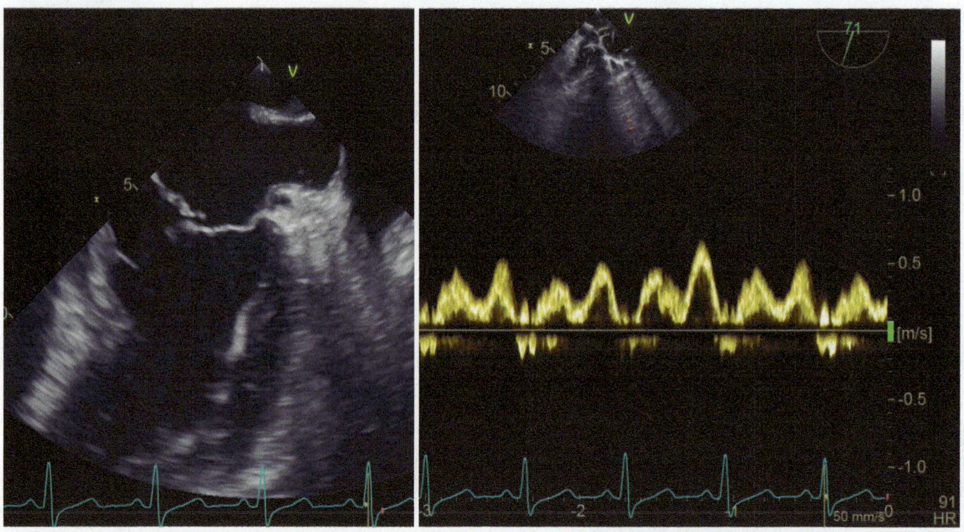

Fig. 21.10 Case 2: Transesophageal image of posterior leaflet prolapse and pulse wave Doppler tracing from superior left pulmonary vein with S/D less than 1 ratio. See also Video 12.4.

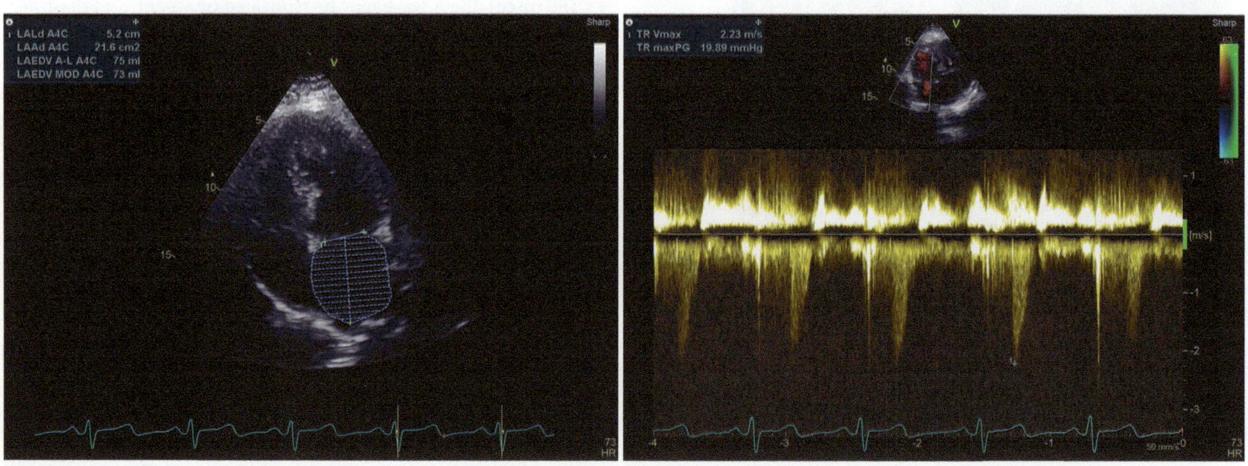

A B

Fig. 21.11 Case 2: Apical four-chamber view. (A) Dilated left atrium = 75 mL = 47 mL/m^2. (B) Continuous wave Doppler of tricuspid regurgitation: Vmax = 2.2 m/sec.

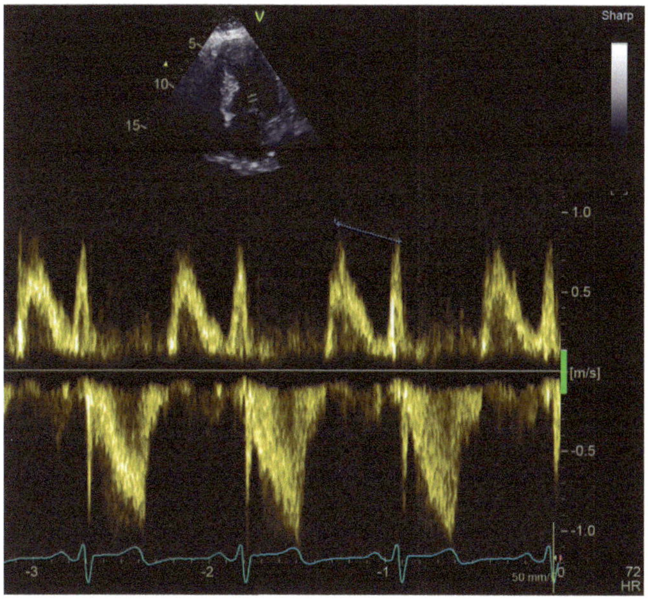

Fig. 21.12 Case 2: Pulse wave Doppler of transmitral inflow. E velocity = 0.92 m/sec, A velocity = 0.82 m/sec.

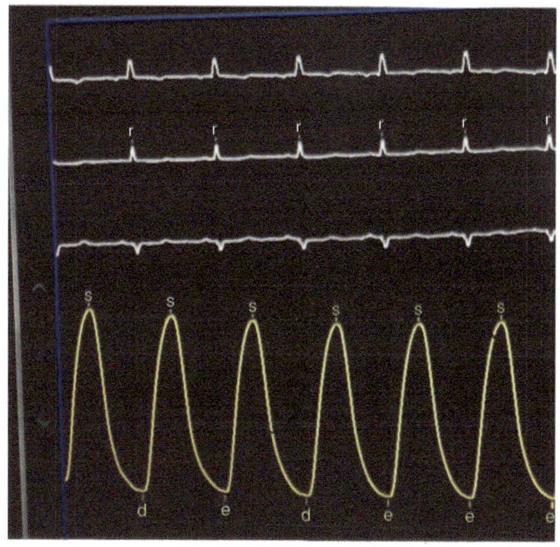

LVEDP 20 mmHg

Fig. 21.14 Case 2: Pressure tracing from the left ventricle (slightly dampened), showing an end-diastolic pressure *(LVEDP)* of 20 mmHg.

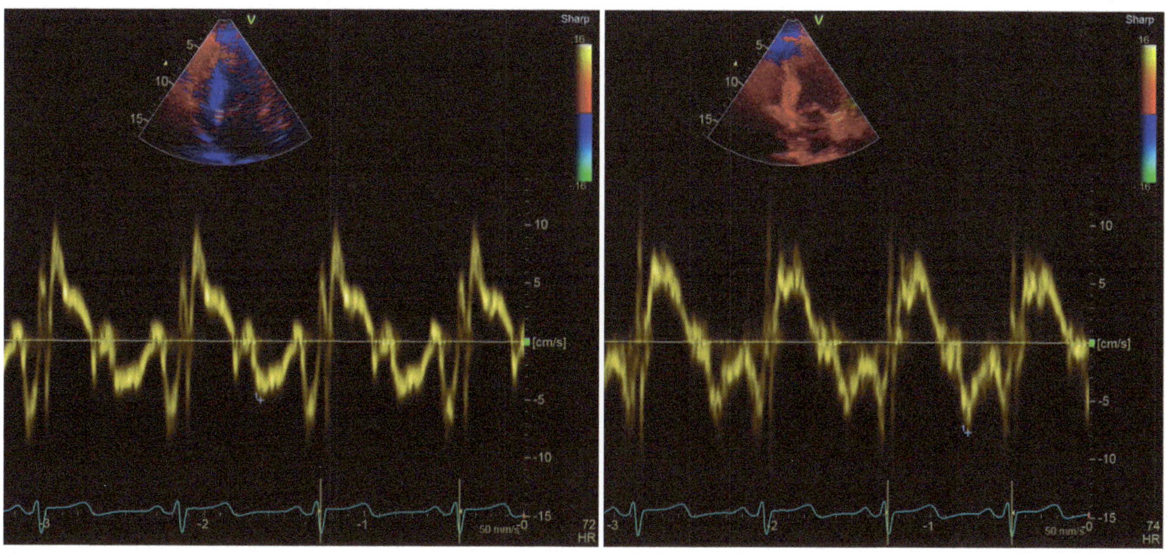

Fig. 21.13 Case 2: Tissue Doppler of the mitral annulus. (A) e′ septal velocity = 5 cm/sec. (B) e′ lateral velocity = 8 cm/sec. E/e′ avg = 18.

of diastolic dysfunction may also be induced by mitral regurgitation per se: increase in LA volume, increase in pulmonary and RV pressures, and increase in E wave velocity due to high LA pressure, often with the development of a restrictive pattern with E greater than A and short deceleration time. Systolic pulmonary venous flow is typically blunted (or even reversed) in severe mitral regurgitation, as it may also be with an increase in LA pressure due to diastolic dysfunction. To separate myocardial diastolic dysfunction from the effects of volume overload may therefore be impossible. In fact, regarding the diagnosis of increased diastolic pressures, one may question how meaningful the separation of the two is. Nevertheless, it has been reported that the difference in duration between transmitral and pulmonary reverse A wave reflects an increase in end-diastolic LV pressures (which when elevated shorten the transmitral A wave).[14] This parameter, however, is not easy to acquire and measure with confidence.

The effect of mitral regurgitation on E/e′ has been evaluated in several relatively small studies. Bruch et al. reported that (septal) E/e′ correlated with LV end-diastolic pressure in functional, but not in primary moderate or severe mitral regurgitation.[15] Conversely, Agricola et al. saw a good correlation of E/e′ with end-diastolic pressure in patients with degenerative mitral regurgitation.[16] Another study investigating patients with both degenerative and functional mitral regurgitation found only a weak correlation between E/e′ and pulmonary capillary pressure.[17] In this study, isovolumic relaxation time (IVRT) and IVRT/$T_{E-e'}$ had the best correlations with pulmonary capillary wedge pressure (PCWP) (r of −0.59 and −0.92, respectively), and this was also true in the subgroup of patients with atrial fibrillation. In the presence of substantial mitral regurgitation, the current guidelines recommend use of (1) a difference in transmitral and pulmonary venous A wave duration of 30 msec or more, (2) IVRT less than 60 msec, and (3) IVRT/$T_{E-e'}$ less than 5.6 for evaluation of diastolic pressures. Average E/e′ greater than 14 is only recommended in patients with impaired ejection fraction.[18] It should be pointed out, however, that the cited parameters are based on small patient numbers, have considerable measurement variability, and thus offer limited help for individual clinical decision making.

Acute mitral regurgitation may occur due to infective endocarditis or ischemic papillary muscle rupture. Hallmarks are very high pulmonary pressures and increased transmitral E/A ratio.

MITRAL ANNULAR CALCIFICATION

Calcification of the mitral annulus is frequent in elderly patients, in particular, those with a history of hypertension (and thus at increased likelihood of diastolic dysfunction). The extent of calcification is best evaluated in parasternal short axis views. The calcific or fibrotic changes decrease the longitudinal motion of the mitral annulus and therefore have a mechanical impact on both lateral and septal e′ that is independent of myocardial function. Thus e′ decreases and E/e′ increases purely due to the effect of annular calcification. A comparative echo catherization study showed weak correlation ($r = 0.42$) between E/e′ and invasively measured filling pressure patients with mitral annular calcification, while E/A and IVRT retained a better correlation ($r = 0.66$ and $r = -0.5$, respectively).[18] The authors recommended using a combination of high (>1.8) E/A ratio and low (<80 msec) IVRT to diagnose elevated filling pressures in the presence of substantial mitral calcification.

MITRAL STENOSIS

A significant reduction in mitral orifice area invariably leads to increased atrial pressure due to obstruction to transmitral flow. Atrial pressure and, by extension, right-sided pressures are therefore not meaningful gauges of LV myocardial diastolic function. Isovolumic relaxation time has been reported to have a modest correlation ($r = -0.62$) and IVRT/$T_{E-e'}$ to have a relatively good correlation (−0.88) with PCWP.[17] Current guidelines in the presence of mitral stenosis recommend use of an IVRT less than 60 msec, IVRT/$T_{E-e'}$ less than 4.2, and a mitral A velocity greater than 1.5 m/sec as signs of diastolic dysfunction, while E/e′ is not recommended.[18]

Nevertheless, conceptually the use of right-sided pressures as a proxy for diastolic function in the presence of mitral stenosis is problematic. Since LV function in mitral stenosis is usually not severely impaired, this dilemma is of negligible clinical importance unless there is coexistence of cardiomyopathy or ischemic heart disease.

PROSTHETIC VALVES

Mitral prostheses hemodynamically are mildly obstructive even if functioning well, leading to transmitral profiles corresponding to (mostly mild) mitral stenosis. Moreover, due to the impact of surgery on the mitral apparatus, a decrease in mitral annular plane mobility is typical, similar to the presence of mitral annular calcification. Usually there is enlargement of the left atrium and increase in right-sided pressures due to the preoperative mitral valve disease. Thus no reliable recommendations for assessment of diastolic function of the left ventricle in this situation can be given, although one modestly sized study with parallel invasive hemodynamic measurements reported fair correlations between changes in IVRT or IVRT/$T_{E-e'}$ and changes in mean PCWP before and after mitral valve repair or replacement in patients with moderate or severe mitral regurgitation.[17] With regard to the effect of percutaneous edge-to-edge repair of mitral regurgitation (MitraClip), increased forward flow, decreased diastolic and systolic LV volumes, and no major changes in ejection fraction have been noted after the procedure. Invasive measurements have shown a clear acute reduction in LA pressure and PCWP after the procedure and a small, but significant decrease in LV end-diastolic pressures.[19] These changes were found after treatment of both degenerative and functional mitral regurgitation. Apart from this, no major impact of this intervention on diastolic LV function has been described.

In the presence of an aortic valve prosthesis, similar concepts apply as to those discussed under aortic stenosis and regurgitation.

TREATMENT

Treatment of diastolic dysfunction in patients with severe valvular heart disease is primarily the treatment of the underlying valvular disease. Apart from this, diuretics may temporarily alleviate diastolic dysfunction symptoms, and achieving as low a heart rate as tolerable increases diastolic filling time and thus may ameliorate symptoms in patients with stenotic lesions. In critically ill patients with systolic LV dysfunction and severe aortic stenosis, short-term intravenous sodium nitroprusside has been given with improvement of cardiac output and LV performance.[20] Besides a beneficial decrease in systemic vascular resistance, a downward shift in the diastolic pressure volume relation improves diastolic function.[21]

The surgical or interventional treatment of severe valve disease leads in most cases to reverse remodeling of the left ventricle and a decrease in myocardial fibrosis, with corresponding hemodynamic improvement. This is typically the case after treatment of aortic stenosis. Additional medical treatment with angiotensin receptor blockers and other drugs has been tried but has not been conclusively shown to be advantageous in this scenario. However, such reverse remodeling after valve intervention does not always ensue. Overall, less reverse remodeling occurs after aortic valve replacement due to aortic regurgitation than after intervention for aortic stenosis. Especially in advanced mitral or aortic regurgitation, there may be only minor or no reverse remodeling at all. In these cases, diastolic dysfunction will persist or worsen.

FUTURE DIRECTIONS

Future research should be focused on identifying the extent of intrinsic myocardial abnormalities in patients with valvular heart disease. Better understanding is needed in regard to when structural changes become irreversible. This should allow to intervene on time and prevent long-term sequelae such as heart failure and atrial fibrillation, comorbidities that occur with frequency in patients with valvular disease and unfortunately often persist following valve repair or replacement.

KEY POINTS

- Best parameters for assessment of diastolic LV function and diastolic pressure in aortic stenosis are E/e′, LA size, TR velocity, and GLS.
- Diastolic dysfunction and end-diastolic LV pressure elevation almost uniformly present in moderate/severe aortic stenosis.
- In aortic regurgitation, best parameters to evaluate diastolic function include E/e′, LA size, and TR velocity.
- In patients with severe mitral annular calcification, best indicators of abnormal diastolic LV function are IVRT less than 80 msec

and E/A greater than 1.8. Association of diastolic pressures with E/e′ is weak.

- Diastolic LV pressure is often elevated in aortic and mitral regurgitation, but diastolic dysfunction is not uniformly present.
- IVRT, IVRT/$T_{E-e'}$, TR velocity, and E/e′ are better validated for . . . elevated PCWP in functional mitral regurgitation than for primary mitral regurgitation.
- In mitral stenosis LA pressure elevation is uniformly present, but there is not necessarily LV diastolic pressure elevation or diastolic dysfunction
- Short IVRT and abnormal IVRT/$T_{E-e'}$ are suggestive of abnormal LV diastolic function in patients with mitral stenosis.

REVIEW QUESTIONS

1. The aortic stenosis patient in Case Study 1 has heart failure symptoms. What is the most likely cause in his case?
   a. Impaired LV systolic function
   b. Mitral stenosis
   c. Impaired LV diastolic function
   d. Impaired RV function
   e. Both a and c
2. The patient in Case Study 1 has grade II diastolic dysfunction. Given that he also has severe symptomatic aortic stenosis, is that important for his prognosis?
   a. No, diastolic dysfunction will disappear after aortic valve intervention.
   b. No, the prognosis depends on systolic pump function (ejection fraction).
   c. Yes, diastolic dysfunction is an independent predictor of the patient's survival.
   d. No, the prognosis depends on pulmonary pressure.
3. This question relates to Case Study 2. The following parameters of diastolic LV function are affected by mitral regurgitation and may have pathologic values even in the absence of myocardial diastolic dysfunction, except
   a. peak E wave velocity, E/A ratio, and E/e′.
   b. LV wall thickness.
   c. RV systolic pressure.
   d. pulmonary venous flow.
   e. LA size.

REFERENCES

1. Villari B, Vassalli G, Monrad ES, Chiariello M, Turina M, Hess OM. Normalization of diastolic dysfunction in aortic stenosis late after valve replacement. *Circulation.* 1995;91:2353–2358.
2. Longhi S, Lorenzini M, Gagliardi C, et al. Coexistence of degenerative aortic stenosis and wild-type transthyretin-related cardiac amyloidosis. *JACC Cardiovasc Imag.* 2016;9:325–327.
3. Lee SP, Lee W, Lee JM, et al. Assessment of diffuse myocardial fibrosis by using MR imaging in asymptomatic patients with aortic stenosis. *Radiology.* 2015;274:359–369.
4. Child N, Suna G, Dabir D, et al. Comparison of MOLLI, shMOLLLI, and SASHA in discrimination between health and disease and relationship with histologically derived collagen volume fraction. *Eur Heart J Cardiovasc Imag.* 2018;19:768–776.
5. Biner S, Rafique AM, Goykhman P, Morrissey RP, Naghi J, Siegel RJ. Prognostic value of E/E′ ratio in patients with unoperated severe aortic stenosis. *JACC Cardiovasc Imag.* 2010;3:899–907.
6. Blair JEA, Atri P, Friedman JL, et al. Diastolic function and transcatheter aortic valve replacement. *J Am Soc Echocardiogr Off Pub Am Soc Echocardiogr.* 2017;30:541–551.
7. Muratori M, Fusini L, Tamborini G, et al. Sustained favourable haemodynamics 1 year after TAVI: improvement in NYHA functional class related to improvement of left ventricular diastolic function. *Eur Heart J Cardiovasc Imag.* 2016;17:1269–1278.
8. Kvernby S, Rönnerfalk M, Warntjes M, et al. Longitudinal changes in myocardial T1 and T2 relaxation times related to diffuse myocardial fibrosis in aortic stenosis; before and after aortic valve replacement. *JMRI.* 2018;doi:10.1002/jmri.25980.
9. Brown J, Shah P, Stanton T, Marwick TH. Interaction and prognostic effects of left ventricular diastolic dysfunction and patient-prosthesis mismatch as determinants of outcome after isolated aortic valve replacement. *Am J Cardiol.* 2009;104:707–712.
10. Villari B, Sossalla S, Ciampi Q, et al. Persistent diastolic dysfunction late after valve replacement in severe aortic regurgitation. *Circulation.* 2009;120:2386–2392.
11. Abudiab MM, Chebrolu LH, Schutt RC, Nagueh SF, Zoghbi WA. Doppler echocardiography for the estimation of LV filling pressure in patients with mitral annular calcification. *JACC Cardiovasc Imag.* 2017;10:1411–1420.
12. Kihara Y, Sasayama S, Miyazaki S, et al. Role of the left atrium in adaptation of the heart to chronic mitral regurgitation in conscious dogs. *Circ Res.* 1988;62:543–553.
13. Corin WJ, Murakami T, Monrad ES, Hess OM, Krayenbuehl H. Left ventricular passive diastolic properties in chronic mitral regurgitation. *Circulation.* 1991;83:797–807.
14. Rossi A, Cicoira M, Golia G, Anselmi M, Zardini P. Mitral regurgitation and left ventricular diastolic dysfunction similarly affect mitral and pulmonary vein flow Doppler parameters: the advantage of end-diastolic markers. *J Am Soc Echocardiogr Off Pub Am Soc Echocardiogr.* 2001;14:562–568.
15. Bruch C, Stypmann J, Gradaus R, Breithardt G, Wichter T. Usefulness of tissue Doppler imaging for estimation of filling pressures in patients with primary or secondary pure mitral regurgitation. *Am J Cardiol.* 2004;93:324–328.
16. Agricola E, Galderisi M, Oppizzi M, Melisurgo G, Airoldi F, Margonato A. Doppler tissue imaging: a reliable method for estimation of left ventricular filling pressure in patients with mitral regurgitation. *Am Heart J.* 2005;150:610–615.
17. Diwan A, McCulloch M, Lawrie GM, Reardon MJ, Nagueh SF. Doppler estimation of left ventricular filling pressures in patients with mitral valve disease. *Circulation.* 2005;111:3281–3289.
18. Nagueh SF, Smiseth OA, Appleton CP, et al. Recommendations for the evaluation of left ventricular diastolic function by echocardiography: an update from the American Society of Echocardiography and the European Association of Cardiovascular Imaging. *Eur Heart J Cardiovasc Imag.* 2016;17:1321–1360.
19. Gaemperli O, Biaggi P, Gugelmann R, et al. Real-time left ventricular pressure-volume loops during percutaneous mitral valve repair with the MitraClip system. *Circulation.* 2013;127:1018–1027.
20. Khot UN, Novaro GM, Popović ZB, et al. Nitroprusside in critically ill patients with left ventricular dysfunction and aortic stenosis. *N Engl J Med.* 2003;348:1756–1763.
21. Popovic ZB, Khot UN, Novaro GM, et al. Effects of sodium nitroprusside in aortic stenosis associated with severe heart failure: pressure-volume loop analysis using a numerical model. *Am J Physiol Heart Circ Physiol.* 2005;288:H416–H423.

22

Stage D Heart Failure With Preserved Ejection Fraction, Heart Transplantation, and Mechanical Circulatory Support

Eiran Z. Gorodeski, Dmitry M. Yaranov, and Randall C. Starling

OUTLINE

DEFINITION OF STAGE D HEART FAILURE

The American College of Cardiology (ACC) and American Heart Association (AHA) guideline for the management of heart failure (HF) classifies disease progression into four stages. Stage A includes patients with risk factors for HF but without structural heart disease, stage B includes those with structural heart disease without HF symptoms, stage C represents symptomatic HF associated with underlying structural heart disease, and stage D reflects refractory symptoms despite guideline-directed medical therapy (GDMT). As opposed to the New York Heart Association (NYHA) functional classification system, whereby patients are grouped by symptom severity and can move from class to class regardless of structural heart disease, this classification emphasizes the natural progression of disease through clinical stages.[1]

While discussion of stage D HF has traditionally been limited to those patients with advanced heart failure with reduced ejection fraction (HFrEF), recognition and understanding of heart failure with preserved ejection fraction (HFpEF) has evolved and with it the need to address the management of patients with stage D HFpEF.[2]

Defining advanced HF, end-stage HF, or stage D HF in a clear manner is important for clinical and research purposes, but it is challenging to do so as the natural history of HF is diverse and its clinical course highly variable.[3] Existing definitions of stage D HF address particular populations but are arguably too imprecise for assessment of individual patients.[4–6] It is usually a cluster of findings that defines stage D HF rather than a single characteristic. A recent consensus document from the Heart Failure Society of America (HFSA) Guidelines Committee suggests that stage D HF be defined by the presence of progressive and/or persistent severe signs and symptoms of HF despite optimized medical, surgical, and device therapy. The definition further includes frequent hospitalizations, severely limited exertional tolerance, and poor quality of life, which are associated with high morbidity and mortality. Importantly, the progressive decline should be primarily driven by the HF syndrome.[4]

HFpEF PHENOTYPES RESULTING IN STAGE D HF

According to ACC/AHA guidelines, HFpEF is defined as the presence of the HF syndrome in an individual with a left ventricular (LV) ejection fraction (EF) of 50% or more.[1] Regardless, HFpEF remains a challenging diagnosis for multiple reasons, including lack of universal definition that unites broad and heterogenic groups of patients. HFpEF is largely the diagnosis of exclusion in patients with clinical symptoms of HF and evidence of preserved or normal EF.[1]

Patients suffering from HFpEF, where LV diastolic dysfunction (DD) predominates, usually also exhibit LV systolic dysfunction as evident by abnormalities of longitudinal strain, LV end-systolic (Ees) stiffness (elastance), ventricular-arterial coupling (Ea/Ees ratio), and vasculoventricular coupling (see Chapter 29).[7–9] In addition, chronotropic incompetence,[10] abnormal vasorelaxation,[11] right heart dysfunction,[12,13] and abnormalities in the periphery[14,15] are also present in patients with HFpEF. Given this complexity and diverse etiology, HFpEF likely represents a group of several pathologies and diagnoses, which are caused by different etiologies but produce the same syndrome.[16–18] A better understanding of this phenotypic heterogeneity, as well as efforts to identify a common denominator for HFpEF, is essential to identify potential therapeutic targets. An ideal HFpEF

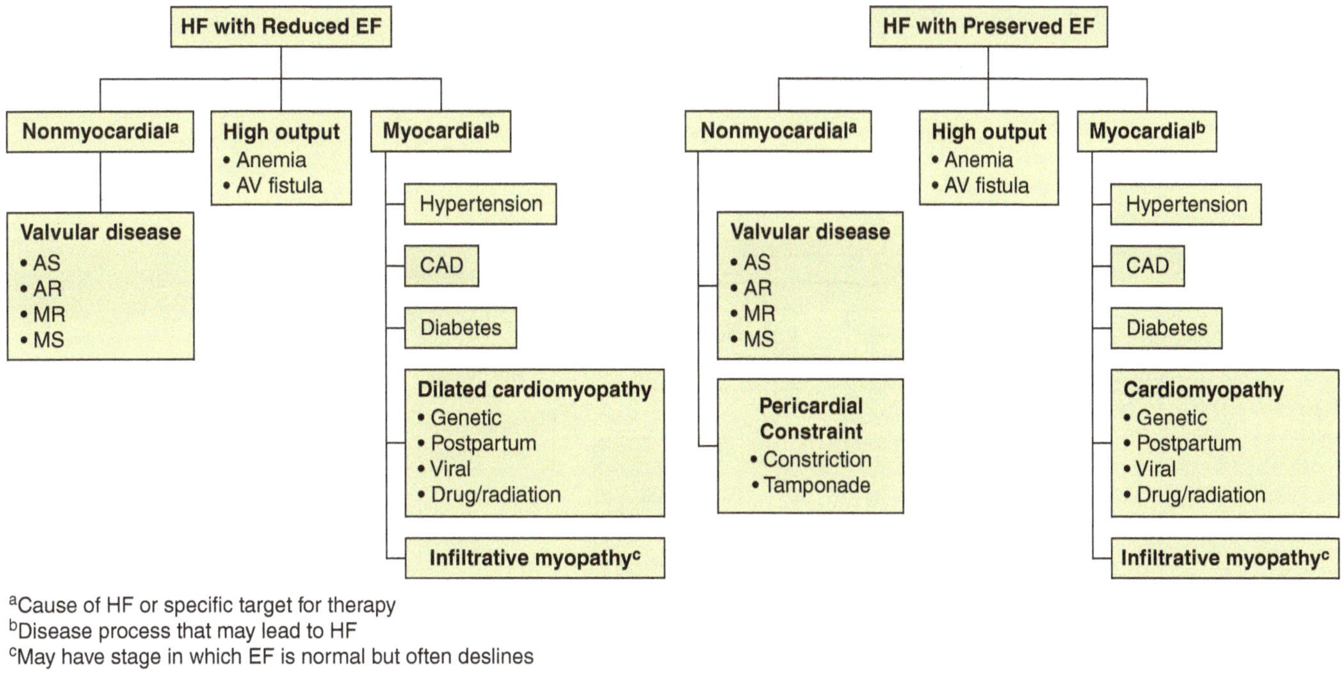

Fig. 22.1 Etiology of heart failure with reduced versus preserved ejection fraction. AS, aortic stenosis; AR, aortic regurgitation; MR, mitral regurgitation; MS, mitral stenosis; CAD, coronary artery disease. (Adapted from Heart Failure Society of America, et al. HFSA 2010 heart failure practice guideline. *J Card Fail.* 2010;16(6):e1-e194. doi:10.1016/j.cardfail.2010.04.004.)

taxonomy system would cluster together pathophysiologically similar individuals who may respond in a more predictable way to treatment.

Exploring the pathophysiology of HFpEF is challenging, and the natural history of clinical progression from the preclinical cardiac dysfunction (stage B) to the final clinical stages of HFpEF (stages C and D) depends on the clinical phenotype. The traditional classification proposed by HFSA guidelines[1,19] divided HFpEF into different groups based on the most likely cause of the disease (Fig. 22.1). Of note, many of the diagnoses in this classification system can be treated, therefore suggesting that progression of HFpEF to stage D HF may be preventable.[19]

Various other classification systems for HFpEF have been proposed. These stratify HFpEF based on clinical variables, physical characteristics, laboratory data, electrocardiogram (ECG) parameters, and/or echocardiographic parameters. A recent analysis of 397 patients with HFpEF utilizing phenomapping (unbiased cluster analysis of dense phenotypic data) identified three clinically relevant categories of patients with HFpEF with significantly different underlying etiology, pathophysiology, and clinical outcomes.[18] However, despite the ability of this analytic approach to separate patients into clusters, there remained a substantial overlap in numerous patients' clinical characteristics, demonstrating the heterogeneous nature of this disease.

Xanthopoulos and Starling (Fig. 22.2) recently proposed a phenotypical classification of HFpEF composed of two groups based on the contribution of hypertension to development of the disease (hypertensive vs nonhypertensive).[17] This hypertension-centric classification system is based on several observations. First, hypertension is the most common comorbidity in patients with HFpEF who otherwise have a single comorbidity, whereas other noncardiac comorbidities are rare in this population. Second, hypertension always preexists HFpEF, whereas virtually all the other noncardiac comorbidities may or may not. Third, comorbidities have minimal contribution to the development of nonhypertensive HFpEF (valvular, cardiomyopathic, and extramyocardial).

EPIDEMIOLOGY

HF is a major public health problem, which is projected to become an epidemic.[20] HF is the most common cause of hospitalization among individuals age 65 years and older.[21] Even though estimates of HFpEF prevalence vary depending on the study population and EF cutoff used, it is believed that half of patients with HF have preserved EF.[22–24] Compared to patients with HFrEF, those with HFpEF are older and more likely to be female.[25–28] The incidence and prevalence of HFpEF increases sharply with age.[29,30] Analysis of age and sex adjusted incidence of HF from 2000 to 2010 in Olmsted County, Minnesota, by Gerber et al. showed the incidence of HF declined for both HFpEF (EF ≥50%) and HFrEF (EF <50%). However, the declines were greater for HFrEF (−45%) than for HFpEF (−28%). The proportion of incident cases of HFpEF increased from 47.8% in 2000–2003 to 52.3% in 2008–2010.[31] In another study, Owan et al. found that the prevalence of HFpEF is increasing relative to HFrEF at a rate of 1% per year, suggesting that HFpEF may become the most common type of HF in the near future.[23] Using the Get With The Guidelines dataset, Steinberg et al. found that the proportion of patients hospitalized with acute HF who had HFpEF increased from 33% in 2005 to 39% in 2010. At the same time the proportion of HF hospitalizations due to HFrEF decreased from 52% to 47% in the United States.[32] These data suggest that the HF landscape is evolving, and it is projected that by the year 2020, 65% of patients hospitalized with HF will have a preserved EF.

The true prevalence of stage D HF, particularly in the HFpEF subgroup, is unknown. Estimates are controversial and based on limited data. Estimates of current theoretical patients with advanced HFpEF ranges between 110,500 and 325,000. Our approach to deriving these estimates are described next.

The current population of the United States is 326 million based on the latest United Nations estimates[33] with 75%[34] being 20 years old or older, thus yielding ~245 million adults. The most recent AHA

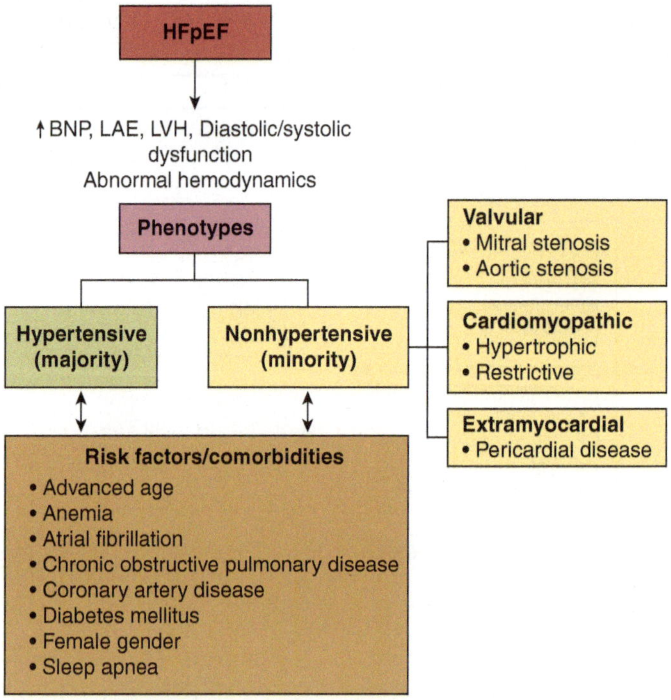

Fig. 22.2 Classification of HFpEF based on phenotype. BNP, brain natriuretic peptide; LAE, left atrial enlargement; LVH, left ventricular hypertrophy. (Adapted from Xanthopoulos A, Triposkiadis F, Starling RC. Heart failure with preserved ejection fraction: classification based upon phenotype is essential for diagnosis and treatment. *Trends Cardiovasc Med.* 2018;28:392–400.)

statistics indicate a HF prevalence of 6.5 million (years 2011–2014) in Americans 20 years of age and older,[21] yielding an estimated HF prevalence of 2.7%.

In 2007 Ammar et al. published a community-based study evaluating the prevalence of HF stages from Olmsted County, Minnesota.[35] Of patients who had HF, ~17% were classified as having HF symptoms (stage C), 3% were further classified as advanced stage C, and ~0.4% were classified as having severe HF (stage D). These estimates are from rural Minnesota, where the population is homogeneous and mostly white, and likely differ from heterogeneous inner-city urban areas that have a high prevalence of African Americans and Hispanics who tend to have higher rates of hypertension. These areas tend to have more individuals with stage D HF, with a prevalence of ~5%.[21,36,37]

IMPLANTABLE HEMODYNAMIC MONITORING IN HFpEF

An important goal in HF management is decongestion: decreasing ventricular filling pressures without compromising cardiac output. Because physical examination findings of congestion are inconsistent, various implantable cardiac filling pressure monitoring devices have been developed in an effort to help clinicians guide HF therapy, prevent exacerbation, and alter natural history of the disease.

Early studies demonstrated the safety and feasibility of long-term right ventricular (RV) pressure monitoring,[38] helping advance knowledge of the pathophysiology of HF, and suggesting that continuous RV pressure monitoring may reduce HF hospitalizations.[39] These discoveries resulted in development of Chronicle (Medtronic, Minneapolis, Minnesota, USA), the first implantable hemodynamic monitor. Chronicle was an implantable RV outflow tract hemodynamic monitor that recorded RV systolic pressure (RVSP), RV diastolic pressure (RVDP), and estimated pulmonary artery pressure (PAP). COMPASS-HF, a randomized clinical trial testing the efficacy of Chronicle, enrolled 301 patients with NYHA Class III-IV symptoms regardless of LV EF,[40] but failed to show any significant effect on hospitalizations as compared to the control group. Secondary analyses of the trial showed a 36% relative risk reduction for first HF readmission, suggesting potential clinical benefit of the implantable hemodynamic monitoring in patients with advanced HF.

Because HF decompensation is characterized by progressive increase in left atrial (LA) pressure, another target for hemodynamic monitoring was development of a permanent implantable direct LA pressure monitoring system. The first to be developed was the HeartPOD (Savacor, a subsidiary of St. Jude Medical, Minneapolis, Minnesota, USA), an implantable transseptal (right atrium to left atrium) sensor lead coupled with a subcutaneous antenna coil. The efficacy of this device was studied in the HOMEOSTASIS[41] pilot study, a prospective uncontrolled cohort, which demonstrated improvements in hemodynamics, symptoms, and outcomes when treatment was guided by LA pressure monitoring. Based on these findings LAPTOP-HF, a large randomized trial designed to test the safety and effectiveness of LA pressure–guided HF therapy, was launched and planned to enroll 730 patients.[42] However, LAPTOP-HF was terminated early by the study's data and safety monitoring board after randomization of only 486 patients because of a high number of implant-related complications.[43]

A further anatomic target for cardiac hemodynamic monitoring in chronic HF is the pulmonary artery (PA). CardioMEMS (St. Jude Medical, Minneapolis, Minnesota, USA) was the first catheter-delivered PAP sensor, implanted via right heart catheterization approach. The device consists of a wireless three-dimensional (3-D) coil and a pressure-sensitive capacitor covered with silicone. The pivotal trial of this device was the CardioMEMS Heart Sensor Allows Monitoring of Pressure to Improve Outcomes in NYHA Class III Heart Failure Patients (CHAMPION) trial,[44] a multicenter, single-blinded, randomized controlled trial of 550 patients with symptomatic HF. In this trial, HF medications were adjusted on the basis of hemodynamic data provided by the sensor. The CHAMPION trial found a 37% reduction in the primary end point of HF-related hospitalization compared to the control group (HR 0.63, 95% confidence interval [CI] 0.52–0.77; P <0.0001). These findings were consistent among those patients who had HFpEF (21% of the cohort), with the rate of HF hospitalization being 46% lower in the treatment group compared with control (incidence rate ratio, 0.54; 95% CI, 0.38–0.70; P <0.0001).[45] Based on the results of the CHAMPION trial in 2014 the US Food and Drug Administration (FDA) approved use of the CardioMEMS sensor in both patients with HFpEF and HFrEF, who had symptomatic HF (NYHA Class III) and were on optimal medical therapy with a history of HF hospitalization within the last year.[46] Follow-up studies to date, including both long-term follow-up of the CHAMPION cohort and postmarketing real-world populations, continue showing the benefit of PA pressure monitoring.[47–49]

Currently ongoing is GUIDE-HF (ClinicalTrials.gov identifier NCT03387813), a randomized clinical trial intended to evaluate the utility of PA pressure monitoring with the CardioMEMS sensor in an expanded patient population, including HF patients outside of the present indication, but at risk for future HF events or mortality. The trial will enroll patients with either HFpEF or HFrEF, and NYHA Class II-IV symptoms who have an elevated N-terminal pro-brain natriuretic peptide (NT-proBNP) and/or a prior HF hospitalization (https://clinicaltrials.gov/ct2/show/NCT03387813). Estimated enrollment will be 3600 participants, with an estimated completion date of April 2023.

INTERATRIAL SHUNT DEVICES IN TREATMENT OF HFpEF

Creation of iatrogenic interatrial shunting has been suggested as a novel therapy for patients with HFpEF and ongoing symptoms despite medical therapy. The potential mechanism of benefit is reduction of LA pressure, particularly during exertion, which relieves pulmonary venous congestion. The preliminary hypothesis for this approach was generated in preclinical computer-based modeling of HFpEF hemodynamics.[50] Currently two devices are available and are being evaluated in ongoing studies in patients with HFpEF. The V-Wave shunt device (V-Wave, Caesarea, Israel)[51] consists of an hourglass-shaped, self-expanding nitinol stent frame, and the Interatrial Shunt Device (IASD II, Corvia Medical Inc., Tewksbury, Massachusetts, USA) is a self-expanding nitinol device (Fig. 22.3).

In a phase I study, the IASD II device led to reduced LA pressures at 6 months and to improved symptoms, quality of life, and functionality as assessed by the 6-minute walk test. There were no device-related complications at 1 year.[52,53] In the REDUCE LAP-HF I phase 2 trial, which enrolled patients with HFpEF and NYHA Class III-IV symptoms, the same device was successfully implanted in over 90% of patients, and no periprocedural complications were observed. At the 1-month follow-up, the IASD resulted in a greater reduction in pulmonary capillary wedge pressure (PCWP) compared with sham controls.[54] Further studies and longer follow-up is necessary to understand if mechanistic effects of such devices will translate into meaningful clinical outcomes improvement.

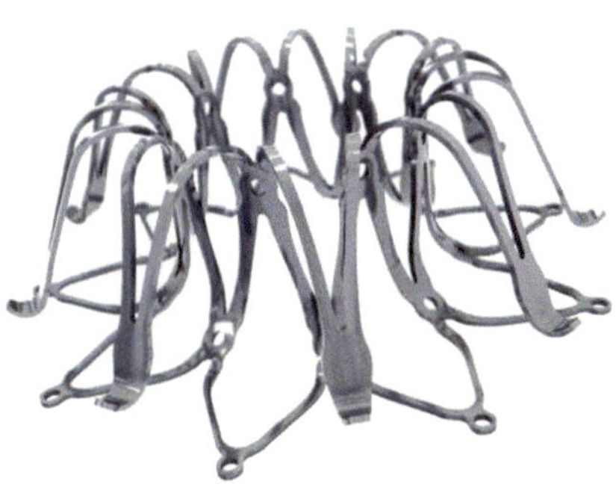

Fig. 22.3 Interatrial Shunt Device IASD II (Corvia Medical, Tewksbury, Massachusetts). Consists of a one-piece self-expanding metal cage that has a double-disc design with an opening (barrel) in the center.

PHARMACOLOGIC MANAGEMENT OF ACUTE AND CHRONIC STAGE D HFpEF

To date no pharmacologic intervention has demonstrated mortality reduction in randomized controlled clinical trials of patients with symptomatic HFpEF. ACC/AHA guidelines recommend the use of diuretics for symptom relief and appropriate management of comorbidities while acknowledging the absence of specific disease-modifying therapies for HFpEF.[1]

Pharmacologic Management in Acute HFpEF

Patients presenting with acute HF (AHF) exacerbation to emergency and hospital settings tend to be treated in similar ways regardless of LV EF. Recent data demonstrate though that the response of patients with HFpEF to these standard treatments may differ, likely related to this population's unique demographic, clinical, and pathophysiologic characteristics.[55]

In the ADHERE AHF registry, patients with HFpEF were more likely to receive intravenous diuretic therapy during the AHF hospitalization compared to those with HFrEF, but had similar weight loss and a similar prevalence of symptom relief at discharge.[56] In the OPTIMIZE-HF registry, patients with HFpEF had slightly less weight loss but slightly more symptomatic improvement than did AHF patients with HFrEF.[27] Patients with HFpEF hospitalized for AHF usually require escalation of loop diuretic doses as well as addition of thiazide diuretics for sequential nephron blockage, especially in those with refractory fluid overload.[57] When these measures fail to relieve congestion, ultrafiltration or other renal replacement approaches may be considered for more aggressive fluid removal. Two major trials investigating ultrafiltration in AHF (CARRESS-HF and UNLOAD) included patients with HFpEF; however, differences in response to ultrafiltration by LV EF were not reported.[58,59] Jeffries et al. found no difference in weight loss, electrolyte perturbations, or in-hospital mortality in patients with HFpEF when compared to patients with HFrEF undergoing ultrafiltration.[60] These limited data suggest that patients with HFpEF and AHF exacerbation respond to standard decongestive therapies in a manner similar to patients with HFrEF experiencing AHF exacerbation.

In patients presenting with AHF exacerbation, reduced capacitance in the venous system and increased arterial stiffness and resistance can worsen acute pulmonary congestion by redistributing fluid to the more compliant pulmonary venous bed.[61] Hypertension is common in patients with HFpEF and AHF exacerbation and may predispose to such shifts. Patients with HFpEF presenting with AHF have higher systolic blood pressure (BP) values than those with HFrEF.[62] Intravenous vasodilator therapy is an important pharmacologic strategy for some patients with AHF and elevated systemic BP; however, there are several caveats to its use in patients with advanced HFpEF.

Schwartzenberg et al. found that patients with HFpEF and AHF have differing hemodynamic responses to treatment with intravenous vasodilators as compared to patients with HFrEF and AHF.[62] The investigators conducted a retrospective study of invasive hemodynamics in 174 patients with HFrEF and 83 with HFpEF that were treated with intravenous nitroprusside, a potent vasodilator. At baseline patients with HFpEF had higher BP, stroke volume, and cardiac output values as compared to those patients with HFrEF, with no differences noted in PCWP and pulmonary artery systolic pressure between the two groups. Treatment with intravenous nitroprusside resulted in greater BP reduction, less enhancement in cardiac output, and greater likelihood of stroke volume drop in HFpEF as compared to HFrEF. These findings suggest fundamental pathophysiologic differences between HFpEF and HFrEF. Careful hemodynamic monitoring is important with intravenous administration of vasodilators in patients with advanced HFpEF and AHF exacerbation to avoid precipitous drops in BP and to avoid hemodynamic instability.[63]

Data from the ADHERE and OPTIMIZE HF registries suggest that as compared to HFrEF clinicians are wary of using various intravenous therapies in patients with HFpEF and AHF in real-world environments.[27,56] In the ADHERE registry, parenteral vasodilators, nesiritide, and inotropes were used infrequently in HFpEF as compared to HFrEF. An exception may be for those patients with advanced HFpEF presenting with signs and symptoms of end-organ hypoperfusion due to decreased forward flow where intravenous inotropes may have a benefit. In these patients rapid improvement of perfusion is needed to prevent irreversible end-organ dysfunction.[56]

Pharmacologic Management in Chronic HFpEF

In the current era the primary goal of pharmacotherapy for ambulatory patients with advanced HFpEF is symptom relief. Overall functional capacity and patient-reported outcomes that reflect the significant day-to-day burden of this syndrome should guide therapy.[64] Unfortunately multiple clinical trials of various pharmacologic agents in HFpEF have failed to demonstrate benefit on functional or symptom outcomes.[65–68] A nonpharmacologic intervention that has demonstrated benefit is exercise training, with improvements in peak oxygen consumption, 6-minute walk distance, and some quality-of-life indexes in elderly women with HFpEF who exercised over a 4-month period.[69] Ongoing trials are testing the impact of newer pharmacologic agents, including soluble guanylate cyclase stimulators, inhaled sodium nitrite, and interleukin-1 blockade, among others.

The Treatment of Preserved Cardiac Function Heart Failure With an Aldosterone Antagonist (TOPCAT) study[70] randomized patients with HFpEF (LV EF ≥45%) to spironolactone or placebo. After 3 years of follow-up there was no difference in the composite end point with spironolactone. A significant reduction in HF hospitalizations, however, was noted in the group of patients treated with spironolactone. A post hoc analysis of TOPCAT revealed significant differences in baseline characteristics and an unusually large difference in the placebo event rates between patients enrolled in the Americas versus those in Russia and Georgia.[71] Further analysis showed that levels of canrenone, the active metabolite of spironolactone, were undetectable in 30% of patients enrolled in Russia and Georgia compared with just 3% in the United States ($P <0.001$).[72] As a result, when looking just at the patients enrolled in the Americas, the use of spironolactone significantly reduced the composite primary end point as well as cardiovascular death and HF hospitalizations. Many researchers have argued that the true therapeutic effect of spironolactone was not reached in the Eastern European population, and thus the original TOPCAT trial results are inconclusive. The most recent ACC/AHA guidelines published this year state that in select patients with HFpEF the use of spironolactone may be considered to reduce hospitalizations (COR IIb, LOA B-R).[1]

Data on use of intravenous chronic inotropes in patients with HFpEF is limited. Chronic home inotrope infusion may be an effective strategy for palliative management of selected end-stage patients with HFpEF. Current ACC/AHA[1] and HFSA[19] guidelines discuss inotropic support and specifically recommend cautious use as "despite improving hemodynamic compromise, positive inotropic agents have not demonstrated improved outcomes in patients with HF in either the hospital or outpatient setting."[1] In the Randomized Evaluation of Mechanical Assistance for the Treatment of Congestive Heart Failure (REMATCH) trial, 72% of patients in the medical arm and 65% of patients in the ventricular assist device arm were on inotropes.[73] Small studies in stage D patients on chronic inotropes demonstrated decrease in repeat hospitalizations[74] and reduction of hospital days.[75] In an adjusted model, continuous milrinone and dobutamine infusions showed equivalent survival rates.[76] However, these studies do not report etiology of cardiomyopathy and proportion of patients with HFpEF enrolled. Patients should be counseled that inotropes are a palliative measure used to facilitate discharge home and improved out-of-hospital functioning in the period before death, but that inotropes are not associated with improved survival.[77]

Recently published small clinical trials investigated the utility of eplerenone,[78] ivabradine,[79] and ranolazine[80] for patients with HFpEF. Some of these newer agents are currently being tested in large randomized clinical trials in this population.

DURABLE MECHANICAL CIRCULATORY SUPPORT IN PATIENTS WITH STAGE D HFpEF

Continuous flow LV assist devices (LVAD) have become the standard of care for eligible patients with end-stage HFrEF.[81,82] Clinical experience with short-term or long-term mechanical circulatory support (MCS) in patients with HFpEF is extremely limited to date and is primarily based on small cohorts of patients or case reports[83–87] (Table 22.1). Indeed, some authors have indicated that HFpEF (nonsystolic HF) is a contraindication for LVAD therapy.[88]

Several investigators reported theoretical benefits of LVAD use in computer models of HFpEF. Those models suggest that MCS for LA and LV unloading would reduce filling pressures and improve total cardiac output, hence improve symptoms and possibly alter the natural progression of the disease.[89,90]

Topilsky et al.[83] were the first to report use of the HeartMate II LVAD (Thoratec Corporation, Pleasanton, California, USA) in patients with advanced HFpEF due to hypertrophic (HCM) or restrictive (RCM) cardiomyopathy. In a cohort of 8 patients these investigators demonstrated the technical feasibility of the implantation procedure and found no differences in mortality compared with patients with HFrEF due to dilated or ischemic cardiomyopathy treated with LVAD. In another publication this same group of investigators reported outcomes in 28 patients with advanced HFpEF due to RCM of various etiologies who underwent LVAD implantation.[91] An echocardiographic analysis of this cohort found that larger LV end-diastolic and end-systolic dimensions are markers of better outcome. LV end-diastolic dimension of 4.6 cm or less was associated with increased mortality post-LVAD implantation. Most of the patients had improvement in their symptom burden as assessed by NYHA class. As compared to those with HFrEF, patients with HFpEF who were supported with an LVAD demonstrated worse RV dysfunction as suggested by increased right atrial (RA) pressure, decreased pump flow, and need for longer inotropic support in the postoperative period.

A case series of three patients with HCM and HFpEF treated with centrifugal continuous flow LVADs demonstrated improvement of hemodynamic parameters and outcomes comparable to patients with dilated cardiomyopathy (DCM) and HFrEF.[84] One of these patients

TABLE 22.1 Published Reports of Stage D HFpEF Patients Supported With LVADs

Year	Authors	Cohort	Outcomes
2011	Topilsky et al.[83]	8 stage D RCM and HCM patients supported with HMII	Mortality comparable to DCM patients, RV failure, prolonged inotropic support, CVL catheters infection is more common.
2013	Swiecicki et al.[87]	9 stage D patients with HFpEF due to amyloidosis supported with HMII	All tolerated implantation well; 2 died prior to discharge; 3 median survival of 13.7 months; 4 alive with a 16–24-month follow-up. GI bleeding is the most common adverse event (3/9 patients).
2013	Muthiah et al.[84]	3 patients with HCM supported with HVAD	One patient "bridged" for 708 days, one patient for 744 days, one died 161 days.
2015	Grupper et al.[91]	28 stage D RCM patients supported with HMII (93%), HVAD (7%)	One-year survival without transplantation 64%, no difference between amyloidosis and nonamyloidosis patients. LV end-diastolic dimension ≤4.6 cm associated with increased mortality. RV failure, requiring short-term medical support is more common.
2017	Patel et al.[92]	198 stage D HFpEF patients due to RCM and HCM from INTERMACS (2008–2014) registry	No statistical difference in survival. Early and late bleeding and late infections are most common complications. Higher mortality with smaller LV cavity (LV end-diastolic dimension <5 cm). No mortality difference between LV EF groups and different INTERMACS profiles.

CVL, Central venous line; *DCM*, dilated cardiomyopathy; *EF*, ejection fraction; *GI*, gastrointestinal; *HCM*, hypertrophic cardiomyopathy; *HFpEF*, heart failure with preserved ejection fraction; *HMII*, HeartMate II; *HVAD*, HeartWare Ventricular Assist Device; *INTERMACS*, Interagency Registry for Mechanically Assisted Circulatory Support; *LV*, left ventricular; *RCM*, restrictive cardiomyopathy; *RV*, right ventricular.

died at 3 months postimplantation due to inlet obstruction leading to transient ischemic attacks and ultimately LVAD pump thrombosis resulting in cardiogenic shock.

Patel et al. reported findings from the Interagency Registry for Mechanically Assisted Circulatory Support Registry (INTERMACS) for patients with HFpEF (RCM or HCM) that underwent continuous flow LVAD implantation between 2008 and 2014.[92] The RCM group included patients with amyloidosis (15.3%), sarcoidosis (16.3%), idiopathic restrictive disease (29.8%), radiation/chemotherapy-induced restrictive disease (15.3%), and others (23%). When compared to patients with DCM and HFrEF, those with the HFpEF phenotypes had significantly higher LV EF and smaller LV end-diastolic dimension. However, overall survival (Fig. 22.4) and event profiles were comparable to those with DCM. Echocardiographic analysis showed that most of the patients had burnt-out cardiomyopathies, and only 5% of the cohort had an LV EF of 40% or more, while 56% had an LV end-diastolic dimension of 6 cm and above. Overall bleeding and infection in the late postimplant period were the only significantly higher adverse events in stage D patients with restrictive cardiomyopathy. Once the non-DCM cohort was analyzed by preimplant LV end-diastolic dimension, those with dimensions less than 5 cm had worse outcomes. However, there was no difference in outcomes regardless of preimplant LV EF.

The major concern with LVAD implantation is obstruction of flow into the LV inflow cannula due to the smaller cavity size and thickness of the LV walls. Patients with HFpEF in the study experienced more frequent and difficult-to-manage suction events. The investigators suggested the need for technical modifications in the surgical procedure. As such they proposed extensive myomectomy[83] prior to placement of the inflow cannula to avoid obstruction of the inflow cannula by muscle bundles, especially in patients with HCM and thickened apex or midventricle.

For both anatomic and physiologic reasons patients with HFpEF may not be ideal candidates for durable MCS. Careful patient selection is key. Further, larger studies are needed to properly assess potential benefits of mechanical circulatory support in patients with stage D HFpEF. As the field of MCS continues to evolve we anticipate that more patients with stage D HFpEF will benefit from durable MCS technologies still under development. The challenge relates to the small size of the left ventricle and limitations based on the inflow cannula. As devices evolve and become smaller it is anticipated more patients with stage D HFpEF will be served.

HEART TRANSPLANTATION FOR STAGE D HFpEF: TRENDS AND NATIONAL OUTCOMES

As discussed earlier, patients with HFpEF have a variety of presentations, with variable progression of disease depending on the underlying etiology. End-stage presentation may be characterized by variable anatomic, physiologic, and hemodynamic characteristics. In general, durable mechanical support options are limited for patients with stage D HFpEF due to inability of cannulas to fit in nondilated ventricles and/or to support biventricular failure.[93] As such heart transplantation is currently the mainstay therapy for patients with end-stage disease.

Prior to 2018, patients with stage D HFpEF in the United States, particularly those with end-stage RCM, HCM, or cardiac amyloidosis, had limited access due to the heart allocation system. The old system allowed higher status listing for patients supported by LVADs, which at the time were almost entirely used in patients with HFrEF or those on continuous inotrope infusion, therefore limiting access to organs for those patients with HFpEF who were lower on the priority list. Partially to address this, a new adult heart allocation system was implemented in the United States in October 2018 (Fig. 22.5). This system was designed to stratify heart transplant candidates according to predicted waiting list mortality. In this new six-tier system, noninotrope-dependent patients with end-stage HFpEF are assigned to status 4—the same status as those patients who are supported by LVADs or continuous inotrope infusion. Patients on the transplant list with HFpEF who deteriorate further and require hemodynamic monitoring in addition to continuous inotrope infusion, or acute mechanical support in an intensive care unit (ICU) setting, are assigned even higher status, thus theoretically giving them similar access to donor hearts. At the time of this writing, the impact of the new US heart allocation system on patients with end-stage HFpEF listed for heart transplantation is not yet known.

HCM and Heart Transplantation

Patients with end-stage HCM have two distinct pathophysiologic presentations. At one end of the spectrum HF is the result of an asymmetric hypertrophied myocardium, causing severe dynamic outflow obstruction.[94,95] This form of HF is generally amendable to septal reduction strategies with improvement of symptoms and quality of life.[94] These patients with obstructive HCM, especially those with a preserved LV EF, represent a minority (<1%) of heart transplant recipients.[96]

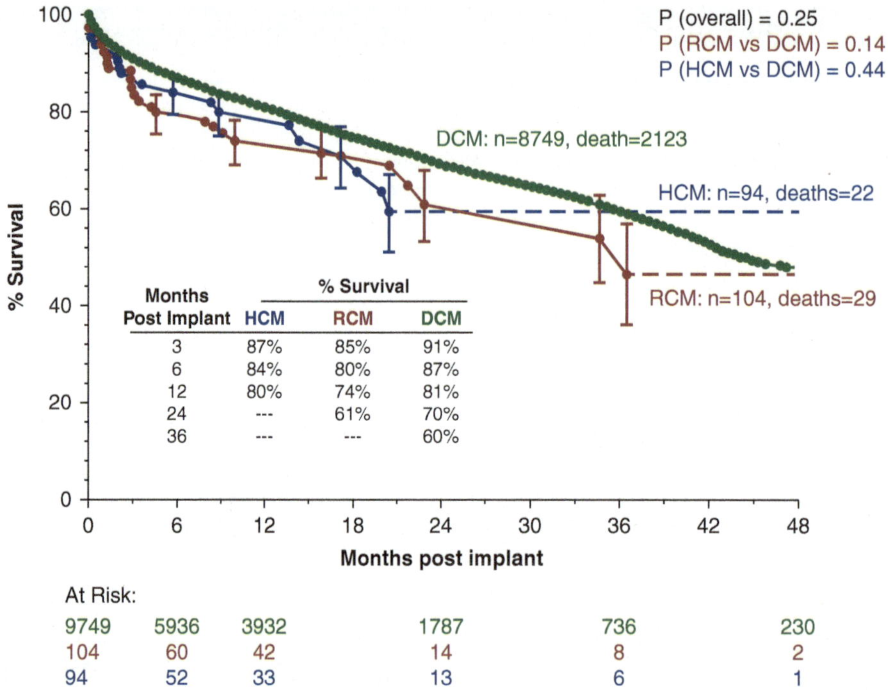

Fig. 22.4 Survival post–continuous flow LVAD implantation for HFpEF (HCM and RCM) compared to DCM cohort. INTERMACS database analysis. *DCM,* Dilated cardiomyopathy; *HCM,* hypertrophic cardiomyopathy; *RCM,* restrictive cardiomyopathy. (From Patel SR, Saeed O, Naftel D, Myers S, Kirklin J, Jorde UP, et al. Outcomes of restrictive and hypertrophic cardiomyopathies after LVAD: an INTERMACS analysis. *J Card Fail.* 2017;23:859–867.)

At the other end of the spectrum are patients with HCM without outflow tract obstruction. These patients can progress to end-stage HF with poor quality of life and debilitating symptoms. Approximately 50% of this population transition from an HFpEF phenotype to an HFrEF phenotype with LV systolic dysfunction and adverse remodeling, including wall thinning and/or ventricular chamber enlargement. The remaining patients with nonobstructive HCM and refractory HF symptoms have preserved systolic function (LV EF >50%) with a nondilated LV cavity associated with impaired cardiac output often associated with impaired LV filling and pulmonary hypertension.[97–104]

Patients with end-stage HCM and preserved LV EF who progress to cardiogenic shock may be initially stabilized with continuous intravenous inotropes while waiting for heart transplantation.[105] Patients who have persistent cardiogenic shock despite inotropic support have limited mechanical support options due to their nondilated ventricles. One durable mechanical support option for patients waiting for heart transplantation may be the total artificial heart (TAH), but this therapy requires significant expertise and is limited to specialized centers.[106]

Maron et al. published the first analysis of the demographic, clinical, and survival outcomes in patients with HCM who underwent heart transplantation, from United Network of Organ Sharing (UNOS) registry over years 1990 to 2004.[96] While the proportion of patients with HCM undergoing heart transplantation in this registry was small (~1%), their outcomes were similar to those patients without HCM. The investigators reported a 10-year survival rate of more than 60% for patients with HCM and a trend toward better survival compared to non-HCM heart transplant recipients. These improved outcomes may be explained by the fact that patients with HCM are typically younger with fewer comorbidities as compared to non-HCM candidates.[96,107] Given the transition of phenotypes in patients with advanced HFpEF, accompanied by LV dilation and remodeling at the time of transplant evaluation and listing, those reports have inherent bias and likely underestimate the actual number of patients with HCM undergoing cardiac transplantation.[96]

RCM and Heart Transplantation

RCM includes a wide spectrum of myocardial pathology, including genetic disorders of the sarcomere and cytoskeleton, infiltrative cardiomyopathies secondary to glycogen storage diseases, radiation/chemotherapy-related cardiomyopathy, amyloid deposition disease, and inflammatory myocardial and endomyocardial disease (see Chapter 23). RCM is characterized by impaired DD, often preserved or mildly depressed LV EF, biatrial enlargement, and nondilated ventricular morphology.[108]

Data in patients with RCM indicate that the RCM diagnosis is a marker for worse waitlist outcomes.[109] DePasquale et al. investigated the outcomes of patients with RCM in the UNOS registry over the years 1987 to 2010.[108] These investigators found that outcomes for patients with RCM following heart transplantation were comparable to those of patients without RCM who underwent transplantation. Among subgroups of patients with RCM those with radiation/chemotherapy-related cardiomyopathy and those with cardiac amyloidosis had worse mortality outcomes as compared to those patients with other forms of RCM.[108]

Successful heart transplantation in patients with AL cardiac amyloidosis depends on timely referrals to transplant centers with appropriate comprehensive diagnostic capabilities for assessment of systemic involvement, timely organ availability, and experience with chemotherapy prior to and shortly after organ transplantation.[110–112] For patients with end-stage AL cardiac amyloidosis, heart transplantation with subsequent autologous stem cell transplantation (ASCT) depends on the amyloid subtype and degree of other system involvement. The development of ASCT has led to improved outcomes and increased numbers of orthotopic heart transplant (OHT) in patients with AL amyloidosis. In small

Status 1
- VA ECMO
- Non-dischargeable, surgically implanted, non-endovascular biventricular support device
- MCSD with life-threatening ventricular arrhythmia

Status 2
- Non-dischargeable, surgically implanted, non-endovascular LVAD
- IABP
- V-tach / V-fib, mechanical support not required
- MCSD with device malfunction/mechanical failure
- TAH, BiVAD, RVAD, or VAD for single ventricle patients
- Percutaneous endovascular MCSD

Status 3
- Dischargeable LVAD for discretionary 30 days
- Multiple inotropes or single high-dose inotrope with continuous hemodynamic monitoring
- VA ECMO after 7 days; percutaneous endovascular circulatory support device or IABP after 14 days
- Non-dischargeable, sugically implanted, non-endovascular LVAD after 14 days
- MCSD with one of the following: device infection, hemolysis, pump thrombosis, right heart failure, mucosal bleeding, aortic insufficiency

Status 4
- Dischargeable LVAD without discretionary 30 days
- Inotropes without hemodynamic monitoring
- Retransplant
- Diagnosis of one of the following: congenital heart disease (CHD), ischemic heart disease with intractable angina, hypertrophic cardiomyopathy, restrictive cardiomyopathy, amyloidosis

Status 5
- On the waitlist for at least one other organ at the same hospital

Status 6
- All remaining active candidates

Fig. 22.5 US adult heart allocation criteria. VA ECMO, venous-arterial extra-corporeal membrane oxygenator; MCSD, mechanical support device; LVAD, left ventricular support device; IABP, intra-aortic balloon pump; TAH, total artificial heart; BiVAD, bi-ventricular assist device; RVAD, right ventricular assist device; VAD, ventricular assist device. (Adapted from US Department of Health and Human Services. Organ Procurement and Transplantation Network Web site. https://optn.transplant.hrsa.gov/learn/professional-education/adult-heart-allocation. Accessed January 9, 2019.)

series, long-term (5-year) survival with combined heart transplantation and ASCT was ~60%. The most common cause of death was the recurrence of light-chain production and end-organ disease and dysfunction, including cardiac amyloid recurrence in transplanted heart.[113–115]

Patients with end-stage transthyretin (TTR) cardiac amyloidosis can be successfully treated with heart transplantation. Combined heart and liver transplantation has been performed in an effort to stop hepatic amyloid production and prevent systemic disease progression. Combined heart and liver transplantation is associated with an excellent outcome, with survival equivalent to heart transplantation alone.[116] Older recipients with primarily cardiac manifestations may benefit from heart transplantation alone, but younger individuals should be considered for combined heart-liver transplantation to prevent systemic progression of the disease.

There is sparse literature on outcomes of patients with radiation-induced cardiomyopathy.[108,117] Overall, posttransplant outcomes in patients with prior radiation appear to be worse than those without prior radiation, mostly related to posttransplant lung cancer and other complications, irrespective of prior restrictive physiology.

PHYSIOLOGY OF THE TRANSPLANTED HEART

With advances in surgical techniques and immunosuppression, the survival rate following OHT significantly exceeds that of medical therapy for advanced HF. Despite anticipated 1-year and 5-year survival rates of 90% and 70%, respectively, acute and chronic allograft rejections have remained major determinants of patient outcome.[118] Other important perioperative issues are pulmonary hypertension and RV dysfunction. As acute rejection is often asymptomatic, regular rejection surveillance is obligatory. For detecting allograft rejection and monitoring immunosuppressive treatment, clinical and laboratory examinations, along with endomyocardial biopsy (EMB), are conducted following a predetermined time schedule.

Despite the inherent limitations and complications associated with biopsy, current noninvasive surveillance methods, though preferable, have yet to match EMBs in terms of sensitivity and specificity. These limitations have fueled the continuing challenge to develop noninvasive methods to detect acute rejection and to monitor response to therapy.

DIASTOLIC FUNCTION AFTER HEART TRANSPLANT

Diastolic dysfunction is common early after transplant, and its incidence decreases during the first year.[119] Immediately after OHT, the heart is relatively noncompliant, with significantly elevated filling pressures and abnormal LV relaxation.[120,121] The early postoperative noncompliance is attributed to factors such as ischemic myocardial injury, high peripheral vascular resistance, denervation, donor-recipient size mismatch, interaction between donor and recipient atria, allograft rejection, preexistent recipient pulmonary hypertension, and volume overload.[122–125] Long-term studies of OHT recipients suggest that these hemodynamics remain mildly abnormal months after the surgery,[126,127] while others with an initial restrictive filling pattern may become nonrestrictive in the first 6 weeks after OHT.[128] Young et al.[129] showed that abnormal PCWP, and RA and PA pressures, improved markedly during the fourth to eighth weeks post OHT. The average PCWP was 19 mmHg immediately after OHT and improved to 12 mmHg at 4 to 8 weeks. In contrast, Greenberg et al. demonstrated that LV filling pressures improved but never completely normalized.[126] At 1 year after OHT, PCWP and RA and PA pressures were elevated in comparison with age-matched controls. Likewise, Valantine et al.[130] found that up to 15% of patients exhibited restrictive physiology at 6 years post-OHT. The significance of these findings is that although the exercise capacity of OHT recipients usually improves in comparison with their pretransplant status, this is only about 60% to 70% of that found in healthy subjects.[131,132] The LV end-diastolic pressure during exercise is often normal or elevated in comparison with control subjects, suggestive of a leftward shift of the pressure-volume curve, which is consistent with DD.[133]

Although uncommon, DD at 1 year is a strong and important predictor of mortality.[119] RV DD, as measured by an elevated RA pressure–to–stroke volume ratio, is shown to be a strong predictor of cardiac mortality. A study by Ross et al.[134] suggests that abnormal diastolic parameters by echocardiographic indexes after the first few weeks after OHT are associated with increased mortality. Similarly, Aziz et al.[135] found that the presence of DD by echography 2 years after transplantation was associated with symptoms of HF and possibly a decreased survival 2 to 5 years after transplantation.

DIASTOLIC FUNCTION IN ALLOGRAFT REJECTION

Despite major improvements in the field of heart transplantation leading to increased survival of organ recipients, acute cardiac allograft rejection remains the most common complication during the first year after OHT. Allograft rejection contributes to ~12% of mortality within the first year post-OHT and is an independent risk factor for developing cardiac allograft vasculopathy.[136]

RV EMB still represents the clinical gold standard in monitoring cardiac allograft rejection. Nevertheless, it is an invasive diagnostic procedure that is uncomfortable and associated with several, albeit rare, major complications such as carotid artery puncture, cardiac tamponade, and heart block. A noninvasive but equally accurate technique to detect rejection is highly desirable.[137,138]

The noninvasive evaluation of the transplanted heart, particularly echocardiographic measures of diastolic function, has become an integral part of long-term follow-up. Changes in myocardial structure caused by rejection-induced edema, lymphocyte infiltration, increased mass, and myocardial necrosis have been shown to compromise myocyte function, resulting in increased myocardial stiffness and abnormal relaxation. With mild or even early rejection, two-dimensional (2-D) echocardiographic changes are subtle and are not accurate or reproducible enough. Pathophysiologically, rejection-induced myocardial edema manifested by an echocardiographically discernible increase in wall thickness is a rather late event. During episodes of rejection, restrictive physiology of the allograft becomes more prominent.[139,140]

Commonly cited Doppler changes in acute rejection include decreased pressure half-time of the early diastolic E wave, decreased isovolumic relaxation time (IVRT), and increased E velocity. Using the patient as his or her own baseline, a significant change—defined as greater than 20% for E velocity and greater than 15% for pressure half-time or IVRT—is fairly consistent with rejection.[141,142] Valantine et al.[143] evaluated 64 patients undergoing hemodynamic and Doppler echocardiographic studies as part of the routine follow-up 1 to 13 years after OHT. Ten patients were found to have strikingly abnormal (restrictive) transmitral flow patterns. This group had a higher incidence of rejection as the only identifiable clinical difference. Restrictive filling pattern was associated with impaired systolic performance, and there was correlation between transtricuspid (RV IVRT) and transmitral (LV IVRT) flow patterns and degree of rejection.

Barba et al.[144] studied 56 OHT recipients 6 weeks postoperatively and found that during acute rejection, LV wall thickness significantly increased compared with negative biopsies, while IVRT and pressure half-time significantly decreased. However, the increase in mitral E velocity was significantly associated with only severe rejection. The progressive shortening of IVRT as a marker of graft rejection showed a high sensitivity (85%) and low specificity (57%). In another prospective study, Berwing et al. reported that parameters of systolic function such as percent fractional shortening and systolic wall thickness of the posterior wall remained without significant changes at moderate (grade II) and severe (grade III) rejections.[145] The same is valid for relaxation parameters such as maximum velocity of posterior wall reduction, the time interval of end systole to maximum velocity of posterior wall reduction (tES-PTR), and IVRT. Although LV filling parameters such as mitral E velocity change significantly between rejection-free interval and advanced grades of rejection, these parameters are too insensitive to diagnose or exclude a moderate or severe acute rejection in the individual case. Analyses of transmitral Doppler and pulmonary venous flow velocity have not lived up to their promise to detect rejection-related diastolic dysfunction for two main reasons. First, transmitral Doppler indices are influenced by variables other than ventricular diastolic function, such as age, heart rate, and (most importantly) ventricular loading conditions.[146] Pulmonary venous flow velocities are particularly variable, even in individuals without heart disease. Second, denervation of the transplanted heart, with its lack of autonomic regulation and the usual sinus tachycardia, leads to a form of restrictive filling pattern that amounts to diastolic dysfunction in the absence of acute rejection.[147]

Tissue Doppler imaging (TDI) and Vp measurements appear promising in allowing earlier and more accurate detection of LV dysfunction in the transplanted heart. Derumeaux et al.[148] found values for sensitivity and specificity of 92% using mitral annular e′ velocity during mild or moderate and severe rejection. With increasing rejection grade, e′ decreased significantly. Puleo et al. tested 121 OHT recipients who underwent TDI at the time of EMB surveillance.[141] These investigators found a significant decrease in mitral annular e′ at the inferior wall during moderate allograft rejection but no change in peak systolic velocity in comparison with nonrejecting allograft recipients, with a sensitivity of 76% and a specificity of 88%.

In 78 OHT recipients, Mankad et al.[131] found a reduction in posterior wall peak systolic and diastolic velocity gradients with rejection, as well as a reduction in mitral annular systolic S′ and diastolic e′ velocities, with a sensitivity of 93% and a specificity of 71%. Dandel et al.[149] also reported that in all patients with acute rejection, a significant reduction in e′ velocity was obtained from the basal LV posterior wall in the short axis. They suggested that absence of such a change could practically exclude acute transplant rejection. In 91.7% of cases, the pulsed Doppler findings reverted completely during antirejection therapy within 65 hours. Stengel et al.[150] found that late diastolic mitral annular a′ velocity and mitral annular systolic S′ velocity were higher in patients with rejection grade less than IIIa compared with those of IIIa or greater. Sensitivity and specificity of a′ less than 8.7 cm/sec in predicting significant allograft rejection were 82% and 53%, respectively. Unlike findings in other studies, neither early diastolic mitral annular e′ velocity nor Vp was associated with the histologic degree of allograft rejection, though there was a trend toward lower e′ values during episodes of rejection. Although an a′ velocity can reliably exclude severe rejection, the fact that the best threshold of an a′ velocity less than 9 cm/sec falsely detected rejection in almost 50% of cases indicates that it is not specific enough and that the pathophysiologic problem of restriction to allograft LV filling impairs the reliability of any tool assessing diastolic function during the early rejection process.

In our own series at the Cleveland Clinic, Sun et al.[151] noted that pericardial effusion, IVRT less than 90 msec, mitral inflow E/A ratio greater than 1.7, diameter of inferior vena cava, and duration of pulmonary vein atrial reversal were independently associated with rejection. However, no single predictor or combination of predictors was powerful enough to eliminate surveillance EMB.

Palka et al.[152] analyzed TDI-derived early diastolic indices of LV and RV function. They found that significant differences in the late isovolumic relaxation myocardial velocity gradient, as well as differences in timing between onsets of mitral E and mitral annular e′ waves and between mitral and tricuspid annular e′, might help identification of those with acute rejection. The sensitivity and specificity of the approach is greater than 0.80. They attributed these differences to altered early diastolic untwisting of the oblique LV fibers and the delay in early diastolic RV relaxation.

FUTURE DIRECTIONS

Treatment of patients with stage D HFpEF is challenging due to lack of proven pharmacologic and interventional modalities. A Class II recommendation for use of spironolactone to reduce risk of HF hospitalization has recently been added to the ACC/AHA HF guidelines, and future randomized trials will be needed to verify this observation and further assess impact on mortality. The utility of interatrial shunt devices for treatment of advanced HFpEF hold promise but remain unclear, with clinical trials testing these technologies ongoing. There is great need to develop novel types of durable mechanical support for patients with advanced HFpEF, specifically pumps or similar technologies that will accommodate smaller LV cavity sizes. Finally, at the time of this writing the impact of the updated 2018 US heart transplant allocation system on transplantation outcomes among patients with advanced HFpEF remains unknown.

KEY POINTS

- Defining advanced HFpEF, end-stage HFpEF, or stage D HFpEF is challenging as the natural history of HF is diverse and its clinical course highly variable. A recent consensus document from the HFSA defines stage D HF by the presence of progressive and/or persistent severe signs and symptoms of HF despite optimized medical, surgical, and device therapy.
- The true prevalence of stage D HF, particularly in the HFpEF subgroup, is unknown. In this chapter we estimate that the number of current theoretical patients in the United States with advanced HFpEF range between 110,500 and 325,000.
- To date there is no pharmacologic therapy that improves mortality in patients with HFpEF. Recent ACC/AHA guidelines state that in select patients with HFpEF the use of spironolactone may be considered to reduce hospitalizations (Class II indication).
- Clinical experience with short-term or long-term mechanical circulatory support in patients with HFpEF is limited. In general, durable mechanical support options are limited for patients with stage D HFpEF due to inability of cannulas to fit in nondilated ventricles and/or to support biventricular failure.
- Prior to 2018, patients with stage D HFpEF in the United States were generally disadvantaged in their access to heart transplantation due to the construct of the heart transplant allocation system. A new adult heart transplant allocation system was implemented in the United States in October 2018. In this new six-tier system, noninotrope-dependent patients with end-stage HFpEF are assigned to status 4—the same status as those patients who are supported by LVAD or continuous inotrope infusion.
- Patients with advanced HFpEF who are active on the heart transplant list and who deteriorate further and require hemodynamic monitoring in addition to continuous inotrope infusion, or acute mechanical support in an ICU setting, are assigned even higher status by exemption, thus giving them similar access to donor hearts.

REVIEW QUESTIONS

1. An 82-year-old female with long-standing hypertension, obesity, type 2 diabetes mellitus, and diagnosis of heart failure with preserved ejection fraction (NYHA Class III) presents with dyspnea on exertion, which has increased over several weeks. She sleeps on two pillows and has significant ankle edema. In the last 3 months she had three admissions for heart failure exacerbation. Current medications include aspirin 81 mg once daily, spironolactone 25 mg once daily, Lasix 40 mg twice daily, metoprolol tartrate 25 mg twice daily, lisinopril 40 mg once daily, lorazepam 2 mg nightly at bedtime, and tramadol 25 mg as needed for back pain. ECG did not demonstrate ischemic changes. Her baseline echocardiogram showed mild LV hypertrophy, with septal and posterior wall thickness of 12 mm and an LV end-diastolic dimension of 4.2 cm, with an EF of 60%. She was admitted to hospital for IV diuresis with Lasix. Which of the following interventions may be beneficial in this patient?
   a. Switch metoprolol tartrate to metoprolol succinate.
   b. Refer for pulmonary artery pressure monitor implant.
   c. Refer for LVAD implantation, as patient is likely reached end-stage HFpEF.
   d. Increase dose of lisinopril to 40 mg twice daily.
2. A 65-year-old female with hypertension and diabetes mellitus presented with progressive dyspnea that now occurs with daily activities. The patient has orthopnea and recurrent episodes of wheezing. By examination, her body mass is 220 lb with a heart rate of 86 bpm and blood pressure of 160/98 mmHg. Jugular venous pressure was 12 cm, and bilateral pitting edema was noted to the knee level. Point of maximum impulse was located in the left fifth intercostal space midclavicular line, and P2 was accentuated. Chest radiograph showed central pulmonary congestion. ECG showed sinus rhythm with voltage criteria for left ventricle. Echocardiogram showed preserved ejection fraction, LV hypertrophy, and grade III diastolic dysfunction. After extensive workup she was diagnosed with HFpEF. Which of the following pharmacologic interventions is recommended by current ACC/AHA guidelines to prevent further readmission to the hospital?
   a. Coreg 25 mg twice daily
   b. Valsartan 160 mg once daily
   c. Spironolactone 25 mg once daily
   d. Digoxin 0.25 mg once daily

3. A 63-year-old male has been under your care for HFpEF during the past 5 years. He has been treated for long-standing hypertension, noninsulin-dependent diabetes, and stasis dermatitis of the left leg. He had extensive workup for HF etiologies but so far results have been unrevealing. Over the course of last year he had four admissions for HF exacerbation, and during his last admission his beta blocker was stopped as his blood pressure could not tolerate it anymore. Today he presents in the office with shortness of breath at rest, complaining of inability of completing any daily activity without shortness of breath. His medications include aspirin 81 mg once daily, spironolactone 25 mg once daily, lisinopril 5 mg once daily, and Lasix 80 mg twice daily. In a recent metabolic stress test, his peak VO_2 was 9.4, resting energy requirement (RER) 1.06. His most recent echocardiogram showed ejection fraction of 40%, LV end-diastolic dimension of 4.2 cm, and LV hypertrophy. Which of the following parameters will be a predictor of higher mortality if long-term durable mechanical support with LV assist device is offered to the patient?
   a. Multiple admissions over the last year
   b. NYHA Class IV symptoms
   c. Inability to tolerate beta blockers
   d. LV end-diastolic dimension of 4.2 cm
   e. LV EF of 40%
4. A 72-year-old woman is evaluated for abnormal ECG. She has noninsulin-dependent diabetes mellitus and essential hypertension controlled with medications. She works as a home attendant and states that she can climb five or six flights of stairs without any symptoms. Her physical exam is unremarkable. A transthoracic echocardiogram (TTE) demonstrates anteroapical hypokinesis with LV EF of 40%. According to the ACC/AHA HF classification, she should be considered in which stage?
   a. Stage A
   b. Stage B
   c. Stage C
   d. Stage D
5. According to ACC/AHA guidelines, the following criteria may be consistent with the diagnosis of HFpEF except
   a. LV GLS = 10%.
   b. Ea/Ees = 0.5.
   c. TAPSE = 10 mm.
   d. LV EF = 45%.
6. When compared to patients with HFrEF, patients with HFpEF
   a. are usually younger.
   b. have higher incidence of HF-related hospital admissions.
   c. are more frequently female.
   d. are declining in prevalence.
7. Which of the following results has been most consistently achieved by the long-term use of implantable intracardiac pressure monitoring?
   a. Worse hemodynamics
   b. Reduced incidence of atrial fibrillation
   c. Reduced rehospitalization rates
   d. Prolonged survival
8. Which of the following is correct regarding the effect of IV nitroprusside in acute decompensated HFpEF, when compared to HFrEF?
   a. It is effective in reducing systolic BP in HFpEF.
   b. It results in greater increase in LV stroke volume.
   c. It is less likely to induce symptomatic hypotension.
   d. It is less likely to induce AKI.

REFERENCES

1. Yancy CW, Jessup M, Bozkurt B, et al. 2017 ACC/AHA/HFSA focused update of the 2013 ACCF/AHA guideline for the management of heart failure: a report of the American College of Cardiology/American Heart Association Task Force on Clinical Practice Guidelines and the Heart Failure Society of America. *J Am Coll Cardiol.* 2017;70:776–803.
2. Fang JC, Ewald GA, Allen LA, et al. Heart Failure Society of America Guidelines C. Advanced (stage D) heart failure: a statement from the Heart Failure Society of America Guidelines Committee. *J Card Fail.* 2015;21:519–534.
3. Gott M, Barnes S, Parker C, et al. Dying trajectories in heart failure. *Palliat Med.* 2007;21:95–99.
4. Bjork JB, Alton KK, Georgiopoulou VV, et al. Defining advanced heart failure: a systematic review of criteria used in clinical rrials. *J Card Fail.* 2016;22:569–577.
5. Stevenson LW, Pagani FD, Young JB, et al. INTERMACS profiles of advanced heart failure: the current picture. *J Heart Lung Transplant.* 2009;28:535–541.
6. Metra M, Ponikowski P, Dickstein K, et al. Advanced chronic heart failure: a position statement from the Study Group on Advanced Heart Failure of the Heart Failure Association of the European Society of Cardiology. *Eur J Heart Fail.* 2007;9:684–694.
7. Borlaug BA, Lam CS, Roger VL, et al. Contractility and ventricular systolic stiffening in hypertensive heart disease insights into the pathogenesis of heart failure with preserved ejection fraction. *J Am Coll Cardiol.* 2009;54:410–418.
8. Tan YT, Wenzelburger F, Lee E, et al. The pathophysiology of heart failure with normal ejection fraction: exercise echocardiography reveals complex abnormalities of both systolic and diastolic ventricular function involving torsion, untwist, and longitudinal motion. *J Am Coll Cardiol.* 2009;54:36–46.
9. Shah AM, Claggett B, Sweitzer NK, et al. Prognostic importance of impaired systolic function in heart failure with preserved ejection fraction and the impact of spironolactone. *Circulation.* 2015;132:402–414.
10. Borlaug BA, Olson TP, Lam CS, et al. Global cardiovascular reserve dysfunction in heart failure with preserved ejection fraction. *J Am Coll Cardiol.* 2010;56:845–854.
11. Borlaug BA, Melenovsky V, Russell SD, et al. Impaired chronotropic and vasodilator reserves limit exercise capacity in patients with heart failure and a preserved ejection fraction. *Circulation.* 2006;114:2138–2147.
12. Melenovsky V, Hwang SJ, Lin G, et al. Right heart dysfunction in heart failure with preserved ejection fraction. *Eur Heart J.* 2014;35:3452–3462.
13. Mohammed SF, Hussain I, AbouEzzeddine OF, et al. Right ventricular function in heart failure with preserved ejection fraction: a community-based study. *Circulation.* 2014;130:2310–2320.
14. Haykowsky MJ, Brubaker PH, John JM, et al. Determinants of exercise intolerance in elderly heart failure patients with preserved ejection fraction. *J Am Coll Cardiol.* 2011;58:265–274.
15. Dhakal BP, Malhotra R, Murphy RM, et al. Mechanisms of exercise intolerance in heart failure with preserved ejection fraction: the role of abnormal peripheral oxygen extraction. *Circ Heart Fail.* 2015;8:286–294.
16. Borlaug BA. Is HFpEF one disease or many?. *J Am Coll Cardiol.* 2016;67:671–673.
17. Xanthopoulos A, Triposkiadis F, Starling RC. Heart failure with preserved ejection fraction: classification based upon phenotype is essential for diagnosis and treatment. *Trends Cardiovasc Med.* 2018;28:392–400.
18. Shah SJ, Katz DH, Selvaraj S, et al. Phenomapping for novel classification of heart failure with preserved ejection fraction. *Circulation.* 2015;131:269–279.
19. Lindenfeld J, Albert NM, Boehmer JP, et al. HFSA 2010 comprehensive heart failure practice guideline. *J Card Fail.* 2010;16:e1–e194.
20. Braunwald E. Shattuck lecture—cardiovascular medicine at the turn of the millennium: triumphs, concerns, and opportunities. *N Engl J Med.* 1997;337:1360–1369.
21. Benjamin EJ, Virani SS, Callaway CW, et al. Heart disease and stroke statistics—2018 update: a report from the American Heart Association. *Circulation.* 2018;137:e67–e492.
22. Owan TE, Redfield MM. Epidemiology of diastolic heart failure. *Prog Cardiovasc Dis.* 2005;47:320–332.

23. Owan TE, Hodge DO, Herges RM, et al. Trends in prevalence and outcome of heart failure with preserved ejection fraction. *N Engl J Med.* 2006;355:251–259.
24. Dunlay SM, Roger VL, Redfield MM. Epidemiology of heart failure with preserved ejection fraction. *Nat Rev Cardiol.* 2017;14:591–602.
25. Bursi F, Weston SA, Redfield MM, et al. Systolic and diastolic heart failure in the community. *JAMA.* 2006;296:2209–2216.
26. Devereux RB, Roman MJ, Liu JE, et al. Congestive heart failure despite normal left ventricular systolic function in a population-based sample: the Strong Heart Study. *Am J Cardiol.* 2000;86:1090–1096.
27. Fonarow GC, Stough WG, Abraham WT, et al. Characteristics, treatments, and outcomes of patients with preserved systolic function hospitalized for heart failure: a report from the OPTIMIZE-HF Registry. *J Am Coll Cardiol.* 2007;50:768–777.
28. Ho JE, Lyass A, Lee DS, et al. Predictors of new-onset heart failure: differences in preserved versus reduced ejection fraction. *Circ Heart Fail.* 2013;6:279–286.
29. Ho JE, Enserro D, Brouwers FP, et al. Predicting heart failure with preserved and reduced ejection fraction: the International Collaboration on Heart Failure subtypes. *Circ Heart Fail.* 2016;:9.
30. Senni M, Tribouilloy CM, Rodeheffer RJ, et al. Congestive heart failure in the community: a study of all incident cases in Olmsted County, Minnesota, in 1991. *Circulation.* 1998;98:2282–2289.
31. Gerber Y, Weston SA, Redfield MM, et al. A contemporary appraisal of the heart failure epidemic in Olmsted County, Minnesota. *2000 to 2010. JAMA Intern Med.* 2015;175:996–1004.
32. Steinberg BA, Zhao X, Heidenreich PA, et al. Trends in patients hospitalized with heart failure and preserved left ventricular ejection fraction: prevalence, therapies, and outcomes. *Circulation.* 2012;126:65–75.
33. United Nations. US population. Worldmeters Web site. http://www.worldometers.info/; 2018.
34. US Census Bureau. Resident population of the United States by sex and age as of July 1, 2016 (in millions). Statica Web site. https://www.statista.com/statistics/241488/population-of-the-us-by-sex-and-age/.
35. Ammar KA, Jacobsen SJ, Mahoney DW, et al. Prevalence and prognostic significance of heart failure stages: application of the American College of Cardiology/American Heart Association heart failure staging criteria in the community. *Circulation.* 2007;115:1563–1570.
36. Loehr LR, Rosamond WD, Chang PP, et al. Heart failure incidence and survival (from the Atherosclerosis Risk in Communities study). *Am J Cardiol.* 2008;101:1016–1022.
37. Bleumink GS, Knetsch AM, Sturkenboom MC, et al. Quantifying the heart failure epidemic: prevalence, incidence rate, lifetime risk and prognosis of heart failure. *The Rotterdam Study. Eur Heart J.* 2004;25:1614–2169.
38. Magalski A, Adamson P, Gadler F, et al. Continuous ambulatory right heart pressure measurements with an implantable hemodynamic monitor: a multicenter. 12-month follow-up study of patients with chronic heart failure. *J Card Fail.* 2002;8:63–70.
39. Adamson PB, Magalski A, Braunschweig F, et al. Ongoing right ventricular hemodynamics in heart failure: clinical value of measurements derived from an implantable monitoring system. *J Am Coll Cardiol.* 2003;41:565–571.
40. Bourge RC, Abraham WT, Adamson PB, et al. Randomized controlled trial of an implantable continuous hemodynamic monitor in patients with advanced heart failure: the COMPASS-HF study. *J Am Coll Cardiol.* 2008;51:1073–1079.
41. Ritzema J, Troughton R, Melton I, et al. Physician-directed patient self-management of left atrial pressure in advanced chronic heart failure. *Circulation.* 2010;121:1086–1095.
42. Maurer MS, Adamson PB, Costanzo MR, et al. Rationale and design of the Left Atrial Pressure Monitoring to Optimize Heart Failure Therapy Study (LAPTOP-HF). *J Card Fail.* 2015;21:479–488.
43. Abraham WT, Adamson PB, Costanzo MR, et al. Hemodynamic monitoring in advanced heart failure: results from the LAPTOP-HF trial. *J Cardiac Fail.* 2016;22:940.
44. Abraham WT, Adamson PB, Bourge RC, et al. Wireless pulmonary artery haemodynamic monitoring in chronic heart failure: a randomised controlled trial. *Lancet.* 2011;377:658–666.
45. Adamson PB, Abraham WT, Bourge RC, et al. Wireless pulmonary artery pressure monitoring guides management to reduce decompensation in heart failure with preserved ejection fraction. *Circ Heart Fail.* 2014;7:935–944.
46. Health. USFaDACfDaR. Access Date Web site. https://www.accessdata.fda.gov/cdrh_docs/pdf10/p100045c.pdf; 2018.
47. Abraham WT, Stevenson LW, Bourge RC, et al. Sustained efficacy of pulmonary artery pressure to guide adjustment of chronic heart failure therapy: complete follow-up results from the CHAMPION randomised trial. *Lancet.* 2016;387:453–461.
48. Desai AS, Bhimaraj A, Bharmi R, et al. Ambulatory hemodynamic monitoring reduces heart failure hospitalizations in "real-world" clinical practice. *J Am Coll Cardiol.* 2017;69:2357–2365.
49. Dickinson MG, Allen LA, Albert NA, et al. Remote monitoring of patients with heart failure: a white paper from the Heart Failure Society of America Scientific Statements Committee. *J Card Fail.* 2018;24:682–694.
50. Kaye D, Shah SJ, Borlaug BA, et al. Effects of an interatrial shunt on rest and exercise hemodynamics: results of a computer simulation in heart failure. *J Card Fail.* 2014;20: 212–221.
51. Del Trigo M, Bergeron S, Bernier M, et al. Unidirectional left-to-right interatrial shunting for treatment of patients with heart failure with reduced ejection fraction: a safety and proof-of-principle cohort study. *Lancet.* 2016;387:1290–1297.
52. Hasenfuss G, Hayward C, Burkhoff D, et al. A transcatheter intracardiac shunt device for heart failure with preserved ejection fraction (REDUCE LAP-HF): a multicentre, open-label, single-arm, phase 1 trial. *Lancet.* 2016;387:1298–1304.
53. Kaye DM, Hasenfuss G, Neuzil P, et al. One-year outcomes after transcatheter insertion of an interatrial shunt device for the management of heart failure with preserved ejection fraction. *Circ Heart Fail.* 2016;9.
54. Feldman T, Mauri L, Kahwash R, et al. Transcatheter interatrial shunt device for the treatment of heart failure with preserved ejection fraction (REDUCE LAP-HF I [Reduce Elevated Left Atrial Pressure in Patients With Heart Failure]): a phase 2, randomized, sham-controlled trial. *Circulation.* 2018;137:364–375.
55. Bishu K, Redfield MM. Acute heart failure with preserved ejection fraction: unique patient characteristics and targets for therapy. *Curr Heart Fail Rep.* 2013;10:190–197.
56. Yancy CW, Lopatin M, Stevenson LW, et al. Clinical presentation, management, and in-hospital outcomes of patients admitted with acute decompensated heart failure with preserved systolic function: a report from the Acute Decompensated Heart Failure National Registry (ADHERE) database. *J Am Coll Cardiol.* 2006;47:76–84.
57. Channer KS, McLean KA, Lawson-Matthew P, et al. Combination diuretic treatment in severe heart failure: a randomised controlled trial. *Br Heart J.* 1994;71:146–150.
58. Bart BA, Goldsmith SR, Lee KL, et al. Ultrafiltration in decompensated heart failure with cardiorenal syndrome. *N Engl J Med.* 2012;367:2296–2304.
59. Costanzo MR, Saltzberg MT, Jessup M, et al. Ultrafiltration is associated with fewer rehospitalizations than continuous diuretic infusion in patients with decompensated heart failure: results from UNLOAD. *J Card Fail.* 2010;16:277–284.
60. Jeffries JL, Bartone C, Menon S, et al. Ultrafiltration in heart failure with preserved ejection fraction: comparison with systolic heart failure patients. *Circ Heart Fail.* 2013;6:733–739.
61. Cotter G, Metra M, Milo-Cotter O, et al. Fluid overload in acute heart failure—re-distribution and other mechanisms beyond fluid accumulation. *Eur J Heart Fail.* 2008;10:165–169.
62. Schwartzenberg S, Redfield MM, From AM, et al. Effects of vasodilation in heart failure with preserved or reduced ejection fraction implications of distinct pathophysiologies on response to therapy. *J Am Coll Cardiol.* 2012;59:442–451.
63. Cotter G, Metzkor E, Kaluski E, et al. Randomised trial of high-dose isosorbide dinitrate plus low-dose furosemide versus high-dose furosemide plus low-dose isosorbide dinitrate in severe pulmonary oedema. *Lancet.* 1998;351:389–393.
64. Udelson JE, Stevenson LW. The future of heart failure diagnosis, therapy, and management. *Circulation.* 2016;133:2671–2686.
65. Kitzman DW, Hundley WG, Brubaker PH, et al. A randomized double-blind trial of enalapril in older patients with heart failure and preserved

ejection fraction: effects on exercise tolerance and arterial distensibility. *Circ Heart Fail.* 2010;3:477–485.
66. Redfield MM, Chen HH, Borlaug BA, et al. Effect of phosphodiesterase-5 inhibition on exercise capacity and clinical status in heart failure with preserved ejection fraction: a randomized clinical trial. *JAMA.* 2013;309:1268–1277.
67. Edelmann F, Wachter R, Schmidt AG, et al. Effect of spironolactone on diastolic function and exercise capacity in patients with heart failure with preserved ejection fraction: the Aldo-DHF randomized controlled trial. *JAMA.* 2013;309:781–791.
68. Redfield MM, Anstrom KJ, Levine JA, et al. Isosorbide mononitrate in heart failure with preserved ejection fraction. *N Engl J Med.* 2015;373:2314–2324.
69. Kitzman DW, Brubaker PH, Morgan TM, et al. Exercise training in older patients with heart failure and preserved ejection fraction: a randomized, controlled, single-blind trial. *Circ Heart Fail.* 2010;3:659–667.
70. Pitt B, Pfeffer MA, Assmann SF, et al. Spironolactone for heart failure with preserved ejection fraction. *N Engl J Med.* 2014;370:1383–1392.
71. Pfeffer MA, Claggett B, Assmann SF, et al. Regional variation in patients and outcomes in the Treatment of Preserved Cardiac Function Heart Failure With an Aldosterone Antagonist (TOPCAT) trial. *Circulation.* 2015;131:34–42.
72. de Denus S, O'Meara E, Desai AS, et al. Spironolactone metabolites in TOPCAT—new insights into regional variation. *N Engl J Med.* 2017;376:1690–1692.
73. Rose EA, Gelijns AC, Moskowitz AJ, et al. Long-term use of a left ventricular assist device for end-stage heart failure. *N Engl J Med.* 2001;345:1435–1443.
74. Hershberger RE, Nauman D, Walker TL, et al. Care processes and clinical outcomes of continuous outpatient support with inotropes (COSI) in patients with refractory endstage heart failure. *J Card Fail.* 2003;9:180–187.
75. Sindone AP, Keogh AM, Macdonald PS, et al. Continuous home ambulatory intravenous inotropic drug therapy in severe heart failure: safety and cost efficacy. *Am Heart J.* 1997;134:889–900.
76. Gorodeski EZ, Chu EC, Reese JR, et al. Prognosis on chronic dobutamine or milrinone infusions for stage D heart failure. *Circ Heart Fail.* 2009;2:320–324.
77. Whellan DJ, Goodlin SJ, Dickinson MG, et al. End-of-life care in patients with heart failure. *J Card Fail.* 2014;20:121–134.
78. Deswal A, Richardson P, Bozkurt B, et al. Results of the Randomized Aldosterone Antagonism in Heart Failure with Preserved Ejection Fraction trial (RAAM-PEF). *J Card Fail.* 2011;17:634–642.
79. Kosmala W, Holland DJ, Rojek A, et al. Effect of If-channel inhibition on hemodynamic status and exercise tolerance in heart failure with preserved ejection fraction: a randomized trial. *J Am Coll Cardiol.* 2013;62:1330–1338.
80. Maier LS, Layug B, Karwatowska-Prokopczuk E, et al. RAnoLazIne for the treatment of diastolic heart failure in patients with preserved ejection fraction: the RALI-DHF proof-of-concept study. *JACC Heart Fail.* 2013;1:115–122.
81. Slaughter MS, Rogers JG, Milano CA, et al. Advanced heart failure treated with continuous-flow left ventricular assist device. *N Engl J Med.* 2009;361:2241–2251.
82. Mehra MR, Naka Y, Uriel N, et al. A fully magnetically levitated circulatory pump for advanced heart failure. *N Engl J Med.* 2017;376:440–450.
83. Topilsky Y, Pereira NL, Shah DK, et al. Left ventricular assist device therapy in patients with restrictive and hypertrophic cardiomyopathy. *Circ Heart Fail.* 2011;4:266–275.
84. Muthiah K, Phan J, Robson D, et al. Centrifugal continuous-flow left ventricular assist device in patients with hypertrophic cardiomyopathy: a case series. *ASAIO J.* 2013;59:183–187.
85. Cho YH, Deo SV, Topilsky Y, et al. Left ventricular assist device implantation in a patient who had previously undergone apical myectomy for hypertrophic cardiomyopathy. *J Card Surg.* 2012;27:266–268.
86. Cevik C, Nguyen HU, Civitello AB, et al. Percutaneous ventricular assist device in hypertrophic obstructive cardiomyopathy with cardiogenic shock: bridge to myectomy. *Ann Thorac Surg.* 2012;93:978–980.
87. Swiecicki PL, Edwards BS, Kushwaha SS, et al. Left ventricular device implantation for advanced cardiac amyloidosis. *J Heart Lung Transplant.* 2013;32:563–568.
88. Lund LH, Matthews J, Aaronson K. Patient selection for left ventricular assist devices. *Eur J Heart Fail.* 2010;12:434–443.
89. Burkhoff D, Maurer MS, Joseph SM, et al. Left atrial decompression pump for severe heart failure with preserved ejection fraction: theoretical and clinical considerations. *JACC Heart Fail.* 2015;3:275–282.
90. Moscato F, Wirrmann C, Granegger M, et al. Use of continuous flow ventricular assist devices in patients with heart failure and a normal ejection fraction: a computer-simulation study. *J Thorac Cardiovasc Surg.* 2013;145:1352–1358.
91. Grupper A, Park SJ, Pereira NL, et al. Role of ventricular assist therapy for patients with heart failure and restrictive physiology: improving outcomes for a lethal disease. *J Heart Lung Transplant.* 2015;34:1042–1049.
92. Patel SR, Saeed O, Naftel D, et al. Outcomes of restrictive and hypertrophic cardiomyopathies after LVAD: an INTERMACS analysis. *J Card Fail.* 2017;23:859–867.
93. Rowin EJ, Maron BJ, Kiernan MS, et al. Advanced heart failure with preserved systolic function in nonobstructive hypertrophic cardiomyopathy: under-recognized subset of candidates for heart transplant. *Circ Heart Fail.* 2014;7:967–975.
94. Maron BJ, Maron MS. Hypertrophic cardiomyopathy. *Lancet.* 2013;381:242–255.
95. Gersh BJ, Maron BJ, Bonow RO, et al. 2011 ACCF/AHA guideline for the diagnosis and treatment of hypertrophic cardiomyopathy: a report of the American College of Cardiology Foundation/American Heart Association Task Force on Practice Guidelines. *Circulation.* 2011;124:e783–e831.
96. Maron MS, Kalsmith BM, Udelson JE, et al. Survival after cardiac transplantation in patients with hypertrophic cardiomyopathy. *Circ Heart Fail.* 2010;3:574–579.
97. Olivotto I, Cecchi F, Poggesi C, et al. Patterns of disease progression in hypertrophic cardiomyopathy: an individualized approach to clinical staging. *Circ Heart Fail.* 2012;5:535–546.
98. Harris KM, Spirito P, Maron MS, et al. Prevalence, clinical profile, and significance of left ventricular remodeling in the end-stage phase of hypertrophic cardiomyopathy. *Circulation.* 2006;114:216–225.
99. Melacini P, Basso C, Angelini A, et al. Clinicopathological profiles of progressive heart failure in hypertrophic cardiomyopathy. *Eur Heart J.* 2010;31:2111–2123.
100. Fernandez A, Vigliano CA, Casabe JH, et al. Comparison of prevalence, clinical course, and pathological findings of left ventricular systolic impairment versus normal systolic function in patients with hypertrophic cardiomyopathy. *Am J Cardiol.* 2011;108:548–555.
101. Thaman R, Gimeno JR, Murphy RT, et al. Prevalence and clinical significance of systolic impairment in hypertrophic cardiomyopathy. *Heart.* 2005;91:920–925.
102. Biagini E, Coccolo F, Ferlito M, et al. Dilated-hypokinetic evolution of hypertrophic cardiomyopathy: prevalence, incidence, risk factors, and prognostic implications in pediatric and adult patients. *J Am Coll Cardiol.* 2005;46:1543–1550.
103. Olivotto I, Cecchi F, Gistri R, et al. Relevance of coronary microvascular flow impairment to long-term remodeling and systolic dysfunction in hypertrophic cardiomyopathy. *J Am Coll Cardiol.* 2006;47:1043–1048.
104. Ho CY, Lopez B, Coelho-Filho OR, et al. Myocardial fibrosis as an early manifestation of hypertrophic cardiomyopathy. *N Engl J Med.* 2010;363:552–563.
105. Rowin EJ, Maron BJ, Abt P, et al. Impact of advanced therapies for improving survival to heart transplant in patients with hypertrophic cardiomyopathy. *Am J Cardiol.* 2018;121:986–996.
106. Arabia FA, Cantor RS, Koehl DA, et al. Interagency registry for mechanically assisted circulatory support report on the total artificial heart. *J Heart Lung Transplant.* 2018;37:1304–1312.
107. Kato TS, Takayama H, Yoshizawa S, et al. Cardiac transplantation in patients with hypertrophic cardiomyopathy. *Am J Cardiol.* 2012;110:568–574.
108. DePasquale EC, Nasir K, Jacoby DL. Outcomes of adults with restrictive cardiomyopathy after heart transplantation. *J Heart Lung Transplant.* 2012;31:1269–1275.

109. Hsich EM, Rogers JG, McNamara DM, et al. Does survival on the heart transplant waiting list depend on the underlying heart disease?. *JACC Heart Fail.* 2016;4:689–697.
110. Gray Gilstrap L, Niehaus E, Malhotra R, et al. Predictors of survival to orthotopic heart transplant in patients with light chain amyloidosis. *J Heart Lung Transplant.* 2014;33:149–156.
111. Varr BC, Liedtke M, Arai S, et al. Heart transplantation and cardiac amyloidosis: approach to screening and novel management strategies. *J Heart Lung Transplant.* 2012;31:325–331.
112. Castano A, Drachman BM, Judge D, et al. Natural history and therapy of TTR-cardiac amyloidosis: emerging disease-modifying therapies from organ transplantation to stabilizer and silencer drugs. *Heart Fail Rev.* 2015;20:163–178.
113. Gillmore JD, Goodman HJ, Lachmann HJ, et al. Sequential heart and autologous stem cell transplantation for systemic AL amyloidosis. *Blood.* 2006;107:1227–1229.
114. Lacy MQ, Dispenzieri A, Hayman SR, et al. Autologous stem cell transplant after heart transplant for light chain (Al) amyloid cardiomyopathy. *J Heart Lung Transplant.* 2008;27:823–829.
115. Dey BR, Chung SS, Spitzer TR, et al. Cardiac transplantation followed by dose-intensive melphalan and autologous stem-cell transplantation for light chain amyloidosis and heart failure. *Transplantation.* 2010;90:905–911.
116. Raichlin E, Daly RC, Rosen CB, et al. Combined heart and liver transplantation: a single-center experience. *Transplantation.* 2009;88:219–225.
117. Uriel N, Vainrib A, Jorde UP, et al. Mediastinal radiation and adverse outcomes after heart transplantation. *J Heart Lung Transplant.* 2010;29:378–381.
118. Lund LH, Edwards LB, Dipchand AI, et al. The registry of the International Society for Heart and Lung Transplantation: thirty-third adult heart transplantation report-2016; focus theme: primary diagnostic indications for transplant. *J Heart Lung Transplant.* 2016;35:1158–1169.
119. Tallaj JA, Kirklin JK, Brown RN, et al. Post-heart transplant diastolic dysfunction is a risk factor for mortality. *J Am Coll Cardiol.* 2007;50:1064–1069.
120. Hausdorf G, Banner NR, Mitchell A, et al. Diastolic function after cardiac and heart-lung transplantation. *Br Heart J.* 1989;62:123–132.
121. Paulus WJ, Bronzwaer JG, Felice H, Kishan N, Wellens F. Deficient acceleration of left ventricular relaxation during exercise after heart transplantation. *Circulation.* 1992;86:1175–1185.
122. Skowronski EW, Epstein M, Ota D, et al. Right and left ventricular function after cardiac transplantation. Changes during and after rejection. Circulation. 1991;84:2409–2417.
123. Frist WH, Stinson EB, Oyer PE, et al. Long-term hemodynamic results after cardiac transplantation. *J Thorac Cardiovasc Surg.* 1987;94:685–693.
124. Braith RW, Mills Jr RM, Wilcox CS, et al. Fluid homeostasis after heart transplantation: the role of cardiac denervation. *J Heart Lung Transplant.* 1996;15:872–880.
125. McClurken JB, Todd BA, Mather PJ, et al. Recipient-donor atrial synchronization benefits acute hemodynamics after orthotopic heart transplantation. *J Heart Lung Transplant.* 1996;15:368–370.
126. Greenberg ML, Uretsky BF, Reddy PS, et al. Long-term hemodynamic follow-up of cardiac transplant patients treated with cyclosporine and prednisone. *Circulation.* 1985;71:487–494.
127. Verani MS, George SE, Leon CA, et al. Systolic and diastolic ventricular performance at rest and during exercise in heart transplant recipients. *J Heart Transplant.* 1988;7:145–151.
128. StGoar FG, Gibbons R, Schnittger I, et al. Left ventricular diastolic function. Doppler echocardiographic changes soon after cardiac transplantation. *Circulation.* 1990;82:872–878.
129. Young JB, Leon CA, Short III HD, et al. Evolution of hemodynamics after orthotopic heart and heart-lung transplantation: early restrictive patterns persisting in occult fashion. *J Heart Transplant.* 1987;6:34–43.
130. Valantine HA, Appleton CP, Hatle LK, et al. A hemodynamic and Doppler echocardiographic study of ventricular function in long-term cardiac allograft recipients. Etiology and prognosis of restrictive-constrictive physiology. *Circulation.* 1989;79:66–75.
131. Mankad JS, Aaronson KD, Mancini DM. Serial assessment of exercise capacity after heart transplantation. *J Heart Lung Transplant.* 1995;14:468–478.
132. Stevenson LW, Sietsema K, Tillisch JH, et al. Exercise capacity for survivors of cardiac transplantation or sustained medical therapy for stable heart failure. *Circulation.* 1990;81:78–85.
133. Kao AC, Van Trigt III P, Shaeffer-McCall GS, et al. Allograft diastolic dysfunction and chronotropic incompetence limit cardiac output response to exercise two to six years after heart transplantation. *J Heart Lung Transplant.* 1995;14:11–22.
134. Ross HJ, Gullestad L, Hunt SA, et al. Early Doppler echocardiographic dysfunction is associated with an increased mortality after orthotopic cardiac transplantation. *Circulation.* 1996;94:II289–II293.
135. Aziz TM, Burgess MI, Haselton PS, et al. Transforming growth factor beta and diastolic left ventricular dysfunction after heart transplantation: echocardiographic and histologic evidence. *J Heart Lung Transplant.* 2003;22:663–673.
136. Lund LH, Khush KK, Cherikh WS, et al. The registry of the International Society for Heart and Lung Transplantation: thirty-fourth adult heart transplantation report-2017; focus theme: allograft ischemic time. *J Heart Lung Transplant.* 2017;36:1037–1046.
137. Baraldi-Junkins C, Levin HR, Kasper EK, et al. Complications of endomyocardial biopsy in heart transplant patients. *J Heart Lung Transplant.* 1993;12:63–67.
138. Spiegelhalter DJ, Stovin PG. An analysis of repeated biopsies following cardiac transplantation. *Stat Med.* 1983;2:33–40.
139. Sagar KB, Hastillo A, Wolfgang TC, et al. Left ventricular mass by M-mode echocardiography in cardiac transplant patients with acute rejection. *Circulation.* 1981;64:II217–II220.
140. Amende I, Simon R, Seegers A, et al. Diastolic dysfunction during acute cardiac allograft rejection. *Circulation.* 1990;81:III66–III70.
141. Puleo JA, Aranda JM, Weston MW, et al. Noninvasive detection of allograft rejection in heart transplant recipients by use of Doppler tissue imaging. *J Heart Lung Transplant.* 1998;17:176–184.
142. Seacord LM, Miller LW, Pennington DG, et al. Reversal of constrictive/restrictive physiology with treatment of allograft rejection. *Am Heart J.* 1990;120:455–459.
143. Valantine HA, Fowler MB, Hunt SA, et al. Changes in Doppler echocardiographic indexes of left ventricular function as potential markers of acute cardiac rejection. *Circulation.* 1987;76:V86–V92.
144. Barba J, Gomez JA, Abecia AC, et al. [Changes in diastolic function in heart rejection: role of Doppler echocardiography]. *Rev Esp Cardiol.* 1992;45:652–656.
145. Berwing K, Friedl A, Schaper J, et al. [Doppler and echocardiography parameters in detection of acute graft rejection after heart transplantation]. *Z Kardiol.* 1994;83:225–233.
146. Seiler C, Aeschbacher BC, Meier B. Quantitation of mitral regurgitation using the systolic/diastolic pulmonary venous flow velocity ratio. *J Am Coll Cardiol.* 1998;31:1383–1390.
147. Hausmann B, Muurling S, Stauch C, et al. Detection of diastolic dysfunction: acoustic quantification (AQ) in comparison to Doppler echocardiography. *Int J Card Imaging.* 1997;13:301–310.
148. Derumeaux G, Douillet R, Redonnet M, et al. [Detection of acute rejection of heart transplantation by Doppler color imaging]. *Arch Mal Coeur Vaiss.* 1998;91:1255–1262.
149. Dandel M, Hummel M, Muller J, et al. Reliability of tissue Doppler wall motion monitoring after heart transplantation for replacement of invasive routine screenings by optimally timed cardiac biopsies and catheterizations. *Circulation.* 2001;104:I184–I191.
150. Stengel SM, Allemann Y, Zimmerli M, et al. Doppler tissue imaging for assessing left ventricular diastolic dysfunction in heart transplant rejection. *Heart.* 2001;86:432–437.
151. Sun JP, Abdalla IA, Asher CR, et al. Non-invasive evaluation of orthotopic heart transplant rejection by echocardiography. *J Heart Lung Transplant.* 2005;24:160–165.
152. Palka P, Lange A, Galbraith A, et al. The role of left and right ventricular early diastolic Doppler tissue echocardiographic indices in the evaluation of acute rejection in orthotopic heart transplant. *J Am Soc Echocardiogr.* 2005;18:107–115.

23

Primary Restrictive, Infiltrative, and Storage Cardiomyopathies

Serge C. Harb, Craig R. Asher, and Allan L. Klein

OUTLINE

INTRODUCTION

A classification serves to bridge the gap between ignorance and knowledge.

J.F. Goodwin[1]

Historically, restrictive cardiomyopathies were among the three primary forms of idiopathic heart muscle diseases, characterized by the World Health Organization as "restrictive filling and reduced diastolic volume of either or both ventricles with normal or near-normal systolic function."[2,3] This early grouping of cardiomyopathies highlighted the readily evident morphologic and functional features of these disorders, which were largely of unknown cause. With advances in diagnostic testing (biochemistry, genetics, immunology, and pathology) and cardiac imaging techniques (echocardiography, computed tomography [CT], magnetic resonance imaging [MRI]), the etiology of many cardiomyopathies can now be identified. The classification proposal of the American Heart Association (AHA) defines primary (involving predominantly the heart) and secondary (related to systemic disorders) cardiomyopathies.[4] Using this classification, except for primary restrictive cardiomyopathy, the entity of "restrictive cardiomyopathy" no longer exists, and most infiltrative and storage disorders are considered specific secondary cardiomyopathies (i.e., amyloid cardiomyopathy). With increasing genetic knowledge and availability of genetic testing, a new phenotype-genotype classification scheme—the MOGE(S) classification—has been endorsed by the World Heart Federation.[5] This system involves notation of five cardiomyopathy characteristics:

- M: Morphofunctional or phenotype
- O: Organ involvement
- G: Genetic transmission
- E: Etiology
- (S): Functional status (This last attribute is optional.)

However, the clinical applicability of this new classification scheme has not yet been established.[6]

From the point of view of the clinician, however they are compiled, these are disorders in which diastolic dysfunction is at least initially the predominant pathophysiologic derangement. They are uncommon diseases, generally with a poor prognosis, and often presenting with advanced right-sided or left-sided heart failure. Much of the data regarding these diseases are based on observational retrospective studies from tertiary centers with little prospective and randomized information. Although a cardiologist will often initiate testing, a multidisciplinary team of geneticists, pathologists, radiologists, hematologists, and oncologists is often required to refine the diagnosis and determine management strategies. Since infiltrative and storage cardiomyopathies occur as part of a multisystem disorder, treatments with chemotherapeutic agents, stem cells, and enzyme replacement are increasingly becoming options.

This chapter will review primary restrictive cardiomyopathy and the most prevalent forms of infiltrative and storage disorders encountered among patients surviving into adulthood. A practical approach to diagnosis, differentiation, and exclusion of other more common disorders with similar pathophysiology and structural appearance will be presented along with current treatment options.

PATHOPHYSIOLOGY

Most primary restrictive cardiomyopathies are characterized by at most mild degrees of increased wall thickness on gross inspection.[7–9] Cardiac biopsy will distinguish whether at the cellular level there is myocyte hypertrophy (increased myocyte diameter and nuclear area), endocardial and interstitial fibrosis (increased collagen to muscle ratio), or both (Fig. 23.1).[10,11] Exclusion of fiber disarray, inflammation, eosinophilia, lymphocytes, amyloid or iron deposits, and pericardial disease via light and electron microscopy is required to distinguish primary restrictive diseases from secondary cardiomyopathies or pericardial diseases that may also manifest with advanced stages of diastolic dysfunction. Absence of an endocardial fibrotic shell with extension into the myocardium excludes endomyocardial disease.

Structural characteristics of primary restrictive cardiomyopathies include (a) biatrial enlargement, (b) nondilated or reduced left ventricular (LV) cavity size, and (c) normal or mildly increased wall thickness.[10] The LV ejection fraction (EF) is usually normal during early stages but often declines with disease progression. Strain imaging also demonstrates abnormal LV and left atrial (LA) contractility almost universally in these patients (see Chapters 4, 12, and 29). The pathogenesis of diastolic impairment may be secondary to myocyte abnormalities, including abnormal calcium handling, accumulation of desmin (a cytoskeletal component), myocyte hypertrophy, and extracellular matrix interstitial fibrosis with proliferation of collagen fibers and elastic elements.[12–14] A marked increase in stiffness of the myocardium or endocardium causes the ventricular pressure to rise dramatically with only small changes in volume, causing an upward shift of the LV pressure-volume relationship and a dip-and-plateau or square-root hemodynamic pattern.[15] Both ventricles are affected by the process, but usually the pressures are higher on the left than the right, which may reflect the relatively decreased compliance of the left ventricle compared with the right ventricle.

Secondary infiltrative and storage cardiomyopathies result from the presence of myocardial cellular or extracellular substances that impair diastolic function. In infiltrative diseases, there is localization to the interstitium (between myocardial cells), as with cardiac amyloidosis; whereas in storage disorders, the deposits are within cells, as with hemochromatosis and Fabry disease.[16] The infiltrative and storage cardiomyopathies may have heterogeneous morphologic and hemodynamic findings, depending on the specific underlying process and the stage of disease, which often involves LV dysfunction, increased wall thickness, and nonrestrictive diastolic filling patterns.

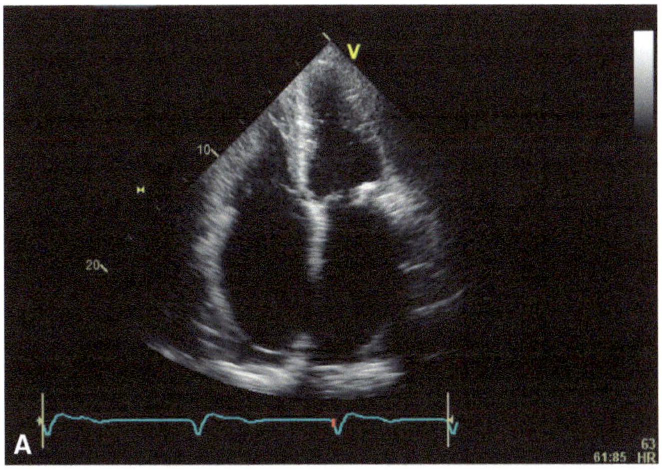

Fig. 23.1A Case Study 1: Apical 4 chamber view of patient with idiopathic restrictive cardiomyopathy demonstrating small left ventricular cavity and severe biatrial enlargement. From Chapter 77, The Dilated, Restrictive and Infiltrative Cardiomyopathies, Rodney H. Falk and Ray E. Hersh 77.8. Elsevier.

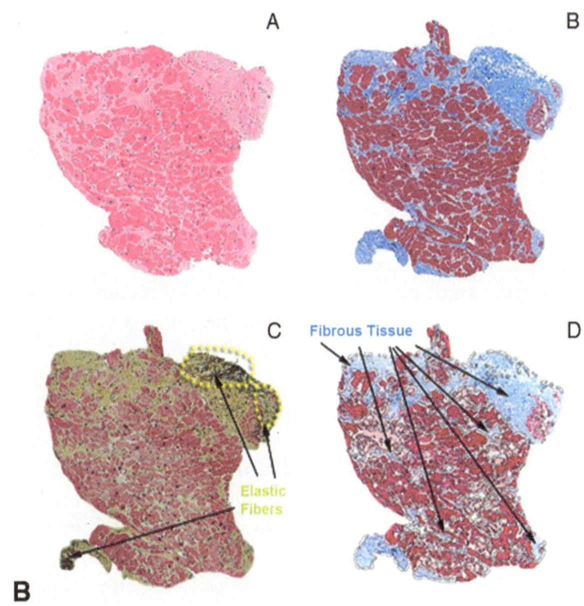

Fig. 23.1B Case Study 1: Light microscopy of endomyocardial biopsy in restrictive cardiomyopathy. **A.** Myocardium showing moderate hypertrophy with myocytes measuring between 30–40 micrometers in average diameter. There is no evidence of storage material in the myocytes' sarcoplasm. The endocardium is thickened and the interstitial space is increased by eosinophilic connective tissue material. (Hematoxylin and eosin, × 100). **B.** Connective tissue stain (trichrome) show dense blue material (fibrosis) which thickens the endocardium and expands the interstitial space surrounding practically every myocyte in the biopsy sample. This forms a restrictive "girdle" that restricts contractility (contraction and relaxation) of the myocytes. (Masson Trichrome stain, ×100). **C.** The fibrous tissue stains yellow in this stain with the same pattern as shown in B. However in this stain there is also accumulation of elastic lamellae in the endocardium consistent with endocardial fibroelastosis in addition to the interstitial fibrosis. (Movat pentachrome, × 100). **D.** This illustration highlights the contours of the myocytes with interstitial fibrous tissue as well as the thickened endocardium in the upper and lower surfaces of the biopsy piece. (Masson trichrome, ×100) With Permission Dr. Rene Rodriguez and Dr. Carmela Tan, Department of Cardiovascular Pathology, Cleveland Clinic, Cleveland, Oh.

CLINICAL RELEVANCE

Primary Restrictive Cardiomyopathies

Case Study 1

A 23-year-old woman presents to her family physician complaining of fatigue, exercise intolerance, muscle aches, and dyspnea with exertion. No other past medical history (PMH) is present. Family history is significant for an aunt with hypertrophic cardiomyopathy (HCM). On examination, she is found to be tachycardic. The cardiac exam is notable for an elevated jugular venous pressure of 10 cm H_2O, an S_3 gallop, and 1+ lower extremity pitting edema. An electrocardiogram (ECG) shows first-degree atrioventricular (AV) block with a P-R interval of 240 msec. A chest x-ray (CXR) shows mild pulmonary congestion. Brain natriuretic peptide (BNP) level is 750 pg/mL, and the creatine phosphokinase (CPK) level is 280 units/L. An echocardiogram shows normal LV and right ventricular (RV) size and function, with moderately dilated atria, grade III diastolic dysfunction (restrictive filling pattern), E/e′ of 15, and a delayed color M mode slope of 35 cm/sec. Cardiac MRI shows normal pericardial thickness and near normal LV wall thickness. Subsequent cardiac catheterization is notable for pressures (mmHg) as follows: right atrial, 15; right ventricular end diastolic, 17; left ventricular end diastolic, 24; pulmonary artery systolic pressure, 55; pulmonary capillary wedge pressure, 25; and cardiac index, 2.3 L/min/m^2. Cardiac biopsy confirms idiopathic restrictive cardiomyopathy and excludes specific infiltrative and storage diseases.

Diagnosis

Primary (or idiopathic) restrictive cardiomyopathy (RCM) is a rare disorder of advanced diastolic impairment, often leading to biventricular diastolic heart failure and sudden cardiac death. It was first described by Benotti et al. in nine patients with heart failure, elevated RV and LV filling pressures, normal systolic function, and dip-and-plateau hemodynamic tracing.[17] In children, the disease is more common in females, and the prognosis is worse compared with adults.[18,19] Familial autosomal dominant transmission and the association with skeletal myopathies (predominantly distal) and heart block have been reported in several generations of families.[10,20,21] Other associations include family members with HCM and Noonan syndrome.[22] Genetic sequence analysis studies in patients with idiopathic RCM have shown mutations in approximately 60% of patients, including in the *MYH7, DES, FLNC, MYBPC3, LMNA, TCAP, TNNI3, TNNT2, TPM1,* and *LAMP2* loci.[23]

The clinical signs and symptoms of primary restrictive cardiac disease relate closely to the degree of LA hypertension required to compensate for reduced ventricular filling.[7,24] Initially, there is exercise intolerance and fatigue, progressing to dyspnea with minimal effort. Exertional chest pain is usually absent. Atrial fibrillation is common due to atrial enlargement. Ventricular arrhythmias or heart block are commonly present in advanced cases and are often the causes of death. Symptoms of proximal or distal myopathy may be present. Cardiac examination may reveal pulmonary congestion, jugular venous distention with a prominent x and y descent, and S_3 depending on the filling characteristics. Right heart failure with hepatomegaly, ascites, peripheral edema, and anasarca are present in advanced cases.[7,25] Kussmaul sign can be detected, while apical retraction (as in constrictive pericarditis) is not seen.

Laboratory testing may provide supportive information. BNP levels are elevated proportional to the degree of elevation in filling pressures and grade of diastolic dysfunction. Elevated BNP levels also may aid in excluding constrictive physiology.[26] CPK levels may be elevated with concomitant myopathy. No data are available on troponin levels in patients with idiopathic restrictive cardiomyopathy.

Echocardiography is often the first-line test and may be virtually diagnostic.[27,28] Atrial enlargement with nondilated ventricles with near normal systolic function is uniformly present on echocardiography. Mild LV dysfunction may develop among patients with advanced disease requiring transplantation. Generally, if hypertrophy is present, it is mild (<15 mm). The pathophysiologic findings of advanced diastolic dysfunction are evident with a comprehensive echocardiographic Doppler study (elevated filling pressures ± restrictive physiology). Restrictive physiology may not be present, depending on the grade of diastolic dysfunction and loading conditions, but abnormal diastolic function should be evident by evaluation of mitral and tricuspid inflow patterns, pulmonary and hepatic venous flows, and isovolumic relaxation time (IVRT).[29,30] Tissue Doppler echocardiography (TDE) e′ and a′ annular velocities are low, with mitral E/e′ annular ratios elevated, consistent with high filling pressures.[29] Concomitantly, the color M mode propagation slope is slow.[31] Tissue Doppler imaging and color M mode, along with pulsed Doppler flow patterns with a respirometer, can help distinguish restrictive from constrictive physiology (see Chapters 10, 11, and 26).

MRI and CT may be useful to exclude increased pericardial thickness, septal bounce, or conical compression.[32,33] Cine MRI may show abnormal filling patterns in early and advanced stages of restrictive cardiomyopathy similar to echocardiography. MRI is capable of distinguishing tissue characteristics and shows a diffuse reduction in signal intensity due to fibrosis in idiopathic restrictive cardiomyopathy, with more specific patterns in other infiltrative processes such as amyloidosis or hemochromatosis.[31]

Cardiac catheterization is often used as a confirmatory test. Using strict criteria, either right-sided or left-sided filling pressures are elevated, with a typical dip-and-plateau RV and LV filling pattern and an M-shaped or W-shaped venous filling pattern with prominent x and y descents.[6] LV diastolic pressures are greater than 5 mmHg more than RV filling pressures. Cardiac index is reduced, and pulmonary artery pressure is greater than 50 mmHg in most patients with a ratio of RV systolic to diastolic pressure greater than 1:3. Often RV endomyocardial biopsy is done at the same time as hemodynamic assessment and importantly excludes other specific etiologies.[9,34]

Management. The prognosis of idiopathic restrictive cardiomyopathy depends most on the age of the patient and presenting hemodynamic factors. Although variable, the course is usually progressive and generally poor among the pediatric population, with survival rates of less than 50% over 2 years, in some studies.[19,35] A serial study of 18 children (9 male; mean age, 4.3 years) evaluated over a course of 31 years at Texas Children's Hospital found that predictors of sudden death included female sex, chest pain, syncope, and ischemia on Holter monitor. The annual mortality rate was 7%, with sudden death occurring in 28% of patients.[34] Other predictors of poor outcome in the pediatric population include decreased cardiac index, pulmonary venous congestion, and elevated pulmonary vascular resistance.[10,20,36,37]

Beta blockers are the primary therapy to reduce the risk of sudden death. Additional medical therapy includes diuretics for symptomatic relief and consideration of antiplatelet agents or anticoagulation, due to the high risk of atrial fibrillation and embolism reported in some series.[33] Vasodilators should be used cautiously unless LV dysfunction is present, since they may cause hypotension. Pacemakers are often required for heart block. Implantable cardioverter-defibrillators are recommended for any patients with ischemic manifestations, along with listing for transplantation.[38] Transplantation can substantially improve survival and is usually required within 4 years of diagnosis, optimally before pulmonary vascular resistance is irreversibly high.[39] Heart-lung transplantation is an option for some children.[39] When concomitant skeletal myopathy is present, the benefits of transplantation may be partial.

Idiopathic restrictive cardiomyopathy may also be diagnosed in adults after exclusion of secondary causes of restrictive physiology. A large series of 94 patients (mean age, 64 years) was identified from 1979 to 1996 at the Mayo Clinic, with typical structural and hemodynamic features of restrictive cardiomyopathy.[40] At follow-up of 68 months, 50% of patients had died, primarily from cardiac causes, and four patients required heart transplantation. Using multivariate analysis, predictors of death included male sex, LA dimension greater than 60 mm, age older than 70 years, and advanced New York Heart Association (NYHA) class (Fig. 23.2).

Infiltrative Cardiomyopathies

Using the AHA classification, cardiac amyloidosis is the most important infiltrative cardiomyopathy in adults. Sarcoidosis has been categorized as a secondary inflammatory disorder.[4] The exceedingly rare infiltrative disorders—Gaucher, Hurler, and Hunter diseases—are familial defects in metabolism that involve multiple systems, including the heart, and will not be discussed in this chapter.

Cardiac Amyloidosis

Case Study 2

A 44-year-old man presents to a cardiologist for a second opinion regarding amyloid cardiomyopathy. He complains of dyspnea with exertion, orthopnea, orthostasis, abdominal distention, and lower extremity swelling and numbness. No other PMH is present. Family history is significant for his father and brother, who died in their 40s with cardiomyopathy. On examination, he appears cachectic and has a supine blood pressure (BP) of 96/64 and upright BP of 80/68 mmHg. The cardiac exam is notable for jugular venous distention to the jaw. There is S_3 gallop, reduced intensity heart sounds, and a II/VI pansystolic murmur at apex. There is ascites and 3+ lower extremity pitting edema. An ECG shows low voltage in the limb leads and an intraventricular conduction delay. CXR shows a globular heart silhouette and mild pulmonary congestion. BNP level is 4000 pg/mL. An echocardiogram shows severely increased biventricular wall thickness with moderately impaired systolic function. The atria are dilated, and the pulmonary artery systolic pressure is 60 mmHg. There is moderate mitral regurgitation. There is grade II diastolic dysfunction E/e′ of 18, with a delayed color M mode slope of 40 cm/sec. There is a moderate-size pericardial effusion. Serum and urine electrophoresis with immunofixation and bone marrow biopsy shows no evidence of abnormal immunoglobulin. A laboratory analysis shows a mutation in transthyretin (TTR) protein, confirming the diagnosis of familial TTR amyloidosis.

Etiology and Classification

Cardiac amyloidosis is the prototype of infiltrative cardiomyopathies and the most frequently encountered in clinical practice.[41–43] There are several types of cardiac amyloidoses, each with its own clinical presentations and prognosis (Table 23.1).[41] Amyloidosis is a multisystem disease in which linear, nonbranching, aggregated protein fibrils with a cross-β pleated configuration are deposited in various organs of the body, including the heart.[44] Within the heart, the amyloid particles can infiltrate the myocardium (atria and ventricles), valves, pericardium, conduction system, and coronary arteries.[42] The fibrils deposit between cells (interstitial), with a replacement of the normal tissue structures. When stained with Congo red, this material shows apple-green birefringence under a polarizing microscope. Alcian blue can also be used to diagnose amyloid.[41,45]

Amyloidosis can be classified by the type of protein deposited. The primary type is the most common form, occurring in 85% of patients with fibrils composed of kappa or lambda immunoglobulin light chains (AL type for amyloid light chain), often associated with a plasma cell dyscrasia such as multiple myeloma.[41,45] AL amyloidosis generally presents in patients from ages 50 to 80 years of age with a mild predilection for males. There may be extracellular deposition of amyloid protein in the kidney, heart, liver, nerves, skin, and tongue, resulting in tissue damage and organ malfunction.[42] The most common manifestations include nephrotic syndrome or renal failure, congestive heart failure, sensorimotor peripheral neuropathy, and orthostatic hypotension. Nearly half of patients have cardiac manifestations, including congestive heart failure; however, the heart is involved in most all patients by pathologic examination.[43] Death from cardiac involvement secondary to congestive heart failure or arrhythmia occurs in greater than 50% of patients with systemic amyloidosis.[46,47]

Familial amyloidosis results from the production of a mutant prealbumin protein (i.e., ATTR-m [a transporter of thyroid hormone and retinol]), and there are different types, which present with cardiomyopathy and peripheral or autonomic neuropathy.[48] ATTR-m is made up of 125 pairs of amino acids, and more than 100 mutations have been recognized.[49] This type of amyloidosis is important to recognize because liver transplantation may be life saving, although optimally it should be performed before cardiac involvement has occurred. Laboratory testing should be performed to test for ATTR if a family history is present or there is no evidence of AL-type amyloid on biopsy. In familial amyloidosis, cardiac involvement occurs in 28% of patients at the time of diagnosis; however, it usually presents later in the course of the disease and has a less ominous prognosis compared with AL (primary) amyloidosis.[48] Peripheral neuropathy may be the presenting feature, but cardiac manifestations may subsequently predominate.[50] The disease was reported over 50 years ago in a Danish family but has also been described in several other

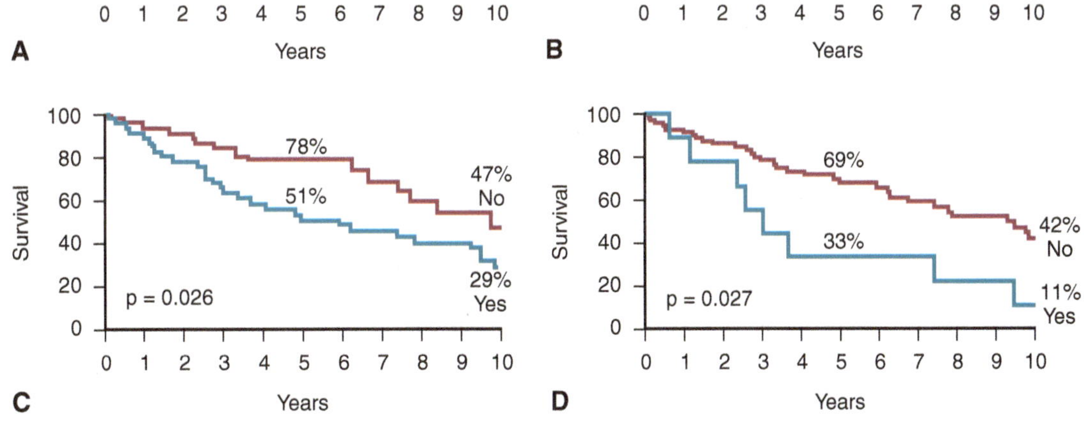

Fig. 23.2 Kaplan-Meier survival curves in relation to **A**, sex; **B**, New York Heart Association functional class; **C**, pulmonary venous congestion; and **D**, left atrial dimension >60 mm. *(From Ammash NM et al: Clinical profile and outcome of idiopathic restrictive cardiomyopathy. Circulation 2000;101:2490–2496.)*

TABLE 23.1 Overview of the Common Forms of Amyloidosis That May Affect the Heart

Amyloid Nomenclature	Precursor Protein	Age Range, yrs	Sex	Clinical Clues	Laboratory Abnormalities
AL	Light chains	50+	Either	Multiorgan involvement. Periorbital bruising or macroglossia are almost pathognomonic of AL in setting of typical MRI or echocardiogram. Severe hypotension with ACE inhibitors	Elevated serum free lambda or kappa, with abnormal ratio. Monoclonal spike in serum and/ or urine. Suppressed immunoglobulins. Proteinuria
ATTRwt	Wild-type (normal) transthyretin	65+	Marked male predominance, >15:1	History of carpal tunnel syndrome 5–10 yrs earlier, with no other organ involvement.	No specific abnormalities. (Normal free light chain values, no proteinuria)
ATTRm	Mutant transthyretin	40+ (mutation dependent). In V122I, the common African-American variant, usual age of clinical onset is 60–65 yrs.	Either, slight male predominance.	African-American/Caribbean origin (for V122I TTR variant).	No specific abnormalities on routine testing. Genetic testing reveals mutation in TTR molecule
AA (Secondary)	Serum amyloid A (an acute phase protein)	May occur in 20s–30s upward with severe inflammatory disease.	Either	Underlying chronic inflammatory disease. Hepatomegaly, splenomegaly. Usually no cardiac involvement, but in rare cases may be severe	High ESR/CRP. Proteinuria.

ACE, Angiotensin-converting enzyme; *CMR,* cardiac magnetic resonance; *CRP,* C-reactive protein; *ECG,* electrocardiogram; *ESR,* erythrocyte sedimentation rate; *LBBB,* left bundle branch block; *TTR,* transthyretin.
Falk RH, Alexander KM, Liao R, Dorbala S. Al (light-chain) cardiac amyloidosis: A review of diagnosis and therapy. J Am Coll Cardiol. 2016;68:1323–1341

families of different ethnic origin and has an autosomal dominant expression.[51,52] Cardiac failure or cardiac arrhythmia is responsible for the deaths in over 50% of patients.[48] Familial amyloidosis has been reported in African Americans as a cause of heart failure secondary to a mutation in ATTR isoleucine-122 (substitution for valine).[53] Approximately 3% to 4% of African Americans or Caribbean blacks harbor this mutation.[54]

Senile systemic amyloidosis (ATTR-wt) occurs predominantly in elderly (>60 years of age) men, but younger individuals and women are increasingly diagnosed. Recent studies of patients undergoing transcatheter aortic valve replacement have found that 20% have ATTR-wt and as a result a less favorable prognosis.[55] ATTR-wt has been associated with congestive heart failure without significant noncardiac involvement.[56,57] Survival is generally better relative to AL.[56,58] There may be extensive deposits in the heart producing congestive heart failure, or there may be minor deposits in the atria with no symptoms. The prevalence of senile amyloid at autopsy appears to be highest in African Americans. It is important to differentiate ATTR-wt from immunoglobulin-derived amyloidosis (AL type) and ATTR-m, because the treatment regimens differ. The better prognosis of ATTR-wt relative to AL is concordant with the accumulating evidence that light chains are responsible for toxicity and poor outcome in AL amyloidosis.[59]

Secondary amyloidosis (AA type) is rare, with the fibrils consisting of protein A, a nonimmunoglobulin acute-phase reactant resulting from a multitude of chronic inflammatory conditions (e.g., tuberculosis, familial Mediterranean fever, rheumatoid arthritis, inflammatory bowel disease).[60] Cardiac involvement is unusual in secondary amyloidosis, with renal manifestations being predominant.[61] Isolated atrial amyloidosis is often found limited to the atria at autopsy in the elderly and derives from atrial natriuretic peptide.[62] It is more common in females and seems to be associated with the presence of atrial fibrillation.[63,64]

Clinical presentation. AL cardiac amyloidosis may present with a spectrum of disease severity.[46,65] In early AL cardiac amyloidosis, patients may be asymptomatic, while those with advanced disease will have the typical evidence of restrictive cardiomyopathy with severe right-heart failure, ascites, and peripheral edema.[66,67] Left-heart failure is a less common manifestation. Additional symptoms include chest pain, presyncope/syncope, and sudden cardiac death. Chest pain resembling angina pectoris may be present despite normal epicardial coronary arteries due to partial obliteration of the distal coronary arteries by amyloid infiltration or intramyocardial vessels.[68,69] Orthostatic hypotension occurs in 10% to 15% of patients secondary to amyloid infiltration of the autonomic nervous system, with symptoms of syncope, diarrhea, lack of sweating, and impotence.[44,70] Renal involvement with nephrotic syndrome and adrenal disease may aggravate postural hypotension. Syncope may be due to postural hypotension or supraventricular or ventricular arrhythmias. Other symptoms may be attributable to peripheral neuropathy, macroglossia, or carpal tunnel syndrome.[41,71]

Physical examination may reveal signs of cardiac cachexia in advanced disease. Low cardiac output may cause decreased blood pressure, and orthostatic hypotension may still occur. Macroglossia, periorbital purpura, petechia, and bruising may be evident on general examination.[41] The cardiac exam may reveal an S_4 (very early disease) or S_3 (advanced disease) on auscultation from either the right or the left heart.[72] Mitral and tricuspid valvular regurgitation may also be present, though usually not severe. There is often evidence of

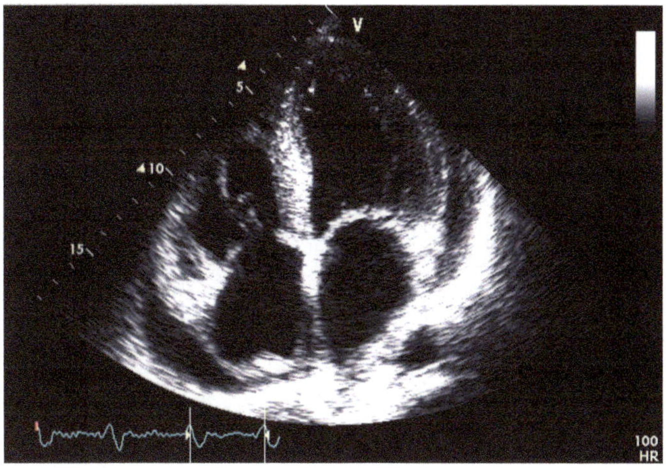

Fig. 23.3 Apical four-chamber view of patient with cardiac amyloidosis demonstrating severe increased wall thickness of the left and right ventricles, dilated atria, and a pericardial effusion.

biventricular heart failure with predominant right-heart failure.[67] The jugular venous pulse will be elevated with a prominent x and y descent, and hepatomegaly, ascites, and peripheral edema will be present, especially in the advanced disease.[41] Neurologic examination may reveal findings consistent with peripheral neuropathy.

The cardiac silhouette on CXR is usually enlarged in patients with advanced disease with evidence of pulmonary congestion or pericardial effusion.[73] The ECG typically has low voltage in the limb leads and shows a pseudoinfarction pattern with Q waves simulating a myocardial infarction in the precordial leads (~50% of patients), but ~16% with LV hypertrophy (LVH).[74,75] More specifically, patients with cardiac amyloidosis have a low ratio of electrocardiographic voltage to LV wall thickness.[76] However, the usefulness of this ratio is limited by the presence of coexisting diseases that may result in reduced voltage. Arrhythmias, especially atrial fibrillation, are common, and sick-sinus syndrome may be present.[41] AV conduction defects may be present, though right and left bundle branch block is less common.[77] Ventricular arrhythmias are not as common as expected and are not usually the cause of sudden cardiac death but, rather, pulseless electrical activity.[78]

Echocardiography. Echocardiography is the test of choice for diagnosis and serial follow-up, of patients with cardiac amyloidosis,[79–86] which gives a distinctive appearance on two-dimensional (2-D) echocardiography and is associated with abnormal LV and RV diastolic function. The findings of a normal or small LV cavity size with markedly thickened myocardium associated with a highly abnormal texture often described as "granular sparkling" in appearance is the classical presentation (Fig. 23.3). Other disorders that cause increased LV wall thickness must be considered (Fig. 23.4). The sparkling appearance is thought to be due to the acoustic mismatch between the highly reflective amyloid deposits in the endocardium, myocardium, and pericardium and the normal tissue.[87,88] Moreover, autopsy and clinical biopsy series have demonstrated the presence of amyloid fibrils in the myocardium at the site of the sparkling echoes. However, the specificity of this finding is limited with the current generation of echocardiographic equipment that routinely incorporates harmonic imaging. Global LV systolic function is usually preserved in early disease, whereas systolic function is usually impaired in advanced disease. The interatrial septum and valve leaflets are thickened. Both atria are enlarged, and small to moderate pericardial effusions are usually present.[84,86]

Cardiac amyloidosis has traditionally been considered to require a restrictive pattern of ventricular filling. However, a spectrum of LV filling abnormalities is detected in patients with cardiac amyloidosis.[73,81,89] In a study of 53 patients with the classic echocardiographic features of cardiac amyloidosis, those with advanced disease demonstrated a mean LV wall thickness greater than 15 mm and a restrictive physiology pattern of LV filling.[72] Furthermore, in serial studies of individual patients, the impaired relaxation pattern gradually evolved into a restrictive pattern through a pseudonormal (intermediate) phase in the progression of the disease.[81] The mechanism for this serial change in LV filling

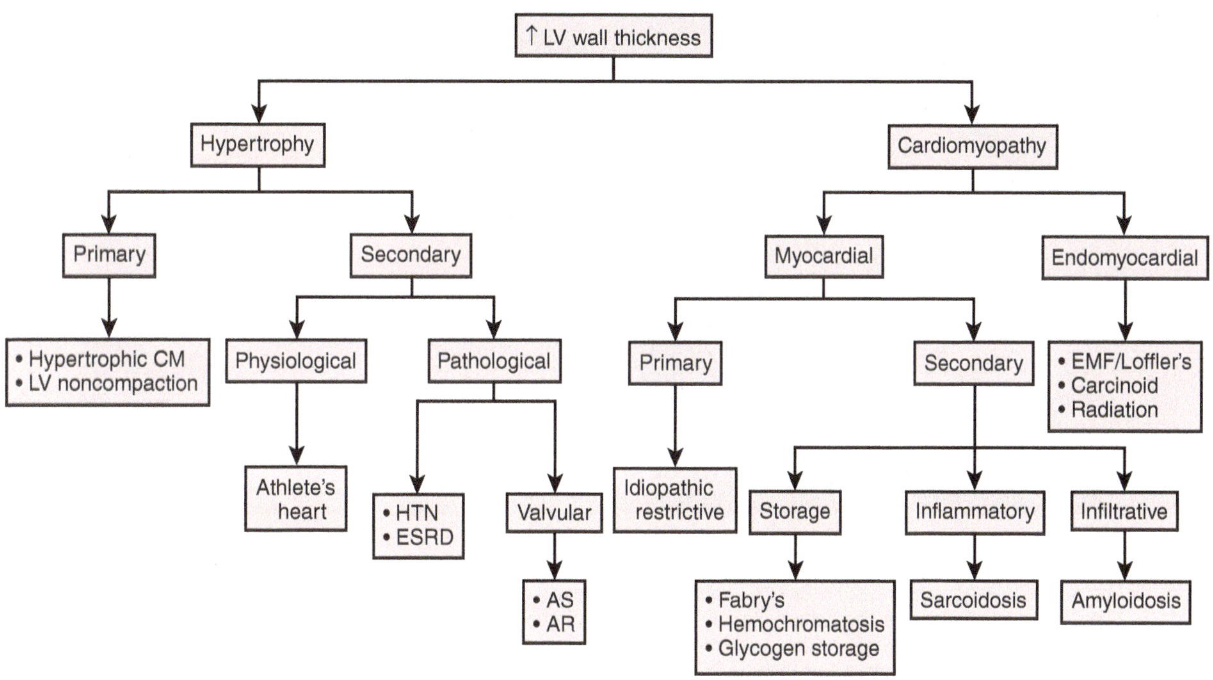

Fig. 23.4 Algorithm with differential diagnosis of increased left ventricular (LV) wall thickness. *CM*, cardiomyopathy; *HTN*, hypertension; *ESRD*, end-stage renal disease; *AS*, aortic stenosis; *AR*, aortic regurgitation; *EMF*, endomyocardial fibrosis.

pattern is thought to be the gradual decrease in the compliance of the left ventricle with progressive deposition of amyloid fibrils in the myocardium, leading to loss of myocardial cells from pressure necrosis.[90] When the duration of the pulmonary venous atrial reversal wave is longer than the mitral A wave duration, LV end-diastolic pressure is elevated, and the disease is progressive with restrictive physiology at the most advanced stages.[91] Eventually the pulmonary atrial reversal wave may be lost due to atrial involvement of amyloid infiltration.

RV diastolic impairment also may occur in patients with cardiac amyloidosis.[80] The RV filling pattern is often similar to that of the left ventricle or may be less advanced. In early cases, there is an RV free wall thickness of less than 7 mm and abnormal relaxation. In advanced cases, the RV wall is greater than 7 mm in thickness, with restrictive physiology present. The systolic forward flows by Doppler echocardiography in the superior vena cava and hepatic veins are also decreased with advanced disease, and the diastolic flow is increased, compatible with restrictive physiology. Pulmonary hypertension occurs as a manifestation of advanced diastolic dysfunction with pulmonary artery systolic pressures generally greater than 50 mmHg.

Speckle tracking echocardiographic strain imaging was first utilized to characterize early systolic dysfunction in patients with cardiac amyloidosis before the onset of congestive symptoms or reduced LV EF.[92,93] Now it is widely utilized for diagnosis. A typical pattern on longitudinal strain is severe impairment of basal and midwall segments with preserved strain in the apical segments.[94] To measure the degree of apical sparing on longitudinal strain and help differentiate cardiac amyloidosis from other causes of LVH, a relative regional strain ratio (RRSR) has been used.[95] This ratio was found to be sensitive and specific in the noninvasive diagnosis of cardiac amyloidosis,[96] and it was also shown to be of prognostic value[97] (Fig. 23.5).

Laboratory testing and biopsy. Cardiac amyloidosis can be diagnosed noninvasively antemortem in most cases from the typical features obtained from the history, examination, ECG, and echocardiogram. However, confirmatory testing is needed before treatment is initiated, and further classification of the subtype of amyloid is necessary. Serum and urine protein immunofixation and serum free light chain assay are recommended to assess for the secretion of a monoclonal protein associated with a plasma cell dyscrasia.[41,45,46,70,98] Although some patients with AL amyloid will have multiple myeloma, a greater proportion may have unassociated monoclonal gammopathies of uncertain significance. Laboratory testing for a TTR mutation and kappa and lambda light chains can be tested for in blood samples. A serum free light chain assay is available to assess the ratio of kappa to lambda free light chains and may be more sensitive than immunofixation.[45,99] A positive serum

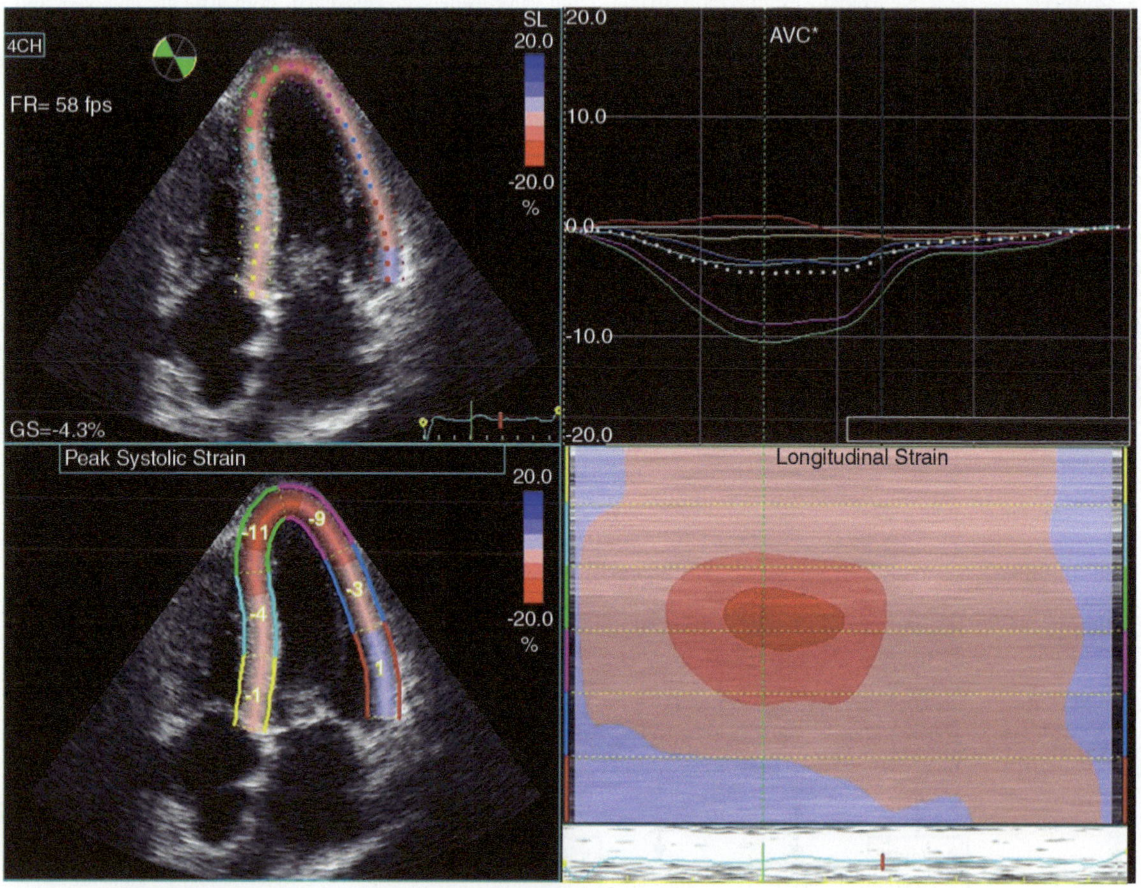

Fig. 23.5 Speckle tracking image of a patient with advanced cardiac amyloidosis showing decreased longitudinal systolic strain. Top left image is from the apical four-chamber view with a *bar* representing a key to the color-coding varying from −20% to 20%. Each apical segment is color coded. The global strain GS is −4.3%. Lower left image shows the actual peak systolic strain values for each segment. For example, the basal septum has a peak strain of −1% ($n = -20\%$). The apical segments have greater peak systolic strain values. Top right image (graph) and lower right image (anatomic M-mode) show decreased peak systolic strain over the cardiac cycle. All the segments in different colors show decreased systolic strain. Basal and midventricular segments have the worst systolic strain, while the apical segment has the best systolic strain. *FR,* frame rate; *fps,* frames per second; *AVC,* aortic valve closure

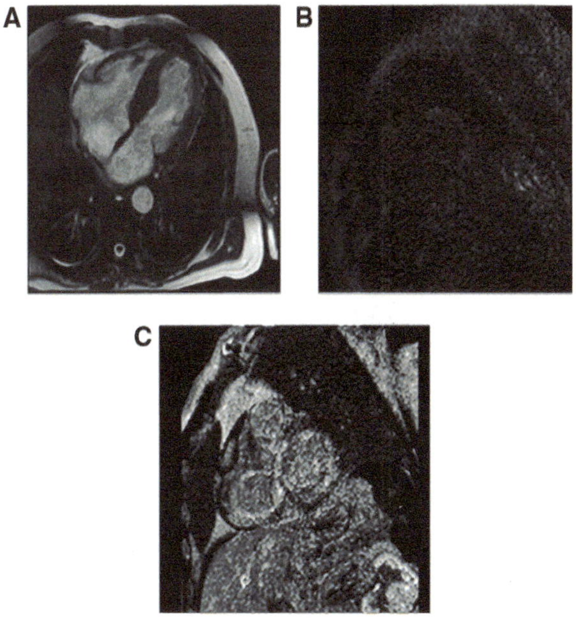

Fig. 23.6 Cardiac magnetic resonance findings in a patient with biopsy proven cardiac amyloidosis. Panel A is a 4 chamber steady-state free precession (SSFP) image showing left ventricular hypertrophy, biatrial enlargement and a trace pericardial effusion. Panel B is the Look-Locker sequence showing the nulling of the myocardium and blood pool at similar timepoints, consistent with abnormal Gadolinium kinetics. Panel C shows delayed enhancement imaging with severe diffuse myocardial enhancement.

immunofixation plus an abnormal kappa/lambda ratio are highly sensitive to diagnose AL amyloidosis.[98]

Noncardiac sites of biopsy can include the bone marrow, fat pad, rectum, gingiva, kidney, and liver, though fat aspirate may detect amyloidosis in ~70% of patients.[46,100,101] If the echocardiogram is not diagnostic or the fat pad aspirate is negative and cardiac amyloidosis is still suspected, an endomyocardial biopsy can be performed to make the diagnosis. A confirmatory cardiac biopsy may be particularly important if there are other confounding causes of increased LV mass, such as LVH or HCM. The presence of low electrocardiographic voltage favors a diagnosis of amyloidosis rather than hypertensive or hypertrophic cardiomyopathy; however, endomyocardial biopsy may be necessary in some cases to give a definitive diagnosis.[102] Although systolic anterior motion (SAM) of the mitral valve on echocardiogram is thought to be pathognomonic of hypertrophic cardiomyopathy, it has also been recognized in a series of patients with cardiac amyloidosis.[103]

Cardiac MRI. Cardiac MRI can be used to identify the increased myocardial thickness and small LV cavity in cardiac amyloidosis and the ancillary findings of biatrial enlargement, pericardial and pleural effusions, and inferior vena cava dilatation, similar to echocardiography. However, it appears to be more sensitive than echocardiography with a distinctive pattern of global LV late gadolinium enhancement (LGE) that matches the deposition of amyloid seen histologically.[104] Myocardial wall thickening due to hypertrophy or amyloid infiltration can be distinguishable.[105–107] A pattern of global and subendocardial LGE and specific features of T1 blood pool kinetics are seen in patients with suspected amyloidosis.[108] Specifically, on Look-Locker images, the blood pool and myocardium null or appear black at similar timepoints due to the slow rate of clearance from the intravascular space. In addition, on T1 and extracellular volume (ECV) mapping, there is typically diffusely higher T1 (>1000 msec) and ECV values (>35%)[109] (Fig. 23.6).

Nuclear Imaging. A potential role for nuclear imaging has emerged for the specific identification of TTR amyloidosis using ^{99m}Tc-3,3-diphosphono-1,2-propanodicarboxylic acid (^{99m}Tc-DPD) in Europe and Tc pyrophosphate in the United States.[110–112] The American Society of Nuclear Cardiology (ASNC) practice points recommend visual grading of myocardial ^{99m}Tc-PYP uptake by comparison to rib uptake and quantitation of cardiac ^{99m}Tc-PYP uptake using heart to contralateral lung (H/CL) ratio. The findings of a myocardial uptake equal to or greater than rib uptake or H/CL ratio above 1.5 strongly suggest TTR amyloidosis (Fig. 23.7).

Fig. 23.8 shows the diagnostic evaluation of suspected amyloidosis.[113]

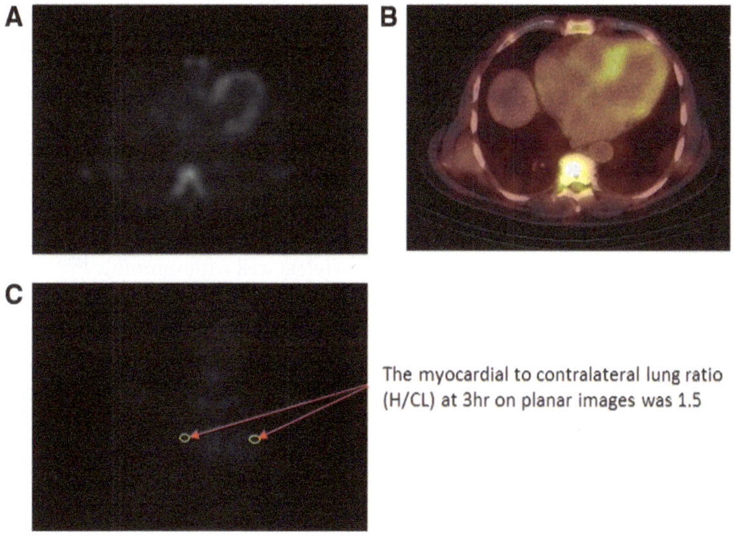

Fig. 23.7 99mTc pyrophosphate imaging in a patient with biopsy proven cardiac amyloidosis. On SPECT imaging (Panel A) and when superimposed on the computed tomogram (Panel B), there is greater myocardial uptake compared to rib uptake by visual analysis. On quantitation (Panel C), the H/CL (myocardial to contralateral lung ratio) is 1.5. These findings are strongly suggestive of TTR amyloidosis.

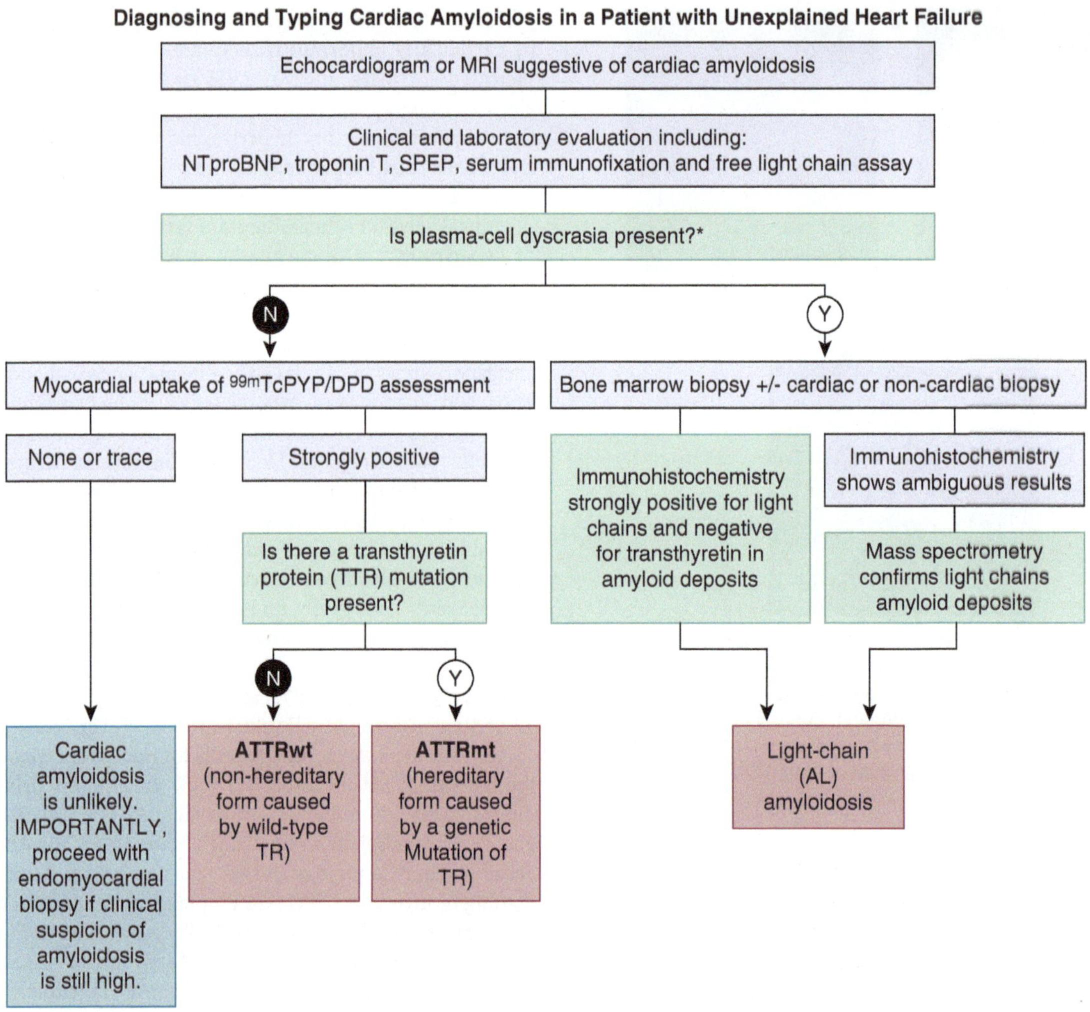

Fig. 23.8 Diagnosing and Typing Cardiac Amyloidosis in a Patient With Unexplained Heart Failure. From Falk RH et al J Am Coll Cardiol 2016;68:1323–4. https://www.onlinejacc.org/content/68/12/1323/F1

Prognosis

The prognosis of cardiac amyloidosis is generally poor, but it depends on the subtype, with AL (primary) amyloidosis having the worst prognosis.[45,46,48,61,64,114] In a study published in the 1990s of over 800 patients with primary amyloidosis over a 10-year period, the median survival was 2.1 years and less than 6 months once congestive heart failure had occurred.[114] More recent data of patients diagnosed between 2010 and 2014 showed a modest improvement with 60% survival at 2 years, particularly in patients in Mayo stage 1 and 2.[115]

Several prognostic indicators have been determined using clinical, imaging, and laboratory criteria. Echocardiographic variables still provide powerful predictive information. Mean LV wall thickness and LV impairment have been suggested as useful variables in assessing the degree of cardiac involvement and prognosis. In a study of 132 patients with biopsy-proven amyloidosis, those with a mean wall thickness of 15 mm had a median survival of 0.4 years compared with 2.4 years for those with a mean wall thickness of 12 mm.[84] Doppler echocardiography has also been shown to be useful in prognostic stratification of patients with cardiac amyloidosis. Patients with a deceleration time of the mitral early filling wave at a baseline study of no greater than 150 msec had significantly reduced survival compared with those whose deceleration time was greater than 150 msec (1-year probability of survival, 49% vs 92%; $p < 0.001$).[82] Bivariate analysis showed that the combination of a shortened deceleration time of no greater than 150 msec and an increased mitral E/A ratio were stronger predictors of cardiac death than were 2-D variables of mean LV wall thickness and fractional shortening. The Tei index, a Doppler echocardiographic-derived parameter that combines systolic and diastolic performance, has been determined to have significant prognostic importance in cardiac amyloidosis.[116] RV enlargement has also been identified as an independent predictor of poor outcome among patients with primary amyloidosis.[47,83]

Both elevated troponin and BNP levels have been associated with a poorer prognosis.[117] A modified prognostic staging system for AL amyloidosis incorporates NT-proBNP, cardiac troponin T (cTNT), and free light chain levels. Patients can be classified in four stages that correlate well with mortality.[118]

Treatment

The mainstay of treatment is relief of symptoms, while efforts are being undertaken to suppress the principal disease process. The definitive treatment for cardiac amyloidosis (AL type) involves antiplasma cell therapy, which stops production of light chains and includes alkylating agents such as melphalan, prednisone, and more recently bortezomib.[41,114,119–121] Autologous stem cell transplantation has shown favorable results mostly in patients without cardiac disease or early cardiac involvement and is the treatment of choice for AL amyloidosis.[122,123] The toxicity of blood cell transplantation, however, limits its use to a minority of patients.

Diuretics are the main drugs used to treat cardiac symptoms. Avoidance or careful use of digoxin has been recommended because of concern for digoxin binding to amyloid fibrils and the risk of arrhythmias.[65,124] Patients with cardiac amyloidosis may also be very sensitive to the negative inotropic effects of calcium channel blockers, either because of their abnormal binding to amyloid fibrils or because of their vasodilator effects.[125] Vasodilator agents such as angiotensin-converting enzyme (ACE) inhibitors or angiotensin-II inhibitors are poorly tolerated, with a risk of significant hypotension.[41] Pacemakers may be useful to treat symptomatic high AV block. Anticoagulation should be considered because of the risk of thrombus formation with atrial amyloid involvement and atrial standstill, even among patients in sinus rhythm.[126,127] Beta blockers have not been shown to provide any specific benefit and should be used with caution because of the tendency for hypotension.

Cardiac transplantation is generally not performed in patients with AL-type amyloid, since systemic involvement of other organs is usually present and may progress.[128–132] It has been considered in select patients without extracardiac disease (<5% of cases), since the transplanted heart is usually not clinically affected.[131,132] In this situation, heart transplantation is coupled to chemotherapy and stem cell transplantation. Still, survival is much lower than for other heart transplant populations.

Liver transplantation has been performed for the familial type (ATTR-m variant), since the circulating ATTR is produced in the liver.[133–135] Thus the new liver will replace the ATTR-m with a normal TTR. Ideally this is performed before cardiac involvement occurs. Nonsteroidal antiinflammatory drugs, such as diflunisal, that can stabilize TTR and prevent the formation of amyloid are being evaluated and have shown promise for stabilizing peripheral neuropathy.[136] Two new agents, patisiran and inotersen, both inhibitors of transthyretin liver synthesis (though by different mechanisms), have been shown to be effective in hereditary TTR amyloidosis.[137,138] Tafamidis, a transthyretin binder, was associated with improved outcomes, including a decrease in all-cause mortality in patients with TTR amyloid cardiomyopathy.[139] There is no specific treatment for the senile type of amyloid, though usually patients can be managed medically with conventional heart failure therapy.

Storage Cardiomyopathies

There has been a growing recognition that cardiac storage disorders often go unrecognized and may be frequent mimics of HCM.[4,140,141] Intracellular accumulation of various substances within myocytes generally results from defects in genes coding for metabolic pathways. It is likely that the list of these disorders continues to expand. Primary cardiomyopathies due to protein kinase AMP-activated gamma-2 (PRKAG2) and lysosomal-associated membrane protein-2 (LAMP2) proteins have been described, and secondary cardiomyopathies include Fabry, Pompe, and Niemann-Pick diseases and hemochromatosis.[4] Fabry disease and the primary cardiomyopathies will be discussed since they are most prevalent in adults. Hemochromatosis, though more likely to manifest as a dilated cardiomyopathy, will also be reviewed.

Fabry Disease

Etiology and presentations. Fabry disease is an uncommon X-linked recessive disorder of metabolism due to gene mutations coding for α-galactosidase A, estimated to occur in 1 in 50,000 individuals. This defect results in a deficiency in the enzyme α-galactosidase A that leads to accumulation of glycosphingolipids, the most common of which is globotriaosylceramide (Gb3), in lysosomes.[142] Although described decades ago, isolated cardiac manifestations have not been widely recognized until the past few decades, and enzyme replacement therapy has only recently become readily available.[143,144] Fabry disease most severely affects homozygous males, with generally milder symptoms occurring in females.[145–148] Abnormal deposition of glycolipid occurs in the cardiovascular system (myocardium, valves, conduction system, blood vessels), nerves, skin, and kidney.[146] Lysosomal inclusions are seen by electron microscopy with vacuolization of myocytes, endothelial, and smooth muscle cells with a concentric lamellar configuration.[148]

The noncardiac manifestations of Fabry disease include angiokeratoma, acroparesthesias, hypohidrosis, and corneal opacities (cornea verticillata).[147–150] Among children in the European Fabry Outcome Survey (FOS), the most frequent symptoms were acroparesthesias, altered temperative sensitivity, gastrointestinal effects, vertigo, tinnitus, and fatigue.[151] Adults may present with microalbuminuria, proteinuria, renal failure, and stroke, though cardiac-related symptoms alone may occur, including dyspnea, chest pain, syncope, and congestive heart failure.[152] Recent prevalence studies have shown that Fabry disease may be the cause of LVH in ~1% of patients carrying a diagnosis of hypertrophic cardiomyopathy.[145,146,153] Furthermore, in one reported series 12% of females (mean age, 51.5 years) with late-onset hypertrophy were demonstrated to have Fabry disease by endomyocardial biopsy, despite electrocardiographic and echocardiographic appearances of HCM (Fig. 23.9).[147] Among female patients with Fabry disease screened for LVH, 63% had evidence of concentric or eccentric hypertrophy, suggesting cardiac involvement.[148]

The diagnosis of Fabry disease in adults is first suspected based on personal and family history. Often the family history may be notable for absence of male-to-male transmission. The ECG may show AV block and a short P-R interval with evidence of LVH.[154] Cardiac manifestations described by echocardiography include increased aortic dimension, mitral regurgitation with mitral valve prolapse, and increased LV wall thickness.[155–160] Although most often the pattern of increased LV wall thickness is concentric hypertrophy or remodeling, asymmetric hypertrophy has been described.[147] The systolic function is usually preserved. SAM of the mitral valve has been described, although more commonly there is no obstruction.[159] Diastolic function, though typically abnormal, is usually not restrictive.[161]

The diagnosis of Fabry disease can be confirmed in males by detection of reduced levels of leukocyte α-galactosidase A levels.[152] Heterozygous females may have normal or mildly decreased levels, and therefore tissue biopsy or gene testing of affected tissue for diagnosis may be required.[147] Efforts have been made to use different imaging modalities to screen patients with LVH for Fabry disease, including echocardiography and MRI, since treatment to reduce the accumulation of cardiac infiltration with glycolipid has become available.[161–163]

Case Study 3

A 48-year-old man presents with dyspnea on exertion. He has been diagnosed with nonobstructive HCM. There is a family history of Fabry disease. On cardiac examination, there is a moderate-intensity ejection murmur that is unchanged with Valsalva. ECG shows a short P-R interval and LVH. Echocardiogram shows severe symmetric hypertrophy (interventricular septum, 1.9 cm; posterior wall, 1.8 cm). There is no SAM of the mitral valve or LV outflow tract gradient at rest or with exercise echocardiogram. A laboratory test for α-galactosidase shows levels below 10%. Genetic testing confirms Fabry disease with a mutation in the gene coding for α-galactosidase A. An endomyocardial biopsy shows inclusion bodies in the sarcoplasmic reticulum. The patient is referred for enzyme replacement therapy.

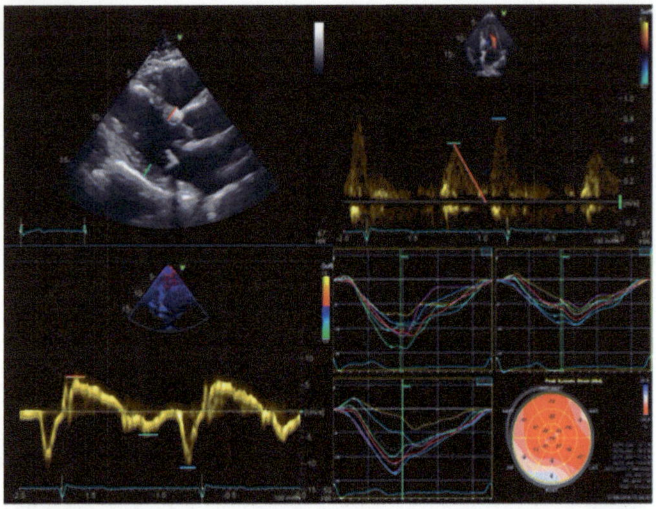

Fig. 23.9 Echocardiographic Images in a Patient with Fabry's Disease. (A) A 2D parasternal long-axis view of increased interventricular septal IVS *(red line)* and posterior wall (PW) thickness *(green line)*. Upper limit of normal for both IVS and PW in males is 1.0 cm and 0.9 cm in females. (B) A pulsed-wave Doppler image of mitral valve inflow from the apical 4D view with E-wave *(green)*. The A-wave is shown in blue and the mitral deceleration time (DT) is shown in red. Normal values for the E:A ratio are 0.8 to 2; and >150 ms for DT. (C) A pulsed-wave tissue Doppler image of the mitral septal annulus with the s′ shown in red, the e′ is shown in green, and the a′ shown in blue. Normal value for the E/e′ ratio (average of septal and lateral e′) is <14. (D) Speckle tracking strain image. Note the reduced strain (shown in blue and with the red arrow) on the bulls-eye map in the basal inferolateral region. A: late diastolic filling velocity; a′: late diastolic tissue Doppler velocity; E: early diastolic filling velocity; e′: early diastolic tissue Doppler velocity; s′: systolic tissue Doppler velocity. (Perry, R, J Am Coll Cardiol Img 2019;12:1230–42).

Echocardiographic screening of mutation-positive patients for Fabry disease, though negative for LVH, has shown reduced tissue Doppler systolic, e′ annular, and a′ annular velocities compared with controls.[161] MRI has also shown abnormalities in patients with Fabry plus LVH with reduced radial and longitudinal strain and strain rate relative to controls and improvement in strain and strain rate with concomitant reduction in wall thickness with treatment.[164] MRI studies show no specific myocardial pattern except a tendency toward midmyocardial posterior-basal late enhancement with gadolinium.[164,165] Also noted are distinctively low native T1 values by MRI.[166] Reduction in radial and longitudinal strain determined echocardiographically in patients with Fabry disease shows a correlation between hypertrophy and late enhancement by MRI.[167]

Once cardiac involvement with Fabry disease has been confirmed, treatment with enzyme replacement (recombinant human α-galactosidase A) can be initiated. Several studies have demonstrated a reduction in LVH and improvement in cardiac function with enzyme replacement particularly if introduced prior to the presence of scar formation.[164,168,169]

Glycogen Storage Disorders

Two gene mutations (PRKAG2 and LAMP2) causing glycogen storage disease have been recognized as rare primary cardiomyopathies mimicking HCM.[140,141] PRKAG2 codes for a regulatory gene for cyclic adenosine monophosphate (cAMP)–activated protein kinase, and LAMP2 (also called Danon disease) codes for a lysosome membrane protein.[4] Neither of these diseases is associated with myocyte disarray or interstitial fibrosis, but rather glycogen-rich vacuoles.

Danon disease occurs as an X-linked dominant gene affecting male children younger than 20 years of age, though females are usually detected as adults. Noncardiac manifestations include skeletal myopathy, mental retardation, behavioral changes, and ocular abnormalities.[125,126] Cardiac manifestations include early onset of HCM, often with extreme hypertrophy, preexcitation, and elevated creatine kinase, troponins, and liver function tests.[140,141] The clinical course progresses rapidly, with premature death often before the age of 25 years.[170]

PRKAG2 deficiency has a dominant inheritance pattern and lesser noncardiac involvement, with patients surviving to adulthood, though often with arrhythmias, skeletal myopathy, and conduction disease.[140]

A study of 50 unselected patients (mean age, 6 years) with the diagnosis of HCM who underwent gene analysis for LAMP2 found 2 (4%) with mutations. Both of these patients had Wolff-Parkinson-White syndrome and skeletal myopathy.[141] A similar study of 75 unselected patients with HCM found 3 (4%) with LAMP2 or PRKAG2 mutations.[140] The same investigators performed a subgroup analysis of 24 patients with LVH and preexcitation and found 11 with mutations in LAMP2 or PRKAG2 with associated findings of LAMP2, including male sex, severe hypertrophy, early onset of HCM, preexcitation, and elevated liver and muscle enzymes. An algorithm for the diagnosis of patients with suspected LAMP2 or PRKAG 2 mutations is proposed in Fig. 23.10.

Hemochromatosis

Case Study 4

A 50-year-old man is undergoing consideration for liver transplantation due to primary hemochromatosis. He has no known cardiac disease and no cardiac risk factors. On examination, his skin is bronze. The cardiac examination is notable for a positive S_4 gallop. ECG shows low voltage in the limb leads. An echocardiogram shows normal LV size and function with abnormal diastolic function (grade 2 filling pattern) and reduced tissue Doppler systolic annular (6 cm/sec) and e′ annular velocities (4 cm/sec). A cardiac MRI is done and shows abnormalities consistent with hemochromatosis. A cardiac biopsy confirms iron overload in the myocardium.

Etiology and presentations. Hemochromatosis is an iron storage disease that affects the heart, pancreas, liver, gonads, joints, and skin.[168] Primary idiopathic hemochromatosis is an autosomal recessive disorder that results in excessive iron absorption.[168,169] It is the most common autosomal recessive disease in Caucasians.[170] Both men and women are affected in middle age (50s–60s), with women usually presenting after menstruation has ceased.[171] Secondary hemochromatosis results from hemoglobin synthesis abnormalities leading to ineffective erythropoiesis, chronic liver disease, excessive intake of iron, or multiple blood transfusions.[169]

Histologically, iron is deposited in the sarcoplasmic reticulum, mostly within the subepicardium and to a lesser extent the subendocardium of the myocardium.[171] Interstitial iron is not seen, characterizing hemochromatosis as a storage, not an infiltrative, disorder.[4] The ventricles and conduction system are most often affected.[171] The degree of myocardial iron correlates with the severity of cardiac dysfunction.[172–77]

Manifestations of cardiac involvement occur when there is a large amount of iron deposited over a long period of time. One-third of patients manifest cardiac symptoms with evidence of congestive heart

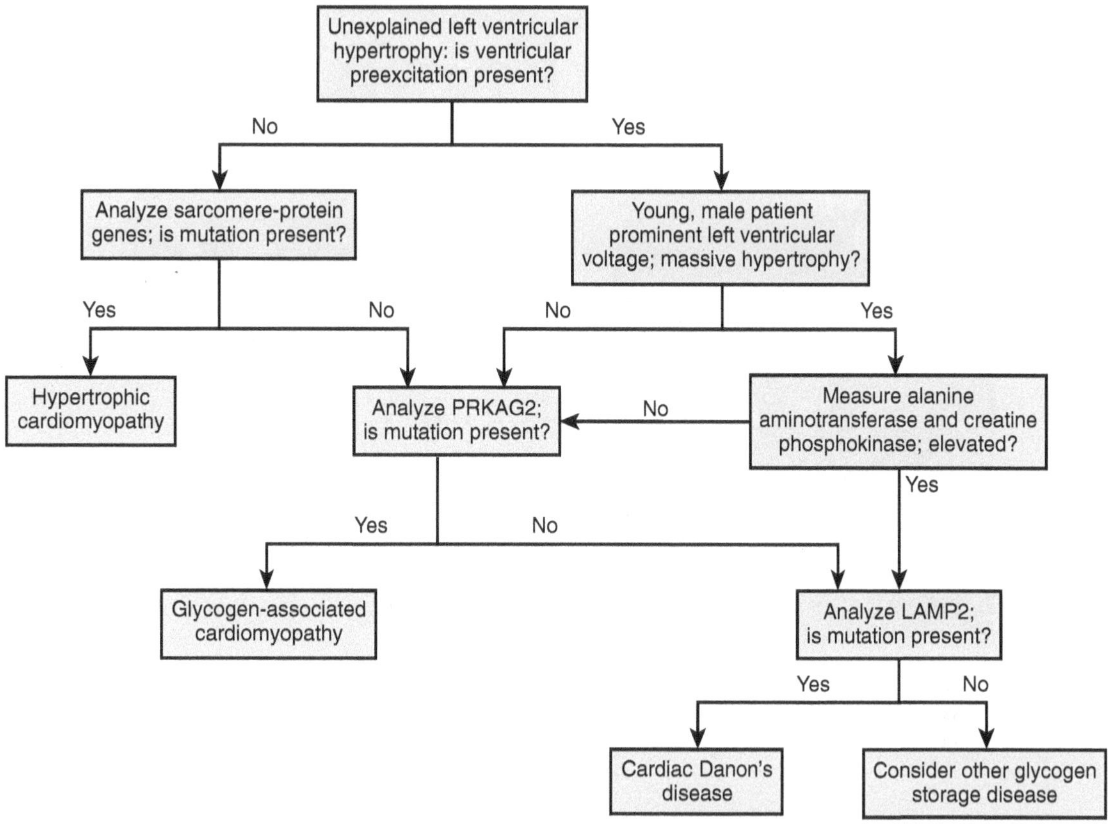

Fig. 23.10 Algorithm for the diagnostic evaluation of patients with unexplained hypertrophy, where hypertrophic cardiomyopathy may not be the etiology. A family history of the dominant inheritance of left ventricular (LV) hypertrophy, unaccompanied by systemic manifestations or electrocardiographic findings of ventricular preexcitation, suggests hypertrophic cardiomyopathy; the identification of a sarcomeric mutation confirms the diagnosis. In young patients with echocardiographic findings of unexplained LV hypertrophy and electrocardiograms with prominent LV voltage and short P-R intervals, delta waves, or both, glycogen storage disease should be suspected. Dominant inheritance and an absence of systemic disease suggest the presence of glycogen-associated cardiomyopathy due to PRKAG2 mutations. Male sex and abnormalities in liver, musculoskeletal, or neurologic function suggest a diagnosis of Danon's disease, although systemic manifestations can be modest or absent in the cardiac form of this disease. When the cause is not established by genetic analyses, a tissue biopsy and a biochemical study may be helpful. (*From Arad M et al: Glycogen storage diseases presenting as hypertrophic cardiomyopathy. N Engl J Med 2005;352:362–372.*)

failure, supraventricular or ventricular arrhythmias, and conduction defects.[168] Cardiac involvement is usually recognized after a noncardiac diagnosis is already known. Less often patients will present with a cardiomyopathy of unknown etiology without known hemochromatosis. Laboratory tests will show an elevated serum ferritin and increased ratio of plasma iron level to total iron binding capacity, urinary iron, liver iron, and saturation of transferrin.[176] Cardiomegaly may be seen on CXR. Electrocardiographic findings have included arrhythmias, conduction disorders, and low voltage. Echocardiography is a useful noninvasive technique in the assessment of cardiac involvement in primary hemochromatosis, detecting clinically occult heart involvement, following patients serially, and assessing LV function after phlebotomy.[175–180]

A retrospective review from the Mayo Clinic described 19 patients with primary hemochromatosis and demonstrated that 7 (37%) had chamber dilatation and systolic dysfunction secondary to hemochromatosis, while 12 patients did not.[181] Increased ventricular wall thickness was not evident in this cohort of patients. Patterns consistent with dilated or restrictive cardiomyopathy or mixed patterns have been described in patients with primary hemochromatosis, though the earliest finding is usually a restrictive pattern.[174,182] Ventricular dysfunction and increased ventricular mass may normalize after successful phlebotomy.[180,183,184] The presence of systolic dysfunction usually signifies a poor prognosis.[175] Manifestations of secondary hemochromatosis in the heart include increased LV wall thickness and mass, increased cavity dimension, and LA enlargement.[185] Specific Doppler filling indexes and tissue Doppler are useful to differentiate patients with hereditary hemochromatosis from normal subjects and therefore may be useful for screening.[186] Exercise radionuclide cine angiography demonstrating exercise-related LV dysfunction in patients with normal baseline function has also been shown to be sensitive to detect preclinical disease.[187]

Myocardial iron deposition can be reproducibly quantified using myocardial T2* (star)[188] (Fig. 23.11). Iron deposition leads to increased magnetic inhomogeneities that reduce myocardial T2* relaxation time. This myocardial T2* time has also been shown to have a prognostic value, with T2* less than 10 msec being associated with a significantly higher risk of developing heart failure.[189] Cardiac MRI can also enable assessment of response to therapy by following myocardial iron content.[190]

Endomyocardial biopsy may be useful to exclude the diagnosis, especially when echocardiographic, magnetic resonance, or clinical features are not evident.[191]

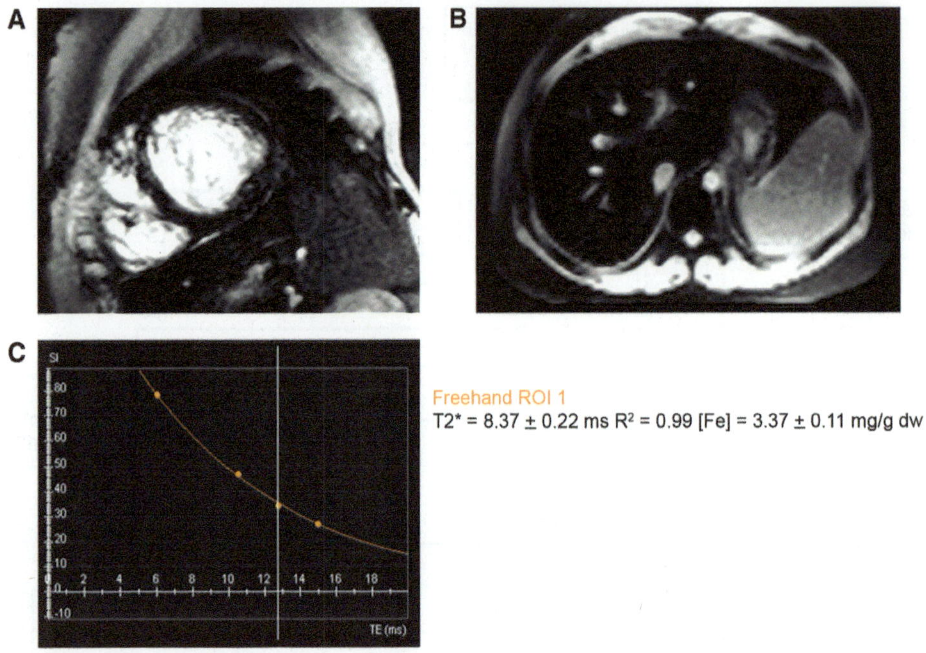

Fig. 23.11 Panel A shows T2* imaging of the myocardium in a patient with hemochromatosis. The myocardium appears abnormally dark, suspicious for iron overload. Panel B is T2* imaging of the patient's liver. It is also abnormally dark consistent with liver iron deposition. On quantitation (Panel C), myocardial T2* was 8.37 ms < 10 ms, consistent with severe myocardial iron overload.

Treatment by repeat phlebotomies in primary hemochromatosis or the use of chelating agents (such as desferoxamine) in secondary hemochromatosis may result in improvement of cardiac involvement, making early diagnosis important.[166–168] Thus cardiac hemochromatosis is a potentially reversible form of cardiomyopathy. Heart transplantation may be considered when the heart involvement is life threatening, or combined heart and liver transplantation may be useful in patients with heart and liver failure.[174,192–194]

FUTURE DIRECTIONS

The AHA and MOGE(S) classifications of cardiomyopathies have shifted the focus toward understanding the genetic and cellular causes of specific heart muscle diseases. Ultimately, the most effective approach to early diagnosis and targeted treatment will be guided by knowledge of the basic underpinnings of the disease processes. Meanwhile, until these advances occur, echocardiography and MRI have risen to the forefront as noninvasive tests with the potential to detect preclinical myocardial disease and differentiate various disorders. These modalities have begun to uncover specific fingerprints for each disease and should continue to be utilized during the evaluation and screening of cardiomyopathies.

Most of the disorders discussed in this review continue to be associated with a poor prognosis and often are managed as palliative diseases. Furthermore, over the past few decades, it is not readily evident to most physicians that progress has occurred. Advances in studying uncommon problems rely on reminding clinicians that experimental investigations are ongoing. Patients and their doctors should be encouraged to pursue evaluations at specialty referral centers, allowing them to receive the latest therapies and to be participants in prospective registries or clinical trials. Many of these centers, such as amyloid or Fabry cardiomyopathy clinics, exist both nationally and internationally and are essential for promoting excellence in care and future research.

At the present time, there is reason for modest optimism. Patients with idiopathic restrictive or amyloid cardiomyopathy without significant noncardiac disease can be considered for cardiac or liver transplantation. Storage cardiomyopathies such as Fabry disease and hemochromatosis may be largely reversible with known accepted therapies. Amyloid cardiomyopathy still presents a difficult challenge; however, a better recognition of non-AL forms of amyloid has allowed more patients to be eligible for treatment.

Although at one time the diseases encompassed by the entity of restrictive cardiomyopathy were considered the topic of case presentations and few therapeutic options, in the future we anticipate earlier diagnosis, enhanced understanding of pathophysiologic mechanisms, and increasing options for treatment and clinical research, with the ultimate goal of improved outcomes.

KEY POINTS

- Restrictive, infiltrative, and storage cardiomyopathies encompass a large variety of disorders in which diastolic dysfunction is at least initially the predominant pathophysiologic derangement. Structural characteristics of these cardiomyopathies typically include biatrial enlargement, nondilated or small LV cavity size, and normal or mildly increased wall thickness.
- Primary (or idiopathic) restrictive cardiomyopathy is a rare disorder of advanced diastolic impairment, often leading to biventricular diastolic heart failure. Cardiac catheterization reveals elevated right-sided or left-sided filling pressures, with a typical dip-and-plateau RV and LV filling pattern and an M-shaped or W-shaped venous filling pattern with prominent x and y descents.
- Cardiac amyloidosis is the prototype of infiltrative cardiomyopathies and the most frequently encountered in clinical practice. It is classified by the type of protein deposited: AL type for amyloid light chain, mutant prealbumin protein for familial amyloidosis, and

wild-type prealbumin protein for senile amyloidosis. Diagnosis often relies on multimodality imaging: echocardiography with strain, nuclear imaging with cardiac ^{99m}Tc-PYP, and cardiac MRI with delayed gadolinium enhancement. The prognosis is generally poor; however, new therapies have been shown to improve outcomes.

- Fabry disease is the prototype for storage cardiomyopathies. It is an X-linked recessive disorder that leads to accumulation of glycosphingolipids. Diagnosis relies on history, physical exam, imaging with echocardiography and cardiac MRI (with distinctively low native T1 values), and reduced levels of leukocyte α-galactosidase A levels in males. In females, tissue biopsy or gene testing may be required.
- Hemochromatosis is a multiorgan iron storage disease that could be primary (idiopathic) or secondary (resulting from ineffective erythropoiesis, chronic liver disease, excessive intake of iron, or multiple blood transfusions). Myocardial iron deposition can be quantified and response to therapy assessed using myocardial T2* (star) by cardiac MRI.

REVIEW QUESTIONS

1. A 42-year-old man presents to cardiology clinic for evaluation of hypertrophic cardiomyopathy (HCM). He was diagnosed with HCM 2 years prior due to an abnormal ECG. He has a history of hypertension, hyperlipidemia, and cataracts. He also has a history of neuropathic pain in his hands and feet. There is no family history of heart disease. Cardiac examination is unremarkable. Skin examination is notable for a rash in the groin region. Labs are notable for a creatinine: 1.4 mg/dL, with 3+ protein in the urine. Echocardiography shows asymmetric septal hypertrophy Interventricular septum (IVS) (2 cm), LV EF 60%. There is no SAM or LV outflow tract (LVOT) obstruction. Grade 2 diastolic dysfunction is present with LA volume index 40 cm/m^2. Global longitudinal strain is −9.6%. What condition does the patient most likely have?
   a. Hypertrophic cardiomyopathy
   b. AL cardiac amyloid
   c. Idiopathic restrictive cardiomyopathy
   d. TTR mutant cardiac amyloid
   e. Fabry disease
2. A 20-year-old man presents with out-of-hospital resuscitated sudden cardiac death. History obtained from his parents notes no significant past medical history but an undiagnosed problem with severe leg cramps limiting his exercise endurance. On ECG in the emergency room there is sinus rhythm with a short P-R interval, delta wave, and LV hypertrophy with repolarization abnormality. Echocardiography shows severe asymmetric septal hypertrophy (3.2 cm) with no LV outflow tract (LVOT) obstruction or SAM. What condition does this patient most likely have?
   a. Hypertrophic cardiomyopathy
   b. Friedreich ataxia
   c. Fabry disease
   d. Danon disease
   e. TTR wild-type cardiac amyloidosis
3. A 17-year-old female presents to a cardiology clinic with exercise intolerance and dyspnea on exertion. She has no other significant past medical history. On cardiac examination, there is an elevated jugular venous pressure of 12 cm H_2O with Kussmaul sign, S_3 gallop, hepatomegaly, and peripheral edema. Laboratory testing is notable for a NT-proBNP level of 1204 pg/mL and troponin I of 0.34 ng/mL. Echocardiography shows LV EF of 60%, maximal wall thickness of 1 cm, LA volume index of 42 mL/m^2, grade 3 diastolic dysfunction with E/e′ 27, and color M mode propagation slope of 30 cm/sec. There is no significant respiratory variation of mitral inflow. The pulmonary artery systolic pressure is 50 mmHg. The hepatic vein Doppler flow shows a blunted systolic wave and prominent atrial reversal waves with inspiration. What is the most likely diagnosis?
   a. Idiopathic constrictive pericarditis
   b. Primary pulmonary hypertension
   c. Hereditary hemochromatosis
   d. Familial cardiac amyloidosis
   e. Idiopathic restrictive cardiomyopathy

REFERENCES

1. Goodwin JF. The frontiers of cardiomyopathy. *Br Heart J.* 1982;48:11–18.
2. Brandenburg RO. Report of the WHO/ISFC task force on the definition and classification of cardiomyopathies. *Br Heart J.* 1980;44:672–673.
3. Richardson P, McKenna W, Bristow M, et al. Report of the 1995 World Health Organization/International Society and Federation of Cardiology Task Force on the definition and classification of cardiomyopathies. *Circulation.* 1996;93:841–842.
4. Maron BJ, Towbin JA, Thiene G, et al. Contemporary definitions and classification of the cardiomyopathies. *Circulation.* 2006;113:1807–1816.
5. Arbustini E, Narula N, Tavazzi L, et al. The MOGE(S) classification of cardiomyopathy for clinicians. *J Am Coll Cardiol.* 2014;64:304–318.
6. Elliott PM. Classification of cardiomyopathies: evolution or revolution?. *J Am Coll Cardiol.* 2013;62:2073–2074.
7. Kushawa SS, Fallon JT, Fuster V. Restrictive cardiomyopathy. *N Engl J Med.* 1997;336:267–276.
8. Keren A, Popp RL. Assignment of patients into the classification of cardiomyopathies. *Circulation.* 1992;86:1622–1633.
9. Siegel RJ, Shah PK, Fishbein MC. Idiopathic restrictive cardiomyopathy. *Circulation.* 1984;70:165–169.
10. Katritsis D, Wilmshurst PT, Wendon JA, et al. Primary restrictive cardiomyopathy: clinical and pathologic characteristics. *J Am Coll Cardiol.* 1991;18:1230–1235.
11. Angelini A, Calzolari V, Thiene G, et al. Morphologic spectrum of primary restrictive cardiomyopathy. *Am J Cardiol.* 1997;80:1046–1050.
12. Hirota Y. Restrictive cardiomyopathy, cardiac amyloidosis and hypereosinophilic heart disease. In: Braunwald E, ed. *Cardiomyopathies, Myocarditis, and Pericardial Disease: Atlas of Heart Diseases.* Philadelphia, PA: Current Medicine; 1995:5.1–5.15.
13. Zhang J, Kumar A, Stalker HF, et al. Clinical and molecular studies of a large family with desmin associated restrictive cardiomyopathy. *Clin Genet.* 2001;59:248–256.
14. Hayashi T, Shimomura H, Terasaki F, et al. Collagen subtypes and matrix metalloproteinase in idiopathic restrictive cardiomyopathy. *Int J Cardiol.* 1998;64:109–116.
15. Abelmann WH, Lorell BH. The challenge of cardiomyopathy. *J Am Coll Cardiol.* 1989;13:1219–1239.
16. Klein AL, Oh JK, Miller FA, et al. Two-dimensional and Doppler echocardiographic assessment of infiltrative cardiomyopathy. *J Am Soc Echocardiogr Off Pub Am Soc Echocardiogr.* 1988;1:48–59.
17. Benotti JR, Grossman W, Cohn PF. Clinical profile of restrictive cardiomyopathy. *Circulation.* 1980;61:1206–1212.
18. Lewis AB. Clinical profile and outcome of restrictive cardiomyopathy in children. *Am Heart J.* 1992;123:1589–1593.
19. Cetta F, O'Leary PW, Seward JB, et al. Idiopathic restrictive cardiomyopathy in childhood: diagnostic features and clinical course. *Mayo Clin Proc.* 1995;70:634–640.

20. Fitzpatrick AP, Shapiro LM, Rickards AF, et al. Familial restrictive cardiomyopathy with atrioventricular block and skeletal myopathy. *Br Heart J.* 1990;63:114–118.
21. Ishiwata S, Nishiyama S, Seki A, et al. Restrictive cardiomyopathy and complete atrioventricular block and distal myopathy with rimmed vacuoles. *Japn Circ J.* 1993;57:928–933.
22. Cooke RA, Chambers JB, Curry PV. Noonan's cardiomyopathy: a non-hypertrophic variant. *Br Heart J.* 1994;71:561–565.
23. Gallego-Delgado M, Delgado JF, Brossa-Loidi V, et al. Idiopathic restrictive cardiomyopathy is primarily a genetic disease. *J Am Coll Cardiol.* 2016;67:3021–3023.
24. Child JS, Perloff JK. The restrictive cardiomyopathies. *Cardiol Clin.* 1988;6:289–316.
25. Ammash NM, Seward JB, Bailey KR, et al. Clinical profile and outcome of idiopathic restrictive cardiomyopathy. *Circulation.* 2000;101:2490–2496.
26. Leya FS, Arab D, Joyal D, et al. The efficacy of brain natriuretic peptide levels in differentiating constrictive pericarditis from restrictive cardiomyopathy. *J Am Coll Cardiol.* 2005;45:1900–1902.
27. Klein AL, Asher CR. Diseases of the pericardium, restrictive cardiomyopathy and diastolic dysfunction. In: Topol EJ, ed. *Textbook of Cardiovascular Medicine.* Philadelphia, PA: Lippincott-Raven; 2004:595–646.
28. Leung DL, Klein AL. Restrictive cardiomyopathy: diagnosis and prognostic implications. In: Otto CM, ed. *The Practice of Clinical Echocardiography.* Philadelphia, PA: WB Saunders; 1996:473–493.
29. Klein AL, Cohen GI, Pietrolungo JF, et al. Differentiation of constrictive pericarditis from restrictive cardiomyopathy by Doppler transesophageal echocardiographic measurements of respiratory variations in pulmonary venous flow. *J Am Coll Cardiol.* 1993;22:1935–1943.
30. Hatle LK, Appleton CP, Popp RL. Differentiation of constrictive pericarditis and restrictive cardiomyopathy by Doppler echocardiography. *Circulation.* 1989;79:357–370.
31. Rajagopalan N, Garcia MJ, Rodriguez L, et al. Apperson-Hansen C, Stugaard M, et al. Comparison of new Doppler echocardiographic methods to differentiate constrictive pericardial heart disease and restrictive cardiomyopathy. *Am J Cardiol.* 2001;87:86–94.
32. Soler R, Rodriguez E, Remuiñán C, et al. Magnetic resonance imaging of primary cardiomyopathies. *J Comput Assist Tomogr.* 2003;27:724–734.
33. Celletti F, Fattori R, Napoli G, et al. Assessment of restrictive cardiomyopathy of amyloid or idiopathic etiology by magnetic resonance imaging. *Am J Cardiol.* 1999;83:798–801.
34. Hosenpud JD, Niles NR. Clinical, hemodynamic and endomyocardial biopsy findings in idiopathic restrictive cardiomyopathy. *West J Med.* 1986;144:303–306.
35. Denfield SW, Rosenthal G, Gajarski RJ, et al. Restrictive cardiomyopathies in childhood: etiologies and natural history. *Tex Heart I J.* 1997;24:38–44.
36. Russo LM, Webber SA. Idiopathic restrictive cardiomyopathy in children. *Heart.* 2005;91:1199–2002.
37. Weller RJ, Weintraub R, Addonizio LF, et al. Outcome of idiopathic restrictive cardiomyopathy in children. *Am J Cardiol.* 2002;90:501–506.
38. Rivenes SM, Kearney DL, Smith EO, et al. Sudden death and cardiovascular collapse in children with restrictive cardiomyopathy. *Circulation.* 2000;102:876–882.
39. Fenton MJ, Chubb H, McMahon AM, et al. Heart and heart-lung transplantation for idiopathic restrictive cardiomyopathy in children. *Heart.* 2006;92:85–89.
40. Ammash NM, Seward JB, Bailey KR, et al. Clinical profile and outcome of idiopathic restrictive cardiomyopathy. *Circulation.* 2000;101:2490–2496.
41. Falk RH, Alexander KM, Liao R, et al. Al (light-chain) cardiac amyloidosis: a review of diagnosis and therapy. *J Am Coll Cardiol.* 2016;68:1323–1341.
42. Gertz MA, Rajkumar SV. Primary systemic amyloidosis. *Curr Treat Option Oncol.* 2002;3:261–271.
43. Kholova I, Niessen HW. Amyloid in the cardiovascular system: a review. *J Clin Pathol.* 2005;58:125–133.
44. Kyle RA, Greipp PR. Amyloidosis (AL): clinical and laboratory features in 229 cases. *Mayo Clin Proc.* 1983;58:665–683.
45. Kyle RA. Amyloidosis. *Circulation.* 1995;91:12769–12771.
46. Gertz MA, Kyle RA. Primary systemic amyloidosis—a diagnostic primer. *Mayo Clin Proc.* 1989;64:1505–1519.
47. Kyle RA, Gertz MA. Primary systemic amyloidosis: clinical and laboratory features in 474 cases. *Semin Hematol.* 1995;32:45–59.
48. Gertz MA, Kyle RA, Thibodeau SN. Familial amyloidosis: a study of 52 North American–born patients examined during a 30-year period. *Mayo Clin Proc.* 1992;67:428–440.
49. Connors LH, Lim A, Prokaeva T, et al. Tabulation of human transthyretin (TTR) variants, 2003. *Amyloid.* 2003;10:160–184.
50. Booth DR, Tan SY, Hawkins PN, et al. A novel variant of transthyretin, 59Thr-- > Lys, associated with autosomal dominant cardiac amyloidosis in an Italian family. *Circulation.* 1995;91:962–967.
51. Fredericksen T, Gotzsche H, Harboe N, et al. Familial primary amyloidosis with severe amyloid heart disease. *Am J Med.* 1962;33:328–348.
52. Benson MD, Wallace MR, Tejada E, et al. Hereditary amyloidosis: description of a new American kindred with late onset cardiomyopathy. *Appalachian amyloid. Arthritis Rheum.* 1987;30:195–200.
53. Jacobson DR, Pastore RD, Yaghoubian R, et al. Variant-sequence transthyretin (isoleucine 122) in late-onset cardiac amyloidosis in black Americans. *N Engl J Med.* 1997;366:466–473.
54. Jacobson DR, Pastore R, Pool S, et al. Revised transthyretin Ile 122 allele frequency in African-Americans. *Human Genet.* 1996;98:236–238.
55. Castano A, Narotsky DL, Hamid N, et al. Unveiling transthyretin cardiac amyloidosis and its predictors among elderly patients with severe aortic stenosis undergoing transcatheter aortic valve replacement. *Eur Heart J.* 2017;38:2879–2887.
56. Kyle RA, Spittell PC, Gertz MA, et al. The premortem recognition of systemic senile amyloidosis with cardiac involvement. *Am J Med.* 1996;101:395–400.
57. Olson LJ, Gertz MA, Edwards WD, et al. Senile cardiac amyloidosis with myocardial dysfunction. Diagnosis by endomyocardial biopsy and immunohistochemistry. *N Engl J Med.* 1987;317:738–742.
58. Ng B, Connors LH, Davidoff R, et al. Senile systemic amyloidosis presenting with heart failure: a comparison with light chain associated amyloidosis. *Arch Intern Med.* 2005;165:1425–1429.
59. Liao R, Jain M, Teller P, et al. Infusion of light chains from patients with cardiac amyloidosis causes diastolic dysfunction in isolated mouse hearts. *Circulation.* 2001;104:1594–1597.
60. Dubrey SW, Cha K, Simms RW, et al. Electrocardiography and Doppler echocardiography in secondary (AA) amyloidosis. *Am J Cardiol.* 1996;77:313–315.
61. Gertz MA, Kyle RA. Secondary systemic amyloidosis: response and survival in 64 patients. *Medicine.* 1991;70:246–256.
62. Pucci A, Wharton J, Arbustini E, et al. Atrial amyloid deposits in the failing human heart display both atrial and brain natriuretic peptide–like immunoreactivity. *J Pathol.* 1991;165:235–241.
63. Goette A, Röcken C. Atrial amyloidosis and atrial fibrillation: a gender-dependent "arrhythmogenic substrate"? *Eur Heart J.* 2004;25:1237–1241.
64. Rocken C, Peters B, Juenemann G, et al. Atrial amyloidosis: an arrhythmogenic substrate for persistent atrial fibrillation. *Circulation.* 2002;106:2091–2097.
65. Gertz MA, Lacy MQ, Dispenzieri A. Amyloidosis. *Hematol Oncol Clin North Am.* 1999;13:1211–1233.
66. Cueto-Garcia L, Tajik AJ, Kyle RA, et al. Callahan JA, et al. Serial echocardiographic observations in patients with primary systemic amyloidosis: an introduction to the concept of early (asymptomatic) amyloid infiltration of the heart. *Mayo Clin Proc.* 1984;59:589–597.
67. Spyrou N, Foale R. Restrictive cardiomyopathies. *Curr Opin Cardiol.* 1994;9:344–348.
68. Barth RF, Willerson JT, Buja LM, et al. Amyloid coronary artery disease, primary systemic amyloidosis and paraproteinemia. *Arch Intern Med.* 1970;126:627–630.
69. Mueller PS, Edwards WD, Gertz MA. Symptomatic ischemic heart disease resulting from obstructive intramural coronary amyloidosis. *Am J Med.* 2000;109:181–188.
70. Bernardi L, Passino C, Porta C, et al. Widespread cardiovascular autonomic dysfunction in primary systemic amyloidosis: does spontaneous

hyperventilation have a compensatory role against postural hypotension?. *Heart.* 2002;88:615–621.

71. Rubinow A, Cohen AS. Skin involvement in generalized amyloidosis. A study of clinically involved and uninvolved skin in 50 patients with primary and secondary amyloidosis. *Ann Intern Med.* 1978;88:781–785.
72. Klein AL, Hatle LK, Burstow DJ, et al. Doppler characterization of left ventricular diastolic function in cardiac amyloidosis. *J Am Coll Cardiol.* 1989;13:1017–1026.
73. Shabetai R. Pathophysiology and differential diagnosis of restrictive cardiomyopathy. *Cardiovasc Clin.* 1988;19:123–132.
74. Dubrey SW, Cha K, Skinner M, et al. Familial and primary (AL) cardiac amyloidosis: echocardiographically similar diseases with distinctly different clinical outcomes. *Heart.* 1997;78:74–82.
75. Murtagh B, Hammill SC, Gertz MA, et al. Electrocardiographic findings in primary systemic amyloidosis and biopsy-proven cardiac involvement. *Am J Cardiol.* 2005;95:535–537.
76. Carroll JD, Gaasch WH, McAdam KP. Amyloid cardiomyopathy: characterization by a distinctive voltage/mass relation. *Am J Cardiol.* 1982;49:9–13.
77. Dubrey SW, Cha K, Anderson J, et al. The clinical features of immunoglobulin light-chain (AL) amyloidosis with heart involvement. *QJM.* 1998;91:141–157.
78. Falk RH, Rubinow A, Cohen AS. Cardiac arrhythmias in systemic amyloidosis: correlation with echocardiographic abnormalities. *J Am Coll Cardiol.* 1984;3:107–113.
79. Klein AL, Oh JK, Miller FA, et al. Two-dimensional and Doppler echocardiographic assessment of infiltrative cardiomyopathy. *J Am Soc Echocardiogr.* 1988;1:48–59.
80. Klein AL, Hatle LK, Burstow DJ, et al. Comprehensive Doppler assessment of right ventricular diastolic function in cardiac amyloidosis. *J Am Coll Cardiol.* 1990;15:99–108.
81. Klein AL, Hatle LK, Taliercio CP, et al. Serial Doppler echocardiographic follow-up of left ventricular diastolic function in cardiac amyloidosis. *J Am Coll Cardiol.* 1990;16:1135–1141.
82. Klein AL, Hatle LK, Taliercio CP, et al. Prognostic significance of Doppler measures of diastolic function in cardiac amyloidosis. A Doppler echocardiography study. *Circulation.* 1991;83:808–816.
83. Patel AR, Dubrey SW, Mendes LA, et al. Right ventricular dilation in primary amyloidosis: an independent predictor of survival. *Am J Cardiol.* 1997;80:486–492.
84. Cueto-Garcia L, Reeder GS, Kyle RA, et al. Echocardiographic findings in systemic amyloidosis: spectrum of cardiac involvement and relation to survival. *J Am Coll Cardiol.* 1985;6:737–743.
85. Falk RH, Plehn JF, Deering T, et al. Sensitivity and specificity of the echocardiographic features of cardiac amyloidosis. *Am J Cardiol.* 1987;59:418–422.
86. Siqueira-Filho AG, Cunha CL, Tajik AJ, et al. M-mode and two-dimensional echocardiographic features in cardiac amyloidosis. *Circulation.* 1981;63:188–196.
87. Chiaramida SA, Goldman MA, Zema MJ, et al. Real-time cross-sectional echocardiographic diagnosis of infiltrative cardiomyopathy due to amyloid. *J Clin Ultrasoun.* 1980;8:58–62.
88. Chandrasekaran K, Aylward PE, Fleagle SR, et al. Feasibility of identifying amyloid and hypertrophic cardiomyopathy with the use of computerized quantitative texture analysis of clinical echocardiographic data. *J Am Coll Cardiol.* 1989;13:832–840.
89. Chew C, Ziady GM, Raphael MJ, et al. The functional defect in amyloid heart disease. The "stiff heart" syndrome. *Am J Cardiol.* 1975;36:438–444.
90. St John Sutton MG, Reichek N, Kastor JA, et al. Computerized M-mode echocardiographic analysis of left ventricular dysfunction in cardiac amyloid. *Circulation.* 1982;66:790–799.
91. Abdalla I, Murray RD, Lee JC, et al. Duration of pulmonary venous atrial reversal flow velocity and mitral inflow a wave: new measure of severity of cardiac amyloidosis. *J Am Soc Echocardiogr.* 1998;11:1125–1133.
92. Koyama J, Ray-Sequin PA, Davidoff R, et al. Usefulness of pulsed tissue Doppler imaging for evaluating systolic and diastolic left ventricular function in patients with AL (primary) amyloidosis. *Am J Cardiol.* 2002;89:1067–1071.
93. Koyama J, Ray-Sequin PA, Falk RH. Longitudinal myocardial function assessed by tissue velocity, strain, and strain rate tissue Doppler echocardiography in patients with AL (primary) cardiac amyloidosis. *Circulation.* 2003;107:2446–2452.
94. Baccouche H, Maunz M, Beck T, et al. Differentiating cardiac amyloidosis and hypertrophic cardiomyopathy by use of three-dimensional speckle tracking echocardiography. *Echocardiography.* 2012;29:668.
95. Phelan D, Thavendiranathan P, Popovic Z, et al. Application of a parametric display of two-dimensional speckle-tracking longitudinal strain to improve the etiologic diagnosis of mild to moderate left ventricular hypertrophy. *J Am Soc Echocardiogr.* 2014;27:888–985. doi: 10.1016/j.echo.2014.04.015.
96. Phelan D, Collier P, Thavendiranathan P, et al. Relative apical sparing of longitudinal strain using two-dimensional speckle-tracking echocardiography is both sensitive and specific for the diagnosis of cardiac amyloidosis. *Heart.* 2012;98:1442–1448. doi: 10.1136/heartjnl-2012-302353.
97. Senapati A, Sperry BW, Grodin JL, et al. Prognostic implication of relative regional strain ratio in cardiac amyloidosis. *Heart.* 2016;102: 748–754.
98. Katzmann JA, Abraham RS, Dispenzieri A, et al. Diagnostic performance of quantitative kappa and lambda free light chain assays in clinical practice. *Clin Chem.* 2005;51:878–881.
99. Abraham RS, Katzmann JA, Clark RJ, et al. Quantitative analysis of serum free light chains. A new marker for the diagnostic evaluation of primary systemic amyloidosis. *Am J Clin Pathol.* 2003;119:274–278.
100. Gertz MA, Lacy MQ, Dispenzieri A. Amyloidosis: recognition, confirmation, prognosis, and therapy. *Mayo Clin Proc.* 1999;74:490–494.
101. Libbey CA, Skinner M, Cohen AS. Use of the abdominal fat tissue aspirate in the diagnosis of systemic amyloidosis. *Arch Int Med.* 1983;143:1549–1552.
102. Ardehali H, Qasim A, Cappola T, et al. Endomyocardial biopsy plays a role in diagnosing patients with unexplained cardiomyopathy. *Am Heart J.* 2004;147:919–923.
103. Oh JK, Tajik AJ, Edwards WD, et al. Dynamic left ventricular outflow tract obstruction in cardiac amyloidosis detected by continuous-wave Doppler echocardiography. *Am J Cardiol.* 1987;59:1008–1010.
104. Syed IS, Glockner JF, Feng D, et al. Role of cardiac magnetic resonance imaging in the detection of cardiac amyloidosis. *JACC Cardiovasc Imag.* 2010;3:155–164.
105. Sechtem U, Higgins CB, Sommerhoff BA, et al. Magnetic resonance imaging of restrictive cardiomyopathy. *Am J Cardiol.* 1987;59: 480–482.
106. von Kemp K, Beckers R, Vandenweghe J, et al. Echocardiography and magnetic resonance imaging in cardiac amyloidosis. *Acta Cardiologica.* 1989;44:29–36.
107. Celletti F, Fattori R, Napoli G, et al. Assessment of restrictive cardiomyopathy of amyloid or idiopathic etiology by magnetic resonance imaging. *Am J Cardiol.* 1999;83:798–801. A10.
108. Maceira AM, Joshi J, Prasad SK, et al. Cardiovascular magnetic resonance in cardiac amyloidosis. *Circulation.* 2005;111:186–193.
109. Haaf P, Garg P, Messroghli DR, et al. Cardiac t1 mapping and extracellular volume (ecv) in clinical practice: a comprehensive review. *J Cardiovasc Magnet Res.* 2016;18:89.
110. Perugini E, Guidalotti PL, Salvi F, et al. Noninvasive etiologic diagnosis of cardiac amyloidosis using 99mTc-3,3-diphosphono-1,2-propanodicarboxylic acid scintigraphy. *J Am Coll Cardiol.* 2005;46:1076.
111. Rapezzi C, Quarta CC, Guidalotti PL, et al. Role of (99m)Tc-DPD scintigraphy in diagnosis and prognosis of hereditary transthyretin-related cardiac amyloidosis. *JACC Cardiovasc Imag.* 2011;4:659.
112. Bokhari S, Castaño A, Pozniakoff T, et al. (99m)Tc-pyrophosphate scintigraphy for differentiating light-chain cardiac amyloidosis from the transthyretin-related familial and senile cardiac amyloidoses. *Circ Cardiovasc Imag.* 2013;6:195–201.
113. Pereira NL, Grogan M, Dec GW. Spectrum of restrictive and infiltrative cardiomyopathies: part 1 of a 2-part series. *J Am Coll Cardiol.* 2018;71:1130–1148.
114. Gertz MA, Kyle RA, Amyloidosis:. prognosis and treatment. *Semin Arthritis Rheum.* 1994;24:124–138.

115. Muchtar E, Gertz MA, Kumar SK, et al. Improved outcomes for newly diagnosed al amyloidosis between 2000 and 2014: cracking the glass ceiling of early death. *Blood.* 2017;129:2111–2119.
116. Tei C, Dujardin KS, Hodge DO, et al. Doppler index combining systolic and diastolic myocardial performance: clinical value in cardiac amyloidosis. *J Am Coll Cardiol.* 1996;28:658–664.
117. Dispenzieri A, Kyle RA, Gertz MA, et al. Survival in patients with primary systemic amyloidosis and raised serum cardiac troponins. *Lancet.* 2003;361:1787–1789.
118. Kumar S, Dispenzieri A, Lacy MQ, et al. Revised prognostic staging system for light chain amyloidosis incorporating cardiac biomarkers and serum free light chain measurements. *J Clin Oncol.* 2012;30:989–995.
119. Muchtar E, Jevremovic D, Dispenzieri A, et al. The prognostic value of multiparametric flow cytometry in al amyloidosis at diagnosis and at the end of first-line treatment. *Blood.* 2017;129:82–87.
120. Kyle RA, Gertz MA, Greipp PR, et al. A trial of three regimens for primary amyloidosis: colchicine alone, melphalan and prednisone, and melphalan, prednisone, and colchicine. *N Engl J Med.* 1997;336:1202–1207.
121. Skinner M, Anderson JJ, Simms R, et al. Treatment of 100 patients with primary amyloidosis: a randomized trial of melphalan, prednisone, and colchicine versus colchicine alone. *Am J Med.* 1996;100:290–298.
122. Skinner M, Sanchorawala V, Seldin DC, et al. High-dose melphalan and autologous stem-cell transplantation in patients with AL amyloidosis: an 8-year study. *Ann Intern Med.* 2004;140:85–93.
123. Comenzo RL, Vosburgh E, Falk RH, et al. Dose-intensive melphalan with blood stem-cell support for the treatment of AL (amyloid light-chain) amyloidosis: survival and responses in 25 patients. *Blood.* 1998;91:3662–3670.
124. Rubinow A, Skinner M, Cohen AS. Digoxin sensitivity in amyloid cardiomyopathy. *Circulation.* 1981;63:1285–1288.
125. Pollak A, Falk RH. Left ventricular systolic dysfunction precipitated by verapamil in cardiac amyloidosis. *Chest.* 1993;104:618–620.
126. Willens HJ, Levy R, Kessler KM. Thromboembolic complications in cardiac amyloidosis detected by transesophageal echocardiography. *Am Heart J.* 1995;129:405–406.
127. Plehn JF, Southworth J, Cornwell III GG. Brief report: atrial systolic failure in primary amyloidosis. *N Engl J Med.* 1992;327:1570–1573.
128. Hosenpud JD, DeMarco T, Frazier OH, et al. Progression of systemic disease and reduced long-term survival in patients with cardiac amyloidosis undergoing heart transplantation. Follow-up results of a multicenter survey. *Circulation.* 1991;84(5):SIII338–SIII343.
129. Dubrey S, Simms RW, Skinner M, et al. Recurrence of primary (AL) amyloidosis in a transplanted heart with four-year survival. *Am J Cardiol.* 1995;76:739–741.
130. Kpodonu J, Massad MG, Caines A, et al. Outcome of heart transplantation in patients with amyloid cardiomyopathy. *J Heart Lung Transplant.* 2005;24:1763–1765.
131. Dubrey SW, Burke MM, Hawkines PN, et al. Cardiac transplantation for amyloid heart disease: the United Kingdom experience. *J Heart Lung Transplant.* 2004;23:1142–1153.
132. Pelosi Jr F, Capehart J, Roberts WC. Effectiveness of cardiac transplantation for primary (AL) cardiac amyloidosis. *Am J Cardiol.* 1997;79:532–535.
133. Suhr OB, Herlenius G, Friman S, et al. Liver transplantation for hereditary transthyretin amyloidosis. *Liver Transplant.* 2000;6:263–276.
134. Skinner M, Lewis WD, Jones LA, et al. Liver transplantation as treatment for familial amyloidotic polyneuropathy. *Ann Intern Med.* 1994;120:133–134.
135. Holmgren G, Ericzon BG, Groth CG, et al. Clinical improvement and amyloid regression after liver transplantation in hereditary transthyretin amyloidosis. *Lancet.* 1993;341:1113–1116.
136. Miller SR, Sekijima Y, Kelly JW. Native state stabilization by NSAIDs inhibits transthyretin amyloidogenesis from the most common familial disease variants. *Lab Invest.* 2004;84:545–552.
137. Adams D, Gonzalez-Duarte A, O'Riordan WD, et al. Patisiran, an RNAi therapeutic, for hereditary transthyretin amyloidosis. *N Engl J Med.* 2018;379:11–21.
138. Benson MD, Waddington-Cruz M, Berk JL, et al. Inotersen treatment for patients with hereditary transthyretin amyloidosis. *N Engl J Med.* 2018;379:22–31.
139. Maurer MS, Schwartz JH, Gundapaneni B, et al. Tafamidis treatment for patients with transthyretin amyloid cardiomyopathy. *N Engl J Med.* 2018;379:1007–1016.
140. Arad M, Maron BJ, Gorham JM, et al. Glycogen storage diseases presenting as hypertrophic cardiomyopathy. *N Engl J Med.* 2005;352:362–372.
141. Yang Z, McMahon CJ, Smith LR, et al. Danon disease as an underrecognized cause of hypertrophic cardiomyopathy in children. *Circulation.* 2005;112:1612–1617.
142. Brady RO, Gal AE, Bradley RM, et al. Enzymatic defect in Fabry's disease. Ceramidetrihexosidase deficiency. *N Engl J Med.* 1967;276:1163–1167.
143. von Scheidt W, Eng CM, Fitzmaurice TF, et al. An atypical variant of Fabry's disease with manifestations confined to the myocardium. *N Engl J Med.* 1991;324:395–399.
144. Eng CM, Guffon N, Wilcox WR, et al. Safety and efficacy of recombinant human alpha-galactosidase a replacement therapy in Fabry's disease. *N Engl J Med.* 2001;345:9–16.
145. Nakao S, Takenaka T, Maeda M, et al. An atypical variant of Fabry's disease in men with left ventricular hypertrophy. *N Engl J Med.* 1995;333:288–293.
146. Sachdev B, Takenaka T, Teraguchi H, et al. Prevalence of Anderson-Fabry disease in male patients with late onset hypertrophic cardiomyopathy. *Circulation.* 2002;105:1407–1411.
147. Chimenti C, Pieroni M, Morgante E, et al. Prevalence of Fabry disease in female patients with late-onset hypertrophic cardiomyopathy. *Circulation.* 2004;110:1047–1053.
148. Kampmann C, Baehner F, Whybra C, et al. Cardiac manifestations of Anderson-Fabry disease in heterozygous females. *J Am Coll Cardiol.* 2002;40:1668–1674.
149. Desnick RJ, Ioannou YA, Eng CM. Alpha-galactosidase a deficiency: Fabry disease. In: Scriver CH, ed. *The Metabolic and Molecular Bases of Inherited Diseases.* New York, NY: McGraw-Hill; 2001:3733–3774.
150. Yousef Z, Elliott PM, Cecchi F, et al. Left ventricular hypertrophy in Fabry disease: a practical approach to diagnosis. *Eur Heart J.* 2013;34:802–808.
151. Ramaswami U, Whybra C, Parini R, et al. Clinical manifestations of Fabry disease in children: data from the Fabry outcome survey. *Acta Paediatrica.* 2006;95:86–92.
152. Desnick RJ, Brady R, Barranger J, et al. Fabry disease, an under-recognized multisystemic disorder: expert recommendations for diagnosis, management, and enzyme replacement therapy. *Ann Intern Med.* 2003;138:338–346.
153. Monserrat L, Gimeno-Blanes JR, Marín F, et al. Prevalence of Fabry disease in a cohort of 508 unrelated patients with hypertrophic cardiomyopathy. *J Am Coll Cardiol.* 2007;50:2399–2403.
154. Pochis WT, Litzow JT, King BG, et al. Electrophysiologic findings in Fabry's disease with a short PR interval. *Am J Cardiol.* 1994;74:203–204.
155. Sakuraba H, Yanagawa Y, Igarashi T, et al. Cardiovascular manifestations in Fabry's disease. A high incidence of mitral valve prolapse in hemizygotes and heterozygotes. *Clin Genet.* 1986;29:276–283.
156. Bass JL, Shrivastava S, Grabowski GA, et al. The M-mode echocardiogram in Fabry's disease. *Am Heart J.* 1980;100:807–812.
157. Cohen IS, Fluri-Lundeen J, Wharton TP. Two dimensional echocardiographic similarity of Fabry's disease to cardiac amyloidosis: a function of ultrastructural analogy?. *J Clin Ultrasoun.* 1983;11:437–441.
158. Linhart A, Palecek T, Bultas J, et al. New insights in cardiac structural changes in patients with Fabry's disease. *Am Heart J.* 2000;139: 1101–1108.
159. Morimoto S, Sugiura A, Iwase M, et al. Relief of left ventricular outflow obstruction by cibenzoline in a patient with Fabry's disease—a case report. *Angiology.* 2006;57:241–245.
160. Goldman ME, Cantor R, Schwartz MF, et al. Echocardiographic abnormalities and disease severity in Fabry's disease. *J Am Coll Cardiol.* 1986;7:1157–1161.
161. Pieroni M, Chimenti C, Ricci R, et al. Early detection of Fabry cardiomyopathy by tissue Doppler imaging. *Circulation.* 2003;107:1978–1984.
162. Pieroni M, Chimenti C, De Cobelli F, et al. Fabry's disease cardiomyopathy: echocardiographic detection of endomyocardial glycosphingolipid compartmentalization. *J Am Coll Cardiol.* 2006;47:1663–1671.

163. Matsui S, Murakami E, Takekoshi N, et al. Myocardial tissue characterization by magnetic resonance imaging in Fabry's disease. *Am Heart J.* 1989;117:472–474.
164. Weidemann F, Breunig F, Beer M, et al. Improvement of cardiac function during enzyme replacement therapy in patients with Fabry disease: a prospective strain rate imaging study. *Circulation.* 2003;108:1299–1301.
165. Moon JC, Sachdev B, Elkington AG, et al. Gadolinium enhanced cardiovascular magnetic resonance in Anderson-Fabry disease: evidence for a disease specific abnormality of the myocardial interstitium. *Eur Heart J.* 2003;24:2151–2155.
166. Liu JM, Liu A, Leal J, et al. Measurement of myocardial native t1 in cardiovascular diseases and norm in 1291 subjects. *J Cardiovasc Magnet Res.* 2017;19:74.
167. Weidemann F, Breunig F, Beer M, et al. The variation of morphological and functional cardiac manifestation in Fabry disease: potential implications for the time course of the disease. *Eur Heart J.* 2005;26:1221–1227.
168. Frustaci A, Chimenti C, Ricci R, et al. Improvement in cardiac function in the cardiac variant of Fabry's disease with galactose-infusion therapy. *N Engl J Med.* 2001;345:25–32.
169. Kalliokoski RJ, Kantola I, Kalliokoski KK, et al. The effect of 12-month enzyme replacement therapy on myocardial perfusion in patients with Fabry disease. *J Inherit Metabol Dis.* 2006;29:112–118.
170. Maron BJ, Roberts WC, Arad M, et al. Clinical outcome and phenotypic expression in lamp2 cardiomyopathy. *JAMA.* 2009;301:1253–1259.
171. Hauser SC. Hemochromatosis and the heart. *Heart Dis Stroke.* 1993;2:487–491.
172. Buja LM, Roberts WC. Iron in the heart. *Etiology and clinical significance. Am J Med.* 1971;51:209–221.
173. Adams PC, Halliday JW, Powell LW. Early diagnosis and treatment of hemochromatosis. *Adv Intern Med.* 1989;34:111–126.
174. Case Records of the Massachusetts General Hospital (Case 31-1994). *N Engl J Med.* 1994;331:460-466.
175. Olson LJ, Baldus WP, Tajik AJ. Echocardiographic features of idiopathic hemochromatosis. *Am J Cardiol.* 1987;60:885–889.
176. Bonkovsky HL, Slaker DP, Bills EB, et al. Usefulness and limitations of laboratory and hepatic imaging studies in iron-storage disease. *Gastroenterology.* 1990;99:1079–1091.
177. Olson LJ, Edwards WD, McCall JT, et al. Cardiac iron deposition in idiopathic hemochromatosis: histologic and analytic assessment of 14 hearts from autopsy. *J Am Coll Cardiol.* 1987;10:1239–1243.
178. Candell-Riera J, Lu L, Serés L, et al. Cardiac hemochromatosis: beneficial effects of iron removal therapy. An echocardiographic study. *Am J Cardiol.* 1983;52:824–829.
179. Short EM, Winkle RA, Billingham ME. Myocardial involvement in idiopathic hemochromatosis. Morphologic and clinical improvement following venesection. *Am J Med.* 1981;70:1275–1279.
180. Rivers J, Garrahy P, Robinson W, et al. Reversible cardiac dysfunction in hemochromatosis. *Am Heart J.* 1987;113:216–217.
181. Olson LJ, Edwards WD, Holmes Jr DR, et al. Endomyocardial biopsy in hemochromatosis: clinicopathologic correlates in six cases. *J Am Coll Cardiol.* 1989;13:116–120.
182. Dabestani A, Child JS, Henze E, et al. Primary hemochromatosis: anatomic and physiologic characteristics of the cardiac ventricles and their response to phlebotomy. *Am J Cardiol.* 1984;54:153–159.
183. Rahko PS, Salerni R, Uretsky BF. Successful reversal by chelation therapy of congestive cardiomyopathy due to iron overload. *J Am Coll Cardiol.* 1986;8:436–440.
184. Easley Jr RM, Schreiner Jr BF, Yu PN. Reversible cardiomyopathy associated with hemochromatosis. *N Engl J Med.* 1972;287:866–867.
185. Henry WL, Nienhuis AW, Wiener M, et al. Echocardiographic abnormalities in patients with transfusion-dependent anemia and secondary myocardial iron deposition. *Am J Med.* 1978;64:547–555.
186. Palka P, Macdonald G, Lange A, et al. The role of Doppler left ventricular filling indexes and Doppler tissue echocardiography in the assessment of cardiac involvement in hereditary hemochromatosis. *J Am Soc Echocardiogr.* 2002;15:884–890.
187. Leon MB, Borer JS, Bacharach SL, et al. Detection of early cardiac dysfunction in patients with severe beta-thalassemia and chronic iron overload. *N Engl J Med.* 1979;21:1143–1148.
188. Anderson LJ, Holden S, Davis B, et al. Cardiovascular T2-star (T2*) magnetic resonance for the early diagnosis of myocardial iron overload. *Eur Heart J.* 2001;22:2171–2179.
189. Kirk P, Roughton M, Porter JB, et al. Cardiac T2* magnetic resonance for prediction of cardiac complications in thalassemia major. *Circulation.* 2009;120:1961–1968.
190. Mamtani M, Kulkarni H. Influence of iron chelators on myocardial iron and cardiac function in transfusion-dependent thalassaemia: a systematic review and meta-analysis. *Br J Haematol.* 2008;141:882–890.
191. Przybojewski JZ. Endomyocardial biopsy: a review of the literature. *Cath Cardiovasc Diag.* 1985;11:287–330.
192. Westra WH, Hruban RH, Baughman KL, et al. Progressive hemochromatotic cardiomyopathy despite reversal of iron deposition after liver transplantation. *Am J Clin Pathol.* 1993;99:39–44.
193. Caines AE, Kpodonu J, Massad MG, et al. Cardiac transplantation in patients with iron overload cardiomyopathy. *J Heart Lung Transplant.* 2005;24:486–488.
194. Ocel JJ, Edwards WD, Tazelaar HD, et al. Heart and liver disease in 32 patients undergoing biopsy of both organs, with implications for heart or liver transplantation. *Mayo Clin Proc.* 2004;79:492–501.

24

Coronary Artery Disease

Lara C. Kovell and Gerard P. Aurigemma

OUTLINE

INTRODUCTION

While coronary artery disease (CAD) and hypertension are common comorbidities in diastolic dysfunction, and heart failure with preserved ejection fraction (HFpEF), relatively less attention has been paid to the interaction between CAD and diastolic dysfunction. This chapter is devoted to reviewing how diastolic dysfunction and coronary disease relate, the assessment of diastolic function in patients with coronary disease, and the role of Doppler echocardiography in elucidating aspects of the pathogenesis of heart failure.

Case Study

A 58-year-old man with a history of inflammatory polyarthritis, hypertension, hyperlipidemia, CAD and status post-coronary artery bypass surgery 18 months prior to admission is taken to the emergency room with acute chest pain and dizziness. He is hypotensive to the 70s and in mild respiratory distress. An electrocardiogram (ECG) is obtained, illustrating diffuse ST-segment depressions (Fig. 24.1). A two-dimensional (2-D) Doppler echocardiogram is performed (Videos 24.1 and 24.2; Figs. 24.2, 24.3, 24.4, and 24.5) while preparations are made for emergent heart catheterization. Table 24.1 summarizes the echo Doppler data obtained shortly before the heart catheterization.

Right and left heart catheterization is performed (Fig. 24.6) showing markedly elevated left ventricular (LV) end-diastolic pressures (EDPs), as well as markedly elevated pulmonary capillary wedge pressure (PCWP). He is found to have occlusion of his bypass grafts and severe ostial stenoses of this proximal left anterior descending and left circumflex coronary arteries. These stenoses are successfully treated with percutaneous coronary intervention.

A LV mechanical assist device is inserted and he is admitted to the coronary care unit for convalescence. The patient is eventually discharged to home.

Diastolic heart failure (we will use the term interchangeably with HFpEF) is a condition characterized by signs and symptoms of heart failure, where "the dominant abnormality resides in diastole."[1] Cross-sectional and population-based studies indicate that ~50% of all patients with congestive heart failure have a normal or near-normal ejection fraction, and that most have diastolic heart failure.[2,3] As is the case with systolic heart failure, the mortality rate of diastolic heart failure is directly related to age and the presence of coronary disease.[1,4] The reported prevalence of diastolic heart failure depends not only on age, but on the diagnostic criteria used to define diastolic dysfunction, the etiology of the disease, and the methods and design of the particular study in question.[1]

The prevalence of coronary disease in patients who develop diastolic heart failure is high, with estimates ranging from 41% to 65% depending on the population. Gottdiener et al. studied over 5000 community-based individuals, age 65 or greater, enrolled in the Cardiovascular Health Study (CHS). Prevalent CAD was associated with more than a threefold higher rate of incident heart failure (41% vs. 15.3%). The population-attributable risk of prevalent CAD in this study was roughly equivalent to that of arterial hypertension.[5] In a subsequent analysis of HF in the CHS database, prevalent coronary heart disease was present in 58% of patients with HFpEF and in 78% of patients with heart failure with reduced ejection fraction (HFrEF).[6]

Similarly, high rates of CAD have been reported in a registry study by Klapholz et al. on clinical characteristics of patients hospitalized with HFpEF,[7] as well as in those enrolled in the Candesartan in Heart Failure: Assessment of Reduction in Mortality and Morbidity (CHARM)–Preserved study.[8] In the study by Klapholz et al., 43% of patients with HFpEF had a history of CAD, defined by chronic angina, stress test positive for ischemia, prior myocardial infarction (MI), coronary stenoses of 50% or more by coronary catheterization, or prior angioplasty or coronary artery bypass surgery.[7] In the CHARM-Preserved trial, roughly 22% had a prior coronary artery bypass graft and 45% had prior MI.[8]

A more contemporary, prospective study of patients admitted for heart failure showed that 65% of patients with HFpEF had significant coronary stenosis, defined as more than 70% or 50% to 70% with a fractional flow reserve (FFR) of 0.8 or less. These high rates were likely related to the mean age of 79 years in the study sample.[9] In a meta-analysis of seven studies of over 30,000 patients with HFpEF, pooled estimated prevalence of CAD in patients with HFpEF was 45.6% using a cutoff of ejection fraction of 50% or more.[10] All of these epidemiologic, clinical trial, and meta-analysis data demonstrate the importance of coronary heart disease in the pathogenesis of diastolic heart failure.

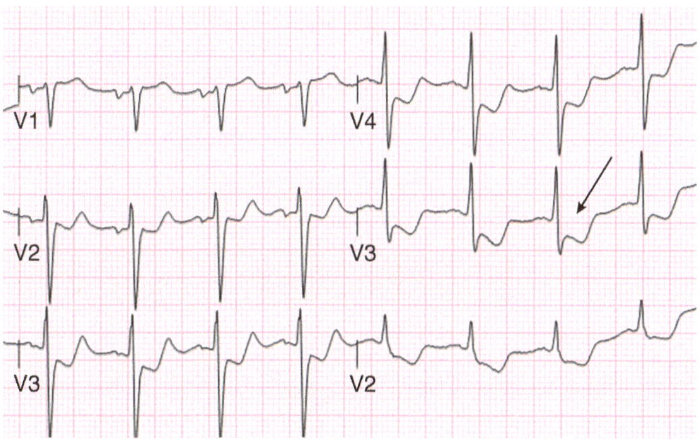

Fig. 24.1 Case study: ECG obtained on admission showing precordial lead abnormalities. There are deep ST-segment depressions present in leads V2 to V6 *(arrow)*.

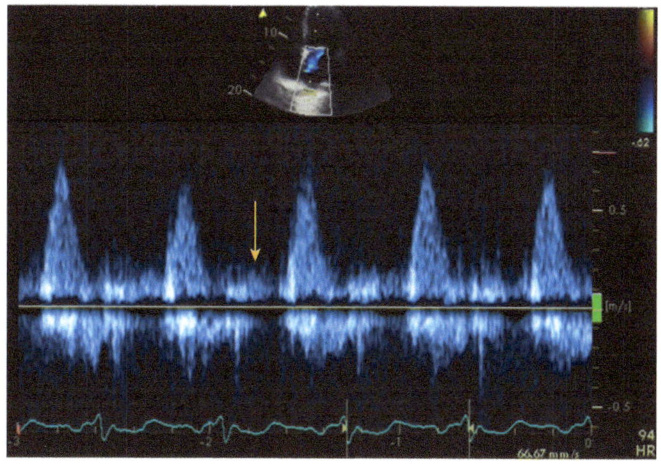

Fig. 24.4 Case study: Pulmonary venous flow velocities; note the very low velocity systolic (S) wave *(arrow)*. In patients without significant mitral regurgitation and who are in normal sinus rhythm, this is a reliable predictor of high LA pressure, which was the case.

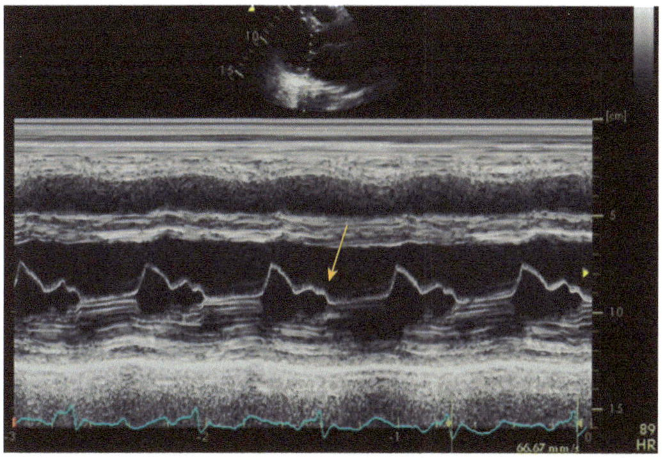

Fig. 24.2 Case study: M mode echo demonstrating an inflection on the closure pattern of the anterior mitral leaflet following atrial systole, the so-called B bump. This is a sign of increased postatrial contraction end-diastolic pressure, which was present in this patient.

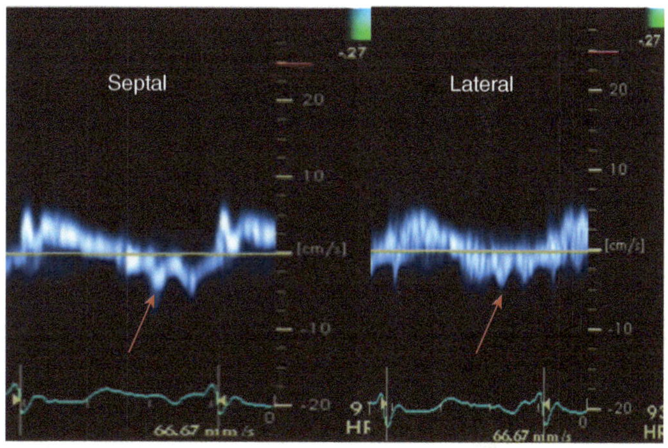

Fig. 24.5 Case study: Septal and lateral tissue Doppler velocities. Tissue Doppler e′ velocities are extremely low *(arrows)*, each below 4 cm/sec.

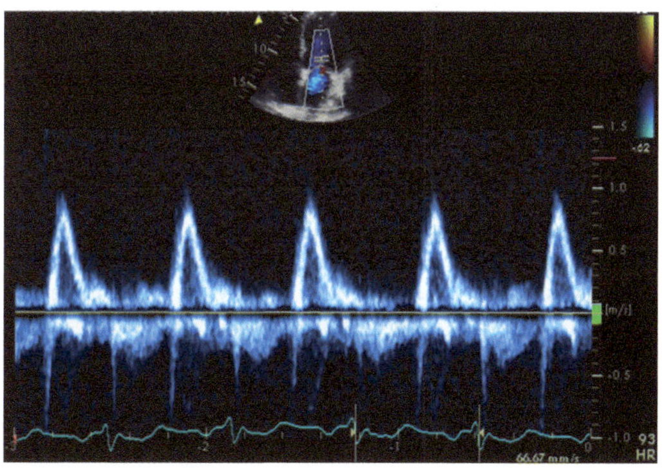

Fig. 24.3 Case study: Transmitral flow pattern. Note the diminutive A wave (see text for speculation).

TABLE 24.1 Case study: Summarization of the Echo Doppler Data Obtained Shortly Before the Heart Catheterization

Parameter	Value
Ejection fraction	40%
E wave (cm/sec)	90
A wave (cm/sec)	20
Pulmonary vein pattern	D dominant
Tissue Doppler e′ (lateral annulus) (cm/sec)	2
Tissue Doppler e′ (septal annulus) (cm/sec)	4
TR velocity (m/sec)	3.2
LA volume index (cc/m^2)	35
E/e′ (average septal and lateral) ratio	30

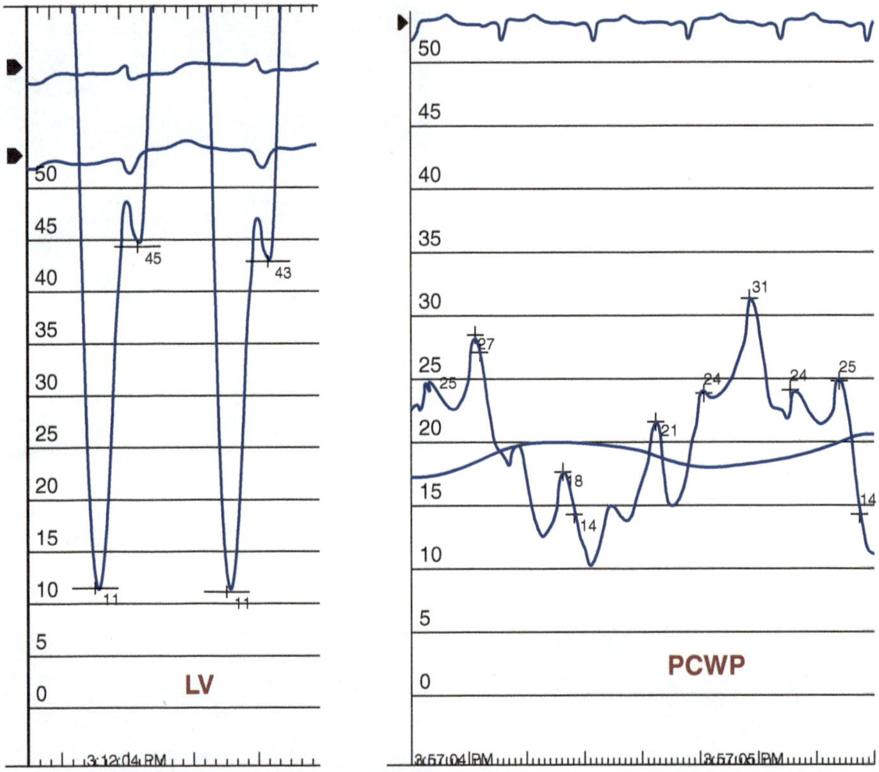

Fig. 24.6 Case study: Left ventricular *(LV, left)* and pulmonary capillary wedge *(right)* tracings demonstrating severe elevations in LV end-diastolic pressure (45 mmHg at end expiration) and elevated mean pulmonary capillary wedge pressure *(PCWP)* (18–20 mmHg).

PATHOPHYSIOLOGY

As reviewed in Chapter 2, diastolic function is determined by the passive elastic properties of the left ventricle and the process of active relaxation.[1,11] Active relaxation is an energy-dependent process that is affected by ischemia. By contrast, abnormal passive elastic properties are generally caused by a combination of increased myocardial mass and alterations in the extramyocardial collagen network.[1] The effects of impaired active myocardial relaxation, caused by acute ischemia, can lead to further stiffness. The interplay between this impaired relaxation and passive stiffness determines LV filling pressure.[1]

Acute Ischemia

It has been demonstrated that acute myocardial ischemia effects changes in both global and regional LV diastolic properties.[12] This point is illustrated in the case study. The results of these alterations include a slower LV pressure decay with a consequent slowing of diastolic filling as intracellular adenosine triphosphate (ATP) is depleted and intracellular calcium rises.[13] Actin-myosin bridges fail to dissociate, and given the persistent attachment, tension is maintained throughout diastole, leading to increased diastolic stiffness and LVEDP.[13–15] These changes in the passive properties of the left ventricle result in an upward shift in the diastolic pressure-volume (P-V) relationship (Fig. 24.7). As a result, the LV diastolic P-V relationship changes: chamber compliance is reduced, the time course is altered, and diastolic pressure is elevated. Under these circumstances, a relatively small increase in central blood volume or an increase in venous tone or arterial stiffness can produce a substantial increase in filling pressures and may result in acute pulmonary edema, as was seen in the case presented.[16] In the patient described in the case study, there was a parallel increase in the PCWP and marked elevation in the LVEDP. These findings were reflected in the high E/e′ ratio, the D-dominant pulmonary vein flow, and even the M mode.

The slowed relaxation following acute ischemia or infarction may persist for days.[17] However, a slower rate of the LV pressure decline is not the only result of direct effects of ischemia on myocardial relaxation. Ischemia may also affect contractility and loading conditions, and may worsen nonuniformity, which may also act to slow the rate of LV pressure decline.[18–20]

Postinfarction LV Remodeling

The subject of post-MI LV remodeling is complicated, and excellent reviews of this topic have been published.[21–23] In the consensus paper by Cohn et al., LV remodeling is defined as "changes in size, shape, and function of the heart after cardiac injury. The process is influenced by hemodynamic load, neurohumoral activation, and other processes."[23] The immediate changes following infarction involve mainly the infarcted region, with infarct expansion observed most frequently after large, transmural infarcts.[21] Subsequently, over weeks to months, further changes occur, and these involve the noninfarcted region.

A review of the mechanisms involved in LV remodeling makes it clear that what may begin as an adaptive process can have detrimental consequences for LV diastolic function. During acute ischemia, myocardial injury and death, and the resultant reduction in systolic function, the region undergoing infarction may develop systolic expansion and perform a reduced amount of effective work.[20,23] Following a large MI, LVEDP remains elevated, and the volume of viable myocardium increases ~30% because of increases in both myocyte cell length and diameter.[20] Given the increased load on the noninfarcted myocardium, eccentric hypertrophy develops and contributes to the increase in LV size.[24] In some instances, the ventricle may undergo progressive infarct expansion, usually within the first 24

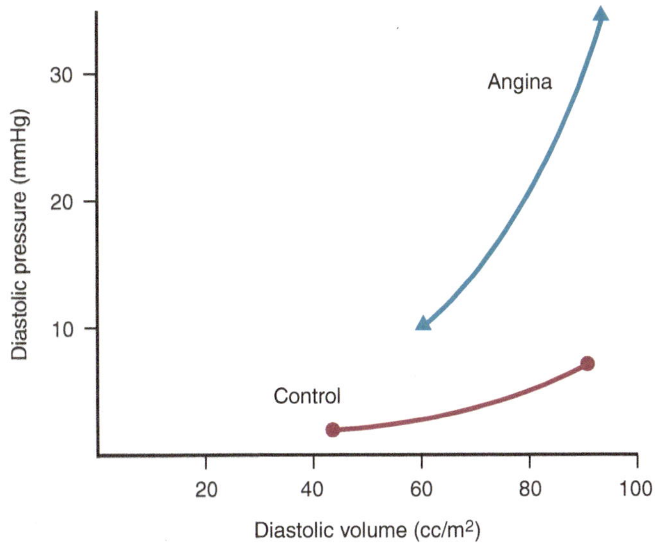

Fig. 24.7 The acute effect of ischemia on the pressure-volume (P-V) relationship. These data are taken from the study of a 60-year-old individual undergoing catheterization. The control diastolic P-V relationship is shown. During the procedure, the patient developed angina; volume assessment and hemodynamic measures were repeated. As can be seen, the P-V relationship shifted dramatically upward, so that at any given diastolic volume, the pressure during the angina episode is higher; note that the ejection fraction has not changed dramatically. (Figure courtesy of Dr. William H. Gaasch.)

to 72 hours. In part, this expansion and volume increase help to compensate for the reduction in effective work via the Frank-Starling mechanism. Even in the absence of acute LV expansion, LV dilation and increased oxygen demand may develop, usually over several months after MI, involving both the infarcted and the noninfarcted regions.[20–24]

Given the curvilinear diastolic P-V relationship, lengthening/dilation of noninfarcted regions is associated with an increase in LVEDP.[20–23] High wall stresses and ventricular remodeling may provide the stimuli for deleterious changes and further remodeling.[22,24] The signal for progressive remodeling in the postinfarction ventricle may be diastolic wall stress, with parallels between this process and what is observed in chronic volume overload due to valvular regurgitation.[22] Myocyte hypertrophy and changes in the extracellular matrix also are part of the remodeling process.[20–23]

Even if systolic function improves post MI, injured areas of the myocardium can demonstrate persistent diastolic dysfunction. In a cardiac magnetic resonance imaging (cardiac MRI) study of dogs undergoing coronary artery occlusion followed by reperfusion, both transmural and subendocardial acute MI segments exhibited significant systolic and diastolic dysfunction compared to remote segments.[25] Reversibly injured regions showed persistent diastolic impairment 24 hours after reperfusion, despite systolic functional recovery.[25]

Persistent diastolic dysfunction post MI can have a detrimental impact on exertional capacity. An invasive hemodynamic exercise study by Andersen et al. looked at post-MI patients with an ejection fraction above 45%, with and without diastolic dysfunction, compared with healthy volunteers.[26] Diastolic dysfunction was defined by left atrial volume index (LAVI) greater than 34 mL/m^2 and E/e′ ratio above 8. At rest, 29% of the patients with diastolic dysfunction had resting PCWP greater than 15 mmHg, while none of those without diastolic dysfunction or the controls had PCWP elevation. The vast majority (94%) of those with diastolic dysfunction had an abnormal rise in PCWP greater than 25 mmHg, compared to 36% of the post-MI patients without diastolic dysfunction. This suggests an explanation for exertional intolerance in post-MI patients with diastolic dysfunction, and the adverse compensatory mechanisms for maintaining cardiac output by increasing LV filling pressures likely contribute to earlier symptomatic heart failure.

CLINICAL RELEVANCE

Diagnosis by Doppler Echocardiography

Doppler echocardiography plays a critical diagnostic role in all patients with heart failure for a variety of reasons. First, diagnostically, it should be emphasized that the physical examination, ECG, and chest x-ray do not reliably distinguish diastolic from systolic heart failure. Second, an accurate ejection fraction determination is essential for the diagnosis of diastolic heart failure. Echocardiography can also rapidly exclude diagnoses such as acute mitral or aortic regurgitation or constrictive pericarditis, conditions also associated with signs and symptoms of heart failure and a normal ejection fraction. Finally, Doppler echocardiography can be used in many instances to reliably estimate filling pressures.

General Principles

As reviewed in Chapter 5, Doppler echocardiography measures the velocity of intracardiac blood flow. Doppler transmitral flow analysis has become the mainstay of the clinical assessment of diastolic function. In normal sinus rhythm, diastolic flow from the left atrium to the left ventricle across the mitral valve occurs in two phases, denoted by two distinct waves: the E wave, which reflects early diastolic filling, and the A wave, in late diastole, which reflects atrial contraction. Because the velocity of blood flow across the mitral valve depends on the transmitral pressure gradient, the E wave velocity is influenced by both the rate of early diastolic relaxation and LA pressure. Alterations in the pattern of these velocities give insight into LV diastolic function and prognosis.[22–25] As pointed out previously (see Chapter 5), standard mitral inflow patterns are extremely sensitive to loading conditions, particularly LA pressure.

Stated another way, early diastolic filling rates might be increased by elevated LA pressure. Therefore, just as a normal ($E > A$) filling pattern does not necessarily indicate normal diastolic function, a reduced E wave velocity and E/A ratio might be found in the presence of elevated filling pressures. As we have come to realize, other data are necessary to give a complete picture of diastolic function. Such other data are generally provided by tissue Doppler analysis and pulmonary artery systolic pressure, and occasionally supplemented by pulmonary vein velocities.[27] Tissue Doppler techniques appear to be somewhat less sensitive to loading conditions than standard Doppler velocities (Fig. 24.8). It is important to bear in mind, in this connection, that the amplitude of the transmitral E wave merely reflects the early diastolic LA-LV gradient. As shown in Fig. 24.9, it is possible that the E wave amplitude and E/A ratio may be low, not necessarily because of low LA pressure but because of a protracted decline in LV diastolic pressure.[28] As we will see, such a protracted decline in diastolic pressure may be caused by acute ischemia.

Acute Effects of Ischemia on Doppler Inflow Patterns

There have been a number of studies of mitral inflow patterns in patients with acute myocardial ischemia (Table 24.2). Labovitz et al. studied functional changes by Doppler echocardiography in 32 patients during transient myocardial ischemia induced by percutaneous coronary interventions (PCIs).[29] Ventricular filling during coronary occlusion showed significant change, evident within 15 seconds of balloon occlusion. There was an acute decrease in peak E velocity as well as

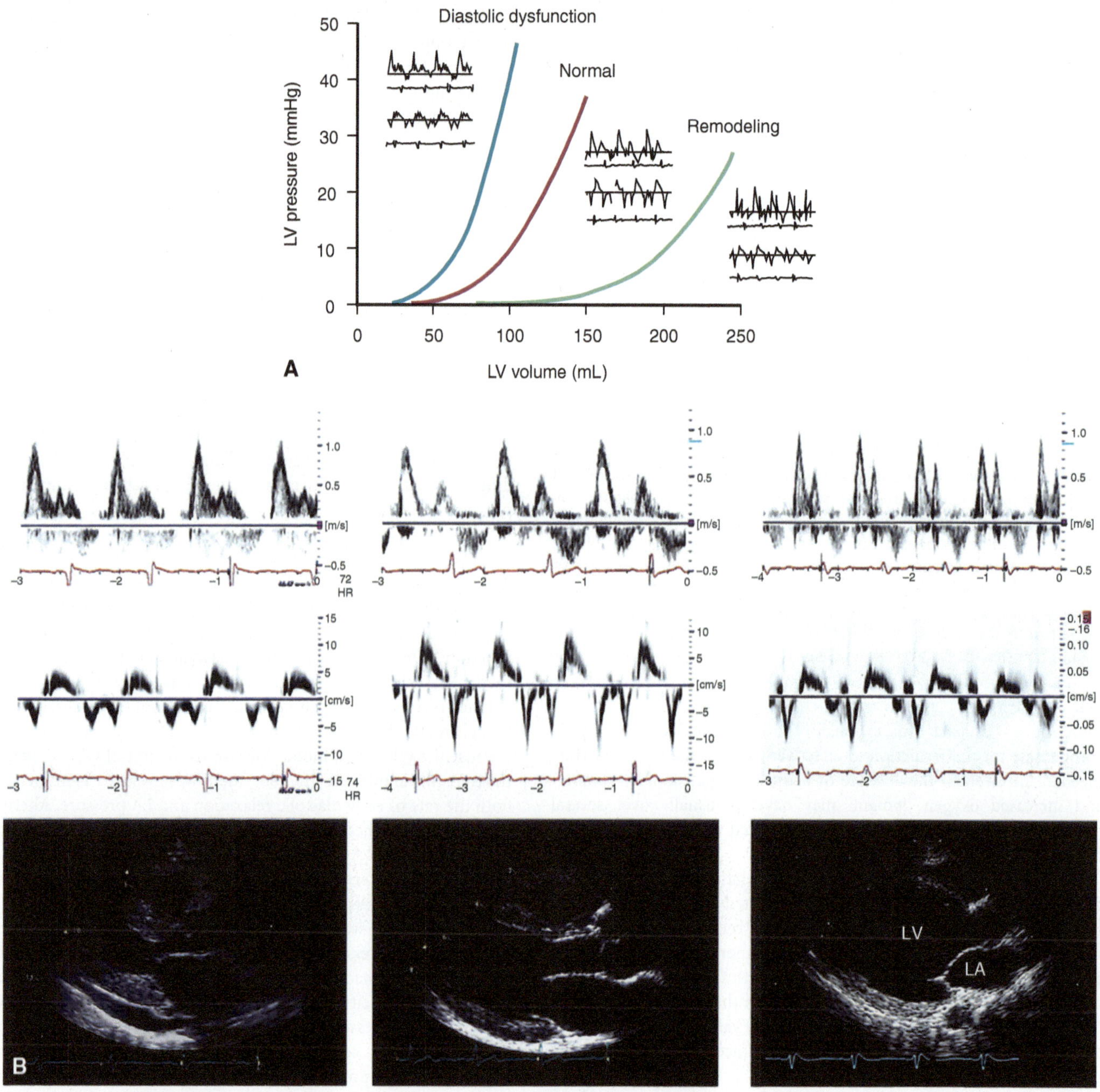

Fig. 24.8 (A) End-diastolic pressure-volume (P-V) relationship curves in normal, diastolic dysfunction, and remodeling groups. Inserted in the figure are the mitral inflow and tissue Doppler recordings for the three groups. The end-diastolic P-V relationship is shifted left-upward for diastolic dysfunction compared with a right-downward shift for a heart that has remodeled. (B) While mitral inflow velocity appears similar in all three groups, mitral annulus tissue Doppler early diastolic velocities are reduced in patients with diastolic dysfunction or remodeling. 2-D echo shows completely normal cardiac structures for the normal subject at the center and increased wall thickness and LA enlargement but normal LV size in the left panel, consistent with diastolic heart failure. On the right is displayed LV enlargement typical of the remodeling heart. (A, Modified from Maurer MS, Spevack D, Burkhoff D, et al. Diastolic dysfunction: can it be diagnosed by Doppler echocardiography? *J Am Coll Cardiol.* 2004;44:1543–1549. B, From Oh JK, Hatle L, Tajik AJ, Little WC. Diastolic heart failure can be diagnosed by comprehensive two-dimensional and Doppler echocardiography. *J Am Coll Cardiol.* 2006;47:500–506.)

E/A ratio (Fig. 24.10), with a return to baseline values within 15 seconds following balloon deflation. The diastolic changes occurred prior to systolic and other clinical changes.[29]

Snow et al. prospectively evaluated 42 patients undergoing elective PCI for severe ischemia (22 patients with unstable angina pectoris and 20 patients with postacute MI ischemia).[30] Doppler echocardiographic studies were performed before (8 ± 5 hours) and after (43 ± 27 hours) post-PCI. Patients with severe ischemia (both the unstable angina and the postinfarction ischemia groups) showed abnormal diastolic filling patterns before PCI, characterized by prolonged isovolumic relaxation time (IVRT) and mitral deceleration time (DT), decreased E/A peak velocity ratio, and increased atrial filling fraction (AFF). Following

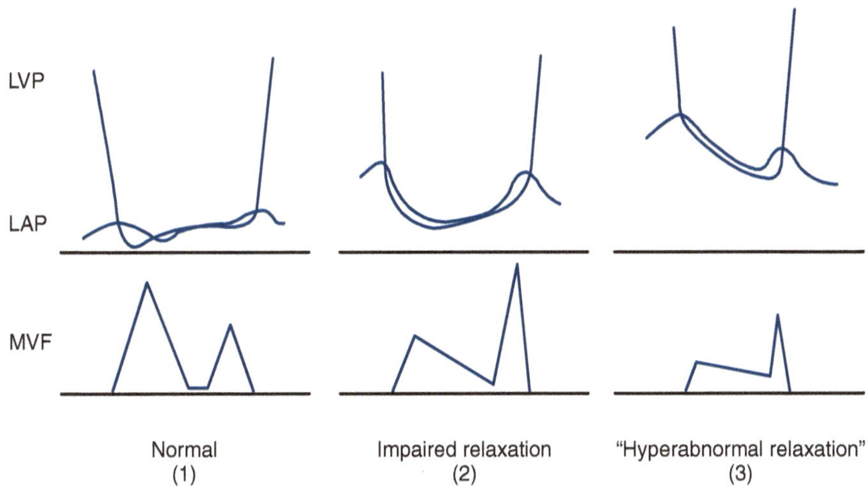

Fig. 24.9 Schematic representation of simultaneous recordings of LV pressure *(LVP)*, left atrial pressure *(LAP)*, and Doppler mitral flow velocity *(MVF)* in (1) a normal subject, (2) a patient with impaired relaxation without clinical heart failure, and (3) a patient with acute heart failure and a delayed relaxation. This figure illustrates that under certain conditions, such as acute ischemia, a low E/A ratio can be associated with elevated filling pressures. (From Bogaty P, Mure P, Dumesnil JG. New insights into diastolic dysfunction as the cause of acute left-sided heart failure associated with systemic hypertension and/or coronary artery disease. *Am J Cardiol*. 2002;89:341–345.)

TABLE 24.2 Transmitral Inflow in Acute Ischemia

Study	Number of patients (n)	Patient population	E	A	E/A	AFF	DT	IVRT
Labovitz et al.[29]	32	Patients undergoing PTCA	N/A	N/A	↓	N/A	N/A	N/A
Snow et al.[30]	22	Patients in the unstable angina group who underwent elective PTCA[a]	N/A	N/A	↔	↔	↓	↓
Iliceto et al.[31]	9	Patients with significant CAD who developed ischemic ECG changes with transesophageal atrial pacing	↓	↑	↓	N/A	N/A	N/A

[a]Doppler echocardiography performed 43 ± 27 hours after PTCA.

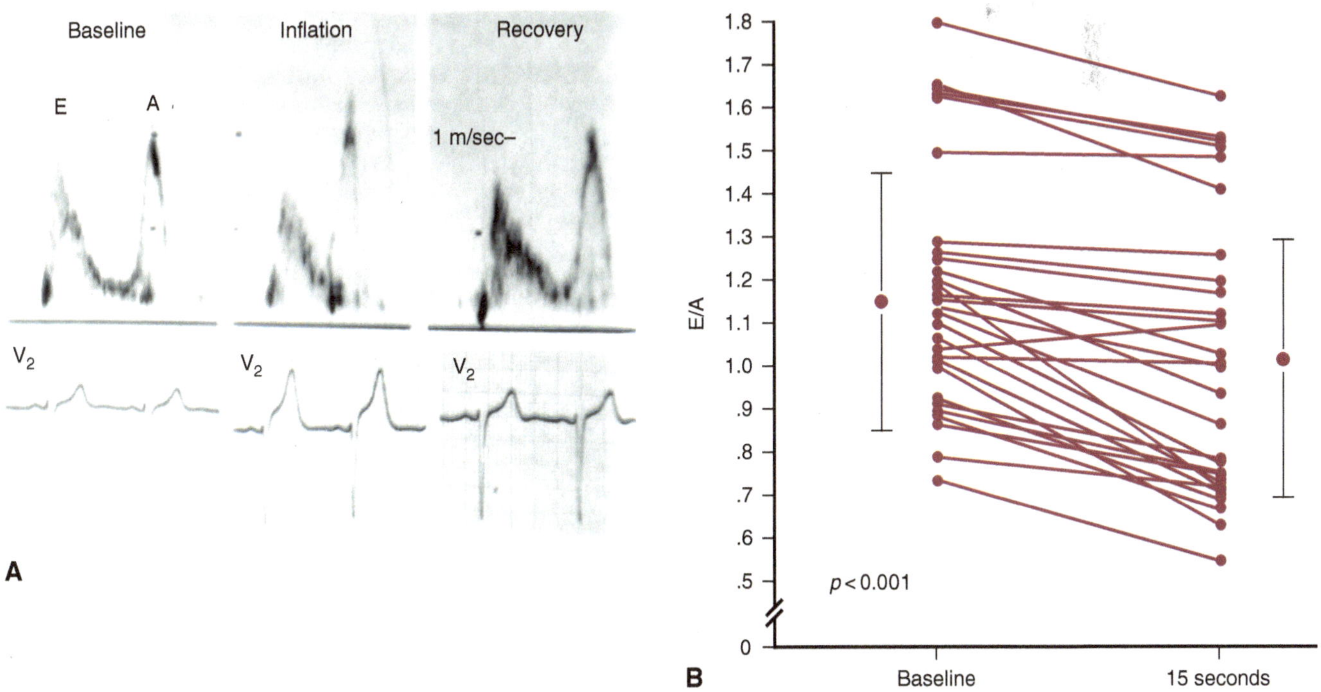

Fig. 24.10 (A) Simultaneous recording of pulsed-wave LV inflow velocities with accompanying electrocardiographic lead V_2 during left anterior descending coronary occlusion/balloon inflation during percutaneous transluminal coronary angioplasty. There is a marked diminution in early (E) and the E/A ratio, which coincides with ST-segment elevation induced by coronary occlusion. The flow profile returned to the baseline state in recovery. (B) There was a significant decrease in the ratio of peak early to peak atrial diastolic velocities (E/A) by 15 seconds after coronary occlusion, with the E/A ratio falling in the vast majority of patients. (From Labovitz AJ, Lewen MK, Kern M, Vandormael M, Deligonal U, Kennedy HL. Evaluation of left ventricular systolic and diastolic dysfunction during transient myocardial ischemia produced by angioplasty. *J Am Coll Cardiol*. 1987;10:748–755.)

PCI, IVRT and DT decreased in both groups, and the decrease in IVRT was significant. After revascularization, the E/A ratio increased, and the AFF decreased in the postacute MI ischemia group at the same time.[30]

It is noteworthy that both studies demonstrated a reduced E/A ratio following acute ischemia, induced by either PCI or the acute ischemic event. The improvement in diastolic function and transmitral flow velocities post-PCI likely reflects early recovery of diastolic determinants, active ventricular relaxation, and compliance. These data may be interpreted in light of the hypothesis of Bogaty[28]: The reduced peak E is probably the result of reduced "driving pressure" between the left atrium and the left ventricle in early diastole. It is conceivable that an acute ischemia–related reduction in peak E is more related to a slow decline in LV diastolic pressure than to reduced LA pressure.

The case study demonstrated a less common finding, likely reflective of ischemia-induced diastolic dysfunction. An inspection of the transmitral Doppler pattern and the ECG shows that despite the presence of sinus rhythm, this patient had very low velocity associated with atrial contraction. We speculate that the very high ventricular diastolic pressures could have presented an afterload mismatch of the atrium, leading to contractile failure.

Iliceto et al.[31] evaluated the effect of atrial pacing-induced ischemia on Doppler-derived LV filling parameters in 17 patients with significant CAD (Fig. 24.11A). The patients were divided into two groups based on ischemic changes on ECG (ST depression >1.5 mm) immediately after cessation of atrial pacing. Group 1 (without ischemic changes) showed no significant changes in LV filling variables, while group 2

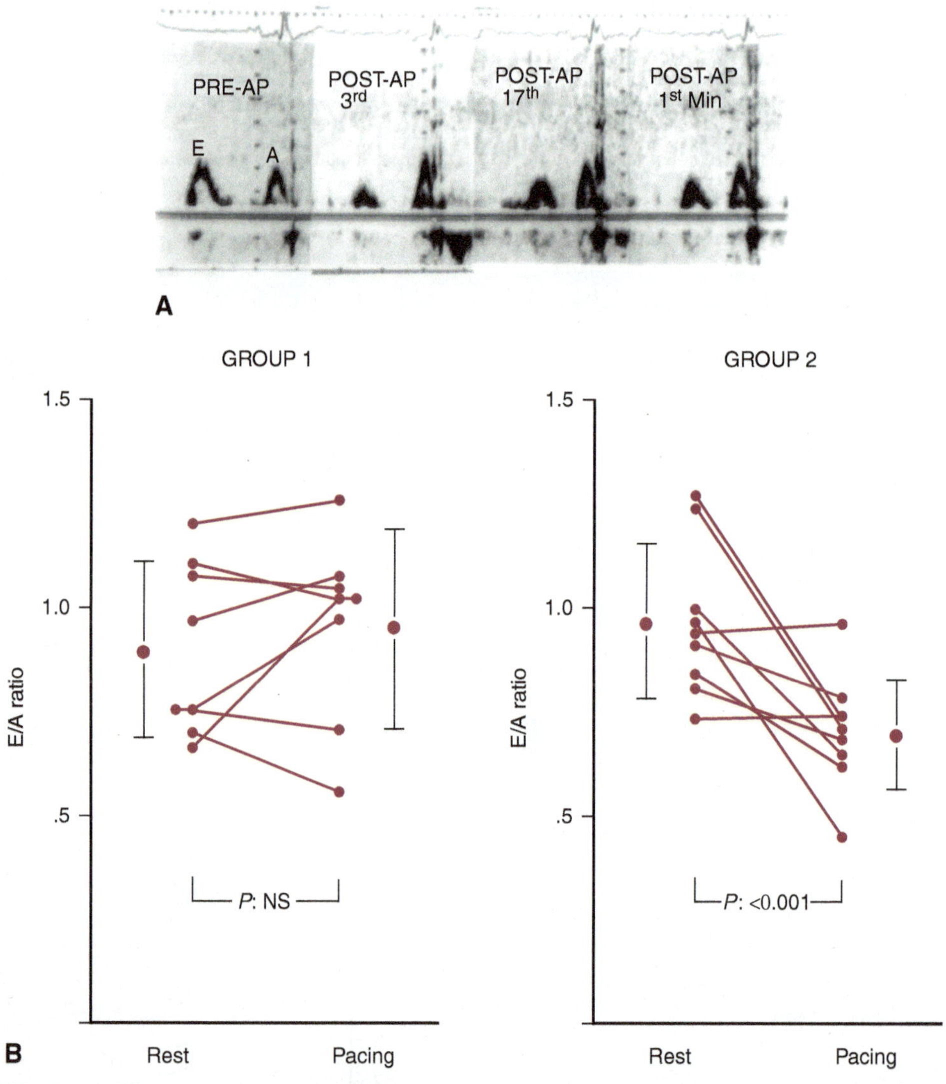

Fig. 24.11 (A) Sequential recording of the transmitral flow velocities before atrial pacing, at the 3rd beat, the 17th beat, and 1 minute postatrial pacing (PAP), demonstrating changes with ischemia and recovery in a patient in group 2 (which developed ischemic electrocardiographic changes on pacing). The first panel at left shows normal LV filling characteristics at rest before atrial pacing (PRE-AP). The next recording *(second panel)*, at the 3rd postatrial pacing beat, shows a significant decrease in the early peak flow velocity, along with an increase in atrial peak flow velocity. At the 17th postatrial pacing beat *(third panel)*, a gradual tendency toward recovery of the LV filling values is observed. At 1 minute after pacing *(fourth panel)*, transmitral flow velocities are very similar to those of the 17th beat. (B) Illustration comparing early/atrial (E/A) peak flow velocity ratio changes with atrial pacing in group 1 (no pacing-induced ischemia) and group 2 (pacing-induced ischemia). Early/atrial peak flow velocity ratio demonstrated a significant decrease in group 2 patients, without any significant change in group 1 patients, paralleling electrocardiographic ischemic changes. (From Iliceto S, Amico A, Marangelli V, D'Ambrosio G, Rizzon P. Doppler echocardiographic evaluation of the effect of atrial pacing-induced ischemia on left ventricular filling in patients with coronary artery disease. *J Am Coll Cardiol*. 1988;11:953–961.)

(with ischemic changes) showed a significant decrease in early peak flow velocity from rest to postpacing, along with a compensatory increase in the atrial component of the mitral inflow velocities. As it was observed in the studies led by Labovitz and Snow, the E/A ratio decreased, and the atrial fraction of the time-velocity integral increased in the group with manifest ischemia. The filling alterations gradually returned to baseline levels 1 minute after cessation of atrial pacing. The changes in LV filling occurring only in group 2 possibly reflect significant ischemia noted by ECG changes and indicate that a threshold for these changes may exist (see Fig. 24.11B).

In an investigation using tissue Doppler imaging (TDI) techniques, Donal et al. studied 28 consecutive patients with acute MI involving either the left anterior descending or the right coronary artery territory treated by primary PCI.[32] Echocardiographic studies were performed within 24 hours of revascularization. A control group comprised 17 individuals with normal coronary angiography and transesophageal echocardiography. The authors recorded systolic (S), early diastolic (E′), late diastolic (A′), isovolumic contraction (IVC), and isovolumic relaxation (IVR) peak velocities by TDI. Not surprisingly, estimated LV filling pressures were significantly higher and the IVR peak velocities were significantly lower in the acute MI populations compared with controls.[32] The combination of IVC greater than 0 and IVR less than 1 separated ischemic from nonischemic segments with 82% sensitivity and 85% specificity. Notably, among the two acute MI groups, even nonischemic segments or walls showed significantly decreased velocities and displacements.[32]

Doppler Filling Profiles in Acute Myocardial Infarction

Doppler echocardiography has been used to estimate prognosis in acute infarction (see Table 24.2). Temporelli et al.[33] showed that DT was a strong prognostic marker both for LV remodeling and for survival following acute MI (Fig. 24.12). A subset of 571 patients with confirmed acute MI and serial Doppler echo at 24 to 48 hours from

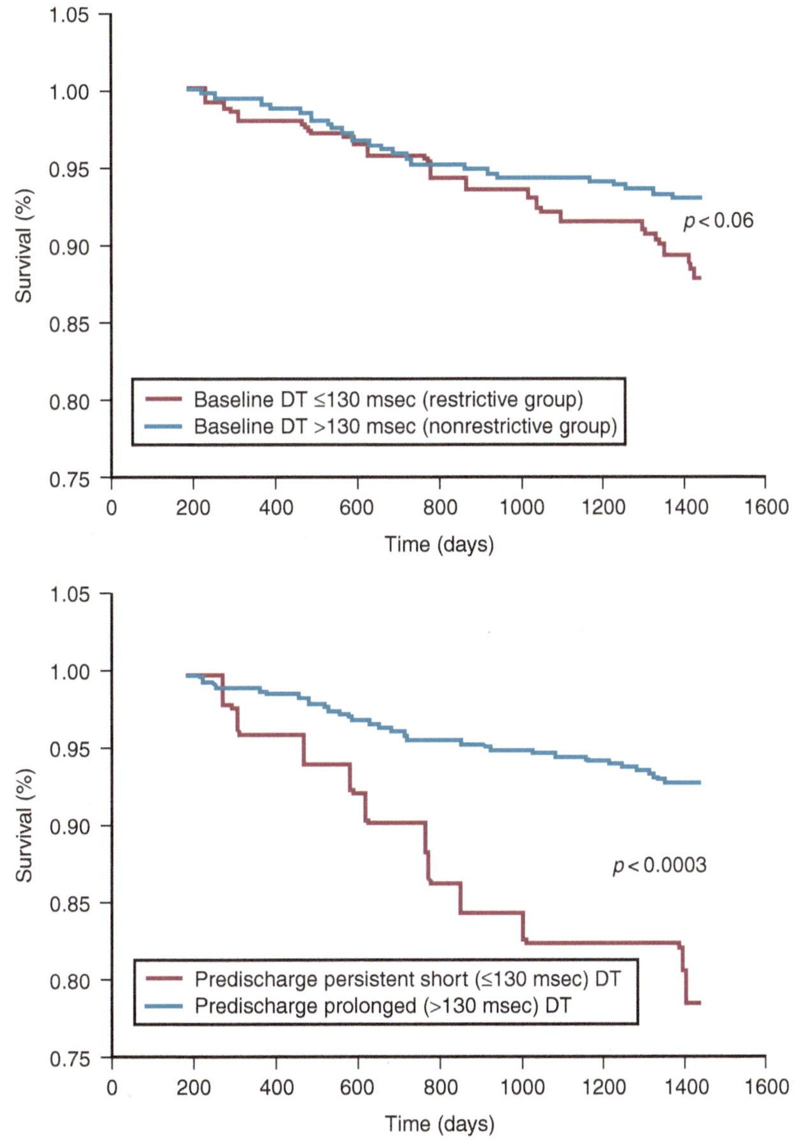

Fig. 24.12 Cumulative survival rates for all-cause mortality according to baseline and predischarge deceleration time *(DT)*. The predischarge persistent short DT predicted a higher mortality. (From Temporelli PL, Gianuzzi P, Nicolosi GL, et al. Doppler-derived mitral deceleration time as a strong prognostic marker of left ventricular remodeling and survival after acute myocardial infarction: results of the GISSI-3 echo substudy. *J Am Coll Cardiol.* 2004;43:1646–1653.)

symptom onset (baseline), at hospital discharge, and at 6 months in the Gruppo Italiano per lo Studio della Sopravvivenza nell'infarto (GISSI-3) substudy formed the basis of the sample. Patients were assigned to two groups based on mitral DT, either restrictive (DT ≤130 msec) or non-restrictive (DT >130 msec). During follow-up, the end-diastolic volume index (EDVI) and the end-systolic volume index (ESVI) increased, and percent of wall motion abnormality decreased in both groups. The magnitude of these changes was more pronounced in patients with a short DT compared with those with a DT greater than 130 msec. A progressive impairment in ejection fraction was limited to patients with restrictive filling. LV dilation was twofold in the baseline restrictive filling group compared with the nonrestrictive filling group.[33] By multivariate analysis, baseline EDVI and the extent of abnormal wall motion, along with predischarge persistent short DT, demonstrated a higher likelihood of severe late LV dilation (an increase in EDVI of >20%).[33] These Doppler parameters also had prognostic importance. Follow-up at 4 years showed that predischarge persistent restrictive filling (DT ≤130 msec) was the best predictor of mortality, compared with other clinical and Doppler echocardiographic variables.[33]

Longitudinal changes and prognostic implications of LV diastolic function in patients with first acute MI were similar in a study by Poulsen et al.[34] They evaluated 58 consecutive patients admitted with first acute MI prospectively by 2-D and Doppler echocardiography, along with clinical evaluation on day 1, day 5, 3 months, and 12 months. The patients were classified into three groups based on the LV diastolic filling pattern at admission: normal, impaired relaxation, and pseudo-normal/restrictive patterns. Heart failure during hospitalization was noted more often in patients with the restrictive pattern than in patients with impaired relaxation at baseline (71% vs. 50%). Those with a restrictive pattern had more severe heart failure by New York Heart Association (NYHA) class compared with normal and impaired relaxation filling patterns. Mitral E wave DT less than 140 msec and age were determined as independent predictors of development of in-hospital heart failure and cardiac death by multivariate regression analysis.[34]

Naqvi et al. evaluated 85 consecutive patients with a first ST-elevation acute myocardial infarction (STEMI), who underwent PCI within 12 hours of hospital admission by echocardiography.[35] The patients were divided into two groups based on development (group A) or no development (group B) of in-hospital events, including cardiac death, heart failure, sustained ventricular tachycardia (VT), and urgent surgical revascularization after primary PCI. Group A had restrictive mitral inflow and lower diastolic mitral annular TDI velocities, resulting in a high E/e′ (mitral inflow peak early velocity/mitral annular peak early velocity of the noninfarct annulus) ratio. Using peak early diastolic velocity of the lateral mitral annulus instead of the averaged peak early diastolic velocity of the noninfarcted annulus resulted in a higher E/e′ in group A versus B.[35] The E/e′ ratio and mitral inflow E wave DT were shown to be independent predictors of an in-hospital event on multivariate stepwise logistic regression analysis. At the 6-month follow-up echocardiographic assessment, baseline mitral inflow DT was an important determinant of later LV EF. The E/e′ ratio, an estimate of myocardial wall relaxation, and DT, an estimate of global LV filling and relaxation, were superior to other echocardiographic parameters in determining in-hospital events and follow-up LV EF at 6 months.[35] A second study of STEMI patients support these findings, showing that low e′ is an independent risk factor for death, heart failure, or a new MI.[36] As is seen in the case study, the tissue Doppler e′ values were extremely low.

Another study of Doppler echocardiography and invasive hemodynamics in patients with STEMI by Prasad et al. showed that abnormal relaxation was the predominant pattern, seen in 50% of the patients, and 25% had restrictive filling.[37] Other findings included reduction of septal e′ velocity at day 3 post-STEMI (5.9 cm/sec from baseline 7.4 cm/sec, $P = 0.002$) and persistently reduced septal e′ at 1-year follow-up, suggesting persistent diastolic dysfunction post-STEMI.[37] Shacham et al. also looked at post-STEMI patients and found that higher time to reperfusion was associated with significantly higher E/e′ ratios and more advanced diastolic grade.[38] This study, along with a second by Remmelink et al., showed elevated LVEDP prior to reperfusion, which improved by 24% postreperfusion along with significant improvements in stiffness and wall stress.[38,39]

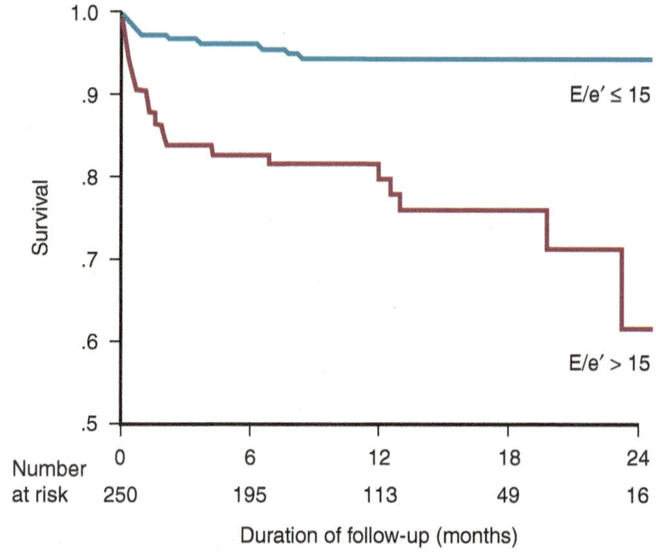

Fig. 24.13 Kaplan-Meier plot demonstrating decreased survival in patients with an E/e′ ratio greater than 15 compared with those with an E/e′ ratio less than 15. (From Hillis GS, Moller JE, Pellikka PA, et al. Noninvasive estimation of left ventricular filling pressure by an E/e is a powerful predictor of survival after acute myocardial infarction. *J Am Coll Cardiol.* 2004;43:360–367.)

A study by Hillis et al. examined the prognostic value of E/e′ in a group of 250 patients who had both Doppler transmitral flow velocities and TDI performed on echo for acute MI at the Mayo Clinic during the index admission.[40] Patients with E/e′ greater than 15 were more often older, female, presenting with heart failure, had diabetes, and had a history of MI. These investigators found that patients with an E/e′ ratio above 15 had lower ejection fraction and a shorter DT. Twenty-nine patients died during a median follow-up period of 13 months, two-thirds of whom had an E/e′ ratio above 15. After stratifying patients based on LV EF, an E/e′ ratio of 15 or more predicted decreased survival in patients with an ejection fraction of 40% or more. When DT was used to further characterize the groups, an E/e′ ratio above 15 was a powerful predictor of mortality only in patients with DT above 140. The E/e′ ratio was the most powerful independent prognostic indicator of survival after acute MI on stepwise multivariate analysis (Fig. 24.13). The E/e′ ratio more importantly complements the prognostic value of a combination of other clinical and echocardiographic parameters.[40]

The same researchers investigated the relationship between echocardiographic indices of acute and chronic LV filling pressures and dilation in 47 patients after their first acute MI.[41] All patients demonstrated a patent infarct-related artery with a thrombolysis in myocardial infarction (TIMI) grade III flow on coronary angiography and akinesia within the same arterial territory on baseline echo.

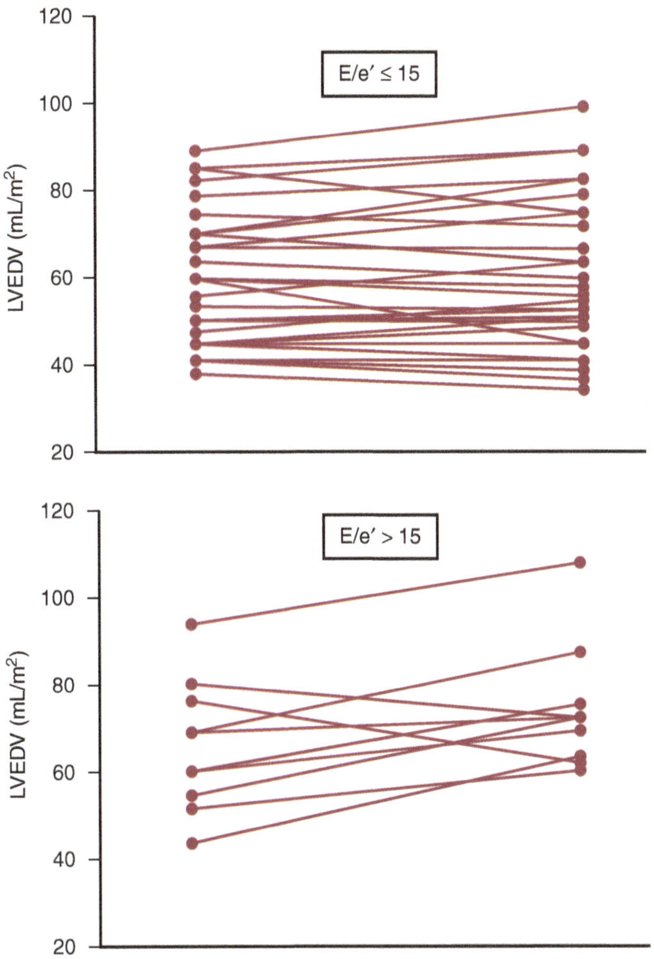

Fig. 24.14 Remodeling described by indexed LV end-diastolic volume (mL/m^2) in patients with early transmitral flow velocity to early mitral annulus velocity ratio (E/E′) of 15 or less compared with those with E/e′ greater than 15. (From Hillis GS, Ujino K, Mulvagh SL, Hagen ME, Oh JK. Echocardiographic indices of increased left ventricular filling pressure and dilation after acute myocardial infarction. *J Am Soc Echocardiogr.* 2006;19:450–456.)

Patients were prospectively designated as remodeling (>15%) and nonremodeling (≤15%) groups based on the increase in indexed LV end-diastolic volume at follow-up echocardiography at ~8 weeks. In this study, E/e′ was higher among the remodeling group, with a moderate correlation between basal E/e′ and changes in indexed LV diastolic volume (Fig. 24.14). Interestingly, LAVI did not predict LV dilation. Both receiver operating characteristic (ROC) curve analysis and multivariate regression analysis confirmed that an E/e′ ratio above 15 was a strong predictor of remodeling.

Estimation of mean left atrial pressure (mLAP) using the E/e′ ratio has also been shown to correlate well with invasive measures of mLAP in patients with acute coronary syndrome (ACS).[42] We have recently published data derived from patients with ACS that compared mLAP measured by Doppler using Nagueh's formula ($1.24 \times [E/e'] + 1.9$) with invasive mLAP by Yamamoto's formula ($1.20 \times MLVDP - 0.82$), with echo and invasive cases performed within 8 hours. In patients with reduced ejection fraction, there was stronger agreement between the two techniques to estimate mLAP compared to the normal EF group.[42]

Sakata et al. investigated the prognostic value of Doppler transmitral flow velocity patterns in acute MI.[43] Over 200 patients with first acute MI recruited to the study underwent 2-D and Doppler echocardiography on admission, and hemodynamic measurements (PCWP and cardiac index) were obtained by using a thermodilution catheter.[43] The A wave velocity was significantly lower in nonsurvivors than in survivors. The E wave velocity and the E/A ratio were significantly higher, while DT was significantly shorter in survivors with heart failure and nonsurvivors than in survivors without heart failure. Comparing patients with low A and those without a low A, the low A group had a significantly higher frequency of mitral regurgitation, incidence of three-vessel coronary disease, PCWP, cardiogenic shock, and a higher mortality after angioplasty or thrombolytic therapy. Cardiac index and LV EF, on the other hand, were significantly lower in the low A group. The low A was strongly associated with heart failure in the acute phase as well as in-hospital mortality. As a predictor of long-term mortality, the low A group had a significantly higher mortality at 5 years.

Other studies have examined LAVI and TDI as predictors of post-MI events.[44] LAVI is a reflection of long-term exposure of the left atrium to abnormal LV diastolic function and filling pressure and is an important indicator of diastolic function. Despite the importance of LAVI in assessing diastolic function, it was not an independent predictor of cardiac events post-MI. However, late diastolic peak velocity (a′) is a reflection of LA function, and the ratio of LAVI/a′ correlated well with brain natriuretic peptide (BNP), and LAVI/a′ of 3.0 or more was able to predict cardiac events in patients with MI ($P = 0.0021$).[44]

A shortened DT in the setting of an acute MI likely reflects either worsened LV compliance or increased LV diastolic volume. An abnormality in compliance may serve to shift the LV P-V curve upward and leftward. Such a shift in the diastolic P-V relationship will lead to a more rapid equilibration of the transmitral pressure gradient and a shortened DT. In later stages of remodeling, the P-V relationship may be shifted to the right. Progressive remodeling and chamber enlargement may be associated with a change in Doppler diastolic filling parameters. The addition of TDI helps distinguish normal from pseudonormal filling patterns (similar to what is shown in Fig. 24.8) and provides pathophysiologic insight into diastolic function in progressive LV remodeling.

Sex Differences in CAD and Diastolic Function

Diastolic heart failure (HFpEF) is common and growing in prevalence, and women make up two-thirds of HFpEF cohorts and 40% of HFrEF.[45] There are few published reports on sex differences in the association between CAD and diastolic function, except from Cho et al. from the Korean Women's Chest Pain Registry. Women and men were compared using propensity matching, and differences in diastolic functional parameters according to CAD severity were only found in women.[46] CAD severity was associated with the presence of diastolic dysfunction only in women, with odds ratio of 1.92 ($P < 0.001$). These authors suggest that myocardial ischemia may be the underlying pathophysiology for the higher prevalence of diastolic dysfunction and HFpEF in women.[46] Although men are more likely to have obstructive coronary lesions, women are more likely to have microvascular disease and endothelial dysfunction, along with thicker arterial walls, nonobstructive CAD, and coronary vasospasm, which can lead to hypertrophy and fibrosis.[45] These mechanisms likely play an important role in the development of HFpEF in women.

CAD as a Distinct HFpEF Phenotype

That there is heterogeneity among HFpEF phenotypes has been deemed to be one of the reasons why there has been difficulty in finding a single effective treatment for HFpEF. Thus far there is limited trial evidence for neurohumoral inhibition improving outcomes in HFpEF. Shah et al. proposed four clinical presentation phenotypes of HFpEF, with CAD one of the phenotypes along with obesity/metabolic syndrome/diabetes, hypertension, and renal dysfunction phenotypes.[47] These people who develop HFpEF with a history of CAD tend to have a greater LV systolic dysfunction, poorer prognosis, and high incidence of sudden cardiac death. Treatment should be tailored to the specific HFpEF phenotype and could include angiotensin-converting enzyme (ACE) inhibitors, complete revascularization, and exercise training in the CAD-HFpEF phenotype.[47]

FUTURE DIRECTIONS

Diastolic heart failure is increasingly being recognized by clinicians, and its role in the pathophysiology, diagnosis, and prognosis of ischemic heart disease is becoming better understood. Diastolic function parameters as determined by Doppler echocardiography and tissue Doppler imaging, including DT, E/e′ ratio, and E and A wave velocity, are associated with LV remodeling and predict acute in-hospital complications and cardiac mortality.

Newer imaging modalities, including speckle strain imaging and three-dimensional echocardiography, may provide additional information and improve understanding of diastolic function in CAD. Further characterization of HFpEF by phenotypes and phenotypic interventions should also help to move forward treatment of this heterogeneous disease.

KEY POINTS

- The prevalence of coronary disease in patients who develop diastolic heart failure is high at ~50%, and coronary disease has a similar population-attributable risk to hypertension.
- Active relaxation is an energy-dependent process that is affected by ischemia. In the setting of ischemia, actin-myosin bridges fail to dissociate, leading to increased diastolic stiffness and LV end-diastolic pressure.
- Diastolic dysfunction contributes to post-MI exertional intolerance, with the majority of those with diastolic dysfunction having an abnormal rise in PCWP greater than 25 mmHg on exercise testing. The adverse compensatory mechanisms for maintaining cardiac output by increasing LV filling pressures likely contributes to earlier symptomatic heart failure.
- The E/e′ ratio, an estimate of myocardial wall relaxation, and DT, an estimate of global LV filling and relaxation, are predictive of in-hospital events and follow-up LV EF at 6 months in post-STEMI patients.
- Women make up two-thirds of HFpEF cohorts and 40% of HFrEF. Women are more likely to have microvascular disease and endothelial dysfunction, along with thicker arterial walls, nonobstructive CAD, and coronary vasospasm, which can lead to hypertrophy and fibrosis.

REVIEW QUESTIONS

1. A 74-year-old woman with a history of hypertension presents with several months of declining activity level leading to 1 day of exertional chest pain, with new dynamic T wave inversions and a troponin I peak of 3.1 ng/mL. Coronary angiography shows severe triple-vessel coronary disease. Transthoracic echo images show normal LV EF at 55% with basal-midinferior hypokinesis, RV dilation and reduced systolic function, a left atrial volume index 39 mL/m^2, and TR peak velocity 2.4 m/sec. Diastolic parameters are shown in the accompanying figure. What is the most appropriate grade of diastolic function?

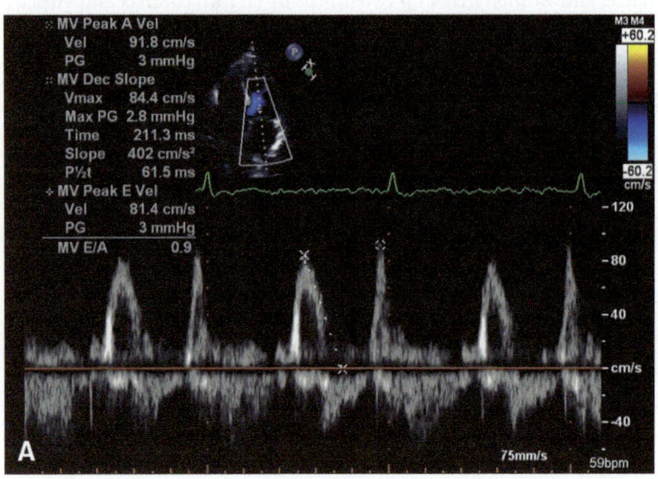

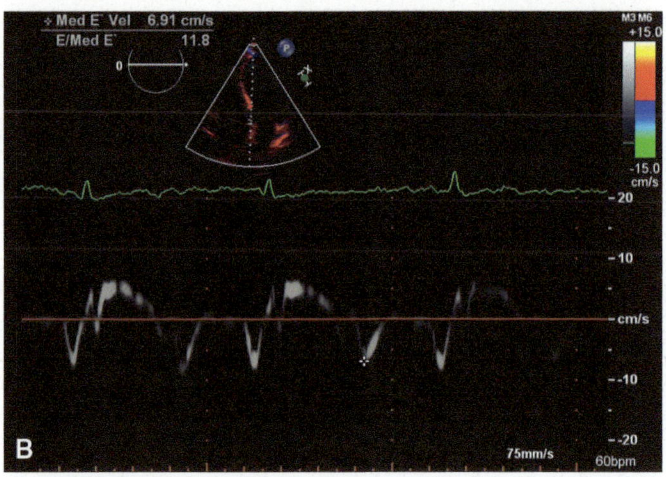

a. Normal diastolic function
b. Grade 1 diastolic dysfunction
c. Grade 2 diastolic dysfunction
d. Grade 3 diastolic dysfunction
e. Indeterminate diastolic grade

2. A 56-year-old man, current daily smoker with known CAD, is admitted to the hospital with worsening shortness of breath. His exam is notable for cool skin, diffuse rales and rhonchi, and diminished pulses below the knees. The ECG shows sinus rhythm with inferolateral ST-segment depressions. The initial troponin I is

1.29 ng/mL. The patient undergoes echocardiography, showing markedly reduced ejection fraction, estimated at 20% with transmitral inflow, pulmonary venous flow, and TDI assessment. Tricuspid regurgitation (TR) jet was incomplete and too indistinct to measure a velocity. The left atrial volume index is 40 mL/m^2. Representative Doppler tracings are shown in the accompanying figures. What can be concluded from the pulmonary venous flow tracing?

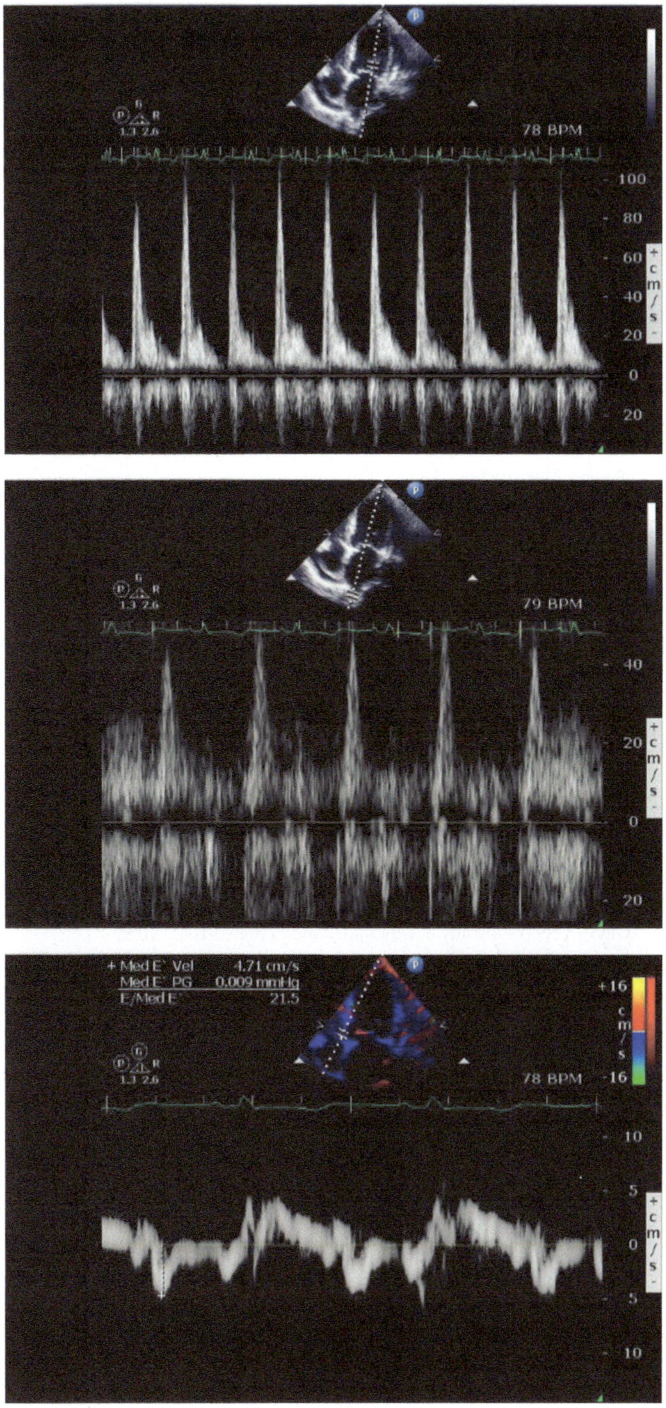

a. The patient has severe mitral regurgitation.
b. The patient is in atrial fibrillation.
c. The patient has high mean LAP.
d. The patient has a high LVEDP.
e. The patient has a high risk of persistent heart failure and cardiac death.

3. The patient in question 2 is treated with diuretics, beta blocker, and nitrates and urgently undergoes successful multivessel PCI with an improvement in symptoms. A subsequent complete echo is performed 3 days later and shows a marked improvement in LV EF, now estimated at 40%. LA size remains enlarged and TR velocity is now 3 m/sec. The accompanying figures are taken from this follow-up Doppler study. What has happened to diastolic function and filling pressures?

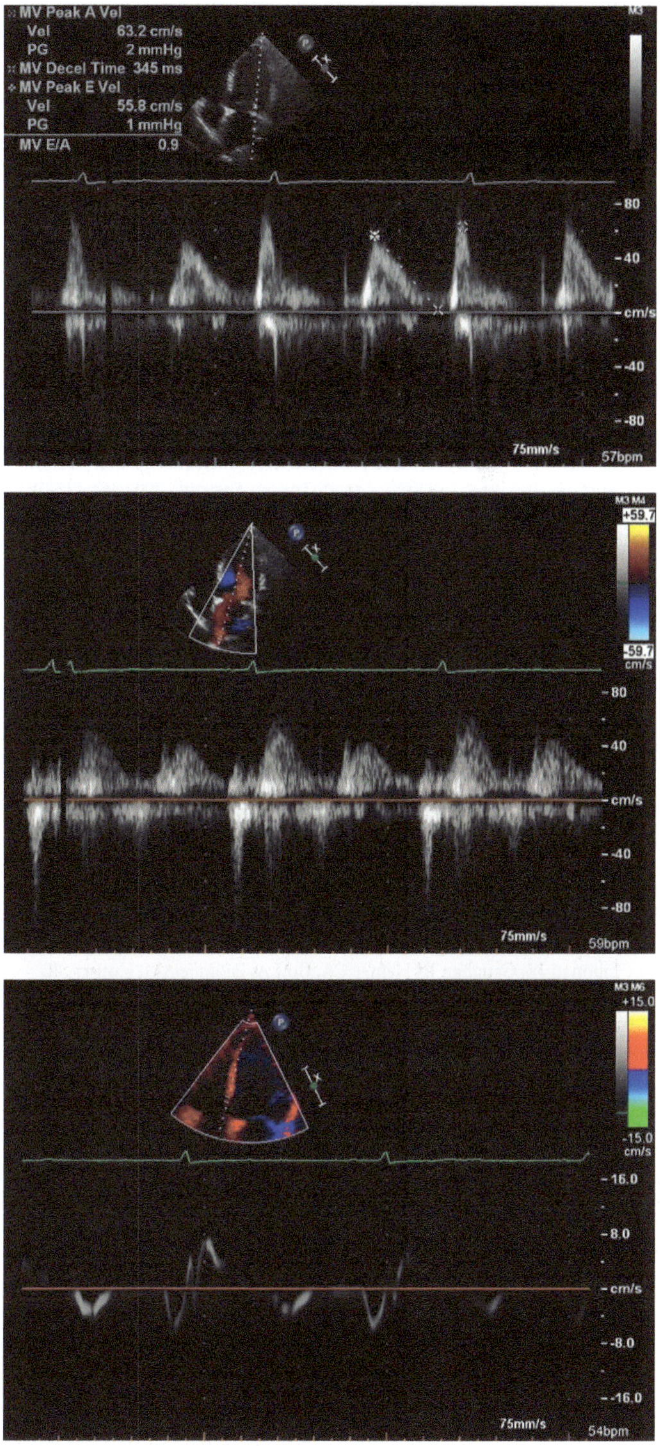

a. Now grade I; filling pressures are normal
b. Now grade I; filling pressures abnormal
c. Still grade III; filling pressures remain abnormal
d. Still grade III; filling pressures higher
e. None of the above

REFERENCES

1. Zile MR, Brutsaert DL. New concepts in diastolic dysfunction and diastolic heart failure: part I: diagnosis, prognosis, and measurements of diastolic function. *Circulation.* 2002;105:1387–1393.
2. Parikh KS, Sharma K, Fiuzat M, et al. Heart failure with preserved ejection fraction expert panel report: current controversies and implications for clinical trials. *JACC Heart Fail.* 2018;6:619–632.
3. Benjamin EJ, Virani SS, Callaway CW, et al. Heart disease and stroke statistics-2018 update: a report from the American Heart Association. *Circulation.* 2018;137(12):e67–e492.
4. Hwang SJ, Melenovsky V, Borlaug BA. Implications of coronary artery disease in heart failure with preserved ejection fraction. *J Am Coll Cardiol.* 2014;63:2817–2827.
5. Gottdiener JS, Arnold AM, Aurigemma GP, et al. Predictors of congestive heart failure in the elderly: the Cardiovascular Health Study. *J Am Coll Cardiol.* 2000;35:1628–1637.
6. Gottdiener JS, McClelland RL, Marshall R, et al. Outcome of congestive heart failure in elderly persons: influence of left ventricular systolic function. *The Cardiovascular Health Study. Ann Intern Med.* 2002;137:631–639.
7. Klapholz M, Maurer M, Lowe AM, et al. Hospitalization for heart failure in the presence of a normal left ventricular ejection fraction: results of the New York Heart Failure Registry. *J Am Coll Cardiol.* 2004;43:1432–1438.
8. Yusuf S, Pfeffer MA, Swedberg K, et al. Effects of candesartan in patients with chronic heart failure and preserved left-ventricular ejection fraction: the CHARM-Preserved Trial. *Lancet (London England).* 2003;362:777–781.
9. Trevisan L, Cautela J, Resseguier N, et al. Prevalence and characteristics of coronary artery disease in heart failure with preserved and mid-range ejection fractions: a systematic angiography approach. *Arch Cardiovasc Dis.* 2018;111:109–118.
10. Zhao J, Zhang Y, He Z, Li N, Liang C. High burden of coronary artery disease in heart failure with preserved ejection fraction. *Arch Cardiovasc Dis.* 2018;111:224–226.
11. Aurigemma GP, Gaasch WH. Clinical practice. *Diastolic heart failure. N Engl J Med.* 2004;351:1097–1105.
12. Carroll J, Carroll E. Exercise-induced angina. In: Gaasch WH, Lewinter MM, eds. *Left Ventricular Diastolic Dysfunction and Heart Failure.* Philadelphia, PA: Lea and Febiger; 1994:259–273.
13. Reger PO, Kolwicz SC, Libonati JR. Acute exercise exacerbates ischemia-induced diastolic rigor in hypertensive myocardium. *SpringerPlus.* 2012;1:46.
14. Jennings RB, Reimer KA. Lethal myocardial ischemic injury. *Am J Pathol.* 1981;102:241–255.
15. Libonati JR, Gaughan JP, Hefner CA, Gow A, Paolone AM, Houser SR. Reduced ischemia and reperfusion injury following exercise training. *Med Sci Sport Exer.* 1997;29:509–516.
16. Gandhi SK, Powers JC, Nomeir AM, et al. The pathogenesis of acute pulmonary edema associated with hypertension. *N Engl J Med.* 2001;344: 17–22.
17. Hess OM, Osakada G, Lavelle JF, Gallagher KP, Kemper WS, Ross J. Diastolic myocardial wall stiffness and ventricular relaxation during partial and complete coronary occlusions in the conscious dog. *Circ Res.* 1983;52:387–400.
18. Pouleur H, Rousseau MF, van Eyll C, Charlier AA. Assessment of regional left ventricular relaxation in patients with coronary artery disease: importance of geometric factors and changes in wall thickness. *Circulation.* 1984;69:696–702.
19. Raya TE, Gay RG, Lancaster L, Aguirre M, Moffett C, Goldman S. Serial changes in left ventricular relaxation and chamber stiffness after large myocardial infarction in rats. *Circulation.* 1988;77:1424–1431.
20. Rockman H, Lew W. Left ventricular remodeling and diastolic dysfunction in chronic ischemic heart disease. In: Gaasch WH, Lewinter MM, eds. *Left Ventricular Diastolic Dysfunction and Heart Failure.* Philadelphia, PA: Lea and Febiger; 1994:306–324.
21. Pfeffer MA, Braunwald E. Ventricular remodeling after myocardial infarction. Experimental observations and clinical implications. *Circulation.* 1990;81:1161–1172.
22. Opie LH, Commerford PJ, Gersh BJ, Pfeffer MA. Controversies in ventricular remodelling. *Lancet (London England).* 2006;367:356–367.
23. Cohn JN, Ferrari R, Sharpe N. Cardiac remodeling--concepts and clinical implications: a consensus paper from an international forum on cardiac remodeling. *Behalf of an International Forum on Cardiac Remodeling. J Am Coll Cardiol.* 2000;35:569–582.
24. Bhatt AS, Ambrosy AP, Velazquez EJ. Adverse remodeling and reverse remodeling after myocardial infarction. *Curr Cardiol Rep.* 2017;19:71.
25. Azevedo CF, Amado LC, Kraitchman DL, et al. Persistent diastolic dysfunction despite complete systolic functional recovery after reperfused acute myocardial infarction demonstrated by tagged magnetic resonance imaging. *Eur Heart J.* 2004;25:1419–1427.
26. Andersen MJ, Ersbøll M, Bro-Jeppesen J, et al. Exercise hemodynamics in patients with and without diastolic dysfunction and preserved ejection fraction after myocardial infarction. *Circ Heart Fail.* 2012;5:444–451.
27. Nagueh SF, Smiseth OA, Appleton CP, et al. Recommendations for the evaluation of left ventricular diastolic function by echocardiography: an update from the American Society of Echocardiography and the European Association of Cardiovascular Imaging. *Eur Heart J Cardiovasc Imag.* 2016;17:1321–1360.
28. Bogaty P, Muré P, Dumesnil JG. New insights into diastolic dysfunction as the cause of acute left-sided heart failure associated with systemic hypertension and/or coronary artery disease. *Am J Cardiol.* 2002;89:341–345.
29. Labovitz AJ, Lewen MK, Kern M, Vandormael M, Deligonal U, Kennedy HL. Evaluation of left ventricular systolic and diastolic dysfunction during transient myocardial ischemia produced by angioplasty. *J Am Coll Cardiol.* 1987;10:748–755.
30. Snow FR, Gorcsan J, Lewis SA, Cowley MJ, Vetrovec GW, Nixon JV. Doppler echocardiographic evaluation of left ventricular diastolic function after percutaneous transluminal coronary angioplasty for unstable angina pectoris or acute myocardial infarction. *Am J Cardiol.* 1990;65:840–844.
31. Iliceto S, Amico A, Marangelli V, D'Ambrosio G, Rizzon P. Doppler echocardiographic evaluation of the effect of atrial pacing-induced ischemia on left ventricular filling in patients with coronary artery disease. *J Am Coll Cardiol.* 1998;11:953–961.
32. Donal E, Raud-Raynier P, Coisne D, Allal J, Herpin D. Tissue Doppler echocardiographic quantification. Comparison to coronary angiography results in acute coronary syndrome patients. *Cardiovasc Ultrasoun.* 2005;3:10.
33. Temporelli PL, Giannuzzi P, Nicolosi GL, et al. Doppler-derived mitral deceleration time as a strong prognostic marker of left ventricular remodeling and survival after acute myocardial infarction: results of the GISSI-3 echo substudy. *J Am Coll Cardiol.* 2004;43:1646–1653.
34. Poulsen SH, Jensen SE, Egstrup K. Longitudinal changes and prognostic implications of left ventricular diastolic function in first acute myocardial infarction. *Am Heart J.* 1999;137:910–918.
35. Naqvi TZ, Padmanabhan S, Rafii F, Hyuhn HK, Mirocha J. Comparison of usefulness of left ventricular diastolic versus systolic function as a predictor of outcome following primary percutaneous coronary angioplasty for acute myocardial infarction. *Am J Cardiol.* 2006;97:160–166.
36. Biering-Sørensen T, Jensen JS, Pedersen S, et al. Doppler tissue imaging is an independent predictor of outcome in patients with ST-segment elevation myocardial infarction treated with primary percutaneous coronary intervention. *J Am Soc Echocardiogr.* 2014;27:258–267.
37. Prasad SB, See V, Tan T, et al. Serial Doppler echocardiographic assessment of diastolic dysfunction during acute myocardial infarction. *Echocardiography (Mount Kisco, New York).* 2012;29:1164–1171.
38. Shacham Y, Steinvil A, Leshem-Rubinow E, et al. Association between time to reperfusion and echocardiography assessed left ventricular filling pressure in patients with first ST-segment elevation myocardial infarction undergoing primary coronary intervention. *Cardiol J.* 2014;21:357–363.
39. Remmelink M, Sjauw KD, Henriques JPS, et al. Acute left ventricular dynamic effects of primary percutaneous coronary intervention from occlusion to reperfusion. *J Am Coll Cardiol.* 2009;53:1498–1502.
40. Hillis GS, Møller JE, Pellikka PA, et al. Noninvasive estimation of left ventricular filling pressure by E/e' is a powerful predictor of survival after acute myocardial infarction. *J Am Coll Cardiol.* 2004;43:360–367.

41. Hillis GS, Ujino K, Mulvagh SL, Hagen ME, Oh JK. Echocardiographic indices of increased left ventricular filling pressure and dilation after acute myocardial infarction. *J Am Soc Echocardiogr.* 2006;19:450–456.
42. Tachjian A, Sanghai S, Stencel J, Parker M, Kakouros N, Aurigemma G. Estimation of mean left atrial pressure in patients with acute coronary syndrome: a Doppler echocardiographic and cardiac catheterization study. *J Am Soc Echocardiogr.* 2019;32(3):365–374. e1.
43. Sakata K, Kashiro S, Hirata S, Yanagisawa A, Ishikawa K. Prognostic value of Doppler transmitral flow velocity patterns in acute myocardial infarction. *Am J Cardiol.* 1997;79:1165–1169.
44. Matsuura H, Yamada A, Sugimoto K, Sugimoto K, Iwase M, Ishikawa T. Clinical implication of LAVI over A' ratio in patients with acute coronary syndrome. *Heart Asia.* 2018;10:e011038.
45. Beale AL, Meyer P, Marwick TH, Lam CSP, Kaye DM. Sex differences in cardiovascular pathophysiology: why women are overrepresented in heart failure with preserved ejection fraction. *Circulation.* 2018;138:198–205.
46. Cho DH, Kim MA, Choi J, et al. Sex differences in the relationship between left ventricular diastolic dysfunction and coronary artery disease: from the Korean women's chest pain registry. *J Womens Health. 2002.* 2018;27:912–919.
47. Shah SJ, Kitzman DW, Borlaug BA, et al. Phenotype-specific treatment of heart failure with preserved ejection fraction: a multiorgan roadmap. *Circulation.* 2016;134:73–90.

25

Hypertrophic Cardiomyopathy

Shemy Carasso, Lynne Williams, Manhal Habib, and Harry Rakowski

OUTLINE

DIASTOLIC FUNCTION IN HYPERTROPHIC CARDIOMYOPATHY

Hypertrophic cardiomyopathy (HCM) is a primary autosomal dominant disorder of the myocardium caused by mutations in several genes encoding cardiac contractile proteins (Fig. 25.1). Alterations in myocardial structure at both a macroscopic and a microscopic level occur in the form of myocardial hypertrophy, fiber disarray, increased loose connective tissue and fibrosis, and abnormalities of the coronary microvasculature, with the net effect of interference with both myocyte force generation and myocardial relaxation[1–3] (Fig. 25.2). While HCM is typically described as a disease of supranormal or hyperdynamic systolic function that leads to left ventricular (LV) outflow tract (LVOT) obstruction, a considerable proportion of patients experience heart failure symptoms in the absence of outflow tract obstruction and a preserved LV ejection fraction (LV EF). In these patients, diastolic dysfunction and microvascular ischemia contribute significantly to symptoms, due to changes in the ventricular myocardium at a molecular, histopathologic, and global structural level.

PATHOPHYSIOLOGY OF DIASTOLIC DYSFUNCTION

Sarcomere Mutations and Their Effects on Calcium Handling

The mutations related to HCM result in the production of abnormal myocardial sarcomeric proteins that have altered contraction and relaxation characteristics. These include changes in the affinity between the various contractile proteins, changes in the sensitivity to Ca^{+2}, the efficiency of energy utilization (from adenosine triphosphate [ATP]), and its expenditure.[4]

In myosin heavy chain (MYH) mutations, the myosin head region is responsible not only for force generation but also hydrolysis of ATP. It also functions as a site for interaction with other sarcomeric proteins, such as the myosin light chains (essential and regulatory), troponin, and actin. Subsequently mutations in this region enhance contractility at the expense of impaired relaxation, and these findings have been demonstrated in ex vivo studies of myofibrillar tissue.[5] During relaxation, pairs of myosins form interacting-heads motif (IHM) structures that when paired with other sarcomeric proteins result in an energy-saving super-relaxed state. In MYH7 mutations, there is a destabilization of IHM interactions and impaired IHM formation, reducing the proportion of myosins in the super-relaxed state. The net effect is a reduction in diastolic relaxation and concomitant increase in energy consumption.[6]

Myosin-Binding Protein C (MYBPC3) Mutations

Unlike the myosin heavy chain, MYBPC does not directly play a role in force generation, but rather acts as a modulator of myocardial contractility via its interactions with myosin filaments and titin. As opposed to the missense mutations seen in other sarcomeric proteins (with the substitution of only one amino acid), mutations in MYBPC3 are typically truncating,[7] often resulting in haploinsufficiency (insufficient functional protein for normal sarcomere performance).[8] MYBPC

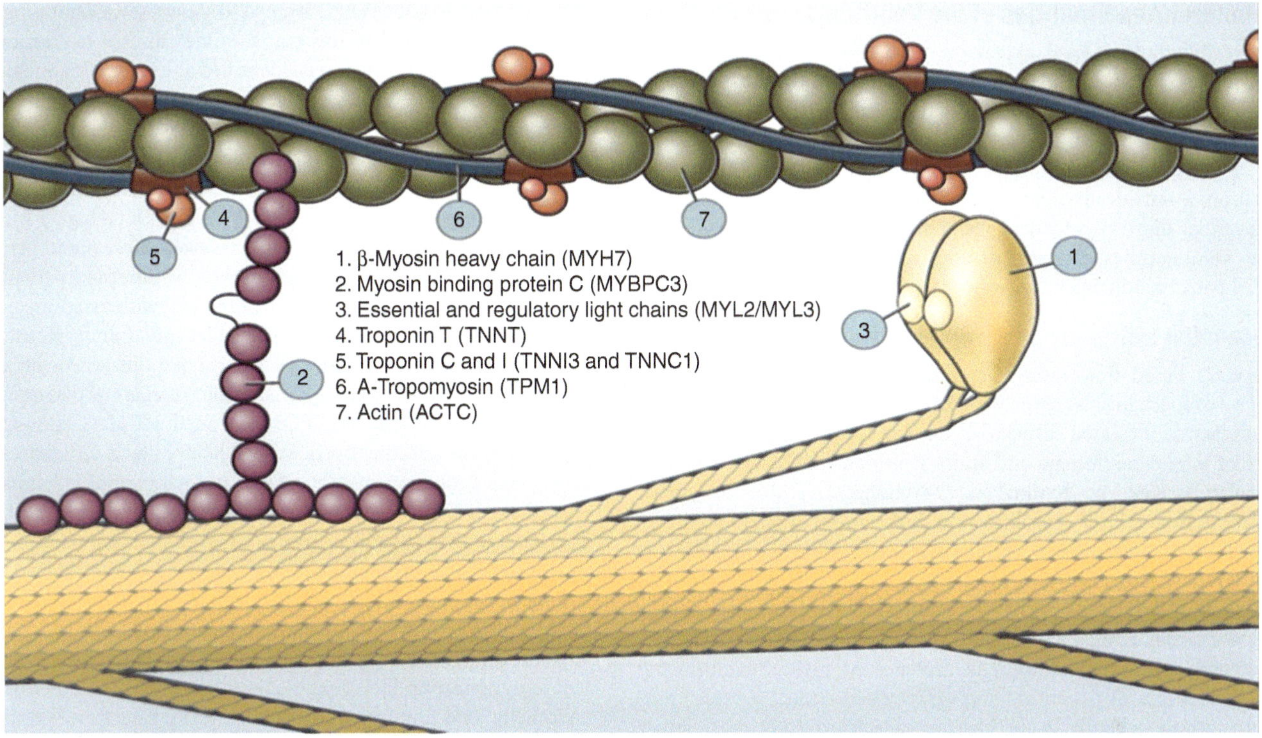

Fig. 25.1 Sarcomeric gene mutations in hypertrophic cardiomyopathy. Cardiac contraction occurs when calcium binds the troponin complex (subunits C, I, and T) and α-tropomyosin, making possible the myosin-actin interaction. Actin stimulates ATPase activity in the globular myosin head and results in the production of force along actin filaments. Cardiac myosin-binding protein C, arrayed transversely along the sarcomere, binds myosin and, when phosphorylated, modulates contraction. In hypertrophic cardiomyopathy, mutations may impair these and other protein interactions, resulting in ineffectual contraction of the sarcomere, and produce hypertrophy and disarray of myocytes. Over 80% of mutations occur in the *MYH7* or *MYBPC3* genes, and double-compound mutations are seen in 3% to 6% of patients.

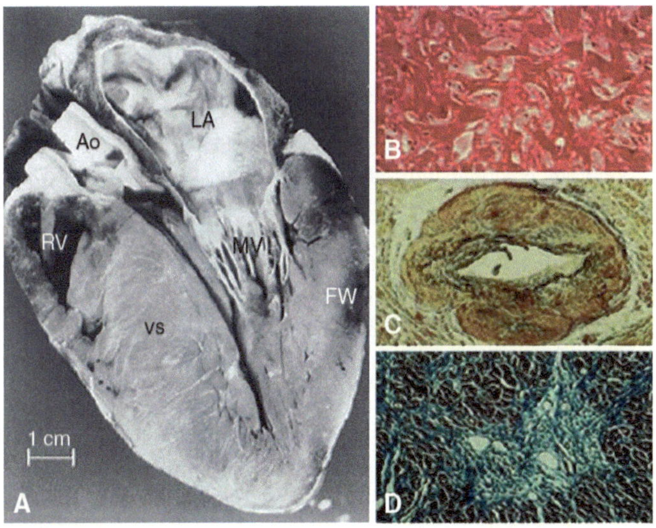

Fig. 25.2 Macroscopic and microscopic pathology of hypertrophic cardiomyopathy. (A) Demonstrates gross hypertrophy of the interventricular septum *(VS)* compared with the ventricular free wall *(FW)*. Histopathology sections demonstrate myocyte disarray (B), medial thickening of the intramural coronary vasculature (C), and vessel luminal obliteration (D). (From Maron BJ. Sudden death in hypertrophic cardiomyopathy. *J Cardiovasc Transl Res.* 2009;2:368–380.)

exerts a stabilizing force on the IHM structures, and as a consequence, reduced levels of functional protein serve to destabilize the IHM and reduce the number of myosins in the super-relaxed state, thereby impacting diastolic relaxation.[9] MYBPC also plays a role in the regulation of sarcomeric calcium levels, and mutations serve to increase myofilament calcium sensitivity and a faster calcium transit decay.[10]

Cardiac Troponin T (TNNT) Mutations

While individual mutations have varying effects on myofilament properties (including increased myofilament calcium sensitivity, decreased maximal force generation, and alterations in binding affinity to the thin filament), all mutations in some way adversely affect diastolic function. Predictable effects include an impairment of myocardial relaxation, a reduction in diastolic chamber compliance, a reduction in contractile reserve, and cardiac dysfunction under inotropic stimulation.[11]

α-Tropomyosin (TPM)

At the low calcium concentrations, seen in diastole in cardiomyocytes, tropomyosin exerts an inhibitory effect on actin-myosin interactions. However, in the presence of a TPM mutation, myofibrillar sensitivity to calcium is increased, and an increase in cycling cross-bridges is seen (resulting in increased tension, stiffness, and an impairment in LV filling).[12]

Structural Abnormalities of the Ventricular Myocardium

At a histopathologic level, hypertrophy, fibrosis, and myocardial fiber disarray are hallmarks of HCM. A recent study has demonstrated significant relationships between maximal LV wall thickness and myocardial fibrosis burden on cardiac magnetic resonance imaging (cardiac MRI) with diastolic function (as assessed by time to peak filling).[13] In addition, a statistically significant relationship between the extent of myocardial disarray and diastolic dysfunction grade and left atrial (LA) volume index has been demonstrated in a pediatric cohort of HCM patients utilizing echocardiography.[14]

Myocardial Ischemia

Coronary blood flow reserve is compromised in HCM through a variety of mechanisms, namely increased myocardial oxygen demand secondary to increased myocardial mass, myocyte disarray, the presence of interstitial fibrosis, and abnormalities of the coronary microvasculature (reduced luminal cross-sectional area due to medial hypertrophy and intimal proliferation, and reduced capillary density).[2] Perfusion abnormalities are common and identifiable using nuclear scintigraphy, cardiac MRI stress imaging, and positron emission tomography.[15] Typically a greater reduction in blood flow occurs in the subendocardial layer, and perfusion abnormalities relate to the degree of hypertrophy. In addition, the presence of myocardial bridging (present in 15% of patients at angiography and 40% at autopsy) may contribute to ischemia in the absence of epicardial coronary artery disease. Ischemia-induced diastolic function occurs at higher heart rates, when a reduction in the diastolic filling period results in an increase in intracavitary pressures, which serves to aggravate subendocardial ischemia further. This is compounded by reduced LV diastolic distensibility during exercise.[16] A recent multicenter study of stress echocardiography in HCM (utilizing the measurement of coronary flow reserve velocity and new wall motion abnormalities as markers of ischemia) has demonstrated that these ischemia-related end points have a greater predictive accuracy for adverse events (both arrhythmia and heart failure related) than hemodynamic end points, such as exercise-induced hypotension and dynamic LVOT obstruction.[17]

CLINICAL PRESENTATION AND PROGNOSIS

Phenotypic Heterogeneity of HCM

HCM is a disease that demonstrates marked phenotypic variation in the degree of hypertrophy, fibrosis, and myocyte disarray. LV hypertrophy (LVH) can range from minimal to severe, with variable morphologic subtypes (of which asymmetric septal hypertrophy is the most common). In some cases, hypertrophy is limited to the apex of the heart. Independent of the degree and pattern of hypertrophy, patients also demonstrate marked phenotypic variability with respect to the hemodynamic consequences of the disease, ranging from nonobstructive HCM to obstructive at the level of either the LVOT, midcavity, or even the right ventricular (RV) outflow tract. While in the majority of cases global LV systolic function is preserved, in a small subset there can be progression to LV dilatation associated with end-stage heart failure (usually referred as burnt-out HCM).[18,19] This represents unfavorable remodeling characterized by loss of function, wall thinning, and chamber dilation causing combined systolic and diastolic dysfunction.

Genotype/Phenotype Relations

The first studies exploring the possibility of mutations holding prognostic importance were derived from small cohorts involving larger families with penetrant disease expression. Initial reports on the clinical expression of MYBPC seemed to show a slower but progressive disease course, with late onset and milder disease expression. The β-MYH7 gene was the first to be identified as a cause of familial HCM, and some mutations are recognized to cause severe hypertrophy that presents clinically early in life with an increased risk for outflow obstruction, heart failure, and sudden death. However, other β-MYH7 mutations may cause less severe clinical disease. Similarly, TNNT2 mutations were associated with less severe LVH but a higher incidence of sudden cardiac death (SCD). However, subsequent genotype-phenotype studies involving large cohorts of unrelated patients have indicated that great caution must be exercised with assigning particular prognostic significance to any particular mutation. A recent multicenter study has shown a lack of phenotypic differences on cardiac MRI or baseline clinical characteristics and markers of disease severity between β-MYH7 and MYBPC3-associated HCM.[20] Although this variation in clinical consequences most likely reflects differences in the biophysical properties of mutant and normal peptides, factors other than these structural changes can also influence disease expression. This clinical diversity is likely related to other genetic phenotypes (epigenetics), environment, gender, and acquired comorbid conditions, and these modifiers account for unfavorable cardiac remodeling and a predisposition to adverse outcomes. Evaluation of candidate molecules as genetic modifiers of HCM, particularly those that influence the extent of hypertrophy, including the renin-angiotensin-aldosterone axis, endothelin, and tumor necrosis factor (TNF), have shown conflicting results. Polymorphisms within the angiotensin-converting enzyme (ACE) gene have been reported to be associated with increased risk for sudden death.[21,22] The complexities of defining genetic modifiers in human HCM populations remain considerable given the substantial heterogeneity of genetic causes that may independently influence hypertrophy.

Origin of Symptoms in HCM

Many patients are either asymptomatic or minimally symptomatic, with severe medically refractory symptoms occurring in only a small proportion.[23–25] Asymptomatic patients may come to attention due to the incidental finding of a heart murmur or an abnormal electrocardiogram (ECG). An increasing number of cases come to attention through family screening of an affected individual. Symptoms leading to considerable disability in HCM patients are typically caused by varying combinations of obstruction, diastolic dysfunction with impaired relaxation and elevated filling pressures, coronary artery disease, mitral regurgitation (MR), and arrhythmia. Dyspnea is a common symptom, predominantly related to the presence of diastolic dysfunction and LVOT obstruction. Worsening dyspnea may be precipitated by either the acute onset of atrial fibrillation (AFib) or more insidiously by the development of LV systolic dysfunction. Chest pain may present as typical angina or atypical pain, but frequently follows a pattern of postprandial exacerbation in patients with obstructive physiology. Patients with nonobstructive HCM present with symptoms less frequently, and usually the symptoms are milder. Congestive heart failure is uncommon in HCM in normal sinus rhythm, but it may be seen with severe obstruction to outflow or severe systolic and/or diastolic dysfunction, and of course it is common in the presence of AFib. Presyncopal and syncopal episodes have a myriad of potential causes, including arrhythmia, outflow tract obstruction, and episodic hypotension secondary to autonomic dysfunction.[26] Palpitations are most commonly associated with the onset of AFib (particularly if paroxysmal). However, nonsustained and sustained ventricular arrhythmias should be considered in the differential diagnosis. Patients with significant diastolic dysfunction develop progressive LA enlargement and an increased risk of incident AFib. Overall, HCM patients appear to have a fourfold to sixfold greater likelihood of developing AFib compared with the general population.[27] The predominance of AFib prevalence increases progressively with age and LA size, which in turn is related to the degree of hypertrophy, severity of MR, and diastolic dysfunction. It is predominant in patients over 60 years of age, but it is not rare in younger patients, in whom it is associated with higher risk for clinical deterioration and HCM-related death. Occasionally an embolic event related to AFib or the presence of a LV aneurysm may result in a stroke as the initial clinical presentation of HCM.

Prognosis

Historically, HCM was felt to be a rare disease with a high risk of adverse events, but with contemporary management strategies, the natural history of the HCM population as a whole is relatively benign, assuming appropriate and timely intervention is offered to those identified to be at an elevated risk of SCD and other complications.[24,25,28] Three distinct modes of death occur: (1) sudden and unexpected (50% of cases), (2) progressive heart failure (30% of cases), and (3) HCM-related ischemic stroke associated with AFib (more commonly seen in elderly patients).[29] SCD remains the most devastating and feared complication of HCM, and in many cases, it may be the initial presentation of disease, with up to two-thirds of patients having no or very little in the way of symptoms prior to death. Over the past decades, the annual risk of SCD has fallen from around 3% to 1%, with a concomitant decrease in all-cause mortality from 5% to 3%.[24,25,28]

DIAGNOSIS OF DIASTOLIC DYSFUNCTION IN HCM

Echocardiography is the imaging modality of choice for the assessment of diastolic function in HCM, although accurate classification of diastolic function grade presents a challenge due to the compounding effects of LVOT obstruction and MR. In addition, HCM is a disease of marked phenotypic heterogeneity in regard to degree of hypertrophy and burden of myocardial scarring and fiber disarray.

CONVENTIONAL TWO-DIMENSIONAL (2-D) TRANSTHORACIC ECHOCARDIOGRAPHY

Mitral and Pulmonary Venous (PV) Flow Velocities

Whereas echocardiography has been successfully utilized for estimation of diastolic function and LV filling pressures in various cardiac disorders, several studies have shown that conventional mitral inflow and PV flow velocities are poorly predictive of LV filling pressures in hypertrophic cardiomyopathy, and these should not be used alone to assess diastolic function in HCM.[30,31] However, multiple echocardiographic measurements have been shown to correlate with LV filling pressures and can be used, among other parameters, for estimation of diastolic function in HCM. The difference between the duration of atrial reversal (Ar), recorded from pulmonary venous flow, and the duration of the transmitral A wave (Ar-A ≥30 msec) has been associated both with an elevation of LV filling pressures[32] and to correlate with abnormal collagen metabolism in patients with HCM.[33]

Myocardial Tissue Doppler Velocities

Assessment of early diastolic longitudinal tissue Doppler velocity at the lateral mitral annulus (e′) is helpful in assessing filling pressures, and it provides additive information regarding functional capacity and prognosis. E/e′ (the ratio of transmitral E wave velocity to e′ velocity) has shown a moderate correlation with invasively measured filling pressures,[31] with functional capacity and exercise tolerance,[34] and has been shown to predict adverse clinical outcomes (including death, cardiac arrest, and ventricular dysrhythmia) in children with HCM.[35] In addition, the E/Vp ratio (the ratio of transmitral E wave velocity to flow propagation velocity of ventricular filling obtained by color M-mode) appears to correlate with invasively measured LV filling pressures.[31]

LA Size and Volume

LA size and, more importantly, LA volumes provide a reflection of the cumulative effects of increased LV filling pressures over time. Increased LA volumes have been shown to correlate with high LV filling pressures,[36] particularly in the absence of significant MR or AFib (as these may lead to LA dilatation even in the presence of a normal LA pressure [LAP]). Assessment of LA volume, indexed to body surface area (LAVI, mL/m^2), is a simple and pivotal parameter to assess diastolic function in HCM patients. A LAVI greater than 34 mL/m^2 has been shown to have significant prognostic implications in HCM and is associated with the risk of progression to heart failure, atrial fibrillation, and increased mortality.[37–40]

Pulmonary Artery Systolic Pressure (PASP)

A significant correlation exists between PASP and LAP, provided pulmonary vascular disease is excluded. A peak velocity of the tricuspid regurgitation (TR) jet greater than 2.8 m/sec supports the presence of increased LAP and LV filling pressures.

ALGORITHM FOR DIASTOLIC FUNCTION ASSESSMENT ON CONVENTIONAL ECHOCARDIOGRAPHY

Given that individual variables have weak correlations with LV filling pressures when used alone in patients with HCM, a comprehensive approach is recommended for assessment of LV diastolic function in this population. In accordance with the recent American Society of Echocardiography/European Association of Cardiovascular Imaging (ASE/EACVI) (see Chapter 19),[41] an integrated four-criteria approach to assess high LV filling pressures in HCM is recommended and should take into consideration the following variables: (1) average E/e′ ratio greater than 14, (2) LA volume index (>34 mL/m^2), (3) pulmonary vein atrial reversal velocity (Ar-A duration ≥30 msec), and (4) peak velocity of TR jet by continuous wave (CW) Doppler greater than 2.8 m/sec (Fig. 25.3). The presence or absence of dynamic obstruction should not affect the application of these parameters for diastolic assessment in HCM. However, in patients with more than moderate MR, only Ar-A duration and peak velocity of TR jet are still valid.

If there is a satisfactory and informative signal in three or four variables, there are two main scenarios: (1) more than half of the variables meet the cutoff values, indicating that LAP is elevated and grade II diastolic dysfunction is present, and (2) if less than half of the variables meet the cutoff values, LAP is normal and grade I diastolic dysfunction is present. In cases of 50% discordance with two or four available variables, findings are inconclusive to estimate LAP. Diastolic function is classified as grade III in the presence of a restrictive filling pattern with abnormally reduced early diastolic mitral annular E′ velocities (septal E′ <7 cm/sec, lateral E′ <10 cm/sec). Estimation of LAP is not recommended if there is only one informative parameter with a satisfactory signal.

EMERGING METHODS FOR THE ASSESSMENT OF DIASTOLIC FUNCTION IN HCM

New imaging technologies can provide crucial structural, physiologic, and diagnostic information related to LV diastolic function in HCM, which cannot be readily or accurately obtained from conventional

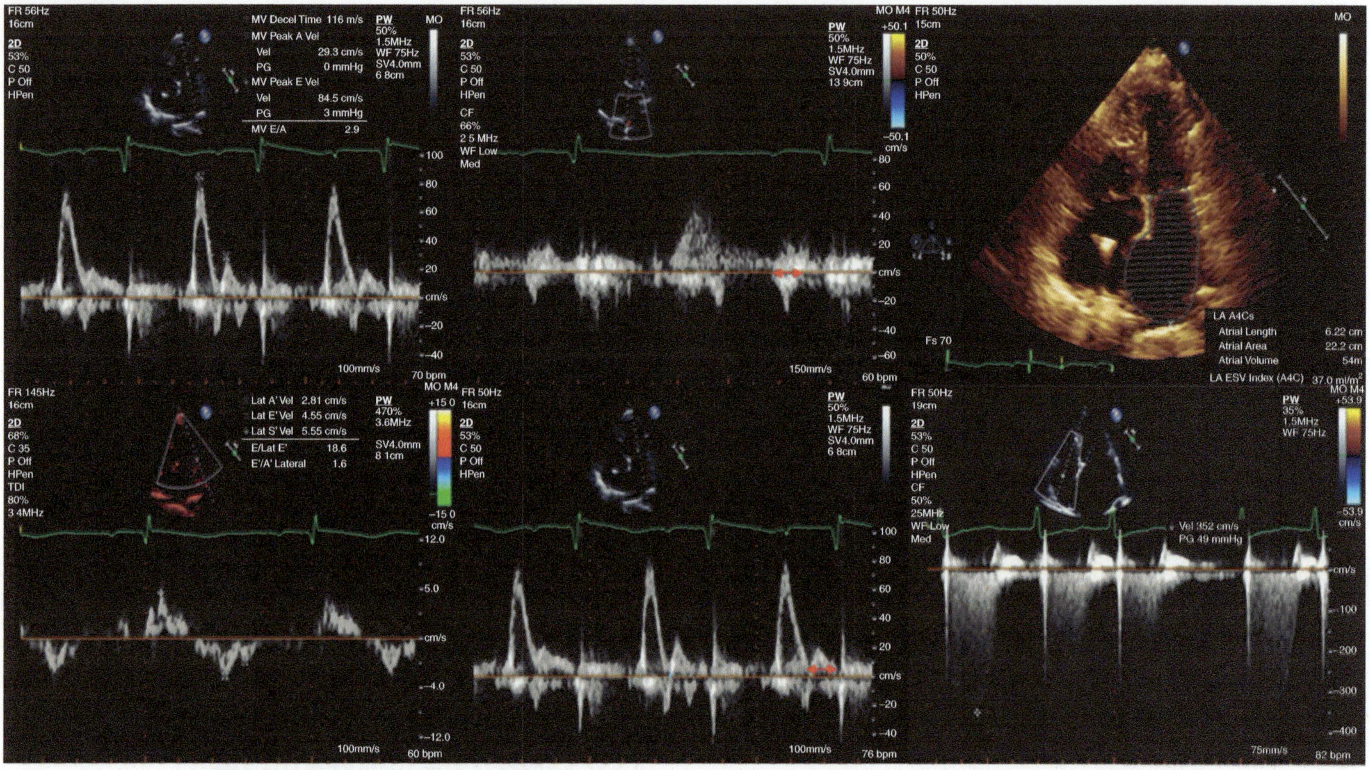

Fig. 25.3 **Algorithm for diastolic function assessment on transthoracic echocardiography.** An integrated four-criteria approach to assess high LV filling pressures in HCM is recommended. In this 45-year-old patient with apical HCM, assessment of these variables demonstrates (1) average E/e′ ratio of 23, (2) LA volume index of 37 mL/m², (3) Ar-A duration of 32 msec, and (4) peak velocity of TR jet by continuous wave Doppler of 3.5 m/sec consistent with grade III diastolic dysfunction.

echocardiographic diastolic parameters. While further large-scale studies are needed to generalize these observations and correlate them with clinical outcomes before they can become integrated into the mainstream assessment of diastolic function, early data suggest a promising role for these new techniques.

Speckle Tracking Echocardiography

2-D speckle tracking represents a new tool to evaluate myocardial mechanics and is more sensitive in the detection of subtle ventricular dysfunction.[42–44] Initially applied on 2-D echocardiography, diastolic parameters, including early and late diastolic myocardial velocity, strain rate, and LV untwisting, have been proposed as new markers of diastolic function.[45–48] LA strain and phasic volumetric quantification has become an important tool for the assessment of LV filling.

LV Strain Rate

LV longitudinal strain rate (Fig. 25.4) has been correlated with various hemodynamic diastolic indices in patients with HCM.[49,50] While commonly measured echocardiographic parameters have not been shown to correlate with LV end-diastolic pressure (LVEDP), the ratio of the transmitral E velocity to the early diastolic strain rate ratio (E/SR_E) demonstrates not only good correlation with LVEDP, but also a higher area under the curve (on receiver operator curve analysis) than either the lateral or septal E/e′ ratio.[50] Taking into account that changes in longitudinal SR_E may at least partly reflect a parallel decrease in longitudinal systolic function, the ratio of SR_E/SR_S (early diastolic strain rate/systolic strain rate) provides additional information regarding the degree of diastolic dysfunction. While in most HCM patients the ratio is less than 1.0, indicating a measure of relaxation delay, SR_E/SR_S was found to positively correlate with LVEDP, with a cutoff value of 0.79 or more, predictive of elevated LVEDP (≥15 mmHg).[49] Conversely, longitudinal peak strain rate at atrial contraction (SR_A) has not been shown to correlate with filling pressures,[49,50] and the clinical significance of SR_A in HCM patients is unclear.

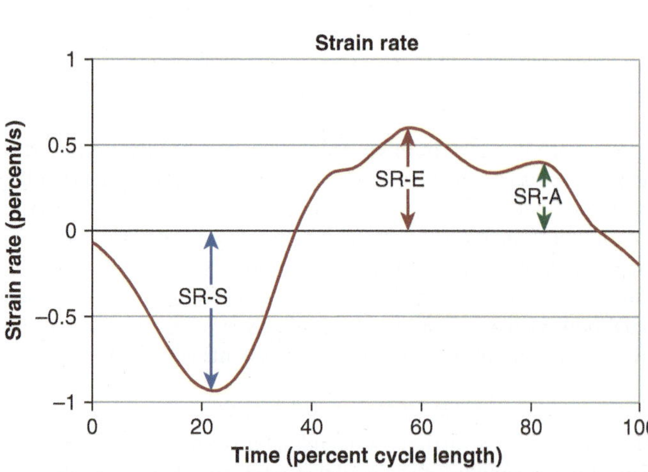

Fig. 25.4 **Left ventricular strain rate analysis for the assessment of diastolic function.** Diastolic parameters can be derived from strain and strain rate evaluation of the left ventricle. A longitudinal strain rate curve is depicted, demonstrating LV systolic strain rate *(SR-S: blue arrow)*, early diastolic strain rate *(SR-E: red arrow)*, and late atrial diastolic strain rate *(SR-A: green arrow)*.

Rotational Mechanics: Fractional Early Apical Reverse Rotation (FEARR) and Untwist Rate

LV systolic torsional (twisting) deformation is one mechanism by which potential energy is stored during ejection, to be later released during diastole and contribute to the creation of suction. In systole, as the base and apex of the heart rotate in opposing directions and generate twisting of the heart muscle, part of the energy used in contraction is stored within the extracellular collagen matrix[51] and compressed titin within the myocytes.[52] During relaxation, this energy is promptly released and manifested by LV untwisting. About 40% of the LV untwisting occurs during isovolumic relaxation,[53,54] and its rate correlates with the time constant of LV pressure decay (τ).[55] Untwisting that occurs during filling can continue to release elastic energy after mitral valve opening, facilitating further filling of the left ventricle. Studies utilizing echocardiographic tissue speckle tracking to assess the untwisting rate have shown it to be proportional to the rate of isovolumic pressure decay[56] and positively associated with the formation and increase of an intraventricular pressure gradient, a marker of diastolic suction during early LV filling. Untwisting provides a temporal link between two crucial diastolic phenomena, relaxation and diastolic suction. In another study, reduced and delayed untwisting of the left ventricle was demonstrated in patients with hypertension and LVH.[57]

In HCM, overall untwisting time (from peak to trough twist) was found to be 28% longer in patients with HCM compared with normal controls and significantly longer in patients with LV outflow obstruction than in patients without such obstruction.[58] Calculation of a FEARR Fraction of Early Apical Reverse Rotation, percent of peak apical rotation angle recovered during the initial phase of diastole, 10% of cycle length (Fig. 25.5) from apical rotation curves was devised to assess initial relaxation and LV suction. Although it has been shown to be similar in normal controls and patients with HCM, it was nearly halved in HCM patients with severe heart failure symptoms, regardless of the presence of LVOT obstruction.[58]

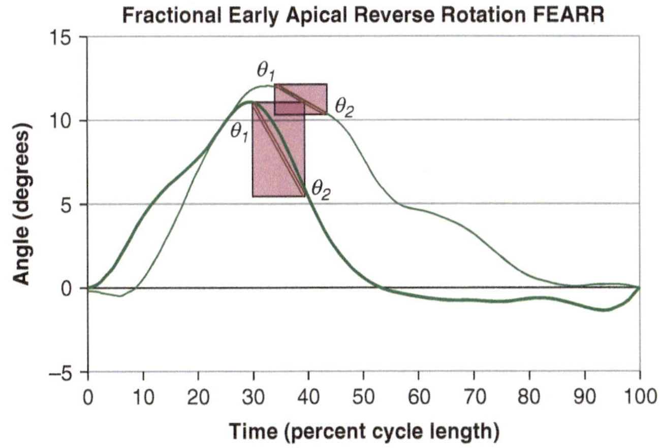

$$\text{FEARR} = \frac{\theta_{peak} - \theta_{t(peak)} + 10\%CL}{\theta_{peak}}$$

Fig. 25.5 Left ventricular untwisting. Apical rotation curves demonstrating counterclockwise (positive) rotation are demonstrated for a healthy control *(thick curve)* and a patient with hypertrophic cardiomyopathy *(thin curve)* is demonstrated. Note that overall untwisting time (from peak to trough twist) is significantly longer in the patient with HCM. Calculation of a fractional early apical rotation fraction (FEARR) is performed by calculating the percentage of peak apical rotation angle recovered during the initial phase of diastole (initial 10% of the cardiac cycle length). FEARR is significantly reduced in the HCM compared with the healthy control.

Phasic LA Volumes and Function

As discussed earlier, LA end-systolic (maximal) size and volume have been shown to be determinants of both exercise capacity and major adverse cardiac and cerebrovascular events in patients with HCM. Despite being validated as a major prognostic marker, LAVI likely reflects the chronic hemodynamic effects of LV diastolic dysfunction. LA phasic emptying volumes are more directly related to LV filling and may provide new insights to LV diastolic function (Table 25.1). Speckle tracking software allows for the assessment of these volumes by tracking changes in LA volume throughout the cardiac cycle. In addition, LA strain and strain rate analysis provide a feasible noninvasive method of assessment of LA function.[59–61] Three distinct phases of atrial function assessed are (1) reservoir function, which represents the storage of pulmonary venous return during ventricular systole and isovolumic relaxation; (2) conduit function, which represents the period of passive emptying of the left atrium down a pressure gradient during early diastole; and (3) booster or active contractile function, which represents intrinsic atrial contractility during which the atria empty before the end of ventricular

TABLE 25.1 A Practical Approach to Echocardiographic Assessment of Diastolic Function in Hypertrophic Cardiomyopathy

	Echocardiographic Modality	Parameters
Two-dimensional echo		LA dimension
		LA volume
Pulsed-wave Doppler	Mitral inflow	E
		A
		IVRT
	Pulmonary veins	S
		D
		A reversal
Tissue Doppler	Mitral annular longitudinal velocity	e′
Multimodality	Left atrial pressure estimation	

A, Late atrial contraction; *D,* diastolic; *E,* early diastolic filling; *e′,* early diastolic longitudinal tissue Doppler velocity; *IVRT,* isovolumic relaxation time; *LA,* left ventricular; *S,* systolic.

From Nagueh SF, et al. Doppler tissue imaging: a noninvasive technique for evaluation of left ventricular relaxation and estimation of filling pressures. *JACC.* 1997;30:1527–1533.

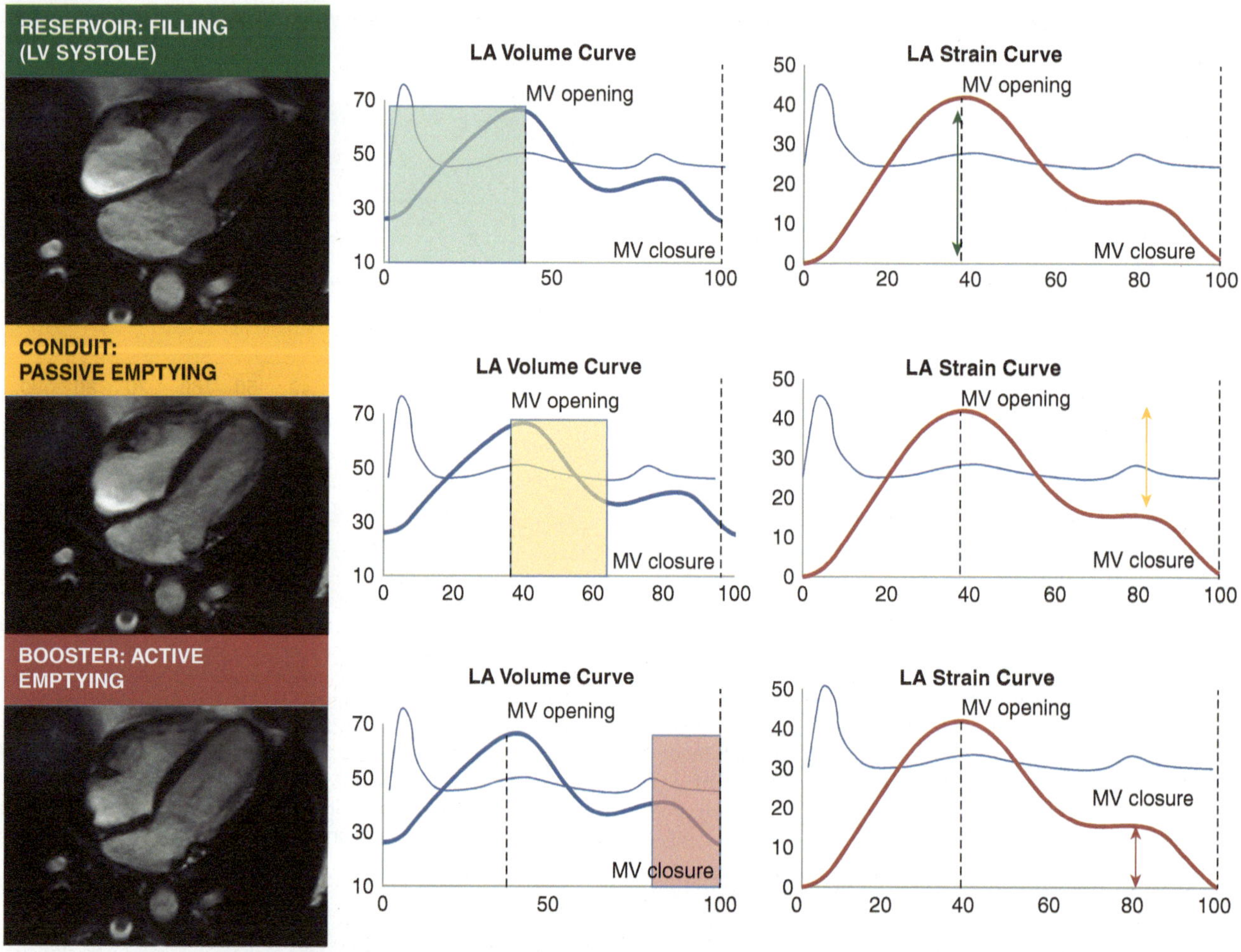

Fig. 25.6 Phasic left atrial function. Three distinct phases of LA function are diagrammatically represented in the form of both LA volume and strain curves: reservoir—the storage of pulmonary venous return during ventricular systole and isovolumic relaxation; conduit—the period of passive emptying of the left atrium down a pressure gradient during early diastole; booster—intrinsic atrial contractility during which the atria empty before the end of ventricular diastole. (From Williams LK, Chan RH, Carasso S, et al. Effect of left ventricular outflow tract obstruction on left atrial mechanics in hypertrophic cardiomyopathy. *Biomed Res Int.* 2015;2015:481245.)

diastole (see Chapters 4 and 12) (Fig. 25.6). In HCM, LA dysfunction and in particular LA booster pump function have been shown to correlate with heart failure symptoms,[62] as well as being a strong predictor for the development of AFib requiring hospitalization.[63] A recent study of a large cohort of HCM patients undergoing cardiac MRI has demonstrated LA EF and minimum LA volumes as predictors of the development of AFib.[64] The relationship between the left ventricle and left atrium is highly dynamic and interdependent, with all phasic aspects of LA function to some degree influenced not only by LV contractility, relaxation, compliance, and filling pressures but also by intrinsic LA contractility, relaxation, and compliance itself. This interdependency has recently been demonstrated in HCM patients, with a significant increase in LA volumes and marked impairment in LA phasic function compared with healthy controls. The presence of LVOT obstruction further increases LA volumes and impairs function, and relief of obstruction and reduction in mitral regurgitation via septal myectomy results in both a significant reduction in LA volume and an improvement in LA function.[65] While there is initially a compensatory increase in LA contractility in response to an increase in LA volumes, eventually further increases in LA volumes will result in a decline in atrial function, as evidenced by the inverse correlation demonstrated between V_{max} and LA EF, reservoir, and booster strain.[65] The increase in LA afterload seen in patients with obstruction is likely to contribute to the greater reduction in LA booster function seen in these patients and may explain the improvement in function seen after septal myectomy. While strain analysis is not yet part of routine clinical practice, the simple addition of measurement of V_{min} to routinely measured V_{max} appears to provide valuable information regarding function. V_{min} demonstrated a stronger correlation with not only measures of global LA function and compliance but also markers of LA contractility (active and booster function).[65] These data suggest that measurement of minimum volume provides a valuable surrogate marker of LA function.

Cardiac MRI T1 Mapping Tensors

Diffusion tensor (DT)–cardiac MRI potentially provides a novel approach for phenotyping through noninvasive interrogation of the three-dimensional (3-D) heart microarchitecture.[66,67] Studies have demonstrated dynamic rearrangement of sheetlets in healthy subjects, as well as changes in HCM consistent with systolic hypercontraction and attenuated diastolic relaxation.[68,69] These observations provided new insight into aberrant dynamics of laminar microstructures in cardiomyopathies and identified distinct mechanisms associated with reduced strain development. Both dilated cardiomyopathy (DCM, low LVEF) and HCM (high LVEF) displayed similarly impaired strain compared to healthy control subjects (normal LV EF). In DCM, a failure to adequately rotate sheetlets to a contracted conformation in systole occurs, whereas in HCM, a failure to adequately rotate sheetlets to a relaxed conformation in diastole predominated. In vivo DT-CMR may provide new mechanistic insights into altered ventricular mechanics, adverse remodeling, and the substrate for arrhythmogenesis in various clinical conditions, including postmyocardial infarction, valvular heart disease, and inherited and congenital cardiac diseases. Other applications include identifying the potential for LV contractile recovery and reverse remodeling, and as a new monitoring marker for interventions to improve contractile function. These data could prove to be useful for modeling the microstructural dynamics of cardiac contraction.

DIFFERENTIAL DIAGNOSES

HCM Versus Hypertensive Heart Disease (HHD)

Arterial hypertension has an estimated prevalence of 28% in North America and 44% in Europe.[70] Given that unexplained LVH has a prevalence of 1:500 in the general population, the coexistence of both disorders can be expected to occur in the order of around 20% of patients, often compounding an accurate diagnosis. Long-standing hypertension (resulting in increased wall stress and an increase in afterload) often results in compensatory hypertrophy, particularly if poorly controlled. Wall stress is inhomogeneous within the left ventricle and greatest in the basal septum, typically resulting in hypertrophy in this region.[71] With time, the typical concentric pattern of hypertrophy becomes more evident. While an absolute wall thickness of 15 mm in any myocardial segment is consistent with a diagnosis of HCM, wall thicknesses can approach this level in HHD, particularly in Afro-Caribbean individuals. Advanced echocardiographic techniques such as tissue Doppler imaging (TDI) and speckle tracking echocardiography are potentially helpful in distinguishing HHD from HCM. Global systolic function remains preserved in most cases of HHD, but regional myocardial deformation (particularly in the basal septum) is often mildly impaired in contrast to the marked reduction in strain in the ventricular septum in HCM.[72] While systolic tissue Doppler velocities are reduced to a similar degree in both HCM and HHD, patients with HCM demonstrate greater reductions in early diastolic velocities (assessed at the medial and lateral mitral annulus).[73]

HCM Versus Athlete's Heart

The accurate diagnosis of HCM in individuals participating in competitive sports is paramount, given the potential risk of SCD. HCM has in most series been identified as the predominant cause of SCD in young athletes. While fewer than 2% of elite athletes develop a maximal wall thickness in the interventricular septum of greater than 12 mm,[74] racial differences exist in the propensity to develop hypertrophy, with as many as 12% of Afro-Caribbean athletes developing wall thicknesses in excess of 12 mm.[75] Asymmetric hypertrophy is rare in response to physiologic adaptation, and hypertrophy is classically concentric and associated with chamber dilatation. As with HHD, there is accumulating evidence to suggest that advanced echocardiographic techniques play a key role in the differentiation of these two conditions. Peak myocardial systolic velocities, strain, and strain rate are typically normal or supranormal in athletes with physiologic hypertrophy in contrast to HCM.[73,76] However, the striking differences in diastolic dysfunction in the two conditions is often more helpful in diagnosis. Diastolic function is preserved (often enhanced) in an athlete's heart, with normal diastolic tissue Doppler velocities and an increase in twist and untwist rates.[73,77] In contrast, the pathologic hypertrophy of HCM is associated with a marked attenuation in diastolic tissue Doppler velocities, delayed untwist, and an increase in LA volumes accompanied by impaired LA function. While mild LA dilatation can be seen in an athlete's heart, LA function is typically preserved.

Subclinical Disease (Genotype Positive Phenotype Negative [GPPN])

With the advent of genetic testing, allowing genetic screening of family members of affected patients, individuals who carry a pathogenic sarcomeric mutation but who have no evidence of LVH can be identified. The effects of sarcomere protein mutations on cardiac contractile function remain incompletely understood. Data from a murine model of disease have demonstrated evidence of diastolic dysfunction and altered cardiac energetics.[78] In GPPN patients there is accumulating data, derived largely from studies using TDI to suggest the presence of abnormal myocardial mechanics prior to the development of overt hypertrophy.[79,80] These initial manifestations of cardiac dysfunction appear to be predominantly related to diastolic dysfunction, while data regarding early systolic dysfunction are conflicting. It is unknown whether the presence of a sarcomeric mutation alone is sufficient to result in abnormalities of myocardial force generation, or whether the characteristic changes in myocardial architecture such as hypertrophy, disarray, and fibrosis are required to impair systolic function.

TREATMENT OF HCM AND EFFECTS ON DIASTOLIC FUNCTION

Medical Therapies

β-Blockers and Calcium Channel Blockers

The presence of symptoms generally warrants the introduction of pharmacologic therapy, typically with agents that exert a negative inotropic and chronotropic effect, regardless of the presence or absence of outflow tract obstruction. Beta blockers and calcium channel blockers have a positive impact on outflow tract obstruction via these effects, but in addition, influence diastolic function. Beta blockers exert their effect via a shortening of relaxation time in a dose-dependent fashion,[81] but they have no impact on diastolic stiffness itself.[82,83] Verapamil demonstrates a less predictable effect on LVOT obstruction due to its potent vasodilator properties, and in some cases it can precipitate a marked increase in outflow tract obstruction and pulmonary edema. Like beta blockers, it has no effect on diastolic stiffness, but augments LV relaxation and mean diastolic filling more consistently than agents such as propranolol.[82,83] Diltiazem, an L-type calcium channel blocker more commonly used in nonobstructive HCM, has been shown to normalize tissue Doppler peak systolic and early diastolic velocities at the lateral mitral annulus in asymptomatic carriers of MYBPC3 mutations.[84]

Disopyramide

Disopyramide is a class IC antiarrhythmic drug, which exerts a potent negative inotropic effect. Its use is predominantly as a second-line agent for the treatment of outflow tract obstruction, and its effects on diastolic function have rarely been studied. However, predominant effects appear to result from an improvement in filling (increased transmitral E wave, transmitral E/A ratio), secondary to reductions in LVOT gradients and a subsequent reduction in LVEDP.[85,86]

Metabolic Modulators

Perhexiline is a metabolic modulator that enhances carbohydrate metabolism in the heart via inhibition of the enzymes responsible for free fatty acid (FFA) uptake into the mitochondria. Glucose metabolism is more metabolically efficient that FFA metabolism, requiring less oxygen requirement to generate an equivalent amount of ATP for contraction and relaxation. In a randomized, double-blind, placebo-controlled trial, perhexiline has shown the capacity to improve cardiac energetics, diastolic function, and exercise capacity.[87]

Late Sodium Current Inhibitors: Ranolazine and Eleclazine

Enhanced activity of the late sodium current I_{NaL} plays a significant role in the pathophysiology of HCM. I_{NaL} is an inward ion current that contributes to the duration of phases 2 and 3 of the cardiac action potential. In HCM the activity is increased severalfold,[88] resulting in abnormalities of repolarization via intracellular sodium overload, a reduction in transmembrane electrical gradient, and cytosolic calcium overload. The net results on increased action duration potential is an increase in diastolic tension and a reduction in diastolic interval, serving to aggravate diastolic dysfunction and microvascular ischemia. Calcium overload not only increases susceptibility to arrhythmia but also increases contractility (aggravating LVOT obstruction). Ranolazine inhibits not only I_{NaL} but also calcium and potassium channels, hence its propensity to cause modest prolongation of the QTc interval. In contrast, eleclazine is a potent selective inhibitor of I_{NaL}. Despite early promise, the results of the recently published RESTYLE-HCM trial, which was a randomized, double-blind, placebo-controlled study of ranolazine, have shown no effect on exercise capacity, plasma brain natriuretic protein (BNP) levels, diastolic function, or quality of life.[89] Similarly, the LIBERTY-HCM trial involving the use of eleclazine has been terminated early,[90] as data did not support continuation of the trial.

INVASIVE SEPTAL REDUCTION THERAPIES

Septal ablation by alcohol and septal myectomy reduce Doppler-estimated τ, increase mitral annulus e′ velocity, and decrease pulmonary artery wedge pressure. Moreover, assessment of mitral inflow velocity propagation (Vp) assessed by color Doppler M-mode has shown an improvement in LV relaxation after septal reduction by increasing the intraventricular pressure gradient or suction during early diastole.[91–93] Tissue Doppler strain rate imaging has shown normalization of diastolic dyssynchrony with septal ethanol ablation.[94] Decreased afterload and an increased cardiac output due to the relief of the obstruction may lead to increased coronary flow and improved myocardial perfusion,[95] which may in turn benefit LV relaxation. Also, the regression of hypertrophy and the changes in LV geometry that occur after septal reduction therapy, as shown in the present and other previous studies,[96,97] may partially explain the improvement in diastolic function.

FUTURE DIRECTIONS

The origin of diastolic dysfunction in HCM is complex and multifactorial. Molecular abnormalities in sarcomeric proteins, derangements of calcium metabolism and sensitivity, abnormal cardiac energetics, structural abnormalities (including hypertrophy, fibrosis, and disarray), and global ventricular geometric abnormalities all serve to increase myocardial stiffness, impair LV relaxation, and increase LA and LV filling pressures. Symptoms in HCM are typically related to LV obstruction, the degree of diastolic dysfunction, and microvascular ischemia. Diastolic dysfunction leads to progressive LA enlargement, which predisposes (in up to 20% of patients) to AFib. AFib decreases effort tolerance dramatically in HCM patients, increases the risk of thromboembolic events, and is responsible for a large part of the morbidity and mortality in this disease.

Conventional methods of assessing diastolic function (mitral inflow and PV velocities) are of limited value in HCM. Assessment of the left atrium is paramount and provides information valuable in predicting the severity of disease and risk of adverse cardiac events. Newer echocardiographic imaging methods, including speckle tracking echocardiography to assess strain, strain rate, rotation, and twist, show promise in better understanding the mechanical origin and degree of diastolic dysfunction and may be linked to prognosis. In addition, much attention is focused on identifying new therapeutic agents to treat diastolic dysfunction and thereby improve symptomatic status and outcomes.

Lately, in the Maverick-HCM study mavacamten, a novel myosin inhibitor treatment in symptomatic patients with non-obstructive HCM demonstrated a significant reduction in NT-proBNP and cTnI, suggesting improvement in myocardial wall stress. By altering the contractile mechanics of the cardiomyocyte, myosin inhibitors have the potential to modify pathophysiology and improve symptoms associated with HCM.

KEY POINTS

- Mutations related to HCM result in the production of abnormal myocardial sarcomeric proteins that have altered contraction and relaxation.
- Coronary blood flow reserve is compromised in HCM through increased myocardial oxygen demand secondary to increased myocardial mass, myocyte disarray, the presence of interstitial fibrosis, and decreased oxygen supply due to abnormalities of the coronary microvasculature.
- Congestive heart failure is uncommon in HCM in normal sinus rhythm, but it may be seen with severe outflow track obstruction, severe systolic and/or diastolic dysfunction, and atrial fibrillation.
- HCM patients have a fourfold to sixfold greater likelihood of developing AFib compared with the general population.
- Conventional mitral inflow and pulmonary venous flow velocities are poorly predictive of LV filling pressures in hypertrophic cardiomyopathy.
- While systolic tissue Doppler velocities are reduced to a similar degree in both HCM and hypertensive heart disease, patients with HCM demonstrate greater reductions in early diastolic velocities.
- Peak myocardial systolic velocities, strain, and diastolic function parameters are preserved in an athlete's heart, when compared to HCM.
- Septal ablation by alcohol and septal myectomy have been shown to reduce Doppler-estimated τ, increase mitral annulus e′ velocity and mitral inflow propagation velocity (Vp), and decrease pulmonary artery wedge pressure.

REVIEW QUESTIONS

1. Which of the following is true regarding the physiologic changes that occur in the presence of myosin heavy chain mutations?
   a. There is decreased myofilament sensitivity to calcium.
   b. Time constant of LV relaxation (τ) shortens.
   c. Myocardial fiber contractility increases.
   d. LV chamber compliance increases.

2. The following mechanisms result in impaired coronary blood flow reserve in HCM, except:
   a. increased myocardial mass.
   b. decreased collagen production.
   c. myocyte disarray.
   d. abnormal coronary vasculature.

3. Which of the following findings reliably distinguishes HCM from physiologic hypertrophy of the athlete?
   a. Increased E/e′
   b. Increased E/A ratio
   c. Eccentric LV hypertrophy
   d. Increased LA volume

REFERENCES

1. Maron BJ. Sudden death in hypertrophic cardiomyopathy. *J Cardiovasc Transl Res.* 2009;2:368–380.
2. Varnava AM, Elliott PM, Sharma S, McKenna WJ, Davies MJ. Hypertrophic cardiomyopathy: the interrelation of disarray, fibrosis, and small vessel disease. *Heart.* 2000;84:476–482.
3. Garfinkel AC, Seidman JG, Seidman CE. Genetic pathogenesis of hypertrophic and dilated cardiomyopathy. *Heart Fail Clin.* 2018;14:139–146.
4. Burke MA, Cook SA, Seidman JG, Seidman CE. Clinical and mechanistic insights into the genetics of cardiomyopathy. *J Am Coll Cardiol.* 2016;68:2871–2886.
5. Spudich JA. Hypertrophic and dilated cardiomyopathy: four decades of basic research on muscle lead to potential therapeutic approaches to these devastating genetic diseases. *Biophys J.* 2014;106:1236–1249.
6. Alamo L, Ware JS, Pinto A, et al. Effects of myosin variants on interacting-heads motif explain distinct hypertrophic and dilated cardiomyopathy phenotypes. *Elife.* 2017;6:e24634.
7. Harris SP, Lyons RG, Bezold KL. In the thick of it: HCM-causing mutations in myosin binding proteins of the thick filament. *Circ Res.* 2011;108:751–764.
8. van Dijk SJ, Dooijes D, dos Remedios C, et al. Cardiac myosin-binding protein C mutations and hypertrophic cardiomyopathy: haploinsufficiency, deranged phosphorylation, and cardiomyocyte dysfunction. *Circulation.* 2009;119:1473–1483.
9. McNamara JW, Li A, Lal S, et al. MYBPC3 mutations are associated with a reduced super-relaxed state in patients with hypertrophic cardiomyopathy. *PLoS One.* 2017;12:e0180064.
10. Fraysse B, Weinberger F, Bardswell SC, et al. Increased myofilament Ca2+ sensitivity and diastolic dysfunction as early consequences of MYBPC3 mutation in heterozygous knock-in mice. *J Mol Cell Cardiol.* 2012;52:1299–1307.
11. Knollmann BC, Potter JD. Altered regulation of cardiac muscle contraction by troponin t mutations that cause familial hypertrophic cardiomyopathy. *Trends Cardiovasc Med.* 2001;11:206–212.
12. Bai F, Weis A, Takeda AK, Chase PB, Kawai M. Enhanced active cross-bridges during diastole: molecular pathogenesis of tropomyosin's hcm mutations. *Biophys J.* 2011;100:1014–1023.
13. Chacko BR, Karur GR, Connelly KA, et al. Left ventricular structure and diastolic function by cardiac magnetic resonance imaging in hypertrophic cardiomyopathy. *Indian Heart J.* 2018;70:75–81.
14. Menon SC, Eidem BW, Dearani JA, Ommen SR, Ackerman MJ, Miller D. Diastolic dysfunction and its histopathological correlation in obstructive hypertrophic cardiomyopathy in children and adolescents. *J Am Soc Echocardiogr.* 2009;22:1327–1334.
15. Maron MS, Olivotto I, Maron BJ, et al. The case for myocardial ischemia in hypertrophic cardiomyopathy. *J Am Coll Cardiol.* 2009;54:866–875.
16. Isobe S, Izawa H, Takeichi Y, et al. Relationship between exercise-induced myocardial ischemia and reduced left ventricular distensibility in patients with nonobstructive hypertrophic cardiomyopathy. *J Nucl Med.* 2003;44:1717–1724.
17. Ciampi Q, Olivotto I, Gardini C, et al. Prognostic role of stress echocardiography in hypertrophic cardiomyopathy: the International Stress Echo Registry. *Int J Cardiol.* 2016;219:331–338.
18. Harris KM, Spirito P, Maron MS, et al. Prevalence, clinical profile, and significance of left ventricular remodeling in the end-stage phase of hypertrophic cardiomyopathy. *Circulation.* 2006;114:216–225.
19. Melacini P, Basso C, Angelini A, et al. Clinicopathological profiles of progressive heart failure in hypertrophic cardiomyopathy. *Eur Heart J.* 2010;31:2111–2123.
20. Weissler-Snir A, Hindieh W, Gruner C, et al. Lack of phenotypic differences by cardiovascular magnetic resonance imaging in MYH7 (beta-myosin heavy chain)- versus MYBPC3 (myosin-binding protein C)-related hypertrophic cardiomyopathy. *Circ Cardiovasc Imaging.* 2017;10(2):e005311.
21. Marian AJ, Yu QT, Workman R, Greve G, Roberts R. Angiotensin-converting enzyme polymorphism in hypertrophic cardiomyopathy and sudden cardiac death. *Lancet.* 1993;342:1085–1086.
22. Lechin M, Quinones MA, Omran A, et al. Angiotensin-I converting enzyme genotypes and left ventricular hypertrophy in patients with hypertrophic cardiomyopathy. *Circulation.* 1995;92:1808–1812.
23. Maron BJ, Rowin EJ, Casey SA, et al. Risk stratification and outcome of patients with hypertrophic cardiomyopathy > = 60 years of age. *Circulation.* 2013;127:585–593.
24. Maron BJ, Rowin EJ, Casey SA, et al. Hypertrophic cardiomyopathy in children, adolescents, and young adults associated with low cardiovascular mortality with contemporary management strategies. *Circulation.* 2016;133:62–73.
25. Maron BJ, Rowin EJ, Casey SA, et al. Hypertrophic cardiomyopathy in adulthood associated with low cardiovascular mortality with contemporary management strategies. *J Am Coll Cardiol.* 2015;65:1915–1928.
26. Williams L, Frenneaux M. Syncope in hypertrophic cardiomyopathy: mechanisms and consequences for treatment. *Europace.* 2007;9:817–822.
27. Guttmann OP, Pavlou M, O'Mahony C, et al. Hypertrophic cardiomyopathy outcomes I. Predictors of atrial fibrillation in hypertrophic cardiomyopathy. *Heart.* 2017;103:672–678.
28. Maron MS, Rowin EJ, Olivotto I, et al. Contemporary natural history and management of nonobstructive hypertrophic cardiomyopathy. *J Am Coll Cardiol.* 2016;67:1399–1409.
29. Maron BJ, Olivotto I, Spirito P, et al. Epidemiology of hypertrophic cardiomyopathy-related death: Revisited in a large non-referral-based patient population. *Circulation.* 2000;102:858–864.
30. Nishimura RA, Appleton CP, Redfield MM, Ilstrup DM, Holmes DR Jr, Tajik AJ. Noninvasive Doppler echocardiographic evaluation of left ventricular filling pressures in patients with cardiomyopathies: a simultaneous Doppler echocardiographic and cardiac catheterization study. *J Am Coll Cardiol.* 1996;28:1226–1233.
31. Nagueh SF, Lakkis NM, Middleton KJ, Spencer III WH, Zoghbi WA, Quinones MA. Doppler estimation of left ventricular filling pressures in patients with hypertrophic cardiomyopathy. *Circulation.* 1999;99:254–261.
32. Nagueh SF, Appleton CP, Gillebert TC, et al. Recommendations for the evaluation of left ventricular diastolic function by echocardiography. *Eur J Echocardiogr.* 2009;10:165–193.
33. Lombardi R, Betocchi S, Losi MA, et al. Myocardial collagen turnover in hypertrophic cardiomyopathy. *Circulation.* 2003;108:1455–1460.
34. Le VV, Perez MV, Wheeler MT, Myers J, Schnittger I, Ashley EA. Mechanisms of exercise intolerance in patients with hypertrophic cardiomyopathy. *Am Heart J.* 2009;158:e27–e34.
35. McMahon CJ, Nagueh SF, Pignatelli RH, et al. Characterization of left ventricular diastolic function by tissue Doppler imaging and clinical status in children with hypertrophic cardiomyopathy. *Circulation.* 2004;109:1756–1762.
36. Appleton CP, Galloway JM, Gonzalez MS, Gaballa M, Basnight MA. Estimation of left ventricular filling pressures using two-dimensional and Doppler echocardiography in adult patients with cardiac disease. Additional value of analyzing left atrial size, left atrial ejection fraction and the difference in duration of pulmonary venous and mitral flow velocity at atrial contraction. *J Am Coll Cardiol.* 1993;22:1972–1982.

37. Nistri S, Olivotto I, Betocchi S, et al. Prognostic significance of left atrial size in patients with hypertrophic cardiomyopathy (from the Italian registry for hypertrophic cardiomyopathy). *Am J Cardiol.* 2006;98:960–965.
38. Losi MA, Betocchi S, Barbati G, et al. Prognostic significance of left atrial volume dilatation in patients with hypertrophic cardiomyopathy. *J Am Soc Echocardiogr.* 2009;22:76–81.
39. Olivotto I, Cecchi F, Casey SA, Dolara A, Traverse JH, Maron BJ. Impact of atrial fibrillation on the clinical course of hypertrophic cardiomyopathy. *Circulation.* 2001;104:2517–2524.
40. Yang H, Woo A, Monakier D, et al. Enlarged left atrial volume in hypertrophic cardiomyopathy: A marker for disease severity. *J Am Soc Echocardiogr.* 2005;18:1074–1082.
41. Nagueh SF, Smiseth OA, Appleton CP, et al. Recommendations for the evaluation of left ventricular diastolic function by echocardiography: an update from the American Society of Echocardiography and the European Association of Cardiovascular Imaging. *J Am Soc Echocardiogr.* 2016;29:277–314.
42. Carasso S, Yang H, Woo A, et al. Systolic myocardial mechanics in hypertrophic cardiomyopathy: novel concepts and implications for clinical status. *J Am Soc Echocardiogr.* 2008;21:675–683.
43. Pirat B, Khoury DS, Hartley CJ, et al. A novel feature-tracking echocardiographic method for the quantitation of regional myocardial function: validation in an animal model of ischemia-reperfusion. *J Am Coll Cardiol.* 2008;51:651–659.
44. D'Hooge J, Heimdal A, Jamal F, et al. Regional strain and strain rate measurements by cardiac ultrasound: principles, implementation and limitations. *Eur J Echocardiogr.* 2000;1:154–170.
45. Dokainish H, Sengupta R, Pillai M, Bobek J, Lakkis N. Usefulness of new diastolic strain and strain rate indexes for the estimation of left ventricular filling pressure. *Am J Cardiol.* 2008;101:1504–1509.
46. Saito M, Okayama H, Nishimura K, et al. Determinants of left ventricular untwisting behaviour in patients with dilated cardiomyopathy: analysis by two-dimensional speckle tracking. *Heart.* 2009;95:290–296.
47. Wang J, Khoury DS, Thohan V, Torre-Amione G, Nagueh SF. Global diastolic strain rate for the assessment of left ventricular relaxation and filling pressures. *Circulation.* 2007;115:1376–1383.
48. Park SJ, Miyazaki C, Bruce CJ, Ommen S, Miller FA, Oh JK. Left ventricular torsion by two-dimensional speckle tracking echocardiography in patients with diastolic dysfunction and normal ejection fraction. *J Am Soc Echocardiogr.* 2008;21:1129–1137.
49. Garceau P, Carasso S, Woo A, Overgaard C, Schwartz L, Rakowski H. Evaluation of left ventricular relaxation and filling pressures in obstructive hypertrophic cardiomyopathy: comparison between invasive hemodynamics and two-dimensional speckle tracking. *Echocardiography.* 2012;29:934–942.
50. Chen S, Yuan J, Qiao S, Duan F, Zhang J, Wang H. Evaluation of left ventricular diastolic function by global strain rate imaging in patients with obstructive hypertrophic cardiomyopathy: a simultaneous speckle tracking echocardiography and cardiac catheterization study. *Echocardiography.* 2014;31:615–622.
51. Waldman LK, Nosan D, Villarreal F, Covell JW. Relation between transmural deformation and local myofiber direction in canine left ventricle. *Circ Res.* 1988;63:550–562.
52. Granzier H, Wu Y, Siegfried L, LeWinter M. Titin: physiological function and role in cardiomyopathy and failure. *Heart Fail Rev.* 2005;10:211–223.
53. Rademakers FE, Buchalter MB, Rogers WJ, et al. Dissociation between left ventricular untwisting and filling. Accentuation by catecholamines. *Circulation.* 1992;85:1572–1581.
54. Notomi Y, Setser RM, Shiota T, et al. Assessment of left ventricular torsional deformation by Doppler tissue imaging: Validation study with tagged magnetic resonance imaging. *Circulation.* 2005;111:1141–1147.
55. Dong SJ, Hees PS, Siu CO, Weiss JL, Shapiro EP. MRI assessment of LV relaxation by untwisting rate: a new isovolumic phase measure of tau. *Am J Physiol Heart Circ Physiol.* 2001;281:H2002–H2009.
56. Notomi Y, Popovic ZB, Yamada H, et al. Ventricular untwisting: a temporal link between left ventricular relaxation and suction. *Am J Physiol Heart Circ Physiol.* 2008;294:H505–H513.
57. Takeuchi M, Borden WB, Nakai H, et al. Reduced and delayed untwisting of the left ventricle in patients with hypertension and left ventricular hypertrophy: a study using two-dimensional speckle tracking imaging. *Eur Heart J.* 2007;28:2756–2762.
58. Carasso S, Yang H, Woo A, Jamorski M, Wigle ED, Rakowski H. Diastolic myocardial mechanics in hypertrophic cardiomyopathy. *J Am Soc Echocardiogr.* 2010;23:164–171.
59. Cameli M, Caputo M, Mondillo S, et al. Feasibility and reference values of left atrial longitudinal strain imaging by two-dimensional speckle tracking. *Cardiovasc Ultrasound.* 2009;7:6.
60. Motoki H, Dahiya A, Bhargava M, et al. Assessment of left atrial mechanics in patients with atrial fibrillation: comparison between two-dimensional speckle-based strain and velocity vector imaging. *J Am Soc Echocardiogr.* 2012;25:428–435.
61. Saraiva RM, Demirkol S, Buakhamsri A, et al. Left atrial strain measured by two-dimensional speckle tracking represents a new tool to evaluate left atrial function. *J Am Soc Echocardiogr.* 2010;23:172–180.
62. Rosca M, Popescu BA, Beladan CC, et al. Left atrial dysfunction as a correlate of heart failure symptoms in hypertrophic cardiomyopathy. *J Am Soc Echocardiogr.* 2010;23:1090–1098.
63. Paraskevaidis IA, Farmakis D, Papadopoulos C, et al. Two-dimensional strain analysis in patients with hypertrophic cardiomyopathy and normal systolic function: a 12-month follow-up study. *Am Heart J.* 2009;158:444–450.
64. Maron BJ, Haas TS, Maron MS, et al. Left atrial remodeling in hypertrophic cardiomyopathy and susceptibility markers for atrial fibrillation identified by cardiovascular magnetic resonance. *Am J Cardiol.* 2014;113:1394–1400.
65. Williams LK, Chan RH, Carasso S, et al. Effect of left ventricular outflow tract obstruction on left atrial mechanics in hypertrophic cardiomyopathy. *Biomed Res Int.* 2015;2015:481245.
66. Basser PJ. Inferring microstructural features and the physiological state of tissues from diffusion-weighted images. *NMR Biomed.* 1995;8:333–344.
67. Basser PJ, Mattiello J, LeBihan D. MR diffusion tensor spectroscopy and imaging. *Biophys J.* 1994;66:259–267.
68. Ferreira PF, Kilner PJ, McGill LA, et al. In vivo cardiovascular magnetic resonance diffusion tensor imaging shows evidence of abnormal myocardial laminar orientations and mobility in hypertrophic cardiomyopathy. *J Cardiovasc Magn Reson.* 2014;16:87.
69. Nielles-Vallespin S, Khalique Z, Ferreira PF, et al. Assessment of myocardial microstructural dynamics by in vivo diffusion tensor cardiac magnetic resonance. *J Am Coll Cardiol.* 2017;69:661–676.
70. Wolf-Maier K, Cooper RS, Banegas JR, et al. Hypertension prevalence and blood pressure levels in 6 European countries, Canada, and the United States. *JAMA.* 2003;289:2363–2369.
71. Baltabaeva A, Marciniak M, Bijnens B, et al. Regional left ventricular deformation and geometry analysis provides insights in myocardial remodelling in mild to moderate hypertension. *Eur J Echocardiogr.* 2008;9:501–508.
72. Kato TS, Noda A, Izawa H, et al. Discrimination of nonobstructive hypertrophic cardiomyopathy from hypertensive left ventricular hypertrophy on the basis of strain rate imaging by tissue Doppler ultrasonography. *Circulation.* 2004;110:3808–3814.
73. Vinereanu D, Florescu N, Sculthorpe N, Tweddel AC, Stephens MR, Fraser AG. Differentiation between pathologic and physiologic left ventricular hypertrophy by tissue Doppler assessment of long-axis function in patients with hypertrophic cardiomyopathy or systemic hypertension and in athletes. *Am J Cardiol.* 2001;88:53–58.
74. Pelliccia A, Maron BJ, Spataro A, Proschan MA, Spirito P. The upper limit of physiologic cardiac hypertrophy in highly trained elite athletes. *N Engl J Med.* 1991;324:295–301.
75. Papadakis M, Carre F, Kervio G, et al. The prevalence, distribution, and clinical outcomes of electrocardiographic repolarization patterns in male athletes of African/Afro-Caribbean origin. *Eur Heart J.* 2011;32:2304–2313.
76. Palka P, Lange A, Fleming AD, et al. Differences in myocardial velocity gradient measured throughout the cardiac cycle in patients with hypertrophic cardiomyopathy, athletes and patients with left ventricular hypertrophy due to hypertension. *J Am Coll Cardiol.* 1997;30:760–768.

77. Kovacs A, Apor A, Nagy A, et al. Left ventricular untwisting in athlete's heart: Key role in early diastolic filling? *Int J Sports Med.* 2014 Mar;35(3):259-64. doi: 10.1055/s-0033-1349076.
78. Spindler M, Saupe KW, Christe ME, et al. Diastolic dysfunction and altered energetics in the alphamhc403/+ mouse model of familial hypertrophic cardiomyopathy. *J Clin Invest.* 1998;101:1775–1783.
79. Ho CY, Sweitzer NK, McDonough B, et al. Assessment of diastolic function with Doppler tissue imaging to predict genotype in preclinical hypertrophic cardiomyopathy. *Circulation.* 2002;105:2992–2997.
80. Nagueh SF, Bachinski LL, Meyer D, et al. Tissue Doppler imaging consistently detects myocardial abnormalities in patients with hypertrophic cardiomyopathy and provides a novel means for an early diagnosis before and independently of hypertrophy. *Circulation.* 2001;104:128–130.
81. Bourmayan C, Razavi A, Fournier C, et al. Effect of propranolol on left ventricular relaxation in hypertrophic cardiomyopathy: an echographic study. *Am Heart J.* 1985;109:1311–1316.
82. Hess OM, Grimm J, Krayenbuehl HP. Diastolic function in hypertrophic cardiomyopathy: Effects of propranolol and verapamil on diastolic stiffness. *Eur Heart J.* 1983;4(F):S47–S56.
83. Doiuchi J, Hamada M, Ito T, Kokubu T. Comparative effects of calcium-channel blockers and beta-adrenergic blocker on early diastolic time intervals and A-wave ratio in patients with hypertrophic cardiomyopathy. *Clin Cardiol.* 1987;10:26–30.
84. McTaggart DR. Diltiazem reverses tissue Doppler velocity abnormalities in pre-clinical hypertrophic cardiomyopathy. *Heart Lung Circ.* 2004;13:39–40.
85. Matsubara H, Nakatani S, Nagata S, et al. Salutary effect of disopyramide on left ventricular diastolic function in hypertrophic obstructive cardiomyopathy. *J Am Coll Cardiol.* 1995;26:768–775.
86. Sumimoto T, Hamada M, Ohtani T, et al. Effect of disopyramide on left ventricular diastolic function in patients with hypertrophic cardiomyopathy: comparison with diltiazem. *Cardiovasc Drugs Ther.* 1992;6:425–428.
87. Abozguia K, Elliott P, McKenna W, et al. Metabolic modulator perhexiline corrects energy deficiency and improves exercise capacity in symptomatic hypertrophic cardiomyopathy. *Circulation.* 2010;122:1562–1569.
88. Coppini R, Ferrantini C, Yao L, et al. Late sodium current inhibition reverses electromechanical dysfunction in human hypertrophic cardiomyopathy. *Circulation.* 2013;127:575–584.
89. Olivotto I, Camici PG, Merlini PA, et al. Efficacy of ranolazine in patients with symptomatic hypertrophic cardiomyopathy: the restyle-HCM randomized, double-blind, placebo-controlled study. *Circ Heart Fail.* 2018;11:e004124.
90. Olivotto I, Hellawell JL, Farzaneh-Far R, et al. Novel approach targeting the complex pathophysiology of hypertrophic cardiomyopathy: the impact of late sodium current inhibition on exercise capacity in subjects with symptomatic hypertrophic cardiomyopathy (liberty-hcm) trial. *Circ Heart Fail.* 2016;9:e002764.
91. Sitges M, Shiota T, Lever HM, et al. Comparison of left ventricular diastolic function in obstructive hypertrophic cardiomyopathy in patients undergoing percutaneous septal alcohol ablation versus surgical myotomy/myectomy. *Am J Cardiol.* 2003;91:817–821.
92. Rovner A, Smith R, Greenberg NL, et al. Improvement in diastolic intraventricular pressure gradients in patients with HOCM after ethanol septal reduction. *Am J Physiol Heart Circ Physiol.* 2003;285:H2492–H2499.
93. Park TH, Lakkis NM, Middleton KJ, et al. Acute effect of nonsurgical septal reduction therapy on regional left ventricular asynchrony in patients with hypertrophic obstructive cardiomyopathy. *Circulation.* 2002;106:412–415.
94. Abraham TP, Nishimura RA, Holmes DR Jr, Belohlavek M, Seward JB. Strain rate imaging for assessment of regional myocardial function: results from a clinical model of septal ablation. *Circulation.* 2002;105:1403–1406.
95. Cannon RO III, McIntosh CL, Schenke WH, Maron BJ, Bonow RO, Epstein SE. Effect of surgical reduction of left ventricular outflow obstruction on hemodynamics, coronary flow, and myocardial metabolism in hypertrophic cardiomyopathy. *Circulation.* 1989;79:766–775.
96. Mazur W, Nagueh SF, Lakkis NM, et al. Regression of left ventricular hypertrophy after nonsurgical septal reduction therapy for hypertrophic obstructive cardiomyopathy. *Circulation.* 2001;103:1492–1496.
97. Quinones JA, DeLeon SY, Vitullo DA, et al. Regression of hypertrophic cardiomyopathy after modified konno procedure. *Ann Thorac Surg.* 1995;60:1250–1254.
98. Ho CY, Mealiffe ME, Bach RG, et al. Evaluation of Mavacamten in Symptomatic Patients With Nonobstructive Hypertrophic Cardiomyopathy. *J Am Coll Cardiol.* 2020;75(21):2649–2660.

26

Pericardial Diseases: Constrictive Pericarditis and Pericardial Effusion

William R. Miranda and Jae K. Oh

OUTLINE

Case Study

A 69-year-old man presented with progressive leg edema, abdominal fullness, shortness of breath, and 30-lb weight gain over the course of 24 months. Past medical history included hypertension and hyperlipidemia on medical therapy. He denied any history of rheumatologic disorder, previous radiation therapy, or cardiothoracic surgery. Physical exam revealed markedly elevated venous pressure (Video 26.1) with prominent x and y descents. Cardiac auscultation showed a high-pitched early diastolic heart sound at the cardiac apex. There was hepatomegaly and bilateral leg edema. Laboratory work revealed normal blood counts, mild elevation in alkaline phosphatase (140 U/L; normal range 40–129), and NT-terminal pro-brain natriuretic peptide (NT-proBNP) (288 pg/mL; reference <97) levels. C-reactive protein level and sedimentation rate were normal. Chest radiography did not show any evidence of pulmonary venous hypertension but revealed calcification of the pericardium. Transthoracic echocardiography (TTE) was performed, showing normal biventricular function and no significant valvular disease. There was severe dilatation of the inferior vena cava (IVC) with minimal inspiratory collapse. Respiratophasic ventricular septal shift (Video 26.2) and expiratory reversals in the hepatic vein pulsed-wave (PW) Doppler were seen. As part of his workup for dyspnea, a chest computerized tomography (CT) was performed; it confirmed the presence of pericardial calcification and revealed marked circumferential thickening of the pericardium (Fig. 26.1A). Cardiac magnetic resonance imaging (MRI) confirmed increased pericardial thickening (maximal thickness 9 mm) (see Fig. 26.1B) without late gadolinium enhancement. The diagnosis of constrictive pericarditis (CP) was made and the patient was referred to surgical pericardiectomy, which was performed without complications.

EPIDEMIOLOGY

CP is a form of diastolic heart failure, secondary to reduced pericardial compliance in the setting of pericardial inflammation and/or fibrosis.[1] The diagnosis of CP in a patient presenting with heart failure is of extreme importance since it is a potentially curable disorder. In addition when left untreated it carries a poor prognosis.[2]

The prevalence of CP is still poorly understood but has been documented in 0.2% to 0.4% of patients following cardiac surgery.[3,4] Over the past half century, the epidemiology of CP has significantly changed.[5] Although tuberculous pericarditis remains the most common cause of CP worldwide,[6,7] its occurrence is now extremely rare in the United States and Europe. Concurrently, the number of iatrogenic CP cases (postcardiac surgery and radiation related) has markedly risen. In a series from our institution,[8] idiopathic and postcardiac surgery accounted for more than 65% of CP cases, followed in frequency by radiation. Similar results have also been published by others.[9,10] Less common causes of CP include connective tissue disorders, malignancy, and trauma.

PATHOPHYSIOLOGY

In CP, diastolic filling is limited due to an inelastic or stiff pericardium.[1,5] Reduced pericardial compliance might be secondary to active inflammation or varying degrees of pericardial fibrosis, scarring, and/or calcification. The development of CP might occur acutely and subacutely, where pericardial inflammation typically prevails, or chronically, in which pericardial fibrosis is the dominant feature. Once felt to be an irreversible condition, it is now well established that a subset of patients with predominantly inflammatory CP can respond to anti-inflammatory

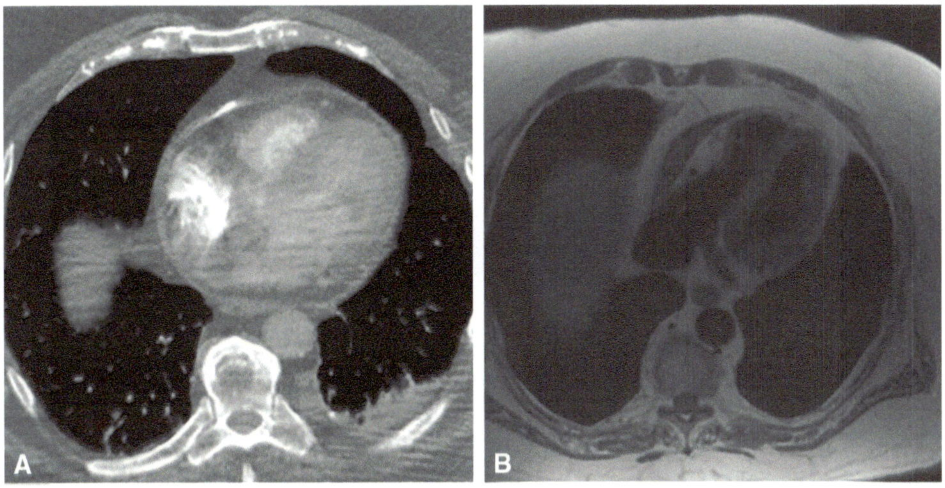

Fig. 26.1 Case study: Computerized tomography and cardiac magnetic resonance imaging findings. Pericardial calcification is seen on CT (A). Cardiac MRI showed marked pericardial thickening.

therapy, thus foregoing the need for surgical treatment, an entity described as transient CP.[11,12]

Pericardial thickening is seen in most (80%) but not all patients with CP[13] (Fig. 26.2A). Although it is still unclear why a subset of patients will develop pericardial constriction following an insult to the pericardium, it is well established that some etiologies (particularly tuberculous pericarditis) carry a high risk of evolving into a constrictive phase. In contrast, the risk of developing CP after idiopathic or postviral pericarditis has been reported to be low, occurring in less than 1% of individuals.[14]

It should be noted that although CP is primarily a disease of the pericardium, in long-standing, chronic isolated CP cases, myocardial atrophy may also develop.[8] Moreover, CP may occur in patients with preexisting underlying myocardial disease, such as those who received radiation therapy or postcardiac surgery. In these patients, features of CP and restrictive cardiomyopathy (RCM) can then coexist, potentially making the recognition and diagnosis of CP more challenging.[15]

Increased ventricular interdependence and dissociation of intrathoracic and intracardiac pressures[1,16] are the two hemodynamic hallmarks of CP. The inelastic, scarred pericardium markedly impairs cardiac distention but also prevents variations in intrathoracic pressures to be fully transmitted to the cardiac chambers.[17] As a consequence, during inspiration, the pressure gradient between the pulmonary veins (which are extrapericardial structures) and the left heart decreases, reducing left atrial filling. Thus left ventricular (LV) filling (and consequently LV output) decreases upon inspiration. The ventricular septum then bows leftward, favoring right ventricular (RV) filling as systemic venous return increases. Upon expiration, the opposite occurs: LV inflow increases, RV filling decreases, and the

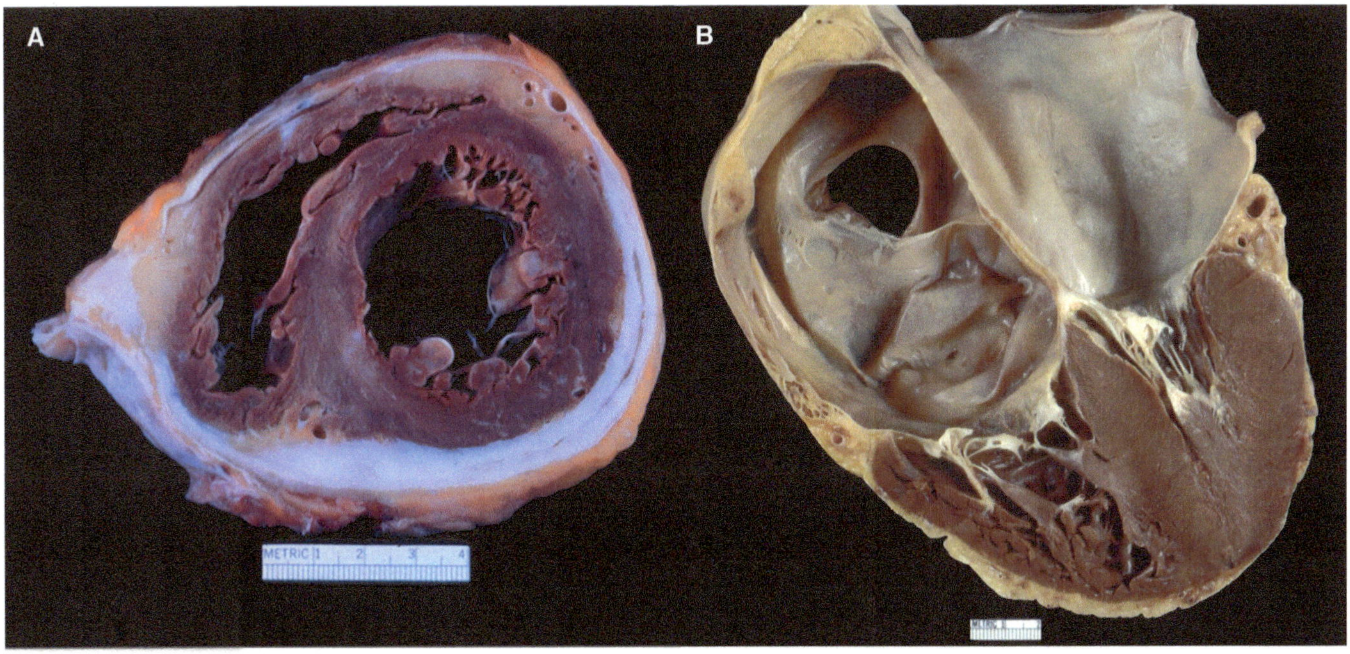

Fig. 26.2 Pathology findings in constrictive pericarditis and restrictive cardiomyopathy. (A) Typical findings of constrictive pericarditis, showing a thickened and fibrotic pericardium. (B) Pathology specimen of idiopathic restrictive cardiomyopathy, showing prominent biatrial enlargement with normal-size ventricles. (A, Courtesy of William D. Edwards, MD; B, Courtesy of Joseph J. Maleszewski, MD).

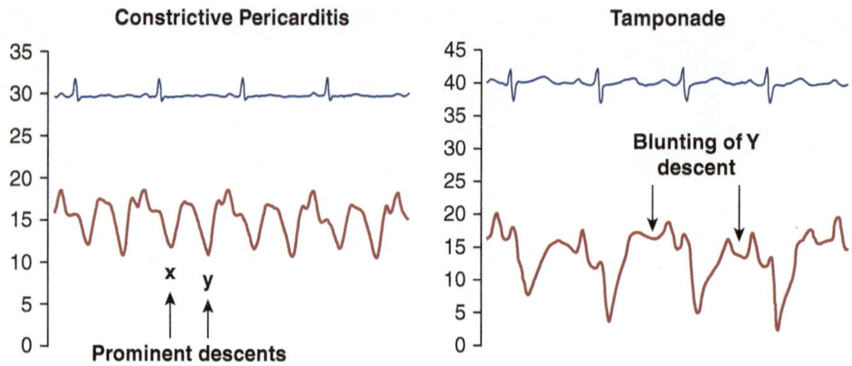

Fig. 26.3 **Right atrial tracings in constrictive pericarditis and cardiac tamponade.** Prominent x and y descents are seen in constrictive pericarditis *(left panel)* in contrast to the typical blunted y descents seen in cardiac tamponade.

septum shifts rightward. Therefore RV and LV volumes and stroke volumes will inversely vary according to phases of the respiratory cycle—the so-called increased ventricular interdependence or enhanced ventricular interaction. Lastly, the significantly elevated right atrial (RA) and left atrial (LA) pressures promote prominent early diastolic flow into the ventricles; however, pericardial reserve volume is rapidly reached, leading to marked diminution of ventricular filling toward mid-late diastole. This is the origin of the rapid filling on invasive ventricular pressure tracings or increased early diastolic velocity (E)/A ratios by Doppler seen in CP.

Although cardiac tamponade also results in severe abnormalities of diastolic function and elevated filling pressures, it is worth highlighting that its underlying hemodynamics markedly differ from CP.[18] In tamponade, the elevated pericardial pressure impairs diastolic filling (particularly in early diastole). This leads to the hallmark feature of cardiac tamponade on cardiac catheterization: blunting of y descents (Fig. 26.3). Thus, early ventricular diastolic filling in classic cardiac tamponade and CP are actually on opposite ends of a spectrum (blunted vs. enhanced, respectively). Some patients with cardiac tamponade might actually develop constrictive features after pericardiocentesis has been performed and cardiac tamponade has been relieved. This clinical entity has been described as effusive-constrictive pericarditis[19–21]; its hemodynamic signature is the persistence of elevated central venous pressures following completed evacuation of the pericardial effusion. The first clue to its diagnosis should be the failure of the jugular venous pressures to normalize following pericardiocentesis, but in these patients features of CP are seen postpericardiocentesis both invasively (cardiac catheterization) and noninvasively (echo Doppler). Clinicians should be aware of the existence of effusive-constrictive pericarditis, as higher rates of pericardiectomy and heart failure hospitalization during follow-up have been described in these patients.

DIAGNOSTIC EVALUATION

Clinical Presentation and Physical Exam Findings

Individuals with CP will typically present with signs and symptoms of right-sided heart failure, such as elevated venous pressure, ascites, and leg edema. Dyspnea can also be present. CP should always be excluded in patient's presenting with heart failure with preserved ventricular function and predominant right-sided failure, as well as in those presenting with progressive heart failure in the setting of previous cardiac surgery.

At bedside, elevation in jugular venous pressure is almost universal, with the typical venous contour of CP, showing prominent x and y descents (see Video 26.1). This pattern is the opposite of what is typically seen in severe tricuspid regurgitation (TR), where a large positive wave (the V wave) instead of a negative wave (i.e., descent) is present. In CP, an increase in venous pressure upon inspiration might also be seen (Kussmaul sign). This, however, is not pathognomonic of CP and can be seen in any pathology resulting in significantly reduced compliance of the right-sided chambers. Cardiac auscultation can reveal a high-pitched apical early diastolic sound, the so-called pericardial knock; this is a specific but not sensitive finding for the presence of CP. Nonpulsatile hepatomegaly and leg edema are also usually present.

Chest Radiography and Electrocardiography

Pericardial calcification on chest radiography may be seen in patients with CP (Fig. 26.4); however, this finding is only seen in approximately one-fourth of patients with CP.[22] Findings of pulmonary venous congestion, cardiomegaly, or massive biatrial enlargement may be a clue to an underlying cardiomyopathic rather than a pericardial process.[23]

Electrocardiography typically shows nonspecific ST-T wave changes. The presence of large P waves similar to those observed in mitral stenosis has also been reported as an electrocardiographic sign of CP.[24] Lastly, the presence of atrial fibrillation is not an uncommon finding among patients with pericardial constriction.

Laboratory Evaluation

Mild elevation in liver enzymes (especially alkaline phosphatase) and creatinine levels are common in CP. Plasma B-type natriuretic peptide levels have been shown to be lower in patients with CP than in those with RCM. However, there can be significant overlap among those with CP and underlying myocardial disease, such those with radiation-induced CP.[25]

Transthoracic Echocardiography

Currently, TTE is the diagnostic modality of choice for the diagnosis of CP.[14] The echocardiographic diagnosis of constrictive physiology is based on the constellation of two-dimensional (2-D) and Doppler abnormalities that will reflect the hemodynamic pillars of CP: enhanced ventricular interaction, dissociation of intrathoracic-intracardiac pressures, and elevation of ventricular filling pressures. The echo Doppler evaluation should always involve a detailed assessment of septal motion, mitral inflow PW and mitral annular tissue Doppler, medial and lateral tissue Doppler of the mitral annulus, evaluation of IVC size/collapsibility, and PW Doppler of the hepatic veins. It should be highlighted that if CP is suspected, the mimickers of CP should be actively sought and excluded by echocardiography.

Abnormal motion of the ventricular septum is one of the first clues to the echocardiographic diagnosis of CP. One of two abnormalities can be seen: respirophasic septal shift or a septal bounce/shudder. The septal

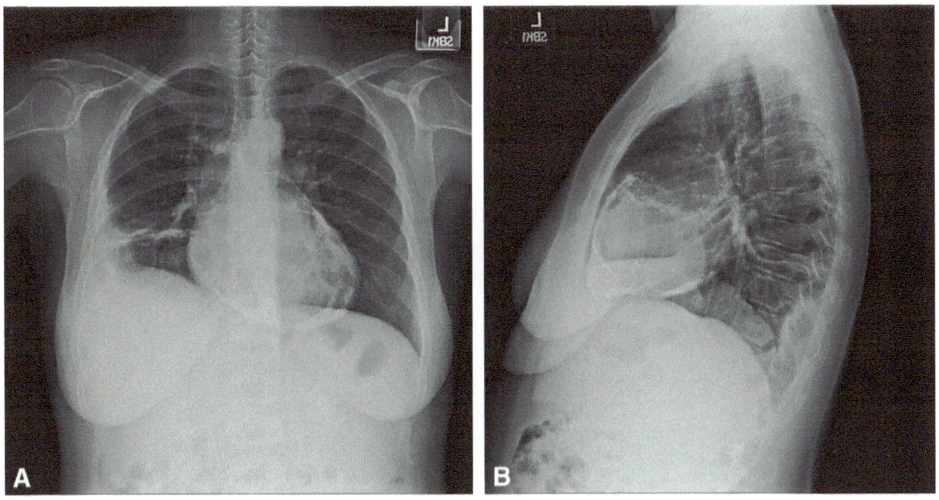

Fig. 26.4 Chest radiography in patients with constrictive pericarditis. Extensive pericardial calcification is seen on posteroanterior (A) and lateral (B) views.

shift is a consequence of the enhanced ventricular interaction and is manifested by respiratory changes in ventricular septal position, with the ventricular septum moving toward the left ventricle during inspiration (as RV volume increases with increased systemic venous return) with opposite motion following expiration (Fig. 26.5; see Video 26.2). The detection of respirophasic septal shift is enhanced when longer clips (10 beat) are recorded. Conversely, this finding can be easily missed when short (1-beat or 2-beat) clips are recorded. In our series,[26] respirophasic septal shift was present in 93% of patients with CP, with a positive predictive value of 92% and a negative predictive value of 74%. The septal

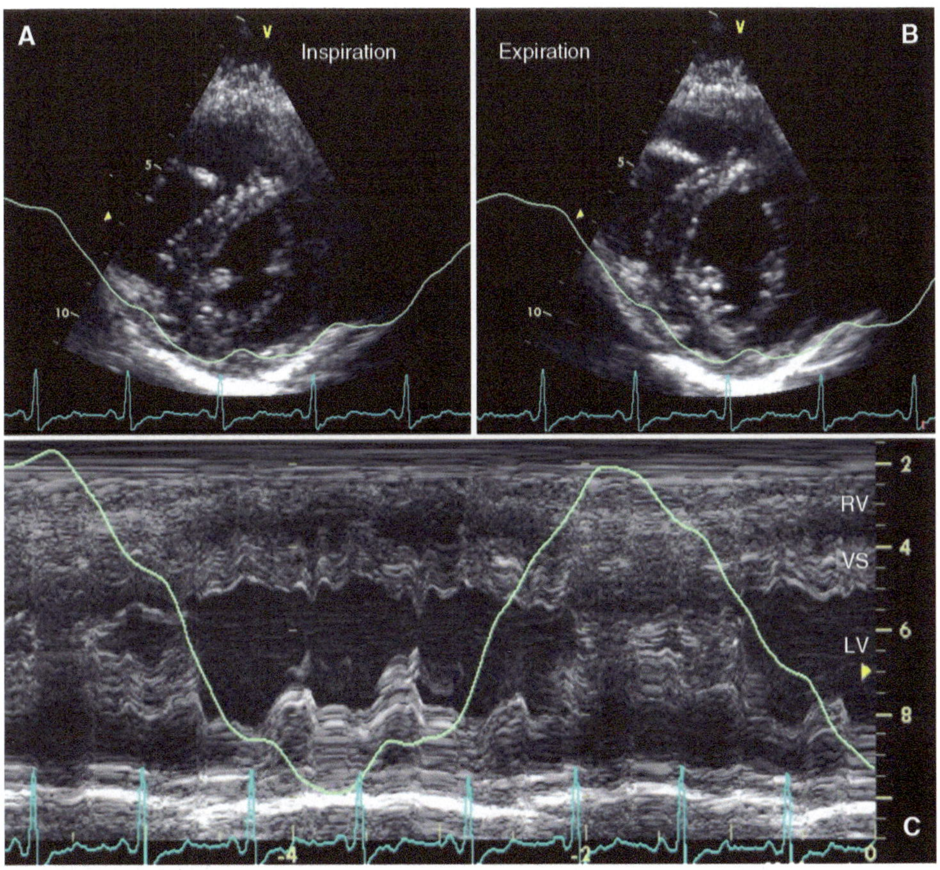

Fig. 26.5 Respirophasic septal shift in patients with constrictive pericarditis. Two-dimensional echocardiography shows septal shift toward the left ventricle during expiration (A) with the opposite occurring during expiration (B). M mode at the midventricular level shows reciprocal inspiratory and expiratory variation in right and left ventricular size and obvious respirophasic septal shift (C). Note the presence the early diastolic septal notch and flattening of LV posterior wall *(best seen on the third beat). LV,* Left ventricle; *RV,* right ventricle; *VS,* ventricular septum.

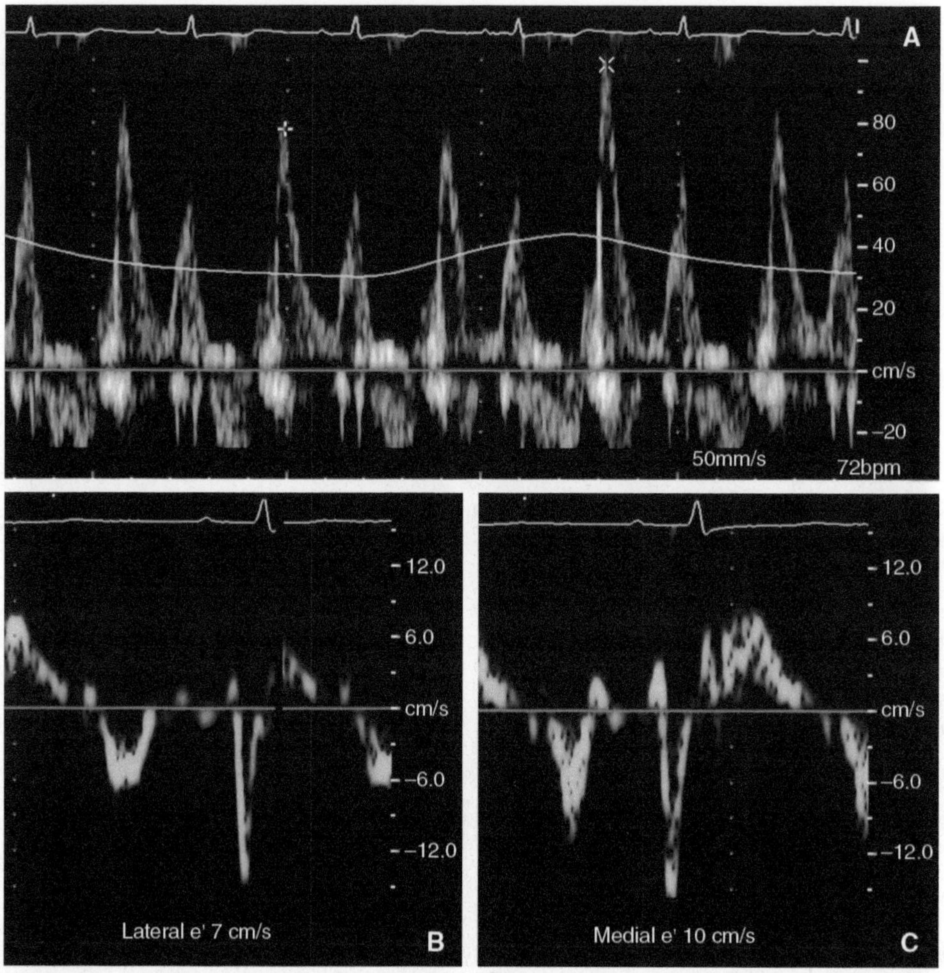

Fig. 26.6 Mitral inflow and annular tissue Doppler in a patient with constrictive pericarditis. Pulsed-wave Doppler of the mitral inflow (A) shows an increased E/A ratio with short deceleration time; note the marked inspiratory decrease in E velocities. Mitral annular tissue Doppler demonstrates an elevated medial e′ velocity (C), higher than the lateral counterpart (B) (i.e., annulus reversus). (*Green tracing* corresponds to simultaneous respirometer; the upward deflect marks the onset of inspiration, whereas the downward deflect marks the onset of expiration.)

bounce results from instantaneous pressure differences between diastolic RV and LV pressures.[27] Although a sensitive finding for CP, it has lower specificity, as it might be challenging to distinguish from abnormal septal motion due to conduction abnormalities or postoperative state.

Attention should then be turned to mitral valve/annular Doppler findings. The presence of elevated (≥9 cm/sec) medial e′ in patients presenting with heart failure should be another clue that CP might be present (Fig. 26.6). Early tissue Doppler velocity is a measure of ventricular relaxation and thus medial e′ velocity is expected to be reduced in patients with intrinsic myocardial disorders.[28] In contrast, due to myocardial tethering to the abnormal pericardium, myocardial velocities at the medial mitral annulus tend to be exaggerated in CP. Noteworthy, only a mildly increased medial e′ might be present in patients with CP following cardiac surgery or radiation therapy given the concomitant myocardial disease. In our experience, patients with radiation-induced CP had a lower septal e′ than patients with primary CP (9.5 cm/sec vs 14.5 cm/sec), with patients with postcardiac surgery CP having intermediate values (11.1 cm/sec).[26] Lastly, also a consequence of LV tethering, mitral lateral e′ might be lower than its medial counterpart, which is the opposite of normal (annulus reversus) (see Fig. 26.6).

As stated in the diastolic function assessment guidelines, mitral inflow PW Doppler typically shows an E/A ratio above 0.8: An expiratory E/A ratio below 1 makes CP extremely unlikely, as it was seen in only 6% of surgically proven CP cases.[29] Inspiratory reduction in PW mitral early diastolic velocities (E) was one of the first echocardiographic features of CP described (see Fig. 26.6), reflecting the underlying dissociation of intrathoracic-intracardiac pressures. Traditionally, inspiratory decreases greater than 25% are suggestive of CP.[30] Although minimal changes in mitral E velocities are present in normal individuals, the degree of respirophasic oscillation in E velocity in patients with CP can be quite variable. Moreover, obesity and primary obstructive pulmonary disorders can also lead to marked variations in mitral E velocities. Thus, although respirophasic variations in mitral E velocities are in keeping with pericardial diseases, its diagnostic yield is limited (a change in mitral E velocity of 15% was found to have a sensitivity of 84% and a specificity of 73% for the diagnosis of CP).[26]

Dilatation of the IVC with abnormal collapsibility is almost a universal finding in CP, and a small-sized IVC should strongly argue against the presence of hemodynamically significant constrictive physiology (an IVC diameter <21 mm or an inspiratory collapse ≥50% was present in only 2% of cases in our CP series).[26] Interrogation of hepatic vein flow by PW Doppler should also be a mandatory step in the echocardiographic evaluation of patients with suspected pericardial disease. The typical feature of CP on hepatic vein Doppler is the

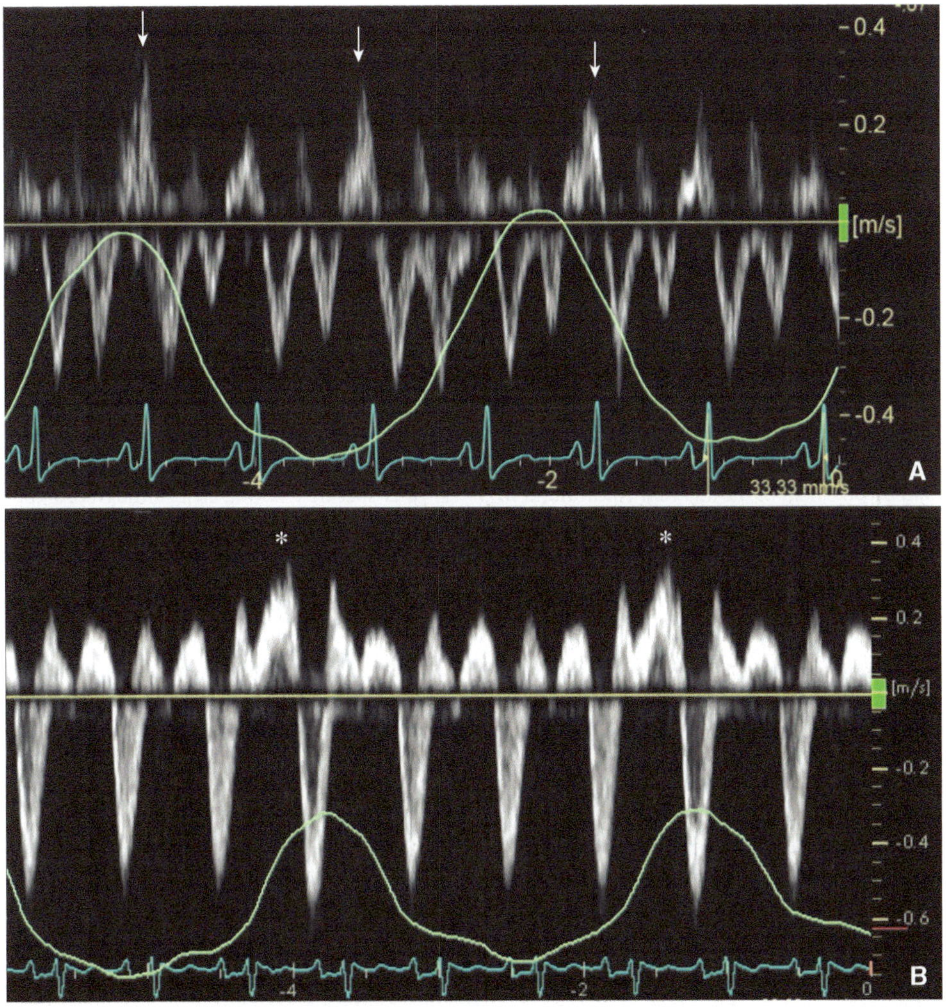

Fig. 26.7 Hepatic vein Doppler in constrictive pericarditis and restrictive cardiomyopathy. Pulsed-wave hepatic vein Doppler (A) shows the typical increased expiratory diastolic flow reversals seen in constrictive pericarditis *(arrows)*. In contrast, in patients with restrictive cardiomyopathy, prominent inspiratory diastolic reversals *(asterisk)* are seen; note the markedly diminished systolic forward flow velocities in this patient, suggesting significantly impaired atrial relaxation/tricuspid annular descent. (*Green tracings* correspond to simultaneous respirometer; the upward deflect marks the onset of inspiration, whereas the downward deflect marks the onset of expiration.)

presence of enhanced expiratory diastolic flow reversals (Fig. 26.7A), with this being the most specific echo Doppler finding for the diagnosis of CP.[26,29] Hepatic vein Doppler is also extremely helpful in identifying conditions that can mimic CP on echocardiography. In RCM, hepatic vein Doppler will show inspiratory increase in diastolic flow reversals[31] (see Fig. 26.7B), reflecting the inability of the noncompliant right ventricle to accommodate the inspiratory increase in venous return, whereas hepatic vein Doppler will show systolic flow reversals when severe TR is present (typically holosystolic in very severe cases).

Lastly, the presence of deformation of the cardiac chambers' contour, tethering of the ventricular walls, or the presence of liver tug (pulling of liver edge by the right ventricle during systole), might provide additional information but should not be used to confirm or refute the diagnosis of CP.

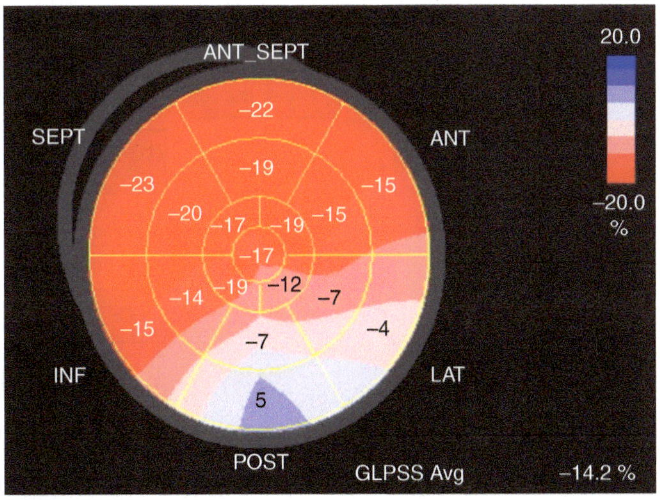

Fig. 26.8 Speckle tracking echocardiography in constrictive pericarditis. Speckle tracking echocardiography shows markedly decreased longitudinal strain in the posterior and lateral wall with increased strain in the septal segments.

Speckle Tracking Imaging

2-D speckle tracking has been suggested to be a useful tool in the assessment of patients with CP and restrictive cardiomyopathy[32] (Fig. 26.8). Global and segmental circumferential strain were found to be lower in CP than in RCM and controls[33]; this was felt to be related

TABLE 26.1 Mayo Clinic Echocardiographic Criteria for the Diagnosis of Constrictive Pericarditis

Criteria	Sensitivity	Specificity	PPV	NPV
1. Ventricular septal shift	93	69	92	74
2. Change in mitral E velocity >14.6%	84	73	92	55
3. Medial e′ velocity ≥9 cm/sec	83	81	94	57
4. Medial e′/lateral e′ ≥0.91	75	85	95	50
5. Hepatic vein diastolic reversal velocity/forward velocity in expiration ≥0.79	76	88	96	49
Criteria 1 and 3	80	92	97	56
Criteria 1 with 3 or 5	87	91	97	65
Criteria 1 with 3 and 5	64	97	99	42

NPV, Negative predictive value; *PPV*, positive predictive value.
From Welch TD, Ling LH, Espinosa RE, et al. Echocardiographic diagnosis of constrictive pericarditis: Mayo Clinic criteria. *Circ Cardiovasc Imag.* 2014;7(3):526–534.

to pericardial restraint and involvement of the adjacent epicardium. In contrast, patients with RCM were also found to have significantly lower global longitudinal strain (GLS) compared to patients with CP, and GLS has been suggested to be of incremental diagnostic value when added to tissue Doppler, respirophasic septal shift, LV ejection fraction, and ventricular mass.[33]

Studies have also demonstrated that strain abnormalities in CP are heterogeneous (reflecting tethering of the myocardium), whereas it tends to be homogeneous in RCM. Kusunose et. al.[34] reported that longitudinal strain was lower in RCM than CP and also noted that this reduction was uniform. In contrast, patients with CP had lower strain in the RV and LV free walls compared to the ventricular septum. Longitudinal and circumferential myocardial strain values were reported to improve following pericardiectomy, particularly in the ventricular free walls.[34]

2-D speckle tracking echocardiography can be particularly helpful in identifying specific etiologies causing hemodynamic derangements, such as amyloid-related RCM or hypertrophic cardiomyopathy leading to restrictive filling patterns.

Diagnostic Algorithm for the Echocardiographic Diagnosis of CP

Our group has proposed a set of diagnostic criteria for the echocardiographic diagnosis of CP (Mayo Clinic criteria).[26] Table 26.1 summarizes sensitivity and specificity of various echo Doppler findings. The presence of respirophasic septal shift accompanied by a medial e′ velocity of 9 cm/sec and above or a hepatic vein Doppler diastolic reversal/forward velocity ratio of 0.79 and above yields a sensitivity of 91% and specificity of 97% for the diagnosis of CP. When all three criteria were met, the sensitivity and specificity were 97% and 99%, respectively. Fig. 26.9 illustrates a proposed approach for the echocardiographic diagnosis of CP.

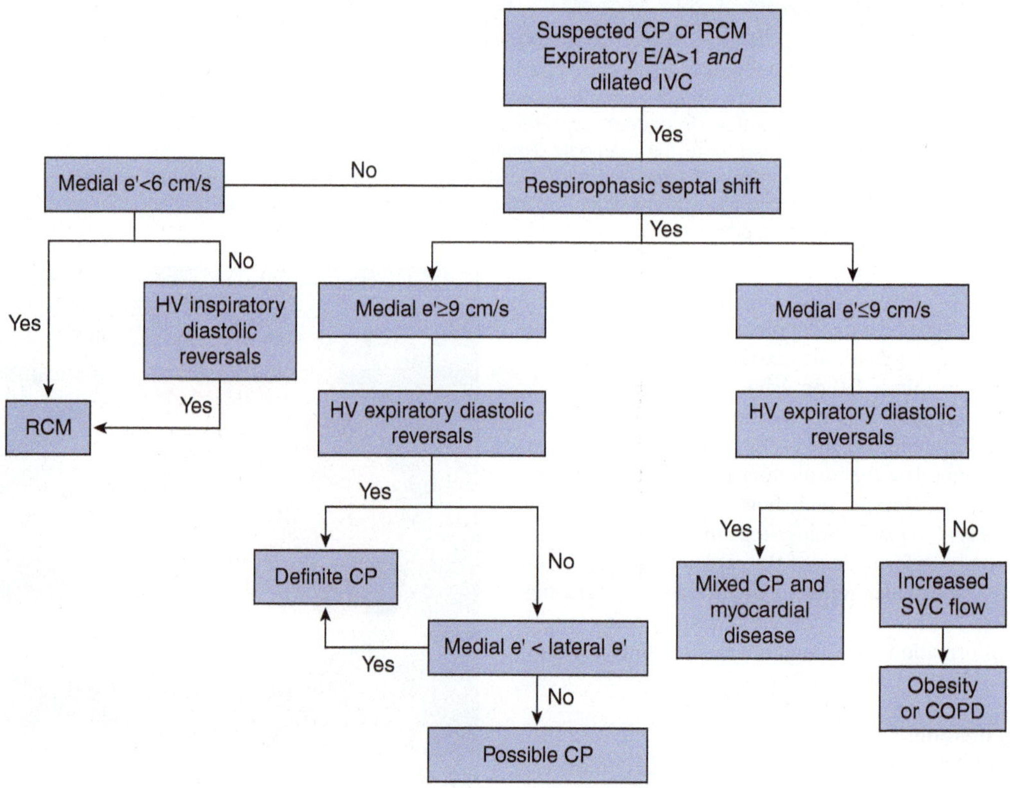

Fig. 26.9 Proposed algorithm for the diagnosis of constrictive pericarditis using echo Doppler. *COPD*, Chronic obstructive pulmonary disease; *CP*, constrictive pericarditis; *HV*, hepatic vein; *IVC*, inferior vena cava; *RCM*, restrictive cardiomyopathy; *SVC*, superior vena cava.

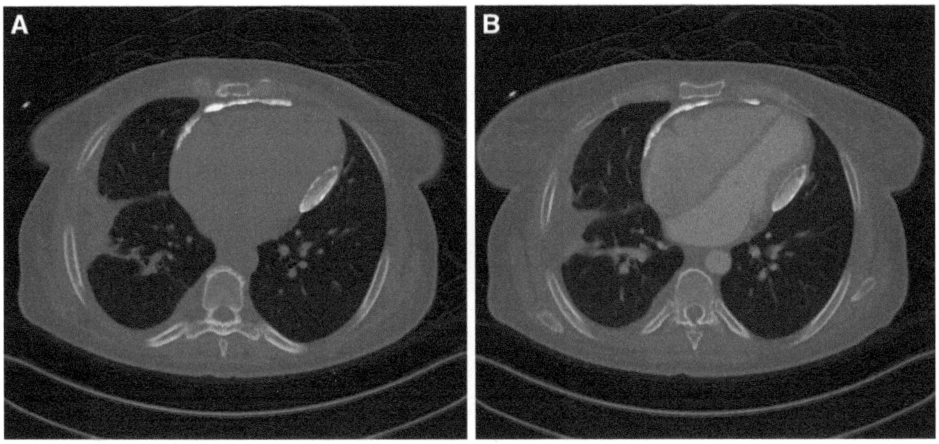

Fig. 26.10 Chest CT in a patient with constrictive pericarditis. Noncontrast study (A) shows extensive calcification of the pericardium anteriorly and posteriorly. Following intravenous contrast administration (B), distortion of the left ventricular contours is seen. (Courtesy of Dr. Nandan Anavekar.)

Computerized Tomography

CT provides great anatomic assessment of the pericardium given its spatial resolution.[15] Findings consistent with CP on CT include increased pericardial thickness, pericardial calcification, deformation of the cardiac contour,[35] and abnormal septal motion on gated cine images[36] (Fig. 26.10). Other supportive findings include dilatation of the IVC, hepatic congestion, and ascites.

Normal pericardial thickness by CT should measure 2 mm or less.[37] The presence of pathologic thickening of the pericardium (>4 mm) is highly suggestive of CP, and pericardial thickness by CT has been correlated with reduced lateral mitral e′ velocities.[38] However, the absence of pericardial thickening does not exclude the presence of constriction; normal pericardial thickness by CT has been reported in 18 of surgically confirmed CP cases.[39] Conversely, the presence of a thickened pericardium should not be seen as pathognomonic for CP, as it can be seen in acute pericarditis in the absence of constrictive features as well as other disorders such as uremia.[35]

CT provides additional information for preoperative planning. Coronary anatomy can be outlined and the presence of significant coronary atherosclerosis ruled out, forgoing the need for routine invasive coronary angiography. In addition, CT outlines thoracic and mediastinal anatomy, which may be critical in patients with prior cardiac operations (e.g., determining the location of the coronary artery bypass grafts). Lastly, it provides important information in patients with prior pericardiectomy, as it demonstrates areas of residual/remaining pericardial tissue.

Cardiac MRI

Cardiac MRI is now an integral diagnostic test in the assessment of patients with pericardial disorders.[40,41] Perhaps the most useful role of cardiac MRI lies in the determination of concomitant pericardial inflammation, but cardiac MRI is also superior to CT in the assessment of pericardial edema and pericardial fluid. The assessment of late gadolinium enhancement is now an integral part in the cardiac MRI assessment of patients with suspected pericarditis as it provides diagnostic and therapeutic information (Fig. 26.11). The presence and extent (both qualitatively[42] and quantitatively[43]) of pericardial late gadolinium enhancement has been shown to predict the response to anti-inflammatory therapy in patients with CP, and this may obviate the need for surgical pericardiectomy. Cardiac MRI might also provide incremental information regarding the presence of an alternative diagnosis based on the presence of extensive myocardial delayed enhancement or typical cardiac MRI features of amyloidosis.

Similar to CT, the presence of pericardial thickening on cardiac MRI is highly suggestive of CP; a thickness greater than 4 mm has been shown to have a 93% diagnostic accuracy when distinguishing CP from restrictive cardiomyopathy.[44] Cardiac MRI provides not only morphologic assessment of the cardiac chambers and pericardium, but also allows for physiologic assessment using free-breathing series. Ventricular septal excursion has been shown to differentiate CP from restrictive cardiomyopathy.[45]

Cardiac Catheterization

Due to advances in echo Doppler as well as cross-sectional imaging, invasive hemodynamic evaluation, once a mandatory step in the diagnostic evaluation of patients with suspected CP, is now reserved for select cases. Since these patients tend to have more complex hemodynamics, commonly having concomitant myocardial and/or valvular disease, it is critical that the invasive assessment is performed by an experienced operator.

Classic diagnostic criteria for CP[16] on cardiac catheterization include elevation of biventricular filling pressures with equalization of end-diastolic pressures (difference within 5 mmHg), rapid diastolic filling waves on RV and LV pressure tracings (square root sign), absence of significant pulmonary arterial hypertension (RV systolic pressure <55 mmHg), and a RV end-diastolic pressure to RV systolic pressure ratio greater than 1:3 (Fig. 26.12).

Dynamic criteria have also been added to invasive diagnostic armamentarium. The presence of ventricular interdependence can be assessed on simultaneous RV and LV tracings, which will show reciprocal respiratory changes in the ratio between RV and LV systolic areas, the so-called ventricular discordance. In contrast, patients with RCM, or with other etiologies for the increase in filling pressures, will typically show concordant respiratory changes in RV and LV pressure systolic areas (ventricular concordance) (see Fig. 26.12). The dissociation of intrathoracic and intracardiac pressures is assessed by analyzing simultaneous LV and pulmonary artery wedge pressure (as it reflects the pressure in the pulmonary veins, which lie outside the pericardial space) and is defined by a difference of 5 mmHg and above between inspiratory and expiratory LV–pulmonary artery pressure wedge

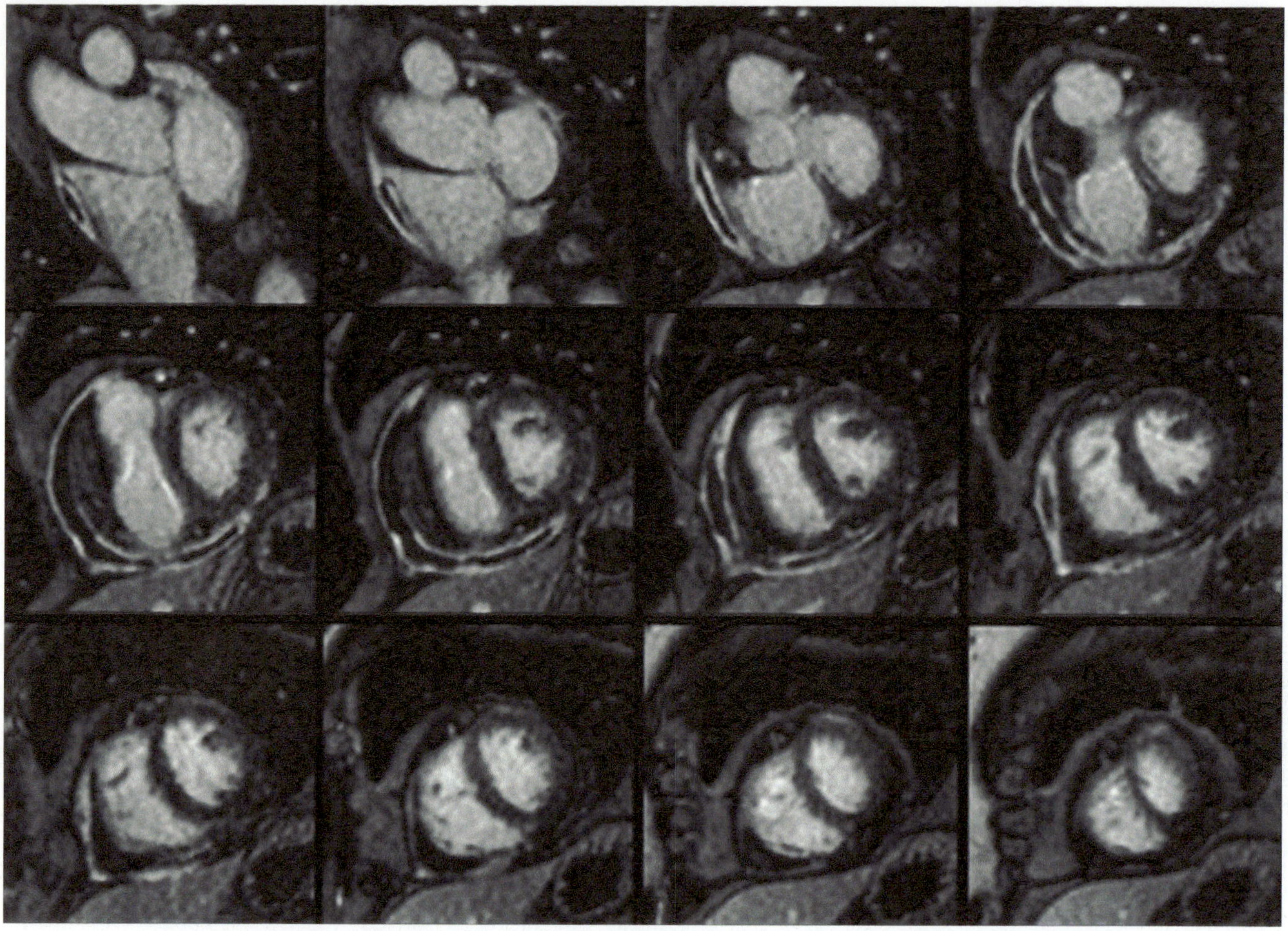

Fig. 26.11 Pericardial Enhancement on Cardiac MRI. Cardiac MRI findings in a patient with constrictive pericarditis showing significant pericardial late gadolinium enhancement with associated pericardial thickening.

gradients (see Fig. 26.11). The presence of ventricular discordance and dissociation of intrathoracic-intracardiac pressures has been shown to be highly sensitive and specific for the diagnosis of CP.[13,17]

It should be noted that all criteria for the invasive diagnosis of CP are load dependent. Therefore patients with RA pressure less than 15 mmHg in the setting of aggressive diuresis should receive a fluid challenge[16] (rapid infusion of 1000 mL normal saline) during the procedure and the hemodynamics reassessed afterward.

Coronary angiography is another diagnostic imaging tool in the assessment of CP, which is sometimes forgotten.[46] Several patients will have undergone coronary angiography as part of their evaluation for heart failure or dyspnea, but if not available, we will typically perform coronary angiography during invasive hemodynamic evaluation of CP. In our experience, the presence of distal fixation of the coronary arteries (Videos 26.3 and 26.4) is a very specific finding for the presence of CP.

Nuclear Imaging

Positron emission tomography (PET) utilizing 18-fluorodeoxyglucose (FDG) provides unique information regarding tissue metabolism, showing increased uptake in areas where inflammation or malignancy is present. Studies have also suggested a role for PET in pericardial disorders; PET can be used to assess pericardial inflammation in various forms of pericarditis,[47,48] but it may also predict the response to the anti-inflammatory therapy in transient constriction.[49]

DIFFERENTIAL DIAGNOSIS

Tricuspid Regurgitation and Restrictive Cardiomyopathy

Traditionally, severe TR and RCM have been described as conditions that mimic CP,[50] given the similarities in clinical presentation. However, after the major advances in echo Doppler, the differentiation between isolated TR and RCM from CP became much easier. In current practice, perhaps the biggest challenge is no longer distinguishing these three clinical entities but trying to identify the predominant hemodynamic lesion when they coexist.

In severe TR, RV enlargement and dilatation of the tricuspid annulus are usually present. In cases of torrential tricuspid insufficiency, color Doppler assessment might be unimpressive due to near equalization of RV and RA pressures. In these circumstances, continuous wave (CW) Doppler usually shows a dagger-shaped, low-velocity systolic Doppler profile. As previously described, in severe TR, systolic reversals on hepatic vein Doppler may be seen, although this is not a sensitive finding. The presence of systolic flow reversals is also useful in recognizing concomitant severe TR in patients with CP. It should be noted that the presence of moderate or more severe TR and CP is not

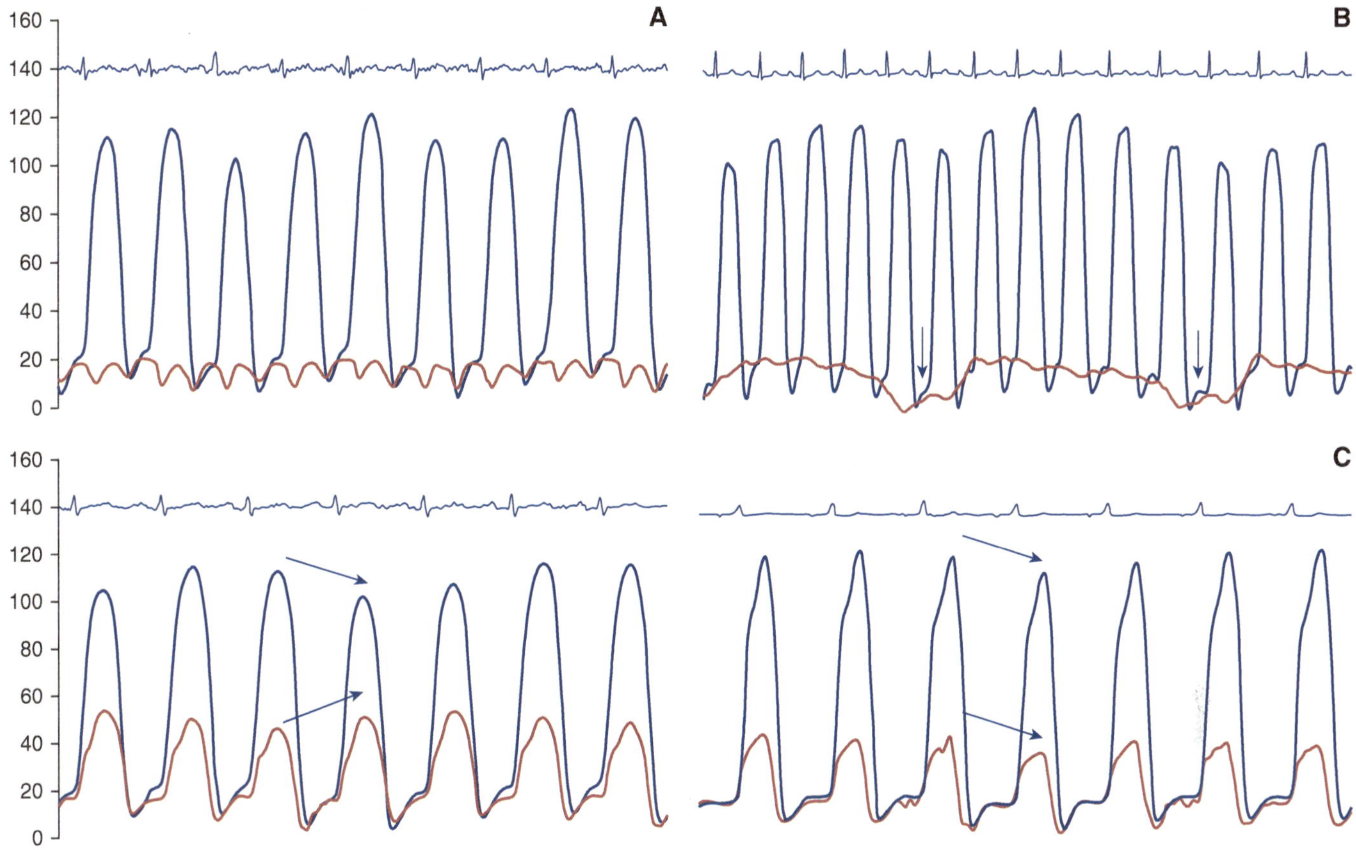

Fig. 26.12 Cardiac catheterization features of constrictive pericarditis. (A) Prominent x and y descents on right atrial tracings *(red)* and equalization of end-diastolic pressures (LV pressure tracings in *blue*). (B) The dissociation of intrathoracic and intracardiac pressures, demonstrating marked decreases in left ventricular *(blue)* and pulmonary artery *(red)* pressures gradients upon inspiration *(arrow)*. (C) Simultaneous left ventricular *(blue)* and right ventricular tracings in constrictive pericarditis *(left)* and restrictive cardiomyopathy *(right)*; note the typical ventricular discordance seen in constriction compared to concordant inspiratory changes seen in restriction.

uncommon and has been described in ~20% of CP patients.[51] These patients will show both systolic and increased expiratory diastolic reversals, a combination of the findings expected in each disease.

Typical features of RCM on echo Doppler include normal-size ventricles with preserved systolic function and massive atrial enlargement[15,50] (Fig. 26.13; see also Fig. 26.2B). Similar to CP, the presence of restrictive mitral inflow and dilatation of the IVC is the rule in RCM, since increases in right and left filling pressure are also commonly present in RCM. Two Doppler findings are very useful in the distinction between RCM and CP: mitral annular tissue Doppler and hepatic vein PW Doppler. In contrast to the elevated early diastolic tissue Doppler velocities seen in CP, in RCM medial and lateral e′ velocities are both reduced with medial mitral e′ sometimes being as low as 2 to 3 cm/sec. Hepatic vein Doppler will show increased inspiratory flow reversals as opposed to the prominent expiratory flow reversals typical of CP. Cardiac catheterization in RCM will show ventricular concordance when simultaneous RV and LV pressures are recorded.

Obesity and Obstructive Lung Disease

Respirophasic septal shift, one of the echocardiographic hallmarks of CP, can also be seen in patients with obstructive lung disease and obese patients. The large swings in intrathoracic pressures lead not only to inspiratory/expiratory changes in septal position but also marked inspiratory variations in mitral inflow. Interrogation of superior vena cava flow by PW Doppler is mandatory in these patients. Patients with CP will show minimal inspiratory increases (or sometimes even diminution) in forward flow velocities, whereas patients with obstructive pulmonary disease or elevated body mass index will show marked increases in systolic flow velocities (>30–40 cm/sec), typically with a monophasic forward flow[52] (Fig. 26.14).

Similarly, respirophasic septal shift can be seen in the presence of significant RV volume overload such as atrial septal defects or tricuspid/pulmonary regurgitation. The associated enlargement of right-sided chambers leads to a degree of pericardial restraint, causing the respirophasic findings. Other features of CP (expiratory diastolic flow reversals on the hepatic veins, annulus reversus, and increased mitral e′ velocities) will, however, be absent in those cases.

Cardiac Tamponade

Pericardial effusions are common in patients with transient CP (present in two-thirds of cases)[12] and are typically small. In addition, by definition, a pericardial effusion prior to pericardiocentesis is always present in patients with effusive-constrictive pericarditis. TTE has largely replaced cardiac catheterization in the hemodynamic evaluation of pericardial effusion. As it is a potentially fatal disorder, the presence of tamponade physiology should be promptly recognized, thus echocardiographers should be familiar with its echo Doppler findings. It should never be forgotten that the size of pericardial

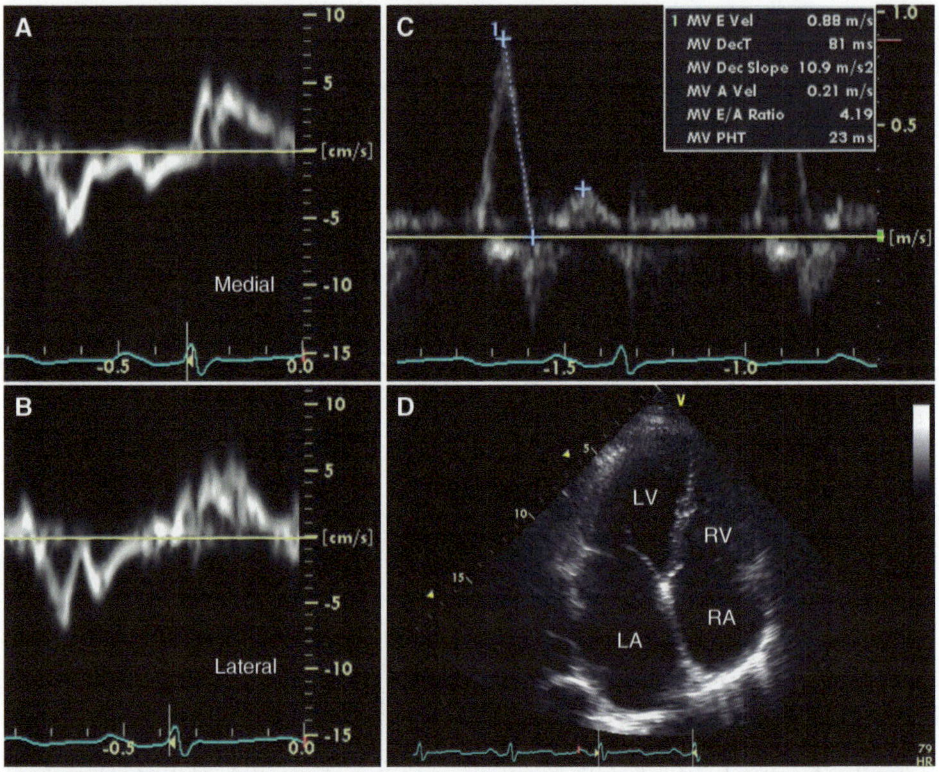

Fig. 26.13 Echo Doppler findings in a patient with idiopathic restrictive cardiomyopathy. Mitral annulus tissue Doppler shows significantly reduced medial and lateral e′ velocities (A, B). Pulsed-wave Doppler of the mitral inflows demonstrates a markedly elevated E/A ratio and short deceleration time (C). Normal-size ventricles with normal wall thickness and massive biatrial enlargement are seen by two-dimensional transthoracic echocardiography (D). *LA*, Left atrium; *LV*, left ventricle; *RA*, right atrium; *RV*, right ventricle.

effusion does not determine its hemodynamic consequences, as slow-growing pericardial effusions are well tolerated, and small acute pericardial effusion (such as those seen during invasive cardiac procedure) can be catastrophic.

The presence of chamber collapse is typically the first clue that a hemodynamically significant pericardial effusion is present. RA and RV collapse/extrinsic compression (best appreciated in the RV outflow tract) are highly sensitive findings[31,53]; in the setting of pulmonary hypertension or increased RA pressure, collapse of right-sided chambers might not be present, and compression of the left atrium or left ventricle might be seen instead. As far as echo Doppler findings, mitral inflow and hepatic vein Doppler will reflect the underlying impairment of early ventricular diastolic filling. Therefore mitral inflow typically shows an E/A ratio less than 1 (with significant respiratory variation in E velocities), whereas hepatic vein Doppler will show marked blunting of diastolic filling with very striking expiratory flow reversals[54,55] (not infrequently holodiastolic). It should be noted that these Doppler findings are in marked contradistinction to those seen in CP, where large mitral E velocities and prominent hepatic vein diastolic forward flow waves are seen.

In effusive-constrictive pericarditis, constrictive physiology will surface after pericardiocentesis has been performed. Therefore typical echo Doppler findings (dilatation of IVC, respirophasic septal shift with inspiratory variation in mitral E velocities, and hepatic vein expiratory reversals) will be seen following pericardial drainage.[20] The presence of echo Doppler of CP postpericardiocentesis appears to be a common finding, and we reported it to be present in 16% of patients undergoing pericardiocentesis.[20] The prognosis of these patients appears to be good, with most patients showing resolution of their constrictive features during follow-up and pericardiectomy only being required in two individuals.

We have also reported that effusive-constrictive pericarditis might be suspected even prior to pericardiocentesis[55]; in patients with a clinical diagnosis of effusive-constrictive pericarditis (defined by persistently elevated jugular venous pressures postpericardiocentesis), preperiocardiocentesis echo Doppler findings are intermediate between the typical features of cardiac tamponade and CP.

TREATMENT

Medical Therapy

Surgical pericardiectomy remains the treatment of choice of most patients with CP. However, as we actively seek evidence of active inflammation (using a combination of laboratory work and cardiac imaging modalities), the number of patients receiving medical therapy for CP has risen. In patients presenting subacutely, we recommend a trial of 8 to 12 weeks of anti-inflammatory prior to pericardiectomy. Elevated serum inflammatory markers and CMR have been shown to identify patients prone to respond to medical therapy.[12] It should also be noted that the degree of response to medical therapy appears to be proportional to the magnitude of late gadolinium enhancement on quantitative analysis.[43]

The therapeutic regimen typically includes a nonsteroidal anti-inflammatory agent or corticosteroids combined with colchicine, unless a contraindication to its use is present. Data on the most appropriate anti-inflammatory agent in transient CP are not available, but some experts favor the use of corticosteroids in more severe cases.

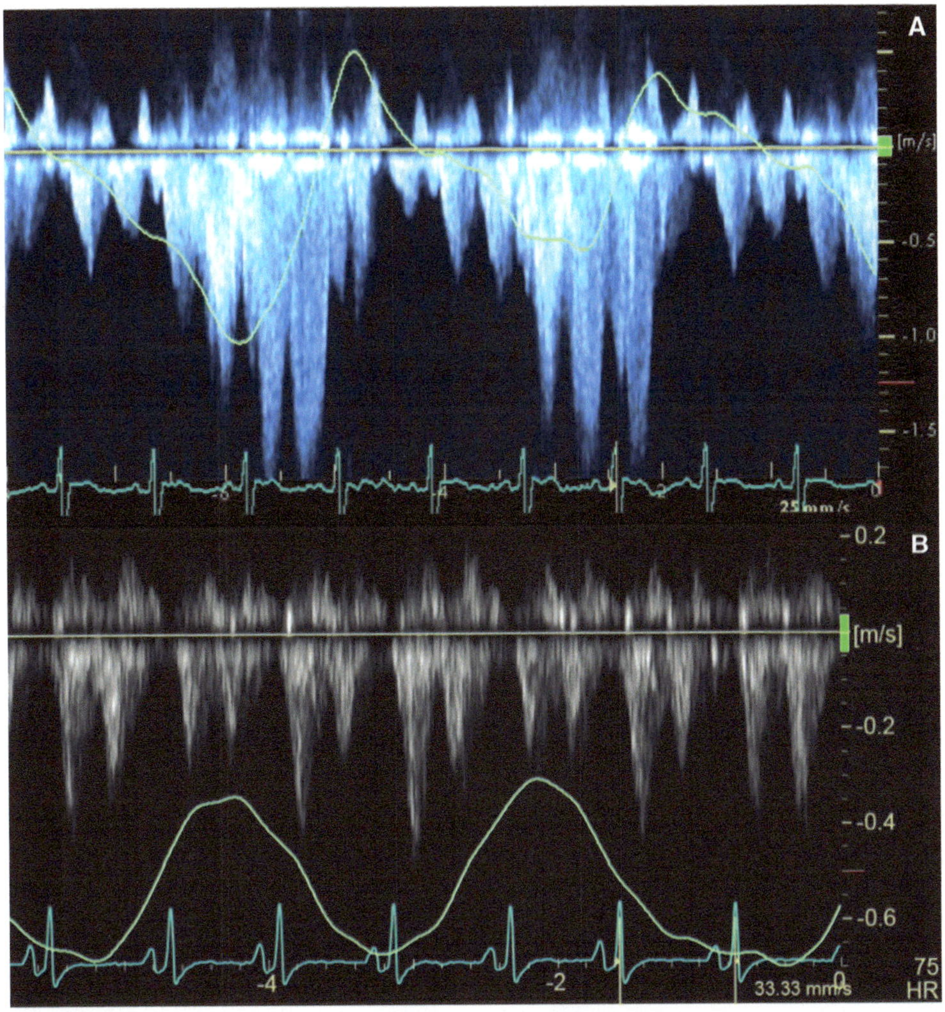

Fig. 26.14 Superior vena cava flow in obesity versus constrictive pericarditis. (A) Pulsed-wave Doppler in an obese patient. Note the striking inspiratory increases in systolic forward flow velocities; similar changes are seen in patients with obstructive lung disease. (B) In contrast, the patient with constrictive pericarditis showed an inspiratory decrease in forward flow velocities. (*Green tracings* correspond to simultaneous respirometer; the upward deflect marks the onset of inspiration, whereas the downward deflect marks the onset of expiration.)

Pericardiectomy

Surgical pericardiectomy provides a potential cure for patients with CP. Radical pericardiectomy should be the treatment of choice in patients with CP,[5,56] including removal of the diaphragmatic portion of the pericardium as well as the pericardial tissue posterior to the left phrenic nerve. Isolated anterior pericardiectomy (also described as phrenic to phrenic) should not be pursued, as it is associated with high rates of recurrent CP.

It is important to note that the mortality associated with pericardiectomy has markedly decreased over the past decades. A recent publication including isolated pericardiectomies performed at our institution between 1993 and 2013 (355 CP cases), reported 2.5% 30-day mortality.[57] Low 30-day mortality rates have also been reported by others.[9] These demonstrate that currently pericardiectomy can be performed at low risk in high-volume centers.

Five- and 10-year survival following pericardiectomy have been reported at 78% and 57%, respectively.[8] Noteworthy, the outcomes postpericardiectomy are directly related to the underlying etiology, with patients with idiopathic CP having the best outcome (88% 7-year survival) compared to 66% in patients with CP postcardiac surgery.[9] Several studies have highlighted the poor long-term prognosis of radiation-induced CP, which has been associated with a higher perioperative mortality.[9]

FUTURE DIRECTIONS

Speckle tracking imaging has been shown to provide incremental prognostic information in several cardiac diseases, including myocardial and valvular disorders; whether strain imaging might provide additional information regarding survival postpericardiectomy (even in patients with idiopathic CP) deserves further investigation. The use of nuclear imaging in myocardial disease has markedly increased in recent years. Whether its routine use can be of value in patients with CP (particularly those with cardiac devices, in which see cardiac MRI sometimes cannot be performed), and whether it may provide additional information regarding a response to anti-inflammatory therapy in transient CP remains to be determined. Similarly, studies on the optimal anti-inflammatory agent for the therapy of transient CP are critically needed. Lastly, the epidemiology, pathophysiology, and natural history of effusive-constrictive pericarditis need better understanding.

KEY POINTS

- Constrictive pericarditis is a curable form of diastolic heart failure.
- Varying degrees of pericardial thickening, calcification, and fibrosis are seen in patients with constrictive pericarditis, but normal pericardial thickness can be present in 20% of patients.
- Idiopathic, postcardiac surgery and radiation are the most common etiologies of constrictive pericarditis in developed countries. Tuberculosis is the most common cause of constrictive pericarditis worldwide.
- Elevated filling pressures, increased ventricular interdependence, and dissociation of intrathoracic-intracardiac pressures are the hemodynamic hallmarks of constrictive pericarditis.
- TTE is the initial diagnostic modality of choice for the diagnosis of constrictive pericarditis.
- Mitral e′ velocities are typically elevated in patients with constrictive pericarditis, but milder increases might be seen in the presence of concomitant myocardial disease.
- Hepatic vein Doppler is an integral component of the echocardiographic assessment of pericardial diseases, also allowing for the differentiation of constrictive pericarditis from its mimickers: restrictive cardiomyopathy and severe tricuspid regurgitation.
- Cardiac MRI provides diagnostic information regarding pericardial thickness and can guide therapy if ongoing pericardial inflammation is present.
- Although surgical pericardiectomy remains the standard therapeutic option, medical therapy with nonsteroidal anti-inflammatory agents or corticosteroids should be attempted if signs of ongoing inflammation are present in those presenting with constrictive features.

REVIEW QUESTIONS

1. A 35-year-old man presents to his primary care physician with a 6-month history of progressive increase in abdominal girth and leg edema. He is otherwise healthy and denies liver disease, thoracic trauma, or any cardiovascular procedures. Physical exam reveals elevated jugular venous pressure. What venous contour should be expected if constrictive pericarditis is present?
   a. Large V waves
   b. Canon A waves
   c. Prominent x and y descents
   c. Blunted y descents
2. A transthoracic echocardiogram was performed. What finding is illustrated in the accompanying figure on this hepatic vein Doppler signal?

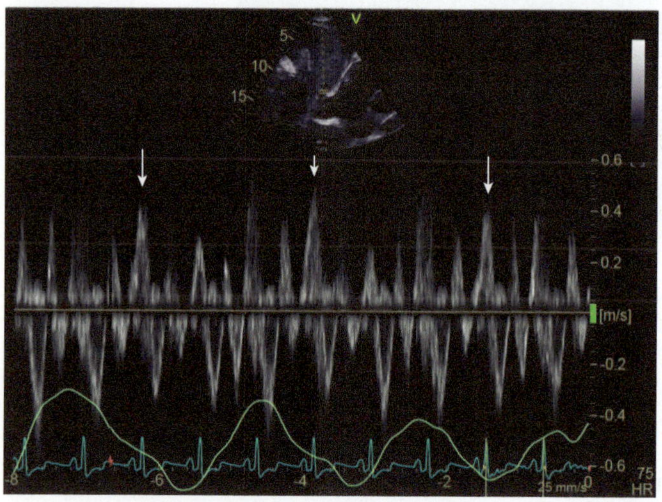

   a. Increased inspiratory diastolic flow reversals
   b. Increased expiratory diastolic flow reversals
   c. Systolic flow reversals
3. The presence of this finding on his transthoracic echocardiogram can be explained by which hemodynamic feature of constrictive pericarditis?
   a. Dissociation of intrathoracic-intracardiac pressures
   b. Elevated filling pressures
   c. Pulsus paradoxus
   d. Increased ventricular interdependence
4. His transthoracic echocardiogram was diagnostic for constrictive pericarditis. A cardiac MRI was then performed and showed a thickened pericardium. In light of the findings shown in the figure, what should be the next step?

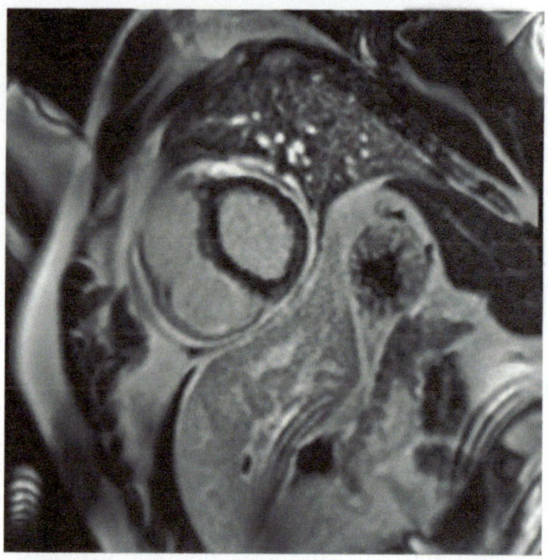

   a. Cardiac catheterization
   b. Anti-inflammatory therapy
   c. Surgical pericardiectomy

REFERENCES

1. Miranda WR, Oh JK. Constrictive pericarditis: a practical clinical approach. *Prog Cardiovasc Dis.* 2017;59(4):369–379.
2. Wood P. Chronic constrictive pericarditis. *Am J Cardiol.* 1961;7:48–61.
3. Im E, Shim CY, Hong GR, et al. The incidence and clinical outcome of constrictive physiology after coronary artery bypass graft surgery. *J Am Coll Cardiol.* 2013;61(20):2110–2112.
4. Matsuyama K, Matsumoto M, Sugita T, et al. Clinical characteristics of patients with constrictive pericarditis after coronary bypass surgery. *Jpn Circ J.* 2001;65(6):480–482.
5. Syed FF, Schaff HV, Oh JK. Constrictive pericarditis—a curable diastolic heart failure. *Nat Rev Cardiol.* 2015;12(12):682.
6. Lin Y, Zhou M, Xiao J, et al. Treating constrictive pericarditis in a Chinese single-center study: a five-year experience. *Ann Thorac Surg.* 2012;94(4):1235–1240.

7. Yetkin U, Kestelli M, Yilik L, et al. Recent surgical experience in chronic constrictive pericarditis. *Tex Heart I J.* 2003;30(1):27–30.
8. Ling LH, Oh JK, Schaff HV, et al. Constrictive pericarditis in the modern era: evolving clinical spectrum and impact on outcome after pericardiectomy. *Circulation.* 1999;100(13):1380–1386.
9. Bertog SC, Thambidorai SK, Parakh K, et al. Constrictive pericarditis: etiology and cause-specific survival after pericardiectomy. *J Am Coll Cardiol.* 2004;43(8):1445–1452.
10. Szabó G, Schmack B, Bulut C, et al. Constrictive pericarditis: risks, aetiologies and outcomes after total pericardiectomy: 24 years of experience. *Eur J Cardiothorac Surg.* 2013;44(6):1023–1028.
11. Gentry J, Klein AL, Jellis CL. Transient constrictive pericarditis: current diagnostic and therapeutic strategies. *Curr Cardiol Rep.* 2016;18(5):41.
12. Haley JH, Tajik AJ, Danielson GK, et al. Transient constrictive pericarditis: causes and natural history. *J Am Coll Cardiol.* 2004;43(2):271–275.
13. Talreja DR, Nishimura RA, Oh JK, et al. Constrictive pericarditis in the modern era: novel criteria for diagnosis in the cardiac catheterization laboratory. *J Am Coll Cardiol.* 2008;51(3):315–319.
14. Adler Y, Charron P, Imazio M, et al. 2015 ESC guidelines for the diagnosis and management of pericardial diseases: the task force for the diagnosis and management of pericardial diseases of the European Society of Cardiology (ESC). Endorsed by the European Association for Cardio-Thoracic Surgery (EACTS). *Eur Heart J.* 2015;36(42):2921–2964.
15. Geske JB, Anavekar NS, Nishimura RA, et al. Differentiation of constriction and restriction: complex cardiovascular hemodynamics. *J Am Coll Cardiol.* 2016;68(21):2329–2347.
16. Nishimura RA. Constrictive pericarditis in the modern era: a diagnostic dilemma. *Heart.* 2001;86(6):619–623.
17. Hurrell DG, Nishimura RA, Higano ST, et al. Value of dynamic respiratory changes in left and right ventricular pressures for the diagnosis of constrictive pericarditis. *Circulation.* 1996;93(11):2007–2013.
18. Holmes DR Jr, Nishimura R, Fountain R, et al. Iatrogenic pericardial effusion and tamponade in the percutaneous intracardiac intervention era. *JACC Cardiovasc Interv.* 2009;2(8):705–717.
19. Hancock EW. Subacute effusive-constrictive pericarditis. *Circulation.* 1971;43(2):183–192.
20. Kim KH, Miranda WR, Sinak LJ, et al. Effusive-constrictive pericarditis after pericardiocentesis: incidence, associated findings, and natural history. *JACC Cardiovasc Imag.* 2018;11(4):534–541.
21. Miranda WR, Oh JK. Effusive-constrictive pericarditis. *Cardiol Clin.* 2017;35(4):551–558.
22. Ling LH, Oh JK, Breen JF, et al. Calcific constrictive pericarditis: is it still with us? *Ann Intern Med.* 2000;132(6):444–450.
23. Kushwaha SS, Fallon JT, Fuster V. Restrictive cardiomyopathy. *N Engl J Med.* 1997;336(4):267–276.
24. Avgoustakis D, Lazarides D, Athanasiades D, et al. The electrocardiogram in constrictive pericarditis before and after radical pericardectomy. *Chest.* 1970;57(5):460–467.
25. Babuin L, Alegria JR, Oh JK, et al. Brain natriuretic peptide levels in constrictive pericarditis and restrictive cardiomyopathy. *J Am Coll Cardiol.* 2006;47(7):1489–1491.
26. Welch TD, Ling LH, Espinosa RE, et al. Echocardiographic diagnosis of constrictive pericarditis: Mayo Clinic criteria. *Circ Cardiovasc Imag.* 2014;7(3):526–534.
27. Coylewright M, Welch TD, Nishimura RA. Mechanism of septal bounce in constrictive pericarditis: a simultaneous cardiac catheterisation and echocardiographic study. *Heart.* 2013;99(18):1376.
28. Nagueh SF, Smiseth OA, Appleton CP, et al. Recommendations for the evaluation of left ventricular diastolic function by echocardiography: an update from the American Society of Echocardiography and the European Association of Cardiovascular Imaging. *J Am Soc Echocardiogr.* 2016;29(4):277–314.
29. Oh JK, Hatle LK, Seward JB, et al. Diagnostic role of Doppler echocardiography in constrictive pericarditis. *J Am Coll Cardiol.* 1994;23(1):154–162.
30. Hatle LK, Appleton CP, Popp RL. Differentiation of constrictive pericarditis and restrictive cardiomyopathy by Doppler echocardiography. *Circulation.* 1989;79(2):357–370.
31. Asher CR, Klein AL. Diastolic heart failure: restrictive cardiomyopathy, constrictive pericarditis, and cardiac tamponade: clinical and echocardiographic evaluation. *Cardiol Rev.* 2002;10(4):218–229.
32. Madeira M, Teixeira R, Costa M, et al. Two-dimensional speckle tracking cardiac mechanics and constrictive pericarditis: systematic review. *Echocardiography.* 2016;33(10):1589–1599.
33. Sengupta PP, Krishnamoorthy VK, Abhayaratna WP, et al. Disparate patterns of left ventricular mechanics differentiate constrictive pericarditis from restrictive cardiomyopathy. *JACC Cardiovasc Imag.* 2008;1(1):29–38.
34. Kusunose K, Dahiya A, Popovic´ ZB, et al. Biventricular mechanics in constrictive pericarditis comparison with restrictive cardiomyopathy and impact of pericardiectomy. *Circ Cardiovasc Imag.* 2013;6(3):399–406.
35. Mahmoud A, Bansal M, Sengupta PP. New cardiac imaging algorithms to diagnose constrictive pericarditis versus restrictive cardiomyopathy. *Curr Cardiol Rep.* 2017;19(5):43.
36. Ghersin E, Lessick J, Litmanovich D, et al. Septal bounce in constrictive pericarditis. Diagnosis and dynamic evaluation with multidetector CT. *J Comput Assist Tomogr.* 2004;28(5):676–678.
37. Bull RK, Edwards PD, Dixon AK. CT dimensions of the normal pericardium. *Br J Radiol.* 1998;71(849):923–925.
38. Choi JH, Choi JO, Ryu DR, et al. Mitral and tricuspid annular velocities in constrictive pericarditis and restrictive cardiomyopathy: correlation with pericardial thickness on computed tomography. *JACC Cardiovasc Imag.* 2011;4(6):567–575.
39. Talreja DR, Edwards WD, Danielson GK, et al. Constrictive pericarditis in 26 patients with histologically normal pericardial thickness. *Circulation.* 2003;108(15):1852–1857.
40. Alajaji W, Xu B, Sripariwuth A, et al. Noninvasive multimodality imaging for the diagnosis of constrictive pericarditis. *Circulation Cardiovascular Imaging.* 2018;11(11):e007878.
41. Klein AL, Abbara S, Agler DA, et al. American Society of Echocardiography clinical recommendations for multimodality cardiovascular imaging of patients with pericardial disease: endorsed by the Society for Cardiovascular Magnetic Resonance and Society of Cardiovascular Computed Tomography. *J Am Soc Echocardiogr.* 2013;26(9):965–1012. e15.
42. Feng D, Glockner J, Kim K, et al. Cardiac magnetic resonance imaging pericardial late gadolinium enhancement and elevated inflammatory markers can predict the reversibility of constrictive pericarditis after anti-inflammatory medical therapy: a pilot study. *Circulation.* 2011;124(17):1830–1837.
43. Cremer PC, Tariq MU, Karwa A, et al. Quantitative assessment of pericardial delayed hyperenhancement predicts clinical improvement in patients with constrictive pericarditis treated with anti-inflammatory therapy. *Circ Cardiovasc Imag.* 2015;8(5):e003125.
44. Masui T, Finck S, Higgins CB. Constrictive pericarditis and restrictive cardiomyopathy: evaluation with MR imaging. *Radiology.* 1992;182(2):369–373.
45. Francone M, Dymarkowski S, Kalantzi M, et al. Assessment of ventricular coupling with real-time cine MRI and its value to differentiate constrictive pericarditis from restrictive cardiomyopathy. *Eur Radiol.* 2006;16(4):944–951.
46. Alexander J, Kelley MJ, Cohen LS, et al. The angiographic appearance of the coronary arteries in constrictive pericarditis. *Radiology.* 1979;131(3):609–617.
47. Ha JW, Lee JD, Ko YG, et al. Images in cardiovascular medicine. Assessment of pericardial inflammation in a patient with tuberculous effusive constrictive pericarditis with 18F-2-deoxyglucose positron emission tomography. *Circulation.* 2006;113(1):e4–e5.
48. Losik SB, Studentsova Y, Margouleff D. Chemotherapy-induced pericarditis on F-18 FDG positron emission tomography scan. *Clin Nuclear Med.* 2003;28(11):913–915.
49. Chang SA, Choi JY, Kim EK, et al. [18F]Fluorodeoxyglucose PET/CT predicts response to steroid therapy in constrictive pericarditis. *J Am Coll Cardiol.* 2017;69(6):750–752.
50. Garcia MJ. Constrictive pericarditis versus restrictive cardiomyopathy? *J Am Coll Cardiol.* 2016;67(17):2061–2076.
51. Góngora E, Dearani JA, Orszulak TA, et al. Tricuspid regurgitation in patients undergoing pericardiectomy for constrictive pericarditis. *Ann Thorac Surg.* 2008;85(1):163–171.

52. Boonyaratavej S, Oh JK, Tajik AJ, et al. Comparison of mitral inflow and superior vena cava Doppler velocities in chronic obstructive pulmonary disease and constrictive pericarditis. *J Am Coll Cardiol.* 1998;32(7):2043–2048.
53. Gillam LD, Guyer DE, Gibson TC, et al. Hydrodynamic compression of the right atrium: a new echocardiographic sign of cardiac tamponade. *Circulation.* 1983;68(2):294–301.
54. Burstow DJ, Oh JK, Bailey KR, Cardiac tamponade: characteristic Doppler observations. *Mayo Clin Proc.* 1989;64(3):312–324.
55. Miranda WR, Newman DB, Sinak LJ, et al. Pre- and post-pericardiocentesis echo-Doppler features of effusive-constrictive pericarditis compared with cardiac tamponade and constrictive pericarditis. *Eur Heart J Cardiovasc Imag.* 2019;20(3):298–306.
56. Hemmati P, Greason KL, Schaff HV. Contemporary techniques of pericardiectomy for pericardial disease. *Cardiol Clin.* 2017;35(4):559–566.
57. Gillaspie EA, Stulak JM, Daly RC, et al. A 20-year experience with isolated pericardiectomy: analysis of indications and outcomes. *J Thorac Cardiovasc Surg.* 2016;152(2):448–558.

27

Diastolic Function in Children and in Children With Congenital Heart Disease

Mark K. Friedberg

OUTLINE

Case Study

A 14-year-old boy presented following a sudden cardiac arrest (likely ventricular fibrillation) and was direct current (DC) cardioverted. Based on his clinical presentation and echocardiogram he was diagnosed with restrictive cardiomyopathy (RCM). Family history was negative. He was assessed for heart transplant, but the family decided not to proceed with transplant. He underwent placement of an intracardiac defibrillator and was started on a beta blocker. His cardiomyopathy workup was unremarkable. Genetic testing revealed several variants of unknown significance. On outpatient follow-up he is clinically well. He participates fully in gym class and reports that his activity and exercise endurance are good.

His echocardiogram showed moderate midseptal and mild apical left ventricular (LV) hypertrophy with good biventricular systolic function. His diastolic function was abnormal with features most consistent with restrictive physiology, although features of delayed relaxation were present. Markedly dilated atria (Fig. 27.1), an increased E/A ratio (Fig. 27.2), and increased pulmonary a-wave reversal duration compared with the mitral A wave duration (Fig. 27.3) were consistent with restrictive diastolic physiology. Conversely, the mitral E wave deceleration time (DT), while short, was not extremely so, likely due to the slow heart rate secondary to beta blockers (see Fig. 27.2), and isovolumic relaxation time was relatively long (Fig. 27.4). The lateral mitral and septal e′ were low for age, and consequently his E/e′ (lateral) ratio is high for age at 110/10 = 11, although intermediate by adult criteria (Fig. 27.5). There was no tricuspid regurgitation (TR) to quantify right ventricular (RV) systolic pressures.

Cardiac catheterization showed LV pressures of 84/18 with a pulmonary capillary wedge pressure (PCWP) of 20 mmHg, an indexed pulmonary vascular resistance of 3.4, RV pressures of 53/10 mmHg, and pulmonary artery pressures of 49/20 mmHg.

INTRODUCTION

Ventricular function is a major determinant of outcomes in children and adults with congenital and acquired heart disease. Evaluation of diastolic function in children, most commonly performed by echocardiography, is strongly linked to clinical outcomes and is therefore important to assess as it provides information with prognostic value.[1] Yet, the clinical assessment of diastolic function, particularly in children, and particularly in those with congenital heart disease (CHD), remains a persistently challenging area. Intrinsic and extrinsic factors affect diastolic performance. Systolic ventricular function, atrial and ventricular compliance, ventricular filling pressures, pericardial constraint, dyssynchrony, ventricular-ventricular interactions, and vascular compliance may each have effects on overall ventricular diastolic performance. Noninvasive evaluation of diastolic function in infants and children is additionally influenced by several factors, including age, heart rate, and respiratory cycle variations.[2–7] This chapter will discuss concepts in diastolic function in pediatric acquired and congenital heart disease and review continuing challenges and efforts regarding the assessment of diastolic performance in this population.

NORMAL DIASTOLIC FUNCTION IN CHILDREN AND DEVELOPMENTAL ASPECTS

The myocardium matures from the fetus through childhood to the young adult, and with this maturation comes changes in its diastolic properties and function. In the fetal myocardium, fetal cardiomyocytes

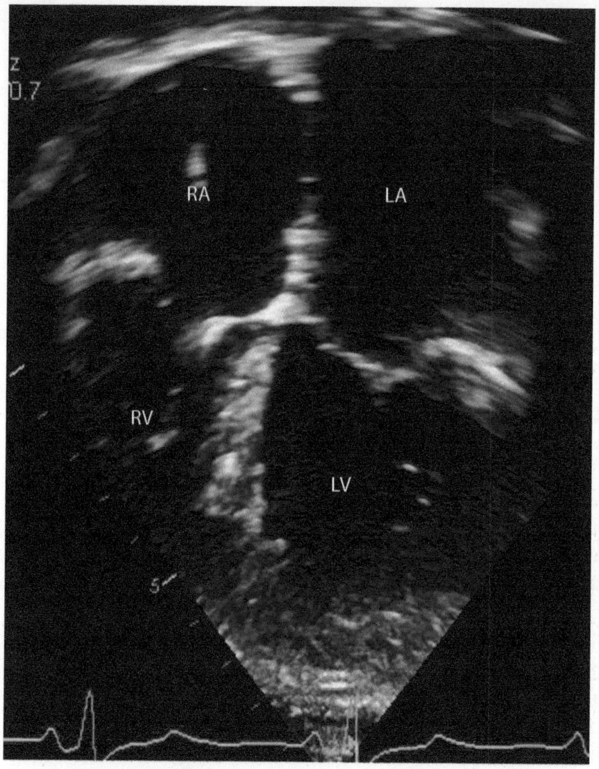

Fig. 27.1 Case study: Markedly dilated atria.

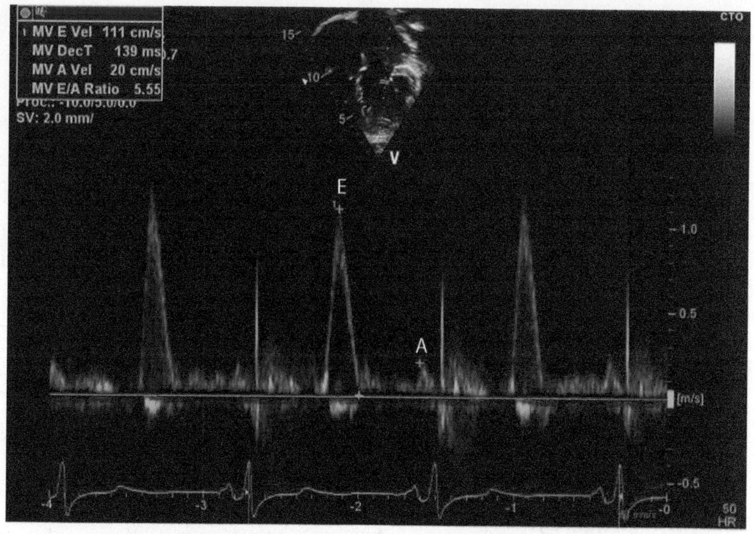

Fig. 27.2 Case study: Increased E/A ratio.

grow by hyperplasia (replication), whereas mature cardiomyocytes grow only by hypertrophy. Energy metabolism differs in that lactate, not long-chain fatty acid, is the primary fuel of the fetal myocardium. Diastolic properties of the fetal myocardium are also significantly different in that myocardial relaxation in the fetus is reduced compared to mature myocardium[8] due to differences in Ca^{2+} handling. Likewise, stiffness is higher due to the larger proportion of noncontractile elements compared to the adult[9] and extrinsic constraint by the pericardium and fluid-filled lungs.[10] Hence the normal fetus, when examined by echocardiography, exhibits a reversed E/A ratio of atrioventricular inflow and tissue Doppler velocities (Fig. 27.6). These would be interpreted as reflecting impaired relaxation if seen in a mature heart. While the influence of extrinsic compression changes dramatically with the newborn's first breaths, the neonate continues to manifest fetal characteristics of reduced early diastolic filling and dominant atrial contribution. These patterns characterize the immature neonatal myocardium for the first few weeks to months after birth, before transitioning to the mature pattern of dominance of early ventricular filling manifested as dominant E and e′ wave velocities and lower atrial contribution, manifested as lower A and a′ wave velocities (Figs. 27.7).

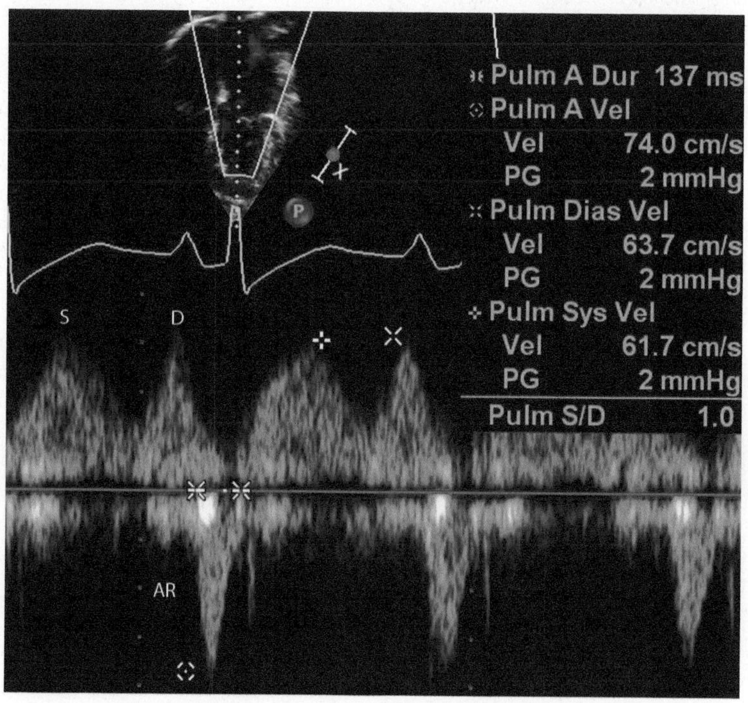

Fig. 27.3 Case study: Increased pulmonary a-wave reversal (AR) duration compared with the mitral A wave duration.

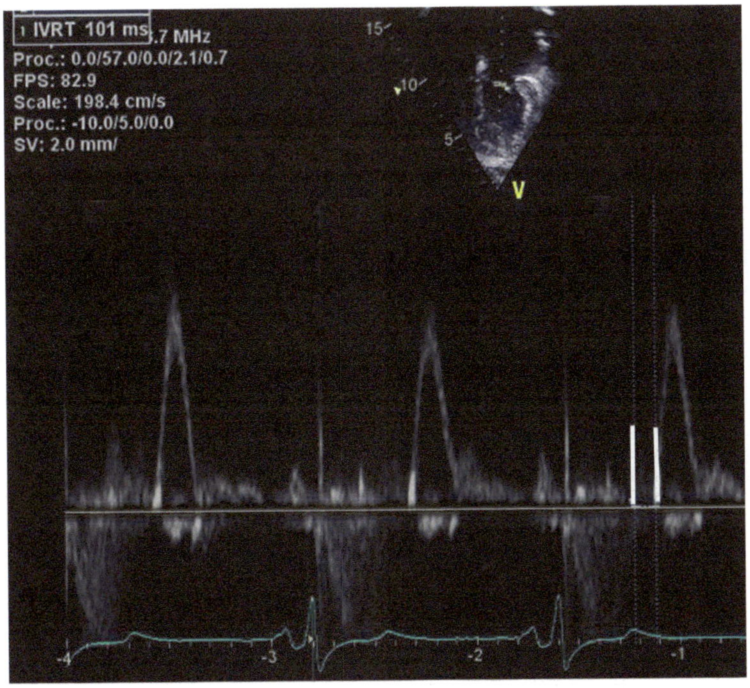

Fig. 27.4 Case study: Isovolumic relaxation time was relatively long.

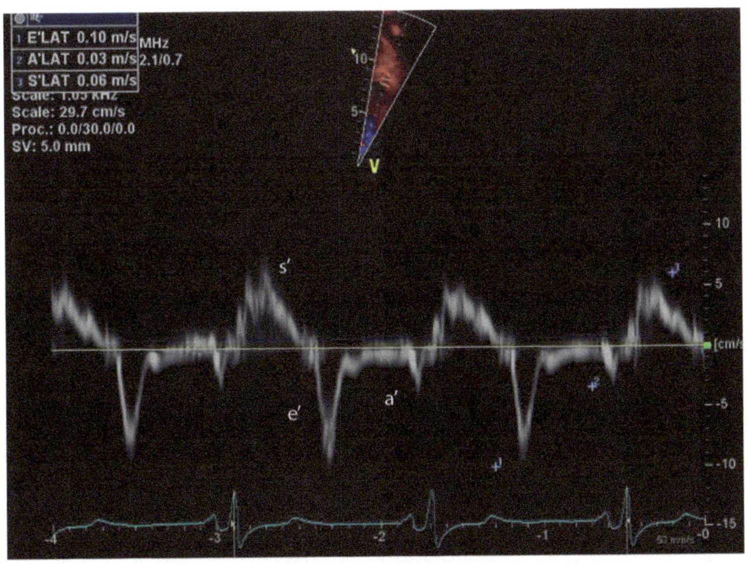

Fig. 27.5 Case study: The lateral mitral and septal e′ were low for age and consequently his E/e′ (lateral) ratio is high for age at 110/10 = 11, although intermediate by adult criteria.

As the normal myocardium matures through childhood and into adolescence, the ventricle displays vigorous relaxation properties. These manifest as dominant early diastolic filling (dominant E and e′ waves), with little contribution left to atrial filling (see Fig. 27.7B). Higher heart rates further contribute to this dynamic physiology. Thus the normal E/A ratio of children and adolescents is often higher than that of adults (and DT shorter) and would be considered to be in ranges indicative of restrictive physiology if judged by adult criteria.

Reference values for diastolic parameters, including tissue Doppler velocity and cardiac time interval parameters, established in sizable cohorts of healthy children, have been available for several years (Tables 27.1, 27.2, and 27.3).[11,12] In general, Doppler parameters linearly increase or decrease over childhood toward adult values at 18 years of age.[11] It is important to note that the normal reference values published in 1998 from the Mayo Clinic database include children from 4 years of age and older, and other studies exclude infants or toddlers, so that overall, normal data from neonates, infants, and toddlers are limited. Inspection of the Mayo Clinic data also shows that confidence intervals become progressively wider as age decreases,[11] introducing further uncertainty for assessment of diastolic function in the already more challenging younger age group.

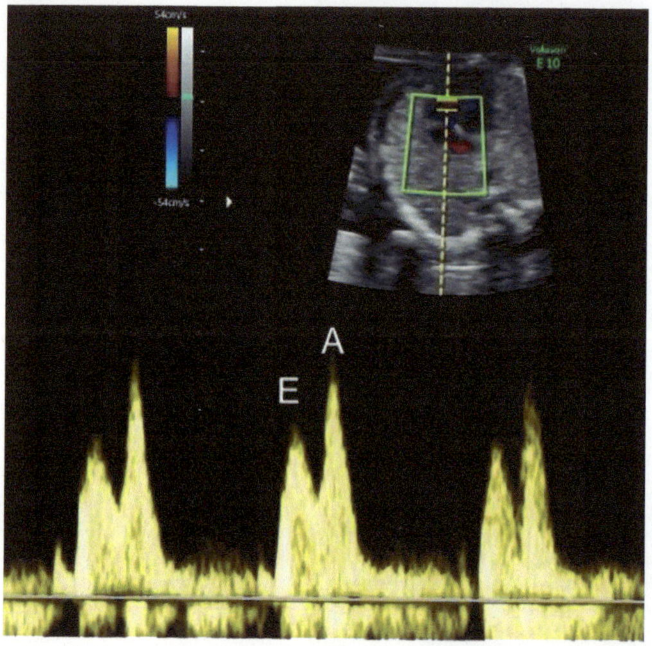

Fig. 27.6 Normal fetal tricuspid valve inflow Doppler. Note the A wave dominance and physiologic E/A reversal.

PATHOPHYSIOLOGY OF DIASTOLIC DYSFUNCTION IN CHILDREN WITH CONGENITAL HEART DISEASE

Diastole is a complex process involving both active and passive components. Abnormalities of relaxation and early rapid filling are often manifested by changes in the rate of relaxation and the amount of early rapid filling. Diastolic dysfunction also is manifested by changes in chamber stiffness, which are traditionally thought to manifest in late diastole. Adverse changes within the myocardium are common in the pathophysiology of congenital and acquired heart disease affecting children, with increases in collagen content and altered extracellular matrix composition leading to altered chamber compliance.

The rate of pressure decline within the ventricular chamber can be determined by invasive methods. Impaired relaxation leads to a decreased rate of ventricular pressure decline. Lengthening of isovolumic relaxation time (IVRT) (defined as the time interval between aortic valve closure and mitral valve opening) is also characteristic of abnormal diastolic filling and can be evaluated noninvasively by M mode or pulse wave (PW) Doppler echocardiography. However, neither IVRT nor tau elucidates whether dysfunction occurs in active or passive relaxation, which act in concert to cause a fall in ventricular pressure and augment filling. As diastolic dysfunction progresses, increased ventricular end-diastolic pressure (EDP) further increases tau and pressure half-time (period of time for LV pressure to fall to 50% of its initial value during isovolumic relaxation), while concomitant changes in atrial compliance and filling pressure act to shorten IVRT duration.

Echocardiography, and in particular Doppler echocardiography, has been an essential noninvasive tool in the quantitative assessment of LV diastolic function. Abnormalities of ventricular compliance and relaxation can be demonstrated by changes in mitral inflow, pulmonary venous Doppler patterns, and tissue Doppler echocardiography as in adults.[13–27] Because diastolic dysfunction may precede systolic dysfunction and is linked to clinical outcomes, assessment of diastolic function is important in the noninvasive characterization and evaluation of children with acquired and congenital heart disease.

In many children with CHD, in utero or early neonatal pathophysiology may lead to myocardial injury and fibrosis and diastolic dysfunction. An example is critical aortic stenosis and other left-sided obstructive lesions, where not only is there LV hypertrophy

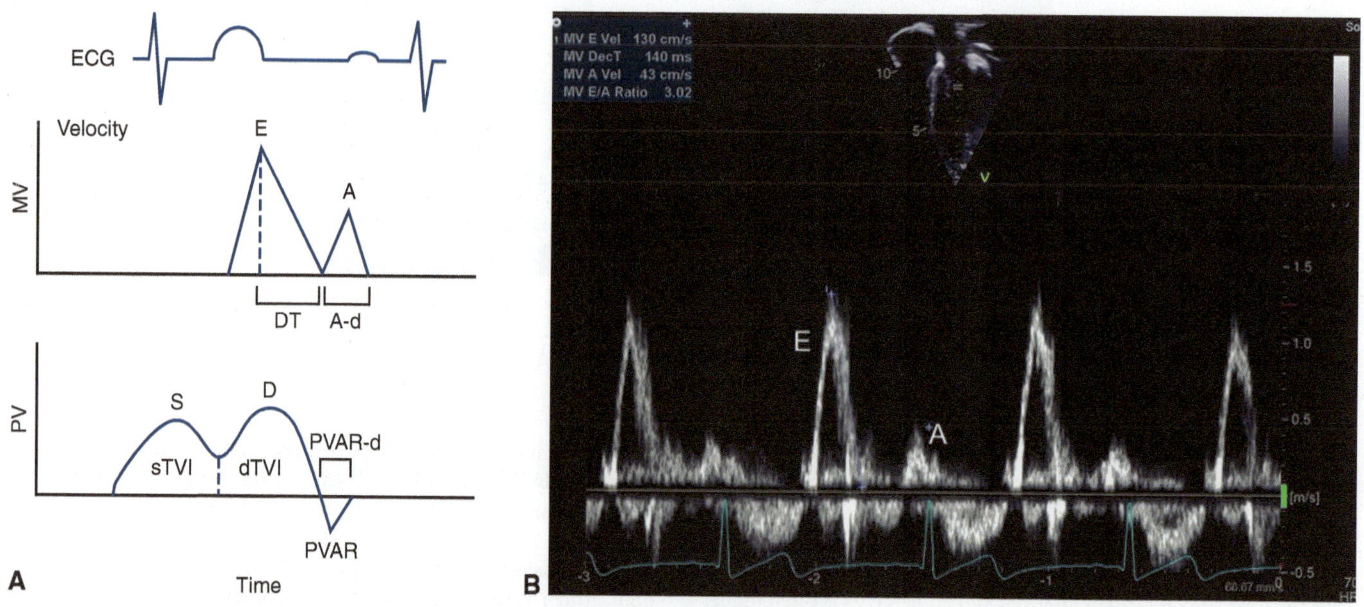

Fig. 27.7 (A) Spectrum of diastolic flow patterns in diastolic dysfunction in children. (B) Doppler of mitral valve inflow in a normal child. Note the marked dominance of early (E wave) over late (A wave) filling, which is normal due to the vigorous ventricular relaxation in children. This ratio is typically higher in normal children than in normal adults. (A, From Olivier M, et al. Serial Doppler assessment of diastolic function before and after the Fontan operation. *J Am Soc Echocardiogr.* 2003;16:1136–1143.)

TABLE 27.1 Normal Doppler Data (*N* = 233): Mitral Valve Flow Variables and Left Ventricular Isovolumic Relaxation Time (Stratified by Age Group)

	3–8 YEARS (*N* = 75)		9–12 YEARS (*N* = 72)		13–17 YEARS (*N* = 76)	
Factor	**Mean**	**1 SD**	**Mean**	**1 SD**	**Mean**	**1 SD**
E velocity (cm/sec)	92	14	86	15	88	14
E TVI (cm)	12.0	2.6	12.3	2.9	14.0	2.9
A velocity (cm/sec)	42	11	41	9	39	8
A TVI (cm)	3.7	1.1	3.7	1.0	3.7	1.1
A duration (msec)	136	22	142	21	141	22
E at A velocity (cm/sec)	16	7	14	5	12	4
E to A velocity ratio	2.4	0.7	2.2	0.6	2.3	0.6
E to A TVI ratio	3.7	2.0	3.7	1.5	4.2	1.7
Deceleration time (msec)	145	18	157	19	172	22
End mitral A to R wave interval (msec)	34	16	29	15	27	19
LV IVRT (msec)	62	10	67	10	74	13

A, Atrial filling wave; *E*, early filling wave; *IVRT*, isovolumic relaxation time; *LV*, left ventricular; *SD*, standard deviation; *TVI*, time velocity integral.
From O'Leary PW, et al. Diastolic ventricular function in children: a Doppler echocardiographic study establishing normal values and predictors of increased ventricular end diastolic pressure. *Mayo Clin Proc.* 1998;73:616–628.

TABLE 27.2 Normal Doppler Data (*N* = 223): Pulmonary Vein Flow Variables

	3–8 YEARS (*N* = 75)		9–12 YEARS (*N* = 72)		13–17 YEARS (*N* = 76)	
Factor	**Mean**	**1 SD**	**Mean**	**1 SD**	**Mean**	**1 SD**
Systolic velocity (cm/sec)	46	9	45	9	41	10
Systolic TVI (cm)	11.1	2.3	11.5	2.2	10.8	2.8
Diastolic velocity (cm/sec)	59	8	54	9	59	11
Diastolic TVI (cm)	8.8	1.8	9.2	2.5	12.1	3.1
Ratio of systolic to diastolic velocity	0.8	0.2	0.8	0.2	0.7	0.2
Ratio of systolic to diastolic TVI	1.3	0.3	1.3	0.4	0.9	0.3
Atrial reversal velocity (cm/sec)	21	4	21	5	21	7
Atrial reversal duration (msec)	130	20	125	20	140	28
Atrial reversal TVI (cm)	1.7	0.5	1.6	0.6	2.0	0.9

SD, Standard deviation; *TVI*, time velocity integral.
From O'Leary PW, et al. Diastolic ventricular function in children: a Doppler echocardiographic study establishing normal values and predictors of increased ventricular end diastolic pressure. *Mayo Clin Proc.* 1998;73:616–628.

and underdevelopment that impede filling, but very commonly endocardial fibroelastosis and myocardial fibrosis, which create a noncompliant ventricle with restrictive filling. Mitral valve hypoplasia and structural abnormalities further impede the ability of the ventricles to fill adequately, and the common presence of an atrial septal defect (ASD) leads to left-to-right shunt at the atrial level and further reduction of LV preload. Hence the progression in the severity of diastolic dysfunction, from delayed relaxation to restrictive filling, typical of adult pathology, may not be applicable to many CHD lesions. Moreover, these abnormalities substantially impede assessment of diastolic function. In other instances, the degree of ventricular loading, over and above myocardial properties per se, is a major determinant of ventricular filling and hence diastolic performance. This will be detailed later, but a prototype example is the preload-restricted Fontan circulation.

DIFFICULTIES IN ASSESSING DIASTOLIC FUNCTION IN CHILDREN AND APPLICABILITY OF ADULT GUIDELINES

While the principles of the pathophysiology of diastolic dysfunction in children, including those with CHD, are similar to adults, the natural history, progression, and echocardiographic manifestations are often different. In many children with heart failure, heart rates are high, resulting in merging of the E and A waves. This complicates use of inflow Doppler to characterize diastolic function. Alterations in ventricular geometry and loading conditions are hallmarks of CHD and complicate the quantitative evaluation of diastolic function. Diastolic parameters, including tissue Doppler velocities and strain imaging, are significantly affected by loading conditions, making determination of diastolic dysfunction using these parameters alone very challenging in

TABLE 27.3 Influences of Age and Heart Rate on Diastolic Doppler Variables in Children

	UNIVARIATE ASSOCIATIONS		BIVARIATE PARTIAL ASSOCIATIONS[a]	
Variable	**Age**	**RR**	**Age**	**RR**
Mitral E velocity	—	↑	↓	↑
Mitral A velocity	↓	↓↓	↑	↓↓
End A to R interval	↑	—	↑	—
Duration of A wave	—	↑	—	—
Mitral deceleration time	↑↑↑	↑↑↑	↑	↑
Mitral E wave TVI	↑↑	↑↑↑	—	↑↑↑
Mitral A wave TVI	—	↓	↑	↓
Mitral E at A velocity	↓	↓↓	—	↓↓
Mitral E to A ratio (velocity)	—	↑↑↑	↓	↑↑↑
Mitral E to A ratio (TVI)	↑	↑↑↑	↓	↑↑↑
LV IVRT	↑↑	↑↑	↑	↑
PV systolic peak velocity	↓	—	↓	—
PV diastolic peak velocity	—	↑	—	↑
Peak PVAR velocity	—	—	—	—
PVAR duration	↑	↑↑	—	↑↑
PV systolic TVI	—	↑	—	↑
PV diastolic TVI	↑↑↑	↑↑↑	↑	↑
PVAR TVI	↑	↑	—	↑
PV systolic to diastolic ratio (velocity)	↓	—	—	—
PV systolic to diastolic ratio (TVI)	↓↓	↓	↓	↓
Ratio of PVAR to mitral A wave duration	—	—	—	—
Ratio of PVAR to mitral A wave TVI	↓	↓↓	—	↓↓

—, No effect; ↑, weak association ($R2 < 0.10$); ↑↑, moderate association ($0.10 < R2 < 0.20$); ↑↑↑, strong association ($R2 > 0.20$); *A*, atrial; *E*, early; *IVRT*, isovolumic relaxation time; *LV*, left ventricular; *PV*, pulmonary vein; *PVAR*, pulmonary vein atrial reversal; *RR*, RR interval; *TVI*, time velocity integral.
[a]Univariate associations column demonstrates the association between age or heart rate (RR interval) and each dependent variable without accounting for other influences. Bivariate partial associations column demonstrates the effect of age or heart rate on each dependent variable after controlling for the influence of the other independent variable (age or heart rate). Upward arrows indicate positive associations between age or RR interval and the measured variable; downward arrows indicate negative associations. The number of arrows shown increases as the degree of association increases.
From O'Leary PW, et al. Diastolic ventricular function in children: a Doppler echocardiographic study establishing normal values and predictors of increased ventricular end diastolic pressure. *Mayo Clin Proc.* 1998;73:616–628.

patients with CHD.[11] Moreover, it is often difficult to apply a dry value from a normal reference to determine whether a given value in a patient is abnormal due to the wide range of normal values in children, changing values with age and heart rate, difficulties in application of adult guidelines to children, absence of guidelines on how to classify diastolic dysfunction in children, presence of often apparently conflicting echo criteria, lack of correlation of echo criteria with invasively measured reference parameters, and the infrequent presence of isolated delayed relaxation in children.[28–30] Our group studied the applicability of adult guidelines to normal children and to those with dilated, hypertrophic, and restrictive cardiomyopathies.[28] Although the adult guidelines have since been updated,[31] our findings remain pertinent. We found that whether using absolute values or abnormal values based on normal pediatric reference data, adult criteria and algorithms were not applicable to children. We found that pediatric reference data successfully defined normal controls, but because of the wide range of normal values, diastolic dysfunction was classified in only a minority of patients with overt, and often severe, cardiomyopathy. Thus our results suggested that current echo criteria are not adequately applicable for the diagnosis and classification of diastolic dysfunction in pediatric cardiomyopathy (and by inference in complex CHD). Our results also showed that when diastolic dysfunction was diagnosed or suspected, discrepancies between diastolic parameters or diagnostic criteria within individual patients are common, adversely affecting interpretation of diastolic dysfunction, the grading thereof, and interobserver agreement. The classification of diastolic dysfunction in adults is based on a paradigm of progression of abnormalities along a continuum of increasing severity from normal, through delayed relaxation, evolving through a phase of pseudonormalization to a pattern of restrictive filling. However, our results showed that criteria consistent with isolated delayed relaxation are distinctly uncommon in children. Only seven hypertrophic cardiomyopathy (HCM) patients (6.4% of the population studied), mostly adolescents, presented with criteria consistent with isolated delayed relaxation, whereas no dilated cardiomyopathy (DCM) or RCM patients had sufficiently concordant criteria to classify delayed relaxation or pseudonormal filling. Of the parameters studied, e′ (especially septal e′), mitral E deceleration time, and left atrial (LA) volume indexed for body surface area seemed best to differentiate children with cardiomyopathy from controls. Yet, even these parameters were often discrepant in the individual child. The E/A ratio, a central parameter in adult paradigms, was not useful in the children studied. Whether the addition of RV systolic pressure, new to the most recent iteration of the American Society of Echocardiography (ASE) adult diastolic guidelines, will be useful in children remains to be studied. It is logical, especially in left-sided obstructive lesions or dysfunction, if there is no RV outflow or pulmonary obstruction. Other studies have mirrored our findings. In a review of 33 original articles, Cantinotti found that in many studies, sample sizes were limited, particularly in the neonatal age range.[32] There was heterogeneity in the methodologies used to perform and normalize measurements and whether results were expressed as normalized by *z* scores, percentiles, or mean values. Although most studies adjusted measurements for age, classification by specific age subgroups varied, and few addressed the relationships of measurements to body size and heart rate. Although reference values were reproducible in older children, they varied significantly in neonates and infants.[32] Thus, as detailed earlier, assessment of diastolic function remains particularly challenging in the youngest children due to lack of normal data, rapid changes with age, and low measurement reproducibility.

Adult-based guidelines aim to classify the severity of diastolic dysfunction and to assess filling pressures. The E/e′ ratio has become an integral component of adult guidelines to assess filling pressures.[28] However, data suggest that this ratio, whether using the lateral mitral or septal E/e′, correlates poorly with invasively measured filling pressures in children.[33] Similarly, in a group of children with RCM, perhaps the hallmark disease of diastolic dysfunction with elevated filling pressures, individual cutoffs for Doppler indices had poor sensitivity in identifying restrictive physiology. The results of these studies, similar to our findings in children with various types of cardiomyopathy, suggested that poor LV compliance is the typical characteristic of RCM in children, even in the presence of what appears to be normal early relaxation and early ventricular filling. Another investigation of pediatric and young adult patients with RCM, lateral a′ velocity, and pulmonary vein a-wave duration, parameters not included in the adult guidelines, predicted elevated LVEDP with over 80% sensitivity and specificity. However, even then, these measurements were only feasible in about half of the patients.[34] Other parameters that are incorporated directly or indirectly in the adult guidelines, such as indexed LA volume and mitral A wave, correlated only moderately with LVEDP.[34] In a study of 61 consecutive pediatric patients, including infants and children with various biventricular heart diseases, LV relaxation, chamber stiffness, and LVEDP were measured using a high-fidelity micromanometer catheter with simultaneous Doppler echocardiography.[35] The E/e′ correlated only moderately with LVEDP with sensitivity of 0.71 and specificity of 0.93 to determine the presence of EDP above the 90th percentile (12.96 mmHg). The e′ and mitral DT correlated weakly with invasive indices of relaxation and stiffness.[35] Similarly, in other studies in children with a biventricular circulation, traditional diastolic parameters did not correlate with LVEDP; only diastolic strain rate parameters correlated, and even then only moderately, with LVEDP.[36] Assessment of filling pressures in children will be detailed further later in the chapter.

ECHOCARDIOGRAPHIC EVALUATION OF DIASTOLIC FUNCTION IN CHILDREN

Echocardiography is the most commonly used tool to noninvasively assess diastolic dysfunction in children, especially for serial assessment. However, from the previous discussion, it is apparent that no single echo parameter is adequate in and of itself to diagnose the severity of diastolic function or quantify filling pressures in children, even in those with a biventricular circulation. At best, single parameters may be sufficiently sensitive to detect diastolic dysfunction, but not to quantify it.[35] Thus it is imperative that a combination of Doppler echocardiographic parameters and clinical criteria is used. In children with restrictive cardiomyopathies, a combination of increased LA size, increased septal E/e′, lack of a mitral A wave, and the presence of a mid-diastolic L′ wave was noted to be useful.[37] Likewise, in our study, a combination of reduced septal e′, decreased mitral E deceleration time, and increased LA volume indexed for body surface area seemed best to differentiate children with cardiomyopathies from controls.[28]

Within these boundaries and limitations, review of individual echo parameters and the progression of diastolic dysfunction in adults is warranted as a basis to using echocardiographic parameters in combination and to their interpretation in children.

Mitral Inflow Doppler

Mitral inflow Doppler reflects the diastolic pressure gradient between the left atrium and the left ventricle (see Fig. 27.7A). The early diastolic filling wave, or E wave, is the dominant diastolic wave in children and young adults and relates to the peak LA-to-LV pressure gradient at the onset of diastole (see Fig. 27.7B). The DT of the mitral E wave reflects the period of time needed for equalization of LA and LV pressures. As such it is influenced by ventricular relaxation and filling pressures. The late diastolic filling wave, or A wave, represents the peak pressure gradient between the left atrium and the left ventricle in late diastole during atrial contraction. Beyond the first months of life, normal mitral inflow Doppler is characterized by a dominant E wave, a smaller A wave, and a ratio of E and A waves (E/A ratio) between 1 and 3.[11,24] Normal durations of mitral DT and IVRT vary with age and have been reported in both pediatric and adult populations.[11,24–26,38,39] As detailed earlier, mitral inflow Doppler velocities are affected not only by changes in LV diastolic function but also by age, altered loading conditions, heart rate, and changes in atrial and ventricular compliance.[24–26,38,40] In the adult population, the earliest stage of LV diastolic dysfunction demonstrated by mitral inflow Doppler is abnormal relaxation. This Doppler pattern represents a mild decrease in the rate of LV relaxation with normal LA pressure. It is characterized by a reduced E wave velocity, increased A wave velocity, decreased E/A ratio less than 1, and a prolonged mitral DT and IVRT (Fig. 27.8). However, as detailed earlier, this pattern is not commonly seen in isolation in children, outside of older children with HCM.

With increased LA pressure, the initial transmitral gradient between the left atrium and the left ventricle increases, producing a pseudonormalized mitral inflow Doppler pattern with increased E wave velocity and E/A ratio and normalized mitral DT and IVRT intervals. This pseudonormal Doppler pattern may be difficult to distinguish from normal mitral inflow Doppler. In older children and adolescents, maneuvers that decrease ventricular preload, such as the Valsalva maneuver, as well as additional evaluation of pulmonary venous inflow and tissue Doppler can help differentiate between pseudonormalized mitral inflow and more advanced LV diastolic dysfunction. However, the Valsalva maneuver may be difficult to perform and interpret in children and is not routinely used in pediatric labs to the extent it is in adults.

Further deterioration of ventricular diastolic function results in further increases in ventricular filling pressures with an additional increase in atrial pressure and a concomitant decrease in ventricular compliance resulting in restrictive ventricular filling. As in adults, the Doppler pattern of restrictive LV filling is characterized by additional increases in E wave velocity, reduction in A wave velocity, an increased E/A ratio, and significant shortening of mitral DT and IVRT.

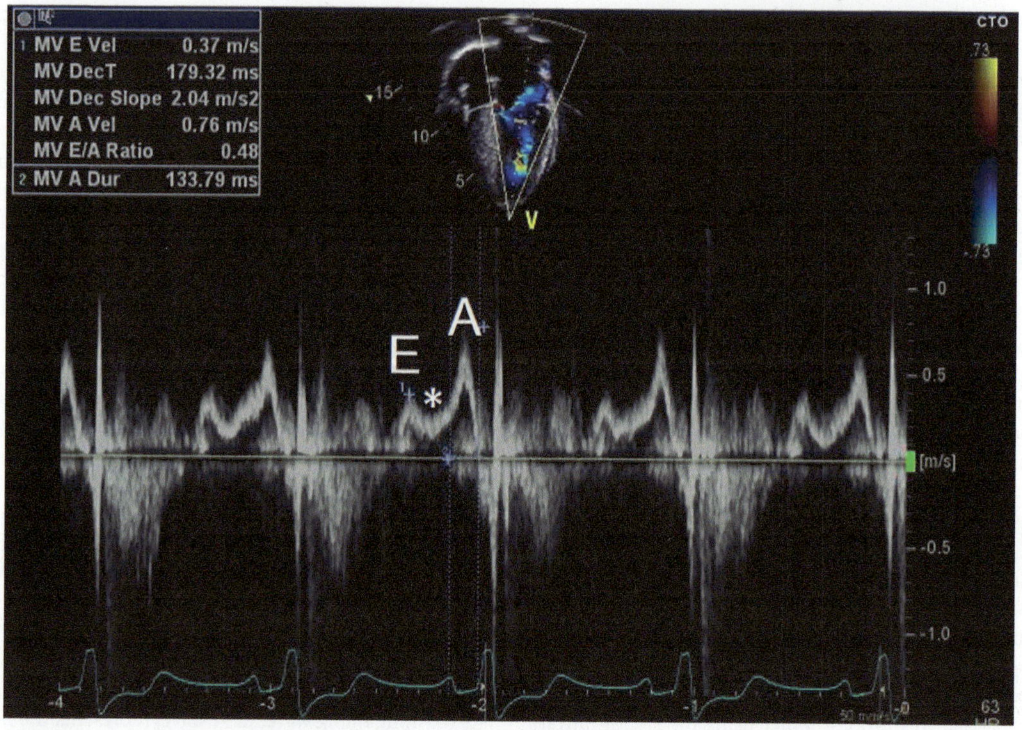

Fig. 27.8 Doppler of mitral valve inflow in a child with hypertrophic cardiomyopathy. Note the lower early *(E)* than late *(A)* diastolic filling wave yielding a reversed E/A ratio. This pattern is typical of impaired relaxation. Note also the prolonged mitral E deceleration time, from the impaired relaxation, which produces an elevated E at A point *(asterisks)*. Thus the ventricle has not adequately relaxed, despite a slow heart rate of 63 bpm, by the time atrial contraction commences. Contrast this to the vigorous relaxation and E over A dominance shown in a normal child in Fig. 27.2B.

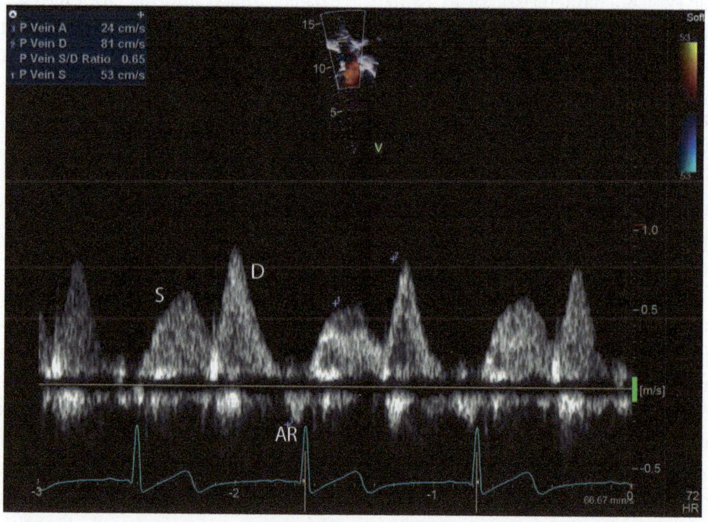

Fig. 27.9 Pulmonary venous Doppler in a normal child showing the systolic *(S)*, diastolic *(D)*, and a-wave reversal *(AR)*. The dominant diastolic wave *(D)* is normal, especially in younger children. More importantly, note that the small a-reversal wave is of short duration.

Pulmonary Venous Doppler

Pulmonary venous Doppler can be combined with mitral inflow Doppler to provide a more comprehensive assessment of LV filling pressures (see Fig. 27.6A).[11,41–44]

Pulmonary venous inflow consists of three distinct Doppler waves: a systolic wave (S wave), a diastolic wave (D wave), and a reversal wave with atrial contraction (a-reversal wave). In adolescents and adults with normal hearts, the characteristic pattern of pulmonary venous inflow consists of a dominant S wave, a smaller D wave, and a small a-reversal wave of low velocity and brief duration. In neonates and younger children, a dominant D wave is often present with a similar brief low-velocity, or even absent, a-reversal wave (Fig. 27.9). Typically, with worsening LV diastolic dysfunction, LA pressure rises, leading to diminished systolic forward flow into the left atrium from the pulmonary veins with relatively increased diastolic forward flow, resulting in a diastolic dominance of pulmonary

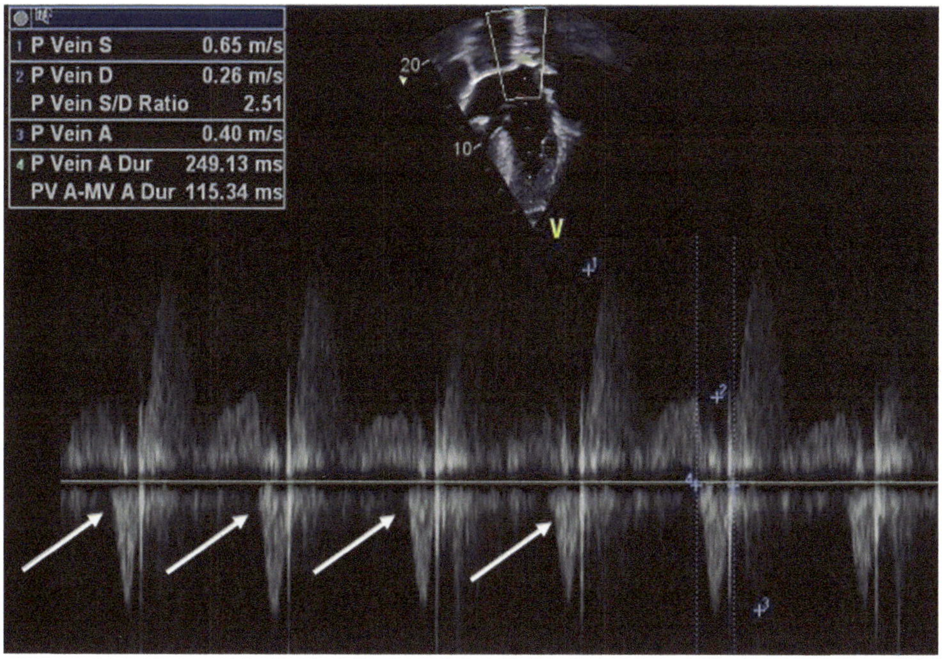

Fig. 27.10 Pulmonary vein Doppler in a child with hypertrophic cardiomyopathy. Flow reversal during atrial contraction (a-wave reversal; *arrows*) is abnormally prominent, both in velocity and in duration, being significantly longer than the mitral A wave duration.

venous inflow. However, we have found the ratio between the pulmonary vein S and D waves quite variable in children and not particularly helpful in diagnosing diastolic dysfunction. Indeed, in a simultaneous echo-cath study in a heterogeneous group of children with biventricular and single-ventricle physiology, the ratio of pulmonary venous S/D flow velocities was not found to be related to invasively measured EDP. In contrast, increased velocity, and in particular increased duration of the pulmonary venous a-reversal wave, is most helpful in suggesting decreased ventricular compliance, particularly when compared to the duration of the mitral inflow A wave (Fig. 27.10). Pediatric and adult studies have demonstrated that an a-reversal wave duration exceeding by 30 msec the corresponding mitral A wave duration or a ratio of pulmonary venous a-reversal wave duration to mitral A wave duration greater than 1.2 is predictive of elevated LV filling pressure.[11,45,46]

Tissue Doppler Velocities

Early (e′) and late (a′) annular or basal wall diastolic velocities can be readily obtained by tissue Doppler echocardiography and mirror the early and late waves of mitral inflow (Fig. 27.11). Similar to systolic tissue Doppler velocities, differences in diastolic velocities exist (1) between the subendocardium and the subepicardium, (2) from cardiac base to apex, and (3) among various myocardial wall segments.[13,14,16,17,20,47–53] Previous studies have reported good correlations between early annular diastolic mitral velocity and invasive measures of diastolic function at cardiac catheterization.[54] As for most parameters, tissue Doppler velocities are influenced by preload[55–57] and afterload.[58–60] This needs to be accounted for when interpreting these velocities. A number of studies have established baseline reference values of tissue Doppler velocities in children (Tables 27.4 and 27.5).[21–23,52,61–63] Additional studies using tissue Doppler have established normal atrioventricular electromechanical coupling intervals.[62] Tissue Doppler velocities vary with age[23,52,63] and heart rate[23,52] (Fig. 27.12). In addition, pulsed-wave tissue Doppler velocities are highly correlated with parameters of cardiac growth, most notably LV end-diastolic dimension and LV mass, with the most significant changes in these velocities occurring during the first year of life.[52]

Tissue Doppler velocities can be helpful in discriminating between normal and pseudonormal transmitral Doppler filling patterns.[15,64–66] In addition to changes incurred by loading conditions, alterations in LA pressure and LV end-diastolic pressure also affect the early transmitral diastolic velocity. However, the corresponding e′ tissue Doppler velocity is typically decreased in patients with pseudonormal filling, allowing differentiation of this abnormal filling pattern from one of normal transmitral Doppler inflow.

The e′ velocity is impacted by myocardial relaxation, restoring forces, and atrial pressure at the time of atrioventricular valve opening.[67] In a small cohort of children, the septal e′ velocity correlated with the invasively measured time constant of relaxation (tau) but with substantial scatter.[68] In a larger study of infants and children, tissue Doppler velocities did not correlate significantly with transmitral inflow Doppler.[52]

Tissue Doppler may also be of clinical value in the differentiation of constrictive from restrictive LV filling (see Chapter 26).[19,69–71] Because the myocardium in patients with constrictive pericarditis is commonly normal, the corresponding tissue Doppler velocities are normal. However, patients with RCM have decreased early diastolic tissue Doppler velocities, allowing separation of these two entities.

The E/e′ Ratio and Measures of Filling Pressures

Filling pressures are strong predictors of outcomes in patients with heart failure and a predictor of death in children with DCM and other conditions.[72] In adults, Nagueh et al. demonstrated a significant correlation of mitral E/e′ with invasively measured mean PCWP.[64] This measure continues to be a central component of adult guidelines for the evaluation of diastolic dysfunction and filling pressures.[31] In various studies, the E/e′ has been reported elevated in diseased pediatric populations, as both components of this ratio are often abnormal. However, as this ratio works predominantly when

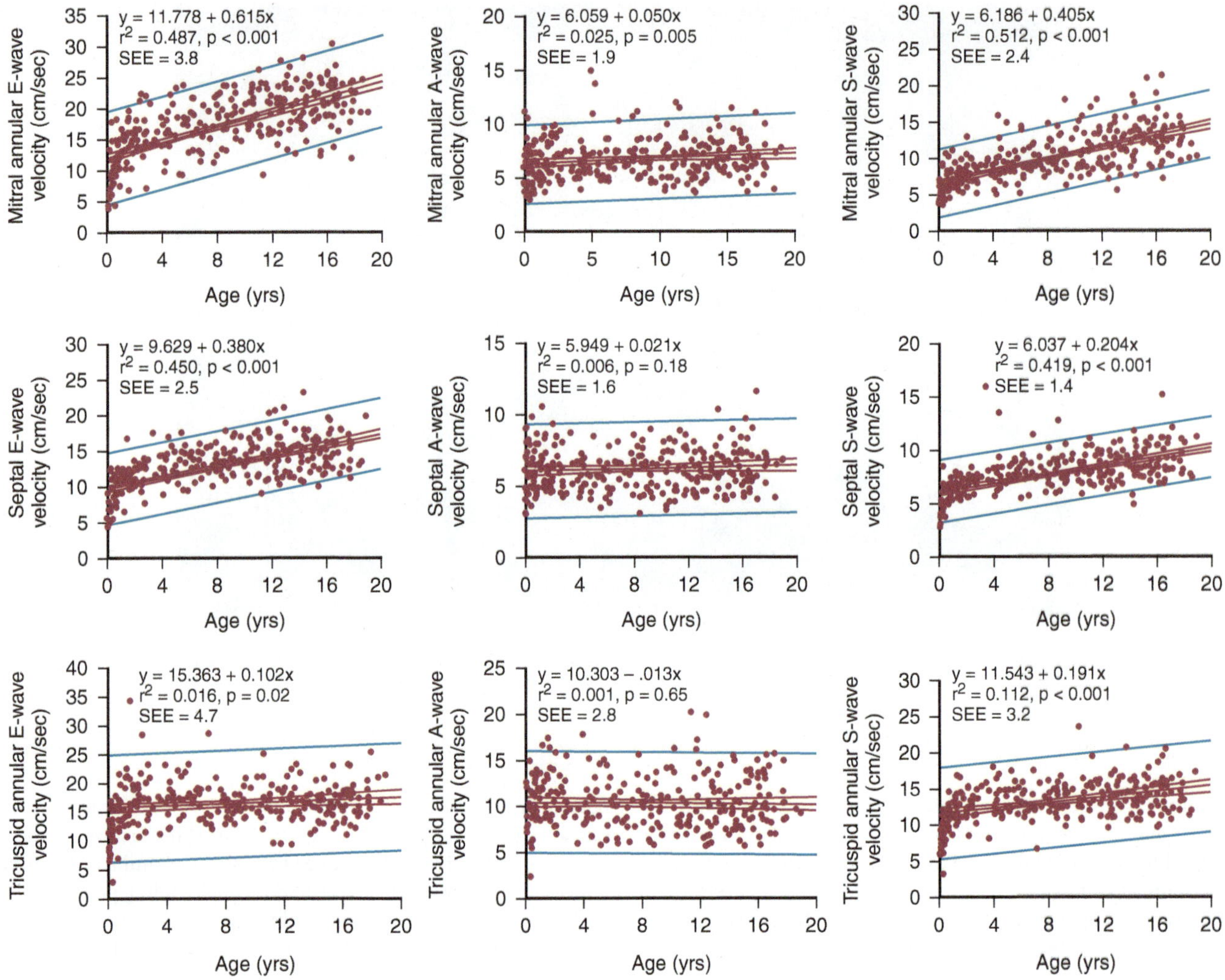

Fig. 27.11 Effect of age on tissue Doppler velocities in healthy children. Data are expressed as mean SD and 95% confidence interval. *(A)*, late diastolic velocity; *(E)*, early diastolic velocity; *(S)*, systolic velocity. (From Eidem BW et al: Impact of cardiac growth on Doppler tissue imaging velocities: A study in healthy children. *J Am Soc Echocardiogr* 2004;17:212–221.)

there is delayed relaxation,[55] which is uncommon in isolation in children, the E/e′ ratio is not a particularly accurate reflector of filling pressures in children.

Normative data for the E/e′ ratio have been reported for children[29,30,52,64,73–75] (Fig. 27.13). These values are significantly altered by age, heart rate, ventricular wall location, and LV dimensions and mass.[52] Values for E/e′ are highest in neonates and decrease with advancing age due primarily to increased e′ velocity. Correlation of the E/e′ ratio to invasively measured filling pressures in children has predominantly been done in children with single-ventricle physiology as these children routinely undergo cardiac catheterization for hemodynamic evaluation before the bicaval pulmonary connection and Fontan procedures. This will be discussed later in the section dealing with evaluation of diastolic function in the functionally single ventricle. In children with biventricular circulation, data are sparse.

In a study of 115 children with heterogeneous single and biventricular heart disease, the E/e′ correlated moderately ($r = 0.54$) with invasively measured EDP in those with biventricular physiology. An E/e′ above 10.7 had 69% sensitivity and 81% specificity for EDP greater than 10 mmHg. In another study in 61 pediatric patients (age 0.4–13 years) who underwent cardiac catheterization for various cardiac pathologies with biventricular circulation, the E/e′ statistically correlated with LVEDP ($r = 0.48$), with an E/e′ above 16.4 having a sensitivity of 0.71 and specificity of 0.93 to determine an EDP greater than 13 mmHg.[35] This E/e′ value is considerably higher than recommended adult cutoffs. Similarly, there was no correlation between EDP and E/e′ in another study of 29 children with heterogeneous biventricular congenital heart disease.[36] Even in a more homogeneous DCM population, the E/e′ correlated weakly with EDP.[33] Similarly, the E/e′ is a poor predictor of EDP in children after heart transplant and was inadequate to predict rejection in these children.[76] Assessment of filling pressures would also be of clinical value in the postoperative intensive care management after surgery for CHD. In a group of 37 infants, an E/e′ cutoff of 15 to predict LA greater than 10 mmHg had a sensitivity of 94% but specificity of only 72%.[77] In a small study of 27 patients, the E/e′ ratio correlated poorly with LA pressure in the immediate postoperative period.[78] Taken together, these studies suggest that a high E/e′ ratio likely indicates that diastolic function is abnormal, but does not accurately ascertain filling pressures in the individual patient. Ezon et al. found only a weak correlation between LVEDP and E/e′ in children with DCM.[33] However, in other studies, the combination of mitral deceleration time and E/e′ improved

TABLE 27.4 **Demographics and Echocardiographic Data in Study Patients**

Demographics	<1 Year	1–5 Years	6–9 Years	10–13 Years	14–18 Years	Total
N	63	68	55	58	81	325
Male	29	39	27	38	44	177
Age (years)	0.40 ± 0.30	3.05 ± 1.51	7.91 ± 1.12	11.99 ± 1.11	16.0 ± 1.40	7.8 ± 6.0
Weight (kg)	6.6 ± 2.7	15.1 ± 5.4	33.8 ± 14.9	47.2 ± 16.3	66.1 ± 15.5	33.3 ± 25.2
BSA (m^2)	0.34 ± 0.08	0.62 ± 0.14	1.07 ± 0.27	1.37 ± 0.29	1.73 ± 0.25	1.0 ± 0.6
HR (bpm)	124 ± 16	105 ± 17	80 ± 11	75 ± 12	69 ± 16	90 ± 26
Echocardiographic						
LVEDD (cm)	2.3 ± 0.3	3.1 ± 0.4	3.9 ± 0.4	4.3 ± 0.4	4.7 ± 0.4	3.6 ± 1.0
LVESD (cm)	1.4 ± 0.2	1.9 ± 0.3	2.4 ± 0.3	2.7 ± 0.3	3.0 ± 0.4	2.3 ± 0.6
LVPWT (cm)	0.4 ± 0.1	0.6 ± 0.1	0.7 ± 0.1	0.8 ± 0.1	0.9 ± 0.2	0.7 ± 0.2
LVSWT (cm)	0.5 ± 0.1	0.6 ± 0.1	0.8 ± 0.1	0.8 ± 0.2	1.0 ± 0.2	0.7 ± 0.2
LV mass (g/m^2)	18.9 ± 6.5	43.6 ± 16.4	82.3 ± 28.3	110.1 ± 32.9	158.4 ± 48.5	81.8 ± 58.9
Mitral E velocity	79.7 ± 18.8	95.2 ± 19.5	94.4 ± 14.8	94.5 ± 16.0	90.3 ± 17.8	90.8 ± 18.5
Mitral A velocity	65.3 ± 13.3	61.3 ± 12.1	49.4 ± 12.5	49.5 ± 13.8	45.5 ± 13.2	54.4 ± 15.0
Mitral E/A ratio	12.4 ± 0.30	1.60 ± 0.46	1.99 ± 0.51	2.02 ± 0.58	2.13 ± 0.65	1.79 ± 0.61
PV S wave velocity	44.6 ± 10.3	48.0 ± 8.9	50.7 ± 11.3	49.0 ± 11.1	47.7 ± 7.3	48.7 ± 9.2
PV D wave velocity	46.0 ± 9.5	54.5 ± 11.0	53.3 ± 11.4	58.4 ± 12.1	57.9 ± 15.0	54.6 ± 12.9
PV A reversal velocity	16.4 ± 6.3	20.6 ± 4.3	20.2 ± 3.8	21.2 ± 4.9	20.0 ± 5.2	20.5 ± 5.1
Tricuspid E velocity	53.3 ± 12.3	61.6 ± 12.5	60.5 ± 13.9	59.6 ± 11.4	60.4 ± 10.9	59.2 ± 12.4
Tricuspid A velocity	53.2 ± 13.0	48.3 ± 12.3	42.4 ± 10.8	39.2 ± 11.3	34.5 ± 11.2	43.3 ± 13.5
Tricuspid E/A ratio	1.01 ± 0.38	1.27 ± 0.31	1.49 ± 0.40	1.61 ± 0.47	1.88 ± 0.56	1.47 ± 0.53
SF (%)	38.9 ± 4.1	38.0 ± 3.6	37.4 ± 3.8	37.4 ± 4.2	36.4 ± 4.3	37.6 ± 4.1
LV MPI	0.33 ± 0.08	0.34 ± 0.07	0.32 ± 0.06	0.34 ± 0.06	0.34 ± 0.08	0.33 ± 0.08
RV MPI	0.29 ± 0.09	0.28 ± 0.07	0.29 ± 0.08	0.28 ± 0.08	0.29 ± 0.08	0.28 ± 0.08

From Eidem BW, et al. Impact of cardiac growth on Doppler tissue imaging velocities: a study in healthy children. *J Am Soc Echocardiogr.* 2004;17:212–221.

BSA: body surface area; HR: heart rate; LVEDD: left ventricular end-diastolic diameter; LVESD: left ventricular end-systolic diameter; LVPWT: left ventricular posterior wall thickness; LVSWT: left ventricualr septal wall thickness, LV: left ventricular; E: pulsed Doppler early velocity; A: pulsed Doppler atrial contraction velocity; PV S: pulmonary venous systolic; PV D: pulmonary venous diastolic; SF: LV shortening fraction; MPI: myocardial performance index; RV: right ventricular.

LVEDP estimation, reinforcing the notion that a more comprehensive approach to diastolic function assessment is needed, rather than reliance on a single measure.[35]

Using similar principles, other echocardiographic measures have been studied in children with various heart diseases to reflect filling pressures, including E/flow propagation velocity (Vp) and E/ early diastolic strain rate.[79] Some of these, especially E/ early diastolic strain rate, have shown better accuracy than the E/e' ratio for prediction of filling pressures or rejection after transplant, but are inadequately validated or accurate and are not as yet routinely used.[36] Clinical implementation is further hampered by the relatively low frame rates of speckle tracking echocardiography in relation to the rapid events of early diastole, especially given the high heart rates of young or sick children. In a small cohort of children undergoing simultaneous cardiac catheterization and transthoracic echocardiography, Border et al.[68] showed a correlation between invasively measured LVEDP and the ratio of peak early transmitral Doppler flow velocity to flow propagation velocity (E/Vp). However, the Vp, despite attractive theoretical and physiologic characteristics, has not gained widespread use in pediatric echo laboratories in part because of low reproducibility when measuring a Doppler slope.

Ryan et al. studied a small group of children with RCM, comparing echo diastolic measures with simultaneously measured LVEDP at cardiac catheterization.[34] Pulmonary vein a-reversal wave duration correlated well with LVEDP, whereas indexed LA volume, mitral valve A wave, lateral e′ velocity, and lateral a′ velocity had only moderate correlations with LVEDP. Of note, lateral a′ velocity of 0.042 m/sec or less and a pulmonary vein AR duration of 156 msec and above had sensitivity and specificity of 80% or more for predicting a LVEDP of 20 mmHg and above.[34]

During mid-diastole (diastasis) there is usually little or no flow from the atrium to the ventricle as pressures in these chambers have equalized. A filling wave in this portion of the cardiac cycle, sometimes termed an L wave, either on inflow Doppler or tissue Doppler, is an important sign of delayed relaxation and increased filling pressures (Fig. 27.14).[37]

Increased atrial volume is a good sign of chronically elevated filling pressures (Fig. 27.15). However, in many cases of CHD this can be difficult to assess due to the confounding presence of atrioventricular valvar stenosis or regurgitation, an atrial or ventricular communication, systemic to pulmonary shunts with volume loading, common atria in some lesions, and/or single-ventricle physiology.

DIASTOLIC DYSFUNCTION IN SPECIFIC CONGENITAL HEART DISEASE

Shunt Lesions: Ventricular Volume Overload

The majority of noninvasive measures of systolic and diastolic ventricular performance are significantly affected by changes in loading conditions. However, studies in children with CHD and associated chronic increases in LV preload have documented minimal changes in tissue Doppler velocities compared with pediatric controls. Harada et al. evaluated 33 children with either ventricular septal defect (VSD) or patent ductus arteriosus (PDA) with increased LV preload using both tissue Doppler and conventional Doppler methodologies compared

TABLE 27.5 **Pulsed-Wave Doppler Tissue Velocities and Time Intervals in Healthy Children by Age Group**

Age Group	N	E* Wave Velocity	A* Wave Velocity	S* Wave Velocity	ICT	IRT	E/E* RATIO
Mitral Annular							
<1 year	63	9.7 ± 3.3 (8.8–10.5)	5.7 ± 1.8 (5.3–6.2)	5.7 ± 1.6 (5.3–6.1)	77.4 ± 18.4 (72.7–82.0)	57.0 ± 14.8 (53.1–60.8)	8.8 ± 2.7 (8.1–9.5)
1–5 yr	68	15.1 ± 3.4[b] (14.3–15.4)	6.5 ± 1.9 (6.1–7.0)	7.7 ± 2.1[b] (7.2–8.2)	76.9 ± 15.9 (72.8–80.9)	62.1 ± 13.2 (58.9–65.4)	6.5 ± 2.0[b] (6.0–7.0)
6–9 yr	55	17.2 ± 3.7[b] (16.2–18.3)	6.7 ± 1.9 (6.2–7.3)	9.5 ± 2.1[b] (8.9–10.1)	77.9 ± 18.9 (72.4–83.4)	62.9 ± 11.9 (59.5–66.3)	5.8 ± 1.9 (5.3–6.4)
10–13 yr	58	19.6 ± 3.4[b] (18.7–20.5)	6.4 ± 1.8 (5.9–6.9)	10.8 ± 2.9[a] (10.0–11.5)	76.6 ± 16.2 (72.4–80.9)	62.6 ± 12.4 (59.4–65.9)	4.9 ± 1.3 (4.6–5.2)
14–18 yr	81	20.6 ± 3.8 (19.7–21.4)	6.7 ± 1.6 (6.3–7.1)	12.3 ± 2.9[b] (11.6–12.9)	78.9 ± 15.4 (75.4–82.3)	69.5 ± 15.5[a] (66.1–73.0)	4.7 ± 1.3 (4.4–5.0)
Total	325	16.5 ± 5.3 (16.0–17.1)	6.4 ± 1.9 (6.2–6.6)	9.3 ± 3.4 (8.9–9.7)	77.5 ± 16.7 (75.7–79.5)	63.2 ± 14.4 (61.7–64.9)	6.1 ± 2.4 (5.9–6.4)
Septal							
<1 year	63	8.1 ± 2.5 (7.5–8.7)	6.1 ± 1.5 (5.7–6.4)	5.4 ± 1.2 (5.1–5.7)	77.5 ± 17.5 (73.0–82.0)	53.0 ± 11.7 (50.0–56.0)	10.3 ± 2.7 (9.7–11.0)
1–5 yr	68	11.8 ± 2.0[b] (11.3–12.3)	6.0 ± 1.3 (5.7–6.4)	7.1 ± 1.5[b] (6.8–7.5)	80.1 ± 15.5 (76.3–83.9)	59.8 ± 12.0 (56.9–62.7)	8.1 ± 1.8[b] (7.7–8.5)
6–9 yr	55	13.4 ± 1.9[b] (12.8–13.9)	5.9 ± 1.3 (5.5–6.3)	8.0 ± 1.3 (7.6–8.4)	82.8 ± 15.3 (78.4–87.2)	65.6 ± 10.7 (62.5–68.7)	7.2 ± 1.6 (6.8–7.7)
10–13 yr	58	14.5 ± 2.6 (13.8–15.2)	6.1 ± 2.3 (5.6–6.7)	8.2 ± 1.3 (7.9–8.5)	87.9 ± 16.4[a] (83.6–92.2)	72.5 ± 12.3 (69.3–75.8)	6.6 ± 1.4 (6.3–7.0)
14–18 yr	81	14.9 ± 2.4 (14.3–15.4)	6.2 ± 1.5 (5.9–6.6)	9.0 ± 1.5 (8.7–9.3)	88.4 ± 15.6 (84.9–91.9)	77.5 ± 14.5 (74.3–80.8)	6.4 ± 1.5 (6.1–6.8)
Total	325	12.6 ± 3.4 (12.2–13.0)	6.1 ± 1.6 (5.9–6.3)	7.6 ± 1.9 (7.4–7.8)	83.5 ± 16.5 (81.7–85.4)	66.1 ± 15.3 (64.4–67.9)	7.7 ± 2.3 (7.5–8.0)
Tricuspid Annular							
<1 year	63	13.8 ± 8.2 (11.7–15.9)	9.8 ± 2.4 (9.1–10.5)	10.2 ± 5.5 (8.8–11.7)	68.7 ± 18.2 (63.9–73.5)	52.0 ± 12.9 (48.5–55.4)	4.4 ± 2.3 (3.8–5.0)
1–5 yr	68	17.1 ± 4.0[b] (16.1–18.1)	10.9 ± 2.7 (10.2–11.6)	13.2 ± 2.0[b] (12.7–13.7)	77.7 ± 15.0 (73.9–81.5)	59.0 ± 13.9 (55.4–62.5)	3.8 ± 1.1 (3.5–4.1)
6–9 yr	55	16.5 ± 3.0 (15.7–17.4)	9.8 ± 2.7 (9.0–10.6)	13.4 ± 2.0 (12.8–14.0)	91.8 ± 21.5[b] (85.5–98.0)	58.5 ± 17.5 (53.4–63.6)	3.6 ± 0.8 (3.4–3.9)
10–13 yr	58	16.5 ± 3.1 (15.7–17.4)	10.3 ± 3.4 (9.3–11.2)	13.9 ± 2.4 (13.2–14.5)	98.1 ± 21.7 (92.2–103.9)	61.7 ± 19.9 (56.4–67.1)	3.5 ± 1.4 (3.2–3.9)
14–18 yr	81	16.7 ± 2.8 (16.0–17.3)	10.1 ± 2.6 (9.5–10.7)	14.2 ± 2.3 (13.7–14.7)	101.9 ± 20.4 (97.2–106.6)	62.9 ± 18.9 (58.5–67.3)	3.7 ± 1.0 (3.5–3.9)
Total	325	16.1 ± 4.7 (15.6–16.7)	10.2 ± 2.8 (9.9–10.5)	13.0 ± 3.4 (12.6–13.4)	88.2 ± 23.1 (85.6–90.8)	59.0 ± 17.2 (57.0–60.9)	3.8 ± 1.4 (3.6–4.0)

A, Late diastolic velocity; *A**, late diastolic annular velocity; *E*, early diastolic inflow Doppler velocity; *E**, early diastolic annular velocity; *ICT*, isovolumic contraction time; *IRT*, isovolumic relaxation time; *S*, systolic velocity; *S**, systolic annular velocity.

Data expressed as mean ± SD (95% confidence interval). Doppler tissue imaging velocities are expressed in cm/sec. Time intervals are expressed in msec.

[a]$P < 0.05$.

[b]$P < 0.01$ compared with proceeding age group.

From Eidem BW, et al. Impact of cardiac growth on Doppler tissue imaging velocities: a study in healthy children. *J Am Soc Echocardiogr.* 2004;17:212–221.

with simultaneous cardiac catherization–derived hemodynamic data.[80] Transmitral early diastolic velocities (E) were significantly increased and correlated directly with increases in LA pressure and pulmonary-to-systemic flow ratios. However, the corresponding early (e′) and late (a′) tissue Doppler velocities were not different compared with controls despite increased LV preload. Following repair, tissue Doppler velocities remained unchanged despite removal of the chronic LV volume overload.[80] Eidem et al. reported similar findings in 94 children with varying sizes of VSDs.[81] The E/e′ ratio was minimally increased compared with controls; however, when divided into subgroups based on VSD size, no significant change in this ratio was demonstrated with increasing LV preload. These data were consistent with previously published invasive hemodynamic data demonstrating normal LV filling pressures in patients with VSDs with otherwise normal LV systolic and diastolic function,[82] as well as with early invasive studies where congestive heart failure from a VSD was attributed to systolic rather than diastolic

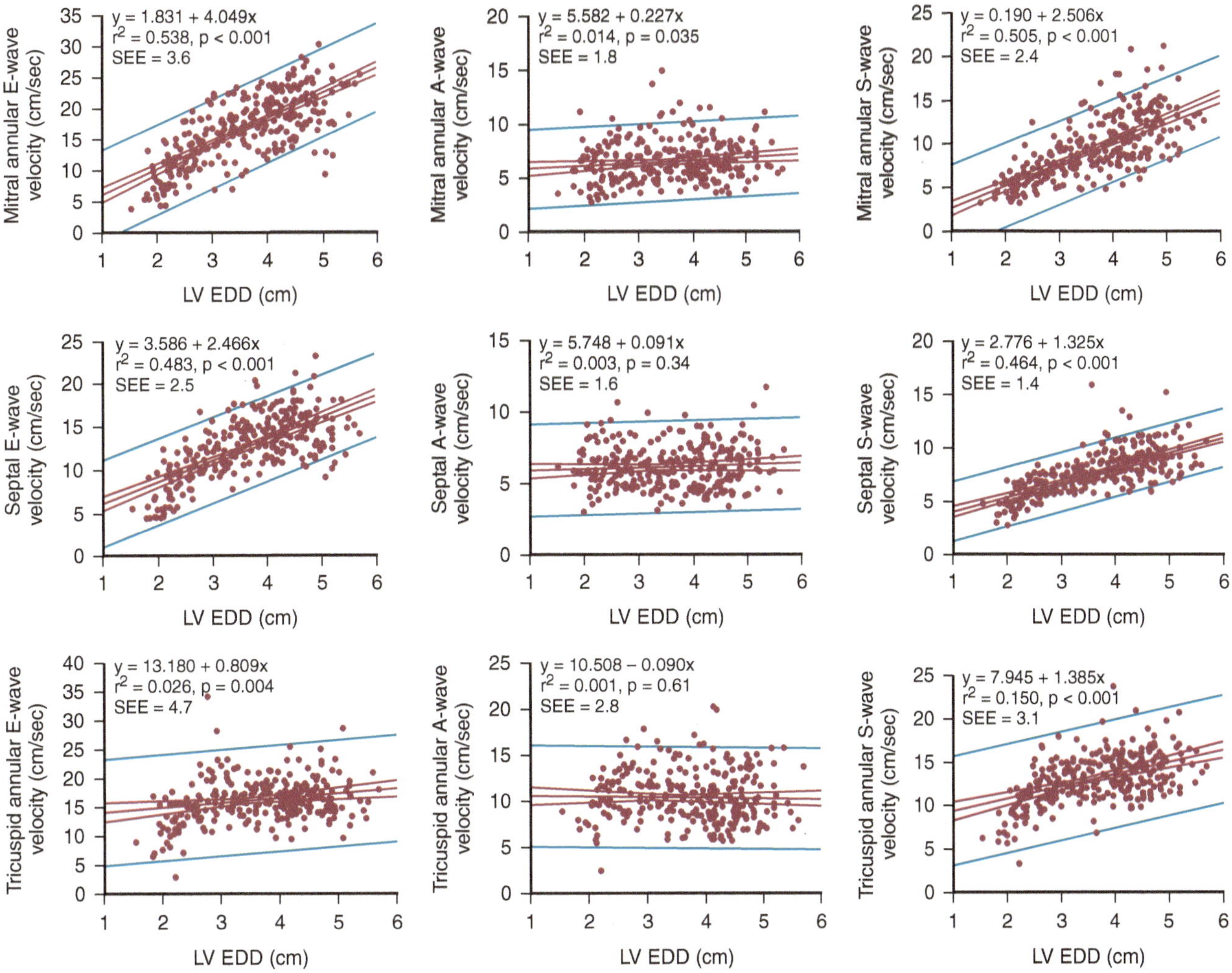

Fig. 27.12 Effect of left ventricular end diastolic dimension (LV EDD) on tissue Doppler velocities in healthy children. Data are expressed as mean SD and 95% confidence interval. *A*, late diastolic velocity; *E*, early diastolic velocity; *S*, systolic velocity. (From Eidem BW et al: Impact of cardiac growth on Doppler tissue imaging velocities: A study in healthy children. *J Am Soc Echocardiogr* 2004;17:212–221.)

dysfunction.[83] Changes in tissue velocities may also be attributable to passive translational cardiac motion or truly reduced motion secondary to ventricular dilatation from increased volume loading.

A proportion of patients with an ASD or VSD repaired in childhood or a small residual VSD not thought to be hemodynamically significant will develop pulmonary hypertension (PH) and abnormally elevated RV systolic pressures (RVSp) during exercise.[84] This has been suggested to possibly be related to abnormal LV diastolic properties rather than abnormal precapillary pulmonary vasoconstriction, as these patients did not decrease RVSp in response to a single dose of sildenafil but demonstrated a steeper RVSp curve during increasing exercise intensity in those patients with lower LV e′ (although E/e′ was not reported).[85] However, this topic remains inconclusive as in contrast to their previous findings, the same group of investigators did not demonstrate changes in RVSp in response to exercise or changes in LV diastolic function (measured as LV e′ and E/e′ ratio) in adults with isolated ventricular septal defect closed in early childhood.[86]

Pauliks et al. evaluated 39 children with atrial septal defects before and after interventional device closure.[87] At baseline, children with ASDs had increased tricuspid and mitral annular velocities compared with controls. Following ASD closure, a transient immediate decrease in tissue Doppler velocities in all myocardial segments was demonstrated, which normalized at 24 hours after the procedure, demonstrating the load dependence of tissue Doppler velocities. Other studies have suggested that the load dependence of tissue Doppler velocities in children with ASD depends on RV size and relative compliance.[88] Cheung et al. evaluated RV function with tissue Doppler imaging (TDI) and showed improved global and regional indices of RV function after interventional device closure of ASDs but not with surgical closure of these defects.[89] Other tissue Doppler studies have demonstrated improvement in LV diastolic function after ASD closure likely related to improved ventricular interaction with decreased RV dilatation and volume overload.[90]

The volume loading imposed by an intracardiac shunt may also provoke dysfunction in a ventricle that is stiff from other reasons such as systemic hypertension. In patients with ASD, echocardiographic evaluations performed before and 2 days after ASD closure, comparing younger versus older patients, e′ was lower in older patients before ASD repair, although after closure, e′ decreased in both groups to a similar degree, regardless of age. However, ASD closure resulted in a greater worsening in measures of LV relaxation and stiffness in older versus younger patients.[91] Nonetheless, other studies have suggested that transcatheter ASD closure is safe and effective in elderly patients even in the presence of overt LV diastolic dysfunction by echocardiography.[92]

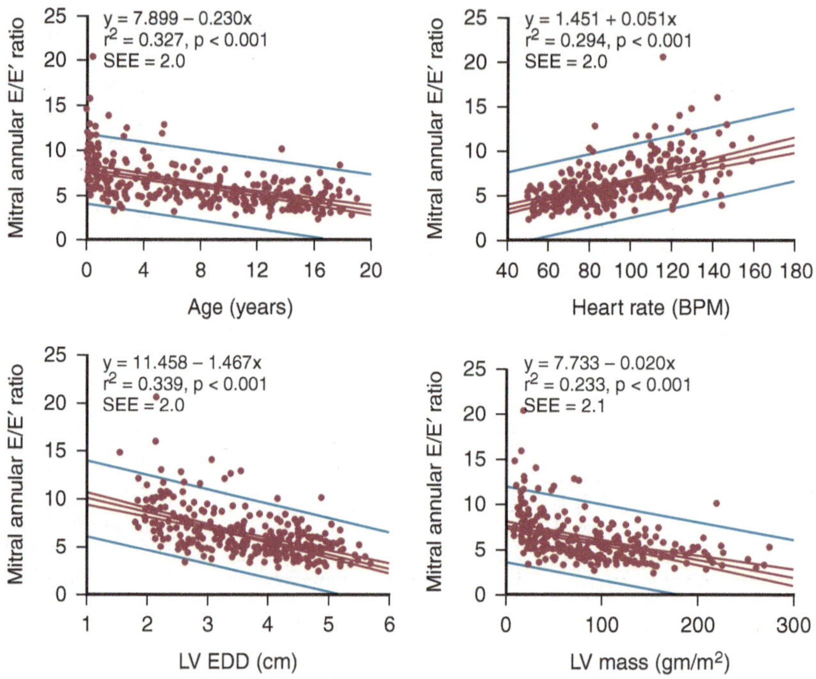

Fig. 27.13 Effect of age, heart rate, left ventricular end-diastolic dimension (*LVEDD*) and LV mass on mitral inflow Doppler early diastolic velocity (*E*)/early mitral annular diastolic tissue Doppler imaging velocity (*E′*) ratio in healthy children. Data are expressed as mean ± SD and 95% confidence interval. (From Eidem BW, et al. Impact of cardiac growth on Doppler tissue imaging velocities: a study in healthy children. *J Am Soc Echocardiogr*. 2004;17:212–221.)

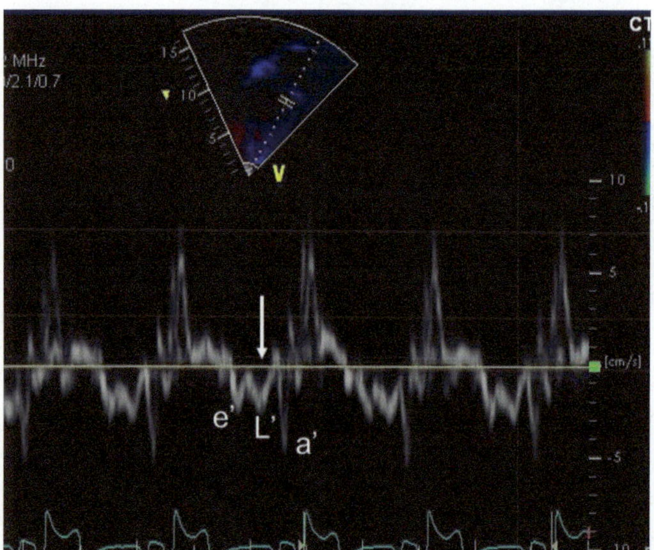

Fig. 27.14 Tissue Doppler imaging in a child with hypertrophic cardiomyopathy. There is a prominent mid-diastolic L wave *(arrow)*, which suggests impaired relaxation and increased filling pressures. Also note the abnormally reversed e′ to a′ ratio with dominance of the a′ wave.

LV Pressure Loading

Children with CHD commonly have myocardial hypertrophy due to increased pressure loading. This can impact diastolic function even prior to overt changes in systolic performance. Children with chronic hypertrophy secondary to aortic stenosis (AS) or hypertension have distinct abnormalities of LV diastolic function when evaluated noninvasively.[93–95] Invasive evaluation of diastolic performance is rarely performed in these patients, but these parameters have also been shown to be abnormal.[96] Banerjee et al. evaluated 10 patients with congenital obstruction of the left ventricular outflow tract (LVOT) (valvular aortic stenosis in 7 children, coarctation of the aorta in 2 children, and supravalvular aortic stenosis in 1 child).[97] Both noninvasive and invasive parameters of LV function were evaluated in these children and compared with normal controls. While systolic parameters, including fractional shortening and end-systolic fiber elastance, were normal, children with LVOT obstruction had prolonged IVRT and time constants of relaxation, although passive diastolic properties, including chamber stiffness and myocardial stiffness, were normal in this small cohort. Decreased tissue Doppler velocities may also reflect diastolic dysfunction,[98,99] although the increased afterload itself may be the cause of lower tissue velocities rather than intrinsic myocardial dysfunction. Indeed, children with the highest aortic valve gradients had the most significant decreases in tissue Doppler velocities.[98] In a study involving children and young adults with AS, aortic regurgitation (AR), or both, mitral inflow E/A and E wave deceleration time, tissue Doppler e′, E/e′, and LA volume were assessed and formulated into a diastolic function score. A higher LV mass *z* score and previous aortic valve balloon dilation were associated with worse diastolic dysfunction.[100] Interestingly, patients with AS or mixed AS and AR had diastolic dysfunction, while those with pure AR were not diagnosed as having diastolic dysfunction.[100]

Chronic elevation of afterload may lead to progressive changes in myocardial architecture, resulting in decreased ventricular compliance and restrictive physiology.[101] This may be related to increased ventricular fibrosis that follows pressure-loading lesions such as aortic stenosis.[102] In a study of 35 children and young adults with congenital aortic stenosis, myocardial extracellular volume fraction (ECV) measured by cardiac magnetic resonance imaging (MRI) was significantly higher in

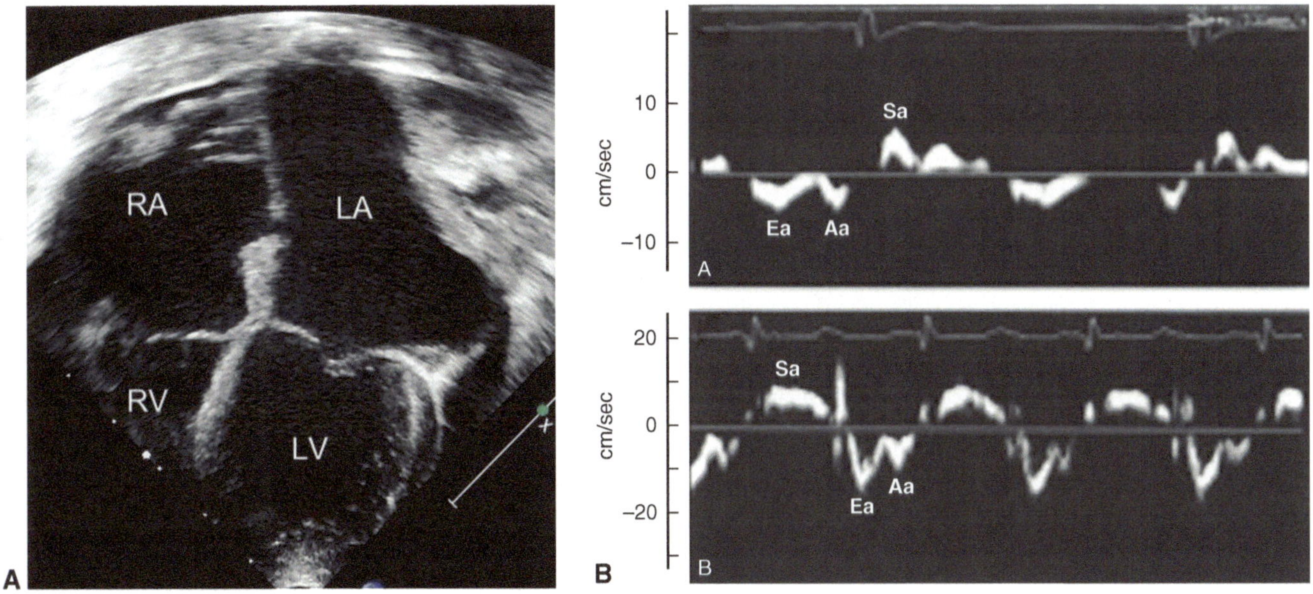

Fig. 27.15 Apical four-chamber view in a child with restrictive cardiomyopathy. There is severe left and right atrial enlargement consistent with increased ventricular filling pressures. *LA*, left atrium; *LV*, left ventricle; *RA*, Right atrium; *RV*, right ventricle.

AS patients compared to normal controls. A higher ECV correlated with echocardiographic indices of diastolic dysfunction, including a higher mitral E wave, E/e′, and indexed LA volume but interestingly not with AS gradient, LV mass, mass/volume ratio (in contrast to studies reviewed earlier), or ejection fraction.[102] Indeed, myocardial ischemia and damage leading to endocardial fibroelastosis with impaired filling and compliance can begin with aortic stenosis in utero.[103] This can manifest in the fetus as fused mitral inflow E and A waves, higher E velocity, shorter mitral inflow time, lower LV lateral and septal e′, and higher E/e′.[103]

After balloon dilatation of aortic stenosis there can be a decrease in LV mass/volume ratio with improved echocardiographic measures of diastolic function, including mitral annular and septal e′ and E/e′ and LVEDP in most patients. One study identified higher pre–balloon aortoplasty LV mass *z* score and worse diastolic function as risk factors for persistent diastolic dysfunction after relief of aortic stenosis, suggesting that severe myocardial damage may be irreversible.[104] Newer modalities, such as strain imaging, may detect more subtle LV diastolic abnormalities in patients with bicuspid aortic valve even without overt stenosis.[105]

CARDIOMYOPATHIES

Hypertrophic and Dilated Cardiomyopathies in Children

Evaluation of diastolic function, especially with the use of TDI, has emerged as a potentially important clinical application to predict clinical outcomes in children with cardiomyopathies.

Molina et al. used the multicenter Pediatric Heart Network data to evaluate echo predictors of disease progression in children with DCM.[106] Mitral inflow parameters and diastolic tissue velocities were significantly associated with disease progression (defined as hospitalization for heart failure, initiation of intravenous inotropic support, transplant listing or increase in listing status, need for mechanical circulatory support, or death). However, many of these parameters were not included in the multivariate analysis because of incomplete separation of early and late diastolic flows or annular motion (Doppler summation waves). This is a common problem in pediatric clinical practice and highlights some of the difficulties in using what seem to be predictive diastolic parameters in children due to the influence, at least in part, of high heart rates. Of note, in this study, the color M mode LV inflow propagation slope was significantly associated with risk for disease progression.[106]

Tissue Doppler velocities have prognostic value for outcomes or disease progression in pediatric cardiomyopathies, including noncompaction, dilated and hypertrophic cardiomyopathies,[1,68,106–112] as well as graft failure in pediatric heart transplant recipients.[113] McMahon et al.[1] prospectively evaluated 54 children with DCM with both conventional echocardiographic indices and tissue Doppler velocities to determine predictors of adverse clinical outcomes (defined as death, cardiac transplantation, or hospitalization). While tissue Doppler velocities, LV and RV myocardial performance index (MPI), RV fractional area change, and LV ejection fraction were all abnormal in DCM patients, only the tricuspid e′ velocity of less than 8.5 cm/sec and LV ejection fraction less than 30% were multivariate predictors of poor clinical outcome.

In various cardiomyopathies, systole, as measured by the duration of mitral or tricuspid regurgitation, prolongs at the expense of a shortened diastolic duration.[114,115] As diastolic duration is exponentially dependent on heart rate, the S/D duration ratio worsens with increasing heart rates, reducing the time available for ventricular filling. In children with DCM, Mondal et al. reported that the tissue Doppler measured S/D duration ratio correlated with need for transplant and mortality, and is thus a potentially useful index for prognostication.[116]

Hypertrophic cardiomyopathy is often considered a disease characterized by diastolic dysfunction. Yet, it is noteworthy that large pediatric studies have not identified diastolic dysfunction, beyond the severity of hypertrophy, as a major risk factor for adverse outcomes, possibly as this was not systematically investigated.[117,118] In a meta-analysis of 25 pediatric HCM studies (patients <18 years of age) that included 3394 patients, LA diameter did not meet the major risk factor criteria for adverse outcome.[119] Earlier studies[108] evaluated LV diastolic function in children with HCM using TDI compared with more traditional echocardiographic parameters, exercise stress testing, and ambulatory Holter monitoring to determine their clinical utility in predicting death or ventricular tachycardia and significant cardiac symptoms. In all, 80 children were prospectively evaluated, with the E/e′ ratio found to be significantly predictive of adverse clinical outcomes. In addition, the E/e′ ratio correlated inversely with peak oxygen consumption obtained during exercise stress testing. While LV ejection fraction, MPI, maximal LV wall thickness, and LA volume were all significantly different compared with controls, none were predictive of the clinical end points. Children with HCM had reduced e′ velocities at the septal and lateral mitral annuli at rest; however, these normalized with exercise while systolic velocities (s′) were normal at rest but failed to augment normally at peak exercise.[120] These results may have stemmed from the increased LVOT gradient found in this study during exercise, but also highlights the relation between systolic and diastolic function as will be discussed later in the chapter.

Diastolic dysfunction as measured by echocardiography has also been found to be impaired in children with HCM associated with Noonan or LEOPARD syndromes.[121] In these patients, the e′ and E/e′ ratios were more impaired in comparison to other pediatric HCM patients. This is important as these syndromic patients may have worse clinical outcomes.

DIASTOLIC FUNCTION IN CONDITIONS PREDOMINANTLY AFFECTING THE RIGHT VENTRICLE

Tetralogy of Fallot

Tetralogy of Fallot (TOF) is the most common cyanotic CHD and the most studied in terms of RV systolic and diastolic function. TOF patients, as with other congenital heart lesions involving the right ventricle, frequently have concomitant changes in ventricular loading conditions, which impact the evaluation of diastolic function. The impact of loading conditions and the difficulty in evaluating diastolic function in congenital RV disease was demonstrated in a small study in asymptomatic children after TOF repair that found the tricuspid E/e′ was not significantly associated with RVEDP or RA pressure, but rather, albeit weakly, with the severity of pulmonary regurgitation (PR).[122] In another study, RV outflow obstruction was associated with lower E/A ratio and antegrade end-diastolic pulmonary flow.[123] Thus the impact of loading conditions should be accounted for when interpreting diastolic function in CHD.

Our group studied RV and LV diastolic function in 53 children after TOF repair in comparison to 49 age-matched controls.[124] TOF patients had more RV diastolic dysfunction in comparison to controls, as manifested by reduced tricuspid valve (TV) E/A ratio, e′ velocity, and longitudinal early diastolic strain rate (see Fig. 27.16). In addition, TOF patients had increased right atrial (RA) volume and TV E/e′ ratio. These results are consistent with the previous discussion that, in children, features consistent with delayed relaxation are often found concomitantly with those characterizing decreased compliance even early in the clinical course (Fig. 27.17). Indeed, more than 20 years ago, Helbing et al. used cardiac MRI to assess RV diastolic function in a small group of children after TOF repair with PR.[125] He found that both impaired filling and restrictive physiology affect RV function in children with repaired tetralogy of Fallot and PR; and that restrictive RV physiology is associated with decreased exercise function.[125] Abnormal early RV diastolic filling is likely related, at least in part, to abnormal systolic function, which is common in repaired TOF. This is because elastic restoring forces play an important role in RV filling, just as they do in the left ventricle.[126] Interestingly, these restoring forces are impacted by septal curvature, which is dependent on pressure gradients between the LV and RV.[126] Thus ventricular-ventricular interactions impact RV diastolic filling through this mechanism, in addition to others. Using cardiac MRI, Sun et al.[127] found that early diastolic dysfunction, as manifested by delayed onset of TV flow, is common after TOF repair and is associated with reduced RV ejection fraction, although not with E/A ratio, ventricular end-diastolic volumes, pulmonary regurgitant fraction, heart rate, or QRS duration. Nonetheless, they attributed this phenomenon to interventricular dyssynchrony.[127]

Beyond RV diastolic abnormalities we found reduced LV early diastolic circumferential strain rate in TOF patients in association with more PR and higher RV volumes suggesting the effect of ventricular-ventricular interactions.[124,128] These were confirmed in a later study from our group in 112 pediatric patients after tetralogy of Fallot repair.[129] In that study, end-diastolic antegrade flow in the main pulmonary artery was associated with larger RV dimensions. Although the presence of end-diastolic forward flow was not associated with other differences in RV diastolic parameters, it was associated with more pronounced pulmonary venous a-reversal and larger LA size. These results suggest that ventricular diastolic interaction affects LV filling pressures.[129] Abnormal LV rotational mechanics and untwisting may also contribute to LV diastolic dysfunction and impaired early diastolic suction in repaired TOF.[130,131]

A multicenter study that included Doppler data from 325 adult-repaired TOF patients assessed the prevalence and clinical implications of LV and RV diastolic dysfunction.[132] LV diastolic dysfunction was defined as mitral lateral e′ less than 10 cm/sec and E/e′ ratio above 9. Abnormal RV diastolic function was defined as tricuspid E/A ratio of 0.8 to 2.1 with E/e′ ratio above 6 or a tricuspid ratio E/A above 2.1 with a deceleration time less than 120 msec. Abnormal LV diastolic Doppler indices, found in 14%, were associated with hypertension, dyslipidemia, three or more cardiac operations, and a history of ventricular tachycardia. In the same population, abnormal RV indices were prevalent in 52% and were associated with hypertension, dyslipidemia, diabetes mellitus, and three or more cardiac operations. Importantly, ventricular tachycardia, an important risk factor for mortality in the TOF population, was more common in those with abnormal RV diastolic function.[132] These results highlight that both ventricles are involved in the pathophysiology of repaired TOF and that in adults, besides the progressive chronicity of the CHD itself, acquired cardiovascular disease becomes significant in adding to the overall burden of disease.

Many studies have used tissue Doppler to investigate diastolic function in repaired TOF. Although the majority of studies have sampled tissue velocities at the base of the heart, some studies have found that regional right ventricular outflow tract (RVOT) diastolic velocities are reduced in TOF patients as compared with controls in relation to RV dilatation.[133] Measuring RVOT properties may be important as abnormal function in this region has been associated with adverse outcomes.[134]

Late diastolic abnormalities have been described after repair of TOF more frequently than in other conditions. The phenomenon of restrictive RV physiology after repair of TOF, as manifested by end-diastolic antegrade pulmonary flow throughout the respiratory cycle, was described over 20 years ago (Fig. 27.18).[135] Initially it was associated with adverse early postoperative course, but was also associated with better long-term outcomes as more restrictive RVs were believed to dilate less in response to chronic PR.[136] Since that time, multiple studies have investigated the significance of so-called restrictive physiology, with variable results.[137] A recent study retrospectively analyzed 399 patients with repaired TOF who had echocardiography and

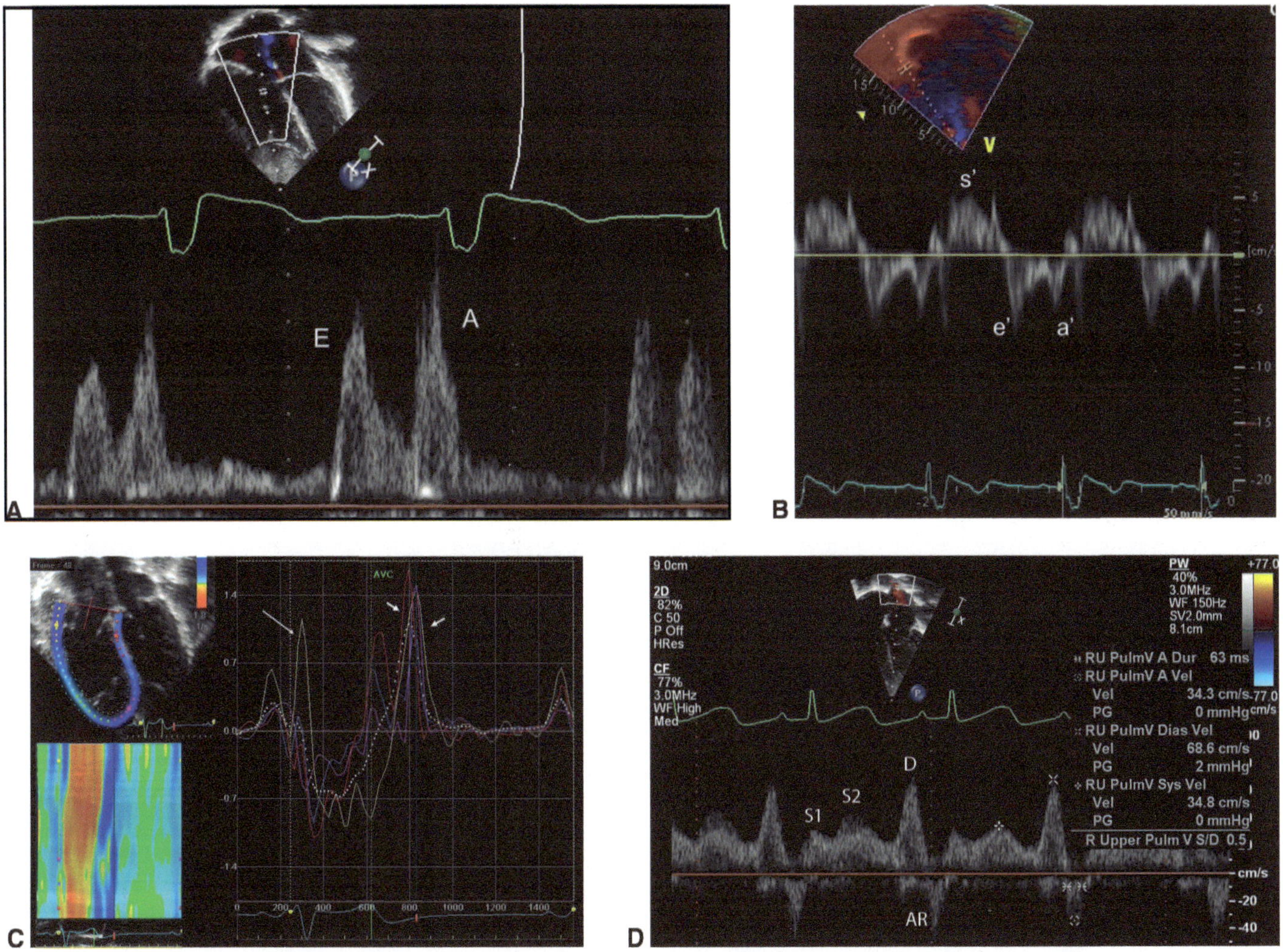

Fig. 27.16 (A) Early right ventricular diastolic abnormalities in a child after tetralogy of Fallot repair, as manifested by reversed tricuspid inflow early *(E)* and late *(A)* Doppler waves. (B) Pulsed-wave Doppler at the tricuspid annulus in an adolescent after repair of tetralogy of Fallot. There are reduced systolic and diastolic velocities and abnormal e′ and a′ ratio, consistent with altered early diastolic right ventricular filling and impaired relaxation. (C) Right ventricular (RV) strain rate imaging in a child after tetralogy of Fallot repair. Segmental and global *(dotted white line)* strain rate values in systole and diastole are abnormally low. In addition to abnormal absolute strain rate values, the mechanical patterns are abnormal. Note the early systolic stretch of the lateral basal RV segment depicted by the yellow curve *(long arrow)*. This stems from electromechanical dyssynchrony induced by early septal activation. The dispersion between right ventricular and septal segments persists into early diastole *(short arrows)* as seen by the delay in peak early diastolic strain rate between the basal septal segment *(red curve)* and basal RV lateral wall *(yellow curve)*. These mechanical abnormalities hinder effective early diastolic relaxation. (D) Early left ventricular diastolic abnormalities are also apparent in this example of pulmonary vein Doppler in another child after repair of tetralogy of Fallot. There is an exaggerated dominance of diastolic *(D)* versus systolic *(S)* flow velocities as well as increased pulmonary a-wave reversal *(AR)*, suggestive of decreased left ventricular compliance. Note the separation of the systolic S1 and S2 waves in this patient.

cardiovascular magnetic resonance.[138] Doppler identified restrictive physiology in 31% of patients. Compared with those without end-diastolic antegrade pulmonary flow, patients with end-diastolic antegrade pulmonary flow were younger, had more PR, and higher RV end-diastolic volume, stroke volume, ejection fraction, and lower LV end-diastolic volume.[138] In contrast, markers of RV restriction such as right atrial size did not differ between the groups. The authors concluded that the clinical significance of RV restrictive physiology remains uncertain.[138] Thus restrictive physiology has been associated with greater RV dilation, but also better exercise capacity despite being related to more RV fibrosis.[139] This seems difficult to reconcile, especially as other diastolic parameters, including diastolic strain rate, were worse in patients with restrictive physiology.[139]

Impaired filling and diastolic function of the RV is also associated with reduced atrial function in repaired TOF patients. Combined echo and cardiac MRI studies have found decreased RA pump and reservoir function in association with decreased RV systolic function.[140] Reduced RA strain was also found in repaired TOF patients.[141] Residua from surgery, including scar tissue and lack of pericardium, may contribute to impaired RA function more than PR and an enlarged right

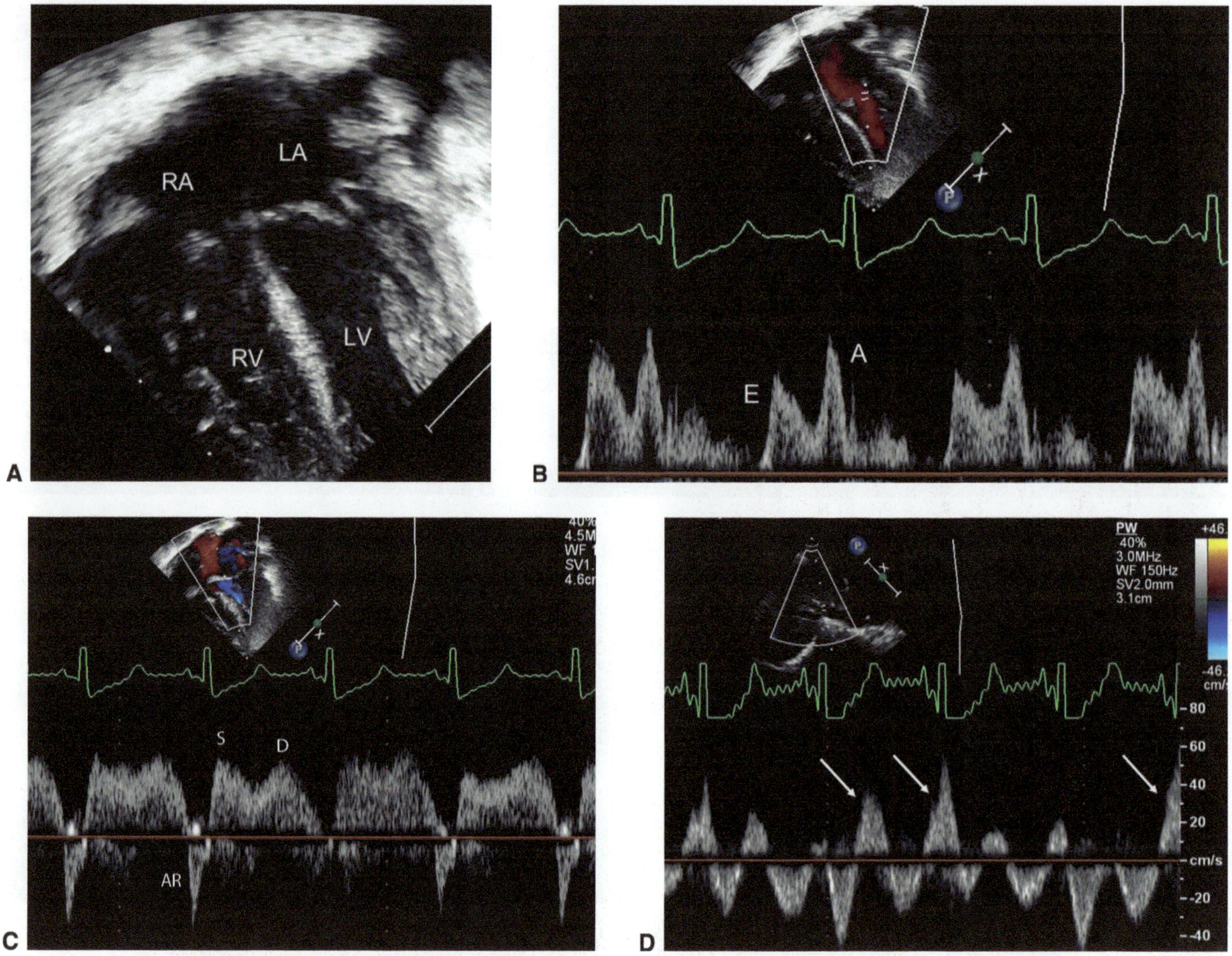

Fig. 27.17 Diastolic dysfunction in an infant after repair of truncus arteriosus. There is biventricular hypertrophy (A). Although still an infant where reversal of early *(E)* and late *(A)* Doppler waves (E/A ratio) may be normal, the prominent mitral valve E/A reversal appears abnormal and is suggestive of impaired relaxation (B). At the same time, prominent pulmonary vein a-wave reversal (AR) is consistent with decreased compliance (C). Thus left ventricular diastolic dysfunction with features of impaired relaxation and decreased compliance is present. Reduced right ventricular compliance is also present as manifested by increased flow reversal in the hepatic vein *(arrows)* (D). *D,* Diastolic; *LA,* left atrium; *LV,* left ventricle; *RA,* right atrium; *RV,* right ventricle; *S,* systolic.

ventricle.[142] LA function can also be impaired in this population in association with clinical outcomes, including occurrence of death, heart failure, hospitalizations, arrhythmia, thromboembolic events, and need for reintervention.[143]

Pediatric Pulmonary Hypertension

Although the overwhelming emphasis has been placed on RV systolic function in PH, diastolic abnormalities are important determinants of outcomes. Similar to well-known findings in adults,[144] we and others showed that RA size, a marker of chronic RV filling pressures, in structurally normal hearts, and in CHD,[145] was associated with greater mortality risk or functional class in children with PH.[146,147] RA area is also predictive of mortality in Eisenmenger syndrome, although it may be influenced by TR commonly found in that lesion.[148] Others have found that early tricuspid annulus diastolic velocities correlate with functional class and mortality in pediatric idiopathic PH.[149] However, echo assessment of RV diastolic function and filling pressures in pediatric PH remains difficult. We studied echo indices acquired simultaneously with high-fidelity catheter reference measures of diastolic function in 16 children undergoing catheter evaluation of PH. Most of these children had CHD.[150] We found overall poor or moderate correlations between echo measures and the reference parameters of the time constant of ventricular relaxation (tau), negative pressure change over time, and EDP.[150] However, correlations were better in patients who did not have an active shunt, influenced perhaps by the load dependence of diastolic evaluation. Tricuspid deceleration time and E/e′ correlated with tau; tricuspid deceleration time, a′, S/D ratio, and global late diastolic strain correlated with dP/dt minimum. These results further demonstrate that diastole cannot be neatly or easily divided into early and late phases in terms of which echo parameters reflect characteristics of early filling versus late diastolic compliance.[150] The good correlation of diastolic strain with invasive parameters in our study suggests that in the future it may be a useful modality to assess myocardial

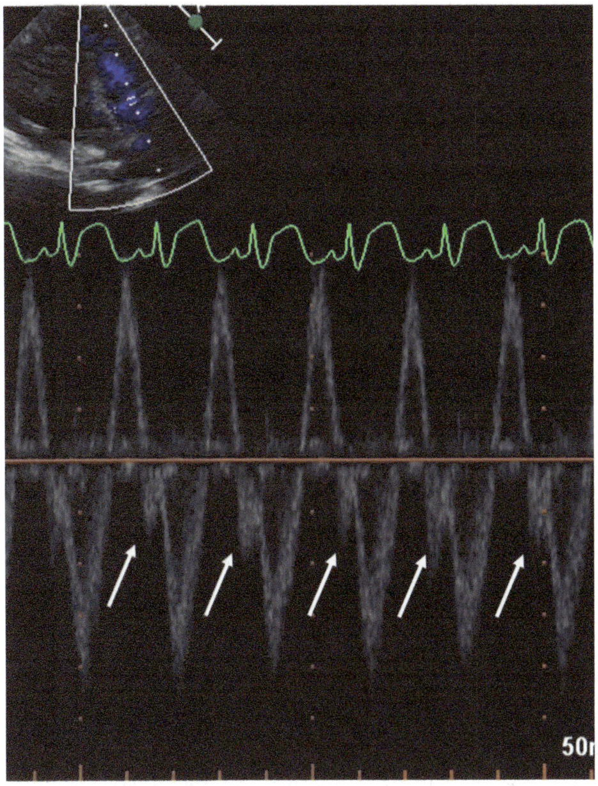

Fig. 27.18 End-diastolic antegrade flow in the main pulmonary artery occurring after atrial contraction and persisting throughout the respiratory cycle *(arrows)*. This phenomenon is thought to reflect restrictive right ventricular physiology. Although most commonly seen after repair of tetralogy of Fallot, this example is from a child who has undergone repair of truncus arteriosus in the past.

diastolic properties. Indeed, in another simultaneous echo–high-fidelity catheter study, Chowdhury et al. found in a heterogeneous population of children undergoing catheterization for CHD or evaluation after heart transplant that RV early diastolic strain rate correlated with invasively measured early active ventricular relaxation at baseline and after changes in preload by administration of a saline bolus, while conventional echocardiographic measures of diastolic function were not predictive of invasively measured diastolic function after preload alteration.[151]

Over and above RV diastolic function, the impact of adverse ventricular-ventricular interactions on diastolic function is particularly prominent in PH.[128,152] The prolonged duration of RV systole manifests as a high S/D duration ratio and impedes RV and LV filling (Fig. 27.19A).[153] Burkett et al. described LV diastolic abnormalities in children with PH studied at the time of cardiac catheterization.[154] The findings were most consistent with impaired early relaxation and filling (see Fig. 27.19B).[154] Thus, although most emphasis is placed on RV systolic function, PH affects both systole and diastole and both the right and left ventricles.[147]

DIASTOLIC ASSESSMENT IN THE FUNCTIONALLY SINGLE VENTRICLE

Diastolic function in single-ventricle physiology impacts outcomes. In a large series of patients with a double inlet left ventricle from the Mayo Clinic, diastolic dysfunction (i.e., elevated LVEDP) was one of two independent risk factors for late death after the Fontan operation.[155] However, assessment and characterization of diastolic function in the individual patient is even more difficult than in biventricular physiology. One of the important considerations is the stage of palliation and its relation to ventricular preload, which affect diastolic parameters. At the first stage of palliation, which, dependent

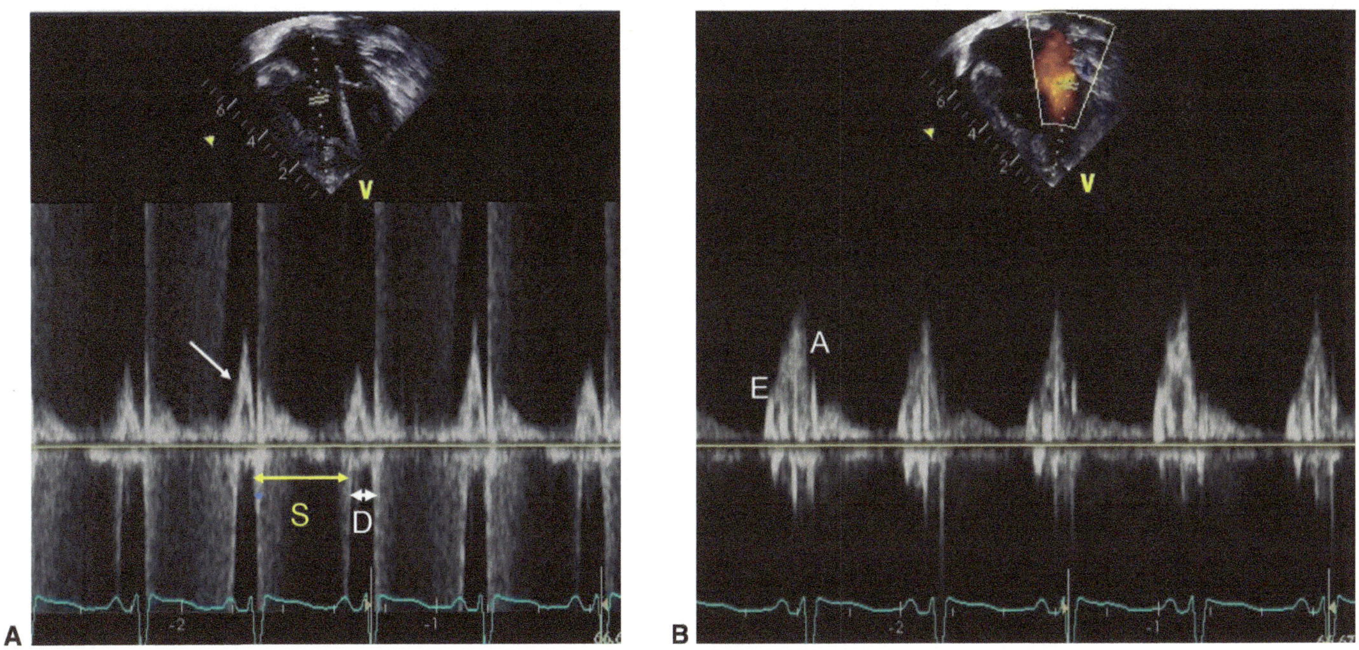

Fig. 27.19 Tricuspid valve regurgitation Doppler in a child with pulmonary hypertension (A). The systolic duration *(S)* is represented by the duration of the tricuspid regurgitant jet *(yellow long double-headed arrow)* and the diastolic duration *(D)* by the interval between regurgitant jets *(white short double-headed arrow)*. Note how the prolonged systolic duration leads to marked shortening of diastolic filling *(arrow)* and a high S/D ratio. This physiology not only reduces RV filling, but due to prolonged leftward septal shift into early LV diastole and reduced LV preload affects LV filling as seen by a short and reversed E/A pattern of the mitral inflow Doppler, a pattern characteristic of delayed relaxation (B).

on the lesion, often consists of a systemic to pulmonary shunt, the ventricle is typically volume overloaded. After the placement of a caval-pulmonary shunt, and after the Fontan procedure, there is a precipitous decrease in ventricular preload and increased mass/volume ratio. Ventricular filling is additionally affected by pulmonary vascular resistance.[156] In this scenario it is often difficult to differentiate preload restriction from intrinsic diastolic dysfunction per se. Whether chronic preload deficiency affects intrinsic myocardial properties in and of itself is an open question. Nonetheless, in aggregate, single-ventricle patients after the Fontan operation appear to have diastolic dysfunction, which may be progressive.

Following this physiology, a high LV mass/volume ratio in the early postoperative period following Fontan palliation (in part due to the reduced preload) may be an indicator of increased early morbidity with pericardial or pleural effusions.[157–159] However, normalization of the mass/volume ratio in Fontan patients may not lead to improved diastolic performance.[160–162] Increased collagen deposition likely contributes to decreased compliance, as demonstrated in other cardiac anomalies.[163] The additional presence of wall motion abnormalities, which are common in these patients, likely contributes further to altered diastology.[164] These patients may show patterns consistent with abnormal relaxation and decreased early diastolic filling with increased compensatory late filling with atrial contraction, prolonged IVRT, and decreased peak early filling velocities,[161,164,165] but also Doppler findings more consistent with decreased ventricular compliance such as shorter inflow deceleration time.[166] Additional findings of mid-diastolic inflow (L wave) also suggest abnormal diastolic function.[166] Thus children with either single or biventricular circulations may have mixed patterns of delayed relaxation and decreased compliance.

Because patients undergo catheter hemodynamic evaluation before stage 2 and 3 surgery in many institutions, there is an opportunity to correlate echocardiographic parameters with catheter hemodynamics in the single-ventricle population. In a small group of children with single-ventricle physiology,[167] tau correlated well with the atrioventricular inflow E/A ratio and IVRT but also with lateral E/e′, which is thought to reflect filling pressures more than early diastolic relaxation.

In a study investigating patients with single right ventricles, ventricular filling pressures correlated significantly with early diastolic strain rate (SRe) and the E/SRe ratio.[168] Conversely, there were no significant correlations between ventricular filling pressures and tissue Doppler measurements. Likewise, in a different study, diastolic strain rate correlated with RVEDP more strongly than Doppler-based parameters.[169] However, results from different studies have been inconsistent. Menon et al. found that in patients with single-ventricle physiology, tissue Doppler velocities and pulmonary vein Doppler correlated, albeit modestly, with direct measurement of ventricular filling pressures. In that study, an E/e′ ratio above 12 was suggestive of ventricular end-diastolic pressures greater than 10.[170] Of note, single left ventricles had better systolic and diastolic function than single right ventricles. This finding concurred with that of a large multicenter study that used mass/volume ratio, peak early diastolic velocity, and E/E′ ratio as well as the Tei index to characterize diastolic function in single ventricles.[171] In a small study, invasively measured tau correlated well with the inflow Doppler E/A ratio, lateral E/e′, and IVRT derived from TDI.[172] Thus there is inconsistency between studies on the correlation of echo parameters with near-simultaneously measured invasive parameters, likely influenced by factors such as small sample sizes, heterogeneous anatomy, physiology, and loading conditions, over and above measurement variability.

Strain and strain rate imaging may also be useful to follow diastolic function over time in the single-ventricle population. Michel et al. found in patients with hypoplastic left heart syndrome after the Fontan procedure that during serial evaluation, global early and late diastolic strain rate progressively decreased while conventional Doppler diastolic parameters did not change, suggesting that these parameters may be more sensitive to detect worsening in diastolic function over time.[79] However, at this time, diastolic strain and strain rate measurements are not used routinely in clinical practice in most pediatric labs given factors such as low frame rates, messy strain rate curves, lack of validation, and lack of experience.

Loss of atrioventricular synchrony can induce failure in patients with a Fontan circulation, consistent with a significant reliance of atrial booster pump function for filling. Studies have shown reduced early atrial emptying and increased contribution from atrial contraction to ventricular filling,[173] consistent with diastolic dysfunction.[174] However, atrial function itself, especially reservoir function, may be impaired and insufficient to compensate for ventricular underfilling. Peak atrial strain (and hence atrial contractile function) correlates with ventricular filling pressures, highlighting atrioventricular interdependence.[175] Thus pulmonary, ventricular, and atrial properties, as well as atrioventricular synchrony, influence diastolic function of the single ventricle.

FUTURE DIRECTIONS

Several emerging areas can potentially add to the assessment of diastolic function. As discussed in the preceding text, assessment of myocardial mechanics in diastole using two-dimensional (2-D) speckle tracking can be done through diastolic strain and strain rate. As noted previously, these are not used routinely in clinical practice in most pediatric labs at this time but may be useful after additional improvement and validation. Lu et al. recently investigated diastolic strain rate in children after orthotropic heart transplant to detect graft dysfunction.[79] They found that an increase in PCWP (reflecting LV filling pressures) of 3 mmHg or more was associated with changes in LA compliance, E/e′ ratio, and the E/LV diastolic strain ratio, which had the highest area under the receiver operating characteristic curve among the various parameters studied. E/LV diastolic strain rate at baseline also significantly differed between children who subsequently developed rejection or coronary artery vasculopathy and those without events.[176] Peak LA systolic strain and distensibility were also found to be more useful surrogates of LV filling pressures than E/e′.[177]

Continuing development of high frame rate ultrasound is expected to improve our ability to characterize the rapid events and myocardial mechanics of early diastole as well as characterization of myocardial stiffness.[178] Concomitantly, the evolution of assessment of extracellular volume noninvasively by cardiac MRI, as a marker of diffuse myocardial fibrosis, will allow comprehensive and complimentary noninvasive assessment by echo and cardiac MRI in terms of fibrosis and its impact on tissue stiffness. This broad topic is beyond the scope of this chapter but will hopefully provide important information that will allow us to define with much better resolution myocardial characteristics, diastolic dysfunction, and their impact on clinical outcomes.

In children with DCM, ventricular mechanical discoordination or dispersion has been described in systole. However, diastolic mechanical dispersion is common in children with DCM and may be worse in those who later undergo transplant or die.[179] The contribution of these mechanical inefficiencies to diastolic dysfunction and patient outcomes requires additional study in children, including in single-ventricle patients as discussed earlier.

Systolic-diastolic coupling is a very well-recognized phenomenon, but not assessed in practice and does not form part of current practice guidelines for assessment of systolic or diastolic function. Systolic and diastolic function are closely linked through the Frank-Starling mechanism, where enhanced filling increases contractility, through elastic recoil and restoring forces in early diastole, and through twist-untwist that promotes intraventricular pressure gradients.[11] We studied systolic-diastolic coupling in children with DCM using tissue Doppler. Systolic-diastolic coupling was found to be weaker in DCM versus controls, in association with ventricular remodeling, suggesting that impaired systolic-diastolic coupling, possibly through abnormal titin or other myocardial properties, may itself contribute to dysfunction.[180] With the advent of TDI and subsequently speckle tracking, ventricular twist-untwist mechanics have been characterized. However, these have not become routine parameters to quantify systolic-diastolic coupling or diastolic function. More work is needed on their utility in the assessment of function in the pediatric population as they may be age related.[181] Twist-untwist and other diastolic abnormalities might be further elucidated by exercise testing. During exercise, diastole shortens, and a key compensatory element to maintain LV filling and stroke volume is increased LV twist and untwist.[182] The use of exercise echo in general in children and specifically for assessment of diastolic function is warranted and requires additional study. Likewise, three-dimensional (3-D) echocardiography and 3-D speckle tracking may facilitate evaluation of torsion mechanics as basal and apical rotation are assessed simultaneously, particularly as frame rates increase with improving technology.

With technological advances and with invasive and surgical procedures that patients with CHD undergo, the use of implanted sensors that transmit continuous hemodynamic data will be helpful to monitor patients for disease progression and understand the relation of diastolic function to symptoms and adverse events. The rapid development of computer learning and big data is expected to enhance the processing and understanding of larger amounts of data, such as that continuously received from implanted devices, thereby enhancing assessment of diastolic function in the individual patient and perhaps allowing development of pediatric-specific diagnostic algorithms for the assessment and classification of diastolic dysfunction.

KEY POINTS

- Myocardial diastolic characteristics and ventricular function evolve over time from fetal life to adulthood.
- While the principles and tools to assess diastolic dysfunction in children are similar to adults, they also differ in important ways. Consequently, adult diagnostic criteria are not readily applicable to children.
- Classification of diastolic function in children is complicated by the wide range of normal values, high heart rates, changing values with age and heart rate, difficulties in application of adult guidelines to children, the presence of often apparently conflicting echo criteria, lack of correlation of echo criteria with invasively measured reference parameters, and influence of loading conditions.
- Outside of adolescents with hypertrophic cardiomyopathy, isolated delayed relaxation in children is uncommon. Echo parameters reflecting delayed ventricular relaxation and decreased ventricular compliance are often found together even early in the clinical course.
- Single echo Doppler parameters may be sufficiently sensitive to detect diastolic dysfunction, but not to quantify it. A combination of echo Doppler indices interpreted in the clinical context is needed to assess diastolic function in children.
- In congenital left-sided obstructive lesions, diastolic dysfunction is common, but mitral abnormalities complicate diastolic assessment.
- In the Fontan circulation, preload restriction affects ventricular filling and limits the assessment of diastolic function.
- The E/e′ ratio, while often abnormal in children due to abnormalities in each of its components, does not reliably reflect ventricular filling pressures, especially in congenital heart disease, including functionally single ventricles.
- Right ventricular diastolic dysfunction is important in diverse pediatric diseases such as dilated cardiomyopathy, repaired tetralogy of Fallot, and pulmonary hypertension.
- Newer and emerging noninvasive technologies that assess myocardial characteristics and function such as strain rate imaging and high frame-rate ultrasound may improve assessment of diastolic function in children.

REVIEW QUESTIONS

1. A newborn with severe aortic stenosis undergoes balloon valvuloplasty but continues to have low cardiac output and requires continuing mechanical ventilation despite relief of the aortic stenosis. Diastolic dysfunction is suspected. Which of the following is most consistent with this scenario?
   a. A merged E and A wave suggests restrictive physiology.
   b. Good LV systolic function makes diastolic function unlikely.
   c. The left atrium is not substantially dilated and therefore filling pressures are low.
   d. Echo signs of endocardial fibroelastosis are consistent with reduced LV compliance.
2. A 15-year-old boy with hypertrophic cardiomyopathy treated with beta blockers with a heart rate of 63 bpm comes for annual outpatient follow-up. Echocardiography shows severe septal hypertrophy, good systolic function, a mitral E/A ratio of 1.7, a deceleration time of 230 msec, a lateral mitral e′ of 4 cm/sec, a septal e′ of 2 cm/sec, and an E/e′ using the lateral mitral annulus e′ of 12 cm/sec. There is increased pulmonary vein A wave reversal velocity and duration (45 cm/sec; 170 msec vs the mitral A wave velocity of 30 msec). A mitral inflow mid-diastolic L wave is seen. The left atrium is dilated with an estimated volume of 58 cm^3. Which of the following is most accurate?
   a. The echo findings suggest delayed relaxation without pseudo-normal physiology.
   b. The echo findings suggest pseudo-nomral physiology without delayed relaxation.
   c. The echo findings suggest delayed relaxation and pseudo-normal physiology.
   d. The relative bradycardia precludes assessment of pseudo-normal physiology.
3. A 12-year-old girl comes for follow-up evaluation after undergoing surgical repair of tetralogy of Fallot in infancy. She is overall well, although cannot keep up with her friends when playing soccer at school. Her right ventricle is dilated with a recent cardiac MRI measured volume of 178 cc/m^2. Which of the following statements is most correct?
   a. Pulmonary regurgitation prolongs with restrictive RV physiology.
   b. Reversed tricuspid inflow E/A ratio, low tricuspid e′, and increased hepatic vein A wave reversal suggest impaired RV relaxation and decreased compliance.
   c. Antegrade end-diastolic flow in the main pulmonary artery throughout the respiratory cycle is highly associated with delayed RV relaxation.
   d. An elevated early tricuspid inflow to early diastolic tricuspid annulus tissue velocity ratio (E/e′ ratio) is highly predictive of RV filling pressures.

REFERENCES

1. McMahon CJ, Nagueh SF, Eapen RS, et al. Echocardiographic predictors of adverse clinical events in children with dilated cardiomyopathy: a prospective clinical study. *Heart.* 2004;90(8):908–915.
2. Johnson GL, Moffett CB, Noonan JA. Doppler echocardiographic studies of diastolic ventricular filling patterns in premature infants. *Am Heart J.* 1988;116(6 Pt 1):1568–1574.
3. Harada K, Takahashi Y, Shiota T, Tamura M, Takada G. Changes in transmitral and pulmonary venous flow patterns in the first day of life. *J Clin Ultrasound.* 1995;23(7):399–405.
4. Harada K, Suzuki T, Tamura M, et al. Role of age on transmitral flow velocity patterns in assessing left ventricular diastolic function in normal infants and children. *Am J Cardiol.* 1995;76(7):530–532.
5. Harada K, Suzuki T, Tamura M, Ito T, Shimada K, Takada G. Effect of aging from infancy to childhood on flow velocity patterns of pulmonary vein by Doppler echocardiography. *Am J Cardiol.* 1996;77(2):221–224.
6. Riggs TW, Snider AR. Respiratory influence on right and left ventricular diastolic function in normal children. *Am J Cardiol.* 1989;63(12):858–861.
7. Riggs TW, Rodriguez R, Snider AR, Batton D. Doppler echocardiographic evaluation of right and left ventricular diastolic function in normal neonates. *J Am Coll Cardiol.* 1989;13(3):700–705.
8. Fisher DJ, Heymann MA, Rudolph AM. Myocardial consumption of oxygen and carbohydrates in newborn sheep. *Pediatr Res.* 1981;15(5):843–846.
9. Friedman WF. The intrinsic physiologic properties of the developing heart. *Prog Cardiovasc Dis.* 1972;15(1):87–111.
10. Grant DA, Maloney JE, Tyberg JV, Walker AM. Effects of external constraint on the fetal left ventricular function curve. *Am Heart J.* 1992;123(6):1601–1609.
11. O'Leary PW, Durongpisitkul K, Cordes TM, et al. Diastolic ventricular function in children: a Doppler echocardiographic study establishing normal values and predictors of increased ventricular end-diastolic pressure. *Mayo Clin Proc.* 1998;73(7):616–628.
12. Dallaire F, Slorach C, Hui W, et al. Reference values for pulse wave Doppler and tissue Doppler imaging in pediatric echocardiography. *Circ Cardiovasc Imag.* 2015;8(2):e002167.
13. Isaaz K, Thompson A, Ethevenot G, Cloez JL, Brembilla B, Pernot C. Doppler echocardiographic measurement of low velocity motion of the left ventricular posterior wall. *Am J Cardiol.* 1989;64(1):66–75.
14. Isaaz K, Munoz del Romeral L, Lee E, Schiller NB. Quantitation of the motion of the cardiac base in normal subjects by Doppler echocardiography. *J Am Soc Echocardiogr.* 1993;6(2):166–176.
15. Farias CA, Rodriguez L, Garcia MJ, Sun JP, Klein AL, Thomas JD. Assessment of diastolic function by tissue Doppler echocardiography: comparison with standard transmitral and pulmonary venous flow. *J Am Soc Echocardiogr.* 1999;12(8):609–617.
16. Galiuto L, Ignone G, DeMaria AN. Contraction and relaxation velocities of the normal left ventricle using pulsed-wave tissue Doppler echocardiography. *Am J Cardiol.* 1998;81(5):609–614.
17. Donovan CL, Armstrong WF, Bach DS. Quantitative Doppler tissue imaging of the left ventricular myocardium: validation in normal subjects. *Am Heart J.* 1995;130(1):100–104.
18. Gulati VK, Katz WE, Follansbee WP, Gorcsan III J. Mitral annular descent velocity by tissue Doppler echocardiography as an index of global left ventricular function. *Am J Cardiol.* 1996;77(11):979–984.
19. Garcia MJ, Rodriguez L, Ares M, Griffin BP, Thomas JD, Klein AL. Differentiation of constrictive pericarditis from restrictive cardiomyopathy: assessment of left ventricular diastolic velocities in longitudinal axis by Doppler tissue imaging. *J Am Coll Cardiol.* 1996;27(1):108–114.
20. Garcia MJ, Rodriguez L, Ares M, et al. Myocardial wall velocity assessment by pulsed Doppler tissue imaging: characteristic findings in normal subjects. *Am Heart J.* 1996;132(3):648–656.
21. Rychik J, Tian ZY. Quantitative assessment of myocardial tissue velocities in normal children with Doppler tissue imaging. *Am J Cardiol.* 1996;77(14):1254–1257.
22. Frommelt PC, Ballweg JA, Whitstone BN, Frommelt MA. Usefulness of Doppler tissue imaging analysis of tricuspid annular motion for determination of right ventricular function in normal infants and children. *Am J Cardiol.* 2002;89(5):610–613.
23. Mori K, Hayabuchi Y, Kuroda Y, Nii M, Manabe T. Left ventricular wall motion velocities in healthy children measured by pulsed wave Doppler tissue echocardiography: normal values and relation to age and heart rate. *J Am Soc Echocardiogr.* 2000;13(11):1002–1011.
24. Nishimura RA, Abel MD, Hatle LK, Tajik AJ. Assessment of diastolic function of the heart: background and current applications of Doppler echocardiography. Part II. Clinical studies. *Mayo Clin Proc.* 1989;64(2):181–204.
25. Myreng Y, Smiseth OA. Assessment of left ventricular relaxation by Doppler echocardiography. Comparison of isovolumic relaxation time and transmitral flow velocities with time constant of isovolumic relaxation. *Circulation.* 1990;81(1):260–266.
26. Appleton CP, Hatle LK, Popp RL. Relation of transmitral flow velocity patterns to left ventricular diastolic function: new insights from a combined hemodynamic and Doppler echocardiographic study. *J Am Coll Cardiol.* 1988;12(2):426–440.
27. Thomas JD, Weyman AE. Echocardiographic Doppler evaluation of left ventricular diastolic function. Physics and physiology. *Circulation.* 1991;84(3):977–990.
28. Dragulescu A, Mertens L, Friedberg MK. Interpretation of left ventricular diastolic dysfunction in children with cardiomyopathy by echocardiography: problems and limitations. *Circ Cardiovasc Imag.* 2013;6(2):254–261.
29. Sundereswaran L, Nagueh SF, Vardan S, et al. Estimation of left and right ventricular filling pressures after heart transplantation by tissue Doppler imaging. *Am J Cardiol.* 1998;82(3):352–357.
30. Nagueh SF, Mikati I, Kopelen HA, Middleton KJ, Quiñones MA, Zoghbi WA. Doppler estimation of left ventricular filling pressure in sinus tachycardia. A new application of tissue doppler imaging. *Circulation.* 1998;98(16):1644–1650.
31. Nagueh SF, Smiseth OA, Appleton CP, et al. Recommendations for the evaluation of left ventricular diastolic function by echocardiography: an update from the American Society of Echocardiography and the European Association of Cardiovascular Imaging. *J Am Soc Echocardiogr.* 2016;29(4):277–314.
32. Cantinotti M, Lopez L. Nomograms for blood flow and tissue Doppler velocities to evaluate diastolic function in children: a critical review. *J Am Soc Echocardiogr.* 2013;26(2):126–141.
33. Ezon DS, Maskatia SA, Sexson-Tejtel K, Dreyer WJ, Jeewa A, Denfield SW. Tissue Doppler imaging measures correlate poorly with left ventricular filling pressures in pediatric cardiomyopathy. *Congenit Heart Dis.* 2015;10(5):e203–e209.
34. Ryan TD, Madueme PC, Jefferies JL, et al. Utility of echocardiography in the assessment of left ventricular diastolic function and restrictive physiology in children and young adults with restrictive cardiomyopathy: a comparative echocardiography-catheterization study. *Pediatr Cardiol.* 2017;38(2):381–389.
35. Masutani S, Saiki H, Kurishima C, Kuwata S, Tamura M, Senzaki H. Assessment of ventricular relaxation and stiffness using early diastolic mitral annular and inflow velocities in pediatric patients with heart disease. *Heart Vessels.* 2014;29(6):825–833.
36. Nadorlik H, Stiver C, Khan S, et al. Correlations between echocardiographic systolic and diastolic function with cardiac catheterization in biventricular congenital heart patients. *Pediatr Cardiol.* 2016;37(4):765–771.
37. Sasaki N, Garcia M, Ko HH, Sharma S, Parness IA, Srivastava S. Applicability of published guidelines for assessment of left ventricular diastolic function in adults to children with restrictive cardiomyopathy: an observational study. *Pediatr Cardiol.* 2015;36(2):386–392.
38. Bryg RJ, Williams GA, Labovitz AJ. Effect of aging on left ventricular diastolic filling in normal subjects. *Am J Cardiol.* 1987;59(9):971–974.
39. Bessen M, Gardin JM. Evaluation of left ventricular diastolic function. *Cardiol Clin.* 1990;8(2):315–332.
40. Stoddard MF, Pearson AC, Kern MJ, Ratcliff J, Mrosek DG, Labovitz AJ. Influence of alteration in preload on the pattern of left ventricular

diastolic filling as assessed by Doppler echocardiography in humans. *Circulation.* 1998;79(6):1226–1236.
41. Klein AL, Tajik AJ. Doppler assessment of pulmonary venous flow in healthy subjects and in patients with heart disease. *J Am Soc Echocardiogr.* 1991;4(4):379–392.
42. Nishimura RA, Abel MD, Hatle LK, Tajik AJ. Relation of pulmonary vein to mitral flow velocities by transesophageal Doppler echocardiography. Effect of different loading conditions. *Circulation.* 1990;81(5):1488–1497.
43. Basnight MA, Gonzalez MS, Kershenovich SC, Appleton CP. Pulmonary venous flow velocity: relation to hemodynamics, mitral flow velocity and left atrial volume, and ejection fraction. *J Am Soc Echocardiogr.* 1991;4(6):547–558.
44. Appleton CP, Gonzalez MS, Basnight MA. Relationship of left atrial pressure and pulmonary venous flow velocities: importance of baseline mitral and pulmonary venous flow velocity patterns studied in lightly sedated dogs. *J Am Soc Echocardiogr.* 1994;7(3 Pt 1):264–275.
45. Appleton CP, Galloway JM, Gonzalez MS, Gaballa M, Basnight MA. Estimation of left ventricular filling pressures using two-dimensional and Doppler echocardiography in adult patients with cardiac disease. Additional value of analyzing left atrial size, left atrial ejection fraction and the difference in duration of pulmonary venous and mitral flow velocity at atrial contraction. *J Am Coll Cardiol.* 1993;22(7):1972–1982.
46. Yamamoto K, Nishimura RA, Chaliki HP, Appleton CP, Holmes Jr DR, Redfield MM. Determination of left ventricular filling pressure by Doppler echocardiography in patients with coronary artery disease: critical role of left ventricular systolic function. *J Am Coll Cardiol.* 1997;30(7):1819–1826.
47. Pai RG, Gill KS. Amplitudes, durations, and timings of apically directed left ventricular myocardial velocities: I. Their normal pattern and coupling to ventricular filling and ejection. *J Am Soc Echocardiogr.* 1998;11(2):105–111.
48. Rodriguez L, Garcia M, Ares M, Griffin BP, Nakatani S, Thomas JD. Assessment of mitral annular dynamics during diastole by Doppler tissue imaging: comparison with mitral Doppler inflow in subjects without heart disease and in patients with left ventricular hypertrophy. *Am Heart J.* 1996;131(5):982–987.
49. Alam M, Wardell J, Andersson E, Samad BA, Nordlander R. Characteristics of mitral and tricuspid annular velocities determined by pulsed wave Doppler tissue imaging in healthy subjects. *J Am Soc Echocardiogr.* 1999;12(8):618–628.
50. Fleming AD, Xia X, McDicken WN, Sutherland GR, Fenn L. Myocardial velocity gradients detected by Doppler imaging. *Br J Radiol.* 1994;67(799):679–688.
51. Uematsu M, Miyatake K, Tanaka N, et al. Myocardial velocity gradient as a new indicator of regional left ventricular contraction: detection by a two-dimensional tissue Doppler imaging technique. *J Am Coll Cardiol.* 1995;26(1):217–223.
52. Eidem BW, McMahon CJ, Cohen RR, et al. Impact of cardiac growth on Doppler tissue imaging velocities: a study in healthy children. *J Am Soc Echocardiogr.* 2004;17(3):212–221.
53. Nii M, Mori K, Kuroda Y. Quantification of the myocardial velocity gradient and myocardial wall thickening velocity in healthy children: a new indicator of regional myocardial wall motion. *J Am Soc Echocardiogr.* 2002;15(6):624–632.
54. Sohn DW, Chai IH, Lee DJ, et al. Assessment of mitral annulus velocity by Doppler tissue imaging in the evaluation of left ventricular diastolic function. *J Am Coll Cardiol.* 1997;30(2):474–480.
55. Firstenberg MS, Greenberg NL, Main ML, et al. Determinants of diastolic myocardial tissue Doppler velocities: influences of relaxation and preload. *J Appl Physiol.* 1985/2001;90(1):299–307.
56. Nagueh SF, Sun H, Kopelen HA, Middleton KJ, Khoury DS. Hemodynamic determinants of the mitral annulus diastolic velocities by tissue Doppler. *J Am Coll Cardiol.* 2001;37(1):278–285.
57. Hung KC, Huang HL, Chu CM, et al. Evaluating preload dependence of a novel Doppler application in assessment of left ventricular diastolic function during hemodialysis. *Am J Kidney Dis.* 2004;43(6):1040–1046.
58. Oki T, Fukuda K, Tabata T, et al. Effect of an acute increase in afterload on left ventricular regional wall motion velocity in healthy subjects. *J Am Soc Echocardiogr.* 1999;12(6):476–483.
59. Müller S, Bartel T, Koopman J, Pandian NG, Erbel R, Pachinger O. Tissue Doppler analysis is hindered in abnormal wall motion and changes in afterload. *Int J Cardiol.* 2003;90(1):81–90.
60. Jacques DC, Pinsky MR, Severyn D, Gorcsan III J. Influence of alterations in loading on mitral annular velocity by tissue Doppler echocardiography and its associated ability to predict filling pressures. *Chest.* 2004;126(6):1910–1918.
61. Kapusta L, Thijssen JM, Cuypers MH, Peer PG, Daniels O. Assessment of myocardial velocities in healthy children using tissue Doppler imaging. *Ultrasound Med Biol.* 2000;26(2):229–237.
62. Swaminathan S, Ferrer PL, Wolff GS, Gómez-Marin O, Rusconi PG. Usefulness of tissue Doppler echocardiography for evaluating ventricular function in children without heart disease. *Am J Cardiol.* 2003;91(5):570–574.
63. Hiarada K, Orino T, Yasuoka K, Tamura M, Takada G. Tissue doppler imaging of left and right ventricles in normal children. *Tohoku J Exp Med.* 2000;191(1):21–29.
64. Nagueh SF, Middleton KJ, Kopelen HA, Zoghbi WA, Quiñones MA. Doppler tissue imaging: a noninvasive technique for evaluation of left ventricular relaxation and estimation of filling pressures. *J Am Coll Cardiol.* 1997;30(6):1527–1533.
65. Garcia MJ, Thomas JD. Tissue doppler to assess diastolic left ventricular function. *Echocardiography.* 1999;16(5):501–508.
66. Rivas-Gotz C, Khoury DS, Manolios M, Rao L, Kopelen HA, Nagueh SF. Time interval between onset of mitral inflow and onset of early diastolic velocity by tissue Doppler: a novel index of left ventricular relaxation: experimental studies and clinical application. *J Am Coll Cardiol.* 2003;42(8):1463–1470.
67. Opdahl A, Remme EW, Helle-Valle T, et al. Determinants of left ventricular early-diastolic lengthening velocity: independent contributions from left ventricular relaxation, restoring forces, and lengthening load. *Circulation.* 2009;119(19):2578–2586.
68. Border WL, Michelfelder EC, Glascock BJ, et al. Color M-mode and Doppler tissue evaluation of diastolic function in children: simultaneous correlation with invasive indices. *J Am Soc Echocardiogr.* 2003;16(9):988–994.
69. Oki T, Tabata T, Yamada H, et al. Right and left ventricular wall motion velocities as diagnostic indicators of constrictive pericarditis. *Am J Cardiol.* 1998;81(4):465–470.
70. Ha JW, Oh JK, Ommen SR, Ling LH, Tajik AJ. Diagnostic value of mitral annular velocity for constrictive pericarditis in the absence of respiratory variation in mitral inflow velocity. *J Am Soc Echocardiogr.* 2002;15(12):1468–1471.
71. Ha JW, Ommen SR, Tajik AJ, et al. Differentiation of constrictive pericarditis from restrictive cardiomyopathy using mitral annular velocity by tissue Doppler echocardiography. *Am J Cardiol.* 2004;94(3):316–319.
72. Hollander SA, Bernstein D, Yeh J, Dao D, Sun HY, Rosenthal D. Outcomes of children following a first hospitalization for dilated cardiomyopathy. *Circ Heart Fail.* 2012;5(4):437–443.
73. Aranda Jr JM, Weston MW, Puleo JA, Fontanet HL. Effect of loading conditions on myocardial relaxation velocities determined by Doppler tissue imaging in heart transplant recipients. *J Heart Lung Transplant Off Pub Int Soc Heart Transplant.* 1998;17(7):693–697.
74. Nagueh SF, Kopelen HA, Quiñones MA. Assessment of left ventricular filling pressures by Doppler in the presence of atrial fibrillation. *Circulation.* 1996;94(9):2138–2145.
75. Nagueh SF, Lakkis NM, Middleton KJ, Spencer III WH, Zoghbi WA, Quiñones MA. Doppler estimation of left ventricular filling pressures in patients with hypertrophic cardiomyopathy. *Circulation.* 1999;99(2):254–261.
76. Savage A, Hlavacek A, Ringewald J, Shirali G. Evaluation of the myocardial performance index and tissue doppler imaging by comparison to near-simultaneous catheter measurements in pediatric cardiac transplant patients. *J Heart Lung Transplant Off Pub Int Soc Heart Transplant.* 2010;29(8):853–858.
77. Larrazet F, Bouabdallah K, Le Bret E, Vouhé P, Veyrat C, Laborde F. Tissue Doppler echocardiographic and color M-mode estimation of left atrial pressure in infants. *Pediatr Crit Care Med J Soc Crit Care Med World Fed Pediat Intensive Crit Care Soc.* 2005;6(4):448–453.

78. Figueras-Coll M, Sanchez-de-Toledo J, Gran F, Abella R, Perez-Hoyos S, Rosés F. Echocardiography in the assessment of left atrial pressure after pediatric heart surgery: a comparison study with measurements obtained from left atrial catheter. *World J Pediatr Congenit Heart Surg.* 2015;6(3):438–442.
79. Lu JC, Magdo HS, Yu S, et al. Usefulness of diastolic strain measurements in predicting elevated left ventricular filling pressure and risk of rejection or coronary artery vasculopathy in pediatric heart transplant recipients. *Am J Cardiol.* 2016;117(9):1533–1538.
80. Harada K, Tamura M, Yasuoka K, Toyono M. A comparison of tissue Doppler imaging and velocities of transmitral flow in children with elevated left ventricular preload. *Cardiol Young.* 2001;11(3):261–268.
81. Eidem BW, McMahon CJ, Ayres NA, et al. Impact of chronic left ventricular preload and afterload on Doppler tissue imaging velocities: a study in congenital heart disease. *J Am Soc Echocardiogr.* 2005;18(8):830–838.
82. Kidd L, Driscoll DJ, Gersony WM, et al. Second natural history study of congenital heart defects. Results of treatment of patients with ventricular septal defects. *Circulation.* 1993;87(2):SI38–SI51.
83. Stewart JM, Hintze TH, Woolf PK, Snyder MS, Seligman KP, Gewitz MH. Nature of heart failure in patients with ventricular septal defect. *Am J Physiol.* 1995;269(4 Pt 2):H1473–H1480.
84. Möller T, Brun H, Fredriksen PM, et al. Right ventricular systolic pressure response during exercise in adolescents born with atrial or ventricular septal defect. *Am J Cardiol.* 2010;105(11):1610–1616.
85. Brun H, Möller T, Fredriksen PM, Thaulow E, Pripp AH, Holmstrom H. Mechanisms of exercise-induced pulmonary hypertension in patients with cardiac septal defects. *Pediatr Cardiol.* 2012;33(5):782–790.
86. Möller T, Lindberg H, Lund MB, Holmstrom H, Dohlen G, Thaulow E. Right ventricular pressure response to exercise in adults with isolated ventricular septal defect closed in early childhood. *Cardiol Young.* 2018;28(6):797–803.
87. Pauliks LB, Chan KC, Chang D, et al. Regional myocardial velocities and isovolumic contraction acceleration before and after device closure of atrial septal defects: a color tissue Doppler study. *Am Heart J.* 2005;150(2):294–301.
88. Pascotto M, Caso P, Santoro G, et al. Analysis of right ventricular Doppler tissue imaging and load dependence in patients undergoing percutaneous closure of atrial septal defect. *Am J Cardiol.* 2004;94(9):1202–1205.
89. Cheung YF, Lun KS, Chau AK. Doppler tissue imaging analysis of ventricular function after surgical and transcatheter closure of atrial septal defect. *Am J Cardiol.* 2004;93(3):375–378.
90. Giardini A, Moore P, Brook M, Stratton V, Tacy T. Effect of transcatheter atrial septal defect closure in children on left ventricular diastolic function. *Am J Cardiol.* 2005;95(10):1255–1257.
91. Masutani S, Taketazu M, Ishido H, et al. Effects of age on hemodynamic changes after transcatheter closure of atrial septal defect: importance of ventricular diastolic function. *Heart Vessels.* 2012;27(1):71–78.
92. Takaya Y, Akagi T, Kijima Y, et al. Echocardiographic estimates of left ventricular diastolic dysfunction do not predict the clinical course in elderly patients undergoing transcatheter atrial septal defect closure: impact of early diastolic mitral annular velocity. *J Interv Cardiol.* 2017;30(1):79–84.
93. Jones M, Ferrans VJ. Myocardial degeneration in congenital heart disease. Comparison of morphologic findings in young and old patients with congenital heart disease associated with muscular obstruction to right ventricular outflow. *Am J Cardiol.* 1997;39(7):1051–1063.
94. Snider AR, Gidding SS, Rocchini AP, et al. Doppler evaluation of left ventricular diastolic filling in children with systemic hypertension. *Am J Cardiol.* 1985;56(15):921–926.
95. Fifer MA, Borow KM, Colan SD, Lorell BH. Early diastolic left ventricular function in children and adults with aortic stenosis. *J Am Coll Cardiol.* 1989;5(5):1147-1154.
96. Sandor GG, Olley PM. Determination of left ventricular diastolic chamber stiffness and myocardial stiffness in patients with congenital heart disease. *Am J Cardiol.* 1982;49(4):771–779.
97. Banerjee A, Mendelsohn AM, Knilans TK, Meyer RA, Schwartz DC. Effect of myocardial hypertrophy on systolic and diastolic function in children: insights from the force-frequency and relaxation-frequency relationships. *J Am Coll Cardiol.* 1998;32(4):1088–1095.
98. Kiraly P, Kapusta L, Thijssen JM, Daniels O. Left ventricular myocardial function in congenital valvar aortic stenosis assessed by ultrasound tissue-velocity and strain-rate techniques. *Ultrasound Med Biol.* 2003;29(4):615–620.
99. Villari B, Vassalli G, Schneider J, Chiariello M, Hess OM. Age dependency of left ventricular diastolic function in pressure overload hypertrophy. *J Am Coll Cardiol.* 1997;29(1):181–186.
100. Friedman KG, McElhinney DB, Rhodes J, et al. Left ventricular diastolic function in children and young adults with congenital aortic valve disease. *Am J Cardiol.* 2013;111(2):243–249.
101. Chan KY, Redington AN, Rigby ML, Gibson DG. Cardiac function after surgery for subaortic stenosis: non-invasive assessment of left ventricular performance. *Br Heart J.* 1991;66(2):161–165.
102. Dusenbery SM, Jerosch-Herold M, Rickers C, et al. Myocardial extracellular remodeling is associated with ventricular diastolic dysfunction in children and young adults with congenital aortic stenosis. *J Am Coll Cardiol.* 2014;63(17):1778–1785.
103. Friedman KG, Schidlow D, Freud L, Escobar-Diaz M, Tworetzky W. Left ventricular diastolic function and characteristics in fetal aortic stenosis. *Am J Cardiol.* 2014;114(1):122–127.
104. Friedman KG, McElhinney DB, Colan SD, et al. Left ventricular remodeling and improvement in diastolic function after balloon aortic valvuloplasty for congenital aortic stenosis. *Circ Cardiovasc Interv.* 2012;5(4):549–554.
105. Kocabay G, Karabay CY, Kalkan S, et al. Relationship between left ventricular diastolic function and arterial stiffness in patients with bicuspid aortic valve. *J Heart Valve Dis.* 2014;23(3):279–288.
106. Molina KM, Shrader P, Colan SD, et al. Predictors of disease progression in pediatric dilated cardiomyopathy. *Circ Heart Fail.* 2013;6(6):1214–1222.
107. Singh TP, Sleeper LA, Lipshultz S, et al. Association of left ventricular dilation at listing for heart transplant with postlisting and early posttransplant mortality in children with dilated cardiomyopathy. *Circ Heart Fail.* 2009;2(6):591–598.
108. McMahon CJ, Nagueh SF, Pignatelli RH, et al. Characterization of left ventricular diastolic function by tissue Doppler imaging and clinical status in children with hypertrophic cardiomyopathy. *Circulation.* 2004;109(14):1756–1762.
109. McMahon CJ, Pignatelli RH, Nagueh SF, et al. Left ventricular non-compaction cardiomyopathy in children: characterisation of clinical status using tissue Doppler-derived indices of left ventricular diastolic relaxation. *Heart.* 2007;93(6):676–681.
110. Garcia MJ, Ares MA, Asher C, Rodriguez L, Vandervoort P, Thomas JD. An index of early left ventricular filling that combined with pulsed Doppler peak E velocity may estimate capillary wedge pressure. *J Am Coll Cardiol.* 1997;29(2):448–454.
111. Takatsuji H, Mikami T, Urasawa K, et al. A new approach for evaluation of left ventricular diastolic function: spatial and temporal analysis of left ventricular filling flow propagation by color M-mode Doppler echocardiography. *J Am Coll Cardiol.* 1996;27(2):365–371.
112. Patel R, Nagueh SF, Tsybouleva N, et al. Simvastatin induces regression of cardiac hypertrophy and fibrosis and improves cardiac function in a transgenic rabbit model of human hypertrophic cardiomyopathy. *Circulation.* 2001;104(3):317–324.
113. Fyfe DA, Ketchum D, Lewis R, et al. Tissue Doppler imaging detects severely abnormal myocardial velocities that identify children with preterminal cardiac graft failure after heart transplantation. *J Heart Lung Transplant Off Pub Int Soc Heart Transplant.* 2006;25(5):510–517.
114. Friedberg MK, Silverman NH. The systolic to diastolic duration ratio in children with heart failure secondary to restrictive cardiomyopathy. *J Am Soc Echocardiogr.* 2006;19(11):1326–1331.
115. Friedberg MK, Silverman NH. Cardiac ventricular diastolic and systolic duration in children with heart failure secondary to idiopathic dilated cardiomyopathy. *Am J Cardiol.* 2006;97(1):101–105.
116. Mondal T, Slorach C, Manlhiot C, et al. Prognostic implications of the systolic to diastolic duration ratio in children with idiopathic or familial dilated cardiomyopathy. *Circ Cardiovasc Imag.* 2014;7(5):773–780.

117. Alexander PMA, Nugent AW, Daubeney PEF, et al. Long-term outcomes of hypertrophic cardiomyopathy diagnosed during childhood: results from a national population-based study. *Circulation.* 2018;138(1):29–36.
118. Lipshultz SE, Orav EJ, Wilkinson JD, et al. Risk stratification at diagnosis for children with hypertrophic cardiomyopathy: an analysis of data from the Pediatric Cardiomyopathy Registry. *Lancet.* 2013;382(9908):1889–1897.
119. Norrish G, Cantarutti N, Pissaridou E, et al. Risk factors for sudden cardiac death in childhood hypertrophic cardiomyopathy: a systematic review and meta-analysis. *Eur J Prevent Cardiol.* 2017;24(11):1220–1230.
120. Ferguson ME, Sachdeva R, Gillespie SE, Morrow G, Border W. Tissue Doppler imaging during exercise stress echocardiography demonstrates a mechanism for impaired exercise performance in children with hypertrophic cardiomyopathy. *Echocardiography.* 2016;33(11):1718–1725.
121. Cerrato F, Pacileo G, Limongelli G, et al. A standard echocardiographic and tissue Doppler study of morphological and functional findings in children with hypertrophic cardiomyopathy compared to those with left ventricular hypertrophy in the setting of Noonan and LEOPARD syndromes. *Cardiol Young.* 2008;18(6):575–580.
122. Hayabuchi Y, Sakata M, Ohnishi T, Inoue M, Kagami S. Ratio of early diastolic tricuspid inflow to tricuspid lateral annulus velocity reflects pulmonary regurgitation severity but not right ventricular diastolic function in children with repaired tetralogy of Fallot. *Pediatr Cardiol.* 2013;34(5):1112–1117.
123. Maskatia SA, Morris SA, Spinner JA, Krishnamurthy R, Altman CA. Echocardiographic parameters of right ventricular diastolic function in repaired tetralogy of Fallot are associated with important findings on magnetic resonance imaging. *Congenit Heart Dis.* 2015;10(3):e113–e122.
124. Friedberg MK, Fernandes FP, Roche SL, et al. Impaired right and left ventricular diastolic myocardial mechanics and filling in asymptomatic children and adolescents after repair of tetralogy of Fallot. *Eur Heart J Cardiovasc Imag.* 2012;13(11):905–913.
125. Helbing WA, Niezen RA, Le Cessie S, van der Geest RJ, Ottenkamp J, de Roos A. Right ventricular diastolic function in children with pulmonary regurgitation after repair of tetralogy of Fallot: volumetric evaluation by magnetic resonance velocity mapping. *J Am Coll Cardiol.* 1996;28(7):1827–1835.
126. Pérez Del Villar C, Bermejo J, Rodríguez-Pérez D, et al. The role of elastic restoring forces in right-ventricular filling. *Cardiovasc Res.* 2015;107(1):45–55.
127. Sun AM, AlHabshan F, Cheung M, et al. Delayed onset of tricuspid valve flow in repaired tetralogy of Fallot: an additional mechanism of diastolic dysfunction and interventricular dyssynchrony. *J Cardiovasc Magn Reson Off J Soc Cardiovasc Magn Reason.* 2011;13:43.
128. Friedberg MK. Imaging right-left ventricular interactions. *JACC Cardiovasc Imag.* 2018;11(5):755–771.
129. Ahmad N, Kantor PF, Grosse-Wortmann L, et al. Influence of RV restrictive physiology on LV diastolic function in children after tetralogy of Fallot repair. *J Am Soc Echocardiogr.* 2012;25(8):866–873.
130. Karnik R, Uppu SC, Tozzi M, et al. Abnormalities in left ventricular rotation are inherent in young children with repaired tetralogy of Fallot and are independent of right ventricular dilation. *Pediatr Cardiol.* 2018;39(6):1172–1180.
131. Kobayashi M, Takahashi K, Yamada M, et al. Assessment of early diastolic intraventricular pressure gradient in the left ventricle among patients with repaired tetralogy of Fallot. *Heart Vessels.* 2017;32(11):1364–1374.
132. Aboulhosn JA, Lluri G, Gurvitz MZ, et al. Left and right ventricular diastolic function in adults with surgically repaired tetralogy of Fallot: a multi-institutional study. *Can J Cardiol.* 2013;29(7):866–872.
133. van der Hulst AE, Westenberg JJ, Delgado V, et al. Tissue-velocity magnetic resonance imaging and tissue Doppler imaging to assess regional myocardial diastolic velocities at the right ventricle in corrected pediatric tetralogy of Fallot patients. *Invest Radiol.* 2012;47(3):189–196.
134. Norgård G, Gatzoulis MA, Moraes F, et al. Relationship between type of outflow tract repair and postoperative right ventricular diastolic physiology in tetralogy of Fallot. Implications for long-term outcome. *Circulation.* 1996;94(12):3276–3280.
135. Cullen S, Shore D, Redington A. Characterization of right ventricular diastolic performance after complete repair of tetralogy of Fallot. Restrictive physiology predicts slow postoperative recovery. *Circulation.* 1995;91(6):1782–1789.
136. Gatzoulis MA, Clark AL, Cullen S, Newman CG, Redington AN. Right ventricular diastolic function 15 to 35 years after repair of tetralogy of Fallot. Restrictive physiology predicts superior exercise performance. *Circulation.* 1995;91(6):1775–1781.
137. Samyn MM, Kwon EN, Gorentz JS, et al. Restrictive versus nonrestrictive physiology following repair of tetralogy of Fallot: is there a difference? *J Am Soc Echocardiogr.* 2013;26(7):746–755.
138. Kutty S, Valente AM, White MT, et al. Usefulness of pulmonary arterial end-diastolic forward flow late after tetralogy of Fallot repair to predict a "restrictive" right ventricle. *Am J Cardiol.* 2018;121(11):1380–1386.
139. Liang XC, Lam WW, Cheung EW, Wu AK, Wong SJ, Cheung YF. Restrictive right ventricular physiology and right ventricular fibrosis as assessed by cardiac magnetic resonance and exercise capacity after biventricular repair of pulmonary atresia and intact ventricular septum. *Clin Cardiol.* 2010;33(2):104–110.
140. Riesenkampff E, Mengelkamp L, Mueller M, et al. Integrated analysis of atrioventricular interactions in tetralogy of Fallot. *Am J Physiol Heart Circ Physiol.* 2010;299(2):H364–H3671.
141. Kutty S, Shang Q, Joseph N, et al. Abnormal right atrial performance in repaired tetralogy of Fallot: a CMR feature tracking analysis. *Int J Cardiol.* 2017;248:136–142.
142. Riesenkampff E, Al-Wakeel N, Kropf S, et al. Surgery impacts right atrial function in tetralogy of Fallot. *J Thorac Cardiovasc Surg.* 2014;147(4):1306–1311.
143. Baggen VJM, Schut AW, Cuypers J, et al. Prognostic value of left atrial size and function in adults with tetralogy of Fallot. *Int J Cardiol.* 2017;236:125–131.
144. Bustamante-Labarta M, Perrone S, De La Fuente RL, et al. Right atrial size and tricuspid regurgitation severity predict mortality or transplantation in primary pulmonary hypertension. *J Am Soc Echocardiogr.* 2002;15(10 Pt 2):1160–1164.
145. Do DH, Therrien J, Marelli A, Martucci G, Afilalo J, Sebag IA. Right atrial size relates to right ventricular end-diastolic pressure in an adult population with congenital heart disease. *Echocardiography.* 2011;28(1):109–116.
146. Kassem E, Humpl T, Friedberg MK. Prognostic significance of 2-dimensional, M-mode, and Doppler echo indices of right ventricular function in children with pulmonary arterial hypertension. *Am Heart J.* 2013;165(6):1024–1031.
147. Ploegstra MJ, Roofthooft MT, Douwes JM, et al. Echocardiography in pediatric pulmonary arterial hypertension: early study on assessing disease severity and predicting outcome. *Circ Cardiovasc Imag.* 2015;8(1):00.
148. Moceri P, Dimopoulos K, Liodakis E, et al. Echocardiographic predictors of outcome in Eisenmenger syndrome. *Circulation.* 2012;126(12):1461–1468.
149. Takatsuki S, Nakayama T, Jone PN, et al. Tissue Doppler imaging predicts adverse outcome in children with idiopathic pulmonary arterial hypertension. *J Pediatr.* 2012;161(6):1126–1131.
150. Okumura K, Slorach C, Mroczek D, et al. Right ventricular diastolic performance in children with pulmonary arterial hypertension associated with congenital heart disease: correlation of echocardiographic parameters with invasive reference standards by high-fidelity micromanometer catheter. *Circ Cardiovasc Imag.* 2014;7(3):491–501.
151. Chowdhury SM, Goudar SP, Baker GH, et al. Speckle-tracking echocardiographic measures of right ventricular diastolic function correlate with reference standard measures before and after preload alteration in children. *Pediatr Cardiol.* 2017;38(1):27–35.
152. Friedberg MK, Redington AN. Right versus left ventricular failure: differences, similarities, and interactions. *Circulation.* 2014;129(9):1033–1044.
153. Alkon J, Humpl T, Manlhiot C, McCrindle BW, Reyes JT, Friedberg MK. Usefulness of the right ventricular systolic to diastolic duration ratio to predict functional capacity and survival in children with pulmonary arterial hypertension. *Am J Cardiol.* 2010;106(3):430–436.

154. Burkett DA, Slorach C, Patel SS, et al. Impact of pulmonary hemodynamics and ventricular interdependence on left ventricular diastolic function in children with pulmonary hypertension. *Circ Cardiovasc Imag.* 2016;9(9):e004612.
155. Earing MG, Cetta F, Driscoll DJ, et al. Long-term results of the Fontan operation for double-inlet left ventricle. *Am J Cardiol.* 2005;96(2):291–298.
156. Gewillig M. The Fontan circulation. *Heart.* 2005;91(6):839–846.
157. Seliem M, Muster AJ, Paul MH, Benson Jr DW. Relation between preoperative left ventricular muscle mass and outcome of the Fontan procedure in patients with tricuspid atresia. *J Am Coll Cardiol.* 1989;14(3):750–755.
158. Kirklin JK, Blackstone EH, Kirklin JW, Pacifico AD, Bargeron Jr LM. The Fontan operation. Ventricular hypertrophy, age, and date of operation as risk factors. *J Thorac Cardiovasc Surg.* 1986;92(6):1049–1064.
159. Mayer Jr JE, Helgason H, Jonas RA, et al. Extending the limits for modified Fontan procedures. *J Thorac Cardiovasc Surg.* 1986;92(6):1021–1028.
160. Gewillig MH, Lundström UR, Deanfield JE, et al. Impact of Fontan operation on left ventricular size and contractility in tricuspid atresia. *Circulation.* 1990;81(1):118–127.
161. Frommelt PC, Snider AR, Meliones JN, Vermilion RP. Doppler assessment of pulmonary artery flow patterns and ventricular function after the Fontan operation. *Am J Cardiol.* 1991;68(11):1211–1215.
162. Fogel MA, Weinberg PM, Chin AJ, Fellows KE, Hoffman EA. Late ventricular geometry and performance changes of functional single ventricle throughout staged Fontan reconstruction assessed by magnetic resonance imaging. *J Am Coll Cardiol.* 1996;28(1):212–221.
163. Iimoto DS, Covell JW, Harper E. Increase in cross-linking of type I and type III collagens associated with volume-overload hypertrophy. *Circ Res.* 1988;63(2):399–408.
164. Penny DJ, Rigby ML, Redington AN. Abnormal patterns of intraventricular flow and diastolic filling after the Fontan operation: evidence for incoordinate ventricular wall motion. *Br Heart J.* 1991;66(5):375–378.
165. Akagi T, Benson LN, Gilday DL, et al. Influence of ventricular morphology on diastolic filling performance in double-inlet ventricle after the Fontan procedure. *J Am Coll Cardiol.* 1993;22(7):1948–1952.
166. Cheung YF, Penny DJ, Redington AN. Serial assessment of left ventricular diastolic function after Fontan procedure. *Heart.* 2000;83(4):420–424.
167. Wang J, Khoury DS, Yue Y, Torre-Amione G, Nagueh SF. Left ventricular untwisting rate by speckle tracking echocardiography. *Circulation.* 2007;116(22):2580–2586.
168. Husain N, Gokhale J, Nicholson L, Cheatham JP, Holzer RJ, Cua CL. Noninvasive estimation of ventricular filling pressures in patients with single right ventricles. *J Am Soc Echocardiogr.* 2013;26(11):1330–1336.
169. Buddhe S, Richmond ME, Gilbreth J, Lai WW. Longitudinal strain by speckle tracking echocardiography in pediatric heart transplant recipients. *Congenit Heart Dis.* 2015;10(4):362–370.
170. Menon SC, Gray R, Tani LY. Evaluation of ventricular filling pressures and ventricular function by Doppler echocardiography in patients with functional single ventricle: correlation with simultaneous cardiac catheterization. *J Am Soc Echocardiogr.* 2011;24(11):1220–1225.
171. Anderson PA, Sleeper LA, Mahony L, et al. Contemporary outcomes after the Fontan procedure: a Pediatric Heart Network multicenter study. *J Am Coll Cardiol.* 2008;52(2):85–98.
172. Chowdhury SM, Butts RJ, Buckley J, et al. Comparison of pressure-volume loop and echocardiographic measures of diastolic function in patients with a single-ventricle physiology. *Pediatr Cardiol.* 2014;35(6):998–1006.
173. Okada DR, Molina MR, Kohari M, Vorovich EE, Owens AT, Han Y. Clinical echocardiographic indices of left ventricular diastolic function correlate poorly with pulmonary capillary wedge pressure at 1 year following heart transplantation. *Int J Cardiovasc Imag.* 2015;31(4):783–794.
174. Sachdeva R, Malik S, Seib PM, Frazier EA, Cleves MA. Doppler tissue imaging and catheter-derived measures are not independent predictors of rejection in pediatric heart transplant recipients. *Int J Cardiovasc Imag.* 2011;27(7):947–954.
175. Khoo NS, Smallhorn JF, Kaneko S, Kutty S, Altamirano L, Tham EB. The assessment of atrial function in single ventricle hearts from birth to Fontan: a speckle-tracking study by using strain and strain rate. *J Am Soc Echocardiogr.* 2013;26(7):756–764.
176. Slørdahl SA, Bjaerum S, Amundsen BH, et al. High frame rate strain rate imaging of the interventricular septum in healthy subjects. *Eur J Ultrasound.* 2001;14(2–3):149–155.
177. D'Alonzo GE, Barst RJ, Ayres SM, et al. Survival in patients with primary pulmonary hypertension. Results from a national prospective registry. *Ann Intern Med.* 1991;115(5):343–349.
178. Villemain O, Correia M, Khraiche D, et al. Myocardial stiffness assessment using shear wave imaging in pediatric hypertrophic cardiomyopathy. *JACC Cardiovasc Imag.* 2018;11(5):779–781.
179. Friedberg MK, Roche SL, Mohammed AF, Balasingam M, Atenafu EG, Kantor PF. Left ventricular diastolic mechanical dyssynchrony and associated clinical outcomes in children with dilated cardiomyopathy. *Circ Cardiovasc Imag.* 2008;1(1):50–57.
180. Menon SC, Eidem BW, Dearani JA, Ommen SR, Ackerman MJ, Miller D. Diastolic dysfunction and its histopathological correlation in obstructive hypertrophic cardiomyopathy in children and adolescents. *J Am Soc Echocardiogr.* 2009;22(12):1327–1334.
181. Courtois M, Kovacs Jr SJ, Ludbrook PA. Transmitral pressure-flow velocity relation. Importance of regional pressure gradients in the left ventricle during diastole. *Circulation.* 1988;78(3):661–671.
182. Prinz C, Faber L, Horstkotte D, et al. Evaluation of left ventricular torsion in children with hypertrophic cardiomyopathy. *Cardiol Young.* 2014;24(2):245–252.

28

Diabetes Mellitus

Harsh V. Thakkar and Kazuaki Negishi

OUTLINE

Case Study

A 65-year-old male presents with exertional dyspnea for investigation. He states his dyspnea worsens when walking up a hill. For history, he has type 2 diabetes (treated with metformin), hypertension, dyslipidemia, and Barrett's esophagus. He previously had an elective percutaneous coronary intervention (PCI) for a positive exercise stress test (indication: exertional dyspnea).

INTRODUCTION

Diabetes is a complex, chronic illness requiring continuous medical care with multifactorial risk-reduction strategies beyond glycemic control.[1] The dynamics of the diabetes epidemic are changing rapidly, once a disease of the West, type 2 diabetes mellitus (T2DM) has now spread to every country in the world. Globally, an estimated 422 million adults were living with diabetes in 2014, compared to 108 million in 1980.[2] This accelerating pandemic comes with high personal and financial costs to the individual, society, and the global economy. Globally, diabetes accounted for at least $376 billion of health expenditure in 2010, and is expected to hit $490 billion in 2030.[3]

Cardiovascular disease remains the principal cause of death and disability among diabetics. Approximately two-thirds of deaths in people with diabetes are attributable to cardiovascular disease: ~40% from ischemic heart disease, followed by ~15% from other heart diseases, principally heart failure (HF), and ~10% from stroke.[4] Although atherosclerotic cardiovascular disease remains the principal cause of death among them, diabetes dramatically increases the incidence of HF with an excess risk of twofold to fivefold, with greater impacts on women.[5] If they are young, the risk is fourfold to eightfold.[5] HF affects approximately one in five diabetic patients.[6] More recently, an epidemiologic study of 1.9 million persons with a median follow-up of 5.5 years found that HF and peripheral arterial disease were the most common initial cardiovascular manifestations in type 2 diabetes.[7]

HF was noted to be a complication of diabetes more than a century ago.[8] Traditionally, the two illnesses have been managed in relative isolation. However, with a high incidence of coexistence of these two chronic conditions, especially with the growing prevalence, clinicians should be more cognizant of the impact each has on the other (i.e., bidirectional effects in terms of causation and outcome). For example, each 1% elevation in hemoglobin A1c (HbA1c) leads to an 8% to 15% increase in the frequency of HF independent of other risk factors.[9,10] Conversely, a 1% reduction of HbA1c levels is associated with a 16% reduced risk of developing HF and worsening outcomes.[11] There is also increasing evidence that HF reciprocally augments the risk of insulin resistance and clinical diabetes.[12] Surprisingly, the link between HF and insulin resistance becomes stronger once the ischemic heart disease is excluded.[10] These pieces of evidence support the existence of diabetic cardiomyopathy as a distinct disease entity, where diastolic dysfunction is the predominant feature of the heart. The postulated mechanism is due to small vessel disease or associated metabolic disturbances (including insulin resistance/hyperinsulinemia). These observations have been confirmed by several subsequent epidemiologic studies. These

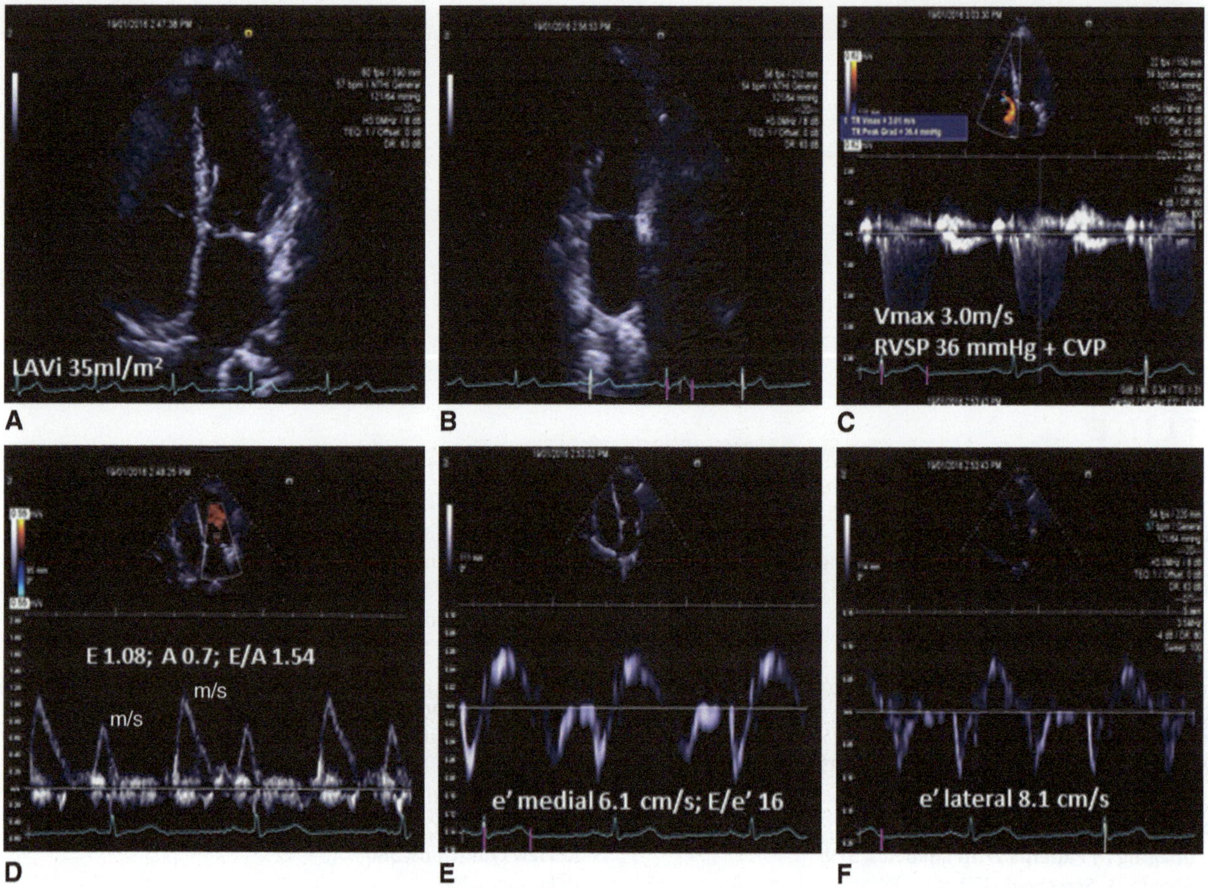

Case 1 Echo Findings. Normal left ventricular (LV) cavity size, but diffuse mild LV hypertrophy. Normal ejection fraction (69% in 3-D echo). Grade 2 diastolic dysfunction with mild left atrial (LA) dilatation (35 mL/m^2), E/e′ 1.54, E/e′ 16, tricuspid regurgitation velocity (TR Vmax) 3.01 m/sec with pulmonary artery systolic pressure (PASP) of 39 mmHg. Grade 2 diastolic dysfunction as evidenced by dilated LA (A, B), transmitral flow showing predominantly passive flow with E/A 1.54 (D), and reduced tissue velocity (e′) (E and F), with pulmonary hypertension (C).

patients have a dismal prognosis, with a 10-fold increase in risk for mortality.[13]

The recent advance in diabetic medication, such as sodium glucose cotransporter-2 (SGLT2) inhibitors, points to a a bright future. The EMPA-REG OUTCOME[14] and the CANVAS Program[15] have demonstrated the beneficial effects of SGLT2 inhibitors in the management of diabetics with HF. Now clinicians have access to effective therapies to prevent cardiovascular morbidity and mortality in these patients. This group of medications has the potential to change the landscape in the treatment of diabetes patients with HF.

MECHANISMS AND PREDICTIVE FACTORS OF DIABETIC CARDIOMYOPATHY

In 1972, Rubler et al. coined the term "diabetic cardiomyopathy," describing diabetic patients developing a specific form of cardiomyopathy in the absence of coronary artery disease (CAD), hypertension, or valvular heart disease, based on autopsy findings.[16] The existence of this entity has been further confirmed by clinical and laboratory studies, which have shed light on pathophysiologic and biochemical mechanisms, which will be discussed in this section. Insulin resistance and/or hyperinsulinemia play a key role in the development of diabetic cardiomyopathy, which is initially characterized by diastolic dysfunction in the absence of CAD and hypertension (Fig. 28.1).[17] They increase systemic metabolic disorders; activate the sympathetic nervous system (SNS); activate the renin-angiotensin-aldosterone system (RAAS); prompt oxidative stress, mitochondrial dysfunction, and endoplasmic reticulum stress; and impair calcium homeostasis. These effects result in cardiac fibrosis, hypertrophy, cardiomyocyte death, dysfunction of the coronary microcirculation, and eventually HF. Furthermore, these pathophysiologic changes in cardiomyocytes underlie the risk factors for insulin resistance and hyperinsulinemia, which can result in a potentially vicious cycle.

INSULIN RESISTANCE AND ALTERED INSULIN SIGNALING IN DIABETES

Insulin resistant states exhibit impaired insulin-mediated glucose uptake in the muscles and adipocytes, impaired suppression of hepatic glucose production, and impaired suppression of lipolysis.[18] There are several mechanisms implicated in the development of insulin resistance. These include increased lipolysis, higher free fatty acid (FFA) release, reduced glucose uptake, decreased secretion of adiponectin (which is an anti-inflammatory adipokine), increased secretion of leptin, and increased secretion of proinflammatory

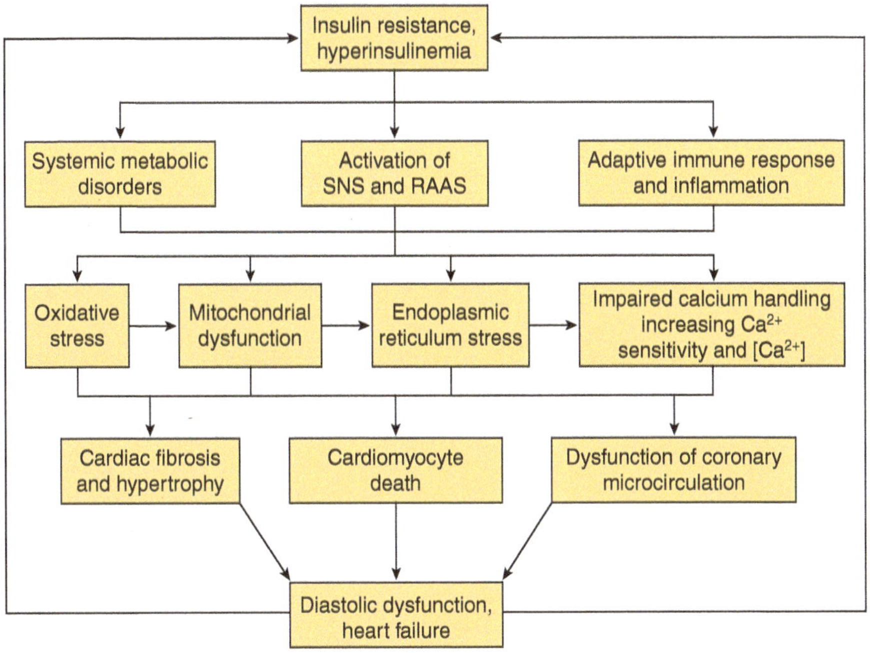

Fig. 28.1 The development and progression of diabetic cardiomyopathy. Insulin resistance and hyperinsulinemia increase systemic metabolic disorders; activate the SNS; activate RAAS; prompt oxidative stress, mitochondrial dysfunction, and endoplasmic reticulum stress; and impair calcium homeostasis. These effects result in cardiac fibrosis, hypertrophy, cardiomyocyte death, dysfunction of the coronary microcirculation, and eventually heart failure. Furthermore, these pathophysiologic changes in cardiomyocytes underlie the risk factors for insulin resistance and hyperinsulinemia, which can result in a potentially vicious cycle. *RAAS*, Renin-angiotensin-aldosterone system; *SNS*, sympathetic nervous system. (Reproduced with permission from Jia DeMarco VG, Sowers JR. Insulin resistance and hyperinsulinaemia in diabetic cardiomyopathy. *Nat Rev Endocrinol.* 2016;12:144–153.)

cytokines. Tumor necrosis factor alpha (TNF-α), interleukin-6 (IL-6), and FFAs activate intracellular kinases that induce serine phosphorylation of insulin receptor substrate-1 (IRS-1), thereby attenuating insulin signaling and inducing insulin resistance.[19] Increased endoplasmic reticulum (ER) stress, increased production of reactive oxygen species, and mitochondrial dysfunction have been suggested to contribute to the development of insulin resistance.[18] Importantly, immune cells infiltrating adipose tissue contribute extensively to the production and secretion of proinflammatory mediators, which in turn exacerbate systemic insulin resistance and contribute to cardiac insulin resistance.[20]

Cellular insulin signaling occurs via two main pathways: one involves IRS-1, an upstream signal activating endothelial nitric oxide synthesis.[21] The other involves mitogen-activated protein (MAP) kinase,[21] which contributes to growth and remodeling responses and the resultant myocardial hypertrophy, myocardial fibrosis, impaired myocardial-endothelial signaling, and death of myocardial and endothelial cells. Insulin-resistant/hyperinsulinemic states exhibit an imbalance between them with MAP kinesis predominating, resulting in myocardial hypertrophy and fibrosis, as well as myocardial and endothelial cell death.

In a rat model of early diabetic cardiomyopathy, an 18-fluorodeoxyglucose (18-FDG) positron emission tomography (PET) study revealed a decrease of myocardial glucose utilization and increased fatty acid oxidation, in association with impaired myocardial function.[22] In T2DM rats, PET showed alterations in myocardial glucose utilization that were linked with cardiac dysfunction.[23] However, 18-FDG itself may constitute a drawback for diabetic patients with impairment in glucose uptake.

METABOLIC FACTORS

Free Fatty Acid Metabolism

The normal heart has remarkable flexibility in switching the fuels depending on the body's nutritional state and physical activity. In a normal heart, more than 95% of adenosine triphosphate (ATP) generated in the heart is derived from oxidative phosphorylation in the mitochondria. Approximately 70% to 90% of the cardiac ATP is produced by the metabolism of the fatty acids and the remainder 10% to 30% is by the metabolism of glucose and lactate, as well as small amounts of amino acids and ketones.[24] FFAs are the preferred energy substrates in the adult heart. They enter the cytosol by passive diffusion or via fatty acid translocase (FAT)/cluster of differentiation 36 (CD36),[25] where insulin also plays an essential role for metabolic homeostasis.[26] The IRS-1 pathway promotes the translocation of FAT/CD36 to the cell membrane causing downstream effects as described earlier. The glucose intake occurs via insulin-stimulating glucose transporter 4 (GULT4). In the state of insulin resistance and hyperinsulinemia, the imbalance between these two results in excessive accumulation of fatty acids in myocytes. The associated lipotoxicity further impairs insulin signaling and reduces physiologic autophagy, which leads to morphologic/structural alterations and impaired myocardial performance.[20]

Calcium Homeostasis

Alteration in calcium homeostasis is the hallmark for the diastolic dysfunction seen in diabetic cardiomyopathy. Sarcoplasmic reticulum plays a key role in excitation-contraction coupling in the heart. During relaxation, Ca^{2+} is transported into the sarcoplasmic reticulum by the sarco/endoplasmic Ca^{2+} ATPase 2a ($SERCA_{2a}$) actively using ATP. The

$SERCA_{2a}$ activity is decreased in the failing diabetic cardiomyocytes,[27] which results in impaired relaxation and active expansion of the left ventricle during early diastole. There is also a diminished calcium sensitivity and alteration in the function of regulatory and contractile proteins caused by the abnormal myocardial metabolism in the diabetic cardiomyocytes.[28]

ALTERED CORONARY MICROCIRCULATION

Impairment in coronary microcirculation occurs frequently in insulin resistance, T2DM, and diabetic cardiomyopathy.[17] This is caused by the decreased levels of bioavailable nitric oxide via the above mentioned IRS-1 pathway.[29] Nitric oxide plays an important role in coronary vascular smooth muscle relaxation, where it activates both guanylyl cyclase, required for synthesis of guanosine monophosphate (GMP), and kinases, which are required for coronary relaxation.[30] When insulin sensitivity is diminished, both reduced production and increased degeneration of nitric oxide take place, resulting in the ambient state of coronary constriction in states.

Insulin resistance and hyperinsulinemia are also associated with increased vascular stiffness, both large and small vessels[31] via the following mechanisms. The increased plasma insulin levels promote the differentiation of vascular smooth muscle cells to an osteoblast-like phenotype, which could contribute to vascular stiffness.[32] Raised insulin levels also increase alkaline phosphatase activity, osteocalcin expression, and the formation of mineralized nodules in vascular smooth muscle cells. Thus impaired vascular smooth muscle cell and endothelial cell function are associated with an elevated afterload and risk of CAD.

MYOCARDIAL FIBROSIS

Myocardial fibrosis and myocyte hypertrophy are among the most frequently proposed mechanisms to explain cardiac changes in diabetic cardiomyopathy. Interstitial fibrosis has been identified in more advanced stages of diabetic cardiomyopathy.[16] Indeed, diffuse fibrosis in myocardium and myocyte hypertrophy are the main histopathologic findings in the end-stage diabetic nephropathy cases by Rubler et al.[16] Accumulation of collagen in the diabetic myocardium may be due partially to hampered collagen degradation resulting from glycosylation of the lysine residues on collagen.[33] Hyperglycemia also leads to increased production of reactive oxygen and nitrogen species, which increase the oxidative stress and cause abnormal gene expression, altered signal transduction, and activation of the pathways leading to apoptosis.[34] This process is associated with glycosylation of p53, resulting in an increase in angiotensin-II synthesis[35] that has dose-dependent effects on collagen secretion and production in cardiac fibroblasts.[36] In addition, chronic metabolic abnormalities present in diabetes lead to modulations in endothelin-1 and its receptors,[37] decreased levels of insulin-like growth factor-I,[38] and increased production of transforming growth factor-β1[39] that result in the promotion of angiotensin-II activity with an increase in myocardial collagen content.

In recent times, with the advent of specialized noninvasive imaging technologies, more detailed information about the structure of the heart can be obtained noninvasively. Studies used cardiovascular magnetic resonance imaging (cardiac MRI) techniques to demonstrate the increase in extracellular volume and myocardial fibrosis in patients with HF.[40] Another study showed a higher median extracellular volume in patients with diabetes as compared to patients without diabetes.[41] The role of fibrosis in myocardial dysfunction is also supported by studies showing a reversal of cardiac fibrosis by the use of short-term pirfenidone and spironolactone, with improvement in diastolic stiffness in diabetic rat models.[42] Alterations in the myocardial structure are minimal in the early stages and may be reversible or partially reversible. As diabetes progresses, the accumulation of collagen becomes more obvious and may play a role in diastolic dysfunction observed in diabetics.

INAPPROPRIATE ACTIVATION OF NEUROHORMONES

Inappropriate activation of the sympathetic nervous system and RAAS further drive the cascade to develop the diabetic cardiomyopathy. The activated sympathetic nervous system stimulates the β1-adrenergic expression and signaling, which promotes myocyte hypertrophy, interstitial fibrosis, and reduced contractile function accompanied by increased myocyte apoptosis.[43] Reduced activation of the parasympathetic system results in altered muscarinic receptor density and composition and decreased acetylcholinesterase activity.[44] Either direct or indirect vagal nerve stimulation has direct beneficial effects on cardiac remodeling and clinical outcomes.[44]

The role of RAAS activation in hyperinsulinemic states leads to the genesis of various cardiovascular disease, including CAD and HF.[17] Furthermore, enhanced activation of angiotensin-I and mineralocorticoid receptor signaling might promote insulin resistance,[45] which leads to a vicious cycle between insulin resistance and RAAS activation, resulting in impaired vascular and cardiac relaxation mediated by nitric oxide[46] as described earlier. In addition, the RAAS activation also promotes vascular oxidative stress via stimulation of nicotinamide-adenine dinucleotide phosphate (NADPH) oxidase activity,[47] and further reduces production of nitric oxide, promotes vascular and cardiac stiffness, and impairs cardiac relaxation.[48] Thus the interaction of insulin resistance with RAAS activation leads to myocardial fibrosis and diastolic dysfunction, which characterize the early stages of diabetic cardiomyopathy.

INTERACTION WITH HYPERTENSION AND CORONARY ARTERY DISEASE

The concomitant prevalence of hypertension and diabetes is rising. In a recent systematic review, the prevalence of hypertension in patients with type 2 diabetes was reported up to 95% depending on the geographic region and the definition of hypertension used.[49] The clinical characteristics and the outcomes are more severe in hypertensive diabetic patients as compared to hypertensive patients or diabetic patients alone. Hypertension and diabetes are independently associated with impaired left ventricular (LV) diastolic function, independent of the effect of obesity, age, LV mass, LV geometry, heart rate, and LV ejection fraction (EF).[50]

The basic atherosclerosis process in patients with diabetes and hypertension appears to have an accelerated development of advanced lesions.[51] The pathophysiologic link between hyperglycemia and macrovascular disease includes direct effects of glucose, activation of protein kinase C, endothelial dysfunction from oxidative stress, activation of athero-inflammatory cytokines, and epigenetic changes.[52,53] In a prospective study conducted in Finland, the risk of CAD-related death was comparable in patients with diabetes and no prior history of myocardial infarction to those without diabetes and prior myocardial infarction.[54] A recent study from Kaiser Permanente Northern California (KPNC) has validated this further. They showed that compared to individuals without a history of diabetes or CAD, prevalent diabetes was associated with approximately double the coronary heart disease risk, and prior CAD was associated with triple the risk.[55]

CARDIAC IMAGING IN PATIENTS WITH DIABETES

This section summarizes cardiac imaging for the assessment of cardiac structure and function in patients with diabetes, especially how to identify the signals, preferably in early stages. HF is a major cardiovascular cause for mortality among the diabetes population,[4] where HF may arise from CAD, but the most common causes are nonischemic.[56] There are four major myocardial signals of diabetic heart disease: abnormal systolic function, diastolic function, and changes in LV geometry and myocardial composition. In this section, we will review who should be screened and how.

Who Should Be Screened?

Persons to be screened include those with symptoms, of course, but also those without symptoms, because, according to the American College of Cardiology/American Heart Association (ACC/AHA) guidelines for HF,[57] patients with diabetes are already in stage A HF, which means they are at high risk for HF, but without structural heart disease or symptoms of HF. However, no one knows whether the patient has stage B HF unless further diagnostic examination is performed. This is important as the recommended managements are different between stages A and B (especially the use of beta blockades). Thus all the patients with diabetes require at least electrocardiogram (ECG) and echocardiography, but there are even higher risks for the development of HF. Our systematic review and meta-analysis with over 1 million diabetes patients determined independent risk factors for HF: age, male gender, body mass index (BMI), HbA1c (per 1% increase as well as >8.0%), fasting glucose, insulin use, and atherosclerotic CAD[58] (Table 28.1).

TABLE 28.1 Risk Factors for Developing Subsequent Heart Failure Among Patients With Type 2 Diabetes Mellitus

Risk Variables	Dichotomous/ Continuous	FULLY ADJUSTED HAZARD RATIO Total (95% CI)	*p*
Age	5-year increase	1.26 [1.13, 1.40]	<0.0001
Gender (male)	Y/N	1.15 [1.00, 1.32]	0.04
BMI	1-unit increase	1.04 [1.01, 1.06]	0.003
Hypertension	Y/N	1.06 [0.81, 1.40]	0.67
HbA1c	1% increase	1.13 [1.12, 1.15]	<0.00001
	6.0%–7.0%	1.02 [0.73, 1.43]	0.89
	7.0%–8.0%	1.29 [0.97, 1.70]	0.08
	8.0%–9.0%	1.10 [1.02, 1.19]	0.02
	9.0%–10.0%	1.31 [1.14, 1.50]	0.0001
	≥10%	1.66 [1.45, 1.89]	<0.00001
Fasting glucose	1 SD increase	1.27 [1.10, 1.47]	0.001
Insulin use	Y/N	1.43 [1.14, 1.79]	0.002
TZDs	Y/N	1.42 [0.79, 2.55]	0.48
Metformin	Y/N	0.92 [0.69, 1.22]	0.55
Sulfonylurea	Y/N	1.14 [0.85, 1.53]	0.37
CAD	Y/N	1.77 [1.31, 2.39]	0.0002

BMI, Body mass index; *CAD,* coronary artery disease; *HbA1c,* hemoglobin A1c; *TZD,* thiazolidinedione.
Adapted from Wang Y, Negishi T, Negishi K, Marwick TH. Prediction of heart failure in patients with type 2 diabetes mellitus—a systematic review and meta-analysis. *Diabetes Res Clin Pract.* 2015;108:55–66.

Imaging for Systolic Function

The European Society of Cardiology (ESC) guidelines recommend transthoracic echocardiography (TTE) for the assessment of myocardial structure and function in subjects with suspected HF (including diabetes mellitus) as a class I indication, where one of the main aims is to assess LV EF to establish a diagnosis of either heart failure with reduced ejection fraction (HFrEF), heart failure with midrange ejection fraction (HFmrEF), or heart failure with preserved ejection fraction (HFpEF).[59] Although the current gold standard for the assessment of EF is cardiac MRI, echocardiography is most widely used and can aid the assessment of the progression of the disease and evaluating the response to therapy.[60] However, most diabetic cardiomyopathy patients present with preserved EF, like the case presented at the beginning who had preserved EF with a normal LV cavity but had evidence of structural changes as depicted by diffuse mild LV hypertrophy, as well as Case 2. Furthermore, among HF patients, the predictive value of EF for mortality is limited,[61] where myocardial strain imaging, especially global longitudinal strain (GLS), has a significant role.

The myocardial strain imaging is a relatively new technique to determine the degree of myocardial deformation (strain and strain rate). In current practice, most are derived from two-dimensional (2-D) speckle tracking echocardiography, but can be derived from three-dimensional (3-D) images as well. Myocardial strain is defined as change in the length of a segment divided by the original length of the segment, whereas the strain rate is the rate at which this deformation occurs during a cardiac cycle. GLS is calculated by averaging the strains of three apical views. Reduced GLS is a sensitive marker of systolic dysfunction, identifying diminished longitudinal deformation even while EF is preserved.

GLS is more sensitive to the conventional strategy for the detection of subclinical systolic dysfunction.[62] Impaired GLS is frequently observed in asymptomatic individuals with diabetes mellitus from 24% up to 45%[63,64] (e.g., Case 3). A study reported that reduced GLS may exist despite normal diastolic function.[63] Importantly, a decrease in GLS was independently associated with all-cause death and hospitalization after adjusting for age, systolic blood pressure (BP), exercise capacity, and HbA1c (HR 1.12 [1.00–1.21]), as well as provided incremental prognostic value up to 10 years after revealing.[64] Abnormal strains were also observed in T1DM.[65,66]

Although hypertension is often concomitantly seen in patients with diabetes mellitus, their effects on myocardial function are not the same. In a cross-sectional study of a stage A HF population, patients with T2DM without hypertension had a significantly lower GLS than those without T2DM and hypertension, but those with hypertension but without T2DM had similar GLS to those with neither.[67]

Cardiac MRI can assess myocardial strain with tagging or feature tracking methods. Tagged MRI indicated higher LV torsion with normal EF and LV mass in well-controlled T1DM patients.[68] Similarly, using tagged-MRI coupled to 3-D echo, circumferential and longitudinal strains and strain rates were found among T2DM patients with poor glycemic control and presence of other cardiovascular risk factors.[69] These data were not confirmed in well-controlled T1DM patients, suggesting a detrimental role of comorbidities and metabolic disturbances in cardiac strain.[68] In experimental T1DM, tagged MRI showed an increase of LV mass and volumes, LV hypertrophy, and fibrosis, in parallel to metabolic alterations.[70,71]

Imaging for Diastolic Function

LV diastolic dysfunction is very common in asymptomatic diabetic patients without other cardiovascular comorbidities, being present in at least 50%.[72] Thus if diastolic dysfunction is mild (i.e., grade I or abnormal relaxation, without raised mean left arterial [LA] pressure),

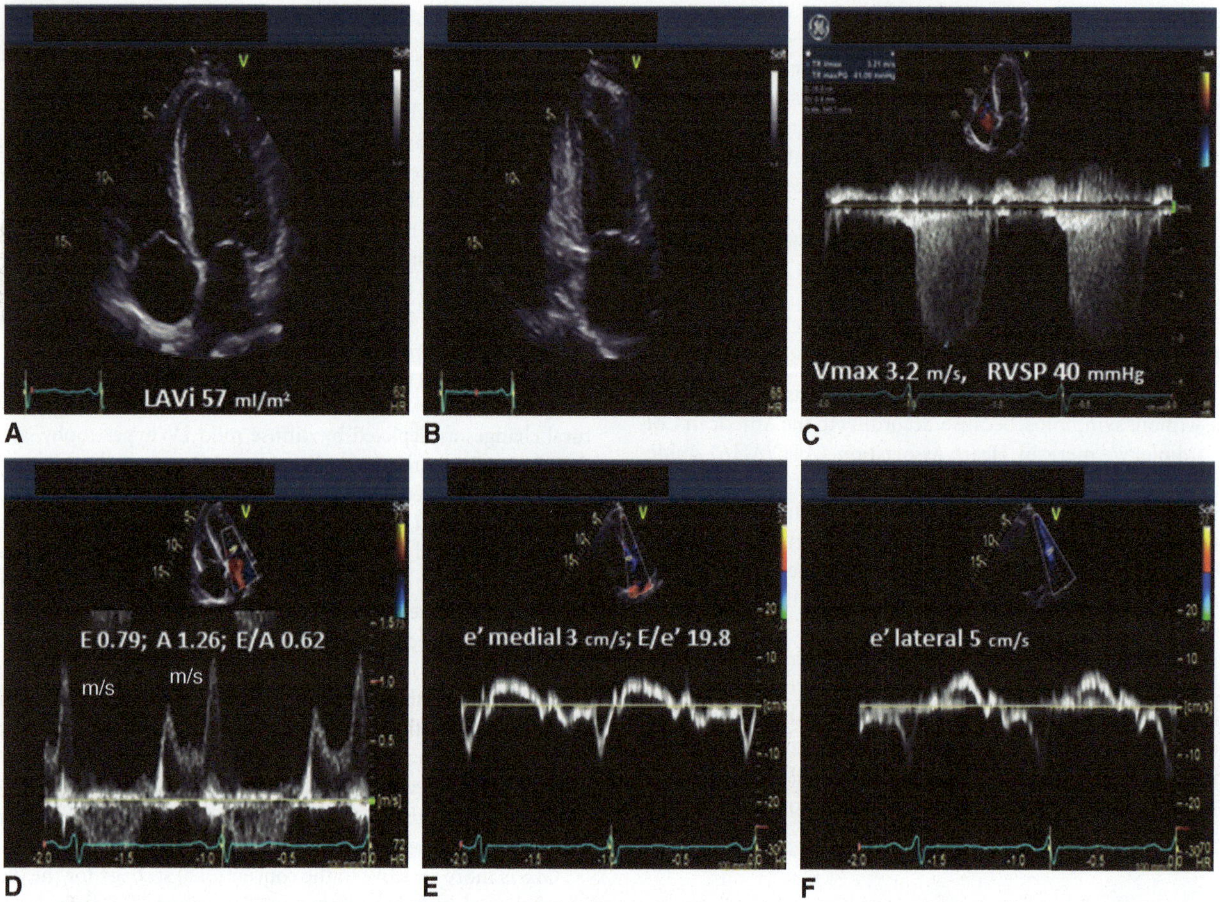
LAVi 57 ml/m²
Vmax 3.2 m/s, RVSP 40 mmHg
E 0.79; A 1.26; E/A 0.62
m/s
m/s
e' medial 3 cm/s; E/e' 19.8
e' lateral 5 cm/s
A
B
C
D
E
F

Case 2.

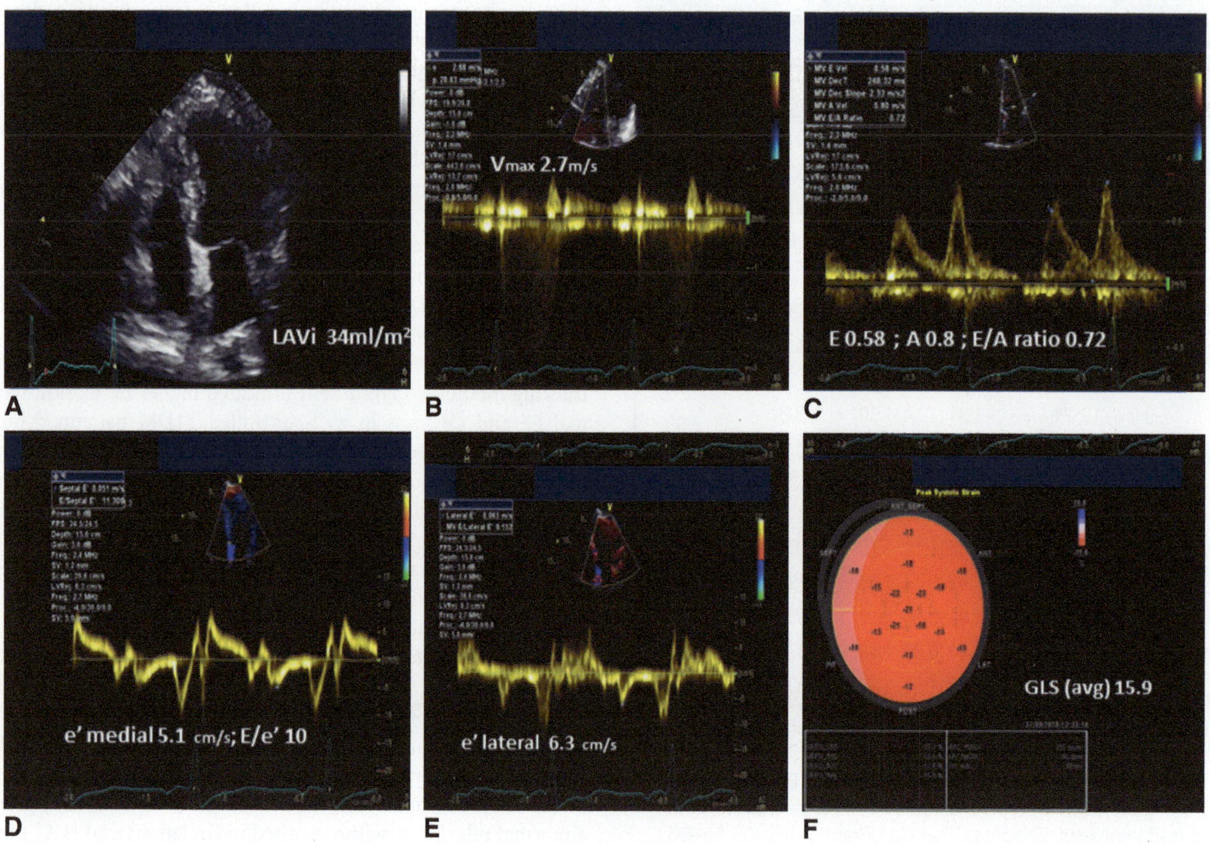
LAVi 34ml/m²
Vmax 2.7m/s
E 0.58 ; A 0.8 ; E/A ratio 0.72
e' medial 5.1 cm/s; E/e' 10
e' lateral 6.3 cm/s
GLS (avg) 15.9
A
B
C
D
E
F

Case 3.

the concern is that this finding is coincidental, such as aging. However, as this disease process progresses, there are symptom developments, mainly dyspnea, as well as changes noted on assessment of diastolic function, as in Cases 1 (grade II) and 2 (grade Ia). There are several recommended methods for diastolic function assessment, especially in diabetes. As the diabetic patients with normal LV EF are frequently associated with diastolic dysfunction,[73] tissue Doppler imaging (TDI), the Valsalva maneuver, and LA volumes should be used. The Valsalva maneuver reduces the LV preload by reverting the LA pressure and unmasks the pseudonormal pattern.[72] A systematic study among type 2 diabetics without any significant cardiovascular comorbidity showed that 46% of patients had diastolic dysfunction when diagnosed by transmitral flow (TMF) alone; this increased to 63% when Valsalva maneuver was used and 74% with TDI.[72] Another study found that using standard TMF alone did not find a significant difference in LV diastolic function between the diabetics and control; however, by using TDI, 50% of diabetic patients who had normal diastolic function by TMF had diastolic dysfunction.[74] In a population of 140 adults (16% diabetic), LA volume index was associated with the degree of diastolic dysfunction, independent of EF, age, gender, and cardiovascular risk score.[75] Diastolic dysfunction in diabetic patients is associated with cardiac autonomic neuropathy as assessed by metaiodobenzylguanidine (MIBG),[76] indicating the link between diastolic dysfunction and altered autonomic nerve activity. Subjects with abnormal e′ have shorter postcontrast T1 values in MRI and higher calibrated integrated backscatter, and they were heavier and had worse exercise capacity, lower insulin sensitivity, and blunted systolic tissue velocity.[77]

More importantly, E/e′ has prognostic implication.[78] Study data from Olmsted County showed that for every 1-U increase in an E/e′ ratio, there was an excess risk of HF by 3% (HR: 1.03; 95% confidence interval [CI]: 1.01–1.06; $p = 0.006$). E/e′ greater than 15 was independently associated with the increased risk of HF (by 61%) after adjustment for age, sex, BMI, hypertension, coronary disease, and echocardiographic parameters (HR: 1.61; 95% CI: 1.17–2.20; $p = 0.003$) (Fig. 28.2) and survival (Fig. 28.3).[78]

Diastolic Stress Test for Diabetes Mellitus

The diagnosis of diabetic cardiomyopathy may be missed in people presenting with unexplained dyspnea if the diagnosis relies exclusively on resting clinical data and echocardiography. This can be problematic as patients develop pathologic elevations in filling pressures only during exercise, in absence of congestion at rest.[79] Patients with diabetes have impaired longitudinal functional reserve in both systolic and diastolic functions.[80] Functional reserve in diabetes mellitus was initially assessed with dobutamine stress echo,[81] where e′ in patients with diabetes mellitus was lower than controls at baseline, low, pre-peak, and peak dose. LV circumferential contractility and longitudinal systolic functional reserves are correlated with stroke index reserve with low-dose dobutamine stress.[82] Exercise stress echocardiography (ExE) would be a preferable option because it will assess the exercise capacity and diastolic functional reserve (Case 4). ExE confirmed diminished systolic and diastolic functional reserve in this population.[83] Noninvasive diastolic stress testing would be most useful in patients with intermediate pretest probability, where the high sensitivity of exercise E/e′ will offer a strong negative predictive value.[84] If this test is negative, the likelihood of the disease would be low, and further testing may not be required. Likewise, in patients with very high or very low pretest probability, noninvasive testing is not required. If the diagnosis has to be confirmed in these patients, then they should be offered invasive exercise stress testing.[84]

Imaging for LV Geometry

The main finding of diabetic cardiomyopathy was LV hypertrophy in the initial autopsy study,[16] where a histopathologic study revealed diffuse fibrosis and myocyte hypertrophy. Using echocardiography, numerous studies, including population-based studies,[85] confirmed LV hypertrophy in a population with diabetes and in prediabetes stage (e.g., impaired glucose tolerance [IGT]).[86] TTE is most widely used as a first imaging tool. LV concentric remodeling represents an early change in myocardial structure, which has been associated

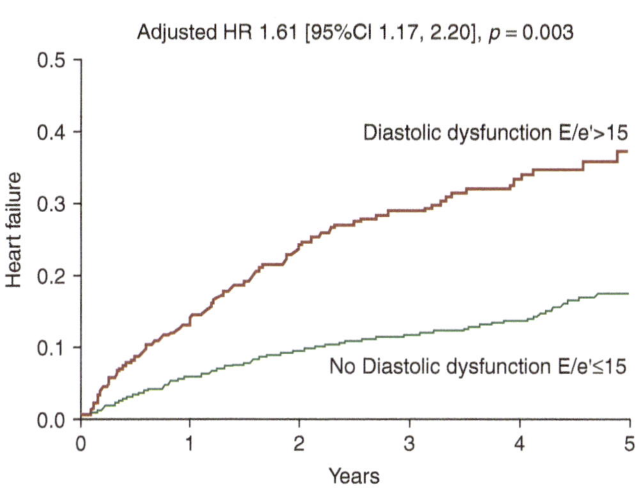

No. at risk

— (E/e'>15)	431	211	91
— (E/e'≤15)	1363	850	413

Fig. 28.2 Diastolic dysfunction and incidence of HF. Diastolic dysfunction defined as the E/e′ ratio ≥ 15 is predictive of HF in Kaplan-Meier analysis. (Reproduced with permission from From AM, Scott CG, Chen HH. The development of heart failure in patients with diabetes mellitus and pre-clinical diastolic dysfunction a population-based study. *J Am Coll Cardiol.* 2010;55:300–305.)

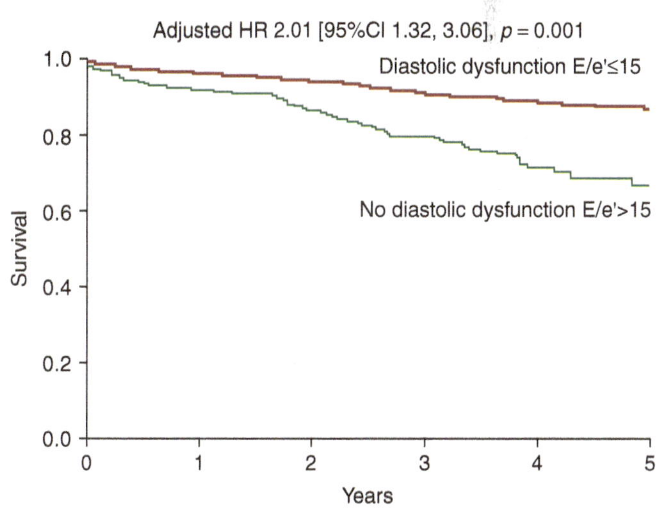

No. at risk

— (E/e'>15)	431	211	90
— (E/e'≤15)	1363	850	413

Fig. 28.3 Diastolic dysfunction and mortality. Diastolic dysfunction defined as the E/e′ ratio ≥15 is predictive for mortality in Kaplan-Meier analysis. (Reproduced with permission from From AM, Scott CG, Chen HH. The development of heart failure in patients with diabetes mellitus and pre-clinical diastolic dysfunction a population-based study. *J Am Coll Cardiol.* 2010;55:300–305.)

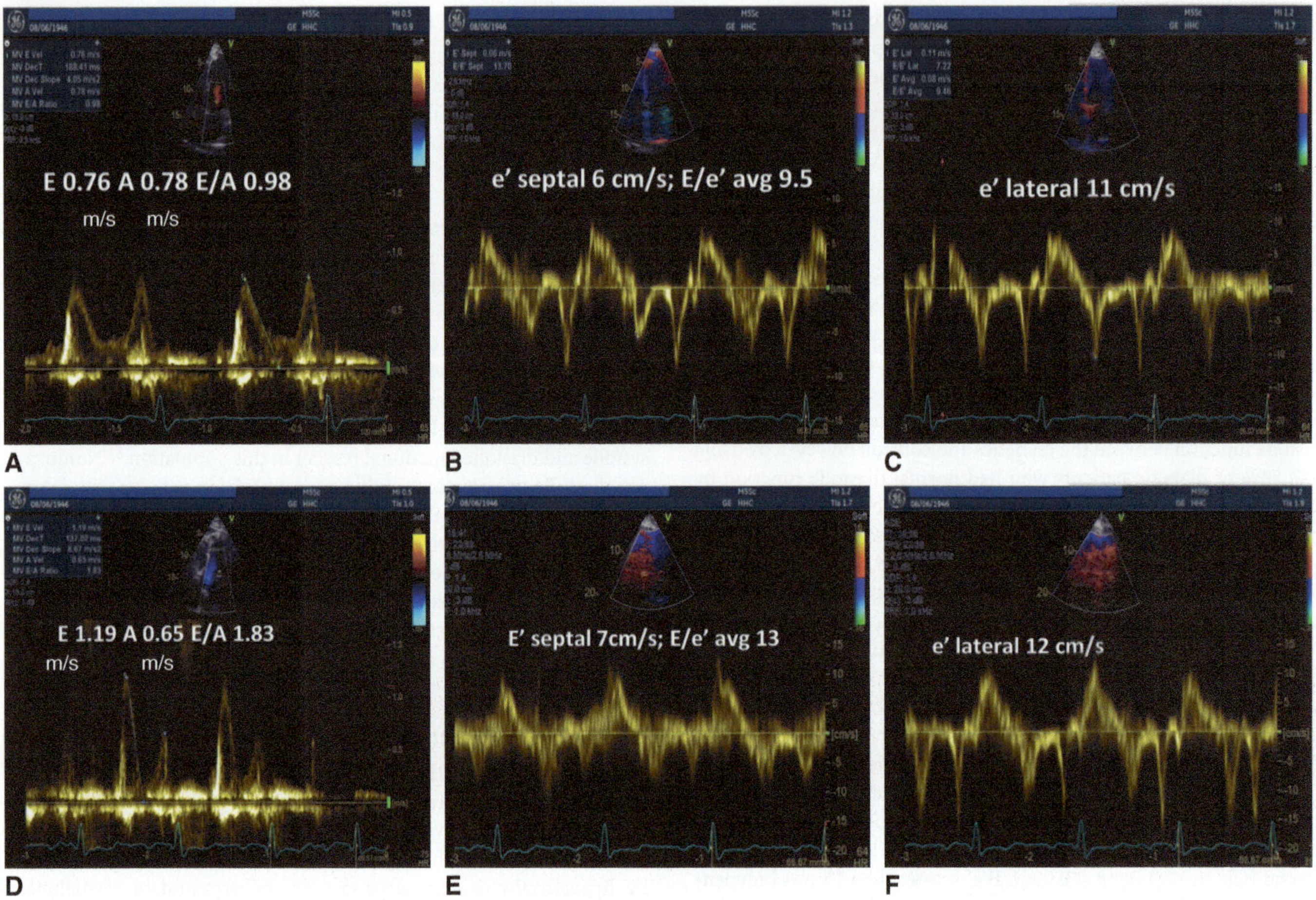

Case 4 Diastolic stress test.

with abnormal function and energetics.[87] The modest level of accuracy of conventional echocardiography for the diagnosis of LV hypertrophy is improved by 3-D imaging[88] or with the use of an ultrasound contrast agent. Cardiac MRI is the gold standard for the assessment of LV geometry because of a greater spatial resolution to evaluate chamber sizes, LV mass, and its distribution. Cine MRI also provides a higher characterization of regional contractility of the left ventricle.[89] It revealed LV dysfunction in well-controlled diabetic normotensive patients.[90,91]

With the combination of the abovementioned systolic/diastolic function and LV geometry, Ernande et al.[92] identified three distinct phenotypes among T2DM patients without overt heart disease using cluster analysis. The three phenotypes are "Cluster 1" as men with preserved systolic and diastolic function, "Cluster 2" as obese and hypertensive women with diastolic dysfunction, and "Cluster 3" as men with LV hypertrophy and systolic dysfunction, where Cluster 1 had a better prognosis than Clusters 2 and 3 in terms of cardiovascular hospitalization and mortality (Fig. 28.4).

Imaging for Myocardial Characterization

Hypertrophy represents an increase in the size of the myocardium, but another component is attributable to increased extracellular volume (ECV), reflecting collagen deposition and fibrosis, which in turn is linked to outcomes.[41] In patients with T2DM with no history of hypertension or CAD, collagen and fat deposits were found in the LV transmural biopsies.[33,93] Due to its invasive nature, it may not be feasible to do routine endomyocardial biopsies in day-to-day clinical practice for the diagnosis of diabetic cardiomyopathy.

MRI provides extra information about myocardial fibrosis and subclinical ischemia, as premature parameters of cardiac dysfunction. T1 mapping by cardiac MRI can provide an alternative method of quantification of diffuse nonspecific fibrosis.[77] In early T2DM subjects with no cardiac symptoms, postcontrast T1 value was associated with diastolic dysfunction, impaired exercise capacity, central adiposity, BP, and insulin sensitivity. The association of T1 time with E/e′ was independent of BP and metabolic disturbance.[77]

MR spectroscopy can assess more precise characteristics of the myocardium, identifying myocardial metabolic changes, such as quantification of the myocardial triglyceride levels. Since there is increasing evidence that myocardial metabolism is altered in T2DM with lipotoxic injury due to lipid oversupply (i.e., myocardial steatosis), it has been demonstrated that myocardial triglyceride content is independently associated with biventricular changes in myocardial systolic and diastolic functions.[94] In another study, myocardial steatosis was independently associated with pronounced impairment of ventricular contractility (evaluated by 2-D speckle tracking imaging) in patients with uncomplicated diabetes mellitus.[95,96]

Other Imaging Techniques for Diabetes Population

Cardiac autonomic dysfunction is another common finding in the early stages of diabetes, which could occur during the impaired glucose

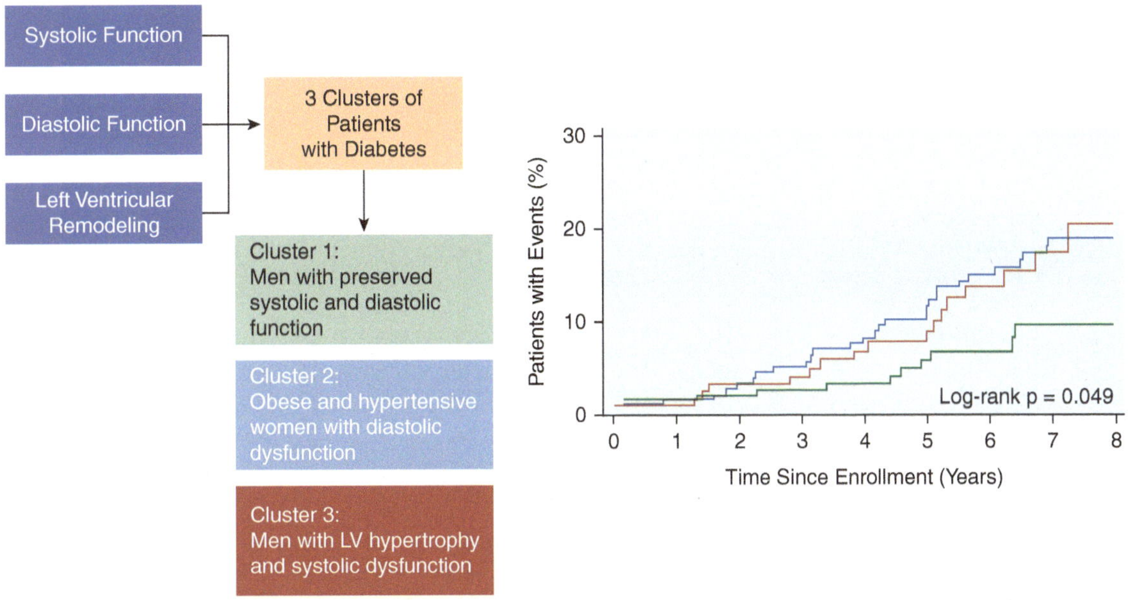

Fig. 28.4 Three cardiac phenotypes in diabetes by cluster analysis. Three distinct phenotypes among T2DM patients without overt heart disease were identified using cluster analysis. The three phenotypes are "Cluster 1" as men with preserved systolic and diastolic function, "Cluster 2" as obese and hypertensive women with diastolic dysfunction, and "Cluster 3" as men with LV hypertrophy and systolic dysfunction, where Cluster 1 had a better prognosis than Clusters 2 and 3 in terms of cardiovascular hospitalization and mortality. (Reproduced from Ernande L, Audureau E, Jellis CL, et al. Clinical implications of echocardiographic phenotypes of patients with diabetes mellitus. *J Am Coll Cardiol.* 2017;70:1704–1716.)

tolerance stage. Among diabetes mellitus patients, HbA1c was independently associated with both early and late heart-to-mediastinum (H/M) ratios.[97]

Similarly, a PET scan determines the metabolic status of the heart. Asymptomatic diabetic patients exhibit an increase in myocardial fatty acid metabolism by PET, though no relation was found between diastolic dysfunction and energy metabolism parameters.[98]

MANAGEMENT

Diabetic cardiomyopathy could manifest as two distinct phenotypes: a restrictive/HFpEF and a dilated cardiomyopathy/HFrEF. Diagnostic strategies and therapeutic algorithms would differ in the two phenotypes. The HFrEF variant can be managed using the standard guideline-based therapy for HFrEF.[57,59] In contrast, management of the HFpEF phenotype has been challenging and mainly involves lifestyle modifications and management of comorbidities, such as hypertension and CAD, lipid-lowering therapies, and the general management of HF because of neutral results from large prospective randomized controlled trials (RCTs). However, newer antidiabetic medications have provided promising results. This section covers the management aspect of diabetes from a cardiac viewpoint.

Lifestyle Modifications

Weight loss, healthier diet, and regular physical activity can positively adjust metabolic abnormalities and improve tissue and systemic insulin resistance by increasing insulin-mediated glucose transport and postreceptor insulin signaling, which seems to be related to facilitated signal transduction at the level of PI3K and insulin receptor substrate.[99,47] Physical activity is associated with a significant reduction in cardiovascular disease and all-cause mortality in patients with diabetes in a recent meta-analysis.[100] Exercise training has been found to be beneficial in reducing the incidence of diabetic cardiomyopathy in both human and animal models.[101,102] Following an exercise program, an exercise-based lifestyle intervention prevented the progression of diastolic dysfunction[103] and raised LV EF by 2% to 3% in patients with obesity and/or diabetes.[104,105] In absence of RCTs, the guidelines committee could not give a high level of recommendation. However, better diabetic control along with physical exercise will have beneficial effects on disease outcomes. Furthermore, maintaining a healthy balanced diet suitable for diabetics will also be expected to offer similar beneficial effects.[106] For example, long-term caloric restriction in patients with obesity and/or diabetes decreased myocyte triglyceride content and improved diastolic dysfunction.[107]

Antidiabetic Medications

A number of clinical trials have been conducted to evaluate the impact of glycemic control on the prevention of cardiovascular events in T2DM. Intensive glycemic control is not necessarily associated with better outcome.[108,109] ACCORD was stopped early because of the significant increase in adverse outcomes.[108] In the ORIGIN trial, the insulin use did not improve the outcome.[109] At the same time, however, several reports demonstrated that intensive glycemic control delays the diabetic cardiomyopathy[110] and even improves cardiac systolic and diastolic functions, indicating reversibility.[111-113] Strict glycemic control mitigates ventricular dysfunction in poorly controlled diabetic patients without CAD in a large prospective study.[111] A longitudinal study demonstrated an improvement in systolic and diastolic functions (including GLS) among patients receiving intensive treatment for diabetes.[112] The mechanism where better glycemic control improves systolic and diastolic function is likely due to more efficient use of myocardial energy substrate and improved microvascular perfusion.[113]

Collectively, how to achieve better glycemic control appears to be key because antidiabetic agents affect patients differently on subsequent HF development (Table 28.2).[114] Metformin and SGLT2i have

TABLE 28.2 Effects of Glucose-Lowering Drugs on HF Outcomes

Glucose-Lowering Agents	Comparator Groups	HF at Baseline	Sample Size	Study Design	Follow-Up (Weeks)	HR (95% CI) for HF Hospitalization	Ref
Metformin	oGLDs (mostly SUs)	100	34,000	Meta-analysis	NA	0.92 (0.86–0.98)	115
	SUs	0	12,272	Retrospective cohort	130	0.83 (0.70–0.99)[a]	116
Insulin	Insulin + SUs vs. metformin + TZDs	7	2,368	RCT	276	16.6% vs. 19.4%, $p = 0.09$	117
	Insulin glargine vs. placebo	NR	12,537	RCT	322.4	0.90 (0.77–1.05)	109
	Insulin vs. oGLDs	NR	554	Retrospective cohort	52	4.3 (1.69–10.94)[b]	118
	Insulin vs. oGLDs	NR	16,417	Retrospective cohort	52	0.96 (0.88–1.05)[c]	119
SUs	Metformin	NR	91,521	Retrospective cohort	369	1.18 (1.04–1.34)	120
	Metformin	NR	17,863	Retrospective cohort	NR	1.24 (1.09–1.36)	121
	oGLDs	0	4,075	RCT	556	0.91 (0.52–1.52)	122
TZDs	Rosiglitazone ± ramipril vs. placebo	0	5,269	RCT	208	7.04 (1.60–31.0)	123
	Rosiglitazone vs. placebo	100	224	RCT	52	7.09 (1.60–30.96)	124
	Pioglitazone vs. placebo	0	5,238	RCT	138	1.49 (1.23–1.80)	125
	Pioglitazone vs. placebo	0§	3,895	RCT	250	3.8% vs. 3.7%, $p = 0.80$[d]	126
DPP-4 inhibitors	Saxagliptin vs. placebo	13	14,735	RCT	109	1.27 (1.07–1.51)	127
	Alogliptin vs. placebo	28	5,380	RCT	72	1.19 (0.89–1.58)	128
	Sitagliptin vs. placebo	18	16,492	RCT	156	1.00 (0.83–1.20)	129
	Vildagliptin vs. placebo	100	253	RCT	52	NR	130
GLP1 receptor agonists	Lixisenatide vs. placebo	22	6,068	RCT	108	0.96 (0.75–1.23)	131
	Liraglutide vs. placebo	17.8	9,340	RCT	198	0.87 (0.73–1.05)	132
	Semaglutide vs. placebo	23.6	3,297	RCT	109	1.11 (0.77–1.61)	133
	Liraglutide vs. placebo	100	300	RCT	26	1.30 (0.89–1.83)	134
	Liraglutide vs. placebo	100	241	RCT	24	10% vs. 3%, $p = 0.04$[e]	135
SGLT2i	Empagliflozin vs. placebo	10	7,020	RCT	161	0.65 (0.50–0.85)	14
	Canagliflozin vs. placebo	14	10,142	RCT	126	0.67 (0.52–0.87)	136
	SGLT2i vs. oGLDs	6	309,056	Retrospective cohort	64	0.61 (0.51–0.73)	137
	SGLT2i vs. placebo	11	34,322	Meta-analysis	NR	0.77 (0.71–0.84)	138

[a]Hazard ratio for death or hospitalization.
[b]Hazard ratio for all-cause mortality.
[c]Not reported, but trial specifically excluded patients with NYHA Class II–IV HF.
[d]Percentage of patients who developed new congestive HF.
[e]Composite of major adverse cardiac events.

DPP-4, Dipeptidyl peptidase; *GLP1,* glucagon-like peptide-1; *HF,* heart failure; *NA,* not available; *NR,* not reported; *oGLDs,* other glucose-lowering drugs; *RCT,* randomized controlled trial; *SGLT2i,* sodium glucose cotransporter-2 inhibitor; *SU,* sulfonylurea; *TZD,* thiazolidinedione.
Adapted and modified from Nassif M, Kosiborod M. Effect of glucose-lowering therapies on heart failure. *Nat Rev Cardiol.* 2018;15:282–291.

protective effects, whereas thiazolidinediones increase HF. Insulin has similar HF incidence with placebo, but increases HF incidence compared with other glucose-lowering drugs. Sulfonylureas are less favorable to metformin. Accordingly, this section will summarize the current evidence of cardio-favorable or at least cardio-safe antidiabetic medications.

Metformin

Metformin has been the first-line medication for T2DM because the UK Prospective Diabetes Study (UKPDS) 34 showed that intensive glucose control with metformin appears to decrease the risk of diabetes-related end points in overweight diabetic patients and is associated with less weight gain and fewer hypoglycemic attacks than are insulin and sulphonylureas.[139] Metformin improves cardiac function by upregulating autophagy[140] and improving insulin resistance of cardiac myocyte by facilitating the uptake of glucose and GLUT-4 translocation.[141,142] Historically, however, metformin had been considered absolutely contraindicated in patients with HF attributable to concerns about lactic acidosis.[143] Recent meta-analysis from nine cohort studies demonstrated the following favorable findings for metformin[115]: It is associated with reduced mortality and all-cause hospitalizations, but it is not associated with an increased risk of lactic acidosis. Metformin did not increase mortality in patients with reduced EF, nor with HF and chronic kidney disease.[115] Although no RCT exists, the totality of the evidence indicates that metformin is at least as safe as other glucose-lowering treatments in patients with diabetes mellitus and HF.[115]

Dipeptidylpeptidase 4 (DPP-4)

DPP-4 inhibitors prolong the effects of endogenous glucagon-like peptide-1 (GLP-1). Agents in this class (e.g., sitagliptin, linagliptin, saxagliptin, vildagliptin) are effective antidiabetic medications. They are weight neutral and are helpful in overweight diabetic patients in combination with metformin. They promote myocardial glucose uptake in patients with nonischemic cardiomyopathy.[144] A recent meta-analysis showed that the overall risk of acute HF was higher in patients treated with DPP-4 inhibitors than in those treated with placebo or active comparators. (Mantel-Haenszel odds ratio [MH-OR] 1.19; $p < 0.05$) without any clear evidence of a difference between drugs of

TABLE 28.3 Summary of Ongoing Cardiovascular Outcome Trials in Type 2 Diabetes Mellitus Registered on Clinicaltrials.gov for SGLT2i and GLP1-RA

Drug Class	Drug Name	Trial Acronym	Duration (years)	Primary End Point	Clinicaltrial.gov Reference
SGLT2i	Ertugliflozin	VERTIS CV	6	3-point MACE	NCT01986881
SGLT2i	Sotagliflozin	SCORED	4.3	3-point MACE	NCT03315143
SGLT2i	Dapagliflozin	DECLARE-TIMI-58	5	CV death or HF hospitalization, 3-point MACE	NCT01730534
SGLT2i	Dapagliflozin	DAPA-HF	2	CV death, HF hospitalization, or urgent HF visit	NCT03036124
SGLT2i	Empagliflozin	EMPEROR-PRESERVED	3	CV death, HF hospitalization	NCT03057951
SGLT2i	Empagliflozin	EMPEROR-REDUCED	3	CV death, HF hospitalization	NCT03057977
SGLT2i	Sotagliflozin	SOLOIST-WHF	3	CV death, HF hospitalization	NCT03521934
GLP1-RA	Albiglutide	HARMONY OUTCOMES	3	3-point MACE	NCT02465515
GLP1-RA	Dulaglutide	REWIND	7	3-point MACE	NCT01394952
GLP1-RA	Semaglutide (oral)	PIONEER 6	1	3-point MACE	NCT02692716

GLP1-RA, Glucagon-like peptide-1 receptor antagonist; *SGLT2i,* sodium glucose cotransporter-2 inhibitor.
Adapted from Das SR, Everett BM, Birtcher KK, et al, 2018 ACC Expert Consensus Decision Pathway on Novel Therapies for Cardiovascular Risk Reduction in Patients With Type 2 Diabetes and Atherosclerotic Cardiovascular Disease. *J Am Coll Cardiol.* 2018 Dec, 72 (24) 3200-3223.

the same class.[145] The possible mechanisms are unclear, but it is important to note that brain natriuretic peptide (BNP) is a substrate for DPP-4 inhibitors. The recently published EXSCEL trial (Exenatide Study of Cardiovascular Event lowering) and TECOS trial (Sitagliptin Cardiovascular Outcomes Study) also did not show any difference in major cardiovascular events between patients who received the active drug and those who received placebo.[129,146]

GLP1-Recepter Agonist (GLP1-RA)

GLP1 is a naturally occurring incretin with potent insulinotropic effects, the action of which is attenuated when glucose levels fall below 4 mmol. GLP1-RA agonists such as liraglutide[132] and semaglutide[133] are newer antidiabetic medications. Both LEADER and SUSTAIN trials showed lower MACE (death from cardiovascular causes, nonfatal myocardial infarction, or nonfatal stroke) in the GLP1-RA group; however, the MACE did not include HF.[132,133] GLP1-RA increases myocardial glucose uptake independently of its ability to enhance insulin secretion and enhanced survival of cardiac cells, improving overall cardiac function.[147] A small study showed that liraglutide improves diastolic function, with increased e′ and reduced E/e′ after 6 months of treatment.[148]

SGLT2i

Sodium glucose cotransporter-2 inhibitor (SGLT2i) is a newer type of agent for glycemic control. Although SGLT2i only modestly reduces HbA1c levels compared with other glucose-lowering agents, it has an entirely insulin-independent mode of action through increase in urinary excretion of glucose.[149] Thus there has been a great expectation SGLT2i might be a superior strategy for glycemic control for patients with HF and T2DM.

A recent meta-analysis summarizing three RCTs (EMPA_REG Outcome,[14] CANVAS Program,[136] and DECLARE-TIMI 58[150]; total $n = 34{,}322$ patients) has demonstrated that SGLT2i has robust benefits on reducing hospitalization for HF (by 23% reduction) and the progression of renal disease (by 45% reduction) regardless of existing atherosclerotic cardiovascular disease or a history of HF. SGLT2i has moderate benefits on atherosclerotic MACE that seem confined to patients with established atherosclerotic cardiovascular disease.[138] There are several trials ongoing and recently completed assessing the benefits of SGLT2i on cardiovascular outcomes and HF in patients with diabetes (Table 28.3).[151] These results will provide further insights and aid better management of diabetic patients.

Cardioprotective Agents

Of note, several cardioprotective agents have shown benefits in diabetics. The effectiveness of angiotensin-converting enzyme (ACE) inhibitors in a population with diabetes has been confirmed to be similar to that of the nondiabetic population in a meta-analysis from 12,586 patients (with diabetes mellitus being 2398) who were enrolled in pivotal RCTs[152] (Table 28.4). Intriguingly, a discrepancy has been found among beta blockers. Favorable effects of carvedilol have been confirmed in this population,[153] whereas metoprolol has a neutral effect so far.[154] Accordingly, ACC/AHA guidelines for HF recommend ACE inhibitors for all diabetes (stage 1, without structural heart disease) and beta blockers for stage 2 HF (structural heart disease but without HF symptoms).[57]

FUTURE DIRECTIONS

Diabetic cardiomyopathy remains a valid challenge in terms of diagnosis and management. Forming appropriate guidelines for this would be preferable, as the incidence of diabetes is increasing worldwide. Diabetic cardiomyopathy is regulated not only by high plasma glucose but also several other factors and mechanisms that contribute to diabetic cardiomyopathy as described in this chapter. The role of hypertension, hyperlipidemia, and oxidative stress also contributes to, and exacerbates, diabetic cardiomyopathy. Early diagnosis is required for preventing and reverting diabetic cardiomyopathy. We will now discuss some new emerging diagnostic and therapeutic options for diabetic cardiomyopathy.

Serologic Markers

Currently, there are no specific serologic biomarkers for a definitive diagnosis of diabetic cardiomyopathy. Some biomarkers might aid in this perspective.

BNP is a helpful biomarker for screening subclinical ventricular diastolic dysfunction in patients with uncontrolled diabetes.[101,102] Epshteyn et al.[155] showed a high positive predictive value of 96% for plasma BNP levels (>90 pg/mL) in diabetic patients for the diagnosis of LV dysfunction with echocardiographic correlation. Matrix metalloproteinases (MMPs) are the enzymes that degrade the extracellular matrix, increase matrix turnover, and change the expression of several micro ribonucleic acids (miRNAs) that induce contractile dysfunction of the myocardium.[156] Elevated levels of MMP, especially MMP-9, and reduced levels of tissue inhibitors of MMPs are observed in myocardial fibrosis.

The clinical usefulness of these new biomolecules for the diagnosis of diabetic cardiomyopathy still needs further evaluation and validation.

TABLE 28.4 Effect of Angiotensin-Converting Enzyme (ACE) Inhibitors on Mortality From Heart Failure in Diabetic and Nondiabetic Patients

	RR[a] ANALYSIS					
Study Name	**Total *N***	**Nondiabetic *N***	**Diabetic *N***	**RR, Nondiabetic (95% CI)**	**RR, Diabetic (95% CI)**	**RRR[b] (95% CI)**
CONSENSUS	253	197	56	0.64 (0.46–0.88)	1.06 (0.65–1.74)	1.67 (0.93–3.01)
SAVE	2,231	1,739	492	0.82 (0.68–0.99)	0.89 (0.68–1.16)	1.09 (0.79–1.50)
SMILE	1,556	1,253	303	0.79 (0.54–1.15)	0.44 (0.22–0.87)	0.56 (0.25–1.22)
SOLVD-Prevention	4,228	3,581	647	0.97 (0.83–1.15)	0.75 (0.55–1.02)	0.77 (0.54–1.09)
SOLVD-Treatment	2,569	1,906	663	0.84 (0.74–0.95)	1.01 (0.85–1.21)	1.21 (0.97–1.50)
TRACE	1,749	1,512	237	0.85 (0.74–0.97)	0.73 (0.57–0.94)	0.87 (0.65–1.15)
Random effects pooled estimate	12,586	10,188	2,398	0.85 (0.78–0.92)	0.84 (0.70–1.00)	1.00 (0.80–1.25)

[a]RR – Relative Risk.
[b]RRR – Relative Risk Reduction.
Adapted from Shekelle PG, Rich MW, Morton SC et al. Efficacy of angiotensin-converting enzyme inhibitors and beta-blockers in the management of left ventricular systolic dysfunction according to race, gender, and diabetic status: a meta-analysis of major clinical trials. *J Am Coll Cardiol.* 2003;41: 1529–1538.

Detection of Metabolic Changes

MR spectroscopy (MRS) may allow the evaluation of metabolic changes noninvasively. It demonstrated that the creatine phosphate (PCr)/ATP ratio (a marker of ATP production [i.e., an indicator of energy change]) is significantly reduced in diabetics, and the ratio is negatively correlated with plasma FFA levels or live triglyceride levels.[95,157] Determining PCr and ATP levels in the human myocardium by a promising novel approach for the diagnosis of diabetic cardiomyopathy is the characterization of metabolic changes in the myocardium using ^{31}P MRS and ^{1}H MRS. The PCr/ATP ratio is reduced in the myocardium of diabetic subjects compared with control patients. Recent studies using ^{1}H MRS showed that an increase in myocardial triglyceride content was associated with diastolic dysfunction in diabetic patients.[158,159]

CONCLUSION

Diabetic cardiomyopathy is no longer a myth, it is recognized as a distinct clinical entity with serious prognostic implications. The underlying pathophysiologic mechanisms include insulin resistance and various cascades of molecular and metabolic disorders and autonomic disturbances. It develops LV hypertrophy, LV diastolic dysfunction, fibrosis, and limited cardiac functional reserve. Given diastolic dysfunction is one of the early manifestations of this condition, its careful assessment is crucial with a diastolic stress test when appropriate. Along with further advances in the diagnostic modalities, novel therapeutic agents such as SGLT2i are expected to change the landscape in the management of diabetic cardiomyopathy as a part of mechanisms explaining the favorable prognostic effect on this population.

KEY POINTS

- Heart failure is common in diabetics (one in five). Hyperglycemia and insulin resistance play key roles in the development of diabetic cardiomyopathy.
- Diastolic dysfunction is one of the early manifestations of diabetic cardiomyopathy. However, grade I diastolic dysfunction is very common but could be coincidental (due to advanced age, etc.). E/e′ above 15 is associated with a poor prognosis in patients with diabetes.
- A diastolic stress test should be considered for the investigation of unprovoked dyspnea with the diabetic patient.
- Myocardial strain is useful and prognostic, and in some cases can be an earlier manifestation of diabetic cardiomyopathy.
- Management is mainly optimization of risk factors, including the concomitant conditions such as hypertension.

REVIEW QUESTIONS

1. The heart failure risk in type 2 diabetes (vs. nondiabetic subjects) is
   a. about the same.
   b. 15% higher.
   c. 60% higher.
   d. 100% higher.
   e. 400% higher.
2. Prevalence of heart failure in diabetic patients is
   a. 1 in 10.
   b. 1 in 5.
   c. 1 in 20.
   d. 1 in 2.
   e. 1 in 15.
3. Which level of HbA1c increases the risk of subsequent heart failure?
   a. More than 5%
   b. More than 6%
   c. More than 7%
   d. More than 8%
   e. More than 10%
4. Each 1% deterioration of GLS is associated with how much increase risk of all-cause mortality and hospitalization?
   a. ~5%
   b. ~10%
   c. ~20%
   d. ~50%
   e. ~100%
5. Which medications have heart failure protective effect (select all)?
   a. Metformin
   b. Insulin
   c. Sulfonylurea
   d. Thiazolidinedione
   e. Sodium glucose cotransporter-2 inhibitor

REFERENCES

1. American Diabetes Association. Introduction: standards of medical care in diabetes—2018. *Diabetes Care.* 2018;41:S1–S2.
2. World Health Organization. Global report on Diabetes. Geneva, Switzerland; 2016.
3. Zhang P, Zhang X, Brown J, et al. Global healthcare expenditure on diabetes for 2010 and 2030. *Diabetes Res Clin Pract.* 2010;87:293–301.
4. Tancredi M, Rosengren A, Svensson AM, et al. Excess mortality among persons with type 2 diabetes. *N Engl J Med.* 2015;373:1720–1732.
5. Kannel WB, McGee DL. Diabetes and cardiovascular disease. The Framingham study. *JAMA.* 1979;241:2035–2038.
6. Nichols MPK, Herbert J, Alston L, Allender S. *Australian Heart Disease Statistics 2015, 2016.* Canberra: National Heart Foundation of Australia; 2018. https://www.heartfoundation.org.au/images/uploads/publications/RES-115-Aust_heart_disease_statstics_2015_WEB.PDF. Accessed on May 30, 2018
7. Shah AD, Langenberg C, Rapsomaniki E, et al. Type 2 diabetes and incidence of cardiovascular diseases: a cohort study in 1.9 million people. *Lancet Diabetes Endocrinol.* 2015;3:105–113.
8. Leyden D. Asthma and diabetes mellitus. *Zeitschrift Klinische Med.* 1881;3:358–364.
9. Iribarren C, Karter AJ, Go AS, et al. Glycemic control and heart failure among adult patients with diabetes. *Circulation.* 2001;103:2668–2673.
10. Witteles RM, Fowler MB. Insulin-resistant cardiomyopathy clinical evidence, mechanisms, and treatment options. *J Am Coll Cardiol.* 2008;51:93–102.
11. Wong AK, AlZadjali MA, Choy AM, Lang CC. Insulin resistance: a potential new target for therapy in patients with heart failure. *Cardiovasc Ther.* 2008;26:203–213.
12. Ashrafian H, Frenneaux MP, Opie LH. Metabolic mechanisms in heart failure. *Circulation.* 2007;116:434–448.
13. Bertoni AG, Hundley WG, Massing MW, Bonds DE, Burke GL, Goff DC Jr. Heart failure prevalence, incidence, and mortality in the elderly with diabetes. *Diabetes Care.* 2004;27:699–703.
14. Zinman B, Wanner C, Lachin JM, et al. Empagliflozin, cardiovascular outcomes, and mortality in type 2 diabetes. *N Engl J Med.* 2015;373:2117–2128.
15. Mahaffey KW, Neal B, Perkovic V, et al. Canagliflozin for primary and secondary prevention of cardiovascular events: results from the CANVAS program (Canagliflozin Cardiovascular Assessment Study). *Circulation.* 2018;137:323–334.
16. Rubler S, Dlugash J, Yuceoglu YZ, Kumral T, Branwood AW, Grishman A. New type of cardiomyopathy associated with diabetic glomerulosclerosis. *Am J Cardiol.* 1972;30:595–602.
17. Jia G, DeMarco VG, Sowers JR. Insulin resistance and hyperinsulinaemia in diabetic cardiomyopathy. *Nat Rev Endocrinol.* 2016;12:144–153.
18. Riehle C, Abel ED. Insulin signaling and heart failure. *Circ Res.* 2016;118:1151–1169.
19. Nishida K, Otsu K. Inflammation and metabolic cardiomyopathy. *Cardiovasc Res.* 2017;113:389–398.
20. Mandavia CH, Aroor AR, Demarco VG, Sowers JR. Molecular and metabolic mechanisms of cardiac dysfunction in diabetes. *Life Sci.* 2013:92:601–608.
21. Dhalla NS, Liu X, Panagia V, Takeda N. Subcellular remodeling and heart dysfunction in chronic diabetes. *Cardiovasc Res.* 1998;40:239–247.
22. van den Brom CE, Huisman MC, Vlasblom R, et al. Altered myocardial substrate metabolism is associated with myocardial dysfunction in early diabetic cardiomyopathy in rats: studies using positron emission tomography. *Cardiovasc Diabetol.* 2009;8:39.
23. Welch MJ, Lewis JS, Kim J, et al. Assessment of myocardial metabolism in diabetic rats using small-animal PET: a feasibility study. *J Nucl Med.* 2006;47:689–697.
24. Doenst T, Nguyen TD, Abel ED. Cardiac metabolism in heart failure: implications beyond ATP production. *Circ Res.* 2013;113:709–724.
25. Palomer X, Salvado L, Barroso E, Vazquez-Carrera M. An overview of the crosstalk between inflammatory processes and metabolic dysregulation during diabetic cardiomyopathy. *Int J Cardiol.* 2013;168:3160–3172.
26. Hotamisligil GS. Inflammation and endoplasmic reticulum stress in obesity and diabetes. *Int J Obesity (London).* 2008;32(7):S52–S54.
27. Belke DD, Dillmann WH. Altered cardiac calcium handling in diabetes. *Curr Hypertens Rep.* 2004;6:424–429.
28. Malhotra A, Sanghi V. Regulation of contractile proteins in diabetic heart. *Cardiovasc Res.* 1997;34:34–40.
29. Zhou X, Ma L, Habibi J, et al. Nebivolol improves diastolic dysfunction and myocardial remodeling through reductions in oxidative stress in the Zucker obese rat. *Hypertension.* 2010;55:880–888.
30. Hayden MR, Habibi J, Joginpally T, Karuparthi PR, Sowers JR. Ultrastructure study of transgenic ren2 rat aorta—part 1: endothelium and intima. *Cardiorenal Med.* 2012;2:66–82.
31. Blaha MJ, DeFilippis AP, Rivera JJ, et al. The relationship between insulin resistance and incidence and progression of coronary artery calcification: the Multi-Ethnic Study of Atherosclerosis (MESA). *Diabetes Care.* 2011;34:749–751.
32. Olesen P, Nguyen K, Wogensen L, Ledet T, Rasmussen LM. Calcification of human vascular smooth muscle cells: associations with osteoprotegerin expression and acceleration by high-dose insulin. *Am J Physiol Heart Circ Physiol.* 2007;292:H1058–H1064.
33. Regan TJ, Wu CF, Yeh CK, Oldewurtel HA, Haider B. Myocardial composition and function in diabetes. The effects of chronic insulin use. *Circ Res.* 1981;49:1268–1277.
34. Frustaci A, Kajstura J, Chimenti C, et al. Myocardial cell death in human diabetes. *Circ Res.* 2000;87:1123–1132.
35. Fiordaliso F, Leri A, Cesselli D, et al. Hyperglycemia activates p53 and p53-regulated genes leading to myocyte cell death. *Diabetes.* 2001;50:2363–2375.
36. Lijnen PJ, Petrov VV, Fagard RH. Induction of cardiac fibrosis by angiotensin II. *Method Find Exp Clin Pharmacol.* 2000;22:709–723.
37. Chen S, Evans T, Mukherjee K, Karmazyn M, Chakrabarti S. Diabetes-induced myocardial structural changes: role of endothelin-1 and its receptors. *J Mole Cell Cardiol.* 2000;32:1621–1629.
38. Kajstura J, Fiordaliso F, Andreoli AM, et al. IGF-1 overexpression inhibits the development of diabetic cardiomyopathy and angiotensin II-mediated oxidative stress. *Diabetes.* 2001;50:1414–1424.
39. Lee AA, Dillmann WH, McCulloch AD, Villarreal FJ. Angiotensin II stimulates the autocrine production of transforming growth factor-beta 1 in adult rat cardiac fibroblasts. *J Mole Cell Cardiol.* 1995;27:2347–2357.
40. Liu S, Han J, Nacif MS, et al. Diffuse myocardial fibrosis evaluation using cardiac magnetic resonance T1 mapping: sample size considerations for clinical trials. *J Cardiovasc Magn Res.* 2012;14:90.
41. Wong TC, Piehler KM, Kang IA, et al. Myocardial extracellular volume fraction quantified by cardiovascular magnetic resonance is increased in diabetes and associated with mortality and incident heart failure admission. *Eur Heart J.* 2014;35:657–664.
42. Miric G, Dallemagne C, Endre Z, Margolin S, Taylor SM, Brown L. Reversal of cardiac and renal fibrosis by pirfenidone and spironolactone in streptozotocin-diabetic rats. *Br J Pharmacol.* 2001;133:687–694.
43. Falcão-Pires I, Leite-Moreira AF. Diabetic cardiomyopathy: understanding the molecular and cellular basis to progress in diagnosis and treatment. *Heart Fail Rev.* 2012;17:325–344.
44. Olshansky B, Sabbah HN, Hauptman PJ, Colucci WS. Parasympathetic nervous system and heart failure: pathophysiology and potential implications for therapy. *Circulation.* 2008;118:863–871.
45. Jia G, Aroor AR, Martinez-Lemus LA, Sowers JR. Overnutrition, mTOR signaling, and cardiovascular diseases. *Am J Physiol Reg Integr Comp Physiol.* 2014;307:R1198–R1206.
46. Kim JA, Jang HJ, Martinez-Lemus LA, Sowers JR. Activation of mTOR/p70S6 kinase by ANG II inhibits insulin-stimulated endothelial nitric oxide synthase and vasodilation. *Am J Physiol Endocrinol Metab.* 2012;302:e201–e208.
47. DeMarco VG, Aroor AR, Sowers JR. The pathophysiology of hypertension in patients with obesity. *Nat Rev Endocrinol.* 2014;10:364–376.
48. Tirosh A, Garg R, Adler GK. Mineralocorticoid receptor antagonists and the metabolic syndrome. *Curr Hypertens Rep.* 2010;12:252–257.
49. Colosia AD, Palencia R, Khan S. Prevalence of hypertension and obesity in patients with type 2 diabetes mellitus in observational studies: a systematic literature review. *Diabetes Metab Syndr Obes.* 2013;6:327–338.
50. Russo C, Jin Z, Homma S, et al. Effect of diabetes and hypertension on left ventricular diastolic function in a high-risk population without evidence of heart disease. *Eur J Heart Fail.* 2010;12:454–461.

51. Nesto RW. Correlation between cardiovascular disease and diabetes mellitus: current concepts. *Am J Med.* 2004;116(5A):S11–S22.
52. Ceriello A, Ihnat MA, Thorpe JE. Clinical review 2: The "metabolic memory": is more than just tight glucose control necessary to prevent diabetic complications? *J Clin Endocrinol Metab.* 2009;94:410–415.
53. Ceriello A. Hyperglycaemia and the vessel wall: the pathophysiological aspects on the atherosclerotic burden in patients with diabetes. *Eur J Cardiovasc Prevent Rehab.* 2010;17(1):S15–S19.
54. Juutilainen A, Lehto S, Rönnemaa T, Pyörälä K, Laakso M. Type 2 diabetes as a "coronary heart disease equivalent": an 18-year prospective population-based study in Finnish subjects. *Diabetes Care.* 2005;28:2901–2907.
55. Rana JS, Liu JY, Moffet HH, Jaffe M, Karter AJ. Diabetes and prior coronary heart disease are not necessarily risk equivalent for future coronary heart disease events. *J Gen Intern Med.* 2016;31:387–393.
56. Marwick TH, Ritchie R, Shaw JE, Kaye D. Implications of underlying mechanisms for the recognition and management of diabetic cardiomyopathy. *J Am Coll Cardiol.* 2018;71:339–351.
57. Yancy CW, Jessup M, Bozkurt B, et al. 2013 ACCF/AHA guideline for the management of heart failure: executive summary: a report of the American College of Cardiology Foundation/American Heart Association Task Force on practice guidelines. *Circulation.* 2013;128: 1810–1852.
58. Wang Y, Negishi T, Negishi K, Marwick TH. Prediction of heart failure in patients with type 2 diabetes mellitus- a systematic review and meta-analysis. *Diabetes Res Clin Pract.* 2015;108:55–66.
59. Ponikowski P, Voors AA, Anker SD, et al. 2016 ESC Guidelines for the diagnosis and treatment of acute and chronic heart failure: The Task Force for the diagnosis and treatment of acute and chronic heart failure of the European Society of Cardiology (ESC), developed with the special contribution of the Heart Failure Association (HFA) of the ESC. *Eur Heart J.* 2016;37:2129–2200.
60. Aneja A, Tang WH, Bansilal S, Garcia MJ, Farkouh ME. Diabetic cardiomyopathy: insights into pathogenesis, diagnostic challenges, and therapeutic options. *Am J Med.* 2008;121:748–757.
61. Park JJ, Park JB, Park JH, Cho GY. Global longitudinal strain to predict mortality in patients with acute heart failure. *J Am Coll Cardiol.* 2018;71:1947–1957.
62. Fang ZY, Schull-Meade R, Leano R, Mottram PM, Prins JB, Marwick TH. Screening for heart disease in diabetic subjects. *Am Heart J.* 2005;149:349–354.
63. Ernande L, Bergerot C, Rietzschel ER, et al. Diastolic dysfunction in patients with type 2 diabetes mellitus: is it really the first marker of diabetic cardiomyopathy? *J Am Soc Echocardiogr.* 2011;24:1268–1275. e1.
64. Holland DJ, Marwick TH, Haluska BA, et al. Subclinical LV dysfunction and 10-year outcomes in type 2 diabetes mellitus. *Heart.* 2015;101: 1061–1066.
65. Geyer H, Caracciolo G, Abe H, et al. Assessment of myocardial mechanics using speckle tracking echocardiography: fundamentals and clinical applications. *J Am Soc Echocardiogr.* 2010;23:351–369. [quiz:453-455].
66. Jędrzejewska I, Król W, Świątowiec A, et al. Left and right ventricular systolic function impairment in type 1 diabetic young adults assessed by 2D speckle tracking echocardiography. *Eur Heart J Cardiovasc Imag.* 2016;17:438–446.
67. Yang H, Wang Y, Negishi K, Nolan M, Marwick TH. Pathophysiological effects of different risk factors for heart failure. *Open Heart.* 2016; 3:e000339.
68. Chung J, Abraszewski P, Yu X, et al. Paradoxical increase in ventricular torsion and systolic torsion rate in type I diabetic patients under tight glycemic control. *J Am Coll Cardiol.* 2006;47:384–390.
69. Fonseca CG, Dissanayake AM, Doughty RN, et al. Three-dimensional assessment of left ventricular systolic strain in patients with type 2 diabetes mellitus, diastolic dysfunction, and normal ejection fraction. *Am J Cardiol.* 2004;94:1391–1395.
70. Al-Shafei AI, Wise RG, Gresham GA, et al. Non-invasive magnetic resonance imaging assessment of myocardial changes and the effects of angiotensin-converting enzyme inhibition in diabetic rats. *J Physiol.* 2002;538:541–553.
71. Loganathan R, Bilgen M, Al-Hafez B, Smirnova IV. Characterization of alterations in diabetic myocardial tissue using high resolution MRI. *Int J Cardiovasc Imag.* 2006;22:81–90.
72. Boyer JK, Thanigaraj S, Schechtman KB, Pérez JE. Prevalence of ventricular diastolic dysfunction in asymptomatic, normotensive patients with diabetes mellitus. *Am J Cardiol.* 2004;93:870–875.
73. Galderisi M. Diastolic dysfunction and diabetic cardiomyopathy: evaluation by Doppler echocardiography. *J Am Coll Cardiol.* 2006;48:1548–1551.
74. Di Bonito P, Moio N, Cavuto L, et al. Early detection of diabetic cardiomyopathy: usefulness of tissue Doppler imaging. *Diabetic Med.* 2005;22:1720–1725.
75. Tsang TS, Barnes ME, Gersh BJ, Bailey KR, Seward JB. Left atrial volume as a morphophysiologic expression of left ventricular diastolic dysfunction and relation to cardiovascular risk burden. *Am J Cardiol.* 2002;90:1284–1289.
76. Sacre JW, Franjic B, Jellis CL, Jenkins C, Coombes JS, Marwick TH. Association of cardiac autonomic neuropathy with subclinical myocardial dysfunction in type 2 diabetes. *JACC Cardiovasc Imag.* 2010;3:1207–1215.
77. Jellis C, Wright J, Kennedy D, et al. Association of imaging markers of myocardial fibrosis with metabolic and functional disturbances in early diabetic cardiomyopathy. *Circ Cardiovasc Imag.* 2011;4:693–702.
78. From AM, Scott CG, Chen HH. The development of heart failure in patients with diabetes mellitus and pre-clinical diastolic dysfunction a population-based study. *J Am Coll Cardiol.* 2010;55:300–305.
79. Borlaug BA, Nishimura RA, Sorajja P, Lam CS, Redfield MM. Exercise hemodynamics enhance diagnosis of early heart failure with preserved ejection fraction. *Circ Heart Fail.* 2010;3:588–595.
80. Negishi K. Echocardiographic feature of diabetic cardiomyopathy: where are we now? *Cardiovasc Diagn Ther.* 2018;8:47–56.
81. Fang ZY, Najos-Valencia O, Leano R, Marwick TH. Patients with early diabetic heart disease demonstrate a normal myocardial response to dobutamine. *J Am Coll Cardiol.* 2003;42:446–453.
82. Palmieri V, Capaldo B, Russo C, et al. Left ventricular chamber and myocardial systolic function reserve in patients with type 1 diabetes mellitus: insight from traditional and Doppler tissue imaging echocardiography. *J Am Soc Echocardiogr.* 2006;19:848–856.
83. Ha JW, Lee HC, Kang ES, et al. Abnormal left ventricular longitudinal functional reserve in patients with diabetes mellitus: implication for detecting subclinical myocardial dysfunction using exercise tissue Doppler echocardiography. *Heart.* 2007;93:1571–1576.
84. Obokata M, Kane GC, Reddy YN, Olson TP, Melenovsky V, Borlaug BA. Role of diastolic stress testing in the evaluation for heart failure with preserved ejection fraction: a simultaneous invasive-echocardiographic study. *Circulation.* 2017;135:825–838.
85. Lee M, Gardin JM, Lynch JC, et al. Diabetes mellitus and echocardiographic left ventricular function in free-living elderly men and women: the cardiovascular health study. *Am Heart J.* 1997;133:36–43.
86. Ilercil A, Devereux RB, Roman MJ, et al. Relationship of impaired glucose tolerance to left ventricular structure and function: the strong heart study. *Am Heart J.* 2001;141:992–998.
87. Levelt E, Mahmod M, Piechnik SK, et al. Relationship between left ventricular structural and metabolic remodeling in type 2 diabetes. *Diabetes.* 2016;65:44–52.
88. Oe H, Hozumi T, Arai K, et al. Comparison of accurate measurement of left ventricular mass in patients with hypertrophied hearts by real-time three-dimensional echocardiography versus magnetic resonance imaging. *Am J Cardiol.* 2005;95:1263–1267.
89. Korosoglou G, Humpert PM. Non-invasive diagnostic imaging techniques as a window into the diabetic heart: a review of experimental and clinical data. *Exp Clin Endocrinol Diabetes.* 2007;115:211–220.
90. Scheuermann-Freestone M, Madsen PL, Manners D, et al. Abnormal cardiac and skeletal muscle energy metabolism in patients with type 2 diabetes. *Circulation.* 2003;107:3040–3046.
91. Diamant M, Lamb HJ, Groeneveld Y, et al. Diastolic dysfunction is associated with altered myocardial metabolism in asymptomatic normotensive patients with well-controlled type 2 diabetes mellitus. *J Am Coll Cardiol.* 2003;42:328–335.

92. Ernande L, Audureau E, Jellis CL, et al. Clinical implications of echocardiographic phenotypes of patients with diabetes mellitus. *J Am Coll Cardiol.* 2017;70:1704–1716.
93. Shimizu M, Umeda K, Sugihara N, et al. Collagen remodelling in myocardia of patients with diabetes. *J Clin Pathol.* 1993;46:32–36.
94. Ng AC, Delgado V, Bertini M, et al. Myocardial steatosis and biventricular strain and strain rate imaging in patients with type 2 diabetes mellitus. *Circulation.* 2010;122:2538–2544.
95. Miki T, Yuda S, Kouzu H, Miura T. Diabetic cardiomyopathy: pathophysiology and clinical features. *Heart Fail Rev.* 2013;18:149–166.
96. Faria A, Persaud SJ. Cardiac oxidative stress in diabetes: mechanisms and therapeutic potential. *Pharmacol Ther.* 2017;172:50–62.
97. Paolillo S, Rengo G, Pagano G, et al. Impact of diabetes on cardiac sympathetic innervation in patients with heart failure: a 123I meta-iodobenzylguanidine (123I MIBG) scintigraphic study. *Diabetes Care.* 2013;36:2395–2401.
98. Rijzewijk LJ, van der Meer RW, Lamb HJ, et al. Altered myocardial substrate metabolism and decreased diastolic function in nonischemic human diabetic cardiomyopathy: studies with cardiac positron emission tomography and magnetic resonance imaging. *J Am Coll Cardiol.* 2009;54:1524–1532.
99. Voulgari C, Papadogiannis D, Tentolouris N. Diabetic cardiomyopathy: from the pathophysiology of the cardiac myocytes to current diagnosis and management strategies. *Vasc Health Risk Manag.* 2010;6: 883–903.
100. Kodama S, Tanaka S, Heianza Y, et al. Association between physical activity and risk of all-cause mortality and cardiovascular disease in patients with diabetes: a meta-analysis. *Diabetes Care.* 2013;36:471–479.
101. Stølen TO, Høydal MA, Kemi OJ, et al. Interval training normalizes cardiomyocyte function, diastolic Ca2+ control, and SR Ca2+ release synchronicity in a mouse model of diabetic cardiomyopathy. *Circ Res.* 2009;105:527–536.
102. Epp RA, Susser SE, Morissette MP, Kehler DS, Jassal DS, Duhamel TA. Exercise training prevents the development of cardiac dysfunction in the low-dose streptozotocin diabetic rats fed a high-fat diet. *Can J Physiol Pharmacol.* 2013;91:80–89.
103. Hare JL, Hordern MD, Leano R, Stanton T, Prins JB, Marwick TH. Application of an exercise intervention on the evolution of diastolic dysfunction in patients with diabetes mellitus: efficacy and effectiveness. *Circ Heart Fail.* 2011;4:441–449.
104. Schrauwen-Hinderling VB, Hesselink MK, Meex R, et al. Improved ejection fraction after exercise training in obesity is accompanied by reduced cardiac lipid content. *J Clin Endocrinol Metab.* 2010;95:1932–1938.
105. Schrauwen-Hinderling VB, Meex RC, Hesselink MK, et al. Cardiac lipid content is unresponsive to a physical activity training intervention in type 2 diabetic patients, despite improved ejection fraction. *Cardiovasc Diabetol.* 2011;10:47.
106. Pappachan JM, Varughese GI, Sriraman R, Arunagirinathan G. Diabetic cardiomyopathy: pathophysiology, diagnostic evaluation and management. *World J Diabetes.* 2013;4:177–189.
107. Hammer S, Snel M, Lamb HJ, et al. Prolonged caloric restriction in obese patients with type 2 diabetes mellitus decreases myocardial triglyceride content and improves myocardial function. *J Am Coll Cardiol.* 2008;52:1006–1012.
108. Ismail-Beigi F, Craven T, Banerji MA, et al. Effect of intensive treatment of hyperglycaemia on microvascular outcomes in type 2 diabetes: an analysis of the ACCORD randomised trial. *Lancet.* 2010;376:419–430.
109. Investigators OT, Gerstein HC, Bosch J, et al. Basal insulin and cardiovascular and other outcomes in dysglycemia. *N Engl J Med.* 2012;367: 319–328.
110. Sharma AK, Srinivasan BP. Triple verses glimepiride plus metformin therapy on cardiovascular risk biomarkers and diabetic cardiomyopathy in insulin resistance type 2 diabetes mellitus rats. *Eur J Pharm Sci.* 2009;38:433–444.
111. Aboukhoudir F, Rekik S. Left ventricular systolic function deterioration during dobutamine stress echocardiography as an early manifestation of diabetic cardiomyopathy and reversal by optimized therapeutic approach. *Int J Cardiovasc Imag.* 2012;28:1329–1339.
112. Leung M, Wong VW, Hudson M, Leung DY. Impact of improved glycemic control on cardiac function in type 2 diabetes mellitus. *Circ Cardiovasc Imag.* 2016;9:e003643.
113. von Bibra H, Hansen A, Dounis V, Bystedt T, Malmberg K, Rydén L. Augmented metabolic control improves myocardial diastolic function and perfusion in patients with non-insulin dependent diabetes. *Heart.* 2004;90:1483–1484.
114. Nassif M, Kosiborod M. Effect of glucose-lowering therapies on heart failure. *Nat Rev Cardiol.* 2018;15:282–291.
115. Eurich DT, Weir DL, Majumdar SR, et al. Comparative safety and effectiveness of metformin in patients with diabetes mellitus and heart failure: systematic review of observational studies involving 34,000 patients. *Circ Heart Fail.* 2013;6:395–402.
116. Eurich DT, Majumdar SR, McAlister FA, Tsuyuki RT, Johnson JA. Improved clinical outcomes associated with metformin in patients with diabetes and heart failure. *Diabetes Care.* 2005;28:2345–2351.
117. Group BDS, Frye RL, August P, et al. A randomized trial of therapies for type 2 diabetes and coronary artery disease. *N Engl J Med.* 2009;360: 2503–2515.
118. Smooke S, Horwich TB, Fonarow GC. Insulin-treated diabetes is associated with a marked increase in mortality in patients with advanced heart failure. *Am Heart J.* 2005;149:168–174.
119. Masoudi FA, Inzucchi SE, Wang Y, Havranek EP, Foody JM, Krumholz HM. Thiazolidinediones, metformin, and outcomes in older patients with diabetes and heart failure: an observational study. *Circulation.* 2005;111:583–590.
120. Tzoulaki I, Molokhia M, Curcin V, et al. Risk of cardiovascular disease and all cause mortality among patients with type 2 diabetes prescribed oral antidiabetes drugs: retrospective cohort study using UK general practice research database. *BMJ.* 2009;339:b4731.
121. Pantalone KM, Kattan MW, Yu C, et al. The risk of developing coronary artery disease or congestive heart failure, and overall mortality, in type 2 diabetic patients receiving rosiglitazone, pioglitazone, metformin, or sulfonylureas: a retrospective analysis. *Acta Diabetologica.* 2009;46:145–154.
122. Turner R, et al. Intensive blood-glucose control with sulphonylureas or insulin compared with conventional treatment and risk of complications in patients with type 2 diabetes (UKPDS 33)UK Prospective Diabetes Study (UKPDS) Group. *Lancet.* 1998;352:837–853.
123. Investigators DT, Dagenais GR, Gerstein HC, et al. Effects of ramipril and rosiglitazone on cardiovascular and renal outcomes in people with impaired glucose tolerance or impaired fasting glucose: results of the diabetes REduction assessment with ramipril and rosiglitazone medication (DREAM) trial. *Diabetes Care.* 2008;31:1007–1014.
124. Dormandy JA, Charbonnel B, Eckland DJ, et al. Secondary prevention of macrovascular events in patients with type 2 diabetes in the PROactive Study (PROspective pioglitAzone Clinical Trial In macroVascular Events): a randomised controlled trial. *Lancet.* 2005;366:1279–1289.
125. Dargie HJ, Hildebrandt PR, Riegger GA, et al. A randomized, placebo-controlled trial assessing the effects of rosiglitazone on echocardiographic function and cardiac status in type 2 diabetic patients with New York Heart Association Functional Class I or II Heart Failure. *J Am Coll Cardiol.* 2007;49:1696–1704.
126. Kernan WN, Viscoli CM, Furie KL, et al. Pioglitazone after ischemic stroke or transient ischemic attack. *N Engl J Med.* 2016;374:1321–1331.
127. Scirica BM, Braunwald E, Raz I, et al. Heart failure, saxagliptin, and diabetes mellitus: observations from the SAVOR-TIMI 53 randomized trial. *Circulation.* 2014;130:1579–1588.
128. Zannad F, Cannon CP, Cushman WC, et al. Heart failure and mortality outcomes in patients with type 2 diabetes taking alogliptin versus placebo in EXAMINE: a multicentre, randomised, double-blind trial. *Lancet.* 2015;385:2067–2076.
129. Green JB, Bethel MA, Armstrong PW, et al. Effect of sitagliptin on cardiovascular outcomes in type 2 diabetes. *N Engl J Med.* 2015;373: 232–242.
130. McMurray JJV, Ponikowski P, Bolli GB, et al. Effects of vildagliptin on ventricular function in patients with type 2 diabetes mellitus and heart failure: a randomized placebo-controlled trial. *JACC Heart Fail.* 2018;6: 8–17.

131. Pfeffer MA, Claggett B, Diaz R, et al. Lixisenatide in patients with type 2 diabetes and acute coronary syndrome. *N Engl J Med.* 2015;373: 2247–2257.
132. Marso SP, Daniels GH, Brown-Frandsen K, et al. Liraglutide and cardiovascular outcomes in type 2 diabetes. *N Engl J Med.* 2016;375:311–322.
133. Marso SP, Bain SC, Consoli A, et al. Semaglutide and cardiovascular outcomes in patients with type 2 diabetes. *N Engl J Med.* 2016;375: 1834–1844.
134. Margulies KB, Hernandez AF, Redfield MM, et al. Effects of liraglutide on clinical stability among patients with advanced heart failure and reduced ejection fraction: a randomized clinical trial. *JAMA.* 2016;316:500–508.
135. Jorsal A, Kistorp C, Holmager P, et al. Effect of liraglutide, a glucagon-like peptide-1 analogue, on left ventricular function in stable chronic heart failure patients with and without diabetes (LIVE)-a multicentre, double-blind, randomised, placebo-controlled trial. *Eur J Heart Fail.* 2017;19:69–77.
136. Neal B, Perkovic V, Mahaffey KW, de Zeeuw D, Fulcher G, Erondu N. Canagliflozin and cardiovascular and renal events in type 2 diabetes. *N Engl J Med.* 2017;377:644–657.
137. Kosiborod M, Cavender MA, Fu AZ, et al. Lower risk of heart failure and death in patients initiated on sodium-glucose cotransporter-2 inhibitors versus other glucose-lowering drugs: the CVD-REAL study (comparative effectiveness of cardiovascular outcomes in new users of sodium-glucose cotransporter-2 inhibitors). *Circulation.* 2017;136:249–259.
138. Zelniker TA, Wiviott SD, Raz I, et al. SGLT2 inhibitors for primary and secondary prevention of cardiovascular and renal outcomes in type 2 diabetes: a systematic review and meta-analysis of cardiovascular outcome trials. *Lancet.* 2019;393:31–39.
139. Turner R, et al. Effect of intensive blood-glucose control with metformin on complications in overweight patients with type 2 diabetes (UKPDS 34)UK Prospective Diabetes Study (UKPDS) Group. *Lancet.* 1998;352: 854–865.
140. Xie Z, Lau K, Eby B, et al. Improvement of cardiac functions by chronic metformin treatment is associated with enhanced cardiac autophagy in diabetic OVE26 mice. *Diabetes.* 2011;60:1770–1778.
141. von Bibra H, St John Sutton M. Impact of diabetes on postinfarction heart failure and left ventricular remodeling. *Curr Heart Fail Rep.* 2011;8:242–251.
142. Wong AK, Symon R, AlZadjali MA, et al. The effect of metformin on insulin resistance and exercise parameters in patients with heart failure. *Eur J Heart Fail. 2012*;14:1303–1310.
143. Inzucchi SE, Masoudi FA, McGuire DK. Metformin in heart failure. *Diabetes Care.* 2007;30:e129.
144. Witteles RM, Keu KV, Quon A, Tavana H, Fowler MB. Dipeptidyl peptidase 4 inhibition increases myocardial glucose uptake in nonischemic cardiomyopathy. *J Card Fail.* 2012;18:804–809.
145. Monami M, Dicembrini I, Mannucci E. Dipeptidyl peptidase-4 inhibitors and heart failure: a meta-analysis of randomized clinical trials. *Nutr Metab Cardiovasc Dis.* 2014;24:689–697.
146. Holman RR, Bethel MA, Mentz RJ, et al. Effects of once-weekly exenatide on cardiovascular outcomes in type 2 diabetes. *N Engl J Med.* 2017;377:1228–1239.
147. Nikolaidis LA, Elahi D, Hentosz T, et al. Recombinant glucagon-like peptide-1 increases myocardial glucose uptake and improves left ventricular performance in conscious dogs with pacing-induced dilated cardiomyopathy. *Circulation.* 2004;110:955–961.
148. Saponaro F, Sonaglioni A, Rossi A, et al. Improved diastolic function in type 2 diabetes after a six month liraglutide treatment. *Diabetes Res Clin Pract.* 2016;118:21–28.
149. Inzucchi SE, Zinman B, Wanner C, et al. SGLT-2 inhibitors and cardiovascular risk: proposed pathways and review of ongoing outcome trials. *Diabetes Vasc Dis Res.* 2015;12:90–100.
150. Wiviott SD, Raz I, Bonaca MP, et al. Dapagliflozin and cardiovascular outcomes in type 2 diabetes. *N Engl J Med.* 2019;380:347–357.
151. Zelniker TA, Braunwald E. Cardiac and renal effects of sodium-glucose co-transporter 2 inhibitors in diabetes: JACC state-of-the-art review. *J Am Coll Cardiol.* 2018;72:1845–1855.
152. Shekelle PG, Rich MW, Morton SC, et al. Efficacy of angiotensin-converting enzyme inhibitors and beta-blockers in the management of left ventricular systolic dysfunction
according to race, gender, and diabetic status: a meta-analysis of major clinical trials. *J Am Coll Cardiol.* 2003;41:1529–1538.
153. Wedel H, Demets D, Deedwania P, et al. Challenges of subgroup analyses in multinational clinical trials:
experiences from the MERIT-HF trial. *Am Heart J.* 2001;142:502–511.
154. El Allaf D, Vandenhoven G., Berthe C., et al. Effect of metoprolol CR/XL in chronic heart failure: Metoprolol CR/XL Randomised Intervention Trial in Congestive Heart Failure (MERIT-HF). *Lancet* 1999;353:2001–2007.
155. Epshteyn V, Morrison K, Krishnaswamy P, et al. Utility of B-type natriuretic peptide (BNP) as a screen for left ventricular dysfunction in patients with diabetes. *Diabetes Care.* 2003;26:2081–2087.
156. Chavali V, Tyagi SC, Mishra PK. Predictors and prevention of diabetic cardiomyopathy. *Diabetes Metab Syn Obesity.* 2013;6:151–160.
157. Rijzewijk LJ, Jonker JT, van der Meer RW, et al. Effects of hepatic triglyceride content on myocardial metabolism in type 2 diabetes. *J Am Coll Cardiol. 2010*;56:225–533.
158. McGavock JM, Lingvay I, Zib I, et al. Cardiac steatosis in diabetes mellitus: a 1H-magnetic resonance spectroscopy study. *Circulation.* 2007;116:1170–1175.
159. Rijzewijk LJ, van der Meer RW, Smit JW, et al. Myocardial steatosis is an independent predictor of diastolic dysfunction in type 2 diabetes mellitus. *J Am Coll Cardiol.* 2008;52:1793–1799.

29

Global and Regional Systolic Function of the Left Ventricle

Cesar J. Herrera and Andrea C. Furlani

OUTLINE

Case Study

An 82-year-old male presents to the office complaining of several months of shortness of breath and cough after walking two blocks or up a flight of stairs. He has also noted leg swelling and occasional palpitations. Past medical history is remarkable for hypertension, type 2 diabetes, lumbar spinal stenosis, and carpal tunnel syndrome. On physical exam, the blood pressure (BP) is 150/90 mmHg and the heart rate (HR) is 84 bpm. He is in no distress. The head exam is unremarkable with a normal tongue on inspection. Lungs are clear, and cardiac auscultation demonstrates a regular rhythm, nondisplaced point of maximum impulse (PMI), normal S_1, S_2 with no murmur, and an S_4 gallop. No jugular venous distention is observed, and all central and distal pulses are felt bilaterally. The abdominal exam is normal, and there is no lower extremity edema.

A surface electrocardiogram (ECG) revealed sinus rhythm, left axis deviation, and minimal voltage criteria for left ventricular hypertrophy (LVH). Echocardiographic images are shown (Figs. 29.1, 29.2, and 29.3). The clinical problem is one of dyspnea on exertion in the setting of multiple risk factors that bring into question the presence of an ischemic equivalent or overt heart failure (HF).

INTRODUCTION

Since the latter half of the 20th century, cardiovascular science has been searching for the still elusive ideal measurement of human left ventricular (LV) function; to that end, ejection fraction (EF) was, and still is, the most commonly used tool to assess what many times has

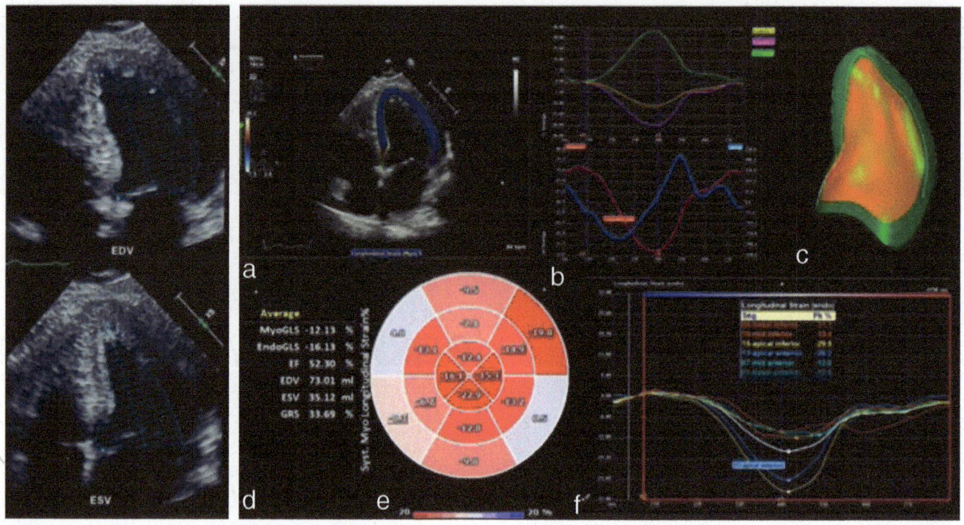

A B

Fig. 29.1 Case study: (A) Simpson biplane method (four-chamber view). EF = 52%. (B) Deformation analysis: *(a)* four-chamber view endocardial and myocardial definition by speckle tracking; *(b)* volume and global strain graphic representation; *(c)* 3-D model of end-diastolic *(green)* and end-systolic volumes; *(d)* ventricular volumes and global speckle tracking-derived strain data; *(e)* bull's eye representation of the 16 LV segments showing preserved strain on apical segments; *(f)* graphic depiction of endocardial longitudinal strain for anterior and inferior segments. *EDV,* End-diastolic volume; *EF,* ejection fraction; *EndoGCS,* endocardial global circumferential strain; *EndoGLS,* endocardial global longitudinal strain; *ESV,* end-systolic volume; *GRS,* global radial strain; *MyoGLS,* myocardial global longitudinal strain.

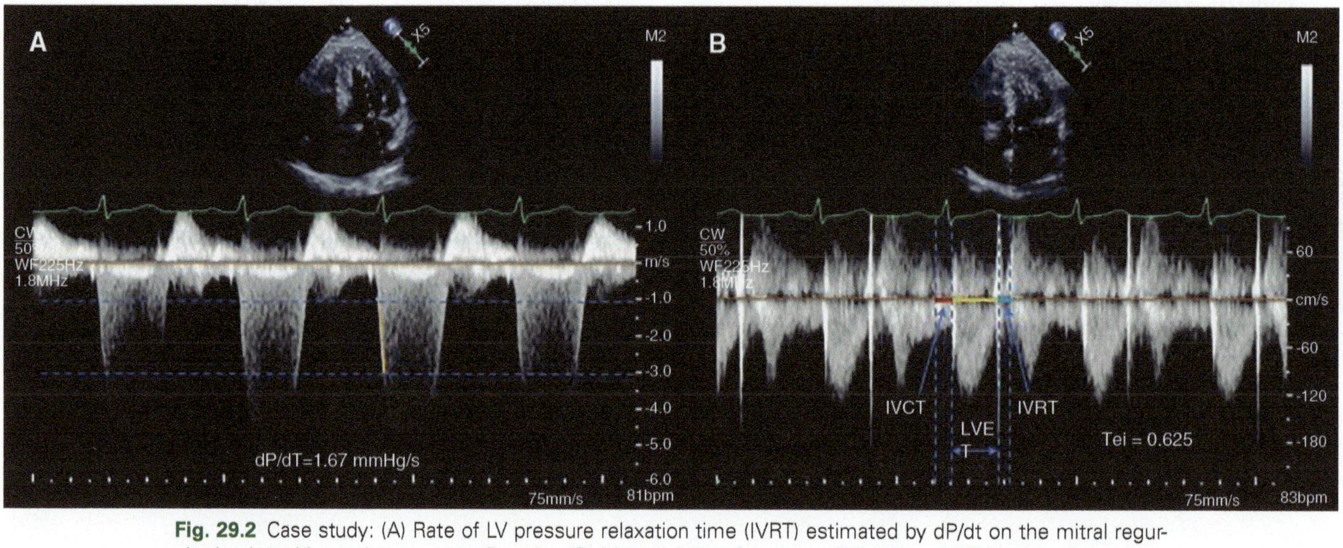

Fig. 29.2 Case study: (A) Rate of LV pressure relaxation time (IVRT) estimated by dP/dt on the mitral regurgitation jet with continuous wave Doppler. (B) Myocardial performance (Tei) index. *IVCT,* Isovolumic contraction time; *IVRT,* isovolumic relaxation time; *LVET,* left ventricular ejection time.

been erroneously described as "myocardial performance," "global systolic function," or "LV contractility."

The (almost intuitive) recognition that ventricular function directly impacts clinical outcomes was confirmed when seminal studies conducted during and after the 1970s demonstrated that EF was indeed an important and often fundamental parameter, both in the selection and adjudication of therapies in conditions such as coronary artery disease (CAD), valvular lesions (particularly aortic stenosis and mitral/aortic regurgitation), and more recently when considering device implantation in HF patients.[1]

Furthermore, the measurement of LV function surpassed the horizon of its historical understanding based on knowledge of systole when, largely thanks to technology, the study of diastole came into play as a critical determinant of cardiac physiology. Presently, practitioners and researchers alike dispose of myriad methodologies that allow quick, reliable, and clinically relevant assessment of LV function making it an almost essential index in modern cardiology and medical practice at large, particularly in the setting of suspected or known HF.

The multiple phenotypes of HF, a syndrome conformed by symptoms of dyspnea, fatigue, and exercise intolerance coupled with

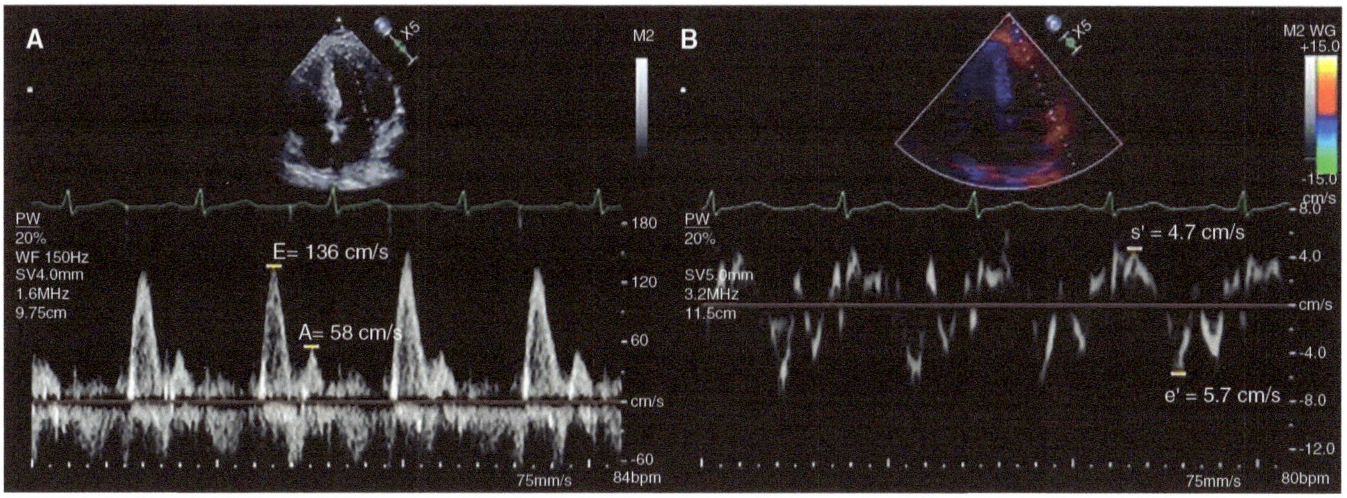

Fig. 29.3 Case study: (A) Transmitral Pulsed-wave *(PW)* Doppler. (B) PW Doppler at the mitral annulus. E/A > 2 and E/e′ = 23 reflect increased LA pressure and grade III diastolic dysfunction. *A*, Late diastolic flow velocity; *E*, early diastolic flow velocity; *e′*, early diastolic velocity; *s′*, systolic velocity.

signs of volume overload (edema, jugular venous distention, or pulmonary congestion) caused by structural/functional impairment of proper diastolic filling and/or cardiac output, have further catapulted basic science and clinical research in this field. Today, and paradoxically as the result of improved outcomes in acute and chronic ischemic heart disease, among other achievements, the diagnosis of HF has reached epidemic proportions both in the United States and worldwide, with several remaining key issues to resolve specially in what has been known as diastolic heart failure (DHF) or HF with preserved ejection fraction (HFpEF), arguably the most common form of HF in the general population, terms that may be used interchangeably through this chapter.[2,3]

Traditionally, HF has been understood as systolic when the EF is less than 40% (HF with reserved EF [HFrEF]) or diastolic when greater than 50% (HFpEF); however, as it will be discussed, questions remain on the proper identification of these patients beyond a simplistic separation based on a single measurement of cardiac activity since many subjects do not necessarily fit in this classification, nor can they always be adequately categorized.[4–10] In addition, observational studies show inconclusive results as far as mortality differences between HFrEF and HFpEF are concerned, though a recent meta-analysis of several publications has demonstrated a lower risk of death among those with better EFs.[11,12] These are some of the very reasons why many question the true nature of HF syndromes as defined based on EF, a parameter that, as this chapter will attempt to demonstrate, may no longer be adequate or sufficient for those purposes.

As it has been alluded to, multiple randomized clinical trials show the unequivocal benefit of several therapeutic modalities in patients affected by HFrEF, not only on functional class or hospitalization rates but also on survival. The same cannot be stated about patients classified as having symptomatic or asymptomatic HFpEF, a group where trials have been difficult to design and/or shown equivocal results at best.

This chapter will review aspects of diastolic parameters relevant to regional and global systolic LV function departing from (1) a critical and historical analysis of EF as an indicator of LV function, (2) current controversies surrounding EF as a fundamental determinant of HF, (3) a review of older and newer tools and technologies available in the pursue of diastolic function, (4) a discussion on the normal physiologic mechanisms of how systole and diastole interact with each other, (5) an analysis of the various hemodynamic parameters obtained by echocardiography and invasive assessment relevant to how systole talks to diastole, and (6) a critical review of the most current literature dealing with the impact of parameters of systolic function in patients with HFpEF. With this, we intend to shed light into the complex process of how regional systolic LV dysfunction and diastolic abnormalities can affect global systolic performance.

HISTORICAL VIEWS OF EF AS AN INDICATOR OF LV FUNCTION

As already stated, there is little doubt that for many decades LV EF measurement has played a fundamental role in modern cardiology, particularly in the decision-making process of therapeutic interventions, to the extent that an unequivocal inverse relationship exists between EF and all-cause mortality once it reaches a point below 40%. The prognosis and management of patients with CAD, cardiomyopathies, HF, arrhythmias, or congenital heart disease rely heavily on the accurate determination of LV size and function. Furthermore, thresholds for the timing of surgical valvular intervention, coronary revascularization, and device therapies have been established based on the volumetric quantification of EF making its precise measurement a matter of critical importance. It is understood then how the preoccupation for an accurate determination of LV EF has haunted clinicians for so long to the point that currently there are at least six clinically available methods for its assessment in humans.

Echocardiography has been the mainstay of EF evaluation despite limitations on image quality, technical and interpretation expertise, equipment variability, and intrinsic errors related to assumptions of LV geometry. Regardless of the technology used, however, the quantification of EF still relies on subjective visual estimation analysis or human-driven quantitative measurements, although more recently machine learning algorithms utilizing either ultrasound, radioisotopes, tomographic data, or invasively obtained angiographic images are beginning to evolve each with their own set of advantages and disadvantages.[13] Visual estimation of EF, while providing a rapid, bedside assessment of global systolic function that can assist on quick clinical decisions, is fraught with the previously stated inconsistencies and, perhaps more importantly, with significant limitations resulting from geometric assumptions, somewhat limited reproducibility, and interobserver variability reported as high as 19%. For these reasons, current guidelines recommend against its use, endorsing instead the biplane rule of discs (modified Simpson method) that although requires tracing of the LV cavity and endocardial border, provides a more accurate assessment of the contribution of longitudinal contraction.[14] The understanding of EF as an indicator of LV performance began decades ago when investigators categorized the basic concept of its calculation as "the central measure of LV function."[15–17] However, the LV EF equation, defined as a fraction of the volume ejected in systole (stroke volume, calculated as the difference between end-diastolic and end-systolic volume) over the LV end-diastolic volume, obviates several important facts that significantly impact its accuracy and true representation of contractility. That is, the change in stroke volume over the end-diastolic volume at a given point assumes a constant load; preload and afterload, important modifiers of EF, are often ignored; and compensatory (or pathologic) structural changes on the left ventricle may significantly alter ventricular volumes. Recently, investigators have gone as far as calling for the removal of EF as the gold standard surrogate of systolic function, while others assert that it has exhausted its usefulness as a presumed marker of contractility. Konstam and Abboud have argued that structural changes in LV end-diastolic volume—provoked by conditions such as remodeling occurring after myocardial infarction, compensatory hypertrophy or dilatation, aging, diabetes, or metabolic syndrome—are characterized by reduction on myocyte contractility/lusitropy that does not necessarily reflect changes on EF.[18,19]

The search for prognostic indicators of potentially devastating conditions such as cardiovascular (CV) disease carries the benefit of risk-stratifying patients and illnesses where either their improved well-being remains a challenge or there is more than one (imperfect) marker under discussion. That is the case of the association between reduction of LV EF and outcomes in the setting of hypertrophy where a large meta-analysis by Kalam et al. has brought some light into the matter by assembling evidence that global longitudinal strain (GLS) represents an accurate predictor of death, malignant arrhythmias, and HF hospitalization superior to EF.[20] After reviewing 16 studies that included nearly 6000 patients with various CV conditions, the authors found that mortality was independently associated with each SD (standard deviation) change in the absolute value of baseline GLS (HR 0.50, 95% confidence interval [CI] 0.36–0.69; $p < 0.002$), and less strongly, with EF (HR 0.81, 95% CI 0.72–0.92; $p = 0.572$). The HR (hazard ratio) per SD change in GLS was associated with a reduction in mortality 1.62 (95% CI 1.13–2.33; $p = 0.009$) times greater than the HR per SD change in LV EF. Justifiably so, these investigators stated that GLS should not only be paired and quoted with LV EF but that perhaps it may even replace it specially on those affected by HFpEF, a population that represents half of all HF cases.[20]

Despite the limitations and controversies just discussed, the understanding and therapeutic approach to HF, the predominant epidemic in North America and one of the most costly conditions in current health care, are precisely largely dependent on a single measurement: the LV EF. We should bear in mind that HF phenotypes are defined based on this rather simplistic index of LV function where preserved EF is only 10 percentage points apart from reduced EF with all the implications that such binary approach implies, let alone the uncertain characterization of those falling within the gray zone of 40% to 49%.

Clearly, the answer to these challenges relies on a more precise understanding of the underlying disease responsible for suspected/confirmed LV systolic dysfunction, the multiple mechanisms involved, and certainly the application of newer tools and evolving concepts on its day-to-day approach.

CURRENT CONTROVERSIES ON EF AS THE FUNDAMENTAL DETERMINANT OF HF

EF by definition is within the normal range in patients labeled as suffering from HFpEF while contractility may not; whether related to microvascular abnormalities, autonomic dysfunction, chronotropic incompetence, calcium metabolic derangements, or abnormal myocardial energetics, it is generally accepted that LV systolic function (contractility) impairment in HFpEF can be demonstrated using volume-dependent and volume-independent markers such as tissue Doppler imaging (TDI) and speckle tracking strain imaging, among others. Even in those with normal or only mildly impaired systolic function it is important to recognize that systolic reserve and peak cardiac output during exercise may also be limited, resulting from abnormal elastic recoil that in turn further impairs diastolic performance.

From the early times of myocardial deformation and diastole imaging, Aurigemma, Gaasch, and others not only alerted to the fact that EF is notably influenced by loading conditions and contractility both acutely and on chronic bases, but also called for a fundamental understanding of the process through which regional systolic function impacts the contractile behavior of the left ventricle in the setting of what was then known as DHF.[21–23] Simply stated, abnormal diastolic behavior is not the exclusive mechanism of DHF since regional and global derangements of LV shortening are present as well, even when the EF is still measured as normal. It has been clear since then that a full comprehension of the contractile behavior of the ventricle requires knowledge of all indices that reflect systolic and diastolic performance, function, and contractility both globally and regionally (Fig. 29.4).

It is worthwhile to revisit the definitions of the various indices of contractile behavior provided by these authors. *Ventricular performance* refers to the pumping ability of the LV assessed by the quantification of the pressure developed by this chamber, the stroke volume ejected, and the stroke work generated by it. *Ventricular function* includes shortening parameters, such as EF and fractional shortening of the minor axis or the apex-to-base long axis. *Ventricular contractility* refers to the inotropic state of the whole ventricle and includes isovolumic and ejection phase indices, as well as those determined at the end of ejection such as end-systolic elastance. Lastly, *myocardial contractility* addresses the intensity of cross-bridge activity, a basic propriety of the human heart muscle that is expressed on the extent and velocity of force development and fiber shortening, independent of loading and remodeling.[21]

For all the previous reasons, it is quite appropriate to question if EF indeed constitutes the fundamental determinant of HF or not; discussing the following dilemmas intends to serve as a departing point that aims at illustrating the understanding of the complex interplay between systole and diastole.

Can the EF Be Normal and Impaired Contractility Still Be Present?

The LV EF can indeed be normal despite changes in cavity dimensions, hypertrophy, or regional systolic dysfunction; although earlier studies had reported the presence of normal systolic performance in HFpEF patients based on EF preservation plus normal systolic elastance and preload-recruitable stroke work, subsequent investigators showed that in reality many patients actually have abnormal longitudinal LV systolic function (as detected by reduced mitral annular systolic velocities and longitudinal strain [LS] on TDI and speckle tracking). Such preservation of EF exists thanks to compensatory conservation of twist that counteracts reduced shortening of the subendocardial fibers and to some extent, at least early on before the appearance of systolic dysfunction, by the compensatory effect of increased radial contraction.[24,25]

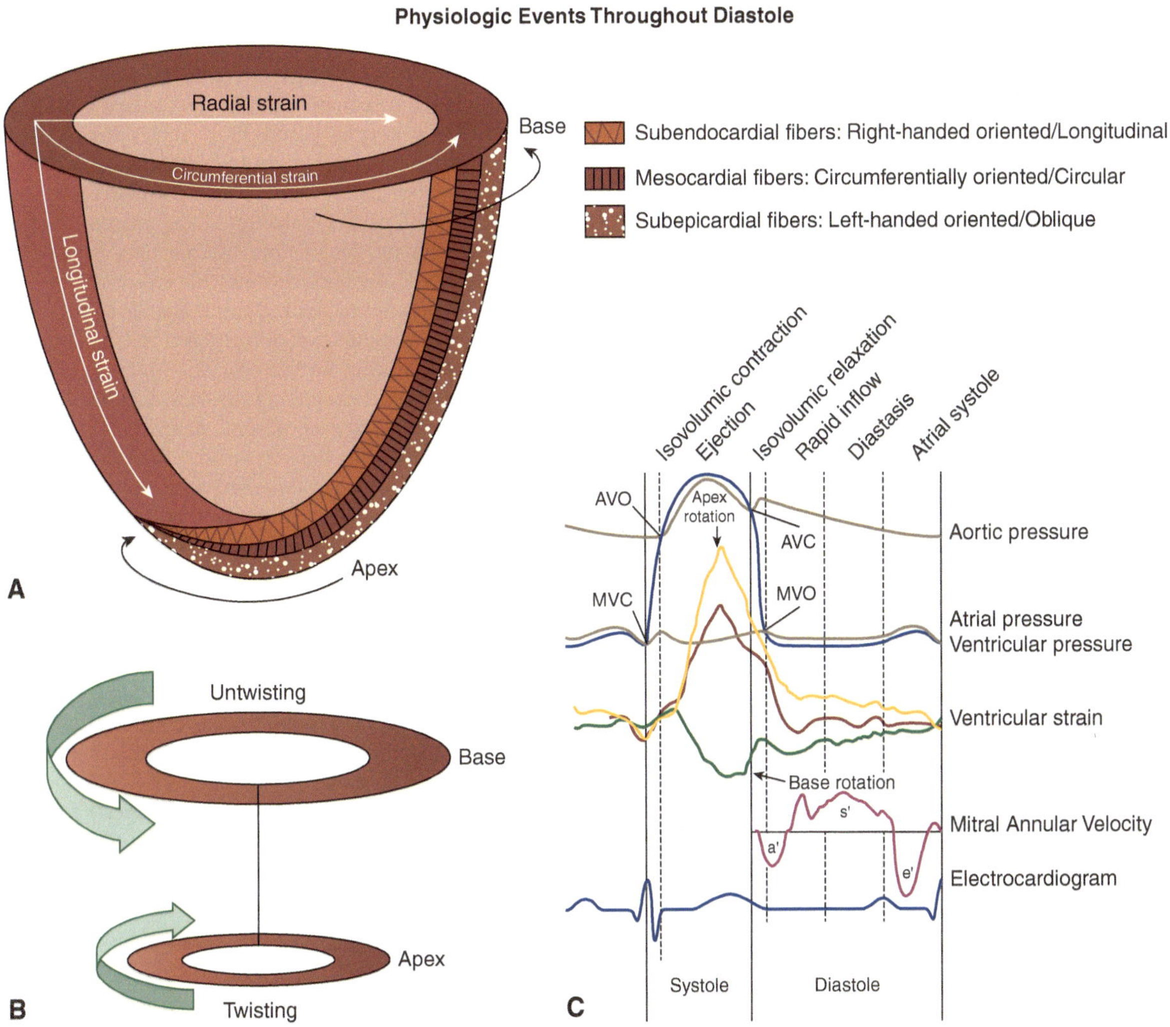

Fig. 29.4 **Graphic depiction of the various events occurring during the cardiac cycle that impact diastole.** (A) Cardiac fiber orientation varies between the three LV layers causing a complex interplay that leads to myocardial deformation. (B) Apex to base twisting and untwisting of the left ventricle. (C) Electric and mechanical phenomenon at the myocyte level and their relationship with cardiac hemodynamics. *AVC,* Aortic valve closure; *AVO,* aortic valve opening; *MVC,* mitral valve closure; *MVO,* mitral valve opening. (Modified from Sengupta PP, et al. Twist mechanics of the left ventricle. Principles and application. *JACC Cardiovasc Imag.* 2008;1(3):366–376. doi:10.1016/j.jcmg.2008.02.006.)

Are There Distinct HFpEF Phenotypes That Obviate the Importance of EF?

Whether utilizing clinical individual parameters/comorbidities or bioinformatics methodologies, grouping and classification of HFpEF patients is currently a rapidly involving area of research that is even applying machine learning algorithms. The hope is that by establishing more precise categorizations, targeted interventions could be attempted in large-scale clinical trials to hopefully shed light into the question of whether HF phenotypes represent a spectrum of the same disease or altogether separate expressions requiring different therapies. Furthermore, phenotyping may not explain all the circumstances surrounding the initial process of asymptomatic diastolic dysfunction nor how it evolves into HFpEF and later into HFrEF, a topic that remains largely undefined.

It is firmly established that the histologic composition of cardiomyocytes of patients with HFpEF versus HFrEF is functionally and structurally different as determined by changes in several parameters mostly related to thickness and filament characteristics. In the former, hypertrophy and preserved myofilament density predominates, whereas in the latter there is minimal or no hypertrophy and significant loss of myofilaments. Despite these differences, as Sanderson and Yip[19] have stated, the separation of HF subjects into clear-cut phenotypes, is contentious,to say the least, for several reasons: Regardless of EF there is similar neuroendocrine activation (brain natriuretic peptide [BNP] and norepinephrine levels), impaired chronotropicity, diastolic dysfunction, and abnormal contractile reserve on exercise among patients with either HFpEF or HFrEF.

For these reasons it is thought that the real difference between HF phenotypes may be the degree of ventricular remodeling and volume changes paralleling the extent of ventricular fibrosis and scarring.[19–24] Figs. 29.5, 29.6, and 29.7 show various two-dimensional (2-D), Doppler, and speckle tracking derived LV myocardial mechanic parameters found in two distinct HF phenotypes.

Is It More Appropriate to Classify HF Based on Etiology and/or Pathophysiology?

Some authors have postulated three distinct mechanisms of HFpEF based on resting parameters: (1) increased myocardial stiffness and

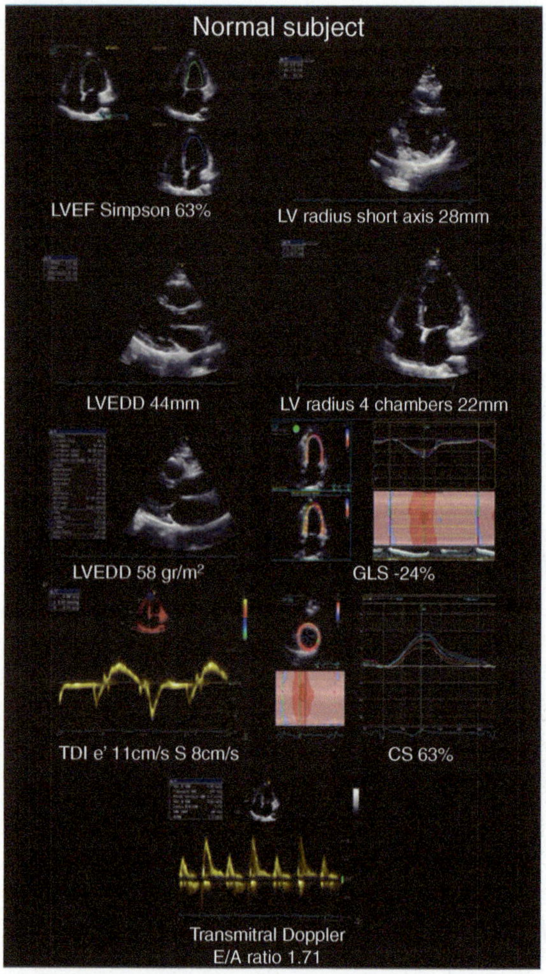

Fig. 29.5 Commonly used and valuable echocardiographic parameters in the assessment of LV function in a normal subject, 2-D, Doppler, and speckle tracking–derived LV myocardial mechanic parameters demonstrate normal ejection fraction, normal LV diastolic diameter and mass, normal GLS and transmitral Doppler index.

impaired diastolic relaxation that leads to high left atrial (LA) pressure predisposing to pulmonary venous congestion and dyspnea; (2) disturbed ventriculo-arterial coupling with increased systolic pressure load, hypertensive response to stress, and load-dependent diastolic dysfunction plus sensitivity of BP to circulating volume (see Chapter 6); and (3) impaired renal function and renal atherosclerosis, particularly among the elderly, causing excessive fluid retention and rapid rise on BP.[26]

Using this concept, one would have the potential advantage of recognizing the most appropriate therapeutic intervention for each physiologic subset. However, since no single, reliable, and reproducible test can fulfill all these requirements, multiple tools would have to be used in the diagnostic process, let alone the fact that such approach will require clinical validation in large-scale series. In consequence, it cannot be overemphasized that since HF shares multiple etiologies and pathophysiologic mechanisms on a given patient, categorizations such as these are quite impractical.

Are Myocardial Deformation Echocardiographic Tools the Answer to Phenotyping?

The recognition that the myocardium is composed of multiple anatomically and functionally separate layers not only brought an unparalleled new understanding of ventricular mechanics but also the promise of a deeper comprehension of HF beyond the use of simple diastolic parameters or EF quantification. As such, departing from anatomic mechanisms and pattern of disease may be a reasonable initial approach to the HF conundrum since it could explain, for example, why CV mortality among HF groups shows such a disparate pattern despite their sharing similar morbidities and predisposing conditions.

In this context, Salem Omar has reviewed three proposed alternative subgroups of HF patients based on LV deformation mechanics: (1) HF with predominant longitudinal dysfunction, where compensatory hypertrophy and unopposed contractile response of the subepicardial layers maintain a normal EF and overall systolic LV performance; (2) HF with transmural dysfunction (longitudinal and circumferential), caused either by simultaneous involvement of both layers or extension of the disease from subendocardium to subepicardium that eventually leads to a fall in EF and LV chamber dilatation; and (3) HF with predominant circumferential dysfunction, in which case the EF is preserved but diastole is impaired due to abnormal twist and suction of the LV.[27]

This mechanistic categorization explains how early subendocardial impairment attenuates LV longitudinal performance, a finding present in many conditions (such as ischemia or hypertension) that initially is compensated by enhanced mechanical deformation in other orientation, in concrete, circumferentially and radially. Should the process continue, particularly with transmural involvement, exhaustion of these mechanisms will invariably lead to chamber dilation and reduction of EF, hallmarks of advanced systolic HF. Furthermore, this myocardial layer approach not only has the advantage of elucidating the various stages of HFpEF that are, at least in part, supported by histologic studies but also could potentially facilitate the identification of cohorts in whom more specific therapies can become effective.

The Use of EF to Distinguish Between Systolic and Diastolic Dysfunction Is Inaccurate

Applying EF measurements to classify HF patients in clinical studies and in the assignment of therapeutic algorithms does not seem to be an ideal conceptualization given the challenges so far described. In fact, some have warned against the common misconception that a reduced EF implies systolic dysfunction and that a preserved EF equates with diastolic dysfunction. That is, to assume that the status of the EF defines the underlying disease mechanism is fraught with potential errors and perhaps has even been responsible for the inconclusive results of many trials. Those authors have gone as far as stating that LV EF exhausted its utility as a presumed marker of contractility and that this practice has hampered the understanding and therapeutic progress of HF as a clinical entity.[18,28,29]

Taking into consideration that myocardial deformation imaging has already reached the bedside and the clinical arena, and recognizing that its different parameters have shown an association with several molecular phenomena (genetic expression, stimulation of β-adrenergic receptors, and messenger ribonucleic acid [mRNA] expression of intracellular calcium ATPase, among others), it appears that the time has come to focus on the underlying myocardial deformation mechanisms involved in HF if a new paradigm is to be established on what arguably represents the most challenging CV epidemic of the millennium.

Should Diastolic Stress Testing Be the Gold Standard Tool When Searching for Diastolic Dysfunction?

Many patients with or without echocardiographically demonstrated diastolic abnormalities at rest may not exhibit symptoms until provoked by effort; evidently, exercise-induced dyspnea is the hallmark of HF, and as such it is only fair to wonder if this largely underutilized testing modality could represent the true index of myocardial performance when confronting a patient with suspected HFpEF.

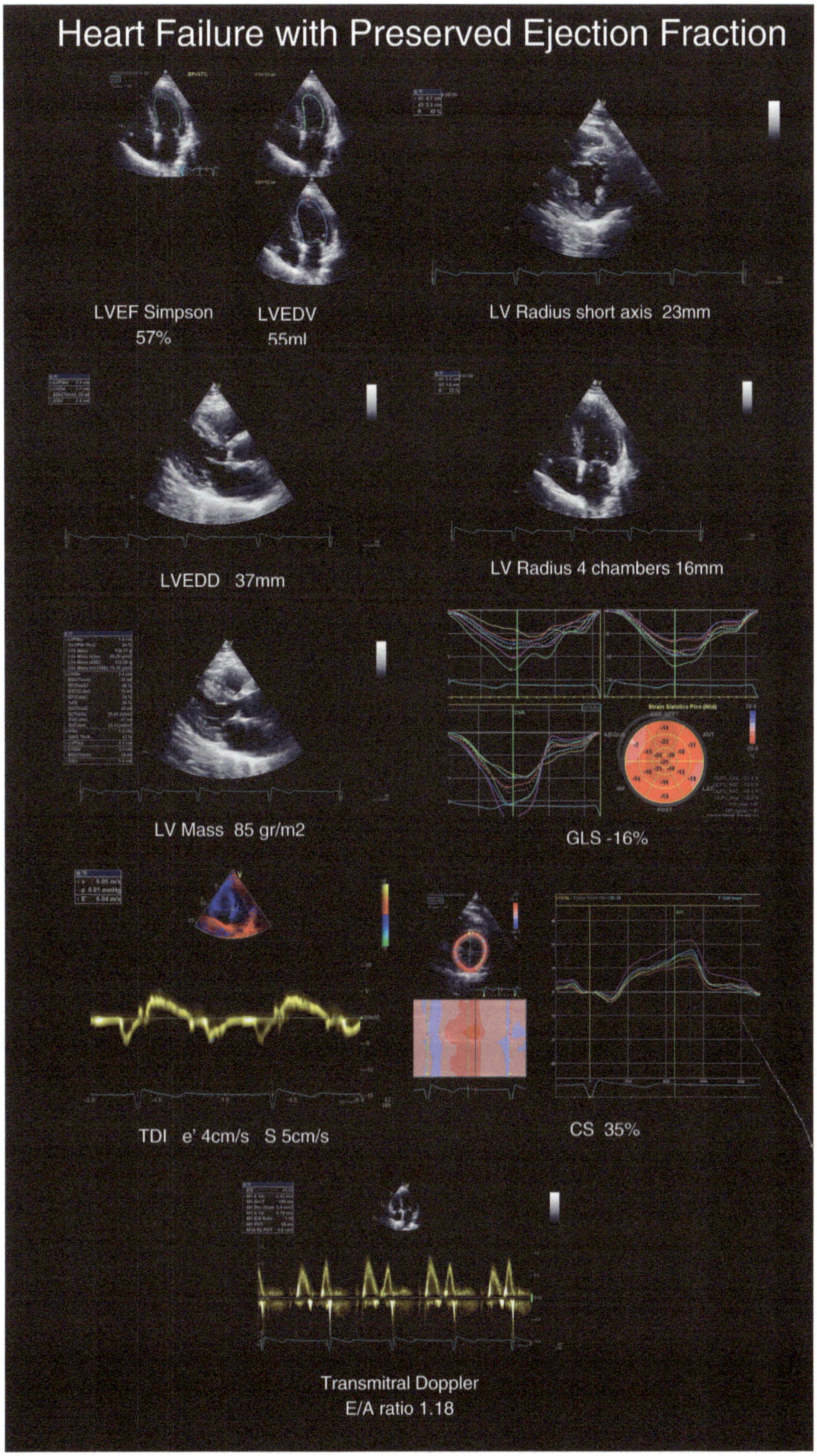

Fig. 29.6 Assessment of LV function in a hypertensive patient with HFpEF, and in HFrEF caused by a nonischemic cardiomyopathy. In the subject with HFpEF. 2-D, Doppler, and speckle tracking–derived LV myocardial mechanic parameters demonstrate increased LA pressure and LV mass, grade II diastolic dysfunction, diminished LV global longitudinal strain *(GLS)*, and compensatory increased circumferential strain *(CS)*.

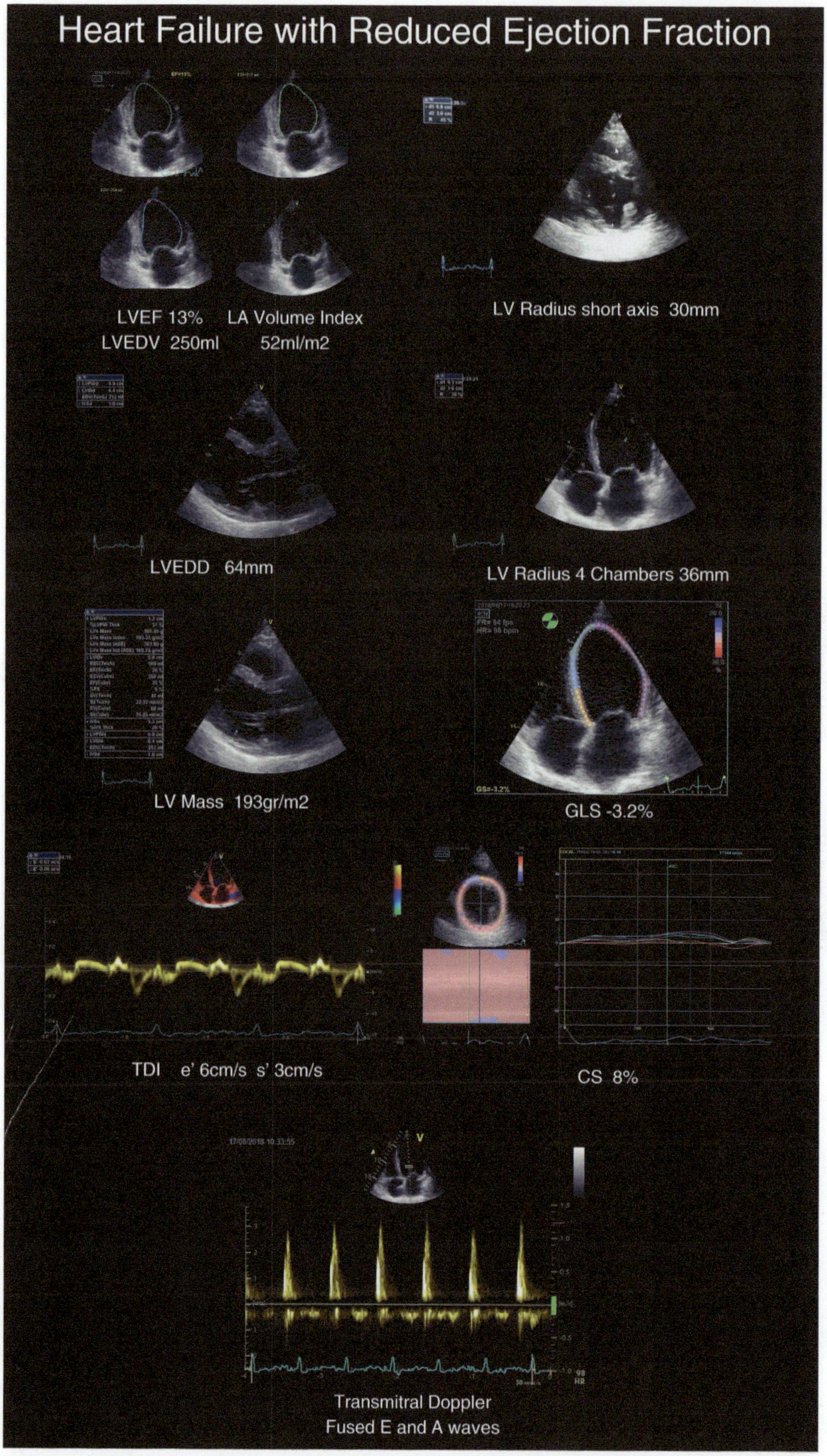

Fig. 29.7 Commonly used and valuable echocardiographic parameters in the assessment of LV function in HFrEF caused by nonischemic cardiomyopathy. 2-D, Doppler, and speckle tracking–derived LV myocardial mechanic parameters demonstrate enlarged LV cavity and increased mass, diminished LV global longitudinal strain *(GLS)*, and decreased circumferential strain *(CS)*.

Under normal physiologic conditions, systolic twisting and early diastolic untwisting of the left ventricle allow the creation of vital negative intracavitary gradients or suction, so that upon increased demand the heart can not only accelerate ejection but also enable rapid filling despite a shortened diastole while keeping a low filling pressure thanks to enhanced myocardial relaxation (shorter tau [τ]).

With exercise, multiple disruptions on the relationship between systole and diastole occur, including reduced mitral annular motion, reduced systolic longitudinal strain, and failure to increase ventricular systolic rotation. LV suction, untwist, and LA function are also compromised and correlate with elevated LV filling pressure, peak VO_2 max, and symptoms, findings that identify a subgroup that carries a higher mortality at least in retrospective series.[30]

Whether using a supine bicycle or posttreadmill images, Doppler signals can be obtained with reasonable success especially after a brief delay following peak exercise; although merging of both mitral E and A waves may occur, tissue Doppler velocities and strain data can be grabbed after stress in most individuals (see Chapter 18). Tan et al. studied subjects diagnosed with HFpEF and with limitations on cardiopulmonary exercise testing, showing reduced radial and longitudinal myocardial systolic strain both at rest and on exercise, reduced systolic and diastolic longitudinal functional reserve (mitral annular velocities failure to rise), impaired ventricular systolic rotation that failed to increase on exercise, and delayed ventricular untwisting with further worsening on exercise associated with diminished LV suction and reduction on stroke volume rise during exercise.[29]

The clinical implications of such findings are that HFpEF does not represent a disorder of diastolic dysfunction or altered stiffness alone, but perhaps more importantly, as the authors state, that given the complex physiologic derangements seen and their link to the most common etiologies behind this disorder (hypertension, diabetes, aging, and the ensuing myocardial hypertrophy/fibrosis) symptoms and outcomes of HF may not change until architectural function of the heart is restored.

Global Longitudinal Speckle Tracking Strain Versus EF?

The already mentioned limitations of EF and the relative ease of performing speckle tracking echocardiography have brought up the question of whether the latter, in concrete GLS, should be a substitute for EF when it comes to the assessment of global LV function. Validated formulae useful in the estimation of EF derived from GLS [$EF = -4.35 \times (GLS + 3.9)4$], and vice versa, in addition to being practical, bring up the notion that GLS could become a better and more reliable parameter of the systolic function.[31]

The first study that compared GLS to conventional measures of LV systolic function, EF, and wall motion score index (WMSI), as a prognosticator of all-cause mortality, showed that in a population with a wide range of EF, it was superior in predicting death. In fact, based on their data, the authors were able to determine that a cutoff of GLS greater than −12% was equivalent to an EF less than 35% concerning outcomes, leading to the conclusion that a GLS less than −12% could be recommended as a threshold for diagnosing severe LV dysfunction.[32] The systematic review of the literature published by Kalam et al. previously discussed found that strong evidence seems to support the notion that the prognostic value of GLS for major adverse cardiac events is indeed superior to EF in a wide range of conditions (Fig. 29.8).[20]

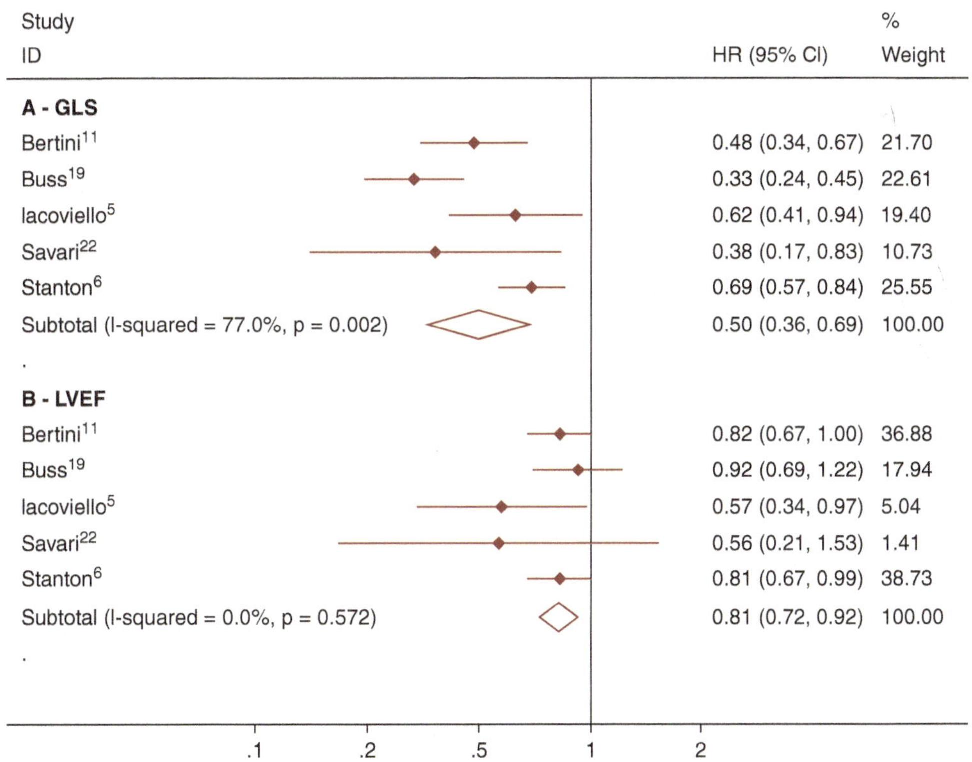

Fig. 29.8 Meta-analysis comparing global longitudinal strain *(GLS)* and LV EF as indicators of all-cause mortality in miscellaneous CV conditions. The prognostic value of GLS for major adverse cardiac events is indeed superior to EF. (Reproduced with permission from Kalam K, et al. Prognostic implications of global LV dysfunction: a systematic review and meta-analysis of global longitudinal strain and ejection fraction. *Heart.* 2014;100(21):1673–1680. doi:10.1136/heartjnl-2014-305538.)

NORMAL PHYSIOLOGY: MECHANISMS SHOWING HOW SYSTOLE AND DIASTOLE TALK TO EACH OTHER

The cardiac cycle is a complex sequence of interactive elements that complement each other and lead to the major events of systole and diastole. Systole begins with the closure of the mitral valve, extending into isovolumetric contraction, aortic valve opening, ejection, and aortic valve closure. Diastole starts when the aortic valve closes and consists of isovolumic relaxation (IVR), mitral valve opening (MVO), early rapid filling, diastasis, late atrial filling, and mitral valve closure. Each of these elements play an important role in the integration of ventricular performance with key fundamental processes that today, thanks to technology, we can assess with great certainty. Fig. 29.4 summarizes graphically the main phenomenon occurring during the various phases of the cardiac cycle relevant to diastole.

Recoil, Stiffness, Relaxation, and Compliance

Stiffness and relaxation are essential ventricular properties derived from myocyte activity and molecular processes. Stiffness is the measurement of the elastic tension of the cardiac muscle. Titin, the giant polypeptide filament responsible for the structural integrity of sarcomeres, and the extracellular matrix (ECM) are the most important determinants of elastic forces in the myocardium. Increased ventricular stiffness is related to a slower relaxation and suboptimal recoil of the left ventricle; it has been shown to be a consequence of changes in the healthy composition of the ECM of the myocardium in addition to higher amounts of collagen-dependent components and abnormal phosphorylation of titin.[33,34]

This resistance to deformation has been previously demonstrated in animal experiments and, more recently, directly measured on biopsy-derived myocardial strips from patients with normal EF and multiple comorbidities, including hypertension and diabetes. Abnormal myocardial stiffness was present only on patients with HF symptoms; in the absence of HF, stiffness and collagen-related components of ECM have been found to be normal. These findings suggest that there are clear structural and functional elements contributing to abnormal myocardial mechanics in HFpEF.[19,35]

During systole, powerful actin-myosin cross-bridges are activated in the myocardium. With the decay of these forces, each cardiac fiber returns to its original state of length on an active process called relaxation, where calcium reuptake, deactivation of the bridge's binding sites, and detachment of the bridge's connections constitute the main components of force decline. The amount of Ca^{2+} actively pumped by the sarcoplasmic reticulum Ca^{2+} ATPase appears to be one of the most crucial determinants of myocyte rate of relaxation. The membrane protein phospholamban exerts an inhibitory effect over sarcoplasmic Ca^{2+} ATPase, and phosphorylation inactivates it, increasing Ca^{2+} uptake and contributing to a higher relaxation rate. Avidity of troponin C for calcium, in addition to the strength and number of attached cross-bridges, also influences the myocardium rate of relaxation. Under ischemia or hypoxia, myocardium calcium reuptake is slower, contributing to a reduced rate of relaxation. The detachment of most active cross-bridges takes place during isovolumic relaxation and depends on adenosine triphosphate (ATP). The affinity of myosin for actin decreases with ATP binding to myosin inducing the cross-bridge to detach, a process regulated by the activity of myosin ATPase.

Moving From Cellular to LV Chamber Mechanics

Torrent-Guasp's model of a helical heart assumes the myocardial structure as a two-loop single muscular band that contracts from the pulmonary artery to the aorta. A basal spiral component loops horizontally around both the right and left ventricles, and a vertical component is responsible for the helical configuration of the band.[36] The sequential electrical activation and contraction of these loops progresses from the right ventricle (close to the pulmonary artery) to the left ventricle (close to the aorta), generating a sequence of LV cavity narrowing (resulting from the basal horizontal loop contraction) and shortening (resulting from contraction of the descendent segment of the vertical loop) that culminates with ventricular ejection. During diastole, in addition to the relaxation mechanisms responsible for cavity distention previously discussed in this chapter, the ascending segment of the vertical loop contracts generating additional lengthening and suction that further facilitates ventricular filling.[36]

LV Strain/Deformation

To better comprehend the strain concept, differences between wall motion and wall deformation must be understood since the myocardial wall can passively change position (displacement) without a change in shape and velocity (deformation). Cardiac strain analysis utilizes the principle of myocardial deformation for global and segmental functional analysis and has demonstrated to be more sensitive to estimate ventricular function than ejection fraction. It is capable of differentiating between active and passive motion of ventricular segments, evaluating longitudinal, circumferential, and radial deformation.[19,37,38] Considering a one-dimensional (1-D) object, the amount of deformation (linear strain) can be explained by the formula $S(\%) = (L - L0)/(L0)$, where S = strain, $L0$ = baseline length, and L = final length or length at the specific time of measurement. Strain rate is the deformation (strain) by a unit of time and is expressed as S-1.

More complex than linear deformation, myocardial contraction occurs in three planes (see Fig. 29.4). During systole, longitudinal and circumferential shortening are expressed as negative strain ($L < L0$), whereas radial thickening is expressed as positive ($L > L0$); during diastole, longitudinal and circumferential lengthening are expressed as positive strain and radial thinning is expressed as negative.[37,39] Despite LV EF being the most widely used measurement of systolic function, its high load dependency and relative inability to detect subtle LV function impairment make strain analysis by speckle tracking echocardiography a powerful tool to complement ventricular function assessment in patients with HFpEF.[35,40] Several studies have demonstrated that compared with healthy subjects and hypertensive controls with diastolic dysfunction, both longitudinal strain and circumferential strain (CS) are significantly impaired in HFpEF. Additionally, a significant and independent association of LS with proBNP levels has been found, raising the notion that LVGLS may act as an independent prognostic factor in this population.[35,41,42] Impaired LS can also be observed in disorders predisposing to HFpEF such as hypertension and diabetes; in this setting, an increased CS is usually present and has been proposed as an important compensatory mechanism to preserve EF. Previous studies have compared CS in asymptomatic patients with normal EF, HFpEF, and HFrEF and demonstrated a progressive decline in this parameter among groups. Therefore the CS may be one key factor to discern asymptomatic subjects with predisposing conditions from those who present with HF.[35,43]

Torsion, Twist/Untwisting, Restoring Forces, and Early Diastolic Load

A crucial spatial element of LV function, torsion results from the myocardial fiber elliptical architecture, which is geometrically oriented to the left in the subendocardium and to the right in the subepicardium.

Despite endocardial forces being stronger, the larger radius of the epicardial fibers produces higher torque dominating the final direction of rotation, thus resulting in counterclockwise apex rotation and clockwise base rotation (see Fig. 29.4).[44] The resultant base-to-apex torsion along the longitudinal axis causes subendocardial fibers to displace toward the ventricular cavity producing wall thickening and reducing volume, while subepicardial basal fibers shorten toward the apex reducing longitudinal cavity length.[45,46] It must be kept in mind that preload, afterload, and contractility exert influence on the degree of LV twist under normal physiologic conditions. As such, inotropic agents like dobutamine, exercise, or biventricular pacing markedly increase LV twist by enhancing contractility and rotation on basal and apical levels.[47] The twisting deformation of myocytes and ECM components generates potential energy (restoring forces) in a degree that is directly related to the extent of myocardial deformation. This energy is subsequently utilized to rebuild myocardial resting configuration causing fibers to return to their original state in a process known as diastolic recoil. Furthermore, LV untwist acts as a link between systolic contraction and diastolic recoil, generating negative transmitral gradients (suction) and efficient early ventricular filling.

An additional important concept—early diastolic load, which is defined as the LV pressure at the time of mitral valve opening—has been demonstrated to be an independent determinant of the peak untwist rate in addition to LV restoring forces and relaxation. Untwist rate is also dependent on systolic LV contraction; accordingly, a poor contraction generates low restoring forces contributing to slow untwisting, low suction, reduced early ventricular filling, and thus high filling pressures and high end-diastolic pressures, which are directly related to exercise intolerance.[47–50]

But how would this be true in HFpEF? For many years LV EF was the only parameter used for evaluating systolic function; however, as will be discussed throughout this chapter, technology clarified that despite a normal EF, segmental and global systolic function can be impaired, impacting on the cycle described earlier.[19,38,51]

Regional (TDI) Versus Global (EF) Contractility

As previously noted, LV EF is typically normal or nearly normal in patients with HFpEF and has been historically assessed by conventional echocardiographic indexes such as M mode, fractional shortening, and the biplane Simpson method. However, additional and newer imaging techniques can demonstrate the presence of otherwise unnoticed global and segmental systolic dysfunction on normal EF patients.

TDI was developed as a quantitative echocardiographic tool to estimate segmental LV wall motion by assessing the velocities of myocardial displacement along the cardiac cycle. Evaluation of regional myocardial displacement utilizing this tool has shown that systolic function can indeed be reduced in patients with HFpEF. Previous studies demonstrated that mitral annulus diastolic e′ wave velocity is closely correlated to ventricular systolic shortening; this implies that a close connection exists between ventricular relaxation velocities and systolic shortening.[50,52]

As far as TDI velocities and their relationship with systolic performance, several concepts must be kept in mind. First, as discussed earlier, satisfactory systolic LV shortening generates enough energy (restoring forces) to optimize relaxation (high myocardial lengthening velocity), which translates on the magnitude of e′. Second, ventricular filling pressures are related to end-diastolic pressure and length, thus, according to the Frank-Starling mechanism, high diastolic pressure generates greater systolic shortening and consequently a high-velocity e′. Lastly, the association between mitral annulus diastolic e′ and ventricular systolic shortening does not imply that e′ is only an indicator of systolic function but instead perhaps it highlights the close connection between elements of systolic and diastolic function.

Systolic longitudinal function by TDI is assessed by the mitral annular motion on the apical window at the septal and lateral levels; considering that contraction takes place on a base-to-apex orientation, the apex remains stationary, while basal displacement can be used as a predictor of global systolic function.[52]

Analysis of mitral annular tissue Doppler in patients with HFpEF demonstrates low systolic velocities in those with pure diastolic dysfunction, a finding that endorses the idea that patients with HF certainly have at least some degree of systolic dysfunction despite normal EF.[40,53] In summary, systole and diastole are two interconnected elements of ventricular function and certainly cannot be untied from each other; this is one of the several reasons proposed by many as to why HFpEF has such a high phenotypic heterogeneity.

INVASIVE HEMODYNAMIC ASSESSMENT

+dP/dt

LV dP/dt is an index that reflects the maximal LV pressure rate of rise during isovolumic contraction; in other words, it indicates the ventricular velocity of contractility. This is the oldest and most widely used parameter to invasively assess LV contractility, and it can be measured by catheterization utilizing a manometer-tipped catheter. dP/dt is largely influenced by preload, afterload, and heart rate; in patients with dyssynchrony, lack of early systolic contractile coordination between opposing walls generates lower forces reducing dP/dt and reflecting abnormal mechanics with underestimation of muscular function.

LV Stroke Work

Stroke work (SW) is defined by the amount of mechanical energy displaced from the ventricle to the arterial system to pump the volume of blood ejected in one cardiac cycle (i.e., stroke volume).

Considering that the intraventricular pressure is the force applied to the amount of blood that will be ejected, LV stroke work can be calculated as the product of stroke volume and mean arterial pressure.

$$SW = SV \times MAP$$

During its invasive assessment, stroke work is reflected in the area inside the pressure-volume loop. Fig. 29.9 represents how it is influenced by preload and afterload.[54]

According to the Frank-Starling mechanism, a preload raise generates a higher stroke volume leading to a higher cardiac output and arterial pressure. Consequently afterload increases, reducing the ejection velocity due to slower myocardial fiber shortening (the ventricle is pumping against a higher resistance). That may increase end-systolic volume slightly, and if preload augmentation is too pronounced it will null the compensatory increment on stroke volume. The opposite effect is seen with preload reduction.

In conditions of increased afterload (i.e., arterial hypertension), the ventricle pumps against a high-resistance system, and the increased end-systolic volume leads to a secondary increase in end-diastolic volume, generating a compensatory rise in the volume ejected. However, ventricles with reduced compliance (e.g., in HFpEF) are unable to accommodate additional blood volume during diastole, therefore progressing to a reduction in stroke volume. On the opposite side, in situations where the end-diastolic volume is already maximized, as in HFrEF patients, any increase in afterload (aortic pressure) may cause a significant reduction in stroke volume.

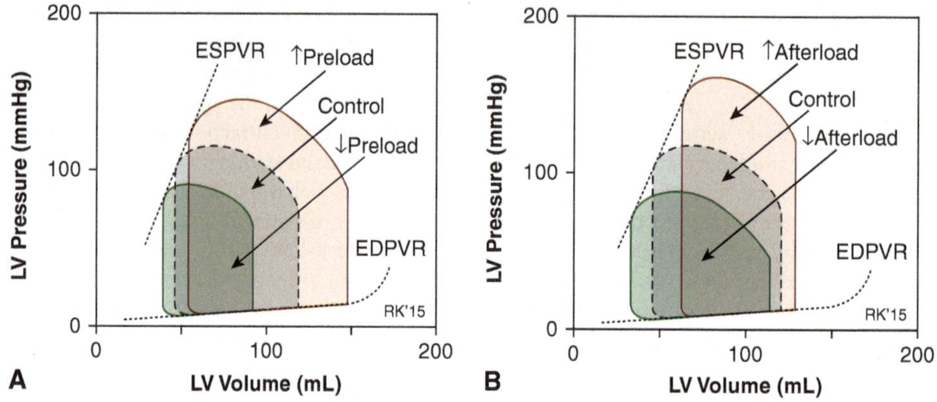

Fig. 29.9 Pressure-volume loop obtained by invasive assessment; stroke work is represented as the area inside the loop. *(A)* Preload and *(B)* afterload influence on stroke volume. *EDPVR,* End-diastolic pressure-volume relationship; *ESPVR,* end-systolic pressure-volume relationship. (Copyright Richard E. Klabunde, cvphysiology.com.)

LV SW can be considered a good measurement of cardiac performance in the absence of acute volume (preload) or pressure (afterload) overload; in such instances, the SW might not reflect the baseline condition of the ventricle (see Fig. 29.9).

Elastance

Elastance reflects the LV-arterial system (AS) coupling through *Emax* (maximal elastance of the left ventricle) and *Ea* (effective elastance of the AS). If systolic and diastolic duration are constant at a given heart rate, arterial end-systolic pressure and stroke volume are grossly linearly related (the end-systolic pressure increases proportionally to the stroke volume). The elastance unit stands for the change in pressure for a specific change in volume (mm/mL).

Emax is utilized as an index of cardiac contractility reflecting the inotropic state of the left ventricle while *Ea* can estimate the hemodynamic properties of the arterial system, considered an elastic chamber. The slope of this interaction can be utilized as a parameter of the resistance that the arterial system imposes to accommodate the stroke flow. The interaction between LV and AS and important aspects of LV-AS coupling can be described by the ratio *Emax/Ea,* named couple index *(k).*[55] Studies have shown that LV and aortic systolic pressures in HFpEF patients are significantly higher than in HFrEF; this is related to the fact that *Emax* is significantly higher in HFpEF as LV contractility (or the inotropic state) is consistently higher in this setting.[56]

ECHOCARDIOGRAPHIC ASSESSMENT

LV Ejection Fraction: 2-D Versus 3-D

Global LV function is usually estimated by the EF, which is measured by the difference between the end-diastolic and end-systolic volumes divided by its end-diastolic volume:

$$EF = EDV - ESV / ED$$

On echocardiographic images, the first frame after mitral valve closure, or the frame in which the LV area is the largest, corresponds to end diastole. End systole corresponds to the first frame after aortic valve closure, or the frame in which the cardiac area is smallest. As will be discussed, LV volume assessment can be done by using 2-D or 3-D echocardiographic imaging; however, since linear measurements do not take in consideration segmental wall motion abnormalities or variations in LV shape, as it occurs in a variety of pathologies, accordingly, they are not adequate for accurate estimation of volumes. For these reasons, the American Society of Echocardiography no longer recommends linear methods such as Teichholz for EF calculation.[17]

2-D Echocardiographic Assessment of EF

2D volumetric measurements derive from tracing the endocardial wall-blood interface and should be obtained on apical four-chamber and two-chamber views. A recurrent challenge on image acquisition is the need to avoid apical foreshortening, which results in an underestimation of volumes; in addition, optimization of settings aiming at high-quality images should always be encouraged since it minimizes errors in endocardial border visualization and tracing.

The biplane method of disks (modified Simpson rule) is the most widely used for 2-D volume calculation and is the one currently recommended. The area-length method assumes the left ventricle to be bullet shaped, which is frequently not true, thus it is advised only when the apical view definition precludes accurate definition of endocardial borders. Bear in mind that this method requires assessment of midcavity LV area on the parasternal short axis and ventricular length on the apical four-chamber view.

The patient in the chapter-opening case study had normal EF by biplane 2-D assessment (see Fig. 29.1).

LV Ejection Fraction by 3-D Echocardiography

The 3-D method of EF quantification does not rely on geometric assumptions for volume determination; however, accurate and reproducible measurements are also dependent on good quality images. Including the whole ventricle within the pyramidal beam is essential for a reliable assessment making foreshortening a less relevant issue.[57] As an additional advantage, the 3-D dataset allows adjustment of the plane, aligning the true long axis and avoiding oblique images.

LV volume assessment by real-time 3-D echocardiography (RT3D) has been shown to be time effective, accurate, and reproducible in various clinical scenarios, and the parameters acquired (LV mass and volumes) positively compare with those obtained from magnetic resonance.[57,58] RT3D echocardiography is also quite reliable in the assessment of LV volumes in remodeled ventricles accurately evaluating wall motion abnormalities and LV dyssynchrony.[57]

For both 2-D and 3-D methods, when the acoustic window is not favorable, the administration of intravenous ultrasound–enhancing contrast agents is useful and recommended for improved endocardial border definition.

Wall Stress

Wall stress is an important determinant of ventricular function and rate of myocardial oxygen consumption, and it has been previously demonstrated to be a sensitive measurement of LV contractility.[59] The noninvasive calculation of wall stress was initially described in the late 1960s and is based on Laplace's law that assumes the ventricle as a spheroid; it has been obtained by numerous different formulas utilizing internal linear measurements or volumes as well as intraventricular pressures.[60] Both end-systolic and end-diastolic wall stress are afterload dependent and therefore technically challenging as the calculation requires simultaneous invasive assessment of intraventricular pressures. Studies have shown a satisfactory correlation when calculating systolic wall stress by replacing intraventricular pressure with mean arterial pressure obtained noninvasively.[61]

In situations of abnormal loading of the heart, wall stress is thought to play the role of a feedback signal to control the extent of ventricular remodeling. Thus if this feedback loop is unbalanced, cardiac decompensation occurs.[41,61] Increased systolic wall stress has been shown to be a determinant of inefficient diastolic function, while increased end-diastolic wall stress is tightly related to LV remodeling and reduced EF. The latter is a physiologically important concept since both major phenotypic variants of HF (reduced or preserved EF) exhibit diverse but common features that cannot be considered as isolated mechanisms.

The echocardiography-based approach for determination of systolic wall stress utilizes measurements of LV cavity (linear/volumes), which are then applied to one of the previously described mathematical formulas to estimate wall stress.[60] The accuracy of this assessment can certainly be improved by applying 3-D techniques.

+dP/dt

This parameter can be estimated by echocardiography utilizing the time interval between 1 and 3 m/sec (time 3-1) measured on the mitral regurgitation velocity curve acquired by continuous wave Doppler. The measurement of this interval is the parameter that best correlates with invasive catheter-derived LV dP/dt.[62] The time obtained is then applied to the formula dP/dt = 32/(time 3-1), where a value greater than 1200 mmHg/sec is considered normal.[62] In sum, dP/dt is closely determined by myocardial contractility and influenced by loading conditions and, when diminished, most likely indicates poor LV systolic function.

A final concept to keep in mind in this context is that considering that systole and diastole coexist in the cardiac cycle, functional and structural abnormalities of intracellular calcium and myofilament mechanics that generate diastolic abnormalities also reflect on systolic function. Accordingly, although dP/dt is a contractility parameter, it is also an important determinant of early diastolic function.[62,63] Lastly, technical limitations encountered in the noninvasive acquisition of dP/dt include the need for the presence of mitral regurgitation, high image quality, and proper alignment of the Doppler signal, all of which can be challenging particularly when eccentric jets are present.

Our patient with HFpEF was found to have a diminished dP/dt indicating suboptimal ventricular contractility (see Fig. 29.2).

MYOCARDIAL PERFORMANCE (TEI) INDEX

The myocardial performance (Tei) index is one of the most commonly used in the calculation of ventricular performance, and it is intended to estimate overall cardiac function combining assessment of systolic and diastolic components.[64] This parameter can be obtained by measuring the isovolumic contraction time (IVCT), which is the interval between mitral valve closure and aortic valve opening, the isovolumic relaxation time (IVRT), the interval between the aortic valve closure and mitral valve opening, and the ejection time (ET), that in turn can be estimated by measuring the duration of flow across the aortic valve, where Tei = (IVCT + IVRT)/ET. Systolic dysfunction prolongs the IVCT as well as shortens the ET, causing the Tei index to increase.

A classic study compared normal subjects with patients with dilated cardiomyopathy and demonstrated that the Tei index is significantly higher as ventricular function worsens (0.39 ± 0.05 for normal subjects; 0.59 ± 0.10 for HFrEF NYHA Class II, EF 30–50%; and 1.06 ± 0.24 for pretransplant patients with EF <30%).[53] In the HFpEF population, both Tei index and BNP serum levels increase with the degree of symptoms (NYHA classification), suggesting that patients with normal EF and heart failure have lower myocardial performance when compared to the general population.[42]

The latter is also true for the patient reported in the chapter-opening case study who had a Tei index of 0.625 compatible with suboptimal myocardial performance overall. He showed abnormal parameters of diastolic function (E/A ratio 2.3, E/e′ ratio 23, and lateral e′ 5.7 cm/sec) indicating diastolic dysfunction with severely increased LA pressure and abnormal systolic function with diminished dP/dt, reduced systolic tissue Doppler velocity, and low GLS[65] (see Figs. 29.2 and 29.3).

TISSUE DOPPLER SYSTOLIC VELOCITIES

Systolic velocities corresponding to mitral annular displacement can be assessed using TDI on apical views, and they play a key role in the evaluation of LV systolic function. Several studies have determined that a cutoff of a mean systolic mitral annular velocity of greater than 7.5 cm/sec (average between six points on the mitral annulus: apical four-chamber, two-chamber, and three-chamber views) can predict normal global LV systolic function with a sensitivity of 79% and a specificity of 88%. Routinely, the average of inferoseptal and lateral velocities are used considering that these are the locations that individually most closely correlate with LV EF measurements.[52]

The acquisition of TDI velocities requires a near perfect longitudinal alignment of the heart in the four-chamber view to obtain the proper sample volume position and therefore a reliable measurement of longitudinal myocardial deformation.

The patient described in the case study presented with reduced mitral annular systolic velocity reflecting poor longitudinal LV displacement despite the presence of a normal EF. This finding indicates decreased myocardial motion on the specific points of sample volume positioning; when a global systolic impairment is present, as in this case, the sampling of all points will also exhibit low velocities. However, a reduced velocity on an isolated point might be encountered in the setting of isolated segmental wall motion abnormalities as well.

MYOCARDIAL STRAIN AND TORSION

LV longitudinal strain was first assessed by TDI; however, the emergence of speckle tracking has allowed state-of-the-art software to detect and trace the endocardial and epicardial borders of the ventricle providing detailed information on longitudinal, circumferential, and radial deformation via global and segmental strain and strain rate measurements, as previously explained in this chapter. Speckle tracking is capable of detecting tissue displacement when evaluating interventricular and intraventricular dyssynchrony; it also makes feasible the evaluation of LV twisting although this application is currently mostly a research tool. Using the short axis views and tracking the endocardial and epicardial borders of the left ventricle, dedicated software detects the rotation of each segment; the twist is then measured in degrees and can be estimated as the difference between the rotation of the basal and apical segments around the longitudinal axis.

Back to the case described at the beginning of the chapter: We observed reduced GLS (−16.13%) and radial strain (32%)—in addition to the dP/dt and Tei index changes mentioned already—indicating that this patient has some degree of global systolic impairment even though the EF was normal. In this example (a known amyloid cardiomyopathy) the patient presents with the typical pattern of relatively preserved apical function demonstrated on the bull's eye indicating normal deformation of that segment compared to the base. This increased apical/basal strain ratio (gradient) has been described in this disease as demonstrative of nonhomogeneous systolic function along myocardial segments reflecting diminished global function despite the presence of regionally preserved function (see Chapter 23).[66]

SYSTOLIC DYSFUNCTION IN HF WITH PRESERVED EF

There is no doubt that many established pharmacologic, surgical, and device therapeutic interventions have benefited mortality, hospitalization rates, and quality of life of patients with HFrEF despite and independent of etiology; intuitively, one would assume that such paradigm is the result of a common unifying mechanism present behind the clinical manifestations and improved outcomes after intervention witnessed in HFrEF today. However, many argue precisely the opposite: that patients with HF either do not share a common pathophysiologic mechanism or that those are yet to be identified. Until that occurs, beneficial treatments for a more complex, less defined group, those with HFpEF, will continue to be limited; in the end, perhaps it will be appropriate to assume that HFpEF represents not a single entity but a range of phenotypes that are just starting to be elucidated based on echocardiographic and clinical features.

With the use of M mode echocardiography, TDI, and strain analysis, many studies conducted over the last 15 years have demonstrated that in subjects categorized as having HFpEF, subtle and not so subtle abnormalities on the regional systolic function of the left ventricle do exist and represent an important concomitant additive negative contributing factor. In addition, the etiologies, clinical morbidities, and comorbidities present in these patients are of varied nature, a fact that makes analytic comparisons difficult.

Therefore it is worthwhile to briefly address in this context the different phenotypes of HFpEF so far identified, prior to discussing how regional performance may affect ventricular function in specific conditions such as acute or chronic HF, hypertension, chemotherapy-induced cardiotoxicity, or severe valvular disease when EF has not yet been impaired.[67–71]

To characterize subgroups of HF patients with preserved EF with the goal of understanding factors related to prognosis and treatment response, Kao et al. cross-analyzed 4113 subjects enrolled in the I-PRESERVE trial as belonging in six different groups. Results were then validated against 3203 patients of the CHARM-PRESERVE study. Of all, two subsets were identified as showing the worse outcomes: (1) elderly women with low body mass index (BMI), renal dysfunction, and anemia, and (2) women with multiple comorbidities such as obesity, diabetes, CAD, and renal failure.[72]

In a smaller series and essentially with the same purposes, Shah et al. defined three HFpEF phenotypes utilizing several statistical learning algorithms applied to 67 continuous variables: (1) younger patients with moderate criteria for diastolic dysfunction and normal BNP, (2) obese diabetics with obstructive sleep apnea and severe impairment on LV relaxation, and (3) elderly subjects with myocardial remodeling, RV dysfunction, pulmonary hypertension, high BNP, and kidney disease. The latter had a 4-fold increased risk of hospitalization and a 1.7-fold risk of death, although important overlap of clinical factors was observed among all phenogroups.[26]

Several additional factors not mentioned so far may impact the physiologic and clinical expression of HFpEF. They are atrial fibrillation, metabolic syndrome, RV impairment, pulmonary hypertension, coexisting chronic pulmonary disease, amyloid deposition, particularly wild-type transthyretin, anemia, and musculoskeletal or autonomic dysfunction. With the goal of teasing these out and addressing whether symptoms can be blamed on abnormal cardiac filling resulting from specific causes, some authors have suggested a schematic diagnostic approach to HFpEF based on their absence (i.e., primary HFpEF) or presence of conditions such as pericardial disease, cardiomyopathy, or severe valvular disease in which case the term *secondary HFpEF* should be used. Once again, as attractive as this scheme may appear, simplification does not imply clarification, let alone beneficial outcomes.[7]

M-Mode Echocardiography, TDI, and Strain Analysis in HFpEF

As early as 2002, several authors had already alerted to the fact that parameters of long axis function were abnormal in patients diagnosed as having DHF. To date, a significant body of literature has accumulated supporting the notion that systolic function (regional or global) is indeed reduced in HFpEF patients independent of EF as measured by M mode mitral annular motion, TDI, and strain analysis, and that these findings are strong independent prognosticators as good as and perhaps superior to EF (Fig. 29.10).

After measuring systolic mitral annular displacement with M mode, Petrie et al. noted that in a series of cases with DHF, 21% to 33% had evidence of "subtle LV systolic dysfunction"; in a similar population, Yip et al. demonstrated reduced mitral annular systolic velocities in 38% of patients compared with controls, while Yu et al. showed similar findings as well.[40,53,73] These studies, however, included cases with already reduced EF and fractional shortening, a limitation not present on a subsequent study published by Vinereanu et al., one of the earliest of its kind, who tested the hypothesis that pure diastolic dysfunction (defined as impaired global diastolic filling with an EF >50%) was associated with longitudinal systolic dysfunction.[74]

In the latter paper, mean mitral annular S velocities, surrogates of longitudinal systolic function, were significantly lower in patients with both asymptomatic diastolic dysfunction and DHF versus controls (8.0 ± 1.2 and 7.7 ± 1.5 cm/sec, respectively, vs 10.1 ± 1.5 cm/sec, p <0.001). These results, confirmed in several other studies and among a wide range of EFs, led the authors to conclude that worsening global LV diastolic dysfunction is associated with a progressive decline in longitudinal systolic function, proposing, nearly 15 years ago, that diagnostic algorithms and definitions of HF needed revision.[74]

Nature, understanding of how vectors of myocardial fiber deformation (i.e., fiber shortening) occurring during the cardiac cycle in the radial, circumferential, and longitudinal planes interact during LV contraction-relaxation (what has come to be known as strain, a dimensionless index of change in length between two points) has expanded our comprehension of HFpEF beyond technology. Currently, robust clinical data support the use of strain in the assessment and perhaps not too far from now in the guidance of the very much needed therapeutic interventions lacking in this elusive syndrome. In the next

CENTRAL ILLUSTRATION: Prognostic and Managment Implications of Abnormal Strain Measurement in Common Clinical Scenarios

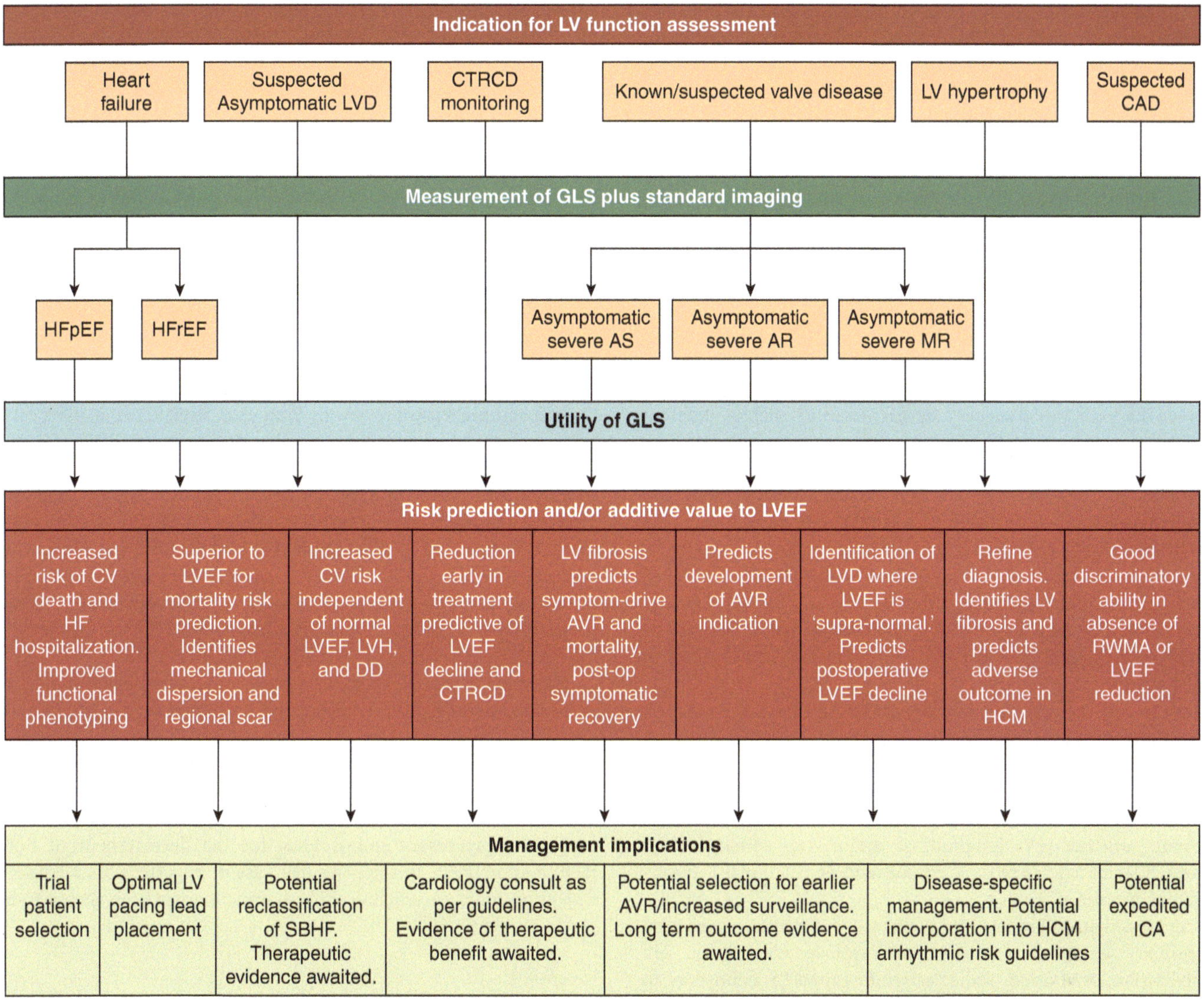

Fig. 29.10 Prognostic and management role of strain measurement in HF and various clinical scenarios. The independent association of reduced GLS with adverse outcomes beyond EF is robust though its impact on management modifications is still being developed. (Reproduced with permission from Potter E, et al. Assessment of left ventricular function by echocardiography. The case for routinely adding global longitudinal strain to ejection fraction. *JACC Cardiovasc Imag.* 2018;11:260–274. doi:10.1016/j.jcmg.2017.11.017.)

paragraphs we review the most pertinent papers that have specifically addressed the role of strain in HFpEF and associated conditions.

Yu et al. performed TDI on 339 subjects, 92 of whom had systolic heart failure (SHF), 73 had DHF, and 68 had isolated diastolic abnormalities diastolic dysfunction (DD); LV myocardial velocities obtained on multiple basal and midsegmental regions showed reduced peak and mean systolic (S) and early diastolic (E) values in most segments: mean S (SHF < DHF < DD < control of 3.3 ± 1.0 < 4.6 ± 1.3 <5.4 ± 1.0 <6.3 ± 1.0 cm/sec; all $p \leq 0.001$) and mean E (SHF = DHF < DD < control of 3.6 ± 1.2 = 3.9 ± 1.3 <5.3 ± 1.6 <7.2 ± 1.7 cm/sec; all $p < 0.001$). A mean S value of 4.4 cm/sec (−2 SD of control subjects) predicted the presence of systolic dysfunction in 92% of patients with SHF, 52% with DHF, and 14% with DD. The authors concluded that abnormalities of systolic function are prevalent in patients previously labeled as having isolated DHF and to a lesser extent DD and that the assessment of S and E velocities, combined with clinical features, allows a more insightful understanding of the severity of ventricular dysfunction and the predominant pathophysiologic mechanism.[73]

In a strong, well-designed, well-conducted seminal paper, Kraigher-Krainer and a group of PARAMOUNT (Prospective Comparison of ARNI (angiotensin receptor-neprilysin inhibitor) With ARB on Management of Heart Failure With Preserved Ejection Fraction Trial) study investigators enrolled 219 patients from this contemporary trial with the goal of determining the frequency and magnitude of impaired systolic deformation present in HFpEF. A control group of normal volunteers and a subgroup of asymptomatic hypertensive subjects with diastolic dysfunction on echocardiography were included for comparison; blind analysis of images was then completed at a single laboratory by a single investigator.[35] Compared to both normal controls and hypertensive heart disease subjects, in this study HFpEF patients demonstrated significantly lower GLS (−20.0 ± 2.1 and −17.07 ± 2.04 vs −14.6 ± 3.3, respectively, $p < 0.0001$ for both) and global circumferential strain (GCS) (−27.1 ± 3.1 and − 30.1 ± 3.5 vs − 22.9 ± 5.9, respectively; $p < 0.0001$ for both); strain was reduced in 50% of HFpEF individuals even after excluding those with CAD or EF less than 55%. Interestingly, in this series only a fraction showed LVH or concentric remodeling, most had LA enlargement, and both GLS and GCS were reduced and not related to standard measures of diastolic function (E′ or E/E′). Lastly, a reduced GLS was significantly and independently associated with NT-proBNP levels, an established prognosticator in HFpEF. These findings once again emphasize the complex, multifactorial pathophysiologic expression of HFpEF and the need for incorporation of strain analysis in its comprehensive noninvasive assessment.[35]

Beware that the study just discussed comprised a series of stable outpatients on appropriate medical therapy with adequate BP control; Park et al.[75] went further and looked at LV deformation in patients presenting with acute decompensated heart failure (ADHF) with a range of EFs attempting to assess the role of GLS as a predictor of 5-year mortality. In what is considered the largest study on the subject, 4172 individuals underwent GLS measurement in the setting of ADHF associated with reduced EF (<40%), midrange EF (40%–49%), and preserved EF (>50%). Mortality by EF was only slightly different among the three groups (41%, 38%, and 39%, respectively, $p = 0.031$), whereas reduced strain conferred a significantly higher mortality independent of EF (49%, 38%, and 34% for severely, moderately, and mildly reduced GLS, respectively, $p < 0.001$) with each 1% in GLS associated with a 5% decrease risk of mortality.

In sum, in this study, almost all patients with ADHF had reduced strain regardless of EF and GLS; a lower strain adjudicated a greater prognostic value than EF implying that deformation should be considered an integral part in the classification and stratification of ADHF patients.[75]

More recently, recognizing that impairment in LV systolic function had been described in HFpEF but that its prognostic relevance was not clearly known, Shah et al.[76] published the largest series on the topic: 447 patients enrolled in the Treatment of Preserved Cardiac Function Heart Failure With an Aldosterone Antagonist (TOPCAT) trial to determine whether LV longitudinal strain was predictive of cardiovascular outcomes beyond clinical and conventional echocardiographic measures.

After a median follow-up of 2.6 years, 115 patients experienced the primary composite outcome of cardiovascular death, HF hospitalization, or aborted cardiac arrest. Impaired LS, defined as an absolute LS less than 15.8%, was present in 52% and was predictive with an adjusted hazard ratio of 2.14; 95% CI, 1.26–3.66; $p = 0.005$). After adjustment for clinical and conventional echocardiographic variables, LS was the strongest predictor of the composite outcome suggesting that it represents a powerful novel imaging marker that can potentially select high-risk groups among the HFpEF universe.[76]

In short, despite normal EF, long axis LV systolic function is not normal in HFpEF patients, which is not a surprising finding since the major determinant of diastolic filling is the power and coordination of the preceding systolic event. Therefore it must be kept in mind that speckle tracking should be routinely used in the clinical decision process of HF patients especially when dealing with complex phenotypes.

Preclinical Diastolic Dysfunction

Nearly a decade ago, the American College of Cardiology/American Heart Association Task Force in Practice Guidelines established an important characterization of HF whereby four different stages were brought into clinical practice for better understanding of this complex syndrome: stage A, defined as the presence of high risk for HF without structural disease or symptoms; stage B, when there are no signs or symptoms but structural heart disease is present; stage C, defined as symptomatic overt HF; and stage D, when treatment-refractory HF is present.[1] When the common scenario of documented abnormal diastolic function on imaging in the setting of normal systolic performance and no symptoms is found, clinicians label it preclinical diastolic dysfunction (PDD), a condition that has been linked to the development of overt HF, reduced quality of life, and increased overall CV risk. Because of the coexistence of diastolic dysfunction with other conditions that may also cause HF symptoms, an accurate diagnosis of PDD is difficult and more so the determination of its real prevalence and true epidemiology.

In the span of a decade (2003–2012), several series that included over 6000 subjects attempted to define the epidemiology of PDD after detailed clinical and Doppler echo assessment was completed. Though it was not clear that all patients were indeed asymptomatic, depending on the severity of diastolic abnormalities found, the estimated prevalence of PDD ranged from 6% to 48% (average 20%–30%), with increasing age, CAD, diabetes, anemia, chronic obstructive pulmonary disease (COPD), and other CV comorbidities appearing as independent risks for the presence of PDD and future development of HFpEF.[77–81]

As a comprehensive review by Wan et al. alerted, two distinct facts limit the understanding of the natural history of PDD: (1) the recognition that many of the comorbidities that accompany this condition are capable of inducing symptoms on their own—the very ones that ultimately determine the development of HFpEF—implying that the evolution of PDD is simply that of the underlying disease that causes diastolic dysfunction, and (2) that whether a linear relationship can be constructed or not remains to be seen. The few studies on the subject though suggest a 3-year cumulative probability of PDD evolving into HF in the range of 6% to 31% (Fig. 29.11).[82,83]

Currently there are two scenarios where measurement of indices of myocardial deformation in the setting of asymptomatic LV diastolic dysfunction may play a clinically relevant role: (1) metabolic disorders such as diabetes, hypertension, obesity, and metabolic syndrome; and (2) cancer therapeutics-related cardiac dysfunction (CTRCD). The first group comprises entities of great epidemiologic impact all considered precursors and/or risks for the development of both HFpEF and HFrEF. In the particular case of hypertension, a reduced GLS as an index of subclinical LV dysfunction has been shown to be

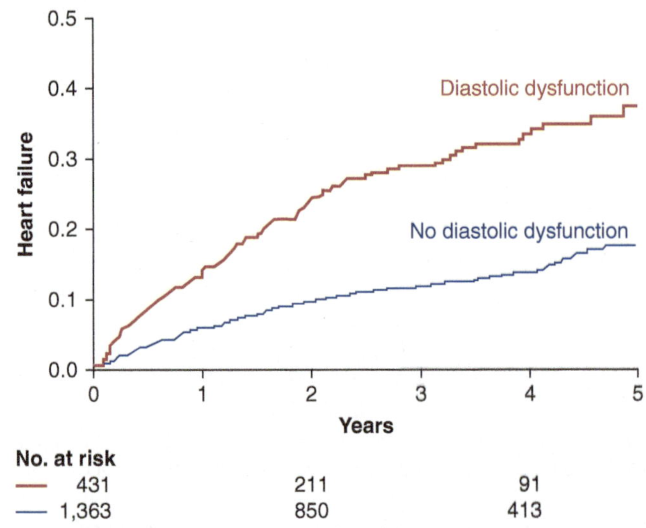

Fig. 29.11 Diastolic dysfunction and subsequent heart failure (HF) in diabetes. Subjects with diabetes and preclinical diastolic dysfunction show a higher cumulative probability of developing HF when compared with those with normal diastolic function. (Reproduced with permission from From AM, et al. The development of heart failure in patients with diabetes mellitus and pre-clinical diastolic dysfunction. A population-based study. *J Am Coll Cardiol.* 2010;55(4):300-305. doi:10.1016/j.jacc.2009.12.003.)

present in hypertensive subjects regardless of concentric hypertrophy and clinical or abnormal diastolic parameters.[84–86] Chronic hypertension is linked not only to myocyte hypertrophy but also to perivascular and myocardial fibrosis with medial thickening that could involve the coronary vessels. These important abnormalities are likely behind the well-known predictive value of hypertension for the development or potentiation of major CV events.[87–89]

To determine the long-term prognostic ability of deformation parameters in asymptomatic hypertensive heart disease, Saito et al. studied 388 subjects and correlated GLS with major adverse cardiovascular events (MACE); not only was there an association of abnormal deformation with adverse outcomes independent of clinical parameters and concentric hypertrophy, but also it was incremental, allowing accurate prediction during follow-up as well (Fig. 29.12). In fact, a combined score of age over 70 years, atrial fibrillation, concentric hypertrophy, and GLS greater than −16% carried a good discriminatory ability for MACE (C statistic of 0.71).[90]

As far as asymptomatic diabetics, in one series nearly half showed evidence of abnormal GLS in the presence of normal diastolic indices and EF, and in two other papers GLS correlated with worse outcomes even in the absence of LV dysfunction or ischemic heart disease.[91–93] Diabetes merits special attention when it comes to PDD since myocardial fibrosis and remodeling (responsible for abnormal diastolic performance) are an intricate part of its evolution and independently related to a poor outcome as proven by Holland et al.'s series (Fig. 29.13).[91]

Fig. 29.11 illustrates data from a well-designed paper that reported findings in Olmsted County, Minnesota, on subjects with PDD followed for 5 years whose 1-year and 5-year cumulative probability of developing HF was 13% and 37%, respectively.[83] Previous studies have shown that an abnormal E/e′ tends to linearly correlate with the development of HF among diabetics; however, contemporary reports have gone further suggesting that strain-defined LV dysfunction is superior in predicting worse outcomes.[51,94]

Although obesity-induced myocardial dysfunction shares common pathophysiologic phenomenon with diabetes cardiomyopathy independent of associated comorbidities, LV mass, blood pressure, or circulating insulin, two distinct features of the increasingly frequent obesity-related HF phenotype are worth noting: (1) sodium retention, with the ensuing increased plasma expansion, and (2) inflammation, a phenomenon that primarily affects adipose tissue, the vascular bed, and myocytes. As a result, LV distensibility (and deformation) is impaired, cardiac volumes increase, filling pressure rises, and clinical HF develops even though systolic performance is not substantially impaired.[95] In fact, in obese individuals strain is reduced parallel to

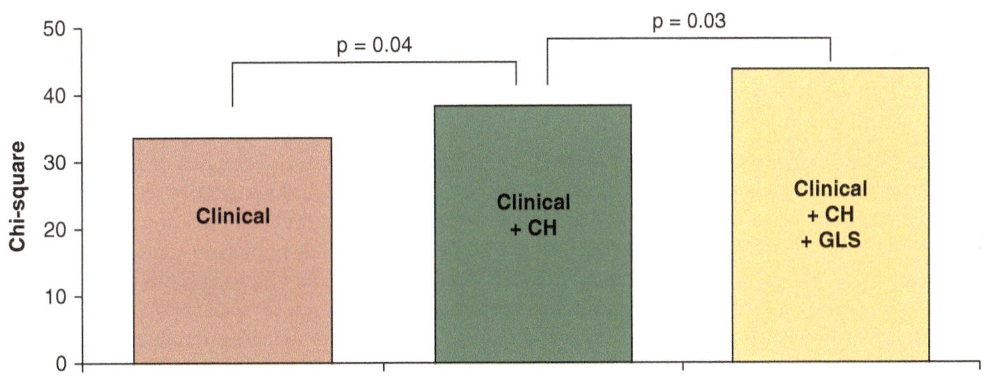

C-statistics	0.64	0.65	0.67
Variable	**Model 1 (Clinical) Chi-square = 33.4 HR (95% CI), p Value**	**Model 2 (Clinical + CH) Chi-square = 38.3 HR (95% CI), p Value**	**Model 3 (Clinical + CH + GLS) Chi-square = 44.0 HR (95% CI), p Value**
Age (per 1 yr increase)	1.03 (1.01-1.06) p < 0.01	1.03 (1.01-1.06) p < 0.01	1.03 (1.01-1.05) p = 0.01
Male	1.11 (0.69-1.78) p = 0.66	1.12 (0.70-1.78) p = 0.65	1.01 (0.62-1.63) p = 0.98
Heart Rate (per 1 mmHg increase)	1.00 (0.99-1.02) p = 0.74	1.00 (0.99-1.02) p = 0.63	1.00 (0.99-1.01) p = 0.94
Systolic Blood Pressure (per 1 mmHg increase)	0.98 (0.97-1.00) p = 0.02	0.99 (0.97-1.00) p = 0.04	0.99 (0.97-1.00) p = 0.03
Atrial Fibrillation	2.15 (1.27-3.63) p < 0.01	2.18 (1.29-3.68) p < 0.01	2.00 (1.17-3.43) p = 0.01
Concentric Hypertrophy		1.68 (1.04-2.73) p = 0.04	1.63 (1.00-3.65) p = 0.051
GLS (per 1% increase)	**heart failure (HF)**		1.08 (1.01-1.16) p = 0.03

Fig. 29.12 Myocardial deformation versus clinical variables in hypertension risk assessment. GLS provides incremental value over clinical parameters and concentric hypertrophy as a correlate of MACE. Reproduced with permission from Saito M, et al. Prognostic implications of LV strain risk score in asymptomatic patients with hypertensive heart disease. *JACC Cardiovasc Imag.* 2016;9(8):911–921. doi:10.1016/j.jcmg.2015.09.027.)

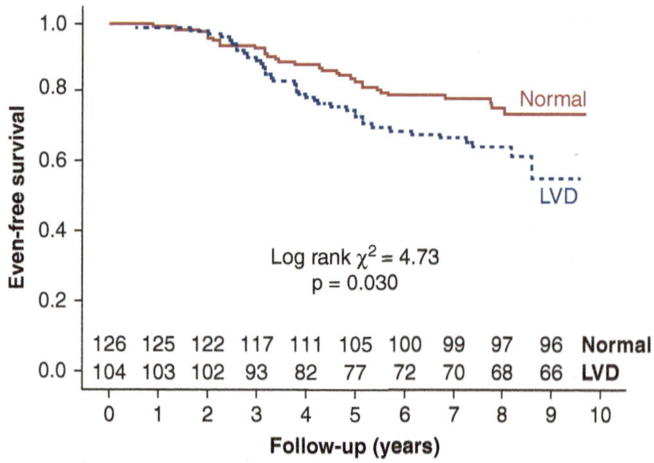

Fig. 29.13 Event-free survival of type 2 diabetes patients based on diastolic function. Subclinical LV dysfunction increases the risk of adverse outcomes (hospitalization and all-cause mortality), especially after 3 years of follow-up. (Reproduced with permission from Holland DJ, et al. Subclinical LV dysfunction and 10-year outcomes in type 2 diabetes mellitus. *Heart* 2015;101(13):1061-1066.doi:10.1136/heartjnl-2014-307391.)

their weight, a finding that makes this parameter a potentially key tool in the assessment and monitoring of weight-reducing therapies. One can only wonder if the institution of early drug interventions may successfully alter the natural history of a process already affecting millions worldwide.[95–98]

Abnormal myocardial deformation in asymptomatic LV dysfunction may play a clinically relevant role in CTRCD (defined as a reduction of >10 EF percentage points to <53%), a setting where impairment in GLS may precede and/or predict EF reduction such that according to American Society of Clinical Oncology Guidelines, a >15% relative reduction in GLS from baseline is considered a cardiotoxic response.

Although is clear that traditional CAD risk factors and comorbidities adjudicate an additive effect to the risk of development of CTRCD, strategies aimed at their modification are yet to be conclusively tested. In fact, judging by the complex interplay between cancer and CV disease risks, it is highly unlikely that definitive answers will be found soon. Therefore efforts aimed at intense risk factor modification affecting cancer patients must continue.[99,100]

A few final words about valvular heart disease. The surgical management of asymptomatic aortic stenosis/insufficiency and mitral regurgitation has traditionally relied on parameters such as the onset of symptoms, chamber enlargement, and EF change.[101] Owing to their subjectivity and unpredictability, a search for more trustworthy and reproducible measurements has remained a challenge, and LV myocardial deformation is beginning to gain a niche in this arena. Current guidelines recommend surgery for asymptomatic severe aortic stenosis if there is a reduction on EF to less than 50%. Unfortunately, it has been shown that postsurgical outcomes, including operative mortality, EF recovery, and long-term prognosis, are worse if patients undergo valve replacement with a lower EF. Meanwhile, a reduction of GLS to less than 15% in the setting of asymptomatic severe aortic stenosis with an EF greater than 50% was associated with mortality and early symptom-driven valve replacement in a series published by Yingchoncharoen. These results imply that a potential role of strain analysis in the selection of patients for intervention does exist and must be explored further.[102]

Of note, GLS has recently been found to correlate with severity of valve dysfunction, exercise tolerance, need for intervention, and ruling out need for surgery not only in aortic stenosis but also in aortic regurgitation where, after adjusting for clinical variables and LV volumes, GLS is independently associated with need for surgery or excludes its need if greater than 19.3%.[51,83,92,93] Finally, in severe primary mitral regurgitation, preoperative GLS reduction (<18%) is a strong independent predictor of postoperative LV dysfunction (EF drop to <50%) regardless of baseline EF as well.[103–109]

The strongest message suggested by the information provided in some of the studies just reviewed is not only is there much to learn about PDD and its link to HF progression but also we now have a clearer understanding of its evolution and hints on better therapies, as suggested by limited trials. It is expected that specific interventions on the horizon will hopefully be used to halt the process of HFpEF particularly in the context of hypertension, metabolic syndrome, and obesity.

In summary, indices of regional systolic performance such as TDI and strain are destined to play a critical role in the characterization and design of the very much needed targeted therapies for HFpEF patients, regardless of their clearly complex phenotypical expressions. The same could be stated about obesity, diabetes, and hypertension, prevalent comorbidities linked to HFpEF and MACE that have reached epidemic proportions worldwide. As suggested by several of the authors cited here, it is time for myocardial deformation parameters to become an integral part of HF registries, trial designs, and the routine echocardiographic evaluation of all patients suspected of or known to have HF, independent of their EF.

FUTURE DIRECTIONS

To a significant degree, progress in CV imaging in general has resulted from technological advancements and their appropriate application in the clinical arena; a few specific instances where further important contributions of various tools are expected to occur in years to come include both cardiac ultrasound and magnetic resonance.

The following represent important concepts relevant to diastology and more specifically to HFpEF, where ongoing and upcoming developments promise to help us better understand the complexities of this syndrome: modifications on speckle tracking technology, reliable and reproducible measurements of elastography, use of machine learning, blood flow visualization, and equipment miniaturization.

A recent review by Collier et al. has summarized some of the progress expected to occur in strain analysis, including full automation and 3-D software consolidation, enhancement of tracking and automatic border detection, reduction on vendor variability, and simultaneous four-chamber strain quantification. All of these will invariably lead to faster, more reliable, and widespread adoption of speckle tracking indices on most clinical laboratories.[38]

As we have seen, LV myocardial stiffness is a key component of the pathophysiology of diastolic dysfunction and HF in several clinical conditions, including hypertensive heart disease and chronic pressure overload; the tools presently available to study the dynamic pressure-related properties of the left ventricle include direct invasive measurements and strain-based indirect myocardial deformation assessment, both of which to some degree possess inaccuracies related to their load-dependent nature. Three techniques appear promising in the young field of elastography: acoustic radiation force impulse (ARFI), shear wave elasticity imaging (SWEI), and supersonic shear imaging (SSI), all using acoustic radiation forces that mechanically stimulate tissues while observing their response.[110]

These acoustic forces are natural, nonthermal biologic consequences of ultrasound generated by dynamic changes in the density of energy, the propagation of sound waves, and their behavior in tissues. By characterizing the slope of the stress-strain curve, ARFI, SWEI, and SSI are capable of directly evaluating tissue stiffness qualitatively and semiquantitatively, and on bovine and rabbit heart experimental models also measure the relaxation time constant (τ). If successfully applied to humans, elastography could become a useful tool in the design of therapeutic models aimed at restoring stiffness in the preclinical stages of diastolic dysfunction.[110]

As Tabassian et al. have recently alerted, both spatial heterogeneity and temporal dyssynchrony of function may contribute to diastolic filling in patients with HFpEF, changes that could be difficult to assess visually because of the limited resolution of human vision. These investigators tested the hypothesis that such alterations are responsible for the impaired global function and exercise capacity exhibited in the early stages of HFpEF and that a machine learning algorithm composed of an unsupervised statistical method and a supervised classifier would be useful in their demonstration during exercise testing protocols.[111]

After analysis of spatiotemporal characteristics of velocity strain and strain rate traces measured echocardiographically from 18 LV segments at rest and during supine bicycle ergometry, the authors were able to allocate subjects into various groups based on strain indices and class (symptomatic and asymptomatic) with adequate accuracy that was enhanced further after the machine learning algorithm was applied ($p < 0.0001$ for classifying subjects into four groups, and larger areas under the curve [0.70–0.89] for discrimination between symptomatic and asymptomatic).

The promise of these findings lays on the automated application of software capable of reducing interobserver and intraobserver variabilities in interpretation; if their accuracy is confirmed they may be useful to predict patient behavior during exercise and by doing so perhaps provide improved classification schemes of HFpEF.[111]

Blood flow through the cardiovascular system is not necessarily smooth and laminar even under normal conditions since it can separate into multiple streams, known as vortices, anywhere within its boundaries. This phenomenon has been linked to intracavitary thrombus formation, ventricular chamber remodeling, and worsening HF symptoms in the setting of systolic dysfunction. Several investigators have shown that abnormal vortical flow patterns can induce deleterious responses on diastole, including LA enlargement, which coupled with the presence of interatrial mechanical delay can further contribute to the occurrence of diastolic dysfunction.[111]

The currently available tools useful in the in vivo study of intracardiac flows, though still experimental, include color Doppler, velocity-encoded cardiac MRI, and echocardiographic contrast particle imaging velocimetry. With the expected technological progress and their future validation in human models, they may facilitate the selection of subgroups where specific therapeutic interventions can be tested even before the onset of symptoms, as has been proposed by Sengupta et al.[112]

Handheld echocardiographic equipment has an already demonstrated reliable diagnostic ability when used by trained noncardiologists and echocardiographers; this field has been successfully applied for some time in the field of trauma and rural pediatric cardiology care. Studies have suggested that the incremental value of point-of-care echocardiography, with or without miniaturized technology, appears to be most useful in the assessment of LV function not only during the initial diagnostic evaluation but also in the serial assessment of HF patients in settings with limited expertise.

To evaluate the usefulness of remote echocardiography in HF subjects, a recent unique trial used cardiologic consultation in addition to robot-assisted remote echo to test in a prospective, randomized, open-label fashion its feasibility and clinical value in a rural area setting. With real-time echocardiography followed by cardiologic consultation at a distance, the total diagnostic process time was substantially reduced, a finding of critical value particularly on those areas/nations where resources are limited the most.[113]

In an era where the use of eHealth solutions has become the norm and where widely available electronic wireless communication could be found everywhere regardless of economic status, these technologies promise to become essential in the evaluation and initial management of HFpEF, particularly in the acute setting.[114]

In conclusion, there is ample evidence that diastolic dysfunction, whichever its clinical manifestations may be, does not represent an isolated condition of only abnormal relaxation and loading where the presence of normal EF constitutes an indication of intact systolic function. Undoubtedly, EF should no longer be considered the only surrogate of favorable prognosis in suspected or known HF, nor can it be the sole target used in clinical trials involving patients with this syndrome. Instead, a combined approach that incorporates indices of myocardial deformation, the presence of structural changes, plus phenotypical characterization ought to become the blueprint where future efforts should concentrate in the search of improved outcomes for patients with HFpEF.[115]

ACKNOWLEDGMENTS

We thank Dr. Pamela Piña and Dr. Amparo Taveras for their invaluable contributions to this manuscript.

KEY POINTS

- Ejection fraction, by definition, is within the normal range in patients labeled as suffering from HFpEF while contractility may be not.
- EF is notably influenced by loading conditions and contractility both acutely and on chronic bases.
- Several studies have demonstrated that compared with healthy subjects and hypertensive controls with diastolic dysfunction, both LS and CS are significantly impaired in HFpEF.
- Strong evidence seems to support the notion that the prognostic value of GLS for major adverse cardiac events is indeed superior to EF in a wide range of conditions
- Indices of regional systolic performance such as TDI and strain are destined to play a critical role in the characterization and design of the very much needed targeted therapies for HFpEF patients.

REVIEW QUESTIONS

1. Choose the correct statement in reference to LV myocardial deformation.
   a. Circumferential deformation in the normal heart is counterbalanced by subendocardial but not subepicardial longitudinal fibers.
   b. Tissue Doppler imaging is harder to obtain and less accurate than speckle tracking when assessing LV deformation in hypertensive subjects.
   c. Abnormal values for GLS are considered so if higher than −20% with SD ± 2%.

   d. Age, gender, volume status, and vendor are generally not considered important sources of variability in the measurement of strain.
2. Select the correct statement about ejection fraction.
   a. It represents the single most reliable parameter to determine the etiology of dyspnea on a given patient.
   b. A reduced EF always equates with systolic dysfunction, and a preserved EF with diastolic dysfunction.
   c. In hypertrophic cardiomyopathy the EF may increase through remodeling and reduced ventricular cavity volume, rather than increased stroke volume or contractility.
   d. Changes in LV volumes generally do not impact EF.
3. Select the best answer regarding exercise testing in suspected LV diastolic dysfunction or overt HFpEF.
   a. Metabolically mediated skeletal abnormalities can interfere with exercise capacity even in the presence of a normal LV EF.
   b. Mitral annular systolic and diastolic velocities do not correlate with peak VO_2 max.
   c. Compromised LV untwisting and reduced GLS during exercise do not correlate with elevated filling pressures.
   d. Exercise testing is not useful to unmask abnormalities in LV mechanics in the presence of normal resting indices.
4. Select the best statement regarding LV systolic function in HFpEF.
   a. In HFpEF the stroke volume is typically very high.
   b. Compared with a normal ventricle, in HFpEF diastolic LV pressure is increased only when volume rises.
   c. In HFpEF the LV diastolic pressure-volume relationship curve is shifted up and to the right.
   d. Patients with HFpEF have a normal EF despite reduced longitudinal strain.

REFERENCES

1. Yancy CW, Jessup M, Bozkurt B, et al. 2013 ACCF/AHA guideline for the management of heart failure. *J Am Coll Cardiol.* 2013;62(16):e147–e239. doi: 10.1016/j.jacc.2013.05.019.
2. Zile MR, Brutsaert DL. New concepts in diastolic dysfunction and diastolic heart failure: part I. *Circulation.* 2002;105(11):1387–1393. doi: 10.1161/hc1102.105289.
3. Garg N, Senthilkumar A, Nusair MB, et al. Heart failure with a normal left ventricular ejection fraction: epidemiology, pathophysiology, diagnosis and management. *Am J Med Sci.* 2013;346(2):129–136. doi: 10.1097/MAJ.0b013e31828c586e.
4. Heidenreich PA, Albert NM, Allen LA, et al. Forecasting the impact of heart failure in the United States. *Circ Heart Fail.* 2013;6(3):606–619. doi: 10.1161/HHF.0b013e318291329a.
5. Ponikowski P, Voors AA, Anker SD, et al. 2016 ESC guidelines for the diagnosis and treatment of acute and chronic heart failure. *Eur Heart J.* 2016;37(27):2129–2200. doi: 10.1093/eurheartj/ehw128.
6. Borlaug BA, Redfield MM. Diastolic and systolic heart failure are distinct phenotypes within the heart failure spectrum. *Circulation.* 2011;123(18):2006–2014. doi: 10.1161/CIRCULATIONAHA.110.954388.
7. Del Buono MG, Buckley L, Abbate A. Primary and secondary diastolic dysfunction in heart failure with preserved ejection fraction. *Am J Cardiol.* 2018;122:1578–1587. doi: 10.1016/J.AMJCARD.2018.07.012.
8. Ambrosio G, Carluccio E. Prognostic role of left ventricular ejection fraction in heart failure: back to the future? *Int J Cardiol.* 2018;273:189–190. doi: 10.1016/j.ijcard.2018.09.025.
9. McMurray JJ. Clinical practice. Systolic heart failure. *N Engl J Med.* 2010;362(3):228–238. doi: 10.1056/NEJMcp0909392.
10. Redfield MM. Heart failure with preserved ejection fraction. Solomon CG, ed. *N Engl J Med.* 2016;375(19):1868–1877. doi: 10.1056/NEJMcp1511175.
11. Meta-analysis Global Group in Chronic Heart Failure (MAGGIC).The survival of patients with heart failure with preserved or reduced left ventricular ejection fraction: an individual patient data meta-analysis. *Eur Heart J.* 2012;33(14):1750–1757. doi: 10.1093/eurheartj/ehr254.
12. Somaratne JB, Berry C, McMurray JJV, et al. The prognostic significance of heart failure with preserved left ventricular ejection fraction: a literature-based meta-analysis. *Eur J Heart Fail.* 2009;11(9):855–862. doi: 10.1093/eurjhf/hfp103.
13. Flachskampf FA, Biering-Sørensen T, Solomon SD, et al. Cardiac imaging to evaluate left ventricular diastolic function. *JACC Cardiovasc Imag.* 2015;8(9):1071–1093. doi: 10.1016/j.jcmg.2015.07.004.
14. Lang RM, Badano LP, Mor-Avi V, et al. Recommendations for cardiac chamber quantification by echocardiography in adults: an update from the American Society of Echocardiography and the European Association of Cardiovascular Imaging. *J Am Soc Echocardiogr.* 2015;28(1):1–39. doi: 10.1016/j.echo.2014.10.003. e14.
15. Folland ED, Parisi AF, Moynihan PF, et al. Assessment of left ventricular ejection fraction and volumes by real-time, two-dimensional echocardiography. A comparison of cineangiographic and radionuclide techniques. *Circulation.* 1979;60(4):760–766.
16. Parisi AF, Moynihan PF, Feldman CL, et al. Approaches to determination of left ventricular volume and ejection fraction by real-time two-dimensional echocardiography. *Clin Cardiol.* 1979;2(4):257–263. doi: 10.1002/clc.4960020404.
17. Starling MR, Crawford MH, Sorensen SG, et al. Comparative accuracy of apical biplane cross-sectional echocardiography and gated equilibrium radionuclide angiography for estimating left ventricular size and performance. *Circulation.* 1981;63(5):1075–1084. doi: 10.1161/01.CIR.63.5.1075.
18. Konstam MA, Abboud FM. Ejection fraction. *Circulation.* 2017;135(8):717–719. doi: 10.1161/CIRCULATIONAHA.116.025795.
19. Yip GW, Frenneaux M, Sanderson JE. Heart failure with a normal ejection fraction: new developments. *Heart.* 2009;95(19):1549–1552. doi: 10.1136/hrt.2009.176222.
20. Kalam K, Otahal P, Marwick TH. Prognostic implications of global LV dysfunction: a systematic review and meta-analysis of global longitudinal strain and ejection fraction. *Heart.* 2014;100(21):1673–1680. doi: 10.1136/heartjnl-2014-305538.
21. Aurigemma GP, Zile MR, Gaasch WH. Contractile behavior of the left ventricle in diastolic heart failure. *Circulation.* 2006;113(2):296–304. doi: 10.1161/CIRCULATIONAHA.104.481465.
22. Baicu CF, Zile MR, Aurigemma GP, et al. Left ventricular systolic performance, function, and contractility in patients with diastolic heart failure. *Circulation.* 2005;111(18):2306–2312. doi: 10.1161/01.CIR.0000164273.57823.26.
23. Carluccio E, Biagioli P, Alunni G, et al. Advantages of deformation indices over systolic velocities in assessment of longitudinal systolic function in patients with heart failure and normal ejection fraction. *Eur J Heart Fail.* 2011;13(3):292–302. doi: 10.1093/eurjhf/hfq203.
24. Wang J, Khoury DS, Yue Y, et al. Preserved left ventricular twist and circumferential deformation, but depressed longitudinal and radial deformation in patients with diastolic heart failure. *Eur Heart J.* 2007;29(10):1283–1289. doi: 10.1093/eurheartj/ehn141.
25. Biering-Sørensen T, Solomon SD. Assessing contractile function when ejection fraction is normal. *Circ Cardiovasc Imag.* 2015;8(11):e004181. doi: 10.1161/CIRCIMAGING.115.004181.
26. Shah SJ, Katz DH, Selvaraj S, et al. Phenomapping for novel classification of heart failure with preserved ejection fraction. *Circulation.* 2015;131(3):269–279. doi: 10.1161/CIRCULATIONAHA.114.010637.
27. Omar AM, Bansal M, Sengupta PP. Advances in echocardiographic imaging in heart failure with reduced and preserved ejection fraction. *Circ Res.* 2016;119(2):357–374. doi: 10.1161/CIRCRESAHA.116.309128.
28. Cikes M, Solomon SD. Beyond ejection fraction: an integrative approach for assessment of cardiac structure and function in heart failure. *Eur Heart J.* 2016;37(21):1642–1650. doi: 10.1093/eurheartj/ehv510.

29. Tan YT, Wenzelburger F, Lee E, et al. The pathophysiology of heart failure with normal ejection fraction: exercise echocardiography reveals complex abnormalities of both systolic and diastolic ventricular function involving torsion, untwist, and longitudinal motion. *J Am Coll Cardiol.* 2009;54(1):36–46. doi: 10.1016/J.JACC.2009.03.037.
30. Dorfs S, Zeh W, Hochholzer W, et al. Pulmonary capillary wedge pressure during exercise and long-term mortality in patients with suspected heart failure with preserved ejection fraction. *Eur Heart J.* 2014;35(44):3103–3112. doi: 10.1093/eurheartj/ehu315.
31. Brown J, Jenkins C, Marwick TH. Use of myocardial strain to assess global left ventricular function: a comparison with cardiac magnetic resonance and 3-dimensional echocardiography. *Am Heart J.* 2009;157(1):102.e1–102.e5. doi: 10.1016/J.AHJ.2008.08.032.
32. Stanton T, Leano R, Marwick TH. Prediction of all-cause mortality from global longitudinal speckle strain. *Circ Cardiovasc Imag.* 2009;2(5):356–364. doi: 10.1161/CIRCIMAGING.109.862334.
33. Zile MR, Baicu CF, Ikonomidis JS, et al. Myocardial stiffness in patients with heart failure and a preserved ejection fraction: contributions of collagen and titin. *Circulation.* 2015;131(14):1247–1259. doi: 10.1161/CIRCULATIONAHA.114.013215.
34. van Heerebeek L, Borbély A, Niessen HWM, et al. Myocardial structure and function differ in systolic and diastolic heart failure. *Circulation.* 2006;113(16):1966–1973. doi: 10.1161/CIRCULATIONAHA.105.587519.
35. Kraigher-Krainer E, Shah AM, Gupta DK, et al. Impaired systolic function by strain imaging in heart failure with preserved ejection fraction. *J Am Coll Cardiol.* 2014;63(5):447–456. doi: 10.1016/j.jacc.2013.09.052.
36. Torrent-Guasp F, Buckberg GD, Clemente C, et al. The structure and function of the helical heart and its buttress wrapping. I. The normal macroscopic structure of the heart. *Semin Thorac Cardiovasc Surg.* 2001;13(4):301–319.
37. Claus P, Omar AMS, Pedrizzetti G, et al. Tissue tracking technology for assessing cardiac mechanics. *JACC Cardiovasc Imag.* 2015;8(12):1444–1460. doi: 10.1016/j.jcmg.2015.11.001.
38. Collier P, Phelan D, Klein A. A test in context: myocardial strain measured by speckle-tracking echocardiography. *J Am Coll Cardiol.* 2017;69(8):1043–1056. doi: 10.1016/j.jacc.2016.12.012.
39. Edvardsen T, Haugaa KH. Imaging assessment of ventricular mechanics. *Heart.* 2011;97(16):1349–1356. doi: 10.1136/hrt.2009.184390.
40. Petrie MC, Caruana L, Berry C, et al. Diastolic heart failure" or heart failure caused by subtle left ventricular systolic dysfunction? *Heart.* 2002;87(1):29–31.
41. Iwanaga Y, Nishi I, Furuichi S, et al. B-type natriuretic peptide strongly reflects diastolic wall stress in patients with chronic heart failure: comparison between systolic and diastolic heart failure. *J Am Coll Cardiol.* 2006;47(4):742–748. doi: 10.1016/j.jacc.2005.11.030.
42. Karasek D, Sinkiewicz W, Błażejewski J. Relationship between B-type natriuretic peptide serum level, echocardiographic TEI index and the degree of diastolic dysfunction in patients with heart failure with preserved systolic function. *Arch Med Sci.* 2011;3:449–456. doi: 10.5114/aoms.2011.23411.
43. Yip GW, Zhang Q, Xie JM, et al. Resting global and regional left ventricular contractility in patients with heart failure and normal ejection fraction: insights from speckle-tracking echocardiography. *Heart.* 2011;97(4):287–294. doi: 10.1136/hrt.2010.205815.
44. Sengupta PP, Korinek J, Belohlavek M, et al. Left ventricular structure and function. *J Am Coll Cardiol.* 2006;48(10):1988–2001. doi: 10.1016/j.jacc.2006.08.030.
45. Chung CS, Shmuylovich L, Kovács SJ. What global diastolic function is, what it is not, and how to measure it. *Am J Physiol Heart Circ Physiol.* 2015;309(9):H1392–H1406. doi: 10.1152/ajpheart.00436.2015.
46. Gaasch WH, Little WC. Assessment of left ventricular diastolic function and recognition of diastolic heart failure. *Circulation.* 2007;116(6):591–593. doi: 10.1161/CIRCULATIONAHA.107.716647.
47. Sengupta PP, Tajik AJ, Chandrasekaran K, et al. Twist mechanics of the left ventricle. Principles and application. *JACC Cardiovasc Imag.* 2008;1(3):366–376. doi: 10.1016/j.jcmg.2008.02.006.
48. Gupta H, Sharifov OF, Schiros CSG, et al. Left ventricular torsion shear angle volume approach for noninvasive evaluation of diastolic dysfunction in preserved ejection fraction. *J Am Heart Assoc.* 2018;69(11):1442. doi: 10.1161/JAHA.117.007039.
49. Opdahl A, Remme EW, Helle-Valle T, et al. Myocardial relaxation, restoring forces, and early-diastolic load are independent determinants of left ventricular untwisting rate. *Circulation.* 2012;126(12):1441–1451. doi: 10.1161/CIRCULATIONAHA.111.080861.
50. Opdahl A, Remme EW, Helle-Valle T, et al. Determinants of left ventricular early-diastolic lengthening velocity. *Circulation.* 2009;119(19):2578–2586. doi: 10.1161/CIRCULATIONAHA.108.791681.
51. Ernande L, Bergerot C, Rietzschel ER, et al. Diastolic dysfunction in patients with type 2 diabetes mellitus: is it really the first marker of diabetic cardiomyopathy? *J Am Soc Echocardiogr.* 2001;24(11):1268–1275. doi: 10.1016/J.ECHO.2011.07.017. e1.
52. Park YS, Park JH, Ahn KT, et al. Usefulness of mitral annular systolic velocity in the detection of left ventricular systolic dysfunction: comparison with three dimensional echocardiographic data. *J Cardiovasc Ultrasound.* 2010;18(1):1–5. doi: 10.4250/jcu.2010.18.1.1.
53. Yip G, Wang M, Zhang Y, et al. Left ventricular long axis function in diastolic heart failure is reduced in both diastole and systole: time for a redefinition? *Heart.* 2002;87(2):121–125.
54. Borlaug BA, Kass DA. Invasive hemodynamic assessment in heart failure. *Heart Fail Clin.* 2009;5(2):217–228. doi: 10.1016/j.hfc.2008.11.008.
55. Chirinos JA. Ventricular-arterial coupling: invasive and non-invasive assessment. *Artery Res.* 2013;7:2–14. doi: 10.1016/j.artres.2012.12.002.
56. Li JK, Atlas G. Left ventricle-arterial system interaction in heart failure. *Clin Med Insights Cardiol.* 2015;9(1):S93–S99. doi: 10.4137/CMC.S18742.
57. Hung J, Lang R, Flachskampf F, et al. 3D echocardiography: a review of the current status and future directions. *J Am Soc Echocardiogr.* 2007;20(3):213–233. doi: 10.1016/j.echo.2007.01.010.
58. Dorosz JL, Lezotte DC, Weitzenkamp DA, et al. Performance of 3-dimensional echocardiography in measuring left ventricular volumes and ejection fraction. *J Am Coll Cardiol.* 2012;59(20):1799–1808. doi: 10.1016/j.jacc.2012.01.037.
59. Reichek N, Wilson J, St John Sutton M, et al. Noninvasive determination of left ventricular end-systolic stress: validation of the method and initial application. *Circulation.* 1982;65(1):99–108.
60. Mosleh W, Elango K, Shah T, et al. Elevated end-diastolic wall stress after acute myocardial infarction predicts adverse cardiovascular outcomes and longer hospital length of stay. *Echocardiography.* 2018;35:1721–1728. doi: 10.1111/echo.14136.
61. Alter P, Rupp H, Stoll F, et al. Increased end diastolic wall stress precedes left ventricular hypertrophy in dilative heart failure—use of the volume-based wall stress index. *Int J Cardiol.* 2012;157(2):233–238. doi: 10.1016/J.IJCARD.2011.07.092.
62. Chung N, Nishimura RA, Holmes Jr DR, et al. Measurement of left ventricular dp/dt by simultaneous doppler echocardiography and cardiac catheterization. *J Am Soc Echocardiogr.* 1992;5(2):147–152. doi: 10.1016/S0894-7317(14)80544-0.
63. Bai XF, Ma AX. Symmetry of cardiac function assessment. *J Geriatr Cardiol.* 2016;13(6):517–520. doi: 10.11909/j.issn.1671-5411.2016.06.014.
64. Tei C, Ling LH, Hodge DO, et al. Rodeheffer RJ, et al. New index of combined systolic and diastolic myocardial performance: a simple and reproducible measure of cardiac function—a study in normals and dilated cardiomyopathy. *J Cardiol.* 1995;26(6):357–366.
65. Nagueh SF, Smiseth OA, Appleton CP, et al. Recommendations for the evaluation of left ventricular diastolic function by echocardiography: an update from the American Society of Echocardiography and the European Association of Cardiovascular Imaging. *J Am Soc Echocardiogr.* 2016;29(4):277–314. doi: 10.1016/j.echo.2016.01.011.
66. Phelan D, Collier P, Thavendiranathan P, et al. Relative apical sparing of longitudinal strain using two-dimensional speckle-tracking echocardiography is both sensitive and specific for the diagnosis of cardiac amyloidosis. *Heart.* 2012;98(19):1442–1448. doi: 10.1136/heartjnl-2012-302353.
67. Espe EKS, Aronsen JM, Eriksen M, et al. Regional dysfunction after myocardial infarction in rats. *Circ Cardiovasc Imag.* 2017;10(9). doi: 10.1161/CIRCIMAGING.116.005997.

68. Aurigemma GP, Silver KH, Priest MA, et al. Geometric changes allow normal ejection fraction despite depressed myocardial shortening in hypertensive left ventricular hypertrophy. *J Am Coll Cardiol.* 1995;26(1):195–202. doi: 10.1016/0735-1097(95)00153-Q.
69. MacIver DH, Adeniran I, Zhang H. Left ventricular ejection fraction is determined by both global myocardial strain and wall thickness. *Int J Cardiol Heart Vasc.* 2015;7:113–118. doi: 10.1016/J.IJCHA.2015.03.007.
70. Nagueh SF, Chang SM, Nabi F, et al. Cardiac imaging in patients with heart failure and preserved ejection fraction. *Circ Cardiovasc Imag.* 2017;10(9):e006547. doi: 10.1161/CIRCIMAGING.117.006547.
71. Reddy YN, Borlaug BA. Heart failure with preserved ejection fraction. *Curr Prob Cardiol.* 2016;41(4):145–188. doi: 10.1016/j.cpcardiol.2015.12.002.
72. Kao DP, Lewsey JD, Anand IS, et al. Characterization of subgroups of heart failure patients with preserved ejection fraction with possible implications for prognosis and treatment response. *Eur J Heart Fail.* 2015;17(9):925–935. doi: 10.1002/ejhf.327.
73. Yu CM, Lin H, Yang H, et al. Progression of systolic abnormalities in patients with "Isolated" diastolic heart failure and diastolic dysfunction. *Circulation.* 2002;105(10):1195–1201. doi: 10.1161/hc1002.105185.
74. Vinereanu D, Nicolaides E, Tweddel AC, et al. "Pure" diastolic dysfunction is associated with long-axis systolic dysfunction. Implications for the diagnosis and classification of heart failure. *Eur J Heart Fail.* 2005;7(5):820–828. doi: 10.1016/j.ejheart.2005.02.003.
75. Park JJ, Park JB, Park JH, et al. Global longitudinal strain to predict mortality in patients with acute heart failure. *J Am Coll Cardiol.* 2018;71(18):1947–1957. doi: 10.1016/J.JACC.2018.02.064.
76. Shah AM, Claggett B, Sweitzer NK, et al. Prognostic importance of impaired systolic function in heart failure with preserved ejection fraction and the impact of spironolactone. *Circulation.* 2015;132(5):402–414. doi: 10.1161/CIRCULATIONAHA.115.015884.
77. Redfield MM, Jacobsen SJ, Burnett Jr JC, et al. Burden of systolic and diastolic ventricular dysfunction in the community. *JAMA.* 2003;289(2):194–202. doi: 10.1001/jama.289.2.194.
78. Lam CS, Lyass A, Kraigher-Krainer E, et al. Cardiac dysfunction and noncardiac dysfunction as precursors of heart failure with reduced and preserved ejection fraction in the community. *Circulation.* 2011;124(1):24–30. doi: 10.1161/CIRCULATIONAHA.110.979203.
79. Mureddu GF, Agabiti N, Rizzello V, et al. Prevalence of preclinical and clinical heart failure in the elderly. A population-based study in Central Italy. *Eur J Heart Fail.* 2012;14(7):718–729. doi: 10.1093/eurjhf/hfs052.
80. Le Jemtel TH, Padeletti M, Jelic S. Diagnostic and therapeutic challenges in patients with coexistent chronic obstructive pulmonary disease and chronic heart failure. *J Am Coll Cardiol.* 2007;49(2):171–180. doi: 10.1016/j.jacc.2006.08.046.
81. Mascarenhas J, Azevedo A, Bettencourt P. Coexisting chronic obstructive pulmonary disease and heart failure: implications for treatment, course and mortality. *Curr Opin Pulm Med.* 2010;16(2):106–111. doi: 10.1097/MCP.0b013e328335dc90.
82. Wan SH, Vogel MW, Chen HH. Pre-clinical diastolic dysfunction. *J Am Coll Cardiol.* 2014;63(5):407–416. doi: 10.1016/j.jacc.2013.10.063.
83. From AM, Scott CG, Chen HH. The development of heart failure in patients with diabetes mellitus and pre-clinical diastolic dysfunction. A population-based study. *J Am Coll Cardiol.* 2010;55(4):300–305. doi: 10.1016/j.jacc.2009.12.003.
84. Drazner MH. The progression of hypertensive heart disease. *Circulation.* 2011;123(3):327–334. doi: 10.1161/CIRCULATIONAHA.108.845792.
85. Messerli FH, Williams B, Ritz E. Essential hypertension. *Lancet (London, England).* 2007;370(9587):591–603. doi: 10.1016/S0140-6736(07)61299-9.
86. Iwashima Y, Horio T, Suzuki Y, et al. Impact of concomitant diabetes and chronic kidney disease on preload-induced changes in left ventricular diastolic filling in hypertensive patients. *J Hypertens.* 2011;29(1):144–153. doi: 10.1097/HJH.0b013e32833f387c.
87. Tocci G, Sciarretta S, Volpe M. Development of heart failure in recent hypertension trials. *J Hypertens.* 2008;26(7):1477–1486. doi: 10.1097/HJH.0b013e3282fe1d3d.
88. Lee WH, Liu YW, Yang LT, et al. Prognostic value of longitudinal strain of subepicardial myocardium in patients with hypertension. *J Hypertens.* 2016;34(6):1195–1200. doi: 10.1097/HJH.0000000000000903.
89. Szelényi Z, Fazakas Á, Szénási G, et al. The mechanism of reduced longitudinal left ventricular systolic function in hypertensive patients with normal ejection fraction. *J Hypertens.* 2013;33(9):1962–1969. doi: 10.1097/HJH.0000000000000624.
90. Saito M, Khan F, Stoklosa T, et al. Prognostic implications of LV strain risk score in asymptomatic patients with hypertensive heart disease. *JACC Cardiovasc Imag.* 2016;9(8):911–921. doi: 10.1016/j.jcmg.2015.09.027.
91. Holland DJ, Marwick TH, Haluska BA, et al. Subclinical LV dysfunction and 10-year outcomes in type 2 diabetes mellitus. *Heart.* 2015;101(13):1061–1066. doi: 10.1136/heartjnl-2014-307391.
92. Kiencke S, Handschin R, von Dahlen R, et al. Pre-clinical diabetic cardiomyopathy: prevalence, screening, and outcome. *Eur J Heart Fail.* 2010;12(9):951–957. doi: 10.1093/eurjhf/hfq110.
93. Miki T, Yuda S, Kouzu H, et al. Diabetic cardiomyopathy: pathophysiology and clinical features. *Heart Fail Rev.* 2013;18(2):149–166. doi: 10.1007/s10741-012-9313-3.
94. Liu JH, Chen Y, Yuen M, et al. Incremental prognostic value of global longitudinal strain in patients with type 2 diabetes mellitus. *Cardiovasc Diabetol.* 2016;15:22. doi: 10.1186/s12933-016-0333-5.
95. Packer M, Kitzman DW. Obesity-related heart failure with a preserved ejection fraction: the mechanistic rationale for combining inhibitors of aldosterone, neprilysin, and sodium-glucose cotransporter-2. *JACC Heart Fail.* 2018;6(8):633–639. doi: 10.1016/J.JCHF.2018.01.009.
96. Obokata M, Reddy YNV, Pislaru SV, et al. Evidence supporting the existence of a distinct obese phenotype of heart failure with preserved ejection fraction. *Circulation.* 2017;136(1):6–19. doi: 10.1161/CIRCULATIONAHA.116.026807.
97. Dornfeld LP, Maxwell MH, Waks A, et al. Mechanisms of hypertension in obesity. *Kidney Int.* 1987;22:S254–S258.
98. John JM, Haykowsky M, Brubaker P, et al. Decreased left ventricular distensibility in response to postural change in older patients with heart failure and preserved ejection fraction. *Am J Physiol Heart Circ Physiol.* 2010;299(3):H883–H889. doi: 10.1152/ajpheart.00332.2010.
99. Plana J, Galderisi M, Barac A, et al. Scherrer-Crosbie M, et al. Expert consensus for multimodality imaging evaluation of adult patients during and after cancer therapy: a report from the American Society of Echocardiography and the European Association of Cardiovascular Imaging from the Cleveland Clinic. *J Am Soc Echocardiogr.* 2014;27:911–939. doi: 10.1016/j.echo.2014.07.012.
100. Armenian SH, Lacchetti C, Barac A, et al. Denduluri N, et al. Prevention and monitoring of cardiac dysfunction in survivors of adult cancers: American Society of Clinical Oncology clinical practice guideline. *J Clin Oncol.* 2017;35(8):893–911. doi: 10.1200/JCO.2016.70.5400.
101. Nishimura RA, Otto CM, Bonow RO, et al. 2014 AHA/ACC guideline for the management of patients with valvular heart disease. *J Thorac Cardiovasc Surg.* 2014;148(1):e1–e132. doi: 10.1016/j.jtcvs.2014.05.014.
102. Yingchoncharoen T, Gibby C, Rodriguez LL, et al. Association of myocardial deformation with outcome in asymptomatic aortic stenosis with normal ejection fraction. *Circ Cardiovasc Imag.* 2012;5(6):719–725. doi: 10.1161/CIRCIMAGING.112.977348.
103. Kearney LG, Lu K, Ord M, et al. Global longitudinal strain is a strong independent predictor of all-cause mortality in patients with aortic stenosis. *Eur Heart J Cardiovasc Imag.* 2012;13(10):827–833. doi: 10.1093/ehjci/jes115.
104. Lafitte S, Perlant M, Reant P, et al. Impact of impaired myocardial deformation on exercise tolerance and prognosis in patients with asymptomatic aortic stenosis. *Eur J Echocardiogr.* 2009;10(3):414–419. doi: 10.1093/ejechocard/jen299.
105. Lancellotti P, Donal E, Magne J, et al. Risk stratification in asymptomatic moderate to severe aortic stenosis: the importance of the valvular, arterial and ventricular interplay. *Heart.* 2010;96(17):1364–1371. doi: 10.1136/hrt.2009.190942.

106. Ewe SH, Haeck ML, Ng AC, et al. Detection of subtle left ventricular systolic dysfunction in patients with significant aortic regurgitation and preserved left ventricular ejection fraction: speckle tracking echocardiographic analysis. *Eur Heart J Cardiovasc Imag.* 2015;16(9):992–999. doi: 10.1093/ehjci/jev019.
107. Mentias A, Naji P, Gillinov AM, et al. Strain echocardiography and functional capacity in asymptomatic primary mitral regurgitation with preserved ejection fraction. *J Am Coll Cardiol.* 2016;68(18):1974–1986. doi: 10.1016/J.JACC.2016.08.030.
108. Mascle S, Schnell F, Thebault C, et al. Predictive value of global longitudinal strain in a surgical population of organic mitral regurgitation. *J Am Soc of Echocardiogr.* 2012;25(7):766–772. doi: 10.1016/J.ECHO.2012.04.009.
109. Witkowski TG, Thomas JD, Debonnaire PJ, et al. Global longitudinal strain predicts left ventricular dysfunction after mitral valve repair. *Eur Heart J Cardiovasc Imag.* 2013;14(1):69–76. doi: 10.1093/ehjci/jes155.
110. Dave JK, Mc Donald ME, Mehrotra P, et al. Recent technological advancements in cardiac ultrasound imaging. *Ultrasonics.* 2018;84:329–340. doi: 10.1016/J.ULTRAS.2017.11.013.
111. Tabassian M, Sunderji I, Erdei T, et al. Diagnosis of heart failure with preserved ejection fraction: machine learning of spatiotemporal variations in left ventricular deformation. *J Am Soc Echocardiogr.* 2018;31(12):1272–1284 doi: 10.1016/j.echo.2018.07.013. 1272-1284.e9.
112. Sengupta PP, Burke R, Khandheria BK, et al. Following the flow in chambers. *Heart Fail Clin.* 2008;4(3):325–332. doi: 10.1016/j.hfc.2008.02.005.
113. Boman K, Olofsson M, Berggren P, et al. Robot-assisted remote echocardiographic examination and teleconsultation: a randomized comparison of time to diagnosis with standard of care referral approach. *JACC Cardiovasc Imag.* 2014;7:799–803. doi: 10.1016/j.jcmg.2014.05.006.
114. Sengupta PP, Pedrizzetti G, Kilner PJ, et al. Emerging trends in CV flow visualization. *JACC Cardiovasc Imag.* 2012;5(3):305–316. doi: 10.1016/j.jcmg.2012.01.003.
115. Potter E, Marwick TH. Assessment of left ventricular function by echocardiography. The case for routinely adding global longitudinal strain to ejection fraction. *JACC Cardiovasc Imag.* 2018;11:260–274. doi: 10.1016/j.jcmg.2017.11.017.

30

Chronotropic Incompetence and Pacing in HPEF Heart Failure with Preserved Ejection Fraction

Cameron T. Lambert and Richard A. Grimm

OUTLINE

Case Study

A 70-year-old female with a history of hypertension, hyperlipidemia, paroxysmal atrial fibrillation (AFib), and complete heart block with a dual chamber permanent pacemaker implanted 10 years prior presented to the cardiology clinic with exertional dyspnea and fatigue for evaluation. Within the last year the patient had received a diagnosis of nonischemic cardiomyopathy (NICM) with an ejection fraction (EF) of 25%. Diagnostic coronary angiogram was normal at an outside hospital. Echocardiogram on the day of her clinic visit confirmed the EF of 25% with global LV hypokinesis and showed a left ventricular (LV) end-diastolic diameter (EDD) of 5 cm, normal RV size and function. Her mitral and tricuspid valves both had trivial regurgitation. Physical exam showed normal vital signs, bilateral lower lobe fine crackles, and mildly elevated jugular venous pressure (JVP). Additionally, her extremities were warm with trace pitting edema to the ankles. Pacemaker interrogation in the office showed a dual-chamber permanent pacemaker with a 99% right ventricular (RV) pacing burden. Given the timeline of events and onset of her cardiomyopathy, a diagnosis of pacing-induced cardiomyopathy was considered.

Based on the working diagnosis and RV pacing burden, she underwent a successful upgrade to a cardiac resynchronization therapy (CRT) capable device and was referred for echocardiogram-guided atrioventricular (AV) optimization. Her underlying rhythm was complete heart block. The initial AV delay was set to 130 msec. Pulsed-wave Doppler sampling from the mitral valve (MV) inflow is seen in Fig. 30.1. The E and A waves were separated; however, the E wave was greater than the A wave. The left ventricular outflow tract (LVOT) velocity time integral (VTI) at this AV delay was ~15 cm. Multiple AV delays were tested during her AV optimization echocardiogram, including 180, 200, 220, and 240 msec. MV inflow and LVOT VTI were assessed at each setting. At 240 msec, the A wave amplitude was significantly greater than the E wave amplitude, and the LVOT VTI increased to ~19 cm. This represented an improvement in her diastolic function from grade III to grade I (Fig. 30.2). Furthermore, AV synchrony improved as the interval between the QRS onset and the end of A wave (QA) duration improved from 120 msec at baseline to 60 msec at the final AV delay of 240 msec.

Six months after her CRT implant and echocardiogram-based AV optimization, the patient presented for follow-up in clinic. She reported New York Heart Association (NYHA) Class I symptoms and an improved exercise tolerance. Her physical exam was significant for clear lung fields, normal central venous pressures, and no lower extremity edema. Follow-up echocardiogram showed an LV EF of 45%, grade I diastolic dysfunction, trace mitral regurgitation (MR), and trace tricuspid regurgitation (TR).

INTRODUCTION

There are approximately 550,000 new cases added to the at least 5 million Americans living with heart failure (HF) each year. Of these cases, approximately 40% to 50% are classified as diastolic HF or more currently heart failure with preserved ejection fraction (HFpEF).[1] HFpEF is defined by abnormalities in LV relaxation, diastolic distensibility, and stiffness.[2,3] Histologically these physiologic abnormalities may manifest as myocyte hypertrophy, increased myofibrillar density, elevated myocyte relative thickness, and increased myofilamentary calcium sensitivity.[3,4] Accurate diagnosis of HFpEF can be difficult, but patients typically have at least one abnormal measurement on hemodynamic heart catheterization or echocardiography supporting this diagnosis.

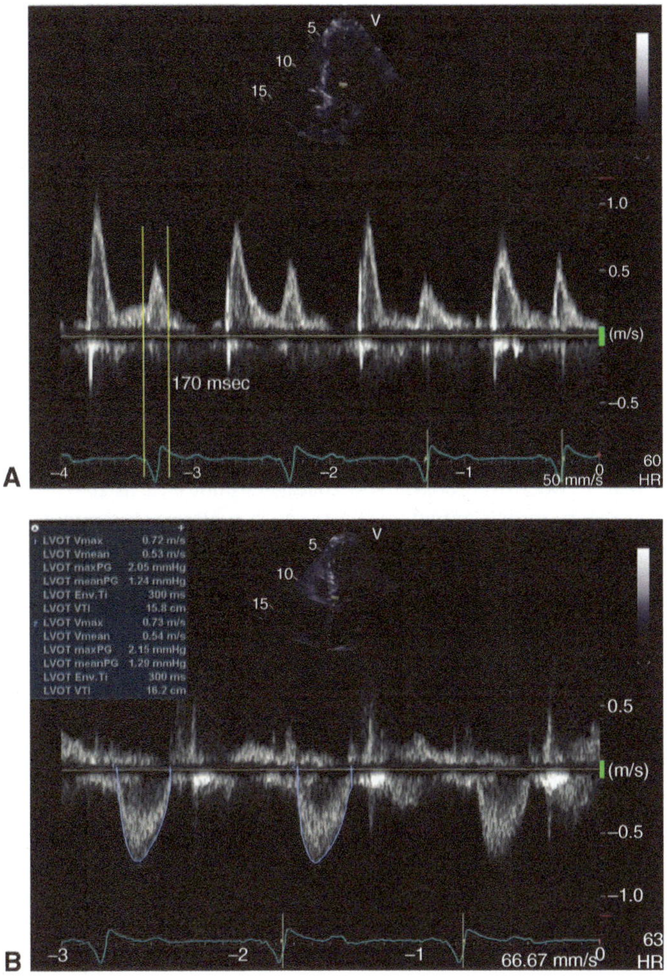

Fig. 30.1 Baseline images obtained with an AV delay of 130 msec. (A) Pulsed-wave Doppler recordings from the level of the mitral valve leaflet tips. Note the E wave peak velocity is significantly greater than the A wave peak velocity. The QA interval (time from onset of QRS to end of A wave) is 170 msec, which is representative of a wasted atrial contribution to ventricular filling. (B) LVOT VTI at this AV delay.

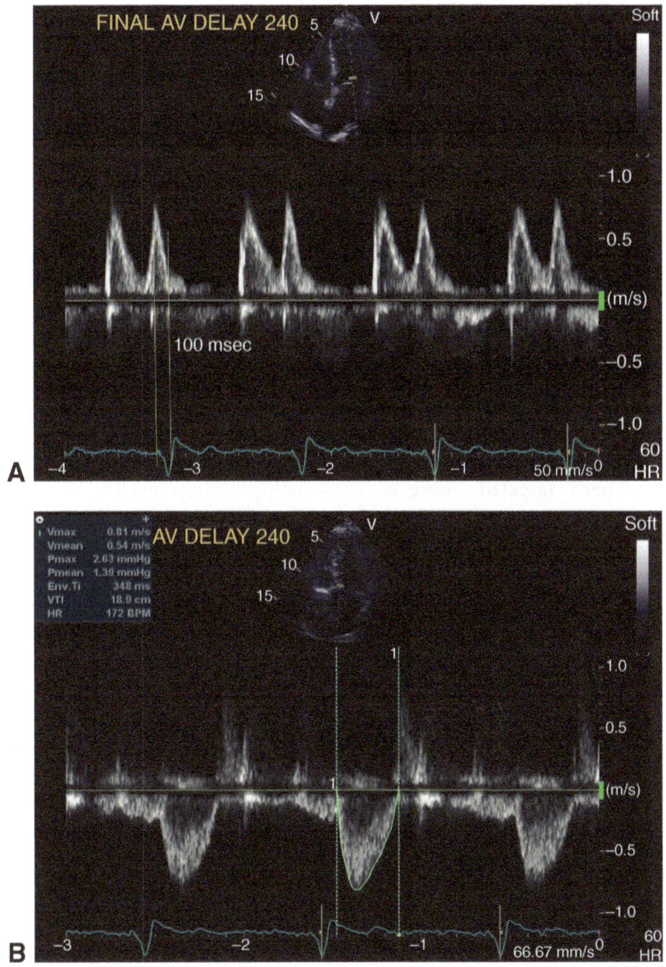

Fig. 30.2 Images obtained with an AV delay of 240 msec. (A) Pulsed-wave Doppler recordings from the level of the mitral valve leaflet tips. Note the E wave peak velocity is nearly equal to the A wave peak velocity. The QA interval has decreased to 100 msec, which is representative of the atrial contraction contributing to ventricular filling. (B) Improved LVOT VTI at this AV delay.

Diastolic filling is influenced by many physiologic variables as briefly mentioned. The cardiac cycle length and the relative timing of atrial and ventricular contractions are also major contributors, to diastolic function. Permanent pacemakers (PPM) influence cardiac cycle timing and have been shown to induce and treat HFpEF. Influencing this relationship are various PPM programming modes and pacing locations. In this chapter the relationship between PPM and diastolic function will be explored with emphasis on the pathophysiology, diagnosis, treatment, and future technologies.

BASIC FUNCTION OF PERMANENT CARDIAC PACEMAKERS

A permanent pacemaker is a system composed of a pulse generator and various forms of leads, which deliver an electrical pulse to the myocardium—within either the endocardium or epicardium. This electrical charge, if above a critical threshold, prompts myocardial cell action potential propagation. This propagation moves away from the electrode in a radial direction. A critical foundational concept is the coupling between electrical and mechanical activation. Myocardial contraction follows electrical stimulation and is impacted by many hemodynamic principles.

The most basic PPM configuration consists of a pulse generator within a prepectoral pocket (typically the patient's left side) and a single lead coursing through the subclavian vein into the right ventricular apex. This configuration leads to a ventricular activation sequence originating in the ventricular apex and coursing posteriorly and toward the base. LV activation occurs after the wave of depolarization traverses the septal myocardium. This sequential (RV followed by LV) activation inherently leads to mechanical dyssynchrony and can affect systolic and diastolic function. An obvious drawback to this configuration of pacing is the lack of attention paid to the atrial activity. Without understanding atrial activity there can be a loss of AV coupling, which can decrease cardiac output by creating suboptimal diastolic filling times, provide an inadequate atrial contribution to LV filling, create poorly tolerated symptoms of palpitations, and predispose the patient to cardiac arrhythmias. Dual-chamber pacemakers circumvent these problems by adding a second lead from the pulse generator, which stimulates the right atrium. There, the lead can sense intrinsic atrial depolarizations and provide AV synchrony with prespecified AV delays.[5]

Cardiac resynchronization therapy pacing adds another dimension to pacing's influence on the cardiac cycle—intraventricular synchrony. CRT requires placement of at least two leads onto the ventricular myocardium. Most commonly a transvenous RV apex lead and a transvenous lead placed onto the LV posterolateral wall via a coronary sinus branch. If coronary sinus anatomy is not favorable or does not permit passage of a lead, epicardial leads can be placed onto the posterolateral LV wall. Historically this technology has been recommended for patients with NYHA Class III/IV symptoms and an LV EF of 35% or less refractory to drug therapy. These patients should have a left bundle branch block (BBB) QRS morphology and a QRS interval of at least 120 msec and preferably more than 150 msec (an indicator of interventricular [VV] dyssynchrony).[4,6] While left BBB has traditionally been targeted with CRT devices, right BBB QRS morphologies have also been targeted, however with disappointing results. Despite some success, there is still a paucity of data in this area.[6] In addition to a wide (QRS >120 msec) and left BBB pattern QRS on electrocardiogram, patients with significant intraventricular and interventricular dyssynchrony can be identified with standard echocardiography. This technology may not only assist in diagnosis but also provides opportunities to refine device settings to optimize both systolic and diastolic function. Data from the Multicenter InSync Randomized Clinical Evaluation (MIRACLE) study group have shown improvements in quality of life, 6-minute walk distances, LV EF, and LV reverse remodeling following the implementation of CRT.[7]

DIASTOLIC DYSFUNCTION

As mentioned earlier, diastolic dysfunction is defined as an abnormality in myocardial relaxation, filling, or distensibility. Diastolic HF requires one of these parameters of diastolic dysfunction and signs or symptoms of HF.[2] The diastolic phase of the cardiac cycle begins with isovolumetric relaxation and ends after the atrial contribution to ventricular filling is completed. On a microscopic level, calcium is taken into the sarcoplasmic reticulum during this phase allowing the relaxation of the myocytes and a rapid decrease in LV pressure. Any aberrancy in these cellular processes causes a decrease in LV preload. According to the Frank-Starling law, this condition yields a decrease in peak pressure and the rate of LV relaxation (lusitropy).[8]

On a more macroscopic level, diastolic dysfunction can be due to abnormal relaxation or an increase in myocardial stiffness. Typically, abnormal relaxation precedes increases in stiffness because stiffness is a marker of a fibrotic ventricle. On a ventricular pressure-volume loop, this is visualized as the slope of the diastolic portion of the loop (changes in LV pressure plotted against changes in diastolic LV volume [dP/dV]).[9] Increased stiffness is inversely proportional to the pressure deceleration time. These measurements and relationships are exploited by echocardiography and assist in accurate diagnosis of variations in diastolic filling parameters.

CHRONOTROPIC INCOMPETENCE IN DIASTOLIC HEART FAILURE

As mentioned, the diastolic phase of the cardiac cycle is complex and depends at least in part on the timing of atrial and ventricular depolarizations. When the speed or timing of the cardiac cycle is inadequate to meet the cardiac output requirements of a patient, they are deemed to have chronotropic incompetence.[10,11] Due to variability in normal values, there are wide ranges in the estimated incidence of chronotropic incompetence (25%–70% of HF patients).[11] This is further impacted by the widespread use of beta blockers, which are now standard of care for HF patients.[12]

Given the complexities associated with normal diastology, it has been difficult to determine the relative contributions of each factor. Chronotropic incompetence is estimated to reduce cardiac output by at least 20%.[11] Kosmala et al. examined 207 patients with stage C HF and 60 patients with stage B HF in an attempt to answer this question.[13] For each study subject, they performed echocardiograms at rest and immediately following a cardiopulmonary exercise test. One of their conclusions was that the development of chronotropic incompetence was an important factor leading asymptomatic patients to symptom development.[13] The severity of diastolic HF correlated to the severity of chronotropic incompetence.

The estimated contribution of chronotropic incompetence is supported by work by Brubaker and colleagues published in 2007.[10] In their report, cardiac output was measured in subjects at rest and during exertion. During exercise, cardiac output was noted to increase nearly 4-fold; of the 4-fold increase, there was a 2.2-fold increase in heart rate (HR), 1.5-fold increase in AV oxygen differences (oxygen extraction), and a 0.3-fold increase in stroke volume. Researchers also measured heart rate recovery (HRR) and linked this to mortality in asymptomatic patients.[10] HRR is defined as the difference in HR between the time of termination of exercise to a prespecified time point following the termination of exercise while supine (1-minute and 2-minute HRR are common). Normal values are at least 12 bpm at 1 minute and at least 42 bpm at 2 minutes.[10] This has also been demonstrated with Framingham data of 3000 patients followed 15 years.[14] Those patients in the top quintile of HRR at 1 minute had the lowest risk of cardiovascular disease (HR 0.61).[14]

PATHOPHYSIOLOGY

Pacing's Impact on Cardiac Function

As demonstrated in the chapter-opening case study, permanent pacing can have deleterious effects on cardiovascular physiology. The mechanisms by which pacing can be detrimental are complex and are dependent on the mode of pacing, site of pacing stimulus delivery, induced dyssynchrony, duration of pacing, and the underlying cardiovascular function. The immediate indications and advantages of pacing must be weighed against these potential adverse outcomes, and steps should be taken to minimize these effects when possible. A detailed overview of pacing's impact on cardiovascular physiology (specifically diastology) can be seen in Tables 30.1 and 30.2.

Pacing's Impact on Diastolic Function

As detailed earlier, pacing can impact all aspects of the cardiac cycle (see Tables 30.1 and 30.2) yielding improvements in NYHA functional class, quality of life (QOL), LV EF, and LV geometry.[8-14,19,21,23,52] While there is significant data available regarding the impact of CRT on systolic function, there is little available regarding the impact of CRT on diastolic function. Critical to the relationship between pacing and CRT on diastolic function is an appropriate AV delay. Optimization of the AV delay maximizes the LV filling time by separating rapid/passive LV filling from the atrial systolic phase of diastole. Additionally, appropriate AV delays shorten the interventricular mechanical delay.[7,53]

Hay et al. examined the short-term effects of RV, biventricular (BiV), and LV free wall pacing in nine patients with HF by examining pressure-volume relationships.[25] They found that only those patients

TABLE 30.1 **Effects of Pacing on Diastolic Parameters**

Atrial Pacing	Right Ventricular Pacing	Biventricular Pacing	Left Ventricular Pacing
• Increase in LVEDP[15] • No significant change in LVEDD and LVESD[16] • Decrease in E wave TVI and increase in pulmonary venous flow in CAD[17] • Decrease in LV (–)dP/dt • Increase in tau[18]	• Minimal change in LVESV[7] • No change in LVEDV and LVESV[19] • Increased myocardial stiffness[20] • Decreased E wave velocity[19] • Decreased LV (–)dP/dt[21] • Increased tau[20] • No significant change in peak LV (–)dP/dt between RVOT and RVA pacing[22]	• Decrease in LVEDV and LVESV[19,23,24] • Increased diastolic filling time[7,25] • Decreased E wave velocity[19] • Decrease in E/A ratio[7,26] • Decrease in E/Vp ratio • Increase in pulmonary S/D flow ratio • Decrease in pulmonary vein atrial reversal velocity • Increase in DT[26] • Lower tau but higher LV (–)dP/dt compared with RVA pacing[25] • Decreased LV (–)dP/dt[21]	Decreased LVEDV[27,28] Decreased LVEDP[21,27] Decreased LVESV[29] Decreased LV (–)dP/dt[21] No significant change in LV (–)dP/dt[27]

LVEDP, Left ventricular end diastolic pressure; *LVEDD*, Left ventricular end diastolic dimension; *LVESD*, Left ventricular end systolic dimension; *TVI*, Time velocity integral; *CAD*, Coronary artery disease; *LVESV*, Left ventricular end systolic volume; LVEDV; Left ventricular end diastolic volume; RVOT, Right ventricular outflow tract; RVA, Right ventricular apex; *DT*, Deceleration time.

TABLE 30.2 **Effects of Pacing Site on Cardiovascular System**

	Dyssynchronous Pacing/RVA Pacing	Synchronous Pacing, BiV Pacing
Cellular level	• Increased tissue norepinephrine level[30] • Asymmetric hypertrophy[31] • Increased stress kinase phosphorylation[32] • Shift in titin isoform[33] • Reduced Ca^{++}-ATPase, phospholamban, and connexin[34,35]	• Increased septal glucose uptake[36] • Decreased interstitial remodeling, TNF-α expression, and apoptosis[37]
Tissue level	• Mismatch of tissue perfusion[30] • Reduction in LV shortening fraction • Chronic LV remodeling[31] • Depressed fiber-sheet extension and wall thickening by epicardial pacing[38] • Prolonged QRS duration	• Correction of LV contractile dysfunction • Reverse remodeling[7] • Increased myocardial efficiency of O_2 use[39,40] • Effect on myocardial perfusion (increase[41]; no change[40])
Organ level	• Increased LAE and LAP[42,43] • Rightward shift of LV ES PVR • Decreased SV and EDV[30] • Upward and left shift of LV end-diastolic P-VR[20] • Reduced cardiac output[44,45] • Increased atrial fibrillation[46,47]	• Increased SBP, SV, dP/dt_{max}, and EF but decreased EDV, ESV, Tei index, and MR[7] • Increased diastolic filling[25,36] • Shortening of IVMD • Increased DT and E-A separation[36] • Increased EF and IVRT[25]
Body level	• Increased risk of HF and death[42,48,46] • Increased incidence of thromboembolism[49]	• Improved NYHA class, quality of life, and 6-min walk[7] • Reduced HF, hospitalization, and mortality[50,51]

RVA, Right ventricular apex; *LV*, Left ventricular; *LAE* = Left atrial enlargement; *LAP*, Left atrial pressure; *LV ES PVR*, left ventricular end systolic pressure volume relation; *SV*, Stroke volume; *EDV*, End diastolic volume; *SBP*, Systolic blood pressure; *ESV*; End systolic volume; *MR*; Mitral regurgitation; *IVMD*, intraventricular mechanical dyssynchrony; *IVRT*, Isovolumic relaxation time; *NYHA*, New York Heart Association; *HF*, Heart failure.

receiving BiV pacing had improvements in diastolic parameters compared to LV only and RV only pacing locations. This work supported a previous study from Auricchio et al. where 27 patients with HF were examined to determine the hemodynamic effects of BiV, RV only, and LV only pacing.[21] In their work, BiV and LV free wall pacing improved LV dP/dt more than RV pacing. This was similar to work by Simantirakis et al. published in 2004 describing 12 patients (6 with preserved LV EF and 6 with decreased EF) who underwent AV node ablation due to AFib. LV filling indices (LV end-diastolic pressure [EDP] and LV end-diastolic volume [EDV]) improved with LV pacing compared to RV pacing, but LV diastolic function indices such as −dP/dt and tau (τ) did not change significantly.[27] This pattern of improved LV diastolic filling indices with little to no change in LV diastolic function markers was also seen in the MIRACLE study.[7,53] This study included 323 patients with moderate to severe HF randomized to either CRT (n = 172) or medical therapy (n = 151). In those patients randomized to have their CRT turned on, LVEDV dimension, LV end-systolic volume (ESV) dimension, and LV EF (increases of 2.6% at 3 months and 3.6% at 6 months) showed improvement. Additionally, there were significant increases in the deceleration time of the E wave at 3 and 6 months in the CRT group. Improved ventricular function was also supported by decreased E wave velocities and myocardial performance index values at follow-up. A wave velocity, E/A ratio, and isovolumic relaxation time (IVRT) showed no significant improvement. The myocardial performance (Tei) index improved with CRT starting at the 3-month follow-up and extending out through the 12-month assessment. The myocardial performance index takes systolic and diastolic performance into consideration by summing the isovolumic contraction time and IVRT and dividing this sum by the ejection time.[52,53]

The abovementioned diastolic parameters affected by pacing can be used to prospectively predict response to CRT. Agacdiken et al. published a report of 23 patients who underwent echocardiographic

TABLE 30.3 Difference Between Responders and Nonresponders to CRT With Respect to Baseline Diastolic and Systolic Parameters

Parameters	Baseline Parameters	Responders ($n = 42$)	Nonresponders ($n = 34$)	p Value
Diastolic parameters	E/A ratio	0.89 ± 0.72	1.29 ± 0.56	<0.05
	Isovolumic relaxation time	131 ± 33	106 ± 37	<0.05
	Mean Em (cm/sec)	3.17 ± 1.72	4.33 ± 1.88	≤0.005
	Mean Am (cm/sec)	4.48 ± 1.54	3.62 ± 1.38	≤0.005
Systolic parameters	SD in Ts, 12 segments (msec)	44.9 ± 9.5	26 ± 11	<0.001
	Septal-to-lateral delay in Ts (msec)	60.9 ± 35.9	23 ± 30	<0.001

SD, Standard deviation; *Ts*, Time to peak myocardial systolic velocity.

examination prior to CRT in addition to 1 and 6 months postimplant.[26] Both responders (EF improvement ≥25%) and nonresponders experienced improvements in diastolic function parameters. In this small group of patients, pulmonary systolic flow to diastolic flow ratio (PVs/PVd) went from 0.9 to 1.3 ($p = 0.02$). Additionally, the early peak velocity to LV flow propagation velocity (E/Vp) decreased from 2.7 to 2 after the first month ($p < 0.002$) and to 1.9 at 6 months postimplant ($p < 0.02$). More important than diastolic measurements, NYHA functional classifications improved in the entire group irrespective of the degree of EF improvement. While there was no direct correlation between the diastology and response to CRT in this study, there was suggestion that responders had a more robust decrease in their restrictive diastology measurements compared to nonresponders.[26]

Waggoner et al.[54] examined the effects of CRT on diastolic filling parameters in a group of HFrEF patients after CRT implantation. They reported improved diastolic filling parameters (mitral E/A, E/e′) in all patients, especially those patients with NICM. These changes were predictive of long-term event rates, including HF hospitalizations.[54] Additional work by Yu et al. examined a group of patients with CRT comparing those who responded to therapy (45%) to those who did not respond favorably (55%).[55] Responders to therapy (reduction in LVESV by ≥15%) had significant decreases in E/e′ (30 to 22, $p < 0.05$) and significant increases in LV filling time (381 msec to 441 msec, $p < 0.05$). Pre-CRT implant relaxation patterns were also shown to predict response to CRT with abnormal initial patterns showing more significant reductions in LV volumes compared to those with pseudonormal patterns (29% vs. 11%, $p < 0.05$). These markers for responders and nonresponders to CRT can be seen in Table 30.3.

ADVERSE EFFECTS OF PACING ON CARDIAC FUNCTION

With an increasing number of patients receiving cardiac implantable electronic devices such as CRT and PPM, interest is growing regarding the adverse effects of pacing on cardiovascular function. Adverse outcomes due to pacing are thought to be due to pacing mode, pacing site, duration of pacing, and the baseline cardiovascular status of the patient.

Pacing Mode

The maintenance of AV synchrony should be the goal of any pacemaker programming. Data show increased burden of MR and TR, elevated risks of AFib, and thromboembolism in patients who lack AV synchrony.[26,42,56] VV synchrony is also an important factor influencing outcomes and will be discussed later.[57]

Early trials such as the Canadian Trial of Physiologic Pacing (CTOPP) published in 2000 showed few benefits to physiologic pacing (pacing that preserves AV synchrony).[58,59] In the CTOPP trial, there was no significant difference in the primary outcome (stroke or death due to cardiovascular causes) among the 1474 patients randomized to a ventricular pacemaker and the 1094 randomized to receive a physiologic pacemaker. Despite the lack of difference in the primary outcome, there were significantly fewer cases of AFib in the group assigned to the physiologic pacemaker compared to the ventricular pacemaker (5.3% vs. 6.6%, $p = 0.05$).

The relationship between pacing mode and outcomes was further explored by Rosenqvist et al. when they compared patients with ventricular-based pacing (VVI) to those with atrial based pacing (AAI) algorithms in 2003.[44] They studied 168 patients over a 2-year follow-up period and showed that HF occurrences (37% vs. 15%, $p < 0.005$) and mortality (23% vs. 8%, $p < 0.05$) were higher in the VVI group compared to the AAI group. They concluded AAI was superior to VVI for patients with chronotropic incompetence, at least in part due to preserved AV synchrony. This was also shown in the Pacemaker Selection in the Elderly (PASE) trial, which followed 407 patients over 65 years of age for 30 months.[60,61] Their results showed improvements in health-related QOL after pacemaker implantation in those patients with chronotropic incompetence. Additionally they showed nonsignificant reductions in death from all causes, stroke or death from any cause, stroke or HF hospitalization or death from any cause, and AFib in those with dual-chamber pacing compared to ventricular-based pacing.[61]

Pacing Site

Any artificial activation of the myocardium can lead to changes in the normal depolarization sequence of the myocardium and create downstream consequences for the patient. RV apical (RVA) pacing leads to the RV apex depolarizing before the left ventricle, resembling left BBB physiology.[34] This form of pacing has been shown to cause decreased regional myocardial perfusion, as well as cellular structure and ventricular geometrical changes.[62-65] Additionally, the QRS prolongation produced by RVA pacing leads to decreased LV function, apical regional wall motion abnormality, and elevated tissue norepinephrine levels and is associated with increased morbidity in HF patients.[28,30,56,66,67]

Early canine studies performed by Prinzen et al. demonstrated worsening of LV function when the dogs' hearts were paced from the RVA compared to the RV septum or left ventricle.[45] These changes in LV function and correlations to electromechanical activation patterns were achieved by creating activation maps and measuring fiber strain within the LV wall. Within the right ventricle there is debate about the most ideal pacing location—RVA or the right ventricular outflow tract (RVOT). Buckingham et al. compared these locations in patients all with EF less than 40%.[22] In their study, EF, peak dP/dt, peak −dP/dt, and relaxation time were used to assess efficacy. The authors concluded that RVOT had a slight advantage over RVA pacing.

More recent work has focused on BiV pacing. In patients with intraventricular dyssynchrony, pacing at the site of latest activation should in theory improve efficiency and volumes, which in turn would improve systolic and diastolic function.[23] Lieberman et al.

studied the impact of pacing site on LV function in 13 patients.[68] This group looked at the differences in LV EF, stroke volume, and dP/dt with LV only, RV, and BiV pacing. They showed that LV and BiV pacing configurations were superior to RV only pacing in all systolic function parameters, and RV only pacing significantly impaired LV relaxation and increased LVEDP.[68] The DECREASE-HF trial examined this same question when they analyzed 306 patients with NYHA Class III or IV symptoms, LV EF of 35% or less, and a QRS duration of 150 msec and more.[69] In their study, LV volumes (LVEDV and LVESV) and LV systolic performance were assessed at baseline, 3 months, and 6 months after enrollment in groups who were LV/RV simultaneous, LV-RV sequential, and LV only paced. The authors concluded that all groups exhibited improvements in LV volumes with BiV pacing showing the greatest improvements. Diastolic function seemed to improve in all groups with BiV showing the greatest reductions in peak E wave velocities and E/A ratios—all suggestive of reduced filling pressures.[69]

Duration of Pacing

The overall amount of time patients are paced is an enormous factor contributing to their systolic and diastolic function. The Dual Chamber and VVI Implantable Defibrillator (DAVID) trial published by Wilkoff et al. examined 506 patients with indications for implantable cardioverter defibrillator (ICD) therapy who did not have an indication for antibradycardia pacemaker therapy and no known persistent atrial arrhythmias.[48] The objective of this study was to determine the impact of dual-chamber pacing compared to ventricular backup pacing. In this study, patients were randomly assigned to have their ICD programmed to a ventricular backup rate of 40 bpm (VVI-40) ($n = 256$) or dual-chamber responsive rate of 70 bpm (DDDR-70) ($n = 250$). Their results showed a significant increase in the composite end point of death or first hospitalization for HF in the DDDR-70 group (HR 1.62, 95% confidence interval [CI] 1.06–2.44). Mortality (HR 1.61, 95% CI 0.84–3.09) and hospitalization for HF (HR 1.54, 95% CI 0.97–2.46) were both independently increased in the DDDR-70 group and trended toward statistical significance. The authors postulated that these increased rates of mortality and HF hospitalization were due to the increased burden of pacing seen in the DDDR-70 group compared to the VVI-40 group (~60% vs. 1% beats paced in the DDDR and VVI groups, respectively). It is very important when considering these results to remember that these patients were being paced from the RVA rather than from a BiV configuration.

These findings confirmed previous results seen in the Multicenter Automatic Defibrillator Implantation Trial II (MADIT II) published by Moss et al. in 2002.[70,71] In their study of 1232 patients with a previous myocardial infarction (MI) and an EF of 30% and less, patients were randomized to receive an ICD or conventional medical therapy. While the patients randomized to ICD lived significantly longer (HR for death from any cause 0.69, 95% CI 0.51–0.93, $p = 0.016$), they had increased rates of HF hospitalizations (19.9% vs. 14.9%, $p = 0.09$). The authors postulated that this increased risk for HF hospitalization was likely due to ventricular dyssynchrony from pacing leading to HF decompensation.

The adverse outcomes associated with ventricular pacing were also explored by Sweeney et al. in the Mode Selection Trial (MOST) published in 2003.[46] In this randomized trial of DDDR versus VVIR pacing in 2010 patients with sinus node dysfunction, the burden of pacing was correlated to the likelihood of HF hospitalization and AFib. For those patients programmed DDDR with a pacing burden greater than 40%, the risk of HF hospitalization was significantly increased (HR 2.99, 95% CI 1.15–7.75). With VVIR and a pacing burden greater than 80%, the risk for HF hospitalization was also significantly increased (HR 2.56, 95% CI 1.48–4.43). The authors concluded that the dyssynchrony induced by ventricular pacing was a significant contributor to the risk of HF decompensation and hospitalization and that the minimization of pacing should be a priority for those patients with depressed EFs and risk for HF.[46,56]

An active BiV pacing configuration was tested by the Multisite Stimulation in Cardiomyopathies (MUSTIC) investigators in 2001.[72] In this study, 48 patients with NYHA Class III HF symptoms and sinus rhythm with a QRS duration greater than 150 msec were enrolled into a single-blind, randomized controlled crossover study where each participant experienced two pacing configurations—passive ventricular backup pacing (40 bpm) or active atriobiventricular pacing. Atriobiventricular pacing improved their 6-minute walk distances by 23% ($p < 0.001$), QOL scores by 32% ($p < 0.001$), peak oxygen uptake by 8% ($p < 0.03$), and hospitalizations by two-thirds ($p < 0.05$). Of patients enrolled in this trial, 85% preferred the atriobiventricular pacing compared to RV pacing.

Taken together, the aforementioned trials suggest nonphysiologic pacing (not BiV) induces dyssynchrony that in some patients may precipitate LV systolic and diastolic dysfunction, which may lead to increased risks for HF. If pacing is required, attempts should be made to minimize the burden of pacing and, when possible, should be performed from a BiV configuration to replicate normal conduction system physiology. More modern pacing modes, such as a managed ventricular pacing (MVP) mode, prioritize atrial pacing (AAI) when AV node function is normal but convert to a ventricular-based (DDD) pacing scheme during periods of AV block. Modes such as this help decrease the cumulative pacing burden to help reduce induced dyssynchrony and downstream sinister effects. Sweeney et al. reported a markedly reduced cumulative pacing burden in patients with a device programmed to the MVP mode (4.1 ± 16.3% vs. 73.8 ± 32.5%, $p < 0.0001$).[73]

Underlying Cardiac Status

As suggested in previous trials such as MOST, the incidence of adverse cardiac events due to pacing corresponds to the patients' underlying cardiovascular status prior to the initiation of pacing. Patients with low EF, history of MI, HF, and an abnormally prolonged QRS had a 42 times higher chance of HF hospitalization compared to those patients without these comorbid conditions.[56] Pediatric studies have also noted this correlation—showing reductions in LV function only in patients who had baseline structural heart disease.[74] In another population described by Iler et al, there was a significant decrease in EF in 29% of patients. Of those patients who experienced a decrease, 33% had a baseline normal EF.[75]

DIAGNOSTIC EVALUATION AND OPTIMIZATION OF DYSSYNCHRONY

The potential pitfalls of pacemaker therapy for chronotropic incompetence and HF are many and are introduced in earlier sections. The chapter-opening case study is a prime example of how many patients present after pacemaker therapy with worsening symptoms due to induced dyssynchrony (either AV or VV dyssynchrony). With better "out of the box" algorithms and programming, many patients do experience robust improvements in their symptoms after pacemaker implant. Despite this, up to one-third of patients who undergo CRT implantation either do not improve or clinically worsen after the implantation of their device.[21,76] Physicians managing these patients must have a systematic approach to evaluation, to optimize outcomes. This systematic approach must consider AV and VV synchrony.

Optimization of the AV Delay

As demonstrated in the case, inappropriate AV delay and resultant diastolic filling can have a tremendous negative impact on a patient's symptom burden and outcomes. The premise for AV optimization is to adjust the device timers to allow for the maximal atrial contribution to ventricular filling during diastole.[21,76,77] These delays should be patient specific.[21] With incomplete atrial emptying, the atrial pressures can rise and create symptoms such as fatigue and dizziness—a constellation of symptoms described as the pacemaker syndrome.[42,43] Without proper AV synchrony, patients can experience increased rates of AV block, atrial fibrillation (due to elevated atrial pressures and subsequent dilation), HF, and even death compared to those patients with optimized AV synchrony.[5,44,49,78] Hemodynamically, the AV delay should allow filling of the left ventricle without interruption of the A wave. An overly short AV delay will lead to ventricular contraction before the atrium is empty, yielding a decreased cardiac output. Accompanying a decreased CO can be a decreased peak dP/dt and increased τ (time constant of isovolumic relaxation).[79] An inappropriately long AV delay could result in wasted diastolic filling time.

The diastolic phase of the cardiac cycle is the period of interest when trying to optimize the AV delay. This period of time is easily assessed using Doppler echocardiography. Efforts should be made to have the end of the A wave occur immediately before the onset of aortic systolic Doppler flow.[80] There have been many AV optimization techniques described, including one by Ritter et al., where an optimization process involves measuring the atrial electrical-mechanical delay (QA interval) at inappropriately short and long AV delays at the beginning of the AV optimization study.[80] This QA interval is measured between the onset of the Q wave and the termination of the mitral A wave. Efforts are made to allow complete atrial emptying (A wave) without truncating its contribution.

Another method involves programming an inappropriately long AV delay. Next, the AV delay is decreased in increments of 20 msec until the A wave truncates (typically down to 60 msec). This is continued until a MV inflow signal is revealed with E and A wave separation and termination of the A wave approximately 40 to 60 msec before the onset of the QRS complex. This pattern would be indicative of stage I diastolic filling—an ideal end point for an AV optimization echocardiogram. Shortening of the QA interval is seen in Figs. 30.1A and 30.2A.

Rokey et al. studied diastolic function using mitral inflow patterns on Doppler echocardiography in patients undergoing AV optimization.[81] Doppler velocities across the mitral valve were measured at AV delays of 75, 150, and 250 msec. Their data showed an inverse correlation between the effectiveness of atrial contraction and early diastolic filling. This, the authors postulated, was due to incomplete atrial contraction with shorter AV delays leading to larger residual atrial volumes and end diastole. During the following systolic period, the left atrial (LA) volume increased even further, which eventually led to an increased transmitral gradient and elevated peak inflow velocity (E wave). Optimized AV delays lead to the opposite—complete atrial filling, lower atrial volumes at end diastole, and lower peak inflow velocities during subsequent diastolic periods.[81]

The utility of AV optimization using pulsed-wave Doppler echocardiography in patients undergoing CRT was studied by Kedia et al.[76] and published in 2006. Following CRT, 50% of patients exhibited grade I diastolic function by pulsed Doppler of the MV inflow, consistent with low atrial filling pressures. Of the remaining 50% with grade II or III diastolic function, 19% demonstrated improved Doppler hemodynamics manifested by an improvement in one diastolic function grade (i.e., III to II or II to I).

Independent predictors of a more prolonged AV delay that resulted in improved hemodynamics by Doppler echocardiography included a paced rhythm, AV block, and an increased LA diameter. Subsequent study of 1951 patients undergoing CRT demonstrated that grade I diastolic dysfunction following an echocardiogram-guided AV delay optimization predicted an improved survival when compared to grade II or III diastolic function graded by pulsed Doppler echocardiography of mitral inflow.[82]

Optimization of the VV Delay

While AV synchrony is important to maximize cardiac output and symptom relief when pacemaker therapies are required, VV synchrony has become an important aspect in the management of patients who have received a CRT capable pacemaker. Optimal VV synchrony is typically defined as the VV delay that produces the maximal systolic function. Apparent benefits to optimized VV synchrony include improvements in LV preload and a reduction in the severity of mitral regurgitation.[83,84] Van Gelder et al.[83] studied patients with severe LV dysfunction who were receiving CRT. With optimal VV synchrony, the authors reported a 3% to 8% increase in dP/dt. This improvement in cardiac function with optimized synchrony was confirmed by the work of Sogaard et al., who noted an increase in EF from 22% to 29% ($p < 0.01$) and a reduction in delayed longitudinal contraction (DLC) from 48% to 23% ($p < 0.01$) in patients with resynchronized ventricular contractions.[85] When CRT was further optimized (sequential RV then LV activation rather than simultaneous LV-RV contraction), DLC improved even more from 33% to 23% ($p < 0.01$) and the EF improved to 33% from 29% ($p < 0.01$). Sequential CRT also improved diastolic filling time when compared to sequential CRT (460 ± 80 msec vs. 430 ± 88 msec, $p < 0.05$).[85]

FUTURE DIRECTIONS

Multisite Pacing in CRT

With clear advantages to AA and VV synchrony, many patients are reaping the benefits of device-based therapies for their cardiovascular diseases. Despite this, there are 30% to 40% of patients who would theoretically benefit from CRT who are unable to receive the treatment due to procedural difficulties. A relatively new area of research is whether the LV leads could be placed outside of the coronary venous system and within the endocardium. In work by Reddy et al., a wireless endocardial electrode was tested in 35 patients who failed traditional CRT implantation.[86] This technology utilizes a subcutaneous phased array ultrasound pulse generator to transmit a signal to an endocardially placed LV electrode. This system requires a traditional transvenous RV pacemaker to provide AV and VV synchrony. The procedure was initially successful in 97% of implants. Within 24 hours of implant, 9% of patients experienced device-related complications with 23% of patients experiencing complications within 1 month. Despite these complications, 66% of patients had an echocardiographic response to therapy (≥5% improvement in EF) with 84.8% of patients reporting clinical improvements. While still in development, these alternative methods to achieve AV and VV synchrony are promising.

Direct His Bundle Pacing

His bundle pacing (HBP) has been discussed since the 1970s but was not described in a human until 2000.[87] By utilizing the heart's intrinsic His-Purkinje conduction system, this mechanism of pacing should in theory preserve systolic and diastolic function, thus avoiding pacing-induced cardiomyopathy. Plagued by early failures due to nonspecialized equipment to insert these complex systems, HBP initially fell out of favor. Now with improved implantation equipment, HBP can be placed successfully in over 90% of cases.[87] Despite these improvements, some series have shown 6.7% of HBP leads will require revision due to loss of capture or increasing thresholds. Despite these complications there is a great deal of interest in this technology based on early work suggesting successful reduction in intraventricular dyssynchrony with HBP when compared to RVA pacing. Catanzariti et al. published a series of patients who experienced reductions in interventricular mechanical delay and left posterior wall motion delays while HBP compared to RVA pacing.[88]

While HBP provides an immediate alternative to traditional CRT and pacing systems by reestablishing intraventricular and interventricular synchrony, some believe HBP may even provide a potential treatment for patients with chronotropic incompetence and diastolic dysfunction. This hypothesis is being tested in the ongoing His Optimized Pacing Evaluated for Heart Failure Trial (HOPE-HF).[89] This multicenter, double-blinded, randomized trial will enroll 160 patients with first-degree AV block, LV EF of 40% and less, and a normal QRS duration. This trial will assess exercise capacity with and without HBP.

KEY POINTS

- Of new HF diagnoses each year, 40% to 50% are classified as HFpEF.
- Traditional pacemaker configurations with a lead in the RV apex lead to an altered ventricular activation sequence, including a late LV activation that leads to dyssynchrony and both systolic and diastolic dysfunction.
- CRT has traditionally been indicated for patients with NYHA Class III/IV symptoms, LV EF of 35% and less, and left bundle branch block with a QRS duration greater than 120 msec.
- Chronotropic incompetence is defined as the inability to meet the cardiac output requirements of a patient due to inappropriately prolonged cardiac cycle length.
- The incidence of chronotropic incompetence is estimated to be 25% to 70% of all HF patients.
- Chronotropy is estimated to provide at least 20% of the overall cardiac output.
- Timing of pacemaker cycles is critical to optimal atrial and ventricular function with inappropriately short atrioventricular delays contributing to abbreviated ventricular filling and decreased cardiac output.
- Studies (MADIT II, DAVID, MOST) have demonstrated decreased HF hospitalizations and mortality when pacing is minimized. If pacing is required, efforts should be made to preserve AV and VV synchrony.
- Many studies have demonstrated an improvement in echocardiographic markers of diastolic function (E/A, E/Em, −dP/dt, Tei, LVEDV, LVESV) in CRT or LV pacing compared to RV pacing.
- Echocardiogram-based AV optimization studies should target a mitral inflow pattern with a distinct A wave (surrogate atrial contribution to ventricular filling).
- Multisite endocardial pacing and His bundle pacing are emerging technologies both aimed at preserving synchrony with preliminary data suggesting improved systolic and diastolic function.

REVIEW QUESTIONS

1. A 49-year-old male smoker with a history of bicuspid aortic valve, peripheral artery disease, coronary artery disease, sinus node dysfunction, and ischemic cardiomyopathy with an EF of 25% is hospitalized due to fatigue and dyspnea. Two years prior to admission he previously underwent an aortic valve replacement (AVR) with concomitant bypass grafting (CABG) to his left anterior descending (LAD) artery and right coronary artery (RCA). Shortly after his AVR/CABG he required implantation of a dual-chamber pacemaker due to high degree AV block.

   Vitals:
   - HR 64 BPM, intermittently dual chamber paced
   - Breaths per minute
   - BP 88/64 mmHg
   - Sa O_2 94%
   - Temp 37 °C

   Physical Exam:
   - Gen: Mild distress due to dyspnea
   - Neck: JVP to angle of jaw at 90 degrees
   - CV: Regular rate and rhythm, S1/S2 present with no appreciate murmurs, rubs, gallops; cool extremities with 1–2+ pitting edema to the level of his thighs
   - Resp: Rales in bilateral bases with diminished air movement in the right lower lobes

   Labwork:
   - Lactate 2.7 units
   - Creatinine 1.8 (baseline 1) units
   - NT-ProBNP 3458 (baseline 400–600) units

   Home Medications:
   - Aspirin 81 mg daily
   - Metoprolol succinate 100 mg daily
   - Lisinopril 10 mg daily
   - Torsemide 20 mg daily

   The patient is admitted to the coronary intensive care unit and a Swan-Ganz catheter is placed. Hemodynamics show an RA pressure of 10 mmHg, RV pressure of 40/12 mmHg, PA pressure of 42/26 mmHg, and a pulmonary capillary wedge pressure (PCWP) of 28 mmHg. Cardiac output is 5.4 L/min with a cardiac index of 1.8.

   The patient improves marginally with the stoppage of his home beta blocker and afterload reduction regimen and with IV infusions of furosemide and nitroprusside but continues to have a chronotropic incompetence less than 2 with elevated lactate.

   What should be done next to acutely improve this patient's hemodynamics?

   a. Immediately insert extracorporeal membrane oxygenation (ECMO).
   b. Insert an intraaortic balloon pump.
   c. Perform urgent bedside echo given concern for aortic valve incompetence.
   d. Program pacemaker basal rate to 90 bpm.
   e. Urgent transplant evaluation.

2. The transmitral Doppler echocardiographic profile of a patient requiring dual-chamber pacemaker therapy is

   a. E = A.
   b. E > A with abbreviated E wave.
   c. E > A with distinct E and A waves.
   d. E < A with abbreviated E wave.
   e. E < A with distinct E and A waves.

3. While technically feasible and theoretically superior to traditional CRT, His bundle pacing has been slow to gain mainstream adoption for patients with chronotropic incompetence due to
   a. increased rates of lead dislodgement compared to traditional PPM leads.
   b. increased rates of tricuspid valve chordal disruption during implant procedures.
   c. implant success rates of only 60% to 70%.
   d. data showing no significant improvement in cardiac function with HBP over RVA pacing.
   e. both a and b.
   f. both b and c.
   g. both a and c.
   h. all of the above.

REFERENCES

1. Zile MR, Gaasch WH, Carroll JD, et al. Heart failure with a normal ejection fraction: is measurement of diastolic function necessary to make the diagnosis of diastolic heart failure? *Circulation.* 2001; 104:779–782.
2. Zile MR, Baicu CF, Gaasch WH. Diastolic heart failure—abnormalities in active relaxation and passive stiffness of the left ventricle. *N Engl J Med.* 2004;350:1953–1959.
3. Van Heerebeek L, Borbély A, Niessen HWM, et al. Myocardial structure and function differ in systolic and diastolic heart failure. *Circulation.* 2006;113:1966–1973.
4. Tracy CM, Epstein AE, Darbar D, et al. 2012 ACCF/AHA/HRS focused update of the 2008 guidelines for device-based therapy of cardiac rhythm abnormalities. *Circulation.* 2012;126:1784–1800.
5. Kindermann M, Fröhlig G, Doerr T, Schieffer H. Optimizing the AV delay in DDD pacemaker patients with high degree AV block: mitral valve Doppler versus impedance cardiography. *PACE.* 1997;20:2453–2462.
6. Auricchio A, Lumens J, Prinzen FW. Cardiac resynchronization therapy has a role in patients with right bundle branch block. *Circ Arrhythm Electrophysiol.* 2014;7:532–541.
7. St. John Sutton MG, Plappert T, Abraham WT, et al. Effect of cardiac resynchronization therapy on left ventricular size and function in chronic heart failure. *Circulation.* 2003;107:1985–1990.
8. Mann D, Zipes D, Libby P, Bonow R. *Braunwald's Heart Disease: A Textbook of Cardiovascular Medicine.* Philadelphia, PA: Elsevier Saunders; 2014.
9. Little WC, Ohno M, Kitzman DW, Thomas JD, Cheng CP. Determination of left ventricular chamber stiffness from the time for deceleration of early left ventricular filling. *Circulation.* 1995;92:1933–1939.
10. Kitzman DW. Chronotropic incompetence: causes, implications, and management. *Dialog Cardiovasc Med.* 2013;18:139–153.
11. Brubaker PH, Kitzman DW. Prevalence and management of chronotropic incompetence in heart failure. *Curr Cardiol Rep.* 2007;9:229–235.
12. Zweerink A, van der Lingen ACJ, Handoko ML, van Rossum AC, Allaart CP. Chronotropic incompetence in chronic heart failure. *Circ Heart Fail.* 2018;11:e004969.
13. Kosmala W, Rojek A, Przewlocka-Kosmala M, Mysiak A, Karolko B, Marwick TH. Contributions of nondiastolic factors to exercise intolerance in heart failure with preserved ejection fraction. *J Am Coll Cardiol.* 2016;67:659–670.
14. Morshedi-Meibodi A, Larson MG, Levy D, O'Donnell CJ, Vasan RS. Heart rate recovery after treadmill exercise testing and risk of cardiovascular disease events (The Framingham Heart Study). *Am J Cardiol.* 2002;90:848–852.
15. Voelker W, Mauser M, Kimmig A, Hoffmeister HM, Overkamp D, Karsch KR. Effect of rapid atrial pacing on left ventricular ejection fraction in patients without organic heart disease. *Zeitschrift Fur Kardiologie.* 1987;76:223–230.
16. Nielsen JC, Kristensen L, Andersen HR, Mortensen PT, Pedersen OL, Pedersen AK. A randomized comparison of atrial and dual-chamber pacing in 177 consecutive patients with sick sinus syndrome: echocardiographic and clinical outcome. *J Am Coll Cardiol.* 2003;42:614–623.
17. Hoffmann R, Lambertz H, Thoennissen G, Flachskampf FA, Hanrath P. Altered left ventricular diastolic function post-atrial pacing in coronary artery disease and left ventricular hypertrophy: further insights by pulmonary venous flow analysis. *Eur Heart J.* 1994;15:1096–1105.
18. Bedotto JB, Grayburn PA, Black WH, et al. Alterations in left ventricular relaxation during atrioventricular pacing in humans. *J Am Coll Cardiol.* 1990;15:658–664.
19. Yu CM, Lin H, Fung WH, Zhang Q, Kong SL, Sanderson JE. Comparison of acute changes in left ventricular volume, systolic and diastolic functions, and intraventricular synchronicity after biventricular and right ventricular pacing for heart failure. *Am Heart J.* 2003;145:846.
20. Bourdillon PD, Lorell BH, Mirsky I, Paulus WJ, Wynne J, Grossman W. Increased regional myocardial stiffness of the left ventricle during pacing-induced angina in man. *Circulation.* 1983;67:316–323.
21. Auricchio A, Stellbrink C, Block M, et al. Effect of pacing chamber and atrioventricular delay on acute systolic function of paced patients with congestive heart failure. *Circulation.* 1999;99:2993–3001.
22. Buckingham TA, Candinas R, Attenhofer C, et al. Systolic and diastolic function with alternate and combined site pacing in the right ventricle. *PACE.* 2006;21:1077–1084.
23. Kass DA, Chen CH, Curry C, et al. Improved left ventricular mechanics from acute VDD pacing in patients with dilated cardiomyopathy and ventricular conduction delay. *Circulation.* 1999;99:1567–1573.
24. Auricchio A, Metra M, Gasparini M, et al. Long-term survival of patients with heart failure and ventricular conduction delay treated with cardiac resynchronization therapy. *Am J Cardiol.* 2007;99:232–238.
25. Hay I, Melenovsky V, Fetics BJ, et al. Short-term effects of right-left heart sequential cardiac resynchronization in patients with heart failure, chronic atrial fibrillation, and atrioventricular nodal block. *Circulation.* 2004;110:3404–3410.
26. Agacdiken A, Vural A, Ural D, et al. Effect of cardiac resynchronization therapy on left ventricular diastolic filling pattern in responder and nonresponder patients. *PACE.* 2005;28:654–660.
27. Simantirakis EN, Vardakis KE, Kochiadakis GE, et al. Left ventricular mechanics during right ventricular apical or left ventricular-based pacing in patients with chronic atrial fibrillation after atrioventricular junction ablation. *J Am Coll Cardiol.* 2004;43:1013–1018.
28. Miyoshi F, Kobayashi Y, Itou H, et al. Prolonged paced QRS duration as a predictor for congestive heart failure in patients with right ventricular apical pacing. *PACE.* 2005;28:1182–1188.
29. Nelson GS, Berger RD, Fetics BJ, et al. Left ventricular or biventricular pacing improves cardiac function at diminished energy cost in patients with dilated cardiomyopathy and left bundle-branch block. *Circulation.* 2000;102:3053–3059.
30. Lee MA, Dae MW, Langberg JJ, et al. Effects of long-term right ventricular apical pacing on left ventricular perfusion, innervation, function and histology. *J Am Coll Cardiol.* 1994;24:225–232.
31. Prinzen FW, Augustijn CH, Arts T, Allessie MA, Reneman RS. Redistribution of myocardial fiber strain and blood flow by asynchronous activation. *Am J Physiol.* 1990;259:H300–H308.
32. Schulz R, Aker S, Belosjorow S, Konietzka I, Rauen U, Heusch G. Stress kinase phosphorylation is increased in pacing-induced heart failure in rabbits. *Am J Physiol Heart Circ Physiol.* 2003;285:H2084–H2090.
33. Bell SP, Nyland L, Tischler MD, McNabb M, Granzier H, LeWinter MM. Alterations in the determinants of diastolic suction during pacing tachycardia. *Circ Res.* 2000;87:235–240.
34. Vassallo JA, Cassidy DM, Miller JM, Buxton AE, Marchlinski FE, Josephson ME. Left ventricular endocardial activation during right ventricular pacing: effect of underlying heart disease. *J Am Coll Cardiol.* 1986;7:1228–1233.

35. Spragg DD, Leclercq C, Loghmani M, et al. Regional alterations in protein expression in the dyssynchronous failing heart. *Circulation.* 2003;108:929–932.
36. St. John Sutton M, Keane MG. Reverse remodelling in heart failure with cardiac resynchronisation therapy. *Heart.* 2007;93:167–171.
37. D'Ascia C, Cittadini A, Monti MG, Riccio G, Saccà L. Effects of biventricular pacing on interstitial remodelling, tumor necrosis factor-α expression, and apoptotic death in failing human myocardium. *Eur Heart J.* 2006;27:201–206.
38. Ashikaga H, Omens JH, Ingels Jr NB, Covell JW. Transmural mechanics at left ventricular epicardial pacing site. *Am J Physiol Heart Circ Physiol.* 2004;286:H2401–H2407.
39. Ukkonen H, Beanlands RSB, Burwash IG, et al. Effect of cardiac resynchronization on myocardial efficiency and regional oxidative metabolism. *Circulation.* 2003;107:28–31.
40. Sundell J, Engblom E, Koistinen J, et al. The effects of cardiac resynchronization therapy on left ventricular function, myocardial energetics, and metabolic reserve in patients with dilated cardiomyopathy and heart failure. *J Am Coll Cardiol.* 2004;43:1027–1033.
41. Knaapen P, van Campen LMC, de Cock CC, et al. Effects of cardiac resynchronization therapy on myocardial perfusion reserve. *Circulation.* 2004;110:646–651.
42. Little RC. Effect of atrial systole on ventricular pressure and closure of the A-V valves. *Am J Physiol.* 1951;166:289–295.
43. Furman S, Cooper JA. Atrial fibrillation during A-V sequential pacing. *PACE.* 1982;5:133–135.
44. Rosenqvist M, Brandt J, Schüller H. Long-term pacing in sinus node disease: effects of stimulation mode on cardiovascular morbidity and mortality. *Am Heart J.* 1988;116:16–22.
45. Prinzen FW, Peschar M. Relation between the pacing induced sequence of activation and left ventricular pump function in animals. *PACE.* 2002;25:484–498.
46. Sweeney MO, Hellkamp AS, Ellenbogen KA, et al. Adverse effect of ventricular pacing on heart failure and atrial fibrillation among patients with normal baseline QRS duration in a clinical trial of pacemaker therapy for sinus node dysfunction. *Circulation.* 2003;107:2932–2937.
47. Nielsen JC, Andersen HR, Thomsen PE, et al. Heart failure and echocardiographic changes during long-term follow-up of patients with sick sinus syndrome randomized to single-chamber atrial or ventricular pacing. *Circulation.* 1998;97:987–995.
48. Wilkoff BL, Cook JR, Epstein AE, et al. Dual-chamber pacing-or ventricular backup pacing in patients with an implantable defibrillator: the Dual Chamber and VVI Implantable Defibrillator (DAVID) trial. *JAMA.* 2002;288:3115–3123.
49. Andersen HR, Thuesen L, Bagger JP, Vesterlund T, Thomsen PEB. Prospective randomised trial of atrial versus ventricular pacing in sick-sinus syndrome. *Lancet.* 1994;344:1523–1528.
50. Bristow MR, Saxon LA, Boehmer J, et al. Cardiac-resynchronization therapy with or without an implantable defibrillator in advanced chronic heart failure. *N Engl J Med.* 2004;350:2140–2150.
51. Cleland JGF, Daubert JC, Erdmann E, et al. The effect of cardiac resynchronization on morbidity and mortality in heart failure. *N Engl J Med.* 2005;352:1539–1549.
52. Persson H, Lonn E, Edner M, et al. Diastolic dysfunction in heart failure with preserved systolic function: need for objective evidence. Results from the CHARM echocardiographic substudy-CHARMES. *J Am Coll Cardiol.* 2007;49:687–694.
53. St. John Sutton MG, Plappert T, Hilpisch KE, Abraham WT, Hayes DL, Chinchoy E. Sustained reverse left ventricular structural remodeling with cardiac resynchronization at one year is a function of etiology: quantitative Doppler echocardiographic evidence from the Multicenter InSync Randomized Clinical Evaluation (MIRACLE). *Circulation.* 2006;113:266–272.
54. Waggoner AD, Rovner A, De Las Fuentes L, et al. Clinical outcomes after cardiac resynchronization therapy: importance of left ventricular diastolic function and origin of heart failure. *J Am Soc Echocardiogr.* 2006;19:307–313.
55. Yu CM, Zhang Q, Yip GWK, et al. Are left ventricular diastolic function and diastolic asynchrony important determinants of response to cardiac resynchronization therapy? *Am J Cardiol.* 2006;98:1083–1087.
56. Sweeney MO, Hellkamp AS. Heart failure during cardiac pacing. *Circulation.* 2006;113:2082–2088.
57. Linde C, Leclercq C, Rex S, et al. Long-term benefits of biventricular pacing in congestive heart failure: results from the MUltisite STimulation In cardiomyopathy (MUSTIC) study. *J Am Coll Cardiol.* 2002;40:111–118.
58. Connolly SJ, Kerr CR, Gent M, et al. Effects of physiologic pacing versus ventricular pacing on the risk of stroke and death due to cardiovascular causes. *N Engl J Med.* 2000;342:1385–1391.
59. Kerr CR, Connolly SJ, Abdollah H, et al. Canadian trial of physiological pacing: effects of physiological pacing during long-term follow-up. *Circulation.* 2004;109:357–362.
60. Newman D. Relationships between pacing mode and quality of life: evidence from randomized clinical trials. *Card Electrophysiol Rev.* 2003;7:401–405.
61. Lamas GA, Orav EJ, Stambler BS, et al. Quality of life and clinical outcomes in elderly patients treated with ventricular pacing as compared with dual-chamber pacing. *N Engl J Med.* 1998;338:1097–1104.
62. Nielsen JC, Bøttcher M, Nielsen TT, Pedersen AK, Andersen HR. Regional myocardial blood flow in patients with sick sinus syndrome randomized to long-term single chamber atrial or dual chamber pacing—effect of pacing mode and rate. *J Am Coll Cardiol.* 2000;35:1453–1461.
63. Karpawich PP, Justice CD, Cavitt DL, Chang CH. Developmental sequelae of fixed-rate ventricular pacing in the immature canine heart: an electrophysiologic, hemodynamic, and histopathologic evaluation. *Am Heart J.* 1990;119:1077–1083.
64. Adomian GE, Beazell J. Myofibrillar disarray produced in normal hearts by chronic electrical pacing. *Am Heart J.* 1986;112:79–83.
65. Van Oosterhout MFM, Prinzen FW, Arts T, et al. Asynchronous electrical activation induces asymmetrical hypertrophy of the left ventricular wall. *Circulation.* 1998;98:588–595.
66. Freeman GL, Little WC, O'Rourke RA. The effect of vasoactive agents on the left ventricular end-systolic pressure-volume relation in closed-chest dogs. *Circulation.* 1986;74:1107–1113.
67. Rosenqvist M, Bergfeldt L, Haga Y, Rydén J, Rydén L, Öwall A. The effect of ventricular activation sequence on cardiac performance during pacing. *PACE.* 1996;19:1279–1286.
68. Lieberman R, Padeletti L, Schreuder J, et al. Ventricular pacing lead location alters systemic hemodynamics and left ventricular function in patients with and without reduced ejection fraction. *J Am Coll Cardiol.* 2006;48:1634–1641.
69. Rao RK, Kumar UN, Schafer J, Viloria E, De Lurgio D, Foster E. Reduced ventricular volumes and improved systolic function with cardiac resynchronization therapy: a randomized trial comparing simultaneous biventricular pacing, sequential biventricular pacing, and left ventricular pacing. *Circulation.* 2007;115:2136–2144.
70. Moss AJ, Zareba W, Hall WJ, et al. Prophylactic implantation of a defibrillator in patients with myocardial infarction and reduced ejection fraction. *N Engl J Med.* 2002;346:877–883.
71. Ellenbogen KA, Thames MD, Mohanty PK. New insights into pacemaker syndrome gained from hemodynamic, humoral and vascular responses during ventriculo-atrial pacing. *Am J Cardiol.* 1990;65:53–59.
72. Cazeau S, Leclercq C, Lavergne T, et al. Effects of multisite biventricular pacing in patients with heart failure and intraventricular conduction delay. *N Engl J Med.* 2001;344:873–880.
73. Sweeney MO, Ellenbogen KA, Casavant D, et al. Multicenter, prospective, randomized safety and efficacy study of a new atrial-based managed ventricular pacing mode (MVP) in dual chamber ICDs. *J Cardiovasc Electrophysiol.* 2005;16:811–817.
74. Shalganov T, Paprika D, Kornyei L, Prodan Z, Bodor G, Szatmari A, Szili-Torok T. Evolution of left ventricular function in pediatric patients with permanent right ventricular pacing with and without structural heart disease. *Europace* 2005;7:292-292.
75. Iler M, Tillan K, Hu T, Chung M. Incidence of left ventricular dysfunction after pacemaker implantation for complete heart block. *J Am Coll Cardiol.* 2006;47:21A.
76. Kedia N, Ng K, Apperson-Hansen C, et al. Usefulness of atrioventricular delay optimization using Doppler assessment of mitral inflow in patients undergoing cardiac resynchronization therapy. *Am J Cardiol.* 2006;98:780–785.

77. Gorcsan J, Abraham T, Agler DA, et al. Echocardiography for cardiac resynchronization therapy: recommendations for performance and reporting-a report from the American Society of Echocardiography Dyssynchrony Writing Group Endorsed by the Heart Rhythm Society. *J Am Soc Echocardiogr.* 2008;21:191–213.
78. Alpert MA, Curtis JJ, Sanfelippo JF, et al. Comparative survival after permanent ventricular and dual chamber pacing for patients with chronic high degree atrioventricular block with and without preexistent congestive heart failure. *J Am Coll Cardiol.* 1986;7:925–932.
79. Ertrophic HY, Nishimura RA, Holmes DR, Ilstrup M, Tajik AJ. Effect of dual-chamber pacing on systolic and diastolic function in patients with hypertrophic cardiomyopathy acute Doppler echocardiographic and catheterization hemodynamic study. *J Am Coll Cardiol.* 1996;27:421–430.
80. Ritter P, Padeletti L, Gillio-Meina L, Gaggini G. Determination of the optimal atrioventricular delay in DDD pacing. Comparison between echo and peak endocardial acceleration measurements. *Europace.* 1999;1:126–130.
81. Rokey R, Quinones MA, Zoghbi WA, Kuo LC, Abinader EG. Influence of left atrial systolic emptying on left ventricular early filling dynamics by Doppler in patients with sequential atrioventricular pacemakers. *Am J Cardiol.* 1988;62:968–971.
82. Koneru S, Popovic Z, Cremer P, et al. PROGNOSTIC value of ECHO-DOPPLER guided AV delay optimization following cardiac resynchronization therapy. *J Am Coll Cardiol.* 2016;7:1491.
83. Van Gelder BM, Bracke FA, Meijer A, Lakerveld LJM, Pijls NHJ. Effect of optimizing the VV interval on left ventricular contractility in cardiac resynchronization therapy. *Am J Cardiol.* 2004;93:1500–1503.
84. Bordachar P, Lafitte S, Reuter S, et al. Echocardiographic parameters of ventricular dyssynchrony validation in patients with heart failure using sequential biventricular pacing. *J Am Coll Cardiol.* 2004;44:2157–2165.
85. Sogaard P, Egeblad H, Pedersen AK, et al. Sequential versus simultaneous biventricular resynchronization for severe heart failure: evaluation by tissue Doppler imaging. *Circulation.* 2002;106:2078–2084.
86. Reddy VY, Miller MA, Neuzil P, et al. Cardiac resynchronization therapy with wireless left ventricular endocardial pacing: the SELECT-LV study. *J Am Coll Cardiol.* 2017;69:2119–2129.
87. Ali N, Keene D, Arnold A, Shun-Shin M, Whinnett ZI, Afzal Sohaib SA. His bundle pacing: a new frontier in the treatment of heart failure. *Arrhythm Electrophysiol Rev.* 2018;7:103–110.
88. Catanzariti D, Maines M, Cemin C, Broso G, Marotta T, Vergara G. Permanent direct his bundle pacing does not induce ventricular dyssynchrony unlike conventional right ventricular apical pacing: an intrapatient acute comparison study. *J Interv Cardiac Electrophysiol Int J Arrhythm Pacing.* 2006;16:81–92.
89. Keene D, Arnold A, Shun-Shin MJ, et al. Rationale and design of the randomized multicentre His Optimized Pacing Evaluated for Heart Failure (HOPE-HF) trial. *ESC Heart Fail.* 2018;5:965–976.

31

Aging and Heart Failure With Preserved Ejection Fraction

James P. MacNamara, Satyam Sarma, and Benjamin D. Levine

OUTLINE

Case Study

A 68-year-old woman with a history of hypertension (HTN) presents to clinic with dyspnea on exertion. She is an avid gardener and has been unable to keep up with her weeding over the past few years. Otherwise, she is mostly sedentary. Her blood pressure (BP) is mildly elevated at 145/70 mmHg, pulse is 75 bpm, and oxygen saturation is 99%. On exam, she has a fourth heart sound, but no peripheral edema or distended neck veins. Transthoracic echocardiogram (TTE) is ordered, and her ejection fraction (EF) is 58%, she has mild left ventricular (LV) hypertrophy, E/A ratio is 0.8, septal e′ is 5.5 cm/sec and lateral e′ is 7.0 cm/sec, average E/e′ is 8, left atrial (LA) volume index is 34.5 mL/m^2, and maximum tricuspid regurgitation velocity could not be measured. Grade I diastolic dysfunction is reported. Having seen her report, she returns to clinic and asks, "Do I have diastolic heart failure?"

From a clinical perspective questions that may be pertinent are, "Does the patient have heart failure with preserved ejection fraction (HFpEF)?" "Based on the reported TTE findings, does the patient have grade I diastolic dysfunction?" "What would be the most comprehensive diagnostic test to evaluate this patient's source of dyspnea?"

INTRODUCTION

Heart failure (HF) with preserved ejection fraction poses a particular challenge for clinicians taking care of seniors: Exertional dyspnea is common, comorbid conditions are diverse, and the treatment options are limited. The incidence of heart failure with preserved ejection fraction (HFpEF) is closely associated with age, and the disease contributes significant morbidity and mortality to the elderly population.[1] Clinically, HFpEF is simply defined as the presence of HF signs and symptoms and a preserved EF; however, the euvolemic HFpEF patient can pose a significant diagnostic challenge. Furthermore, dyspnea on exertion is often multifactorial in the elderly. Finally, the cardiovascular changes associated with aging are complex and affected by multiple factors of a person's life.

Aging in itself is not the same for everyone. A 60-year-old obese patient with hypertension (HTN) and diabetes may have a cardiovascular system akin to 90 years of aging, whereas a 60-year-old top athlete may have the heart of a 40-year-old. A sedentary lifestyle and comorbidities, such as metabolic syndrome and kidney disease, likely synergize with aging to impact LV relaxation and compliance. It remains unknown how these changes cross over to the pathologic condition of HFpEF. Furthermore, it is unknown if aging alone is sufficient. If humans live long enough, will they all eventually develop HFpEF?

This chapter aims to critically evaluate the epidemiology and pathophysiology of HFpEF and the aging heart. The first objective of this chapter is to describe the clinical course of HFpEF in the elderly, specifically the challenges in diagnosing the disease in elderly patients. The second objective is to evaluate which aspects of aging are responsible for changes in cardiac function that may lead to HFpEF, with particular attention to changes that are related to not only aging but also how one ages. The final objective will be to explore future avenues of research for HFpEF, diastolic dysfunction, and the elderly, specifically in regard to diagnosis and prevention. Overall, this chapter is meant to help clinicians distinguish between expected aging and pathologic findings when they evaluate elderly patients with dyspnea.

HFpEF AND THE ELDERLY

Epidemiology of HFpEF in Seniors

As the population ages, the rates of cardiovascular diseases increase, including HTN, coronary artery disease (CAD), and congestive heart failure (CHF).[2] Currently CHF affects over 6.5 million adults with annual health care costs of $24 billion, and half of CHF cases are patients with a preserved EF.[2–5] HFpEF is particularly prevalent among seniors with a mean age of +70 and affecting 13% of persons +80 years of age.[6,7] By 2050, the senior population is estimated to exceed 86 million individuals.[8] Clinicians must be prepared to evaluate, diagnose, and treat various causes of dyspnea and differentiate them from expected physiologic changes due to aging.

Elderly patients with HFpEF are a particularly vulnerable population. CHF is the leading cause of hospitalization in patients over age 65 years, and over half of these admissions are HFpEF.[9] An evaluation of elderly hospitalized HF patients found impaired quality of life and depression symptoms to be more prevalent in HFpEF compared to heart failure with reduced ejection fraction (HFrEF), while physical limitation and impaired cognition were similar.[10] In the Cardiovascular Health Study, frailty was found in 6.9% of participants over the age of 65.[11] Frailty has been proposed as a syndrome of unintentional weight loss, exhaustion, weakness, slow walking speed, and low physical activity. In TOPCAT, the presence of frailty was associated with higher risk of HF hospitalization as well as mortality for patients with HFpEF.[12] In HFpEF, patient-centered outcomes are either similar to or worse than HFrEF, and the morbidity of the disease in the elderly is increased when combined with frailty. It is important for clinicians caring for these patients to recognize elderly HFpEF patients as high risk for poor outcomes.

The role HFpEF plays in the death of seniors remains unclear, and there is a higher burden of cardiovascular death in this syndrome than previously thought.[13] Two clinical trials of elderly patients with HFpEF, TIME-CHF and PEP-CHF, reported a cardiovascular cause of death in 60% and 70% of total deaths, though a subanalysis of TIME-CHF demonstrated higher rates of non-CV death in subjects with HFpEF compared to HFrEF.[14,15] Over 300,000 deaths in the United States per year are attributed to HFpEF, and the mortality rates in HFpEF remain steady, in contrast to HFrEF where mortality has started to decline.[7,16] The body of literature regarding the mode of death in HFpEF is heterogeneous, and competing risks play a role that needs to be further defined.

The Role of Comorbidities

While chronologic age can be measured easily, biologic aging may be more relevant for development of HFpEF in a senior population. Increasing age is associated with many of the comorbidities associated with HFpEF, including HTN, diabetes, CAD, renal dysfunction, and atrial fibrillation (AFib).[2] Each of these comorbidities is known to negatively impact diastolic function, and each is highly prevalent in HFpEF (Box 31.1; Tables 31.1 and 31.2). In clinical practice, it is likely that both chronologic aging and biologic aging contribute to development of HFpEF in the elderly as the cardiovascular system takes multiple hits (Fig. 31.1). This multiple hit hypothesis may be what transitions seniors from changes of diastolic function to pathologic HFpEF. Most of the studies discussed in this chapter attempt to separate the effects of aging from the effects of comorbidities by excluding subjects with known comorbid conditions. While helpful when addressing the cardiovascular changes attributable to solely aging, in practice the presence of cardiovascular comorbidities should increase the index of suspicion for HFpEF in the elderly.

BOX 31.1 Proposed Mechanisms of Structural and Cellular Cardiovascular Changes With Aging

Biologic Aging of the Cardiovascular System[1]

- Structural changes
- Arterial stiffening
- Loss of cardiomyocytes
- Hypertrophy
- Ischemic changes
- Cardiac stiffening

Cellular changes

- Molecular signaling changes
- Smooth muscle dysfunction
- Cardiac fibrosis
- Impaired adaptability of autonomic nervous system

TABLE 31.1 Cardiovascular Effects of Common Co-morbidities Over Time

Comorbidity	Cardiovascular Effect Over Time
Diabetes	Increased left ventricular stiffness $SERCA_{2A}$ dysfunction
Hypertension	Left ventricular hypertrophy Increased left ventricular stiffness
Obesity	Concentric remodeling Systemic inflammation Epicardial fat deposits
Chronic kidney disease	Chronic volume overload
Atrial fibrillation	Atrial cardiomyopathy Impaired atrial contraction
Coronary artery disease	Endocardial ischemia

There are many proposed mechanisms for each comorbidity and while this list is not exhaustive, it highlights the potential pathologic cardiovascular effects of comorbidities commonly associated with heart failure with preserved ejection fraction.

AFib in particular is a defining comorbidity of HFpEF. AFib is highly prevalent in HFpEF and associated with similar risk factors and comorbidities.[17–20] In a subanalysis of the CHARM-Preserved trial, AFib coexisted with HFpEF in 29% of subjects and was negatively associated with cardiovascular mortality and hospitalization.[21] In AFib trials, HFpEF is present in 8% to 24% of subjects.[17] This relationship is more challenging in clinical practice, since patients without true HFpEF may have dyspnea on exertion or even pulmonary edema when ventricular rates are rapid, but once their rhythm is controlled, their symptoms improve. Yet AFib begets HFpEF, which begets AFib. For example, chronically elevated LA pressures cause LA dilation, remodeling, and then an atrial cardiomyopathy.[22,23] This pathology in turn creates a favorable substrate for AFib. Furthermore, obesity, HTN, and diabetes are associated with atrial and ventricular remodeling that may lead to both AFib and HFpEF. Finally, AFib impairs late ventricular filling and is thought to impair hemodynamics in HFpEF, though clinical studies are lacking to evaluate this theory. Given their similarities in presentation and risk factors, the presence of either AFib or HFpEF in an elderly patient with other typical comorbidities should raise the clinical suspicion for the other.

Clinical Course of HFpEF in Seniors

The most common clinical presentation of HFpEF in seniors is fatigue and exertional dyspnea.[24] However, there are many conditions that may lead to dyspnea or fatigue, some pathologic, some the result of aging. For example, there is an expected decline in maximal oxygen uptake (VO_2max), the body's ability to utilize oxygen, which is seen with each decade of life.[25] Furthermore, seniors have been shown to have decreased muscle mass, oxygen-carrying capacity of the blood, and lung function.[26,28] Like VO_2max, forced expiratory volume in 1 sec (FEV1) decreases with each decade of life.[28] Several pathologic conditions, such as obstructive CAD, intrinsic lung disease, depression, or

TABLE 31.2 PREVALENCE OF CONDITIONS KNOWN TO NEGATIVELY IMPACT DIASTOLIC DYSFUNCTION IN HFpEF SAMPLES (% of total patients)

(% OF TOTAL PATIENTS)	Olmsted County	ADHERE	Ancillary DIG Trial	CHARM-Preserved Trial
Number of patients	4596	26322	988	3023
Hypertension, %	63	77	60	23
Hx MI or CAD, %	53	50	50	45
Diabetes, %	33	45	29	28
Atrial fibrillation, %	41	21	No data	29

Prevalence of Co-morbidities in HFpEF, trials and studies demonstrating the high association of hypertension, CAD diabetes and atrial fibrillation in HFpEF. HFpEF, Heart Failure with Preserved ejection Fraction; ADHERE, *Acute Decompensated HEart Failure National REgistry;* DIG, *Digitalis Investigation Group;* CHARM, *Candesartan in Heart Failure: Assessment of Reduction in Mortality and Morbidity;* Hx, *history;* MI, *myocardial infarction;* CAD, *coronary artery disease.*

Adapted from Owan TE, et al. Trends in prevalence and outcome of heart failure with preserved ejection fraction. *N Engl J Med.* 2006;355(3):251–259; Yancy CW, et al. Clinical presentation, management, and in-hospital outcomes of patients admitted with acute decompensated heart failure with preserved systolic function: a report from the Acute Decompensated Heart Failure National Registry (ADHERE) database. *J Am Coll Cardiol.* 2006;47(1):76–84; Yusuf S, et al. Effects of candesartan in patients with chronic heart failure and preserved left-ventricular ejection fraction: the CHARM-Preserved trial. *Lancet.* 2003;362(9386):777–781; Ahmed A, et al. Effects of digoxin on morbidity and mortality in diastolic heart failure: the ancillary digitalis investigation group trial. *Circulation.* 2006;114(5):397–403.

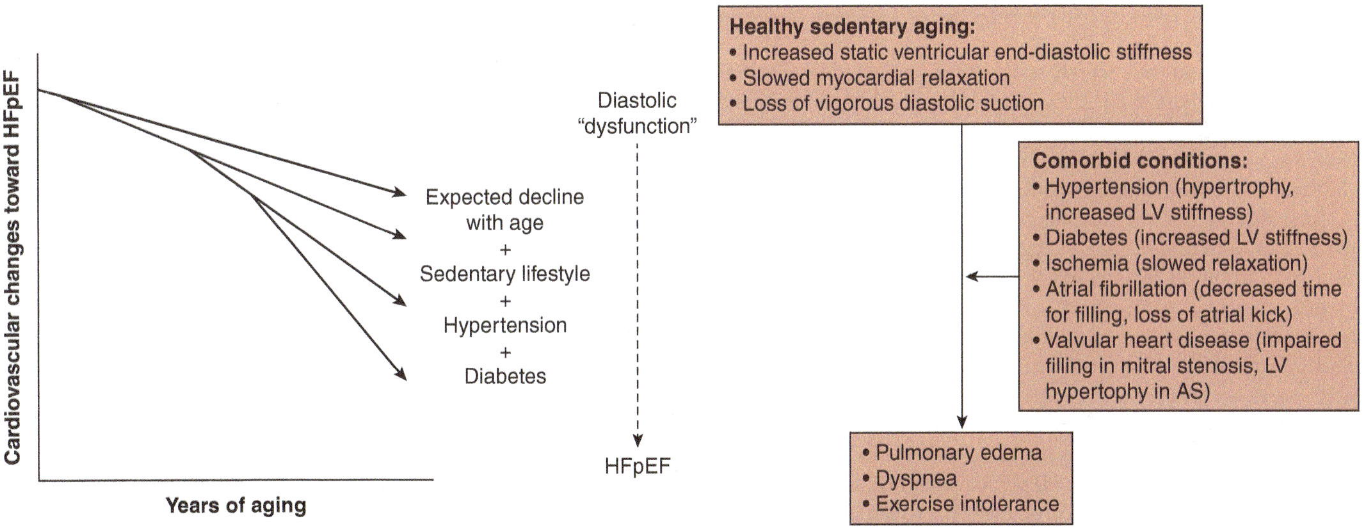

Fig. 31.1 Proposed paradigm by which aging and comorbid conditions overlaid on a substrate of slowed relaxation and decreased compliance could result in heart failure with preserved ejection fraction *(HFpEF). AS,* Aortic stenosis; *LV,* left ventricular.

systemic illnesses may also present with exertional dyspnea or fatigue and are common among seniors.[2,29–32] While a variety of diseases cause dyspnea, HFpEF is a common culprit. HFpEF generally presents later in life, and the incidence of HFpEF overtakes HFrEF in the seventh decade of life.[33] HFpEF makes up 90% of incident CHF diagnoses in elderly women.[34] A prototypical elderly HFpEF patient is female and likely to have HTN, obesity, diabetes, or AFib,[35] but there is great diversity in the disease. Thus a clinician must approach dyspneic patients with a broad perspective to appropriately identify the source.

Diagnosis of HFpEF in Seniors

The American Heart Association/American College of Cardiology (AHA/ACC) definition from 2013 consists of symptoms of HF (Box 31.2) and an EF of 50% and above[36] (Box 31.3). The AHA/ACC guidelines do not specify measures of diastolic function or left venticular (LV) filling pressures. In contrast, the European Society of Cardiology (ESC) guidelines recommend evaluating filling pressures either invasively through pulmonary capillary wedge pressure (PCWP) or LV end-diastolic pressure (EDP) or by estimating volume overload through elevated E/e′ ratio or elevated brain natriuretic protein (BNP).[37] Neither guideline refers to graded diastolic dysfunction as defined by the American Society of Echocardiography (ASE), though this classification is what is reported to many clinicians.[38] The formal diagnostic criteria for HFpEF are no different for seniors than other populations.

For decompensated HFpEF patients with acute congestion and a preserved EF, the diagnosis is straightforward. However, many patients with early stages of HFpEF may present with dyspnea on exertion without clear physical evidence to suggest HF. For these patients, the diagnosis can be challenging. The most reliable method to establish the diagnosis is invasive hemodynamic exercise testing, where a pathologic increase in LV filling pressure is detected with a right heart catheter during exercise.[39] Alternatively, a noninvasive diastolic stress test can be performed to estimate elevated LV filling pressures with exercise,[40] though such markers are imprecise (see Chapter 18). Recently, Reddy et al. proposed a diagnostic score, call the H2FPEF, which combines a number of clinical and echocardiographic characteristics to identify those at risk for HFpEF.[41] Age over 60 years is one of the

BOX 31.2 Framingham Heart Failure Criteria

Framingham Heart Failure Criteria[11]

Diagnosis of HF requires 2 major criteria OR 1 major and 2 minor criteria.

Major Criteria

Acute pulmonary edema
Cardiomegaly
Hepatojugular reflux
Neck vein distention
Paroxysmal nocturnal dyspnea or orthopnea
Pulmonary rales
Third heart sound (S_3 gallop rhythm)
Weight loss >4.5 kg in 5 days in response to treatment

Minor Criteria

Ankle edema
Dyspnea on exertion
Hepatomegaly
Nocturnal cough
Pleural effusion
Tachycardia (HR >120)

BOX 31.3 AHA/ACC and ESC Diagnostic Guidelines for HFpEF

AHA/ACC Definition

1. EF ≥50%
2. Also referred to as diastolic HF. Several different criteria have been used to further define HFpEF. The diagnosis of HFpEF is challenging because it is largely one of excluding other potential noncardiac causes of symptoms suggestive of HF. To date, efficacious therapies have not been identified

ESC Definition

Three conditions must be satisfied:

1. Symptoms or signs of HF
2. Normal or near normal systolic function, EF >50%, in the absence of ventricular dilatation
3. Evidence of elevated filling pressures: pulmonary capillary wedge pressure >12 mmHg, left ventricular end-diastolic pressure >16 mmHg, echocardiographic Doppler E/E′ >15, or B-type natriuretic peptide >200

AHA; American Heart Association
ACC: American College of Cardiology
ESC: European Society of Cardiology
EF: Ejection Fraction
HF: Heart Failure
HFpEF: Heart Failure with Preserved Ejection Fraction

scoring markers and thus corresponds with increased odds of having HFpEF in their cohort. While the widespread applicability of this score for diagnosing HFpEF is unknown, it has strong potential to identify those who warrant further evaluation, particularly among the elderly who are likely to have a higher score.

Currently, the ASE diastolic function guidelines do not have a formal role in detecting or diagnosing HFpEF, even though abnormal diastolic function is a hallmark of the disease. There are many reasons for this omission, but primarily it highlights the complex nature of diastolic function and the transition to a disease state. The 2016 ASE guidelines focus on using echocardiographic markers specifically to detect increased LA pressures in patients with myocardial pathology.[38] Yet decompensated HFpEF patients, where this approach is most apt, are diagnosed clinically with relative ease. With the focus on elevated resting LA pressures, euvolemic HFpEF patients may not be detected by an echo performed at rest. Three analyses of HFpEF clinical trials confirm that when diastolic function is assessed by an echo in clinically adjudicated HFpEF patients, upwards of 30% have normal diastolic function (Fig. 31.2).[42–44] The progression from normal cardiac function to decompensated HFpEF is likely a gradual decline that involves multiple cardiac and noncardiac mechanisms.[45] The individual components of diastolic function that can ultimately lead to HFpEF are each impacted by aging differently.

CARDIOVASCULAR AGING, DIASTOLIC DYSFUNCTION, AND HFpEF

The cardiovascular changes in HFpEF are primarily subclinical systolic dysfunction, decreased cardiac compliance, and abnormal lusitropy or relaxation of the left ventricle.[46–48] Aging by itself is associated with a slowing in relaxation and a decline in ventricular compliance, though there are many factors that influence how aging leads to cardiovascular

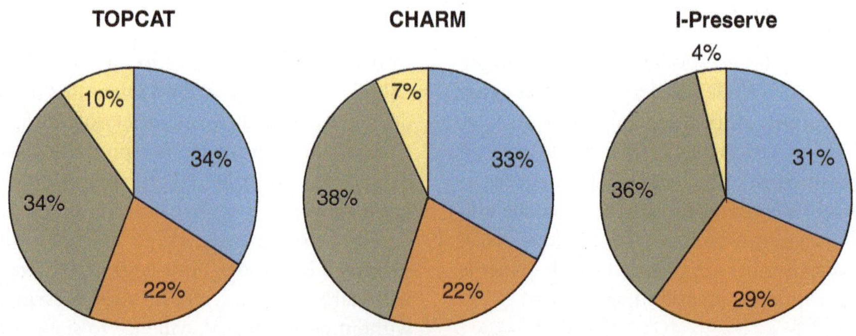

Fig. 31.2 Application of diastolic guidelines to three clinical trials of ajudicated HFpEF patients. All three demonstrate ~33% of HFpEF patients have normal diastolic function by echocardiography. (Data from Zile MR, et al. Prevalence and significance of alterations in cardiac structure and function in patients with heart failure and a preserved ejection fraction. *Circulation.* 2011;124(23):2491–2501; Persson H, et al. Diastolic dysfunction in heart failure with preserved systolic function: need for objective evidence: results from the CHARM Echocardiographic Substudy-CHARMES. *J Am Coll Cardiol.* 2007;49(6):687–694; Shah AM, et al. Cardiac structure and function in heart failure with preserved ejection fraction: baseline findings from the echocardiographic study of the Treatment of Preserved Cardiac Function Heart Failure with an Aldosterone Antagonist trial. *Circ Heart Fail.* 2014;7(1):104–115.)

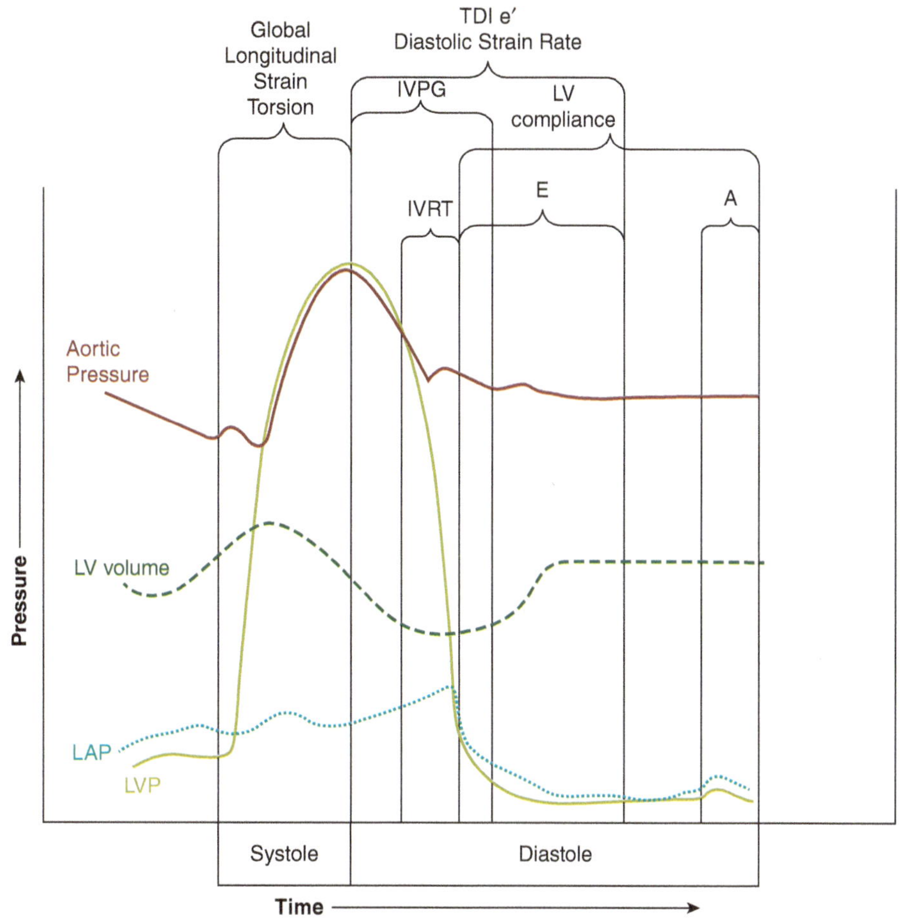

Fig. 31.3 Pressure curve throughout the cardiac cycle representing left ventricular pressure *(LVP)*, left atrial pressure *(LAP)*, left ventricular *(LV)* volume, and aortic pressure. Surrogates for systole, relaxation, and compliance are marked during their respective period of the cardiac cycle. The purpose of this section is to review the changes attributable to aging on LV systolic function, relaxation, and compliance. *A,* Late diastolic mitral inflow; *E,* early diastolic mitral inflow; *e′,* early diastolic mitral annular velocity; *IVPG,* intraventricular pressure gradient; *IVRT,* isovolumetric relaxation time; *TDI,* tissue Doppler imaging. (Adapted from Prasad A, et al. The effects of aging and physical activity on Doppler measures of diastolic function. *Am J Cardiol.* 2007;99(12):1629–1636.)

changes. Most notably, sedentary aging has been repeatedly associated with decline in cardiac function, compared to lifelong exercise.[49–51] The presence of comorbidities, such as the metabolic syndrome, also influences these changes. Therefore it becomes challenging to differentiate what changes are attributed to aging itself as opposed to inactivity or cardiovascular damage from comorbid pathologic states.

Are the cardiovascular changes of aging normal? This question underscores the complex nature of the processes underlying diastolic function and HFpEF. Some age-related changes in the human body can be considered normal, such as the graying of hair. This cannot be prevented (though it can be hidden) and does not precede a pathologic state for most people. The cardiovascular changes with age do not follow the same pattern. Perhaps fitness is an apt model: As stated earlier, a person's maximal oxygen uptake declines with each decade of life. If a healthy 70-year-old's VO_2max is 20 mL/kg/min and a healthy 30-year-old's is 40 mL/kg/min, the difference is an expected aspect of aging, but the 70-year-old is still less fit. In turn, if a 70-year-old's heart is less compliant and relaxes slower than a 30-year-old's, the change is expected but not normal, or at least not youthful.

It is currently unknown exactly how decreases in systolic function, relaxation, and compliance coalesce into the disease state of HFpEF. In seniors it is likely that a combination of expected changes with aging, prior exercise, and presence of comorbidities combine to push the heart first into an asymptomatic disease state with subclinical structural abnormalities (stage B HFpEF) and then into a symptomatic phase over time.[45] Understanding these changes is critical to understanding the development of HFpEF in seniors and may hold the key to identifying preventative strategies. This section will focus on the three critical cardiovascular alterations in HFpEF: subclinical systolic dysfunction, slowed ventricular relaxation, and decreased ventricular compliance. Over the past 30 years a variety of techniques have been used to assess these phases of the cardiac cycle (Fig. 31.3; Table 31.3). Aging is associated with clear patterns of decline in multiple aspects of cardiac function, but their relationship to pathology, such as the development of HFpEF, is less clear.

Systolic Function (Fig. 31.4)

Diastole begins in systole as the systolic excursion engages compressive forces (e.g., titin and the connective tissue matrix) and primes the ventricle for early relaxation (see Chapters 1 and 30). Thus to understand age's effect on cardiac function and a person's risk for HFpEF, systolic function must be considered. EF is generally preserved with healthy aging, but advances in noninvasive imaging over the past 20 years have enabled a more thorough analysis of systolic function. Modern markers

TABLE 31.3 Representative Examples of Surrogates for Various Aspects of Cardiac Function

Systolic Function	Relaxation	Compliance
TDIs′	Tau	Stiffness index
MAPSE	Isovolumetric relaxation time	
Global longitudinal strain	TDIe′	
Torsion	Intraventricular pressure gradient	

TDI: Tissue Doppler Imaging
MAPSE: Mitral Annular Planar Excursion

of subclinical systolic function target the motion of the left ventricle, as opposed to EF, which is a measure of volumes (see Chapter 10). Global longitudinal strain and mitral annular excursion measure longitudinal motion as the mitral annulus moves toward the apex during systole. Torsion represents the twisting of the ventricle during systole and has been shown to increase with age.[52] In a study of 313 healthy subjects, Kaku et al. demonstrated an increase in global three-dimensional (3-D) strain from −36.3% in subjects aged 20 to 29 years to −39.0% in subjects aged over 60 years though the consequence of this difference is unclear.[53] Limited studies suggest that overall systolic mechanics do not decrement with age.

With aging, the heart undergoes alterations that may compromise longitudinal function, such as myocardial remodeling and becoming more spheroid. In 1998, Wandt et al. described a 20% decrement in mitral annular excursion from the third to the eighth decade of life.[54] More recent studies have demonstrated that multiple factors influence the assessment of longitudinal motion, including BP (i.e., afterload), imaging technique, and regular exercise training. A **cardiac** magnetic resonance imaging (MRI) analysis of subjects aged 50 to 79 years (48 healthy, 40 with HTN) did not demonstrate a significant decrease in longitudinal shortening with age but did find a decrease in patients with HTN, highlighting the importance of afterload in the assessment of longitudinal systolic function.[55] Howden et al., using speckle tracking echocardiography, found reduced longitudinal strain in sedentary seniors compared to sedentary young participants, but this difference was ameliorated in seniors with a committed level of lifelong exercise[56] (Fig. 31.5). It is likely that structural adaptations of a sedentary lifestyle and increases in BP and arterial stiffness (see Chapter 6) are responsible for diminished longitudinal motion with aging. Differences among measurement techniques complicate definitive conclusions.[57] Further studies, as well as an identification of a gold standard reference, are needed to further elucidate changes in cardiac motion with aging, its overall impact to cardiac performance, and its contribution to HFpEF.

LV Relaxation (Fig. 31.6)

Elevated LV filling pressures are a clinical hallmark of HFpEF and are primarily due to alterations in both LV relaxation and compliance. LV relaxation refers to the early diastolic period when the ventricle is recoiling from systolic contraction creating a suction effect and pressure gradient from the left atrium into the left ventricle[58,59] (see Chapter 2). Relaxation can be assessed through a variety of invasive and noninvasive

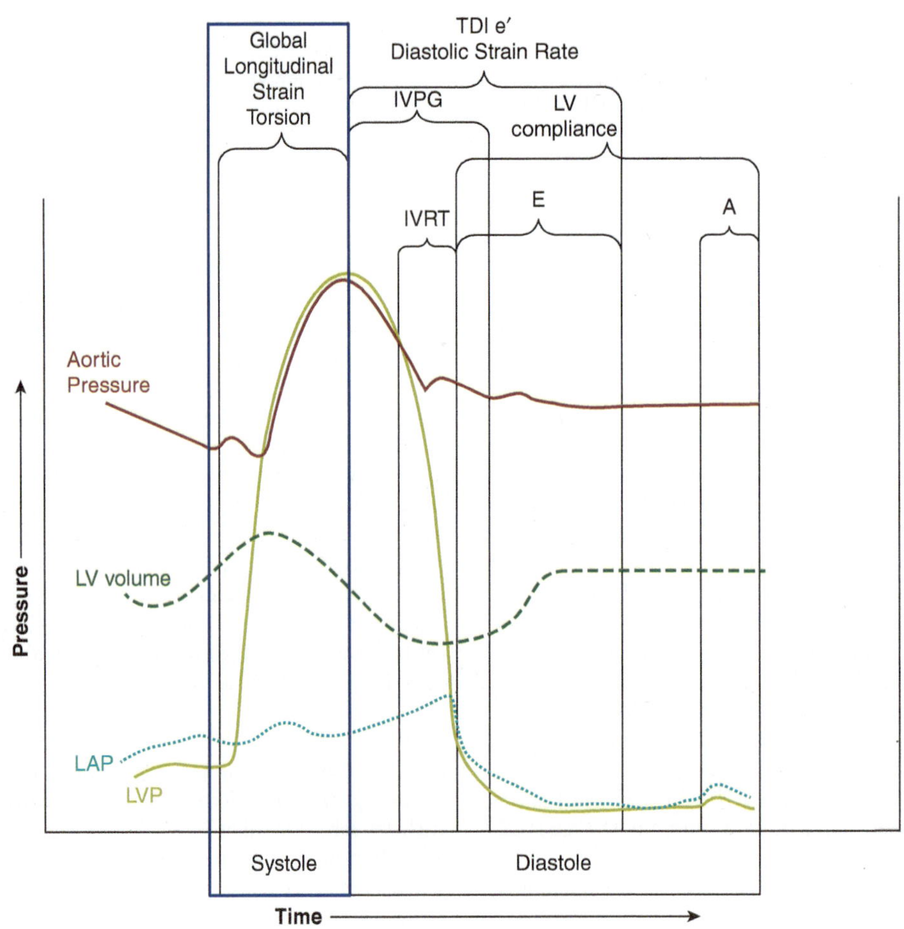

Fig. 31.4 Systolic function.

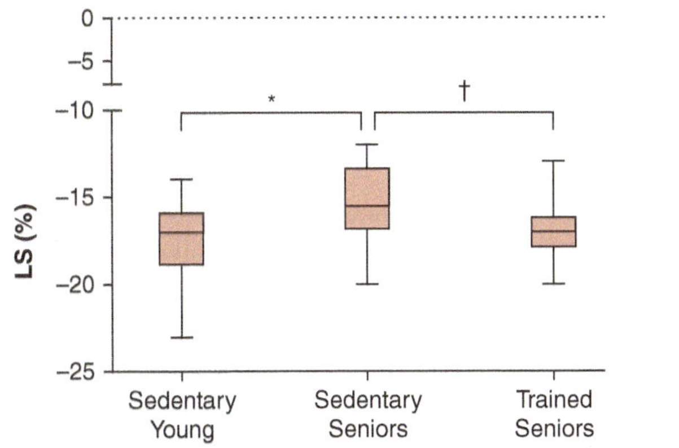

Fig. 31.5 Longitudinal strain *(LS)* in sedentary young controls, sedentary seniors, and lifelong exercisers. Sedentary seniors have a significantly lower (less negative) strain than their fit peers. *, $p < 0.05$; †, $p < 0.05$. (From Howden EJ, et al. Effects of sedentary aging and lifelong exercise on left ventricular systolic function. *Med Sci Sports Exerc.* 2018;50(3):494–501.)

surrogates. Invasively, relaxation is best represented as a time constant (tau [τ]), the logarithmic pressure decay within the left ventricle after aortic valve closure.[60] τ is calculated either from a directly measured LV pressure curve or extrapolated from systolic BP, PCWP, and isovolumetric relaxation time (IVRT). Using echocardiography, there are several markers of ventricular relaxation. Early diastolic velocity of the mitral annulus measured by tissue Doppler imaging (e′) is the most frequently used marker of relaxation and tracks the longitudinal velocity of the ventricular base through early diastole. IVRT is a measure of ventricular relaxation prior to diastolic filling, and propagation velocity of early mitral inflow (Vp) is dependent on the intrinsic ventricular relaxation and diastolic suction (see Chapters 9, 10 and 11). This section will evaluate the current state of evidence for the effect of aging and fitness on ventricular relaxation.

Invasive Markers of Relaxation

Few studies have evaluated the change of relaxation with aging invasively. In 1980, Hirota et al. performed one of the first studies to suggest alterations in LV relaxation were associated with aging.[61] They examined LV pressure decline in 18 subjects, 4 of whom were older than 60 years, referred for diagnostic catheterization. Despite small numbers, they found a modest but significant correlation between τ and age (Fig. 31.7). Other studies are equally small and have found inconsistent relationships between aging and τ. Unpublished data from our lab using systolic BP, PCWP, and IVRT to calculate τ also demonstrate a modest prolongation of τ with increasing age. Approximately 3.5 τ are needed for the heart to fully relax. If τ is prolonged and the heart rate increases, the ventricle may not have time to completely relax, which may contribute to HFpEF patients' pathologic increase in filling pressure during exercise.[58]

Noninvasive Markers of Relaxation

Given the sparsity and inconsistency of invasive data, the relationship between relaxation and aging has been established primarily by

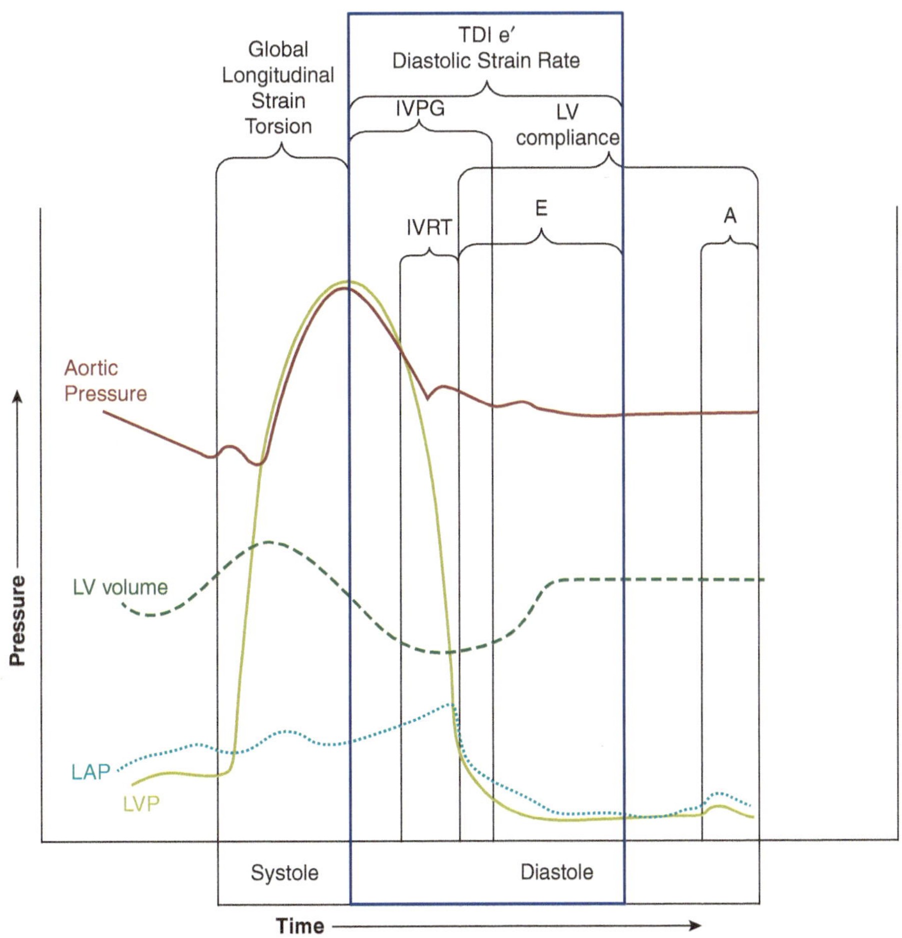

Fig. 31.6 Left ventricular relaxation.

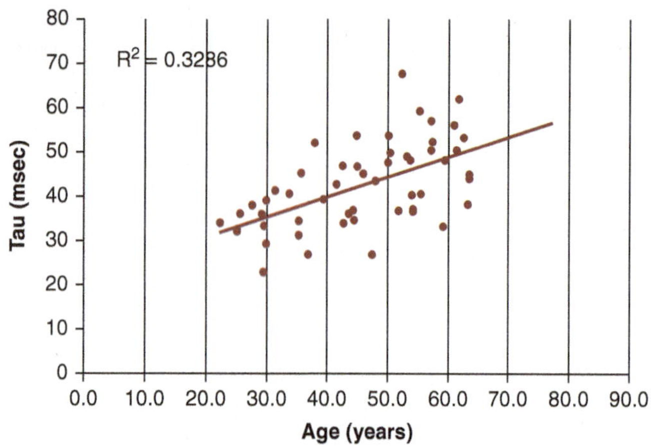

Fig. 31.7 Linear regression of cross-sectional data of 53 healthy subjects who underwent right heart catheterization for various studies (unpublished data). This represents modest prolongation of τ with increased age of the subject.

noninvasive means. Early diastolic velocity (e′) is an imperfect surrogate for myocardial relaxation but has been shown repeatedly to decrease with age[50,62–65] (Fig. 31.8). Popovic et al. found that intraventricular pressure gradient (IVPG), a marker of early diastolic suction, is lower in sedentary seniors compared to young controls.[66] Interestingly, top athletes had similar IVPGs to their sedentary peers. Early diastolic strain rate measures the velocity of ventricular recoil using speckle tracking and has been shown to be inversely associated with aging.[67] While none of these markers perfectly represents relaxation, the bulk of evidence suggests that LV filling during early diastole diminishes with age.

Prasad et al.[7] sought to determine if these age-related changes in relaxation are solely due to aging or are related to fitness and sedentary aging. To answer this question, 13 healthy, sedentary seniors (aged 70 ± 4 years), 12 top athletes (aged 68 ± 3 years), and 12 young subjects (aged 32 ± 9 years) underwent evaluation of their diastolic function at rest and under various loading parameters using saline infusion and lower body negative pressure (LBNP).[50] Fit seniors' e′ was lower than young controls but significantly higher than sedentary seniors. Furthermore, IVRT was similar between top athletes and sedentary seniors. In this case, an active lifestyle blunted the decline in relaxation but did not completely prevent it. Furthermore, this study evaluated the effects of cardiac loading, a key influence on diastolic performance, by measuring and manipulating LA pressure with saline loading and LBNP. During maximal unloading with LBNP, the fit seniors' e′ normalized and became similar to young controls, but the sedentary seniors remained lower. In conclusion, LV relaxation appears to decline steadily with age, and while this may be slowed with lifelong exercise it cannot be prevented.

LV Compliance (Fig. 31.9)

In addition to abnormal relaxation, elevated cardiac pressure during exercise is a downstream effect of ventricular compliance (see Chapter 2). Compliance is the inverse of stiffness and describes how easily the heart expands when filled with blood. As the ventricular filling increases, higher filling pressures develop for a given volume in a nonlinear fashion. Instantaneous compliance itself is the change in volume divided by the change in pressure (dV/dP) and can be represented over a range of pressures as an exponential pressure-volume (P-V) curve.[49,68] Compliance can be calculated for the overall LV chamber (chamber compliance) by using PCWP or myocardial compliance by using transmural pressure. Transmural pressure is the difference between the LA (pulmonary capillary wedge) pressure and right atrial (RA) pressure and accounts for the effects of pericardial constraint on the P-V relationship. When compared to age-matched healthy controls, patients with HFpEF have decreased distensibility (higher pressure for a given volume) but similar overall compliance.[47]

There are two invasive methods to assess LV compliance (see Chapter 8). A LV conductance catheter can be placed directly in the left

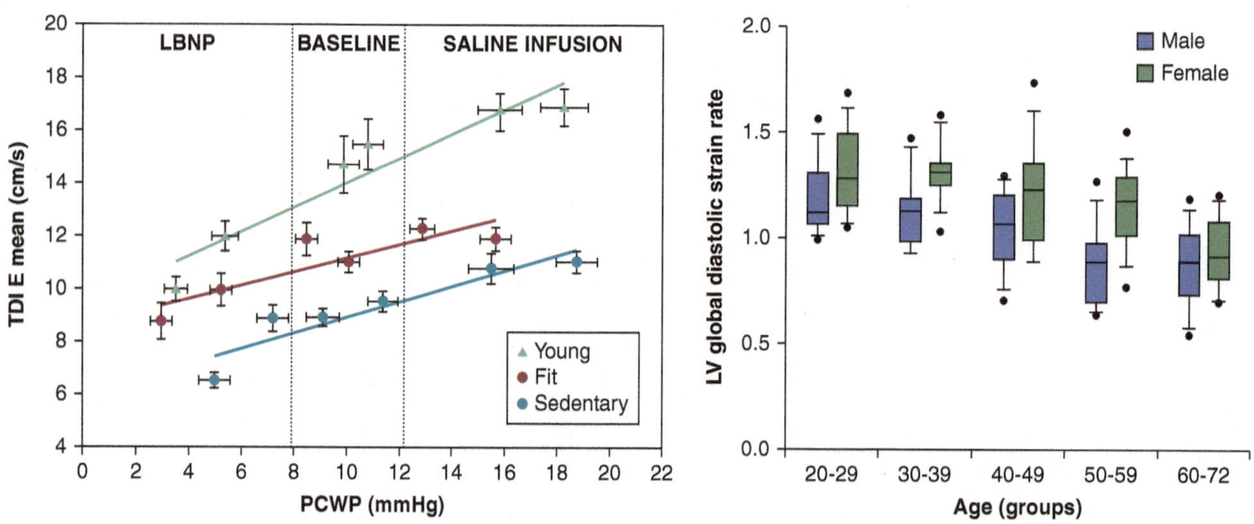

Fig. 31.8 Two studies demonstrating decline in markers of relaxation with increasing age of the subject. The left panel shows the effect of age and loading on the early diastolic tissue Doppler velocity of the mitral annulus. E′ is lowest in sedentary seniors (circle) compared to fit seniors (open circle) and young adults loaded (triangles). Early diastolic strain rate by speckle tracking (right) declines in 147 healthy Dutch volunteers aged 20-72 years in both men (purple) and women (female). (Left panel: from Prasad, A., et al., The effects of aging and physical activity on Doppler measures of diastolic function. *Am J Cardiol*, 2007. 99(12): p. 1629-36., Right panel: from van Grootel, R.W.J., et al., Influence of age and sex on left ventricular diastolic strain analysis. *Int J Cardiovasc Imaging*, 2019. 35(3): p. 491–498.)

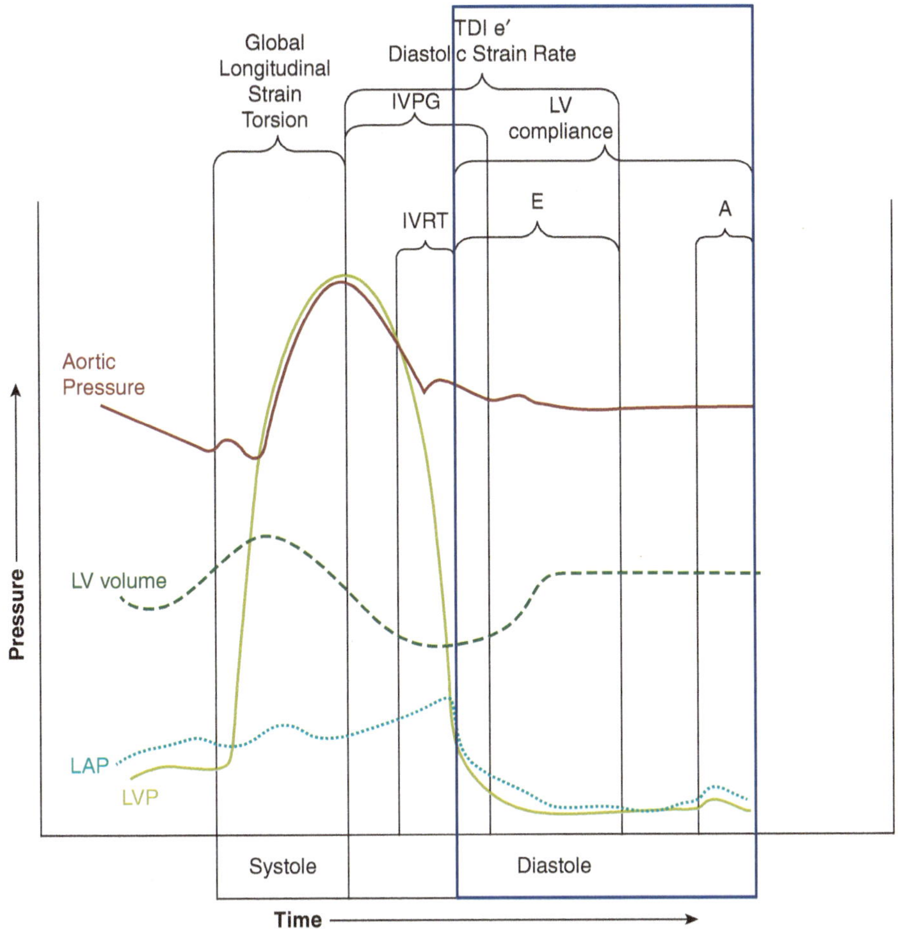

Fig. 31.9 Left ventricular compliance.

ventricle; electrical signals emitted from either end of the catheter are sensed by electrodes in between to determine volumetric changes of the ventricle in real time.[69,70] This technique has the advantage of measuring EDP and volumes simultaneously but has risks of arterial access and LV manipulation. A safer method for research volunteers combines a right heart catheter and echocardiography.[49,51,71,72] The right heart catheter provides RA pressure and PCWP. Echocardiography measures the end-diastolic volume (EDV). From baseline, loading parameters can be manipulated using lower body negative pressure and saline infusion to decrease and increase cardiac filling, respectively. These points create an end-diastolic P-V curve for the participant that represents LV compliance.

Animal models have shown decreases in left compliance with aging, but as with all other measures it was unclear if aging was the true culprit. Arbab-Zadeh et al. measured LV P-V curves and Starling curves in 12 healthy but sedentary seniors (mean age 70 years), 12 top athletes (mean age 68 years), and 14 young sedentary controls using the methods described earlier to evaluate if decrease in LV compliance is an unavoidable result of aging.[9,49] The results (Fig. 31.10) show the opposite. While there was a significant increase in LV stiffness in healthy seniors compared to young controls, the top athletes' ventricles were much more compliant than their sedentary senior counterparts, almost mirroring the young controls. This experiment suggests that LV stiffness is a result of sedentary aging rather than aging alone and prompts the question if exercise can prevent or even reverse the decrease in LV compliance seen with aging.

Mitral Inflow

Mitral inflow patterns have been a critical aspect of the evaluation of diastolic function for over 50 years but are a great source of confusion in the elderly (see Chapter 9). Traditionally an inverted E/A ratio (<1) had been deemed impaired relaxation. More recent guidelines have used other parameters, such as tissue Doppler and LA size, to detect diastolic dysfunction before stratifying the grade using inflow.[38] Age-related changes in mitral inflow patterns have long been recognized, but the mechanism of these changes remains unclear. The mitral inflow is a pulse wave Doppler signal at the level of the mitral valve leaflets and represents flow into the left ventricle during early diastole (E wave) and late diastole (A wave).[73] The mitral inflow occurs throughout the diastolic phase and is driven by pressure gradients between the left ventricle and left atrium, which are in turn influenced by LV relaxation and compliance. Therefore the alterations in mitral inflow with aging are a complex combination of aging, fitness, and hemodynamic circumstances.

Due to mitral inflow's widespread clinical use there has been considerable interest in evaluating the changes with age. In 1987, Bryg et al. found a considerably higher E/A ratio in young subjects compared to older subjects.[74] In 1991, Kitzman et al. demonstrated similar mitral inflow differences between the age groups despite similarities in LV mass, volumes, EF, LA size, BP, and PCWP.[75] The Cardiovascular Health Study demonstrated in 5000 men and women in a community-based population study that E wave progressively decreased and A wave progressively increased with age independent of gender, race, and

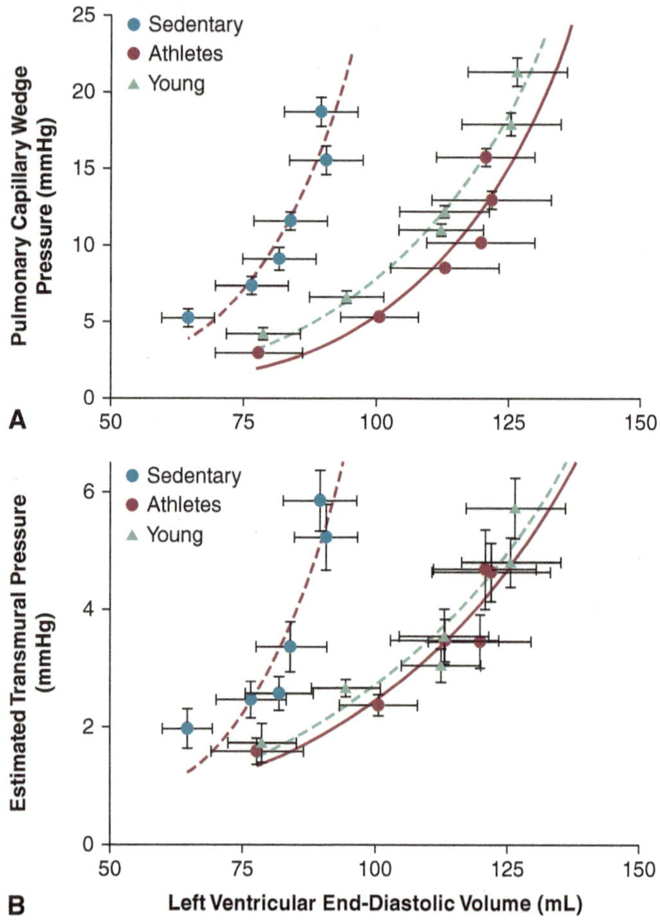

Fig. 31.10 Compliance curves for top athletes *(open circle)*, healthy sedentary seniors *(closed circles)*, and young controls *(triangles)*. As a heart stiffens, the compliance curve moves leftward (more pressure for less volume). Sedentary seniors had compliance curves significantly shifted leftward, whereas top athletes' compliance curves are superimposable on young controls. Cardiac compliance can be represented as a function of pulmonary capillary wedge pressure (PCWP) *(top)*, or isolated LV compliance can be determined by evaluating the transmural pressure (PCWP − right atrial pressure) *(bottom)*. (From Arbab-Zadeh A, et al. Effect of aging and physical activity on left ventricular compliance. *Circulation*. 2004;110(13):1799–1805.)

presence of certain cardiovascular diseases such as HTN and CAD.[76] Finally, Prasad et al. showed sedentary seniors were not able to achieve an E/A ratio greater than 1 even during rapid saline infusion causing increased LA pressures[50] (Fig. 31.11). At baseline, top athletes had E/A ratios between their sedentary peers and young controls, but across different loading parameters their E/A ratios were more similar to their sedentary peers. In conclusion, the E/A ratio declines with age independent of cardiac parameters, comorbidities, and fitness and should not be used in isolation as a marker of pathology, such as grade I diastolic dysfunction (Fig. 31.12).

LV Filling Pressure

If relaxation prolongs with aging and compliance diminishes with sedentary aging, do these changes result in higher LV filling pressures in the elderly compared to the young? In 2017, Wolsk et al. studied 62 healthy participants, evenly distributed for age from 20 to 80 years, to determine if hemodynamic profiles at rest and during exercise varied by age.[77] The subjects were rigorously screened and determined to be healthy by history, echocardiography, exercise test, electrocardiogram (ECG), and spirometry. In the supine position, their hemodynamic profile was assessed by right heart catheterization at rest, with passive leg raise, and incremental exercise. Resting filling pressures were similar in all age groups, but during leg raise and exercise PCWPs trended up and cardiac output trended down significantly with age. During supine exercise testing, 30% of healthy seniors aged 60 to 80 ($n = 18$) mounted a wedge pressure greater than 25 mmHg (Fig. 31.13). This study demonstrates age-related alterations in LV filling with stress, such as leg raise or moderate exercise, even in subjects as young as age 40. Of note, these subjects' hearts were already loaded in the supine position, and thus it is unknown if these differences would have manifested during upright exercise. As would be suspected when comparing age groups, the seniors had higher BP and lower VO_2max than young subjects. As fitness and age are also associated, it becomes challenging to distinguish which is primarily responsible for the abnormalities seen in this study. In conclusion, while sedentary aging is associated with adverse changes in relaxation and compliance, an elevated LV filling pressure at rest should be considered pathologic.

FUTURE DIRECTIONS

Is the Problem Aging or Sedentary Aging?

A major goal of this chapter is distinguishing expected changes in diastolic function from pathologic changes in the elderly. It is clear that diastolic function declines with age and the incidence of HFpEF increases with age, but the connection between these phenomena is still being defined and probed for potential areas of intervention. As discussed, the age-associated decline in some measures of diastolic dysfunction, including LV compliance, is not seen in lifelong athletes and top athletes. On the other end, obesity and low physical activity demonstrate a dose-dependent association with the development of HF, particularly HFpEF. Therefore a lack of physical fitness and exercise contributes to the decline in diastolic function and likely the development of HFpEF in the elderly.

In the elderly patient at risk for or who has developed HFpEF, the future will need improvement in three areas: diagnosis, prevention, and therapy. The need for a novel, effective therapy in HFpEF is not unique to the elderly and is discussed in other chapters. Given the alterations in noninvasive measures of diastolic function, there is an effort to find age-specific cutoffs for diastolic parameters, though this approach has proved challenging. Finally, data compiled from the past two decades suggest that a lack of physical fitness negatively contributes to both measures of LV compliance and lifetime risk of HFpEF. In this section we examine efforts to redefine diastolic dysfunction and HFpEF in a manner that considers age, as well as recent epidemiologic and experimental data that demonstrate exercise can prevent pathologic changes associated with aging and HFpEF.

The New Normal

Cutoffs that define when a metric has passed from normal to abnormal are clinically expedient but fraught with physiologic limitations. As discussed in the prior section, there is an expected decline in relaxation with age that appears independent from fitness and comorbidities. It remains unclear if this decline should be considered normal. The case of e′ and the push to define age-specific cutoffs highlight this conundrum. The 2016 ASE guidelines use a septal and lateral e′ velocity cutoff of 7 cm/sec and 10 cm/sec, respectively, but they are likely too high to apply to elderly patients.[38] These cutoffs were based on test performances across a wide variety of healthy people. The Cardiovascular Healthy Study, among others, has demonstrated a progressive

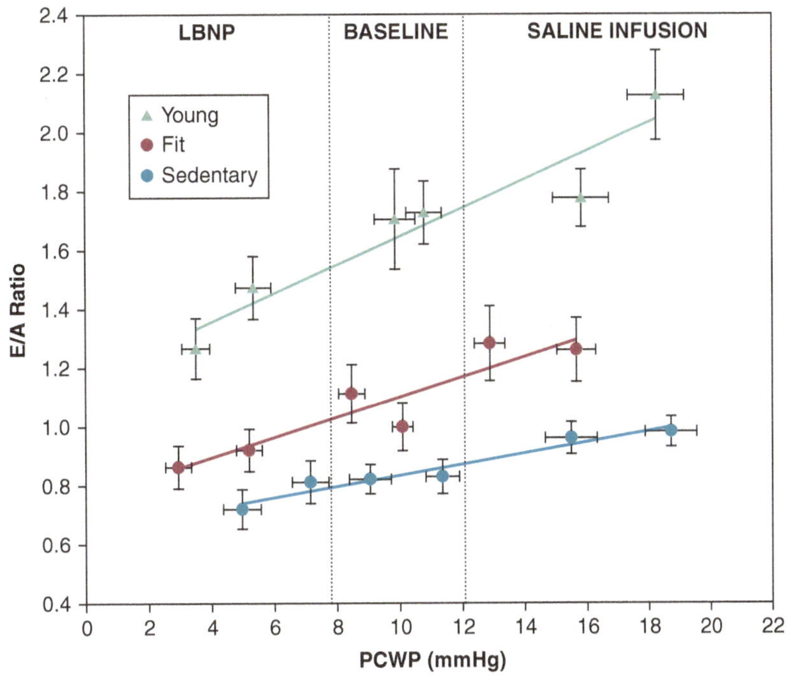

Fig. 31.11 **The E/A ratios in young subjects (triangles), sedentary seniors (closed circles), and top athletes (open circles) are different across loading conditions.** Despite differences in fitness, the two senior groups are distinctly lower in all loading conditions from the young controls. *LBNP*, Lower Body Negative Pressure; *PCWP*, pulmonary capillary wedge pressure. (From Cleland JG, et al. The perindopril in elderly people with chronic heart failure (PEP-CHF) study. *Eur Heart J.* 2006;27(19):2338–2345.)

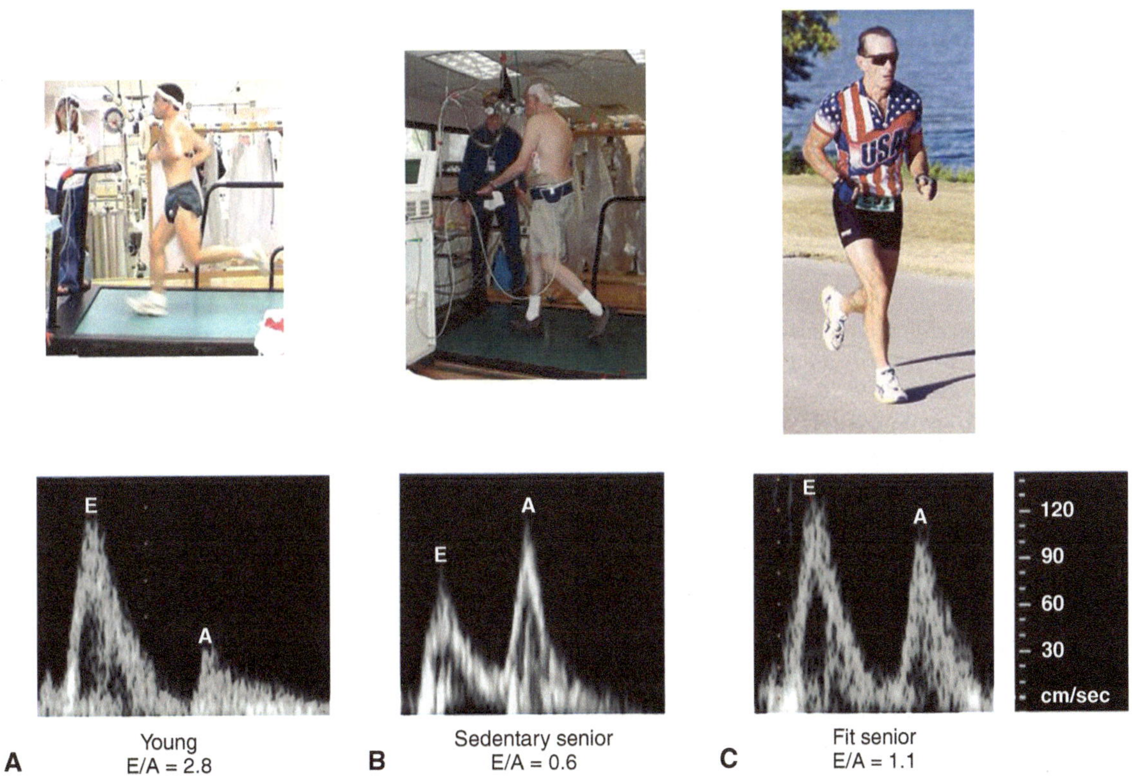

Fig. 31.12 **Examples for how aging and fitness impact resting mitral inflow pattern in young controls (A), sedentary seniors (B), and top athletes (C).** The sedentary senior (B) has an E/A ratio less than 1, while the top athlete's inflow pattern is higher than sedentary seniors (C vs. B) but not as high as young controls (C vs A). These patterns suggest that alterations in relaxation can be attenuated by lifelong exercise but not prevented. (Modified from Prasad A, et al. The effects of aging and physical activity on Doppler measures of diastolic function. *Am J Cardiol.* 2007;99(12):1629–1636.)

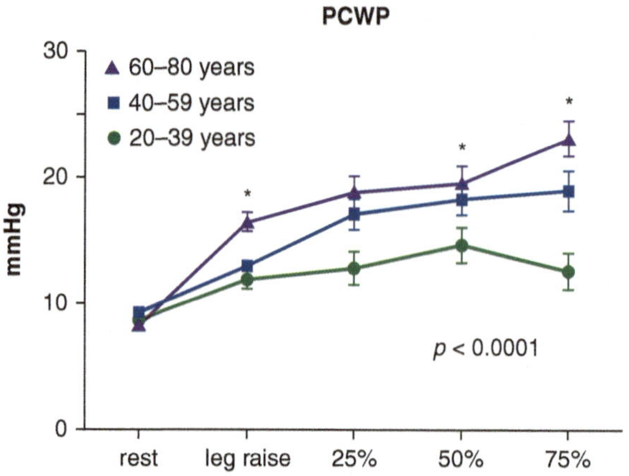

Fig. 31.13 Pulmonary capillary wedge pressure *(PCWP)* measured across age groups at rest and supine graded exercise. Percentages represent exercise at labeled percentage of VO_2max. PCWP is similar at rest, but during exercise PCWP increase more in seniors *(purple)* and middle-aged subjects *(blue)* than young subjects *(green)*. (From Wolsk E, et al. The influence of age on hemodynamic parameters during rest and exercise in healthy individuals. *JACC Heart Fail.* 2017;5(5):337–346.)

decline in e′ with age across a large population.[76] Given the expected decline in e′ with age, these cutoffs have come under scrutiny.

In 2016, Shah et al. analyzed the Atherosclerosis Risk in Communities (ARIC) study to establish reference ranges for diastolic parameters as well as the risk of HF or death.[78] ARIC is a large, multiple-community prospective epidemiologic study designed to evaluate cardiovascular disease and risk factors. To establish reference limits, continuous associations between diastolic parameters (e′, LA volume index [LAVi], E/e′ ratio) and NT-proBNP and incident HF hospitalization or death were established in 5801 subjects aged 67 to 90 years. The 10th and 90th percentile limits for these measures were established in a low-risk, healthy reference subgroup of approximately 400 subjects. Using ASE guideline cutoffs, the investigators found that 82% of subjects had an abnormal septal e′ and 91% had an abnormal lateral e′. Additionally, neither measure demonstrated an association with incident HF hospitalization or death (HR 1.11 [074–1.68], HR 0.80 [0.49–1.30], respectively). Using the lower 10th percentile cutoff of the reference subgroup, only 21% and 18% of subjects in the broader cohort had abnormal values. Yet in the validation cohort, the inflection point for incident HF appears higher, closer to 6 cm/sec septal and 8 cm/sec for lateral e′ (Fig. 31.14). Markers of increased LA pressure, E/e′ ratio, and LAVi also were associated with the development of HF in this population. In conclusion, the e′ thresholds in the current ASE guidelines are not predictive for development of HF in an older population. The true age-related cutoff, if one actually exists, remains a goal of future clinical guidance. The challenge for further evaluation is to refine what clinical parameters are normal, which are abnormal but expected for age, and which are pathologic.

Exercise for Prevention

Regular physical activity plays a key role in the cardiovascular changes seen with aging, and fitness has salutary effects.[79,80] Physical activity has been associated with a declining risk of several cardiovascular risk factors, including HTN, diabetes, and obesity.[81,82] As an epidemic and major consequence of sedentary lifestyle, obesity has been repeatedly associated as a risk factor for the development of HFpEF.[56] Furthermore, low leisure time physical activity has been associated with the future development of HFpEF.[83] In the Framingham Heart Study, there was an inverse association between physical activity and HFpEF, but not HFrEF. In a cross-sectional analysis of the Cooper Clinic Longitudinal Study (CCLS), Brinker et al. demonstrated an inverse association between fitness and diastolic dysfunction as well as abnormal concentric remodeling.[84] In another analysis of the CCLS, participants who increased their fitness by 1 MET over 4.4 years demonstrated a 17% reduction in development of HF.[85]

In an effort to determine whether exercise training may prevent HFpEF, Fujimoto et al. in 2013 randomized healthy seniors aged 67 ± 6 years in 2 × 2 fashion to 1 year of exercise training and alagebrium, a thiazolium derivative that breaks advanced glycation end-product crosslinks and prevents the accumulation of collagen. P-V curves quantifying the degree of LV stiffness were established for each subject before and after their training intervention. Ultimately 1 year of training did not impact the subject's compliance.[72] When alagebrium and exercise were combined, ventricular compliance was modestly improved, suggesting that when structural affects are addressed, exercise is effective. It is possible that there is a point of no return when cardiac plasticity is insufficient to reverse the effects of sedentary aging. Given that a middle-aged population has more remodeling reserve, Howden et al. performed a similar trial in middle-aged subjects with a longer duration of training.[71] They recruited 61 healthy participants (53 ± 5 years) and randomized them to 2 years of exercise training or yoga as a control. Exercise training demonstrated both an increase in fitness (VO_2max), LVEDV, as well as improvement in LV stiffness (Fig. 31.15). This study was the first of its kind to demonstrate reversal of age-related stiffness in healthy subjects. As stiffness is a known and essential component of the pathology of HFpEF, the potential to reverse it has implications in the prevention of HFpEF. Future studies are needed to determine the dose of exercise required, determine if this point of no return is directly related to the risk of HFpEF, and if possible demonstrate a reduction in HFpEF incidence.

CONCLUSIONS

The diagnosis of HFpEF should be considered for any elderly patient with dyspnea, and stage B HFpEF is a potential source for the dyspnea that the patient experienced in the chapter-opening case study. In this patient's case, her resting evaluation is insufficient to diagnose or exclude the disease. Her echo parameters, particularly the e′, were close to or below the clinical cutoffs but also are not beyond the expected decline with age and are not predictive of HF. A cardiopulmonary exercise test (CPET) is able to evaluate for cardiac, pulmonary, or muscular sources of dyspnea and fatigue. Her CPET demonstrated a diminished VO_2max but no clear or excessive cardiac or pulmonary limitations. She was diagnosed with deconditioning and given an exercise routine to improve her functional capacity and reduce her dyspnea. Other patients may require a right heart catheterization during exercise to secure the diagnosis.

In conclusion, HFpEF occurs commonly in the elderly and carries a high risk for morbidity and mortality. The confluence of the expected cardiovascular changes with age and other cardiac and non-cardiac insults contribute to this association. Great care must be taken when evaluating seniors with exertional dyspnea as many diseases may present similarly, and the echocardiogram is fraught with limitations for defining diastolic dysfunction. Future research should be directed at better defining which elderly patients are at risk for developing HFpEF and tailor the noninvasive assessment to help clinicians recognize these patients. Furthermore, exercise training can reverse the negative effects of sedentary aging up to a certain point. While challenging to implement over a lifetime, it is critically important that clinicians and patients do not neglect routine exercise in an effort to prevent the growing epidemic of HFpEF.

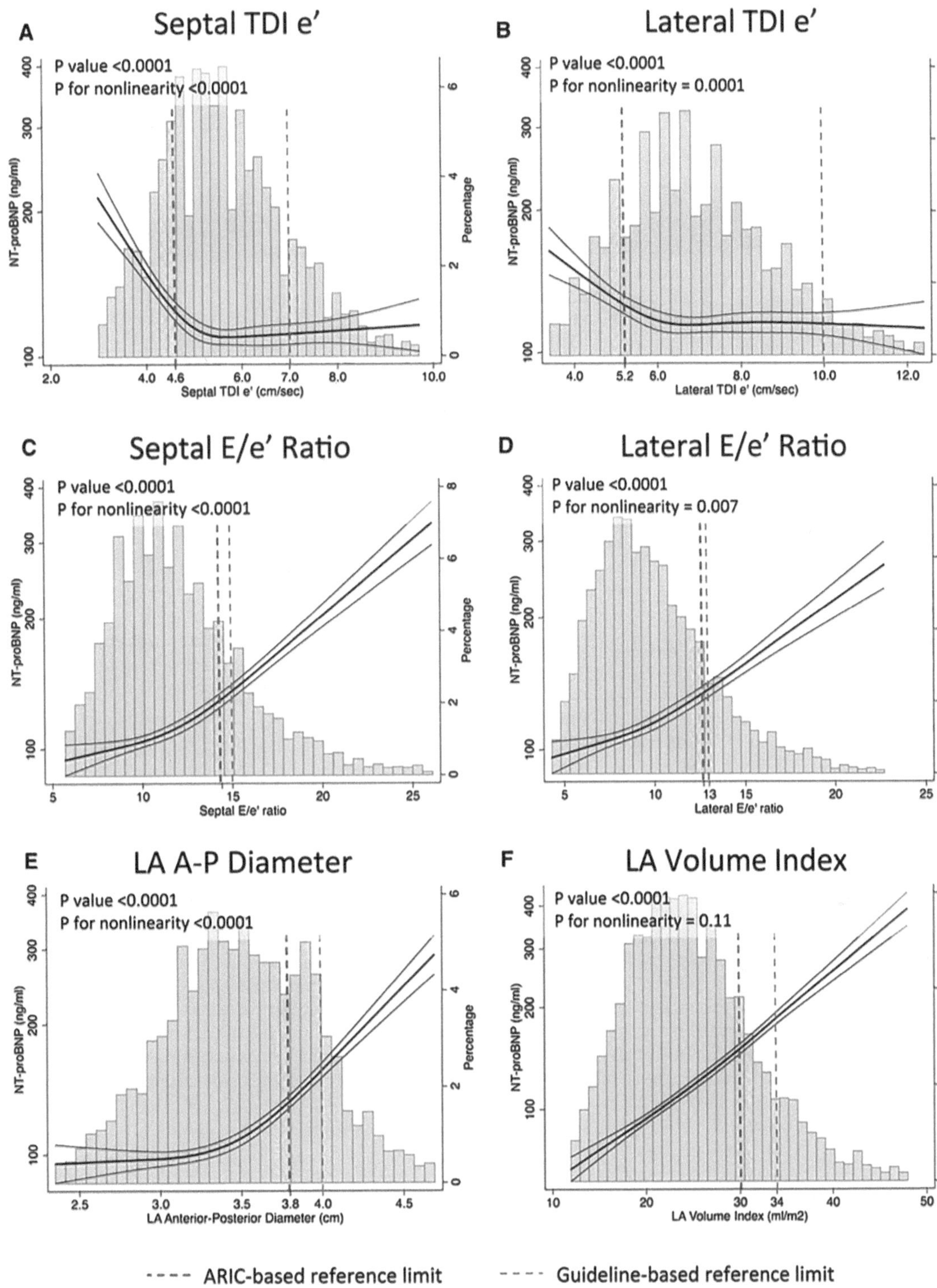

Fig. 31.14 Performance of clinically used parameters of diastolic function. Restricted cubic splines showing relationship between early diastolic velocities of the septal (A) and lateral (B) mitral annulus *(X-axis)* and incident heart failure hospitalization or death *(Y-axis)*. The prevalence of each value *(gray bar)* in ARIC cohort is shown. The *ASE* recommended cutoffs *(red line)* and ARIC based cutoffs *(blue line)* are shown. A majority of healthy seniors have e' values below the *ASE* recommendations without subsequent increase in HF hospitalization or death. The ARIC derived cut-off is beyond the inflection point where risk increases. In contrast, the E/e' ratio and markers of left atrial size were predictive of incident HF (C-F).

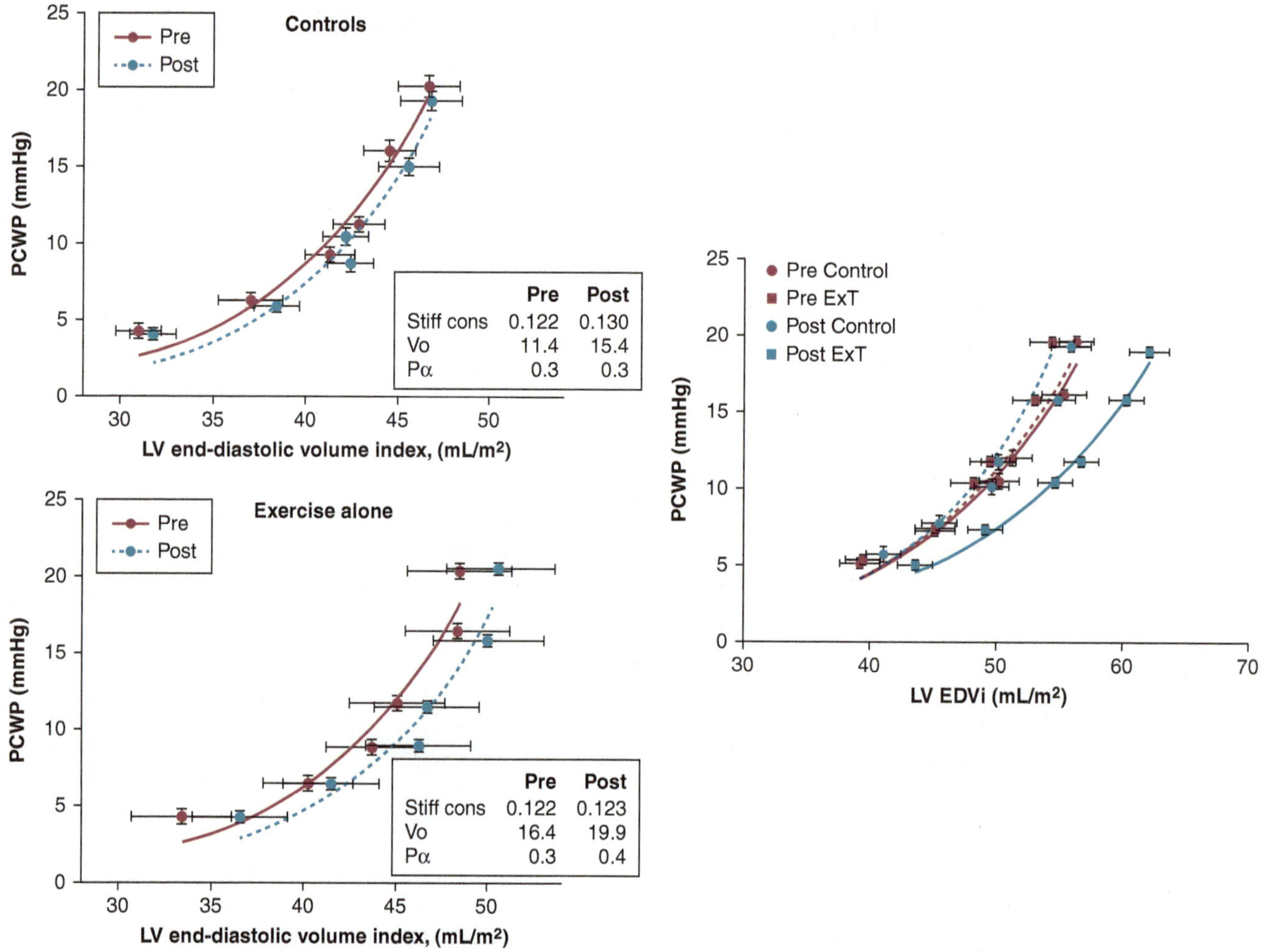

Fig. 31.15 Results of two training studies showing the impact of age and exercise on LV compliance. Exercise training did not improve LV compliance in elderly subjects (aged 67 ± 6 years) *(left)*. Subsequently, 61 healthy middle-aged subjects (53 ± 5 years) were randomized to high-intensity exercise versus placebo *(right)*. The exercise group *(red curve)* improved their compliance after 2 years of exercise *(curve shifted to the right)*, whereas control group *(black curve)* showed no improvement. These studies suggest that while cardiac plasticity exists, age-related declines in compliance can be reversed with exercise. (Adapted from Fujimoto N, et al. Cardiovascular effects of 1 year of alagebrium and endurance Exercise Training (ExT) in healthy older individuals. *Circ Heart Fail.* 2013;6(6):1155–1164; Howden EJ, et al. Reversing the cardiac effects of sedentary aging in middle age—a randomized controlled trial: implications for heart failure prevention. *Circulation.* 2018;137(15):1549–1560.)

KEY POINTS

- The incidence of HFpEF is closely associated with age, and the syndrome contributes significant morbidity and mortality to the elderly population.
- Dyspnea on exertion in the elderly is often multifaceted and can arise from a number of pathologic conditions and expected physiologic changes with aging. A careful evaluation is required to identify sources of dyspnea in these patients.
- Diastolic function is a complex combination of systolic function, LV relaxation, and LV compliance. The individual impact of aging on each of these components helps shed light of how aging, along with lifestyle and comorbidities, ultimately contributes to the syndrome of HFpEF.
- Current echocardiographic diastolic function guidelines are insufficient to identify seniors at risk for HF or death. Efforts to create age-specific cutoffs are ongoing but struggle to capture the complexity of diastolic function.
- Systolic function does not decline with age, though more studies are needed to understand the full effect of aging on systolic cardiac motion, such as strain and torsion.
- LV relaxation decreases with age. Lifelong aerobic exercise can attenuate but not entirely prevent the age-associated decline in diastolic function.
- LV compliance declines with sedentary aging, but exercise can prevent this decline. During middle age, high-intensity exercise can reverse the decline in compliance due to sedentary aging. At older ages, exercise may not improve compliance due to lack of cardiac plasticity.

REVIEW QUESTIONS

1. Does the patient in the case study have HFpEF?
   a. Yes
   b. No
   c. "Need more information"
2. Does the patient in the case study have grade I diastolic dysfunction?
   a. Yes
   b. No, this is a normal echocardiogram for her age.
   c. No, she has more advanced diastolic dysfunction.
3. What would be the most comprehensive diagnostic test to evaluate the source of dyspnea in the patient described in the case study?
   a. Exercise treadmill test (ETT)
   b. Cardiopulmonary exercise test
   c. Cardiac MRI
   d. Coronary angiogram
4. What percentage of subjects over the age of 65 have abnormal e′ velocities as defined by the American Society of Echocardiography diastolic function guidelines?
   a. 0%–25%
   b. 25%–50%
   c. 50%–75%
   d. 75%–100%
5. What aspect of cardiac function declines with age even in lifelong exercisers?
   a. LV systolic function
   b. LV relaxation
   c. LV compliance
6. What is an expected age-associated physiologic change with age that could result in fatigue on exertion?
   a. Decreased EF
   b. Increased VO_2max
   c. Decreased muscle mass
   d. Elevated resting cardiac filling pressures
7. At what decade of life does the incidence of HFpEF overtake HF with reduced EF?
   a. 40–49 years
   b. 50–59 years
   c. 60–69 years
   d. 70–79 years
8. The following echocardiographic findings are commonly found in healthy elderly sedentary subjects, except
   a. increased LA volume.
   b. increased longitudinal strain.
   c. increased mitral A velocity.
   d. increased IVRT.

REFERENCES

1. Upadhya B, Kitzman DW. Heart Failure with Preserved Ejection Fraction in Older Adults. *Heart Fail Clin.* 2017;13:485–502.
2. Benjamin EJ, Virani SS, Callaway CW, Chamberlain AM, Chang AR, Cheng S, Chiuve SE, Cushman M, Delling FN, Deo R, de Ferranti SD, Ferguson JF, Fornage M, Gillespie C, Isasi CR, Jimenez MC, Jordan LC, Judd SE, Lackland D, Lichtman JH, Lisabeth L, Liu S, Longenecker CT, Lutsey PL, Mackey JS, Matchar DB, Matsushita K, Mussolino ME, Nasir K, O'Flaherty M, Palaniappan LP, Pandey A, Pandey DK, Reeves MJ, Ritchey MD, Rodriguez CJ, Roth GA, Rosamond WD, Sampson UKA, Satou GM, Shah SH, Spartano NL, Tirschwell DL, Tsao CW, Voeks JH, Willey JZ, Wilkins JT, Wu JH, Alger HM, Wong SS, Muntner P. American Heart Association Council on E, Prevention Statistics C and Stroke Statistics S. Heart Disease and Stroke Statistics-2018 Update: A Report From the American Heart Association. *Circulation.* 2018;137:e67–e492.
3. Gerber Y, Weston SA, Redfield MM, Chamberlain AM, Manemann SM, Jiang R, Killian JM, Roger VL. A contemporary appraisal of the heart failure epidemic in Olmsted County, Minnesota, 2000 to 2010. *JAMA Intern Med.* 2015;175:996–1004.
4. Heidenreich PA, Albert NM, Allen LA, Bluemke DA, Butler J, Fonarow GC, Ikonomidis JS, Khavjou O, Konstam MA, Maddox TM, Nichol G, Pham M, Pina IL, Trogdon JG. American Heart Association Advocacy Coordinating C, Council on Arteriosclerosis T, Vascular B, Council on Cardiovascular R, Intervention, Council on Clinical C, Council on E, Prevention and Stroke C. Forecasting the impact of heart failure in the United States: a policy statement from the American Heart Association. *Circ Heart Fail.* 2013;6:606–619.
5. Go AS, Mozaffarian D, Roger VL, Benjamin EJ, Berry JD, Blaha MJ, Dai S, Ford ES, Fox CS, Franco S, Fullerton HJ, Gillespie C, Hailpern SM, Heit JA, Howard VJ, Huffman MD, Judd SE, Kissela BM, Kittner SJ, Lackland DT, Lichtman JH, Lisabeth LD, Mackey RH, Magid DJ, Marcus GM, Marelli A, Matchar DB, McGuire DK, Mohler 3rd ER, Moy CS, Mussolino ME, Neumar RW, Nichol G, Pandey DK, Paynter NP, Reeves MJ, Sorlie PD, Stein J, Towfighi A, Turan TN, Virani SS, Wong ND, Woo D, Turner MB. American Heart Association Statistics C and Stroke Statistics S. Heart disease and stroke statistics--2014 update: a report from the American Heart Association. *Circulation.* 2014;129:e28–e292.
6. Writing Group M, Lloyd-Jones D, Adams RJ, Brown TM, Carnethon M, Dai S, De Simone G, Ferguson TB, Ford E, Furie K, Gillespie C, Go A, Greenlund K, Haase N, Hailpern S, Ho PM, Howard V, Kissela B, Kittner S, Lackland D, Lisabeth L, Marelli A, McDermott MM, Meigs J, Mozaffarian D, Mussolino M, Nichol G, Roger VL, Rosamond W, Sacco R, Sorlie P, Roger VL, Thom T, Wasserthiel-Smoller S, Wong ND, Wylie-Rosett J. American Heart Association Statistics C and Stroke Statistics S. Heart disease and stroke statistics--2010 update: a report from the American Heart Association. *Circulation.* 2010;121:e46–e215.
7. Owan TE, Hodge DO, Herges RM, Jacobsen SJ, Roger VL, Redfield MM. Trends in prevalence and outcome of heart failure with preserved ejection fraction. *N Engl J Med.* 2006;355:251–259.
8. Wan He MS VV, DeBarros KA. 65 in the United States: 2005. U.S. Census Bureau. U.S. Government Printing Office. 2005.
9. Zannad F, Agrinier N and Alla F. Heart failure burden and therapy. *Europace.* 2009; 11 Suppl 5:v1-9.
10. Warraich HJ, Kitzman DW, Whellan DJ, Duncan PW, Mentz RJ, Pastva AM, Nelson MB, Upadhya B, Reeves GR. Physical Function, Frailty, Cognition, Depression, and Quality of Life in Hospitalized Adults >/ = 60 Years With Acute Decompensated Heart Failure With Preserved Versus Reduced Ejection Fraction. *Circ Heart Fail.* 2018;11:e005254.
11. Fried LP, Tangen CM, Walston J, Newman AB, Hirsch C, Gottdiener J, Seeman T, Tracy R, Kop WJ, Burke G, McBurnie MA, Cardiovascular Health Study Collaborative Research G. Frailty in older adults: evidence for a phenotype. *J Gerontol A Biol Sci Med Sci.* 2001;56:M146–M156.
12. Sanders NA, Supiano MA, Lewis EF, Liu J, Claggett B, Pfeffer MA, Desai AS, Sweitzer NK, Solomon SD, Fang JC. The frailty syndrome and outcomes in the TOPCAT trial. *Eur J Heart Fail.* 2018;20:1570–1577.
13. Vaduganathan M, Patel RB, Michel A, Shah SJ, Senni M, Gheorghiade M, Butler J. Mode of Death in Heart Failure With Preserved Ejection Fraction. *J Am Coll Cardiol.* 2017;69:556–569.
14. Cleland JG, Tendera M, Adamus J, Freemantle N, Polonski L, Taylor J, Investigators P-C. The perindopril in elderly people with chronic heart failure (PEP-CHF) study. *Eur Heart J.* 2006;27:2338–2345.
15. Rickenbacher P, Pfisterer M, Burkard T, Kiowski W, Follath F, Burckhardt D, Schindler R, Brunner-La Rocca HP, Investigators T-C. Why and how do elderly patients with heart failure die? Insights from the TIME-CHF study. *Eur J Heart Fail.* 2012;14:1218–1229.
16. Liao L, Allen LA, Whellan DJ. Economic burden of heart failure in the elderly. *Pharmacoeconomics.* 2008;26:447–462.
17. Kotecha D, Lam CS, Van Veldhuisen DJ, Van Gelder IC, Voors AA, Rienstra M. Heart Failure With Preserved Ejection Fraction and Atrial Fibrillation: Vicious Twins. *J Am Coll Cardiol.* 2016;68:2217–2228.

18. Reddy YNV, Obokata M, Gersh BJ, Borlaug BA. High Prevalence of Occult Heart Failure With Preserved Ejection Fraction Among Patients With Atrial Fibrillation and Dyspnea. *Circulation.* 2018;137:534–535.
19. Cikes M, Claggett B, Shah AM, Desai AS, Lewis EF, Shah SJ, Anand IS, O'Meara E, Rouleau JL, Sweitzer NK, Fang JC, Saksena S, Pitt B, Pfeffer MA, Solomon SD. Atrial Fibrillation in Heart Failure With Preserved Ejection Fraction: The TOPCAT Trial. *JACC Heart Fail.* 2018;6:689–697.
20. Vermond RA, Geelhoed B, Verweij N, Tieleman RG, Van der Harst P, Hillege HL, Van Gilst WH, Van Gelder IC, Rienstra M. Incidence of Atrial Fibrillation and Relationship With Cardiovascular Events, Heart Failure, and Mortality: A Community-Based Study From the Netherlands. *J Am Coll Cardiol.* 2015;66:1000–1007.
21. Olsson LG, Swedberg K, Ducharme A, Granger CB, Michelson EL, McMurray JJ, Puu M, Yusuf S, Pfeffer MA, Investigators C. Atrial fibrillation and risk of clinical events in chronic heart failure with and without left ventricular systolic dysfunction: results from the Candesartan in Heart failure-Assessment of Reduction in Mortality and morbidity (CHARM) program. *J Am Coll Cardiol.* 2006;47:1997–2004.
22. Melenovsky V, Borlaug BA, Rosen B, Hay I, Ferruci L, Morell CH, Lakatta EG, Najjar SS, Kass DA. Cardiovascular features of heart failure with preserved ejection fraction versus nonfailing hypertensive left ventricular hypertrophy in the urban Baltimore community: the role of atrial remodeling/dysfunction. *J Am Coll Cardiol.* 2007;49:198–207.
23. Knackstedt C, Gramley F, Schimpf T, Mischke K, Zarse M, Plisiene J, Schmid M, Lorenzen J, Frechen D, Neef P, Hanrath P, Kelm M, Schauerte P. Association of echocardiographic atrial size and atrial fibrosis in a sequential model of congestive heart failure and atrial fibrillation. *Cardiovasc Pathol.* 2008;17:318–324.
24. Esposito F, Mathieu-Costello O, Shabetai R, Wagner PD, Richardson RS. Limited maximal exercise capacity in patients with chronic heart failure: partitioning the contributors. *J Am Coll Cardiol.* 2010;55:1945–1954.
25. Betik AC, Hepple RT. Determinants of VO2 max decline with aging: an integrated perspective. *Appl Physiol Nutr Metab.* 2008;33:130–140.
26. Haykowsky MJ, Ezekowitz JA, Armstrong PW. Therapeutic exercise for individuals with heart failure: special attention to older women with heart failure. *J Card Fail.* 2004;10:165–173.
27. Ershler WB, Sheng S, McKelvey J, Artz AS, Denduluri N, Tecson J, Taub DD, Brant LJ, Ferrucci L, Longo DL. Serum erythropoietin and aging: a longitudinal analysis. *J Am Geriatr Soc.* 2005;53:1360–1365.
28. Ware JH, Dockery DW, Louis TA, Xu XP, Ferris Jr BG, Speizer FE. Longitudinal and cross-sectional estimates of pulmonary function decline in never-smoking adults. *Am J Epidemiol.* 1990;132:685–700.
29. Hasin DS, Goodwin RD, Stinson FS, Grant BF. Epidemiology of major depressive disorder: results from the National Epidemiologic Survey on Alcoholism and Related Conditions. *Arch Gen Psychiatry.* 2005;62:1097–1106.
30. Fiske A, Wetherell JL, Gatz M. Depression in older adults. *Annu Rev Clin Psychol.* 2009;5:363–389.
31. Thannickal VJ, Murthy M, Balch WE, Chandel NS, Meiners S, Eickelberg O, Selman M, Pardo A, White ES, Levy BD, Busse PJ, Tuder RM, Antony VB, Sznajder JI, Budinger GR. Blue journal conference. Aging and susceptibility to lung disease. *Am J Respir Crit Care Med.* 2015;191:261–269.
32. Akgun KM, Crothers K, Pisani M. Epidemiology and management of common pulmonary diseases in older persons. *J Gerontol A Biol Sci Med Sci.* 2012;67:276–291.
33. Tribouilloy C, Rusinaru D, Mahjoub H, Souliere V, Levy F, Peltier M, Slama M, Massy Z. Prognosis of heart failure with preserved ejection fraction: a 5 year prospective population-based study. *Eur Heart J.* 2008;29:339–347.
34. Gottdiener JS, Arnold AM, Aurigemma GP, Polak JF, Tracy RP, Kitzman DW, Gardin JM, Rutledge JE, Boineau RC. Predictors of congestive heart failure in the elderly: the Cardiovascular Health Study. *J Am Coll Cardiol.* 2000;35:1628–1637.
35. Bhatia RS, Tu JV, Lee DS, Austin PC, Fang J, Haouzi A, Gong Y, Liu PP. Outcome of heart failure with preserved ejection fraction in a population-based study. *N Engl J Med.* 2006;355:260–269.
36. Yancy CW, Jessup M, Bozkurt B, Butler J, Casey Jr DE, Drazner MH, Fonarow GC, Geraci SA, Horwich T, Januzzi JL, Johnson MR, Kasper EK, Levy WC, Masoudi FA, McBride PE, McMurray JJ, Mitchell JE, Peterson PN, Riegel B, Sam F, Stevenson LW, Tang WH, Tsai EJ, Wilkoff BL. 2013 ACCF/AHA guideline for the management of heart failure: executive summary: a report of the American College of Cardiology Foundation/American Heart Association Task Force on practice guidelines. *Circulation.* 2013;128:1810–1852.
37. Paulus WJ, Tschope C, Sanderson JE, Rusconi C, Flachskampf FA, Rademakers FE, Marino P, Smiseth OA, De Keulenaer G, Leite-Moreira AF, Borbely A, Edes I, Handoko ML, Heymans S, Pezzali N, Pieske B, Dickstein K, Fraser AG, Brutsaert DL. How to diagnose diastolic heart failure: a consensus statement on the diagnosis of heart failure with normal left ventricular ejection fraction by the Heart Failure and Echocardiography Associations of the European Society of Cardiology. *Eur Heart J.* 2007;28:2539–2550.
38. Nagueh SF, Smiseth OA, Appleton CP, Byrd 3rd BF, Dokainish H, Edvardsen T, Flachskampf FA, Gillebert TC, Klein AL, Lancellotti P, Marino P, Oh JK, Popescu BA, Waggoner AD. Recommendations for the Evaluation of Left Ventricular Diastolic Function by Echocardiography: An Update from the American Society of Echocardiography and the European Association of Cardiovascular Imaging. *J Am Soc Echocardiogr.* 2016;29:277–314.
39. Maron BA, Cockrill BA, Waxman AB, Systrom DM. The invasive cardiopulmonary exercise test. *Circulation.* 2013;127:1157–1164.
40. Ha JW, Andersen OS, Smiseth OA. Diastolic Stress Test: Invasive and Noninvasive Testing. *JACC Cardiovasc Imaging.* 2019;13:272–282.
41. Reddy YNV, Carter RE, Obokata M, Redfield MM, Borlaug BA. A Simple, Evidence-Based Approach to Help Guide Diagnosis of Heart Failure With Preserved Ejection Fraction. *Circulation.* 2018;138:861–870.
42. Zile MR, Gottdiener JS, Hetzel SJ, McMurray JJ, Komajda M, McKelvie R, Baicu CF, Massie BM, Carson PE, Investigators IP. Prevalence and significance of alterations in cardiac structure and function in patients with heart failure and a preserved ejection fraction. *Circulation.* 2011;124:2491–2501.
43. Persson H, Lonn E, Edner M, Baruch L, Lang CC, Morton JJ, Ostergren J, McKelvie RS, Investigators of the CES-C. Diastolic dysfunction in heart failure with preserved systolic function: need for objective evidence:results from the CHARM Echocardiographic Substudy-CHARMES. *J Am Coll Cardiol.* 2007;49:687–694.
44. Shah AM, Shah SJ, Anand IS, Sweitzer NK, O'Meara E, Heitner JF, Sopko G, Li G, Assmann SF, McKinlay SM, Pitt B, Pfeffer MA, Solomon SD, Investigators T. Cardiac structure and function in heart failure with preserved ejection fraction: baseline findings from the echocardiographic study of the Treatment of Preserved Cardiac Function Heart Failure with an Aldosterone Antagonist trial. *Circ Heart Fail.* 2014;7:104–115.
45. Kosmala W, Marwick TH. Asymptomatic Left Ventricular Diastolic Dysfunction: Predicting Progression to Symptomatic Heart Failure. *JACC Cardiovasc Imaging.* 2019.
46. Borlaug BA, Paulus WJ. Heart failure with preserved ejection fraction: pathophysiology, diagnosis, and treatment. *Eur Heart J.* 2011;32:670–679.
47. Prasad A, Hastings JL, Shibata S, Popovic ZB, Arbab-Zadeh A, Bhella PS, Okazaki K, Fu Q, Berk M, Palmer D, Greenberg NL, Garcia MJ, Thomas JD, Levine BD. Characterization of static and dynamic left ventricular diastolic function in patients with heart failure with a preserved ejection fraction. *Circ Heart Fail.* 2010;3:617–626.
48. DeVore AD, McNulty S, Alenezi F, Ersboll M, Vader JM, Oh JK, Lin G, Redfield MM, Lewis G, Semigran MJ, Anstrom KJ, Hernandez AF, Velazquez EJ. Impaired left ventricular global longitudinal strain in patients with heart failure with preserved ejection fraction: insights from the RELAX trial. *Eur J Heart Fail.* 2017;19:893–900.
49. Arbab-Zadeh A, Dijk E, Prasad A, Fu Q, Torres P, Zhang R, Thomas JD, Palmer D, Levine BD. Effect of aging and physical activity on left ventricular compliance. *Circulation.* 2004;110:1799–1805.
50. Prasad A, Popovic ZB, Arbab-Zadeh A, Fu Q, Palmer D, Dijk E, Greenberg NL, Garcia MJ, Thomas JD, Levine BD. The effects of aging and physical activity on Doppler measures of diastolic function. *Am J Cardiol.* 2007;99:1629–1636.
51. Fujimoto N, Hastings JL, Bhella PS, Shibata S, Gandhi NK, Carrick-Ranson G, Palmer D, Levine BD. Effect of ageing on left ventricular compliance and distensibility in healthy sedentary humans. *J Physiol.* 2012;590:1871–1880.

52. Yoneyama K, Gjesdal O, Choi EY, Wu CO, Hundley WG, Gomes AS, Liu CY, McClelland RL, Bluemke DA, Lima JA. Age, sex, and hypertension-related remodeling influences left ventricular torsion assessed by tagged cardiac magnetic resonance in asymptomatic individuals: the multi-ethnic study of atherosclerosis. *Circulation.* 2012;126:2481–2490.
53. Kaku K, Takeuchi M, Tsang W, Takigiku K, Yasukochi S, Patel AR, Mor-Avi V, Lang RM, Otsuji Y. Age-related normal range of left ventricular strain and torsion using three-dimensional speckle-tracking echocardiography. *J Am Soc Echocardiogr.* 2014;27:55–64.
54. Wandt B, Bojo L, Hatle L, Wranne B. Left ventricular contraction pattern changes with age in normal adults. *J Am Soc Echocardiogr.* 1998;11: 857–863.
55. Parikh JD, Hollingsworth KG, Wallace D, Blamire AM, MacGowan GA. Left ventricular functional, structural and energetic effects of normal aging: Comparison with hypertension. *PLoS One.* 2017;12:e0177404.
56. Howden EJ, Carrick-Ranson G, Sarma S, Hieda M, Fujimoto N, Levine BD. Effects of Sedentary Aging and Lifelong Exercise on Left Ventricular Systolic Function. *Med Sci Sports Exerc.* 2018;50:494–501.
57. Mangion K, Clerfond G, McComb C, Carrick D, Rauhalammi SM, McClure J, Corcoran DS, Woodward R, Orchard V, Radjenovic A, Zhong X, Berry C. Myocardial strain in healthy adults across a broad age range as revealed by cardiac magnetic resonance imaging at 1.5 and 3.0T: Associations of myocardial strain with myocardial region, age, and sex. *J Magn Reson Imaging.* 2016;44:1197–1205.
58. Hay I, Rich J, Ferber P, Burkhoff D, Maurer MS. Role of impaired myocardial relaxation in the production of elevated left ventricular filling pressure. *Am J Physiol Heart Circ Physiol.* 2005;288:H1203–H1208.
59. Zile MR, Brutsaert DL. New concepts in diastolic dysfunction and diastolic heart failure: Part I: diagnosis, prognosis, and measurements of diastolic function. *Circulation.* 2002;105:1387–1393.
60. Weiss JL, Frederiksen JW, Weisfeldt ML. Hemodynamic determinants of the time-course of fall in canine left ventricular pressure. *J Clin Invest.* 1976;58:751–760.
61. Hirota Y. A clinical study of left ventricular relaxation. *Circulation.* 1980;62:756–763.
62. Alam M, Wardell J, Andersson E, Samad BA, Nordlander R. Characteristics of mitral and tricuspid annular velocities determined by pulsed wave Doppler tissue imaging in healthy subjects. *J Am Soc Echocardiogr.* 1999;12:618–628.
63. Munagala VK, Jacobsen SJ, Mahoney DW, Rodeheffer RJ, Bailey KR, Redfield MM. Association of newer diastolic function parameters with age in healthy subjects: a population-based study. *J Am Soc Echocardiogr.* 2003;16:1049–1056.
64. Okura H, Takada Y, Yamabe A, Kubo T, Asawa K, Ozaki T, Yamagishi H, Toda I, Yoshiyama M, Yoshikawa J, Yoshida K. Age- and gender-specific changes in the left ventricular relaxation: a Doppler echocardiographic study in healthy individuals. *Circ Cardiovasc Imaging.* 2009;2:41–46.
65. Daimon M, Watanabe H, Abe Y, Hirata K, Hozumi T, Ishii K, Ito H, Iwakura K, Izumi C, Matsuzaki M, Minagoe S, Abe H, Murata K, Nakatani S, Negishi K, Yoshida K, Tanabe K, Tanaka N, Tokai K, Yoshikawa J. and Japanese Normal Values for Echocardiographic Measurements Project Study I. Gender differences in age-related changes in left and right ventricular geometries and functions. Echocardiography of a healthy subject group. *Circ J.* 2011;75:2840–2846.
66. Popovic ZB, Prasad A, Garcia MJ, Arbab-Zadeh A, Borowski A, Dijk E, Greenberg NL, Levine BD, Thomas JD. Relationship among diastolic intraventricular pressure gradients, relaxation, and preload: impact of age and fitness. *Am J Physiol Heart Circ Physiol.* 2006;290:H1454–H1459.
67. van Grootel RWJ, Kauling RM, Menting ME, McGhie J, Roos-Hesselink JW, van den Bosch AE. Influence of age and sex on left ventricular diastolic strain analysis. *Int J Cardiovasc Imaging.* 2019;35:491–498.
68. Dauterman K, Pak PH, Maughan WL, Nussbacher A, Arie S, Liu CP, Kass DA. Contribution of external forces to left ventricular diastolic pressure. Implications for the clinical use of the Starling law. *Ann Intern Med.* 1995;122:737–742.
69. Baan J, Jong TT, Kerkhof PL, Moene RJ, van Dijk AD, van der Velde ET, Koops J. Continuous stroke volume and cardiac output from intra-ventricular dimensions obtained with impedance catheter. *Cardiovasc Res.* 1981;15:328–334.
70. Baan J, van der Velde ET, de Bruin HG, Smeenk GJ, Koops J, van Dijk AD, Temmerman D, Senden J, Buis B. Continuous measurement of left ventricular volume in animals and humans by conductance catheter. *Circulation.* 1984;70:812–823.
71. Howden EJ, Sarma S, Lawley JS, Opondo M, Cornwell W, Stoller D, Urey MA, Adams-Huet B, Levine BD. Reversing the Cardiac Effects of Sedentary Aging in Middle Age-A Randomized Controlled Trial: Implications For Heart Failure Prevention. *Circulation.* 2018;137:1549–1560.
72. Fujimoto N, Hastings JL, Carrick-Ranson G, Shafer KM, Shibata S, Bhella PS, Abdullah SM, Barkley KW, Adams-Huet B, Boyd KN, Livingston SA, Palmer D, Levine BD. Cardiovascular effects of 1 year of alagebrium and endurance exercise training in healthy older individuals. *Circ Heart Fail.* 2013;6:1155–1164.
73. Appleton CP, Hatle LK, Popp RL. Relation of transmitral flow velocity patterns to left ventricular diastolic function: new insights from a combined hemodynamic and Doppler echocardiographic study. *J Am Coll Cardiol.* 1988;12:426–440.
74. Bryg RJ, Williams GA, Labovitz AJ. Effect of aging on left ventricular diastolic filling in normal subjects. *Am J Cardiol.* 1987;59:971–974.
75. Kitzman DW, Sheikh KH, Beere PA, Philips JL, Higginbotham MB. Age-related alterations of Doppler left ventricular filling indexes in normal subjects are independent of left ventricular mass, heart rate, contractility and loading conditions. *J Am Coll Cardiol.* 1991;18:1243–1250.
76. Gardin JM, Arnold AM, Bild DE, Smith VE, Lima JA, Klopfenstein HS, Kitzman DW. Left ventricular diastolic filling in the elderly: the cardiovascular health study. *Am J Cardiol.* 1998;82:345–351.
77. Wolsk E, Bakkestrom R, Thomsen JH, Balling L, Andersen MJ, Dahl JS, Hassager C, Moller JE, Gustafsson F. The Influence of Age on Hemodynamic Parameters During Rest and Exercise in Healthy Individuals. *JACC Heart Fail.* 2017;5:337–346.
78. Shah AM, Claggett B, Kitzman D, Biering-Sorensen T, Jensen JS, Cheng S, Matsushita K, Konety S, Folsom AR, Mosley TH, Wright JD, Heiss G, Solomon SD. Contemporary Assessment of Left Ventricular Diastolic Function in Older Adults: The Atherosclerosis Risk in Communities Study. *Circulation.* 2017;135:426–439.
79. Fleg JL, Cooper LS, Borlaug BA, Haykowsky MJ, Kraus WE, Levine BD, Pfeffer MA, Pina IL, Poole DC, Reeves GR, Whellan DJ, Kitzman DW, National Heart L, Blood Institute Working G. Exercise training as therapy for heart failure: current status and future directions. *Circ Heart Fail.* 2015;8:209–220.
80. Pandey A, Parashar A, Kumbhani D, Agarwal S, Garg J, Kitzman D, Levine B, Drazner M, Berry J. Exercise training in patients with heart failure and preserved ejection fraction: meta-analysis of randomized control trials. *Circ Heart Fail.* 2015;8:33–40.
81. Kitzman DW, Brubaker PH, Herrington DM, Morgan TM, Stewart KP, Hundley WG, Abdelhamed A, Haykowsky MJ. Effect of endurance exercise training on endothelial function and arterial stiffness in older patients with heart failure and preserved ejection fraction: a randomized, controlled, single-blind trial. *J Am Coll Cardiol.* 2013;62:584–592.
82. Turner MJ, Spina RJ, Kohrt WM, Ehsani AA. Effect of endurance exercise training on left ventricular size and remodeling in older adults with hypertension. *J Gerontol A Biol Sci Med Sci.* 2000;55:M245–M251.
83. Pandey A, Darden D, Berry JD. Low Fitness in Midlife: A Novel Therapeutic Target for Heart Failure with Preserved Ejection Fraction Prevention. *Prog Cardiovasc Dis.* 2015;58:87–93.
84. Brinker SK, Pandey A, Ayers CR, Barlow CE, DeFina LF, Willis BL, Radford NB, Farzaneh-Far R, de Lemos JA, Drazner MH, Berry JD. Association of cardiorespiratory fitness with left ventricular remodeling and diastolic function: the Cooper Center Longitudinal Study. *JACC Heart Fail.* 2014;2:238–246.
85. Pandey A, Patel M, Gao A, Willis BL, Das SR, Leonard D, Drazner MH, de Lemos JA, DeFina L, Berry JD. Changes in mid-life fitness predicts heart failure risk at a later age independent of interval development of cardiac and noncardiac risk factors: the Cooper Center Longitudinal Study. *Am Heart J.* 2015;169:290–297. e1.

32

Perioperative Assessment of Diastolic Function

Stephen H. Gregory and Madhav Swaminathan

OUTLINE

Case Study

A 75-year-old female presents for coronary artery bypass grafting (CABG) for treatment of unstable angina secondary to severe three-vessel coronary artery disease. The patient reports a history of hypertension, hyperlipidemia, and diabetes mellitus. Preoperative transthoracic echocardiogram demonstrated normal left ventricular (LV) and right ventricular (RV) systolic function, left atrial (LA) enlargement, mild mitral regurgitation (MR), and no evidence of pulmonary hypertension. Preoperative laboratory assessment is notable for a serum creatinine of 0.8 mg/dL and hemoglobin of 12.7 g/dL. The Society of Thoracic Surgeons risk calculator predicts a 1.3% risk of in-hospital or 30-day mortality.

INTRODUCTION

The assessment and utilization of diastolic function in the perioperative care of patients undergoing cardiac surgery remains controversial. The most recent American Society of Echocardiography/European Association of Cardiovascular Imaging (ASE/EACVI) guidelines on the evaluation of LV diastolic function cautions that diastolic assessment may not necessarily be applicable in the perioperative setting.[1] Nevertheless there is a significant body of literature examining the utility of perioperative diastolic assessment, and a large percentage of cardiac anesthesiologists assess diastolic function as part of their standard perioperative transesophageal echocardiogram (TEE) exam.[2] This chapter discusses the approach to the intraoperative assessment of diastolic function in patients undergoing cardiac surgery.

CURRENT GUIDELINES FOR DIASTOLIC ASSESSMENT

The intraoperative assessment of diastolic function largely mirrors that of the patient undergoing assessment outside of the surgical setting with some notable differences.[1,3] Similar to the assessment of diastolic function in other settings, multiple measurement techniques should be utilized with underlying patient age, pathology, heart rate, ventricular loading conditions, and other factors (as discussed in the chapter) helping to contextualize the results of echocardiographic analysis.

The 2016 ASE/EACVI guidelines for the assessment of diastolic function in patients with normal ejection fraction (EF) advocate using annular e′ velocity, the E/e′ velocity (with e′ measured as an average of the septal and lateral annular velocities), the LA maximum volume index, and the peak velocity of the tricuspid regurgitation jet.[1] Conservative cutoffs for diastolic dysfunction are used to try to improve diagnostic specificity (Table 32.1). While assessment of transmitral flow, tricuspid regurgitation, and tissue Doppler velocities of the mitral annulus is readily accomplished via TEE, reliable assessment of LA volume is challenging given the proximity of the TEE probe to the left atrium, and TEE assessment typically underestimates the LA volume by ~9% when compared to standardized assessment by transthoracic echocardiography.[4]

In patients with reduced LV EF and myocardial pathology, determination of diastolic dysfunction can be accomplished using an algorithm that utilizes the E/e′ velocity, LA maximum volume index, and peak tricuspid regurgitation velocity, but also utilizes the ratio of transmitral E wave velocity to the transmitral A wave velocity (E/A ratio) and the maximum velocity of the transmitral E wave to help

TABLE 32.1 Measurements and Cutoff Values Used for Determination of Diastolic Function in Patients With a Normal Left Ventricular (LV) Ejection Fraction[a]

	Measurement	Abnormal Cutoff
1	Average E/e′	>14
2	Septal e′ velocity	<7 cm/sec
	Lateral e′ velocity	<10 cm/sec
3	Tricuspid regurgitation velocity	>2.8 m/sec
4	Left atrial volume index	>34 mL/m^2

[a]Patients meeting >2 of these criteria are categorized as having LV diastolic dysfunction.

Adapted from Nagueh SF, et al. Recommendations for the evaluation of left ventricular diastolic function by echocardiography: an update from the American Society of Echocardiography and the European Association of Cardiovascular Imaging. *J Am Soc Echocardiogr.* 2016;29(4):277–314.

with additional characterization (Fig. 32.1). The limited ability of TEE to optimally assess LA volume remains a barrier to directly applying this algorithm in the intraoperative setting.

The assessment of diastolic function in the perioperative period differs from other arenas in a number of ways. Perioperative diastolic assessment is performed almost exclusively via TEE. Additionally, hemodynamic factors, such as ongoing bleeding, positive pressure ventilation, and changing patient position, may complicate assessment. Anesthetic medications that alter contractility, heart rate, and afterload may also influence measures of diastolic function. An understanding of the influence of the perioperative period on echocardiographic assessment of diastolic function is important to allow for appropriate characterization of LV filling pressures that in turn influences hemodynamic management for optimizing cardiac output.

In the chapter-opening case study, intraoperative TEE assessment confirmed normal LV systolic function and mild mitral regurgitation (MR). Diastolic assessment was performed with the chest closed prior to surgical incision with the patient in the supine position (Fig. 32.2). Transmitral flow demonstrated an E/A ratio of approximately 1.8. Tissue Doppler imaging (TDI) demonstrated a lateral e′ velocity of 9.5 cm/sec and an E/e′ ratio of 7.8 (see Fig. 32.2). Tricuspid regurgitation velocity was 2.0 m/sec. Given the patient's normal E/e′ ratio and normal E/A ratio, she was judged to have normal LAP.

Additional assessment to further characterize the patient's diastolic function was performed, including LV inflow propagation velocity (Vp) and pulmonary vein pulse wave Doppler assessment. Vp was 57 cm/sec and pulmonary vein flow assessment showed an S wave to D wave ratio greater than 1. Both measurements were consistent with normal LV filling pressures, confirming normal diastolic function.

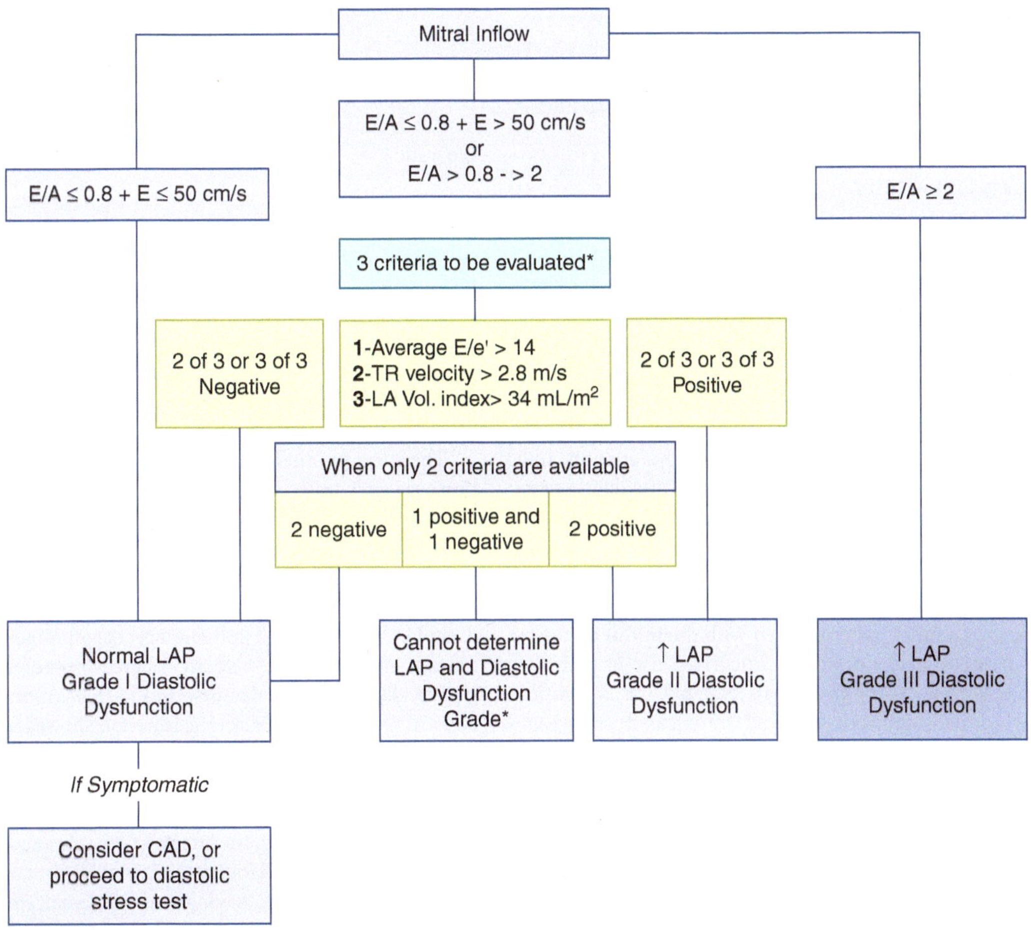

Fig. 32.1 Algorithm for the assessment of LV diastolic function in patients with myocardial pathology including decreased LV EF undergoing transthoracic echocardiography. *CAD,* Coronary artery disease; *E/A,* ratio of transmitral E wave to transmitral A wave velocity as measured by pulse wave Doppler; *E/e′,* ratio of transmitral E wave velocity to tissue Doppler e′ velocity measured as an average of the medial and lateral mitral annular e′; *EF,* ejection fraction; *LA,* left atrium; *LAP,* left atrial pressure; *LV,* left ventricular; *TR,* tricuspid regurgitation. (From Nagueh SF, Smiseth OA, Appleton CP, et al. Recommendations for the evaluation of left ventricular diastolic function by echocardiography: an update from the American Society of Echocardiography and the European Association of Cardiovascular Imaging. *J Am Soc Echocardiogr.* 2016;29(4):277–314.)

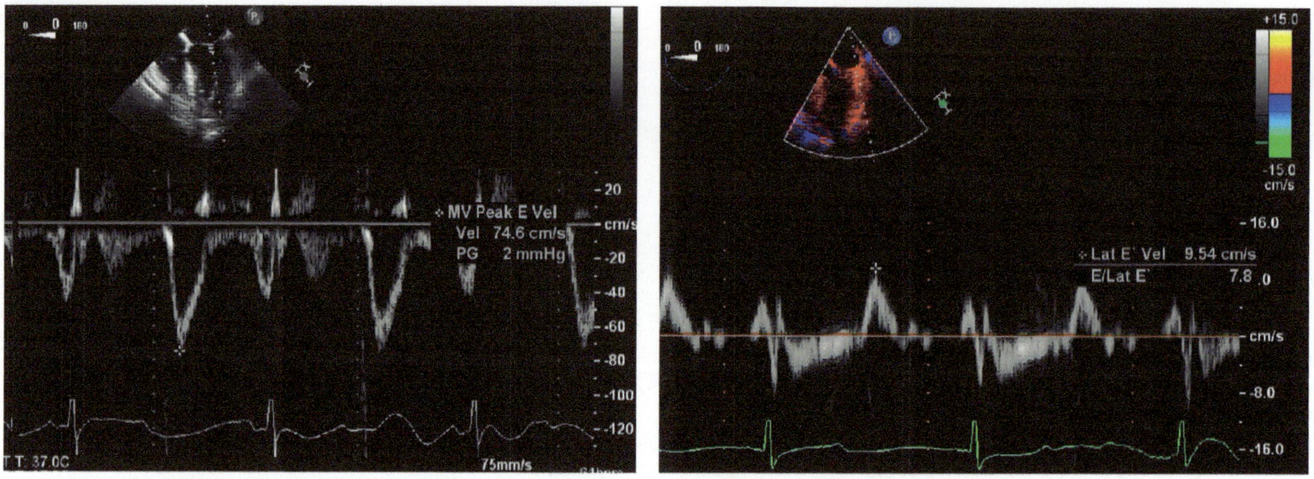

Fig. 32.2 Diastolic assessment of introductory case. (A) Transmitral pulsed-wave Doppler analysis demonstrates an E/A ratio of approximately 1.8. (B) Lateral mitral annular e′ velocity is 9.54 cm/sec with an E/e′ ratio of 7.8 with normal TR velocity. This is consistent with normal left atrial pressure.

THE EFFECT OF THE PERIOPERATIVE PERIOD ON THE ASSESSMENT OF LV DIASTOLIC DYSFUNCTION

Perioperative hemodynamic perturbations can have a significant effect on the assessment of diastolic function. Changes associated with general anesthesia may complicate the accurate assessment and classification of diastolic dysfunction in this patient population.

Intravascular Volume Status

Cardiac surgery typically involves substantial fluctuations in intravascular volume status, with bleeding, ongoing resuscitation, and surgical manipulation of the heart or chest wall resulting in rapid and variable shifts in myocardial preload. Changes in preload are known to have a significant effect on measures of diastolic function, including transmitral E wave velocities and the e′ value.

The response of the transmitral E wave velocity and E/A ratio to changes in ventricular preload is dependent on the underlying degree of diastolic dysfunction.[5] In patients with diastolic dysfunction, increases in preload increase the peak E wave velocity (thus increasing the E/A ratio), and decreases in preload tend to decrease the velocity (decreasing the E/A ratio).[3] In healthy patients with normal diastolic function, E wave velocity also increases with increasing preload, but the E/A ratio is not significantly affected as the A wave velocity simultaneously increases.[6] A similar pattern is seen with the mitral annular e′ velocity, with increases in the e′ with a concurrent rise in preload and decreases in e′ with a decline in preload. Notably, the E/e′ ratio does not appear to be significantly altered by preload changes.[6] Though propagation velocity appears to be mostly unaffected by changes in preload, the utility of this measurement in quantifying diastolic function is limited by technical challenges in obtaining the measurement and its inability to effectively discriminate between grades of diastolic dysfunction.[7,8]

Mechanical Ventilation and Patient Position

Patients undergoing general anesthesia almost always require invasive mechanical ventilation to maintain oxygenation and ventilation. Evidence suggests that patient position and the level of positive end-expiratory pressure (PEEP) both have a significant effect on indices of diastolic function.[9,10] Two prior studies have evaluated the influence of incremental PEEP application on diastolic assessment in patients undergoing cardiac surgery. Increasing PEEP is associated with a significant decrease in the lateral mitral annular e′ velocity with a concomitant reduction in transmitral E wave velocity[9]. Notably, this study did not find a major difference in the ratio of E/e′ (with e′ assessed using either the lateral mitral annulus alone or as an average of the lateral and septal mitral annulus e′ values) with changes in PEEP. Similarly, Trendelenburg position was associated with an increase in the septal and lateral e′ values as well as transmitral E wave velocity with no significant change in the E/e′ ratio.

Anesthetic Agents

Anesthetic agents appear to have different degrees of influence on the measurement of indices of diastolic function. Unfortunately, direct comparison of these agents is difficult, as studies examining the influence of anesthetic agents on diastolic function have focused on heterogeneous diastolic indices and have examined a diverse population, ranging from healthy volunteers to patients with known diastolic dysfunction.

The effect of inhaled anesthetic gas and propofol on diastolic function was previously investigated in both healthy volunteers and patients with preexisting diastolic dysfunction undergoing aortic valve replacement.[11,12] Both studies evaluated the effect on mitral annular e′ velocity, and the study examining healthy patients also assessed isovolumic relaxation time (IVRT). In patients without preexisting diastolic dysfunction, halothane and sevoflurane did not have a significant effect on the e′ velocity, whereas propofol caused a small but statistically significant decrease in e′ (18.0 cm/sec vs. 16.8 cm/sec).[12] Patients with impaired diastolic function showed an increase in e′ during spontaneous ventilation, which returned to baseline following the initiation of positive pressure ventilation and did not differ from the propofol group.[11] These findings have not been consistently replicated in other studies examining the effects of volatile anesthetics and propofol on diastolic function. Houltz et al. previously described both isoflurane and halothane as having a detrimental effect on LV diastolic function, whereas Gare et al. described no significant change in LV diastolic function with either propofol or midazolam sedation, in contrast to the findings of Filipovic (discussed earlier).[5,13,14]

The effect of remifentanil on systolic and diastolic function was assessed in healthy patients with no known diastolic dysfunction undergoing minor surgery.[15] In this study, remifentanil was not associated with worsening of transmitral E wave velocity or e′ and did not appear to affect systolic function. In contrast, the administration of dexmedetomidine appears to significantly worsen indices of both LV diastolic and systolic performance. A study examining the impact of dexmedetomidine in patients with preexisting diastolic dysfunction demonstrated a significant increase in the LV and RV E/e′ ratios as well as an increase in myocardial performance index.[16]

In summary, the effect of anesthetic agents on diastolic function remains poorly defined, and data on any effect, either positive or negative, are inconclusive. It is unclear whether the changes in indices of diastolic function observed in patients under anesthesia represent a true physiologic decline in diastolic function or are simply a result of transient alterations in loading conditions or other influences. The echocardiographer should be aware of the potential influence of anesthetic agents on diastolic function to contextualize diastolic assessment.

DISEASE-SPECIFIC ASSESSMENT OF DIASTOLIC DYSFUNCTION

Mitral Valve Disease

Assessment of LV diastolic function can be challenging in patients with mitral valve disease (see Chapter 21). Many indices of LV diastolic function rely on inferring LV filling pressures from LA hemodynamic measurements (i.e., pulmonary venous flow, transmitral flow, TDI of the mitral annulus, and propagation velocity). The presence of significant mitral valve disease may alter the reliability of these measurements.

In patients with mitral stenosis, diastolic function cannot be reliably assessed based on transmitral flow patterns or mitral annular e′ velocity. Patterns of transmitral flow are predominantly a result of mitral disease and not LV filling dynamics. Similarly, the mitral annulus may be mechanically restricted in mitral stenosis, especially in patients with mitral annular calcification. There are a limited number of echocardiographic assessments that may provide some insight into LV filling pressures in patients with mitral stenosis. A delay in onset between the transmitral E wave and the e′ wave can suggest LV diastolic dysfunction. The E/e′ ratio should not be used to quantify diastolic function in this patient population due to the previously mentioned restriction of the mitral annulus.[1]

Mitral regurgitation also complicates assessment of diastolic function. Hemodynamic assessments that rely on LA pressure as a means to evaluate LV diastolic function are compromised by the presence of significant MR. Transmitral E wave velocity tends to be higher, and pulmonary venous flow shows systolic blunting or even reversal in patients with MR.[17] E/e′ ratio is of unclear reliability in patients with MR. In patients with secondary MR, an E/e′ ratio greater than 15 has been associated with elevated LV filling pressures, and an E/e′ ratio greater than 13.5 has been associated with an increase in the incidence of rehospitalization, worsening heart failure (HF), and mortality.[18,19] In contrast, E/e′ ratio does not appear to reliably predict LV filling pressures in patients with primary MR.[19]

Atrial Fibrillation

Assessment of diastolic function in patients with atrial fibrillation (AFib) in the perioperative period can be challenging and often requires the use of atypical indices and cutoff values to characterize diastolic dysfunction. There is no significant difference between the approach to diastolic assessment during and outside of the perioperative period in patients with AFib.[1]

In patients with depressed LV EF, the transmitral E wave deceleration time appears to reliably predict the presence of elevated LV filling pressures. Temporelli et al. evaluated a series of patients with severely decreased LV EF and found deceleration time to be the sole independent predictor of pulmonary capillary wedge pressure (PCWP).[20] In patients with a normal LV EF, an E/e′ ratio greater than 11 reliably predicts elevated LV filling pressures in AFib.[21,22] As with many Doppler parameters, deceleration time, transmitral E wave velocity, and mitral annular e′ velocity are all vulnerable to variability in the R-R ratio seen in AFib. Therefore these calculations should be performed using an average of multiple measurements over time, typically 10 cardiac cycles.

Generally the perioperative assessment of diastolic function in AFib is complicated by the frequent requirement for indices not routinely acquired and the inability to effectively grade the degree of diastolic dysfunction in the typical hemodynamic environment of cardiac surgery. The authors of this chapter do not routinely perform intraoperative diastolic assessment in patients with AFib.

Hypertrophic Cardiomyopathy

As mentioned elsewhere in this book (Chapter 25), the assessment of diastolic function and concomitant LV filling pressures in patients with hypertrophic cardiomyopathy (HCM) is nuanced, as some indices of diastolic function may only weakly correlate with invasive evaluation of diastolic function in this patient population.[23] Notably, the use of transmitral E/A ratio and deceleration time do not seem to reliably predict LA pressure in patients with HCM.[24] In contrast, less load-dependent indices of diastolic function, such as the E/e′ ratio, appear to correlate with invasive measurements of diastolic function, though with less accuracy than in the general population.[25] In the outpatient setting, diastolic assessment may have some prognostic value, with an association between elevated E/e′ ratio and an elevated risk of death, cardiac arrest, ventricular tachycardia, and decreased functional status.[26] In the perioperative setting, the poor correlation between echocardiographic and invasive indices of diastolic function combined with the variability in loading conditions under anesthesia leaves room for significant error in the interpretation of diastolic function in patients with HCM. Consequently, routine intraoperative assessment of diastolic function in patients with HCM is likely not beneficial.

A subset of patients with HCM that is refractory to medical management may present for invasive alcohol septal ablation or septal myectomy to alleviate dynamic left ventricular outflow tract (LVOT) obstruction. Following septal myectomy, there is typically a reduction in LV septal thickness and systolic LVOT gradient. Interestingly, myectomy may also be associated with reverse remodeling, resulting in a gradual improvement in LV diastolic function in patients with HCM.[27] There appears to be a consistent reduction in LA volume index, with some studies demonstrating an increase in lateral e′ velocity and a decrease in the E/e′ ratio, consistent with an overall reduction in LA pressure and reduced clinical HF symptoms.[27] Studies using speckle tracking echocardiography to evaluate diastolic function have demonstrated similar improvement in peak strain rate during isovolumic relaxation and peak early diastolic strain rate following alcohol septal ablation in patients with HCM.[28]

LV Assist Devices

Patients presenting with end-stage HF are increasingly being treated with the implantation of a continuous flow left ventricular assist device (LVAD). By the nature of their severe LV dysfunction, all of these patients will have concomitant LV diastolic dysfunction prior to LVAD implantation.[1] Understanding of the utility of diastolic assessment of patients with continuous flow LVADs is still evolving. Current data focus primarily on echocardiographic assessment as a means to estimate PCWP in LVAD patients.[29–32]

Estep et al. evaluated 50 patient with prior Heartmate II (Abbott Laboratories, Chicago, IL) LVAD implantation presenting with

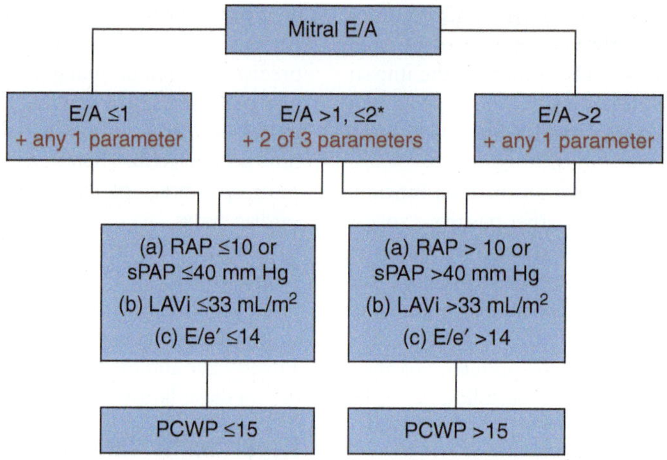

Fig. 32.3 Algorithm for the estimation of pulmonary capillary wedge pressure in patients with left ventricular assist devices. *E/A,* Ratio of transmitral E wave velocity to transmitral A wave velocity; *LAVi,* left atrial volume index; *PCWP,* pulmonary capillary wedge pressure; *RAP,* right atrial pressure; *sPAP,* systolic pulmonary artery pressure. (From Estep JD, Vivo RP, Krim SR, et al. Echocardiographic evaluation of hemodynamics in patients with systolic heart failure supported by a continuous-flow LVAD. *J Am Coll Cardiol.* 2014;64(12):1231–1241.)

symptoms of congestive heart failure (CHF) and attempted to correlate echocardiographic measures of diastolic function with invasive assessment of elevated mean PCWP.[31] Based on their analysis, they proposed an algorithm for estimating PCWP based on the evaluation of transmitral inflow E wave and A wave velocity, estimated systolic pulmonary artery pressure, echocardiographically estimated RA pressure, LA volume index, and the ratio of transmitral E wave velocity to mitral annular tissue velocity (e′) (Fig. 32.3). Longitudinal studies examining changes in indices of diastolic function following LVAD implantation have not clearly demonstrated any significant improvement in intrinsic LV diastolic function. However, there has been some improvement shown in Doppler parameters of diastolic function, likely as a result of LV unloading with LVAD implantation.[32]

ECHOCARDIOGRAPHIC PREDICTORS OF SURGICAL OUTCOME

Systolic Function

Preoperative systolic function has been shown to strongly predict perioperative and long-term mortality following a number of cardiac surgical operations, and evaluation of systolic function plays a major role in risk stratification and decision making in cardiac surgery. Furthermore, correlation of EF with the presence or absence of HF symptoms is more strongly predictive of mortality than examining EF alone.[33] Recently, a large nationwide cohort study examined the role of EF and HF in predicting mortality following CABG. When adjusted for comorbidities, patients with an EF of 30% to 50% were 1.75 times as likely to die within 30 days when compared to patients with a normal EF. Patients with an EF of less than 30% had an adjusted mortality six times higher than the control.[33] This trend in postoperative mortality with decreased EF has been well described across the cardiac surgical population, including patients having valve replacement, CABG, and transcatheter valve procedures.[34–39] Accordingly, EF is a component of both the Society of Thoracic Surgeons (STS) and European System for Cardiac Operative Risk Evaluation (EuroSCORE) scoring systems for prediction of postoperative morbidity and mortality following cardiac surgery.

Beyond assessment of EF, the impact of global longitudinal strain (GLS) in detecting subtle myocardial dysfunction and predicting postoperative outcome has been examined in multiple recent studies. In general, it appears that GLS analysis provides some incremental predictive value following cardiac surgery, especially in patients with normal EF. In a cohort of patients undergoing CABG, mitral valve, and aortic valve surgery, ~40% of patients with normal EF showed a decrease in their GLS. These patients showed a 2.4-fold increase in their risk for postoperative death compared to patients with normal GLS measurements. These patients also demonstrated an increase in N-terminal pro-brain natriuretic peptide (NT-proBNP) levels, worse HF symptoms, and an increase in the need for postoperative inotropic support.[40] Similarly, other studies have found that decreased GLS is an independent predictor of postoperative low cardiac output syndrome in cardiac surgery and positively predicts prolonged hospitalization after surgical aortic valve replacement for aortic stenosis, though the overall benefit of adding this analysis to existing predictive models is modest.[41,42]

Diastolic Function

In patients undergoing CABG, a simplified assessment of diastolic function utilizing only the transmitral E wave velocity and lateral mitral annular e′ velocity, as assessed by tissue Doppler, has been found to strongly predict the incidence of postoperative major adverse cardiac events[43] (Fig. 32.4). Interestingly, this approach appears to be superior in predicting outcome when compared to a comprehensive intraoperative assessment of diastolic function based on the 2009 ASE recommendations for the assessment of diastolic function.[44] Similarly, a study of patients with severely reduced LV EF (<35%) demonstrated that the presence of restrictive diastolic dysfunction was correlated with a dramatic increase in postoperative mortality and a decrease in improvement of measures of LV systolic function following CABG.[45] Patients undergoing combined mitral valve repair and CABG show comparable results, with an increase in postoperative morbidity and mortality and an increase in recurrence of significant MR in patients with restrictive diastolic dysfunction.[46]

In addition to its role in predicting postoperative mortality there is emerging evidence that LV diastolic dysfunction correlates strongly with the development of postoperative AFib. In patients undergoing CABG or valve surgery with no history of AFib, those with LV diastolic dysfunction, as graded by preoperative echocardiography, were 5 to 28 times more likely to develop postoperative AFib than patients with

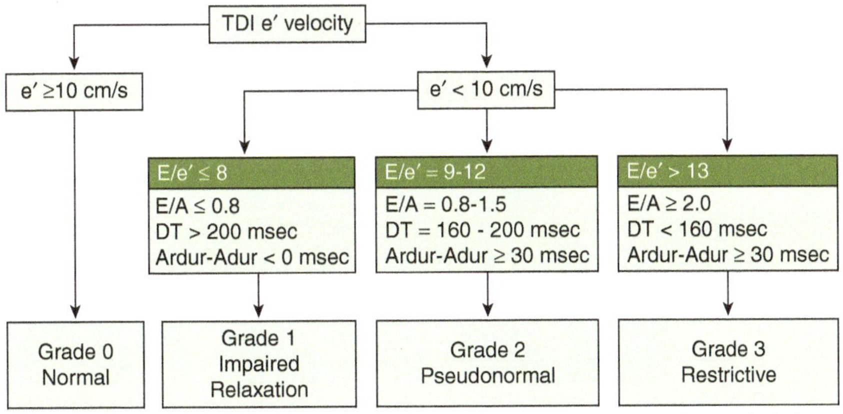

Fig. 32.4 **Algorithm used for grading diastolic dysfunction in the perioperative period, based on the 2009 recommendations for the evaluation of left ventricular diastolic function by echocardiography.** A simplified assessment can be performed utilizing only the e′ velocity and the E/e′ ratio *(denoted in grey)*. *A,* Transmitral diastolic A wave; *Adur,* transmitral A wave duration; *Ardur,* pulmonary vein flow A reversal wave duration; *DT,* E wave deceleration time; *E,* transmitral early wave; *e′,* lateral mitral annular early diastolic tissue velocity; *TDI,* tissue Doppler imaging. (From Swaminathan M, Nicoara A, Phillips-Bute BG, et al. Utility of a simple algorithm to grade diastolic dysfunction and predict outcome after coronary artery bypass graft surgery. *Ann Thorac Surg.* 2011;91(6):1844–1850.)

normal preoperative diastolic function.[47] The increase in LA wall stress and LA pressure in patients with LV diastolic dysfunction is postulated to be responsible for the increased risk of AFib in this population.[3]

DIASTOLIC ASSESSMENT IN THE POSTOPERATIVE CARDIAC SURGERY PATIENT

In the early postoperative period there are a number of potential hemodynamic factors that may confound diastolic assessment, including ongoing volume resuscitation and the need for mechanical ventilation (discussed earlier), pacing, inotropic support, an open pericardium, and a recent ischemic insult secondary to aortic cross-clamping and arrest of the heart to facilitate surgical repair. In general, diastolic function appears to worsen in the immediate postoperative period following cardiac surgery and is an important and often unrecognized cause of congestive HF symptoms in the perioperative period.[48–50] Recognition of the presence and causes of diastolic dysfunction in the perioperative period is useful to help tailor postoperative management.

A large percentage of patients undergoing cardiac surgery will require epicardial pacing in the immediate postoperative period. The effect of pacing on intrinsic diastolic function and diastolic assessment is complex. Most studies examining the hemodynamic effects of pacing have focused on patients with implanted pacemaker leads, whereas patients undergoing cardiac surgery will typically have leads placed on the epicardium.[51–53] In general, it appears that atrial pacing alone does not significantly affect assessment of diastolic function.[1] In contrast, ventricular pacing appears to have a significant deleterious effect on measures of LV diastolic function, though studies have shown variable effects depending on the specific site of pacing.[51,54,55] In one analysis, Mitov et al. found that patients undergoing pacing originating from the RV apex had no significant change in their diastolic assessment, whereas patients having pacing originating in the right ventricular outflow tract (RVOT) seemed to have worsening of diastolic dysfunction.[51] Similarly, a study of patients undergoing RV apical pacing showed that a transition from ventricular sensing to ventricular pacing was associated with a significant reduction in the tissue Doppler e′ velocity (as well as s′ velocity), especially in patients with preexisting diastolic dysfunction.[55] Though data are limited with regard to epicardial pacing it can be inferred that ventricular pacing likely has a deleterious effect on diastolic function.

This interaction is made increasingly complex by the interplay of pacing, heart rate, and the surgical opening of the pericardium during the procedure. A small study of 21 patients undergoing CABG examined systolic and diastolic function prior to and following pericardiotomy and with atrial pacing at and 30 bpm above the native heart rate.[56] The authors did not note any changes in diastolic function with pericardiotomy or with atrial pacing at the native rate, but an increase in the heart rate was associated with a decrease in the E/A ratio and shortened deceleration time, which were interpreted as representative of worsening of diastolic function. Paradoxically, the propagation velocity increased with increasing heart rate. Notably, this study did not utilize tissue Doppler in its assessment of LV diastolic function.

Inotropic therapy is frequently used to augment cardiac output in the postoperative period following cardiac surgery. The effect of inotropic medications on LV diastolic function is likely minimal but may potentially worsen hemodynamic status in patients with preexisting diastolic dysfunction by promoting tachycardia and decreasing LV diastolic filling time.[48] There is evidence that the B-type natriuretic peptide nesiritide may improve echocardiographic measures of diastolic function, but the use of this medication is limited given the current lack of evidence for clinical benefit in patients with acute decompensated HF and concerns about hypotension and renal dysfunction.[48,57]

In general it should be expected that diastolic function will decline in the period immediately following cardiac surgery. Unfortunately, reproducible assessment may be difficult in the setting of rapidly changing hemodynamic and volume status, need for pacing, and levels of inotropic support. Careful attention to these changes can help better contextualize postoperative diastolic assessment.

HOW TO APPROACH DIASTOLIC ASSESSMENT IN THE PERIOPERATIVE PERIOD

Similar to the assessment of diastolic function in the awake patient presenting for transthoracic echocardiography, the perioperative assessment of diastolic function is nuanced and requires consideration of multiple patient and surgical factors. Due to the significant and often

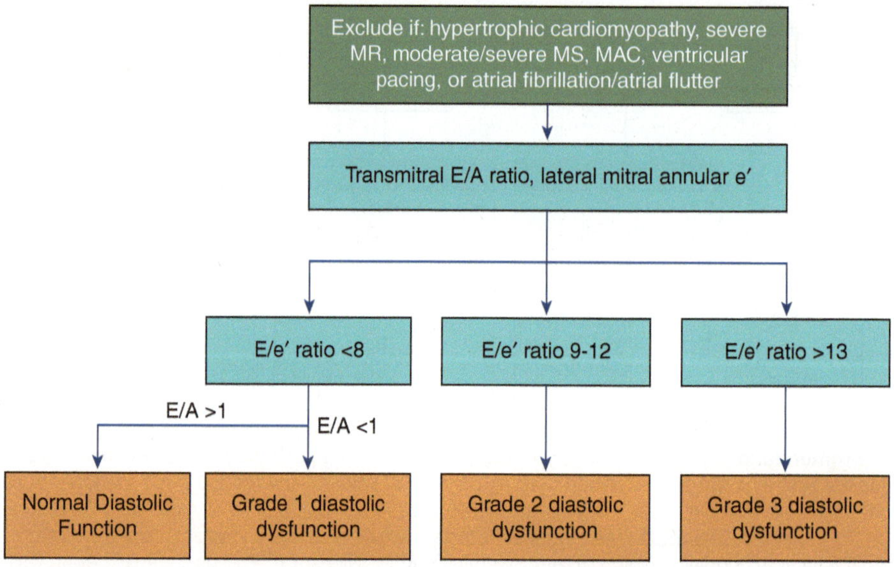

Fig. 32.5 Proposed algorithm for the perioperative assessment of diastolic function. *E/A,* Ratio of transmitral E wave to transmitral A wave velocity; *MAC,* mitral annular calcification; *MR,* mitral regurgitation; *MS,* mitral stenosis.

competing effects of mechanical ventilation, positioning, anesthetic drugs, and other perioperative events, it is important to recognize the limitations of the various indices of diastolic assessment and to tailor echocardiographic assessment to these limitations. The ideal measurement used for diastolic assessment in a patient undergoing TEE during a surgical procedure should be (a) easily and quickly performed, (b) load independent, (c) not significantly altered by changes in position or by anesthetic medications, (d) not influenced by pacing, (e) minimally affected by underlying patient pathology, and (f) useful in either patient management or prognostication. Unfortunately, there is no single assessment or combination of assessments that fulfills all of these criteria.

There is a subset of patients for whom diastolic assessment in the perioperative period may be misleading or unhelpful. Notably, patients with hypertrophic cardiomyopathy, significant mitral valve pathology, and patients who are receiving ventricular pacing may have echocardiographic measures of diastolic function that do not necessarily correlate with their intrinsic degree of diastolic dysfunction. Furthermore, patients with AFib may undergo diastolic assessment, but the methods recommended for diastolic assessment in patients with AFib are not well validated in the perioperative setting and may be unreliable.

In general it appears that the most effective measurement of diastolic function that is least affected by the physiologic changes encountered in the perioperative period is the ratio of transmitral E wave to mitral annular e′ velocity (E/e′ ratio). The transmitral E/A ratio also appears to be relatively preserved and can provide useful information in the perioperative period. The authors recommend primarily using a combination of these two measurements to attempt to estimate diastolic function in the perioperative period (Fig. 32.5). There are a number of other measurements that may be helpful in focusing diastolic assessment (Table 32.2), although their utility in the perioperative environment is less well defined. A pragmatic approach to the evaluation of perioperative diastolic function is presented in Fig. 32.5.

TABLE 32.2 **Supplemental Measurements for Assessment of Left Ventricular Diastolic Function in the Perioperative Period**
Tricuspid regurgitation velocity
Transmitral E wave deceleration time
Propagation velocity
Mitral annular e′ velocity
Pulmonary venous S/D ratio
Isovolumetric relaxation time
Myocardial performance index

CONCLUSIONS

The utility of diastolic assessment in the perioperative period is limited by a number of patient and procedure-specific factors, and the rigid application of current guidelines for assessment of diastolic function is limited during perioperative TEE. With that in mind, perioperative diastolic assessment has important implications for patient management. It can direct risk stratification for major postoperative outcomes, including death and AFib, and may be used to guide perioperative volume management. Focusing on load-independent indices to classify diastolic function likely provides the best insight into the degree of preexisting diastolic dysfunction in the perioperative period. Further research is necessary to better characterize changes in diastolic function in response to perioperative interventions and attempt to delineate (a) whether diastolic function is modifiable and (b) whether improvements in diastolic function can be used to drive improvements in patient outcome following cardiac surgery.

FUTURE DIRECTIONS

There is emerging interest in the use of diastolic strain quantification in the prognostication of patients in a variety of cardiac diseases, including CHF, amyloidosis, and valvular heart disease.[58–60] Similarly, diastolic strain can be assessed utilizing three-dimensional (3-D) echocardiography and has been demonstrated to effectively predict LV filling pressures.[61] For both two-dimensional (2-D) and 3-D diastolic strain assessment, in-depth assessment of their prognostic or therapeutic utility in the perioperative period is lacking. To date there has been minimal application of this technology in the perioperative environment, but this may serve as a potential future target to improve prognostication and diastolic assessment during the perioperative period.

KEY POINTS

- Assessing diastolic function in the perioperative period with certainty is challenging, and a strict application of the ASE/EACVI guidelines is difficult given the need to assess LA volume index using TEE.
- Physiologic perturbations typical of the perioperative period, including hemodynamic changes, mechanical ventilation, fluid shifts, and positioning for surgery, may alter the interpretation of echocardiographic variables.
- The E/e′ ratio and transmitral E/A ratio appear to be the diastolic indices least affected by the hemodynamic changes in the perioperative period.
- Anesthetic agents may also affect diastolic function, but it is unclear whether these changes under anesthesia are a result of direct pharmacologic effects on the myocardium or alterations in ventricular loading conditions.
- Current evidence suggests that perioperative LV diastolic assessment is most likely useful in prognosticating mortality and new AFib following CABG.
- In patients with HCM, severe mitral valve disease, significant mitral annular calcification, and AFib, classification of LV diastolic function is challenging and may not correlate with invasive measurements of LV filling pressures. Furthermore, ventricular pacing may negatively impact indices of diastolic function.

REVIEW QUESTIONS

1. A 59-year-old man presents to the operating room for CABG surgery. In which of the following concurrent cardiac pathologies would intraoperative TEE be most accurate for estimating LV filling pressures?
   a. Mitral annular calcification
   b. Degenerative mitral regurgitation
   c. Tricuspid regurgitation
   d. Hypertrophic cardiomyopathy
2. A 68-year-old man presents for CABG. Intraoperative transesophageal echocardiography reveals grade III diastolic dysfunction. The presence of grade III diastolic dysfunction most strongly predicts which of the following postoperative complications?
   a. Acute kidney injury
   b. Atrial fibrillation
   c. Ventricular tachycardia
   d. Stroke
3. A 57-year-old woman is in the intensive care unit 6 hours following CABG. She has an epicardial pacemaker in place pacing her heart at 90 bpm. Diastolic assessment will be the most accurate while using which of the following pacing modes?
   a. AAI
   b. DDD
   c. DOO
   d. VVI

REFERENCES

1. Nagueh SF, Smiseth OA, Appleton CP, et al. Recommendations for the evaluation of left ventricular diastolic function by echocardiography: an update from the American Society of Echocardiography and the European Association of Cardiovascular Imaging. *J Am Soc Echocardiogr.* 2016;29(4):277–314.
2. Dobbs HA, Bennett-Guerrero E, White W, et al. Multinational institutional survey on patterns of intraoperative transesophageal echocardiography use in adult cardiac surgery. *J Cardiothorac Vasc Anesth.* 2014;28(1):54–63.
3. Nicoara A, Whitener G, Swaminathan M. Perioperative diastolic dysfunction: a comprehensive approach to assessment by transesophageal echocardiography. *Semin Cardiothorac Vasc Anesth.* 2014;18(2):218–236.
4. Block M, Hourigan L, Bellows WH, et al. Comparison of left atrial dimensions by transesophageal and transthoracic echocardiography. *J Am Soc Echocardiogr.* 2002;15(2):143–149.
5. McIlroy DR, Lin E, Durkin C. Intraoperative transesophageal echocardiography: a critical appraisal of its current role in the assessment of diastolic dysfunction. *J Cardiothorac Vasc Anesth.* 2015;29(4):1033–1043.
6. Firstenberg MS, Levine BD, Garcia MJ, et al. Relationship of echocardiographic indices to pulmonary capillary wedge pressures in healthy volunteers. *J Am Coll Cardiol.* 2000;36(5):1664–1669.
7. Garcia MJ, Smedira NG, Greenberg NL, et al. Color M-mode Doppler flow propagation velocity is a preload insensitive index of left ventricular relaxation: animal and human validation. *J Am Coll Cardiol.* 2000;35(1):201–208.
8. Moller JE, Poulsen SH, Sondergaard E, Egstrup K. Preload dependence of color M-mode Doppler flow propagation velocity in controls and in patients with left ventricular dysfunction. *J Am Soc Echocardiogr.* 2000;13(10):902–909.
9. Juhl-Olsen P, Hermansen JF, Frederiksen CA, Rasmussen LA, Jakobsen CJ, Sloth E. Positive end-expiratory pressure influences echocardiographic measures of diastolic function: a randomized, crossover study in cardiac surgery patients. *Anesthesiology.* 2013;119(5):1078–1086.
10. Chin JH, Lee EH, Kim WJ, et al. Positive end-expiratory pressure aggravates left ventricular diastolic relaxation further in patients with pre-existing relaxation abnormality. *Br J Anaesth.* 2013;111(3):368–373.
11. Filipovic M, Michaux I, Wang J, Hunziker P, Skarvan K, Seeberger M. Effects of sevoflurane and propofol on left ventricular diastolic function in patients with pre-existing diastolic dysfunction. *Br J Anaesth.* 2007;98(1):12–18.
12. Filipovic M, Wang J, Michaux I, Hunziker P, Skarvan K, Seeberger MD. Effects of halothane, sevoflurane and propofol on left ventricular diastolic function in humans during spontaneous and mechanical ventilation. *Br J Anaesth.* 2005;94(2):186–192.
13. Gare M, Parail A, Milosavljevic D, Kersten JR, Warltier DC, Pagel PS. Conscious sedation with midazolam or propofol does not alter left ventricular diastolic performance in patients with preexisting diastolic dysfunction: a transmitral and tissue Doppler transthoracic echocardiography study. *Anesth Analg.* 2001;93(4):865–871.
14. Houltz E, Caidahl K, Adin C, Gustavsson T, Ricksten SE. Effects of halothane and isoflurane on left ventricular diastolic function during surgical stress in patients with coronary artery disease. *Acta Anaesthesiol Scand.* 1997;41(7):931–938.
15. Bolliger D, Seeberger MD, Kasper J, et al. Remifentanil does not impair left ventricular systolic and diastolic function in young healthy patients. *Br J Anaesth.* 2011;106(4):573–579.
16. Lee SH, Na S, Kim N, Ban MG, Shin SE, Oh YJ. The effects of dexmedetomidine on myocardial function assessed by tissue Doppler echocardiography during general anesthesia in patients with diastolic dysfunction: a CONSORT-Prospective, Randomized, Controlled Trial. *Medicine (Baltimore).* 2016;95(6):e2805.

17. Zoghbi WA, Adams D, Bonow RO, et al. Recommendations for noninvasive evaluation of native valvular regurgitation: a report from the American Society of Echocardiography developed in collaboration with the Society for Cardiovascular Magnetic Resonance. *J Am Soc Echocardiogr.* 2017;30(4):303–371.
18. Bruch C, Klem I, Breithardt G, Wichter T, Gradaus R. Diagnostic usefulness and prognostic implications of the mitral E/E′ ratio in patients with heart failure and severe secondary mitral regurgitation. *Am J Cardiol.* 2007;100(5):860–865.
19. Bruch C, Stypmann J, Gradaus R, Breithardt G, Wichter T. Usefulness of tissue Doppler imaging for estimation of filling pressures in patients with primary or secondary pure mitral regurgitation. *Am J Cardiol.* 2004;93(3):324–328.
20. Temporelli PL, Scapellato F, Corra U, Eleuteri E, Imparato A, Giannuzzi P. Estimation of pulmonary wedge pressure by transmitral Doppler in patients with chronic heart failure and atrial fibrillation. *Am J Cardiol.* 1999;83(5):724–727.
21. Kusunose K, Yamada H, Nishio S, et al. Clinical utility of single-beat E/e′ obtained by simultaneous recording of flow and tissue Doppler velocities in atrial fibrillation with preserved systolic function. *JACC Cardiovasc Imaging.* 2009;2(10):1147–1156.
22. Sohn DW, Song JM, Zo JH, et al. Mitral annulus velocity in the evaluation of left ventricular diastolic function in atrial fibrillation. *J Am Soc Echocardiogr.* 1999;12(11):927–931.
23. Nagueh SF, Bierig SM, Budoff MJ, et al. American Society of Echocardiography clinical recommendations for multimodality cardiovascular imaging of patients with hypertrophic cardiomyopathy: endorsed by the American Society of Nuclear Cardiology, Society for Cardiovascular Magnetic Resonance, and Society of Cardiovascular Computed Tomography. *J Am Soc Echocardiogr.* 2011;24(5):473–498.
24. Nishimura RA, Appleton CP, Redfield MM, Ilstrup DM, Holmes Jr DR, Tajik AJ. Noninvasive doppler echocardiographic evaluation of left ventricular filling pressures in patients with cardiomyopathies: a simultaneous Doppler echocardiographic and cardiac catheterization study. *J Am Coll Cardiol.* 1996;28(5):1226–1233.
25. Geske JB, Sorajja P, Nishimura RA, Ommen SR. Evaluation of left ventricular filling pressures by Doppler echocardiography in patients with hypertrophic cardiomyopathy: correlation with direct left atrial pressure measurement at cardiac catheterization. *Circulation.* 2007;116(23):2702–2708.
26. Rakowski H, Carasso S. Quantifying diastolic function in hypertrophic cardiomyopathy: the ongoing search for the holy grail. *Circulation.* 2007;116(23):2662–2665.
27. Tower-Rader A, Furiasse N, Puthumana JJ, et al. Effects of septal myectomy on left ventricular diastolic function and left atrial volume in patients with hypertrophic cardiomyopathy. *Am J Cardiol.* 2014;114(10):1568–1572.
28. Chen S, Duan F, Yuan J, et al. Effect of septal ablation on regional diastolic dysfunction and diastolic asynchrony in patients with hypertrophic obstructive cardiomyopathy: a follow-up study using speckle tracking echocardiography. *Echocardiography.* 2013;30(5):564–571.
29. Moon MR, DeAnda A, Castro LJ, Daughters II GT, Ingels Jr NB, Miller DC. Effects of mechanical left ventricular support on right ventricular diastolic function. *J Heart Lung Transplant.* 1997;16(4):398–407.
30. Herod JW, Ambardekar AV. Right ventricular systolic and diastolic function as assessed by speckle-tracking echocardiography improve with prolonged isolated left ventricular assist device support. *J Card Fail.* 2014;20(7):498–505.
31. Estep JD, Vivo RP, Krim SR, et al. Echocardiographic evaluation of hemodynamics in patients with systolic heart failure supported by a continuous-flow LVAD. *J Am Coll Cardiol.* 2014;64(12):1231–1241.
32. Chapman CB, Allana S, Sweitzer NK, et al. Effects of the HeartMate II left ventricular assist device as observed by serial echocardiography. *Echocardiography.* 2013;30(5):513–520.
33. Dalen M, Lund LH, Ivert T, Holzmann MJ, Sartipy U. Survival after coronary artery bypass grafting in patients with preoperative heart failure and preserved vs reduced ejection fraction. *JAMA Cardiol.* 2016;1(5):530–538.
34. Barili F, Pacini D, Grossi C, Di Bartolomeo R, Alamanni F, Parolari A. Reliability of new scores in predicting perioperative mortality after mitral valve surgery. *J Thorac Cardiovasc Surg.* 2014;147(3):1008–1012.
35. Capodanno D, Barbanti M, Tamburino C, et al. A simple risk tool (the OBSERVANT score) for prediction of 30-day mortality after transcatheter aortic valve replacement. *Am J Cardiol.* 2014;113(11):1851–1858.
36. Goldberg JB, DeSimone JP, Kramer RS, et al. Impact of preoperative left ventricular ejection fraction on long-term survival after aortic valve replacement for aortic stenosis. *Circ Cardiovasc Qual Outcomes.* 2013;6(1):35–41.
37. Pieri M, Belletti A, Monaco F, et al. Outcome of cardiac surgery in patients with low preoperative ejection fraction. *BMC Anesthesiol.* 2016;16(1):97.
38. Ranucci M, Castelvecchio S, Conte M, et al. The easier, the better: age, creatinine, ejection fraction score for operative mortality risk stratification in a series of 29,659 patients undergoing elective cardiac surgery. *J Thorac Cardiovasc Surg.* 2011;142(3):581–586.
39. Sannino A, Gargiulo G, Schiattarella GG, et al. Increased mortality after transcatheter aortic valve implantation (TAVI) in patients with severe aortic stenosis and low ejection fraction: a meta-analysis of 6898 patients. *Int J Cardiol.* 2014;176(1):32–39.
40. Ternacle J, Berry M, Alonso E, et al. Incremental value of global longitudinal strain for predicting early outcome after cardiac surgery. *Eur Heart J Cardiovasc Imaging.* 2013;14(1):77–84.
41. Amabili P, Benbouchta S, Roediger L, et al. Low cardiac output syndrome after adult cardiac surgery: predictive value of peak systolic global longitudinal strain. *Anesth Analg.* 2018;126(5):1476–1483.
42. Sonny A, Alfirevic A, Sale S, et al. Reduced left ventricular global longitudinal strain predicts prolonged hospitalization: a cohort analysis of patients having aortic valve replacement surgery. *Anesth Analg.* 2018;126(5):1484–1493.
43. Swaminathan M, Nicoara A, Phillips-Bute BG, et al. Utility of a simple algorithm to grade diastolic dysfunction and predict outcome after coronary artery bypass graft surgery. *Ann Thorac Surg.* 2011;91(6):1844–1850.
44. Nagueh SF, Appleton CP, Gillebert TC, et al. Recommendations for the evaluation of left ventricular diastolic function by echocardiography. *J Am Soc Echocardiogr.* 2009;22(2):107–133.
45. Vaskelyte J, Stoskute N, Kinduris S, Ereminiene E. Coronary artery bypass grafting in patients with severe left ventricular dysfunction: predictive significance of left ventricular diastolic filling pattern. *Eur J Echocardiogr.* 2001;2(1):62–67.
46. Gelsomino S, Lorusso R, Bille G, et al. Left ventricular diastolic function after restrictive mitral ring annuloplasty in chronic ischemic mitral regurgitation and its predictive value on outcome and recurrence of regurgitation. *Int J Cardiol.* 2009;132(3):419–428.
47. Melduni RM, Suri RM, Seward JB, et al. Diastolic dysfunction in patients undergoing cardiac surgery: a pathophysiological mechanism underlying the initiation of new-onset post-operative atrial fibrillation. *J Am Coll Cardiol.* 2011;58(9):953–961.
48. Alsaddique AA, Royse AG, Royse CF, Fouda MA. Management of diastolic heart failure following cardiac surgery. *Eur J Cardiothorac Surg.* 2009;35(2):241–249.
49. Imamura T, Kinugawa K, Shiga T, et al. An elevated ratio of early to late diastolic filling velocity recovers after heart transplantation in a time-dependent manner. *J Cardiol.* 2012;60(4):295–300.
50. McKenney PA, Apstein CS, Mendes LA, et al. Increased left ventricular diastolic chamber stiffness immediately after coronary artery bypass surgery. *J Am Coll Cardiol.* 1994;24(5):1189–1194.
51. Mitov V, Perisic Z, Jolic A, et al. The effect of right ventricle pacemaker lead position on diastolic function in patients with preserved left ventricle ejection fraction. *Hell J Nucl Med.* 2013;16(3):204–208.
52. Simantirakis EN, Vardakis KE, Kochiadakis GE, et al. Left ventricular mechanics during right ventricular apical or left ventricular-based pacing in patients with chronic atrial fibrillation after atrioventricular junction ablation. *J Am Coll Cardiol.* 2004;43(6):1013–1018.
53. Tops LF, Schalij MJ, Holman ER, van Erven L, van der Wall EE, Bax JJ. Right ventricular pacing can induce ventricular dyssynchrony in patients with atrial fibrillation after atrioventricular node ablation. *J Am Coll Cardiol.* 2006;48(8):1642–1648.

54. Chiladakis JA, Koutsogiannis N, Kalogeropoulos A, Zagli F, Arvanitis P, Alexopoulos D. Unfavourable effects of continuous, atrial-synchronised ventricular pacing on ventricular systolic and diastolic function in patients with normal left ventricular ejection fraction: usefulness of tissue and colour Doppler echocardiography. *Hellenic J Cardiol.* 2007;48(6):335–340.
55. Fang F, Zhang Q, Chan JY, et al. Deleterious effect of right ventricular apical pacing on left ventricular diastolic function and the impact of pre-existing diastolic disease. *Eur Heart J.* 2011;32(15):1891–1899.
56. Royse CF, Royse AG, Wong CT, Soeding PF. The effect of pericardial restraint, atrial pacing, and increased heart rate on left ventricular systolic and diastolic function in patients undergoing cardiac surgery. *Anesth Analg.* 2003;96(5):1274–1279.
57. O'Connor CM, Starling RC, Hernandez AF, et al. Effect of nesiritide in patients with acute decompensated heart failure. *N Engl J Med.* 2011;365(1):32–43.
58. Dahl JS, Barros-Gomes S, Videbaek L, et al. Early diastolic strain rate in relation to systolic and diastolic function and prognosis in aortic stenosis. *JACC Cardiovasc Imaging.* 2016;9(5):519–528.
59. Liu D, Hu K, Stork S, et al. Predictive value of assessing diastolic strain rate on survival in cardiac amyloidosis patients with preserved ejection fraction. *PLoS One.* 2014;9(12):e115910.
60. Ohtani T, Mohammed SF, Yamamoto K, et al. Diastolic stiffness as assessed by diastolic wall strain is associated with adverse remodelling and poor outcomes in heart failure with preserved ejection fraction. *Eur Heart J.* 2012;33(14):1742–1749.
61. Shin SH, Park SD, Woo SI, Kim DH, Park KS, Kwan J. Utility of global strain by two-dimensional and three-dimensional speckle tracking for assessing left ventricular diastolic function: comparison with pressure wire analysis. *Korean Circ J.* 2013;43(9):615–621.

33

Pulmonary Hypertension in Heart Failure With Preserved Ejection Fraction

Garvan C. Kane

OUTLINE

ABBREVIATIONS

HFpEF	heart failure with preserved ejection fraction
HFrEF	heart failure with reduced ejection fraction
mPAP	mean pulmonary arterial pressure
PA	pulmonary arterial/artery
PCWP	pulmonary capillary wedge pressure
PH	pulmonary hypertension
PVR	pulmonary vascular resistance
RV	right ventricle / right ventricular
TAPSE	tricuspid annular plane systolic excursion

Case Study

A 66-year-old woman with long-standing systemic hypertension, obstructive sleep apnea, coronary artery disease, atrial fibrillation, and chronic kidney disease is referred for evaluation. She had a pulmonary vein isolation procedure 10 years prior but had recurrent atrial fibrillation and 5 years ago underwent surgical maze at the time of coronary artery bypass grafting. She presents now with a 12-month history of progressive dyspnea, lower extremity edema, and weight gain. She has functional Class III symptoms of exertional dyspnea. She denies chest pain, palpitations, or syncope.

On physical examination her pulse is 80 bpm and irregular, blood pressure (BP) is 108/70 mmHg, respiration rate is 20/min, body weight is 131 kg, body mass index (BMI) is 52 kg/m^2, and O_2 saturation at rest is 90%. Her cardiovascular exam is remarkable for an elevation in her jugular venous pressure to the angle of the jaw and an accentuated pulmonic component of S_2 and III/VI holosystolic murmur best heard at the lower left sternal border. Her abdomen is obese and nontender. There is marked bilateral edema. Laboratory tests: creatinine (Cr) = 2.5 mg/dL. Transthoracic echocardiogram was obtained and representative images are shown (Videos 33.1, 33.2, 33.3, and 33.4; Figs. 33.1, 33.2, and 33.3).

The patient is prescribed a low sodium diet, nocturnal positive airway pressure (PAP) therapy with O_2 supplementation, furosemide 80 mg twice daily, and leg wraps and abdominal massage three times a week at the lymphedema clinic. However, over the following 3 weeks despite increasing her furosemide to 160 mg twice daily she becomes wheelchair bound with functional Class IV dyspnea, her weight rises to 136.8 kg, and her creatinine increases from 2.5 to 2.8 mg/dL.

She is referred for a right heart catheterization. Her hemodynamics are as follows:

- Mean right atrial (RA) pressure: 21 mmHg
- Pulmonary artery pressures (S/D/m): 71/30/49 mmHg
- Pulmonary capillary wedge pressure (PCWP): 29/38/24 mmHg
- Cardiac output: 5 L/min
- Pulmonary arteriolar resistance: 5 Wood units (WU)

DEFINITION AND CLASSIFICATION OF PH

Pulmonary hypertension (PH) is not in of itself a diagnosis or disease but a syndrome characterized by an elevation in pulmonary arterial (PA) pressure, traditionally defined as a mean PA pressure (mPAP) assessed by right heart catheterization, of 25 mmHg or higher.[1] Pulmonary pressure can be further classified based on the PCWP. The PH is precapillary if the PCWP is less than or equal to 15 mmHg and postcapillary when the PCWP is greater than 15 mmHg (Fig. 33.4).[2] Pulmonary vascular resistance (PVR) is defined as the (mPAP – PCWP) divided by the cardiac output. Put simply, a PVR less than 3 Wood units (WU) is consistent with postcapillary PH, and a PVR of 3 WU or greater is consistent with precapillary PH.[3] PH is most often due to left-sided heart disease; however, many patients with left heart disease have PH,

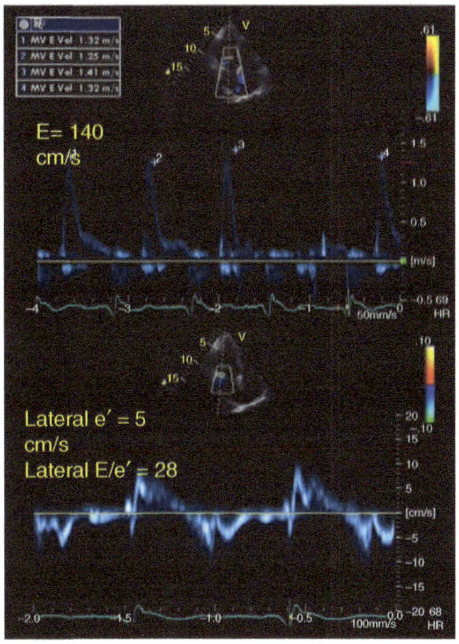

Fig. 33.1 Case study: Echo Doppler data from patient. The upper panel demonstrates a mitral inflow pattern in atrial fibrillation with an E velocity of 140 cm/sec and a short deceleration time. The lower panel shows an average lateral e' velocity to be reduced at 5 cm/sec resulting in a markedly elevated E/e' ratio of 28.

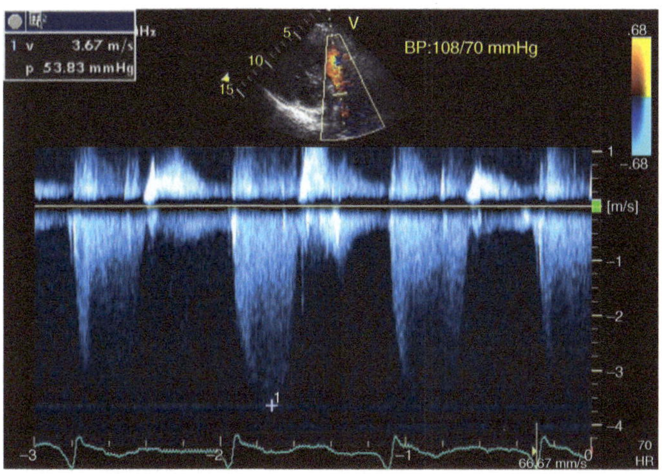

Fig. 33.2 Case study: Echo Doppler data from patient. Doppler profile of the tricuspid regurgitation signal with a peak velocity of 3.7 m/sec.

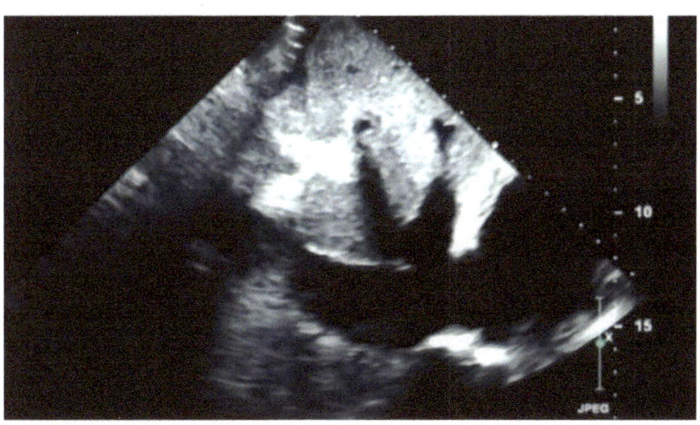

Fig. 33.3 Case study: Still 2-D image of the very dilated inferior vena cava from the patient's echo.

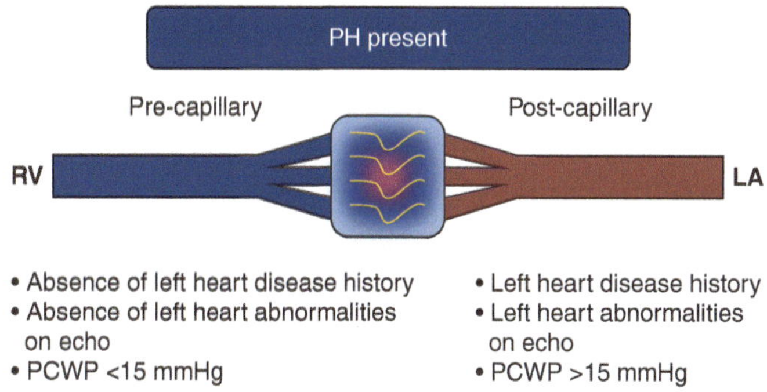

Fig. 33.4 Types of pulmonary hypertension. Pulmonary hypertension *(PH)* can be classified as precapillary or postcapillary. Precapillary PH patients tend to lack a history of left heart disease, have no left heart abnormalities on echocardiography, and at catheterization have a pulmonary capillary wedge pressure *(PCWP)* less than 15 mmHg. "Used with permission of Mayo Foundation for Medical Education and Research, all rights reserved.

an elevated PCWP, and an elevated PVR. This condition has been variably described as "out-of-proportion PH" or "mixed PH."[3,4] The proposed mechanism is that a chronic elevation in pulmonary venous pressure leads to pulmonary vascular vasoconstriction or pulmonary vascular remodeling. Other measures to characterize this mixed PH syndrome include PH with a high transpulmonary gradient (i.e., a difference between the mPAP and the PCWP of ≥10–12 mmHg). The 2015 guidelines[5] preferred the use of the diastolic pressure gradient (the absolute difference between the PCWP and the diastolic PAP). A diastolic pressure gradient of less than 7 mmHg and a PVR less than 3 WU in the setting of a PCWP over 15 mmHg and an mPAP of 25 mmHg and above characterizes an isolated postcapillary PH. Whereas PH is defined as mixed or combined precapillary and postcapillary when the PCWP is greater than 15 mmHg, and the diastolic pressure gradient is 7 mmHg and above and the PVR over 3 WU. However, in isolation the diastolic pressure gradient is imprecise,[6] and the clinician should factor in the PCWP, the diastolic pressure gradient, and the PVR.

Recently guidelines addressing PH in left heart disease were published as part of the Sixth World Symposium on Pulmonary Hypertension.[7] The panel reviewed the evidence concerning patient populations with isolated postcapillary PH (IpcPH) and those with combined postcapillary and precapillary PH (CpcPH).[7] While discussing the value of various hemodynamic variables, including PVR, transpulmonary gradient, and the diastolic pressure gradient, they recognized that no one variable accurately characterizes a particular phenotype and all have potential limitations.[7,8] They also underscored the importance of an accurate PCWP measurement.[7]

Epidemiology

Heart failure with preserved left ventricular (LV) ejection fraction (HFpEF), defined as symptomatic left heart failure occur in the setting of a LV EF that is normal (≥50%), is responsible for close to half of all HF hospitalizations and is a significant cause for postcapillary, or group 2, PH.[9] The diagnosis of postcapillary PH is usually straightforward. Discerning the etiology of PH occurring in the context of severe left-sided valvular disease or a dilated left ventricle with reduced EF is typically not challenging. However, the patient with PH and HFpEF may be harder to assess clinically. Typically these patients may not have marked pulmonary congestion, at least at rest, and have features of right heart failure and left-sided abnormalities that may be underappreciated on imaging. Many of these patients may have normal or borderline LV filling pressures at rest making even the hemodynamic catheterization difficult.

TABLE 33.1 Epidemiology of Heart Failure With Preserved Ejection Fraction and Pulmonary Hypertension

	Prevalence of PH in HFpEF		EF	PA pressure	Other
Lam et al.[10]	83%	Echo	≥50%	PASP >35 mmHg	Elevated E/e′ ratio
Shah et al.[16]	36%	Echo	≥45%	TR velocity >2.9 m/sec	Heart failure history
Vanhercke et al.[17]	51%	Echo	≥50%	TR velocity >2.75 m/sec	≥75 years
Benza et al.[18]	47%	RHC	≥40%	PAmP ≥25 mmHg	
Leung et al.[15]	53%	RHC	≥50%	PAmP >25 mmHg	PAWP ≥15
Hurdman et al.[19]	62%	RHC	≥45%	PAmP >25 mmHg	PAWP ≥15
Gerges et al.[20]	54%	RHC	≥40%	PAmP ≥25 mmHg	
Borlaug et al.[21]	88%	RHC	≥50%	PAmP ≥30 mmHg with exercise	PAWP ≥15 at rest PAWP ≥25 with exercise

E′, Early diastolic annular tissue velocity; *E/e′*, the ratio of the peak early diastolic mitral inflow velocity to E′; *EF*, ejection fraction; *HFpEF*, heart failure with preserved ejection fraction, *PAmP*, pulmonary artery mean pressure; *PAWP*, pulmonary artery wedge pressure; *PH*, pulmonary hypertension; *RHC*, right heart catheterization; *TR*, tricuspid regurgitant Doppler.

A high clinical index of suspicion is required to ensure that these patients are not misclassified as having pulmonary arterial hypertension (PAH).

PH in the setting of HFpEF is common and is associated with worse exercise capacity and worse clinical outcomes.[10–12] However, the true prevalence of PH in HFpEF is challenging as studies vary based on differences in severities of HFpEF, the definition of PH used, the mechanism of PAP measurement (right heart catheterization or echocardiography), and the recognition that variations within patients of PAP hour-to-hour and day-to-day are common due to changes in volume status, stress, and systemic BP.[2,13] Studies have demonstrated the presence of PH in HFpEF to be between 35% and 80% (Table 33.1).[10,14,15] In a community-based study of 244 patients with HFpEF, Lam et al. identified PH as defined by an echo-derived PA systolic pressure over 35 mmHg, to be present in 83% of patients.[10] In comparison, PH was present in only 8% of hypertensive controls. An E/e′ ratio and a PA systolic pressure were the best echo parameters for the diagnosis of heart failure, with PA systolic pressure elevation being the best predictive measure on receiver operating characteristic curve analysis.[10]

While common in HFpEF, PH has various phenotypes. This spans HFpEF patients with earlier stages of disease without any evidence of PH or those that display abnormal pulmonary vasodilatation only with exercise, and some developing PH with exercise.[16,17] Then there are those with PH at rest but due solely to passive elevation in downstream left heart filling pressures and then those displaying features of coexisting pulmonary vascular disease, potentially sharing some pathophysiologic overlap with pulmonary arterial hypertension[11,18–21] (Fig. 33.5).

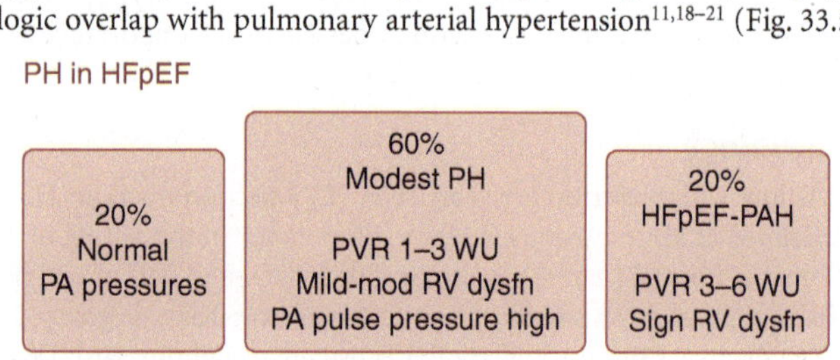

Fig. 33.5 Pulmonary hypertension in heart failure with preserved ejection fraction *(HFpEF)*. Approximately 20% of patients with HFpEF have normal pulmonary artery *(PA)* pressures, 60% have a modest elevation in PA pressures, typically with a normal pulmonary vascular resistance *(PVR)* and mild or mild-moderate right ventricular *(RV)* dysfunction. Only 20% of patients with HFpEF have an elevated PVR, marked RV dysfunction. *PAH*, Pulmonary arterial hypertension; *PH*, pulmonary hypertension; *WU*, Wood units. "Used with permission of Mayo Foundation for Medical Education and Research, all rights reserved.

Prognosis of PH in HFpEF

A consistent finding in the literature is that the presence of PH in the setting of patients with HFpEF is associated with increased all-cause mortality.[10,12,15,22] Rates of death in HFpEF patients with PH are in a similar range to those patients with heart failure with a reduced ejection fraction (HFrEF) and PH.[23] Whether PH is an independent marker of poor prognosis is unclear as it may simply be a marker of the degree of elevation in LV filling pressures. An impairment in diffusion capacity on pulmonary function testing, likely a marker of pulmonary vascular disease, is firmly associated with mortality in patients with HFpEF and PH.[24] An elevation in pulmonary pressures is also typically associated with the degree of right ventricular (RV) dysfunction. The contribution of the RV dysfunction to prognosis is also likely significant. Whether it is genuinely the elevation in pulmonary pressure, in isolation of the RV dysfunction, that conveys higher risk is not well established.[10,14,15,25,26] Likely measures of the degree of RV-PA uncoupling may better reflect the severity of disease and prognosis in these patients,[27] with measures such as PA capacitance being predictive,[28] as is seen in pulmonary arterial hypertension.[29]

Pathophysiology

The pathophysiology of PH in patients with HFpEF is complex. The hallmark of group 2 PH is an elevation in left atrial (LA) pressure leading to pulmonary venous hypertension and pulmonary venous congestion. However, many patients, in addition, develop significant functional and structural abnormalities of the pulmonary vasculature.[30] In principle, when the PH is solely due to passive pulmonary venous hypertension, the hemodynamic profile is one of an elevated PCWP and a proportional increase in PAP.[31,32] Typically in these cases the transpulmonary gradient and PVR are both normal. In these patients, a reduction in LA pressure should bring about a proportional reduction and normalization of mPAP. However, likely brought about by increased severity and chronicity of pulmonary venous hypertension, but also perhaps other clinical or genetic characteristics, some patients develop PAP elevation out of proportion to the pulmonary venous pressures, due to pulmonary vasoconstriction and pulmonary artery remodeling.[33,34] These patients represent a significant proportion of HF patients who undergo invasive hemodynamic catheterization.[35] One also recognizes that an increase in pulmonary vascular stiffness and pulmonary artery pressure occurs with age, even in the absence of an elevation in LV filling pressure.[36]

It has long been demonstrated that pressure elevations in the pulmonary capillary beds lead to disturbance of the alveolar and

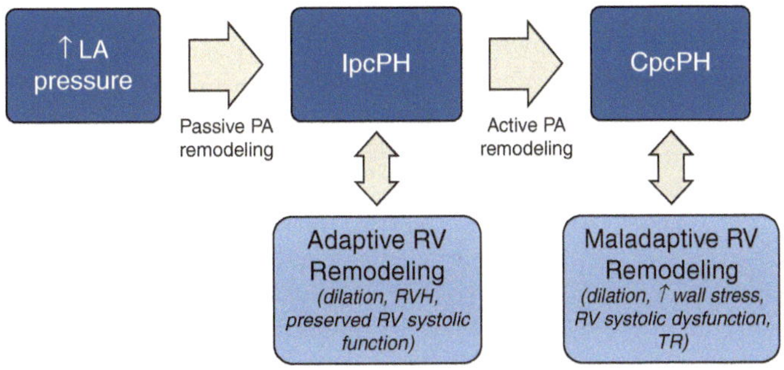

Fig. 33.6 Pathophysiology of pulmonary hypertension in heart failure with preserved ejection fraction *(HFpEF)*. All PH starts with an elevation in left atrial *(LA)* pressure. This leads to pulmonary artery *(PA)* vasoconstriction and passive remodeling and isolated postcapillary pulmonary hypertension *(IpcPH)*. With progression of the disease there develops active structural PA remodeling with the development of combined precapillary and postcapillary PH. IpcPH tends to be associated with mild adaptive changes of the right ventricle with mild dilation, a modest degree of right ventricular *(RV)* wall hypertrophy *(RVH)*, and a preservation of RV systolic function; CpcPH, on the other hand, tends to be associated with a greater degree of more maladaptive remodeling with a typical phenotype of marked RV dilation, significant tricuspid valve regurgitation *(TR)*, and marked RV systolic dysfunction. *CpcPH*, Combined precapillary pulmonary hypertension.

endothelial cell membranes and over time to thickening and weakening of the extracellular matrix.[37,38] In response to the chronic elevations in hemodynamic pressure there is progressive remodeling of the vascular wall with vessel hypertrophy and fibrosis, indeed, structural changes that bear similarities to those that occur in pulmonary arteriopathies. In a detailed histopathologic study of patients with heart failure, PH was associated with global pulmonary vascular remodeling. The severity of PH most strongly correlated with intimal thickening of small vessels.[30] Patients with group 2 PH similarly develop significant endothelial dysfunction.[34] As with patients with pulmonary arterial hypertension, there is a relative deficiency in the production of nitric oxide as well as elevated levels of the pulmonary vasoconstrictor endothelin. Deficiencies in nitric oxide and elevations in endothelin have been demonstrated to cause hypertrophy by inducing the growth of pulmonary vascular smooth muscle cells analogous to that seen in pulmonary arterial hypertension. These may also be pathogenic in the development of pulmonary vascular remodeling in patients with PH and HFpEF. These similarities of the pulmonary vascular bed[19,20] have led to attempts at targeting these pathways in patients with group 2 PH, with variable results (see Management section later in the chapter).

In addition to pulmonary vascular changes, the impact on RV structure and systolic function is also an area of intense investigation. In response to PA pressure elevation, the RV hypertrophies and dilates. However, changes in the RV systolic function frequently do not track in tandem with increases in pulmonary vascular load (Fig. 33.6). This PA-RV uncoupling correlates with impaired exercise capacity, right heart failure, and prognosis.[17,39–42]

Clinical Assessment and Diagnosis

While right heart catheterization remains a critical test in the assessment of precapillary versus postcapillary PH, it is "not sufficient to make a clear distinction between idiopathic pulmonary arterial hypertension and PH due to left heart disease."[7] The workup of the patient with PH requires a comprehensive assessment with history, physical examination, and both noninvasive and, when required, invasive testing. In essence, the patient with precapillary PH should have the absence of left heart disease by history and examination, the absence of left heart abnormalities on echocardiography, and a PCWP that is normal on invasive testing (see Fig. 33.4). Patients with left heart disease by history or examination and left heart abnormalities on echocardiography should be considered as having postcapillary PH regardless of the PCWP and right heart catheterization.[43]

Clinical History and Examination

The risk factors for PH in patients with HFpEF (Table 33.2) include female sex, advancing age, systemic hypertension, coronary artery disease, obesity, and diabetes.[44] As these are also risk factors for the development of HFpEF itself, one may speculate that they may be markers of severity of HFpEF with the associated development of PH rather than markers of PH per se. A contemporary history of a sleep-related breathing disorder, such as obstructive sleep apnea, is common in patients with PH in the setting of HFpEF as is atrial fibrillation.[45] On examination HFpEF patients with PH tend to have an increased accentuation of the pulmonary component of the second heart sound and evidence of elevated central venous pressure.

Laboratory Testing

No laboratory test identifies an elevation in pulmonary pressure, but rather several measures that have been reported in HFpEF patients with PH are those that likely reflect a degree of RV dysfunction or an elevation in central venous pressure. These include hyponatremia, an elevation in plasma brain natriuretic peptide (BNP) or

TABLE 33.2 Clinical Features and Risk Factors of Pulmonary Hypertension Due to Heart Failure With Preserved Ejection Fraction and Pulmonary Arterial Hypertension

PH Due to HFpEF	Pulmonary Arterial Hypertension
Older age	Younger age
Systemic hypertension	Connective tissue disease
Diabetes	Liver disease
Obesity	Congenital heart disease
Atrial fibrillation	History of appetite suppressants or amphetamines
Coronary artery disease	HIV
History of orthopnea	
Pulmonary congestion	

HFpEF, Heart failure with preserved ejection fraction; *HIV,* human immunodeficiency virus; *PH,* pulmonary hypertension.

TABLE 33.3 Electrocardiogram Features of Pulmonary Hypertension Due to Heart Failure With Preserved Ejection Fraction and Pulmonary Arterial Hypertension

PH due to HFpEF	Pulmonary Arterial Hypertension
Left axis deviation	Right axis deviation
Left atrial enlargement	Right atrial enlargement
Left ventricular hypertrophy	Right ventricular hypertrophy
Atrial fibrillation	

HFpEF, Heart failure with preserved ejection fraction; *PH,* pulmonary hypertension.

the N-terminal proBNP (NT-proBNP), and signs of renal or hepatic dysfunction.[44,46,47]

12-Lead Electrocardiogram

The 12-lead electrocardiogram (ECG) in patients with HFpEF more likely displays left axis deviation, LA enlargement, and/or LV hypertrophy (Table 33.3).[48] The presence of atrial fibrillation significantly suggests left heart disease rather than replace with PAH. A patient with replace with PAH typically has right axis deviation, RA enlargement, and evidence of RV hypertrophy on ECG.[49,50]

Transthoracic Echocardiography

Echocardiography is a crucial test that can discriminate precapillary from postcapillary PH. However, unlike in PH related to severe left-sided valve disease or in the setting of a depressed LV EF, the echocardiographic characteristics of patients with HFpEF and PH, as opposed to those with PAH, may be more subtle. Both groups of patients will have evidence of PH, a normal LV EF, and the absence of significant aortic and mitral valve disease. Most patients will have evidence of right atrial and ventricular enlargement, may have tricuspid valve regurgitation, and RV systolic dysfunction. No one parameter helps distinguish these two entities, but a comprehensive echocardiogram in light of clinical characteristics can generally suggest one phenotype over the other. As outlined in Table 33.4 there are a variety of characteristics that make a precapillary more likely than a postcapillary mechanism. Patients with PH due to HFpEF are more likely to have LA enlargement and less often have significant RA enlargement compared to those patients with PAH.[44] LA volume by magnetic resonance imaging (MRI) also separates HFpEF from idiopathic PAH.[51] A degree of RV hypertrophy is related to the severity of PH, but the presence of increased LV wall thickness strongly suggests a postcapillary mechanism for the PH. Diastolic function parameters can be helpful, although abnormalities of mitral inflow and early diastolic mitral annular tissue medial (E′) Doppler velocities have been recognized in patients with significant precapillary PH and RV dysfunction. Scalia et al. have proposed the echocardiographic pulmonary to left atrial ratio (ePLAR), which is the maximum tricuspid regurgitant Doppler velocity divided by the mitral E/e′ ratio, as a measure to discriminate precapillary from postcapillary PH.[52] Notching of the right ventricular outflow tract (RVOT) profile, a feature characteristic of an elevation in PVR in patients with precapillary PH,[53] less frequently is present in patients with PH due to HFpEF.[54]

In patients with early stages of HFpEF, LV filling pressures are typically not markedly elevated at rest, indeed often are normal at rest and only unmasked with exercise.[55] Hence rest echocardiography may not show evidence of elevated E/e′ at rest. Typically these patients have a delayed relaxation mitral inflow pattern. Exercise echocardiography has an emerging role in identifying patients whose filling pressures are normal at rest but increase with exercise. An E/e′ ratio of 15 and above with exercise has an excellent correlation with an elevated PCWP with exercise.[55,56]

In patients with later stages of HFpEF and PH, significant RV dilatation is common. It is this cohort of patients that may be confused with PA hypertension. It is recognized that patients with significant RV dilatation and dysfunction may have a reduction in medial e′ velocities that reflect RV rather than LV septal disease. Hence, in these patients, the lateral e′ should be used rather than the medial e′ velocity for the estimation of LV filling pressures. This cohort of patients typically has a significant elevation in LV filling pressures at rest. Hence lateral E/e′ ratios are typically elevated in HFpEF patients and normal in patients with precapillary PH. In keeping with characteristics of an elevation in LV filling pressure the mitral inflow pattern is typically pseudonormal or restrictive (i.e., grade 2–3 diastolic dysfunction). A delayed relaxation or grade 1 pattern is uncommon in patients with elevated filling pressures at rest. However, this pattern may be seen in patients with normal LV filling pressures but significant RV dysfunction. In these patients it is assumed that the significant RV dysfunction leads to underfilling of the left atrium, a low LA pressure, and hence a delayed relaxation mitral inflow pattern. Studies in PAH have identified a cohort of patients with a delayed relaxation mitral inflow pattern that is

TABLE 33.4 Echocardiographic Features in the Setting of Pulmonary Hypertension That Favor an Etiology of Heart Failure With Preserved Ejection Fraction or Pulmonary Arterial Hypertension

Echo Variables	PH due to HFpEF	PAH
Left atrial size	Enlarged	Normal/small
LV mass	Increased	Normal
RA to LA size ratio	LA > RA	RA > LA
Intraatrial septum	Bows to the right	Bows to the left
Mitral inflow pattern	Restrictive	Normal/delayed relaxation pattern
Medial E′	Low	Normal or low
Lateral E′	Low	Normal
E/e′ with exercise	>15	<8–10
ePLAR (TRV / E/e′)	<0.3	>0.3
Echo PVR	Not helpful in distinguishing etiology of PH	

E′, Early diastolic annular tissue velocity; *E/e′,* the ratio of the peak early diastolic mitral inflow velocity to E′; *ePLAR,* echocardiographic pulmonary to left atrial ratio; *HFpEF,* heart failure with preserved ejection fraction; *LA,* left atrial; *LV,* left ventricle; *PH,* pulmonary hypertension; *PAH,* pulmonary arterial hypertension; *PVR,* pulmonary vascular resistance; *RA,* right atrial.

associated with small left atria and ventricles, lower LA pressures, more severe elevations in PVR, and right heart dysfunction.[57]

Exercise Testing

A measure of exercise capacity plays a definite role in quantifying the severity of disease in both patients with PAH and PH due to HFpEF. Both cohorts of patients may display an impaired exercise capacity, RV dysfunction with exercise, and evidence of the abnormal pulmonary vasodilatory response.[17,58] The performance of cardiopulmonary assessment with exercise allows an assessment of ventilator efficiency, although abnormalities have been seen in both precapillary and post-capillary patients with abnormalities more likely in HF patients with a component of pulmonary vascular disease.[59] Some studies have suggested a lower end-tidal CO_2 level in patients with PA hypertension rather than PH due to heart failure[60]; however, in isolation cardiopulmonary exercise testing may not be able to differentiate PA hypertension from HFpEF.[71,61] An elevated VE/VCO_2 slope is a marker of more severe disease and worse prognosis in patients with HFpEF, PH, and elevated PVR.[62] As discussed earlier, echo Doppler with measurement of E/e′ ratio and tricuspid regurgitant velocity may be of value in discriminating patients who do not appear to have evidence of elevated filling pressures at rest.[55,56]

Composite Scores

No one singular variable is generally adequate in most patients to make a diagnosis of PH due to HFpEF rather than due to PAH. Instead, a summation of various clinical factors allows the provider to determine a preinvasive test probability of group 2 PH. Various composite scores have been proposed that integrate clinical history, examination, and noninvasive testing results to favor a diagnosis of HFpEF in patients with dyspnea or HFpEF versus precapillary PH in patients with PH.[45,54,63–66]

Right Heart Imaging

Right heart dysfunction is a well-recognized prognostic factor in patients of left-sided heart disease. Emerging studies have characterized the importance of the assessment of RV systolic dysfunction in patients with HFpEF.[67] Those HFpEF patients with PH, particularly those with elevated PVR, predispose to more significant right heart dysfunction. The severity of right heart dysfunction likely contributes to patient's symptoms both in terms of a limitation cardiac output and symptoms of systemic congestion.[17] Quantitation of RV systolic function is an emerging prognostic indicator in patients with HFpEF.[42] Echocardiographic measures of longitudinal function appear to best reflect RV contractility in patients with PH, and it is likely (as with precapillary PH) measures of RV longitudinal systolic strain better reflect disease severity than measures of annular excursion, whether tricuspid annular plane systolic excursion (TAPSE) or S′.[42,68,69] Fractional area change has also been shown to predict future hospitalization for right heart failure as well as all-cause mortality in HFpEF patients with PH.[26,40] Integration of the assessment of RV systolic function with pulmonary hemodynamics (i.e., an integrated assessment of RV-PA coupling) likely provides incremental insight into the pathophysiology and disease severity of HFpEF.[17,42] Accurate quantitation of RV volumes and EF can be obtained from cardiac MRI or by three-dimensional (3D) echocardiography.

Right Heart Hemodynamic Assessment

Invasive right heart catheterization is an important test to help distinguish PH due to HFpEF from forms of precapillary PH. In principle, patients with HFpEF have an elevation in PCWP to greater than or equal to 15 mmHg. PCWP should be measured in the resting state at passive end expiration with the tracing measured at end ventricular diastole. An elevated PCWP should be confirmed to be a true wedge tracing, rather than a dampened PA tracing, by determination of blood O_2 saturation. Any concern of the validity of the PCWP tracing should prompt a direct LV end-diastolic pressure (EDP) measurement. A finding of an elevated PCWP in excess of 15 mmHg, an elevation in mPAP proportional to the PCWP, and a PVR less than 3 WU in the setting of a normal LV EF and in the absence of significant left-sided valvular disease would confirm the diagnosis of PH due to HFpEF. However, a number of other hemodynamic profiles may occur. Work by Borlaug and others has characterized that upwards of 50% of patients with HFpEF do not have an elevation in PCWP at rest.[55,70] If these patients have a standard hemodynamic assessment in the resting state, many patients will be mischaracterized. Furthermore, many patients with HFpEF do not have evidence of an elevation in pulmonary pressures at rest but develop exercise-induced PH. Hence dynamic exercise (e.g., with supine cycle ergometry) provides significant insight into the pathophysiology of patients with HF with significant underappreciation if only the rest hemodynamics are assessed.[71]

Other clues to the presence of a postcapillary mechanism for PH may include large v waves on the wedge tracing in the absence of mitral regurgitation or a paradoxical increase in PCWP with a pulmonary vasodilator challenge. However, the operator should have a high index of suspicion and have a low threshold for challenging the patient with either saline loading or exercise. Particularly in patients with a higher clinical pretest probability (i.e., older age, diabetes, hypertension, and/or obesity) the operator should not settle for a normal PCWP at rest but rather challenge the patient to see if he or she can bring out the phenotype of HFpEF. A variety of protocols have been used; however, it is the practice in our laboratory to perform supine lower extremity bike exercise with assessment of PCWP. Interpretation of the waveforms is more challenging with exercise due to the swings in intrathoracic pressure. However, a PCWP over 25 mmHg with exercise is diagnostic for HFpEF. For those invasive laboratories that are unable to perform exercise hemodynamics, an acute intravenous saline load has been proposed as an alternative.[72] Current data suggest that a PCWP over 18 to 20 mmHg immediately after an infusion of 500 mL of saline over 5 minutes is abnormal.[7,71–75]

One must also recognize that patients with PAH and markedly abnormal right ventricles, particularly in the setting of systemic volume overload, may have mild increases in left-sided filling pressures due to ventricular interdependence. In short, distinguishing PH due to HFpEF from precapillary PH should not be based solely on a PCWP measurement but rather on thorough integration of clinical, echocardiographic, and hemodynamic evaluation, commonly requiring exercise noninvasive or invasive hemodynamic assessment (Fig. 33.7).

Management

The mainstay of treatment of PH due to HFpEF should be directed toward optimizing management of the underlying cardiac dysfunction, including optimized volume assessment. Approaches for management are discussed in detail elsewhere in this book. In the presence of concomitant right heart dysfunction, management of volume overload is of particular value to reduce ventricular wall stress, the impact of RV enlargement and interventricular septal shift on LV filling, and the negative impact of central venous pressure elevation on hepatic congestion, renal perfusion, and neurohormonal activation. Aldosterone antagonists may have an incremental benefit over loop diuretics in both HFpEF and RV dysfunction.[76] Addressing potential contributing factors, including systemic hypertension, sleep-related breathing disorders, and obesity, are likely of value.

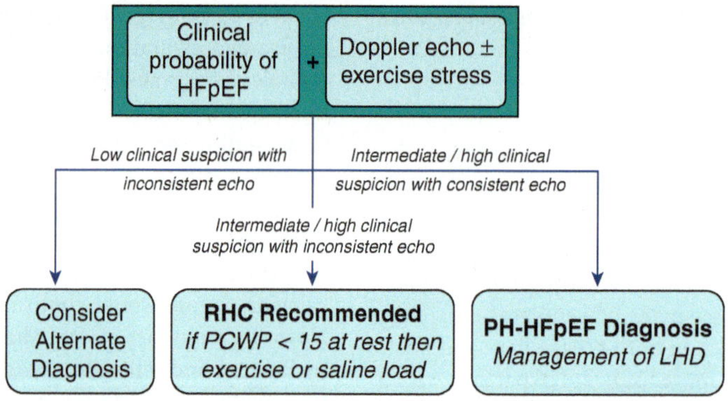

Fig. 33.7 Suggested algorithm for the evaluation of the patient suspected with pulmonary hypertension *(PH)* in the setting of heart failure with preserved ejection fraction *(HFpEF)*. The diagnostic assessment should involve the integration of the clinical history and examination with Doppler echocardiography. Doppler stress echocardiography should be considered in patients with predominantly exercise-induced symptoms. Right heart catheterization *(RHC)* should be considered for patients with intermediate or high clinical suspicion of HFpEF-PH with an indeterminate echo evaluation. In these patients, if rest RHC demonstrates a pulmonary capillary wedge pressure *(PCWP)* less than 15 mmHg, an exercise or saline challenge should be considered.

While there is some evidence that pulmonary vascular targeted therapy might be of benefit in some patients with HFpEF and PH,[81] many studies have failed to show consistent benefit. Furthermore, many have shown a propensity to increased pulmonary congestion presumably related to increased pulmonary blood flow in the setting of LV diastolic dysfunction.[78]

Studies that have assessed endothelin receptor antagonists in patients with HF have, in general, yielded neutral or negative results.[79–82] Indeed the propensity of these agents to lead to systemic volume retention likely underscores their potential for exacerbation of left heart failure. However, endothelin-A antagonism may have a role in selected patients with HFpEF[83]; particularly in those with early stages of disease, evaluation is ongoing. One multicenter trial to evaluate the efficacy of endothelin receptor antagonist macitentan is currently being tested in patients with a phenotype of pulmonary vascular disease and HFpEF. This study aims to exclude patients who developed volume overload with the initiation of endothelin antagonism (SERENADE; NCT03153111).

Most studies to date have involved heterogeneous patient populations with HFpEF patients with varying degrees of PH and pulmonary vascular disease (Table 33.5). The only study of a phosphodiesterase-5 (PDE5) inhibitor in patients with HFpEF with PH, pulmonary vascular disease, and RV dysfunction was the single-center study by Guazzi, which suggested benefit.[77] Other studies to date typically enrolled a different patient phenotype, with normal PVR and minimal to no RV dysfunction (see Table 33.5). The focus of future studies will be on the subset of patients with HFpEF who have evidence of a significant precapillary component (i.e., with PH apparently out of proportion to the elevation in PCWP with elevated PVR) (Table 33.6). To date, though, there are no randomized multicenter trial data that support the use of pulmonary vascular-targeted therapies in any form of PH in the setting of HFpEF that is of clinic benefit. Use of these therapies, outside of clinical trials, is not recommended.[7]

In contrast to HF patients with reduced LV EF in whom chronic nitrate therapy can help with pulmonary congestion and functional capacity, long-acting nitrates do not appear to be of benefit in patients

TABLE 33.5 Studies of Sildenafil in Patients With Heart Failure With Preserved Ejection Fraction and Pulmonary Hypertension

Study	Therapy	Average mPAP, mmHg	RA pressure	RV systolic function	PVR	Results
Redfield et al.[84]	Sildenafil 20 mg TID × 12 weeks, then 60 mg TID × 12 weeks	25 mmHg	Normal	Normal function	Normal	No benefit
Borlaug et al.[85]	Sildenafil 20 mg TID × 12 weeks, then 60 mg TID × 12 weeks	25–30 mmHg	Normal	Mild dysfunction	Normal	No benefit
Hoendermis et al.[86]	Sildenafil 60 mg TID × 12 weeks	30 mmHg	Normal	Mild dysfunction	Normal	No benefit
Hussain et al.[27]	Sildenafil 20 mg TID × 12 weeks, then 60 mg TID × 12 weeks	25–30 mmHg		Reduced TAPSE, low TAPSE/RVSP ratio	Probably normal	No benefit
Guazzi et al.[77]	Sildenafil 50 mg TID × 52 weeks	40 mmHg	Very high	Moderate-severe dysfunction	4–5	Benefit

mPAP, Mean pulmonary arterial pressure; *PVR,* pulmonary vascular resistance; *RA,* right atrial; *RV,* right ventricular; *RVSP,* right ventricular systolic pressure; *TAPSE,* tricuspid annular plane systolic excursion; *TID,* three times daily.

TABLE 33.6 Current Trials of Pulmonary Vascular Therapies Enrolling Patients With Heart Failure With Preserved Ejection Fraction and Pulmonary Hypertension

Trial	Therapy Versus Placebo	Study Subject Characteristics
DYNAMIC (NCT 02744339)	Riociguat 1.5 mg three times daily	HFpEF, mPAP >25 mmHg, PCWP >15 mmHg
Oral Treprostinil (NCT 03037580)	Oral treprostinil	HFpEF
PASSION (EudraCT: 2017-003688-37)	Tadalafil 40 mg once daily	HFpEF, mPAP >25 mmHg, PCWP >15 mmHg, PVR >3 WU
SERENADE (NCT 03153111)	Macitentan 10 mg once daily	HFpEF, PCWP >15 mmHg, pulmonary vascular disease or RV dysfunction

HFpEF, Heart failure with preserved ejection fraction; *mPAP,* mean pulmonary artery pressure; *PCWP,* pulmonary capillary wedge pressure; *PVR,* pulmonary vascular resistance; *RV,* right ventricular.

with HFpEF.[84] Hence routine use of nitrates in this patient population is not recommended.

To continue with the patient in our chapter-opening case study, metolazone was added and the fluid began to come off. Over 1 month the patient lost 25 lb, creatinine improved to 2.5 mg/dL, and she began to be able to walk. The patient was tried on sildenafil (against guideline recommendations) and within 5 days of starting sildenafil, 10 mg three times daily, the patient gained 10 lb, had worsening dyspnea, and was hospitalized for intravenous diuresis. Sildenafil was stopped and diuresis resumed.

At 3 months her weight was down to 106 kg (BMI 42 kg/m^2) predominantly due to diuresis. Her creatinine improved to 2.0 mg/dL. At 4 months her weight was down to 101 kg (BMI 38 kg/m^2) and creatinine was stable at 2.1 mg/dL. She had repeat right heart catheterization, and the results were very similar: RA mean pressure 32 mmHg; mPAP 50 mmHg; mean PCWP 26 mmHg, and CO 5.7 L/min for a PVR of 4.2 WU.

Twelve months after diagnosis her weight was 92 kg, BMI 36 kg/m^2, and creatinine 2.1 mg/dL. She was taking 100 mg of oral furosemide twice daily and metolazone 2.5 mg once a week, and she was participating in cardiopulmonary rehabilitation three times a week. One year later, weight was 85 kg and creatinine 2.1, and she could walk 2 to 3 miles. Sildenafil was retried. Within 2 weeks she was hospitalized with decompensated biventricular heart failure. Sildenafil was stopped and after diuresis she did well.

FUTURE DIRECTIONS

Current investigation points toward characterization of the cause and significance of a normal pulmonary vascular remodeling in patients with HFpEF, recognizing that RV pulmonary arterial uncoupling may provide novel targets in the management of these complex patients. Whether therapies will best target the abnormal pulmonary vascular remodeling or the right heart dysfunction, or both, is unclear. Studies are underway to assess conventional pulmonary vascular targeted therapies in patients with heart failure, PH, and elevated PVR. However, further studies are required to understand the optimal candidate targets in these tissue beds better.

KEY POINTS

- The majority of patients with HFpEF have PH.
- Most PH in HFpEF is modest and is not associated with significant right heart dysfunction.
- Approximately 20% of patients with HFpEF develop a PH syndrome with mixed postcapillary and precapillary features.
- Both the presence and severity of PH pertain a poorer prognosis in HFpEF.
- The diagnosis of PH in HFpEF requires an integration of the history, physical examination, and Doppler echocardiography. Right heart catheterization is needed in some patients.
- Approximately 50% of patients with HFpEF have normal LV filling pressures at rest. Exercise with echo or catheterization is frequently required in the evaluation.
- Pulmonary vascular targeted therapies, including PDE5 inhibitors (e.g., sildenafil), have a role in the management of patients with PH in the setting of HFpEF.

REVIEW QUESTIONS

1. Based on the echocardiogram, which of the following statements is likely true about the patient in the case study?
   a. Left and right atrial pressure are normal
   b. Left atrial pressure is elevated and right atrial pressure is normal
   c. Left atrial pressure is normal and right atrial pressure is elevated
   d. Left and right atrial pressures are both elevated
2. The hemodynamics of the patient in the case study are consistent with which diagnosis?
   a. Pulmonary arterial hypertension
   b. Isolated postcapillary pulmonary hypertension
   c. High output heart failure
   d. Combined postcapillary and precapillary pulmonary hypertension
3. Which therapeutic intervention is the next best step for the patient described in the case study?
   a. Add metolazone
   b. Add metoprolol
   c. Add sildenafil
   d. Ultrafiltration

REFERENCES

1. Badesch DB, Champion HC, Sanchez MA, et al. Diagnosis and assessment of pulmonary arterial hypertension. *J Am Coll Cardiol.* 2009;54(1):S55–S66.
2. McLaughlin VV, Archer SL, Badesch DB, et al. ACCF/AHA 2009 expert consensus document on pulmonary hypertension a report of the American College of Cardiology Foundation Task Force on Expert Consensus Documents and the American Heart Association developed in collaboration with the American College of Chest Physicians; American Thoracic Society, Inc.; and the Pulmonary Hypertension Association. *J Am Coll Cardiol.* 2009;53(17):1573–1619.
3. Galiè N, Hoeper MM, Humbert M, et al. Guidelines for the diagnosis and treatment of pulmonary hypertension: the Task Force for the Diagnosis and Treatment of Pulmonary Hypertension of the European Society of Cardiology (ESC) and the European Respiratory Society (ERS), endorsed by the International Society of Heart and Lung Transplantation (ISHLT). *Eur Heart J.* 2009;30(20):2493–2537.
4. Fang JC, DeMarco T, Givertz MM, et al. World Health Organization pulmonary hypertension group 2: pulmonary hypertension due to left heart disease in the adult—a summary statement from the Pulmonary Hypertension Council of the International Society for Heart and Lung Transplantation. *J Heart Lung Transplant.* 2012;31(9):913–933.
5. Simonneau G, Gatzoulis MA, Adatia I, et al. Updated clinical classification of pulmonary hypertension. *J Am Coll Cardiol.* 2013;62(25):D34–D41.
6. Tampakakis E, Leary PJ, Selby VN, et al. The diastolic pulmonary gradient does not predict survival in patients with pulmonary hypertension due to left heart disease. *JACC Heart Fail.* 2015;3:9–16.
7. Vachiéry JL, Tedford RJ, Rosenkranz S, et al. Pulmonary hypertension due to left heart disease. Proceedings of the 6th World Symposium on Pulmonary Hypertension. *Eur Respir J.* 2019;53:1801897. doi: 10.1183/13993003.01897–2018.
8. Naeije R, Gerges M, Vachiery JL, Caravita S, Gerges C, Lang IM. Hemodynamic phenotyping of pulmonary hypertension in left heart failure. *Circ Heart Fail.* 2017;10:e004082.
9. Hansdottir S, Groskreutz DJ, Gehlbach BK. WHO's in second? A practical review of World Health Organization Group 2 pulmonary hypertension. *Chest.* 2013;144(2):638–650.
10. Lam CS, Roger VL, Rodeheffer RJ, Borlaug BA, Enders FT, Redfield MM. Pulmonary hypertension in heart failure with preserved ejection fraction: a community-based study. *J Am Coll Cardiol.* 2009;53:1119–1126.
11. Borlaug BA, Obokata M. Is it time to recognize a new phenotype? Heart failure with preserved ejection fraction with pulmonary vascular disease. *Eur Heart J.* 2017;38:2874–2878.
12. Vanderpool RR, Saul M, Nouraie M, Gladwin MT, Simon MA. Association between hemodynamic markers of pulmonary hypertension and outcomes in heart failure with preserved ejection fraction. *JAMA Cardiol.* 2018;3:298–306.
13. Benza RL, Raina A, Abraham WT, et al. Pulmonary hypertension related to left heart disease: insight from a wireless implantable hemodynamic monitor. *J Heart Lung Transplant.* 2015;34:329–337.
14. Ghio S, Gavazzi A, Campana C, et al. Independent and additive prognostic value of right ventricular systolic function and pulmonary artery pressure in patients with chronic heart failure. *J Am Coll Cardiol.* 2001;37(1):183–188.
15. Leung CC, Moondra V, Catherwood E, Andrus BW. Prevalence and risk factors of pulmonary hypertension in patients with elevated pulmonary venous pressure and preserved ejection fraction. *Am J Cardiol.* 2010;106(2):284–286.
16. Lewis GD, Bossone E, Naeije R, et al. Pulmonary vascular hemodynamic response to exercise in cardiopulmonary diseases. *Circulation.* 2013;128:1470–1479.
17. Borlaug BA, Kane GC, Melenovsky V, Olson TP. Abnormal right ventricular-pulmonary artery coupling with exercise in heart failure with preserved ejection fraction. *Eur Heart J.* 2016;37:3293–3302.
18. Shah SJ, Kitzman DW, Borlaug BA, et al. Phenotype-specific treatment of heart failure with preserved ejection fraction: a multiorgan roadmap. *Circulation.* 2016;134:73–90.
19. Assad TR, Hemnes AR, Larkin EK, et al. Clinical and biological insights into combined post- and pre-capillary pulmonary hypertension. *J Am Coll Cardiol.* 2016;68:2525–2536.
20. Opitz CF, Hoeper MM, Gibbs JS, et al. Pre-capillary, combined, and post-capillary pulmonary hypertension: a pathophysiological continuum. *J Am Coll Cardiol.* 2016;68. 368–337.
21. Gorter TM, van Veldhuisen DJ, Voors AA, et al. Right ventricular-vascular coupling in heart failure with preserved ejection fraction and pre- vs. post-capillary pulmonary hypertension. *Eur Heart J Cardiovasc Imag.* 2018;19:425–432.
22. Gorter TM, Hoendermis ES, van Veldhuisen DJ, et al. Right ventricular dysfunction in heart failure with preserved ejection fraction: a systematic review and meta-analysis. *Eur J Heart Fail.* 2016;18:1472–1487.
23. Damy T, Goode KM, Kallvikbacka-Bennett A, et al. Determinants and prognostic value of pulmonary arterial pressure in patients with chronic heart failure. *Eur Heart J.* 2010;31:2280–2290.
24. Hoeper MM, Meyer K, Rademacher J, Fuge J, Welte T, Olsson KM. Diffusion capacity and mortality in patients with pulmonary hypertension due to heart failure with preserved ejection fraction. *J Am Coll Cardiol Heart Fail.* 2016;4:441–449.
25. Shah AM, Shah SJ, Anand IS, et al. Cardiac structure and function in heart failure with preserved ejection fraction: baseline findings from the echocardiographic study of the treatment of preserved cardiac function heart failure with an aldosterone antagonist trial. *Circ Heart Fail.* 2014;7:104–115.
26. Burke MA, Katz DH, Beussink L, et al. Prognostic importance of pathophysiologic markers in patients with heart failure and preserved ejection fraction. *Circ Heart Fail.* 2014;7:288–299.
27. Hussain I, Mohammed SF, Forfia PR, et al. Impaired right ventricular-pulmonary arterial coupling and effect of sildenafil in heart failure with preserved ejection fraction. *Circ Heart Fail.* 2016;9:e002729.
28. Adir Y, Guazzi M, Offer A, Temporelli PL, Cannito A, Ghio S. Pulmonary hemodynamics in heart failure patients with reduced or preserved ejection fraction and pulmonary hypertension: similarities and disparities. *Am Heart J.* 2017;192:120–127.
29. Mahapatra S, Nishimura RA, Sorajja P, Cha S, McGoon MD. Relationship of pulmonary arterial capacitance and mortality in idiopathic pulmonary arterial hypertension. *J Am Coll Cardiol.* 2006;47(4):799–803.
30. Fayyaz AU, Edwards WD, Maleszewski JJ, et al. Global pulmonary vascular remodeling in pulmonary hypertension associated with heart failure and preserved or reduced ejection fraction. *Circulation.* 2018;137:1796–1810.
31. Melenovsky V, Hwang SJ, Redfield MM, Zakeri R, Lin G, Borlaug BA. Left atrial remodeling and function in advanced heart failure with preserved or reduced ejection fraction. *Circ Heart Fail.* 2015;8:295–303.
32. Rossi A, Gheorghiade M, Triposkiadis F, Solomon SD, Pieske B, Butler J. Left atrium in heart failure with preserved ejection fraction: structure, function, and significance. *Circ Heart Fail. 2014*;7:1042–1049.
33. Gerges C, Gerges M, Lang MB, et al. Diastolic pulmonary vascular pressure gradient: a predictor of prognosis in "out of proportion" pulmonary hypertension. *Chest.* 2013;143:758–766.
34. Delgado JF, Conde E, Sánchez V, et al. Pulmonary vascular remodeling in pulmonary hypertension due to chronic heart failure. *Eur J Heart Fail.* 2005;7:1011–1016.
35. Schwartzenberg S, Redfield MM, From AM, Sorajja P, Nishimura RA, Borlaug BA. Effects of vasodilation in heart failure with preserved or reduced ejection fraction implications of distinct pathophysiologies on response to therapy. *J Am Coll Cardiol.* 2012;59(5):442–451.
36. Kane GC, Sachdev A, Villarraga HR, et al. Impact of age on pulmonary artery systolic pressures at rest and with exercise. *Echo Res Pract.* 2016;3:53–61.
37. Lee YS. Electron microscopic studies on the alveolar-capillary barrier in the patients of chronic pulmonary edema. *Japn Circ J.* 1979;43(10):945–954.

38. Tsukimoto K, Mathieu-Costello O, Prediletto R, Elliott AR, West JB. Ultrastructural appearances of pulmonary capillaries at high transmural pressures. *J Appl Physiol.* 1985/1991;71:573–582.
39. Andersen MJ, Hwang SJ, Kane GC, et al. Enhanced pulmonary vasodilator reserve and abnormal right ventricular: pulmonary artery coupling in heart failure with preserved ejection fraction. *Circ Heart Fail.* 2015;8:542–550.
40. Melenovsky V, Hwang SJ, Lin G, Redfield MM, Borlaug BA. Right heart dysfunction in heart failure with preserved ejection fraction. *Eur Heart J.* 2014;35:3452–3462.
41. Mohammed SF, Hussain I, AbouEzzeddine OF, et al. Right ventricular function in heart failure with preserved ejection fraction: a community-based study. *Circulation.* 2014;130:2310–2320.
42. Bosch L, Lam CSP, Gong L, et al. Right ventricular dysfunction in left-sided heart failure with preserved versus reduced ejection fraction. *Eur J Heart Fail.* 2017;19:1664–1671.
43. Shapiro BP, McGoon MD, Redfield MM. Unexplained pulmonary hypertension in elderly patients. *Chest.* 2007;131(1):94–100.
44. Thenappan T, Shah SJ, Gomberg-Maitland M, et al. Clinical characteristics of pulmonary hypertension in patients with heart failure and preserved ejection fraction/clinical perspective. *Circ Heart Fail.* 2011;4(3):257–265.
45. Berthelot E, Montani D, Algalarrondo V, et al. A clinical and echocardiographic score to identify pulmonary hypertension due to HFpEF. *J Card Fail.* 2017;23:29–35.
46. Rabinovitz A, Raiszadeh F, Zolty R. Association of hyponatremia and outcomes in pulmonary hypertension. *J Card Fail.* 2013;19: 550–556.
47. Carlsen CM, Bay M, Kirk V, Gøtze JP, Køber L, Nielsen OW. Prevalence and prognosis of heart failure with preserved ejection fraction and elevated N-terminal pro brain natriuretic peptide: a 10-year analysis from the Copenhagen Hospital Heart Failure Study. *Eur J Heart Fail.* 2012;14:240–247.
48. McMurray JJ, Carson PE, Komajda M, et al. Heart failure with preserved ejection fraction: clinical characteristics of 4133 patients enrolled in the I-PRESERVE trial. *Eur J Heart Fail.* 2008;10(2):149–156.
49. Bossone E, Paciocco G, Iarussi D, et al. The prognostic role of the ECG in primary pulmonary hypertension. *Chest.* 2002;121:513–518.
50. McGoon MD, Kane GC. Pulmonary hypertension: diagnosis and management. *Mayo Clin Proc.* 2009;84(2):191–207.
51. Crawley SF, Johnson MK, Dargie HJ, Peacock AJ. LA volume by CMR distinguishes idiopathic from pulmonary hypertension due to HFpEF. *JACC Cardiovasc Imag.* 2013;6:1120–1121.
52. Scalia GM, Scalia IG, Kierle R, et al. ePLAR—the echocardiographic pulmonary to left atrial ratio—a novel non-invasive parameter to differentiate pre-capillary and post-capillary pulmonary hypertension. *Int J Cardiol.* 2016;212:379–386.
53. Takahama H, McCully RB, Frantz RP, Kane GC. Unraveling the RV ejection doppler envelope: insight into pulmonary artery hemodynamics and disease severity. *J Am Coll Cardiol Cardiovasc Imag.* 2017;10:1268–1277.
54. Opotowsky AR, Ojeda J, Rogers F, et al. A simple echocardiographic prediction rule for hemodynamics due to HFpEF. *JACC Cardiovasc Imag.* 2012;5:765–775.
55. Obokata M, Kane GC, Reddy YN, Olson TP, Melenovsky V, Borlaug BA. Role of diastolic stress testing in the evaluation for heart failure with preserved ejection fraction: a simultaneous invasive-echocardiographic study. *Circulation.* 2017;135:825–838.
56. Kane GC, Oh JK. Diastolic stress test for the evaluation of exertional dyspnea. *Curr Cardiol Rep.* 2012;14:359–365.
57. Hardegree EL, Sachdev A, Fenstad ER, et al. Impaired left ventricular mechanics in pulmonary arterial hypertension: identification of a cohort at high risk. *Circ Heart Fail.* 2013;6(4):748–755.
58. Grewal J, McCully RB, Kane GC, Lam C, Pellikka PA. Left ventricular function and exercise capacity. *JAMA.* 2009;301(3):286–294.
59. Guazzi M. Exercise VE/VCO2 slope: an endurance marker of prognosis also in patients with HFpEF and pulmonary hypertension, at least! *J Card Fail.* 2017;23:783–785.
60. Hemnes AR, Pugh ME, Newman AL, et al. End tidal CO(2) tension: pulmonary arterial hypertension vs pulmonary venous hypertension and response to treatment. *Chest.* 2011;140(5):1267–1273.
61. Gorter TM, Obokata M, Reddy YNV, Melenovsky V, Borlaug BA. Exercise unmasks distinct pathophysiologic features in heart failure with preserved ejection fraction and pulmonary vascular disease. *Eur Heart J.* 2018;39:2825–2835.
62. Klaassen SHC, Liu LCY, Hummel YM, et al. Clinical and hemodynamic correlates and prognostic value of VE/VCO2 slope in patients with heart failure with preserved ejection fraction of pulmonary hypertension. *J Card Fail.* 2017;23:777–782.
63. Bonderman D, Wexberg P, Martischnig AM, et al. A noninvasive algorithm to exclude pre-capillary pulmonary hypertension. *Eur Respir J.* 2011;37:1096–1103.
64. D'Alto M, Romeo E, Argiento P, et al. Echocardiographic prediction of pre- versus postcapillary pulmonary hypertension. *J Am Soc Echocardiogr.* 2015;28:108–115.
65. Jacobs W, Konings TC, Heymans MW, et al. Noninvasive identification of left-sided heart failure in a population suspected of pulmonary arterial hypertension. *Eur Respir J.* 2015;46:422–430.
66. Reddy YNV, Carter RE, Obokata M, Redfield MM, Borlaug BA. A simple, evidence-based approach to help guide diagnosis of heart failure preserved ejection fraction. *Circulation.* 2018;138:861–870.
67. Gorter TM, van Veldhuisen DJ, Bauersachs J, et al. Right heart dysfunction and failure in heart failure with preserved ejection fraction: mechanisms and management. Position statement on behalf of the Heart Failure Association of the European Society of Cardiology. *Eur J Heart Fail.* 2018;20:16–37.
68. Sachdev A, Villarraga HR, Frantz RP, et al. Right ventricular strain for prediction of survival in patients with pulmonary arterial hypertension. *Chest.* 2011;139(6):1299–1309.
69. Fine NM, Chen L, Bastiansen PM, et al. Outcome prediction by quantitative right ventricular function assessment in 575 subjects evaluated for pulmonary hypertension. *Circ Cardiovasc Imag.* 2013;6(5):711–721.
70. Borlaug BA, Nishimura RA, Sorajja P, Lam CS, Redfield MM. Exercise hemodynamics enhance diagnosis of early heart failure with preserved ejection fraction. *Circ Heart Fail.* 2010;2:588–595.
71. Obokata M, Nagata Y, Kado Y, et al. Ventricular-arterial coupling and exercise-induced pulmonary hypertension during low-level exercise in heart failure with preserved or reduced ejection fraction. *J Card Fail.* 2017;23:216–220.
72. Andersen MJ, Olson TP, Melenovsky V, Kane GC, Borlaug BA. Differential hemodynamic effects of exercise and volume expansion in people with and without heart failure. *Circ Heart Fail. 2015*;8:41–48.
73. Fujimoto N, Borlaug BA, Lewis GD, et al. Hemodynamic responses to rapid saline loading: the impact of age, sex, and heart failure. *Circulation.* 2013;127:55–62.
74. D'Alto M, Romeo E, Argiento P, et al. Clinical relevance of fluid challenge in patients evaluated for pulmonary hypertension. *Chest.* 2017;151: 119–126.
75. Robbins IM, Hemnes AR, Pugh ME, et al. High prevalence of occult pulmonary venous hypertension revealed by fluid challenge in pulmonary hypertension. *Circ Heart Fail.* 2014;7:116–122.
76. Xiang Y, Shi W, Li Z, et al. Efficacy and safety of spironolactone in the heart failure with mid-range ejection fraction and heart failure with preserved ejection fraction: a meta-analysis of randomized clinical trials. *Medicine (Baltimore).* 2019;98(13):e14967.
77. Guazzi M, Vicenzi M, Arena R, Guazzi MD. Pulmonary hypertension in heart failure with preserved ejection fraction: a target of phosphodiesterase-5 inhibition in a 1-year study. *Circulation.* 2011;124:164–174.
78. Bermejo J, Yotti R, García-Orta R, et al. Sildenafil for improving outcomes in patients with corrected valvular heart disease and persistent pulmonary hypertension: a multicenter, double-blind, randomized clinical trial. *Eur Heart J.* 2018;39:1255–1264.
79. Lüscher TF, Enseleit F, Pacher R, et al. Hemodynamic and neurohumoral effects of selective endothelin a (et(a)) receptor blockade in chronic heart

failure: the heart failure et(a) receptor blockade trial (heat). *Circulation.* 2002;106:2666–2672.
80. Anand I, McMurray J, Cohn JN, et al. Long-term effects of darusentan on left-ventricular remodelling and clinical outcomes in the endothelina receptor antagonist trial in heart failure (earth): randomised, double-blind, placebo-controlled trial. *Lancet.* 2004;364:347–354.
81. Packer M, McMurray JJV, Krum H, et al. Long-term effect of endothelin receptor antagonism with bosentan on the morbidity and mortality of patients with severe chronic heart failure: primary results of the enable trials. *JACC Heart Fail. 2017*;5:317–326.
82. Vachiéry JL, Delcroix M, Al-Hiti H, et al. Macitentan in pulmonary hypertension due to left ventricular dysfunction. *Eur Respir J.* 2018;51:1701886.
83. Zile MR, Bourge RC, Redfield MM, Zhou D, Baicu CF, Little WC. Randomized, double-blind, placebo-controlled study of sitaxsentan to improve impaired exercise tolerance in patients with heart failure and a preserved ejection fraction. *JACC Heart Fail.* 2014;2:123–130.
84. Redfield MM, Anstrom KJ, Levine JA, et al. Isosorbide mononitrate in heart failure with preserved ejection fraction. *N Engl J Med.* 2015;373:2314–2324.
85. Borlaug BA, Lewis GD, McNulty SE, et al. Effects of sildenafil on ventricular and vascular function in heart failure with preserved ejection fraction. *Circ Heart Fail.* 2015;8:533–541.
86. Hoendermis ES, Liu LC, Hummel YM, et al. Effects of sildenafil on invasive haemodynamics and exercise capacity in heart failure patients with preserved ejection fraction and pulmonary hypertension: a randomized controlled trial. *Eur Heart J.* 2015;36:2565–2573.

34

General Treatment of Heart Failure With Preserved Ejection Fraction and Randomized Trials

Michael Chetrit and Hisham Dokainish

OUTLINE

Case Study

A 45-year-old male presents for a 1-month follow-up visit after an index hospitalization for dyspnea and peripheral edema, at which time he was found to be hypertensive. He has no known diabetes or coronary artery disease (CAD). His only medication is amlodipine 5 mg daily. On physical examination, body mass index (BMI) is 38 kg/m^2, blood pressure 160/88 mmHg, and heart rate 90 and regular. Jugular venous pressure is 6 cm above the angle of Louis. Heart sounds reveal normal S_1 and S_2, with an S_4 but no murmur. Chest examination is unremarkable. There is mild lower-extremity pitting edema. Serum creatinine level is 1.9 mg/dL, and the N-terminal pro-brain natriuretic peptide (NT-proBNP) level is 9476 pg/mL. Echocardiography reveals moderate concentric left ventricular hypertrophy (LVH) with LV ejection fraction (EF) of 55% and left atrial (LA) dilation (volume index 40 mL/m^2). Cardiac magnetic resonance imaging (MRI) confirms a concentrically thickened left ventricle and is negative for all suspected cardiomyopathies. He is ultimately diagnosed with heart failure with preserved ejection fraction (HFpEF).

Question: How would you manage this patient?

INTRODUCTION

Heart failure (HF) with preserved left ventricular (LV) ejection may constitute up to 50% of HF cases and is increasing in prevalence.[1] Patients with this syndrome also suffer substantial morbidity and mortality. HFpEF is characterized by a morphologically normal, enlarged, and/or hypertrophied left ventricle with EF of 50% and above, impairment to diastolic filling, increasing LV stiffness resulting in elevated left ventricular filling pressures (LVFP), and signs and symptoms of clinical HF.[2] In general, HFpEF excludes HF associated with significant valve disease. Given the absence of specific evidence-based therapy for HFpEF, treatment is geared toward management of volume overload and comorbidities, including hypertension, CAD, diabetes, obesity, sleep apnea, atrial fibrillation (AFib), and renal dysfunction.[3] The reasons why standard therapies effective in HF with reduced EF (HFrEF)—angiotensin-converting enzyme (ACE) inhibitors, angiotensin receptor blockers (ARBs), beta blockers, and mineralocorticoid inhibitors (MRAs)—have not been shown to reduce major cardiovascular (CV) events in HFpEF patients remain unclear. Ongoing phase III trials of newer drugs such as the angiotensin receptor neprilysin inhibitor (ARNI) sacubitril/valsartan[4] and the sodium glucose cotransporter-2 (SGLT2) inhibitor empagliflozin may identify, at last, effective targeted therapies for HFpEF.

BACKGROUND

HFpEF is a diagnosis that can be challenging to definitively make. It requires the clinician to establish that signs and symptoms of HF indeed exist, along with corroboration using the following criteria: LV EF of 50% and above, morphologic abnormalities consistent with the diagnosis (LV hypertrophy and/or LA enlargement), and documentation of elevated LV filling pressures (by echocardiography or cardiac catheterization and/or elevated natriuretic peptides).[3] Other causes of HF such as pericardial disease, valvular disease, and high-output HF are usually excluded. In addition, mimickers of HFpEF must be excluded, such as lung disease, obesity, sleep apnea, renal failure, precapillary pulmonary hypertension, and hematologic or metabolic abnormalities.[1]

Earlier placebo-controlled randomized controlled trials (RCTs) in HFpEF patients include the Candesartan in Heart Failure: Assessment of Reduction in Mortality and Morbidity (CHARM)–Preserved trial,[5] the Digitalis Investigation Group (DIG) ancillary trial,[6] and the Perindopril in Elderly People with Heart Failure (PEP-CHF) trial.[7] These trials did not demonstrate lower primary end points in the treatment compared to placebo arms; however, some secondary end points (such as HF hospitalization) were decreased in the CHARM trial. The Study of the Effects of Nebivolol Intervention on Outcomes and Rehospitalization in Seniors with Heart Failure (SENIORS) trial[8] did demonstrate a reduction in the primary end point in the treatment arm, but in patients with LVEF greater than 35%, and was a subanalysis of a larger trial. More recent RCTs of medical therapy in HFpEF patients include the Irbesartan in Heart Failure with Preserved Ejection Fraction Study (I-PRESERVE) trial,[9] the Japanese Diastolic Heart Failure Trial (J-DHF),[10] the Aldosterone Antagonist Therapy for Adults with Heart Failure and Preserved Systolic Function (TOPCAT) trial,[11] and the Inorganic Nitrite Delivery to Improve Exercise Capacity in HFpEF (INDIE) trial.[12] However, none of these trials demonstrated a difference in the primary outcome in treatment compared to placebo arms. Potential reasons these trials were negative include (1) patients were enrolled who did not truly have HFpEF, (2) the therapy was not effective, (3) the numerous comorbidities common in HFpEF patients and their associated adverse outcomes diluted any potential therapeutic effect, (4) the pathophysiology of HFpEF is not well understood and thus treatments targeted at specific disease mechanisms remain elusive, and (5) heterogeneity in HFpEF subtypes may respond differently to therapy. Further complicating the landscape is that different trials used different LV EF cutoff values to connote preserved LV EF (e.g., LV EF $\geq$35% in SENIORS, $\geq$40% in CHARM, and $\geq$45% in I-PRESERVE and TOPCAT).

Therefore current guidelines[3] focus on stages: stage A (prevention of HF), generally with a healthy lifestyle, control of hypertension, and prevention of coronary disease, although newer therapies show promise in reducing the incidence of HF in patients at risk[13]; for stage C (symptomatic HF), coronary revascularization, treatment of AF, and treatment of hypertension. Regarding specific therapies there are weak recommendations for MRAs (in HFpEF patients fulfilling specific criteria) or ARBs for the goal of reducing HF hospitalizations. Fortunately, there are several phase III RCTs, likely to report results in 1 to 2 years, which may provide targeted therapies to improve clinical outcomes in patients with HFpEF.

PATHOPHYSIOLOGY

HFpEF also can be referred to as heart failure with normal EF and diastolic HF. The choice of term sheds much light on the pathophysiology of this syndrome. While the main pathology of HFpEF is impairment to diastolic filing and increased ventricular stiffness (lower ventricular compliance), there is also evidence that systolic function is impaired. Studies with speckle tracking echocardiography have shown impaired longitudinal and circumferential myocardial systolic function in HFpEF patients.[14] Thus even though LV EF is preserved ($\geq$50%), many HFpEF patients demonstrate abnormalities in systolic function. Nevertheless, there is general agreement that upward and leftward shift of the LV pressure-volume curve is one of the main pathophysiologic abnormalities in HFpEF patients. This results in higher LV pressure for a given volume and leads to elevated LA pressures and pulmonary congestion and/or effort intolerance.[1] To date, RCTs have focused therapy on treating volume overload and ventricular stiffness but have not yet yielded strong results.

It has recently been suggested that phenotyping in HFpEF patients is necessary as heterogeneity in HFpEF is common, and this may be one of the reasons that helps explain lack of response to prior RCTs. A study utilizing machine learning has identified three phenotypes: (1) younger patients with moderate diastolic dysfunction with relatively normal natriuretic peptide levels, (2) obese, diabetic patients with a high prevalence of obstructive sleep apnea with the poorest LV relaxation, and (3) older patients with chronic kidney disease, electrical and myocardial remodeling, pulmonary hypertension, and right ventricular dysfunction.[15] Outcomes (including hospitalization and death) have been shown to vary by phenogroup, with an increase in risk from group 1 to group 3, suggesting different therapy may work for different phenotypes.[16]

In addition, an emerging pathophysiologic model that has been proposed for HFpEF suggests that a proinflammatory condition exists, leading to systemic microvascular endothelial inflammation, increases in oxidative stress, decreases in nitric oxide–cyclic guanosine monophosphate, microvascular dysfunction, and rarefaction.[1] These processes result in increased myocyte stiffness, cardiomyocyte hypertrophy, and fibrosis, leading to global cardiac remodeling and dysfunction, impaired coronary flow reserve, impaired oxygen delivery, uptake, and utilization in skeletal muscle signaling.[1]

For future HFpEF therapies to show promise it is possible that they may need to be targeted to a specific HFpEF phenotype and/or target the proinflammatory process (and its downstream effects) in HFpEF patients.

GENERAL TREATMENT GUIDELINES

Currently, the principles underlining the management of patients presenting with HFpEF involve identification and treatment of the underlying etiology, treatment of comorbid conditions that may play a role in both the development and the exacerbation of HF symptoms, and a focus on symptom management.[17] Patient education is also paramount, with instruction on the importance of self-care, weight management, aerobic exercise programs, sodium restriction and fluid status, and regular clinical follow-up being emphasized.[1,18]

Optimization of fluid status is an initial focus of therapy (Class of Recommendation [COR] Ia, Level of Evidence [LOE] C) in current guidelines[3]. Aside from decreasing pulmonary venous congestion and LV filling pressures, diuretic therapy prevents plasma volume expansion, which has been implicated in the pathophysiology of patients with HFpEF.[19] In a cohort of patients with HFpEF it was shown that capillary wedge pressure increases with plasma volume expansion.[20] This phenomenon is thought to be secondary to pericardial restraint from right heart dilation and/or increased total heart volumes. Loop diuretic therapy remains the most effective therapy to optimize fluid status and avoid plasma volume expansion. Diuretic therapy should be tailored to the patient's body weight, symptoms, and electrolyte status.[1,18] The CardioMEMS Heart Sensor Allows Monitoring of Pressure to Improve Outcomes in NYHA Class III Heart Failure Patients (CHAMPION) trial was designed to investigate the utility of noninvasive LV filling pressure monitors in a group of HF patients, 20% of whom had preserved EF. Optimal filling pressures were achieved primarily with increasing doses of both loop and thiazide diuretics and resulted in a reduction in HF hospitalizations.[21] The addition of thiazide and thiazide-like diuretics, administered before the dose of loop diuretics, can be a helpful addition in patients with excessive volume overload or diuretic resistance. Careful monitoring should be applied when considering adjunctive diuretics as volume depletion, loss of urinary electrolytes, and renal dysfunction can occur.[1] Although evidence is limited, restricting dietary sodium to less than 2 g per day is currently recommended by most guidelines.[3] Further, sodium restriction may play a more significant role in patients with recurrent episodes of refractory episodes of volume overload. In the Empagliflozin Cardiovascular Outcome Event Trial in Type 2 Diabetes Mellitus Patients (EMPA-REG) trial of 7020 diabetic patients without clinical HF, randomization to empagliflozin (an SGLT2 inhibitor) was associated with a relative risk reduction of 35% in HF hospitalization, which may at least in part be due to the osmotic diuresis.[22] Diuretic therapy to optimize volume status and maintain euvolemia plays a central role in symptom management and is a reasonable first step in improving the functional status in patients with HFpEF.

TREATMENT OF COMORBIDITIES

Comorbid conditions are highly prevalent in HFpEF patients. Comorbidities, including CAD, hypertension, diabetes, renal dysfunction, and others, contribute to the underlying physiopathology of HFpEF; in addition, the absolute number of comorbidities has been associated with an increased risk of all-cause hospitalization.[23] Thus treatment of these comorbidities plays a key role in the management of HFpEF patients. These comorbidities are reviewed in detail in other chapters but are briefly covered here.

Hypertension

Control of hypertension is a major focus in treatment of HFpEF patients. Given hypertension is associated with an increase in LV diastolic pressures and delays early diastolic filling that contributes to an increase in LA pressure, poorly controlled blood pressure exacerbates HFpEF symptoms. The traditional model for HFpEF development involves chronic systolic hypertension, which leads to LVH, impaired LV compliance, and a stiff ventricle.[24,25] Antihypertensive therapy has been associated with LVH regression with an improvement in diastolic performance and LV distensibility.[25] A meta-analysis of 80 clinical trials, including 3767 patients, showed that antihypertensive drug classes had differing effects on LV mass reduction. ARBs produced a 13% reduction of LV mass index; calcium channel blockers (CCBs), 11%; ACE inhibitors, 10%; diuretics, 8%; and beta blockers, 6%.[26] In the Losartan Intervention For Endpoint Reduction in Hypertension (LIFE) study, regression of LVH was associated with 37% reduction in cardiovascular death, stroke, or myocardial infarction (MI) and a 28% reduction in all-cause mortality.[27] The Systolic Blood Pressure Intervention (SPRINT) trial, which randomized 9361 patients with cardiovascular disease to aggressive hypertensive treatment or standard therapy (target systolic blood pressure <120 mmHg vs. <140 mmHg, respectively), demonstrated improved overall survival and a reduction in HF hospitalizations with aggressive blood pressure (BP) control.[28] Similar findings were seen in the Treatment of Hypertension in Patients 80 Years of Age or Older (HYVET) trial.[29] Consequently, control of hypertension is recommended in current guidelines (COR 1a, LOE B),[3] and strategies should be in agreement with the Eighth Joint National Committee guidelines for the management of BP.[30]

Coronary Artery Disease

CAD is common in HFpEF patients, with a reported prevalence ranging from 35% to 53%.[31–33] Moreover, the presence of CAD among patients with HFpEF has been associated with worse outcomes.[34,35] Observational data in patients with HFpEF have suggested less deterioration in LV EF and lower mortality in HFpEF patients who underwent complete coronary revascularization.[31] Therefore current guidelines recommend revascularization of clinically significant CAD in HFpEF patients (COR IIa, LOE C).[3] Primary prevention of CAD in HFpEF patients, however, remains controversial. While the benefit of statin therapy for primary prevention has been demonstrated, the use of a statin for the prevention of HF (independent of CAD) has not. The effect of rosuvastatin in patients with chronic HF (GISSI-HF) trial was a double-blinded, placebo-controlled trial involving 4574 HF patients (450 had an EF >40%). When compared to a placebo arm, in the patients randomized to rosuvastatin, there was no significant difference in mortality (adjusted hazard ratio [HR] 1.00 [95.5% confidence interval (CI) 0.898–1.122], $p = 0.943$) or hospitalizations (adjusted HR 1.01 [99% CI 0.908–1.112], $p = 0.903$).[36] Observational studies looking specifically at HFpEF cohorts have suggested a possible benefit of statin therapy, but randomized trials are needed to confirm these preliminary findings.[37,38] Thus there is currently no role for statins for primary prevention of CAD in HFpEF patients nor is there a role for widespread routine catheterization to detect subclinical CAD.[3]

Diabetes Mellitus

Diabetes mellitus is an established HF risk factor, independent of CAD,[31] with an average prevalence of 45% among HFpEF patients.[39] It is also associated with a nearly twofold increase in morbidity and mortality in HFpEF patients.[33] In both the DIG trial[40] and the I-PRESERVE trial,[41] which enrolled patients with an EF greater than 45%, diabetes was associated with increased risk of hospitalization and death. Patients with HFpEF and diabetes were typically younger, with a higher BMI, and a history of hypertension and CAD.[39] Diabetes and impaired glucose metabolism have been suggested to contribute to arterial stiffness and LVH. More specifically, diabetes promotes myocardial fibrosis with subsequent diastolic dysfunction along with worsened renal and endothelial function, which can lead to HFpEF; this syndrome is known as diabetic cardiomyopathy.[42,43] Other suggested pathophysiologic mechanisms include sodium retention and volume overload through activation of the renin-angiotensin-aldosterone system (RAAS) and activation of systemic inflammation. More recently, SGLT2 inhibitors have been associated with a relative risk reduction of 38% for all-cause mortality and 35% for HF hospitalization in diabetic patients.[14] This class of drug is currently undergoing trials in the HFpEF population and may be a useful therapy should studies be positive.[39]

Obesity

Obesity is a worldwide epidemic and a modifiable risk factor for the development of HFpEF.[44] Obesity has been associated with LVH, diastolic dysfunction, volume expansion, systemic inflammation, and other deleterious effects of obesity on the cardiovascular system.[45] In the I-PRESERVE trial, 34% had BMI of 35 kg/m^2 and above. In this subgroup of obese patients, 40% underwent coronary angiography and had documented increased LV filling pressures without any objective occlusive CAD,[46] suggesting obesity may, in addition to other comorbidities, contribute to both diastolic dysfunction and its symptoms. In 100 obese patients with HFpEF randomized to either exercise, exercise and diet, or both, caloric restriction resulted in improvements in exercise capacity and reduction in fat mass.[47] In smaller studies, exercise improved exercise capacity and quality of life, and reduced symptoms.[47,48] While exercise is currently recommended in current HFpEF guidelines (COR 1, LOE A), there is currently no clear recommendation for weight loss in this patient population.

Sleep Apnea

HFpEF is also associated with obstructive sleep apnea (OSA), a condition known to result in increased LV afterload, diastolic dysfunction, and dyspnea.[49] Repetitive arousals and hypoxia throughout the duration of sleep result in increased sympathetic activity, endothelial dysfunction, and major swings in intrathoracic pressures, causing increased afterload and systolic and diastolic LV dysfunction.[50] Common risk factors for the development of OSA include excessive weight, hypertension, smoking, diabetes, retrognathia, macroglossia, and a large neck circumference.[51] Studies have evaluated diastolic function in obese patients with severe OSA, all finding abnormal diastolic function and increased LA volume index in these patients compared to obese patients without OSA.[49] In a study of 45 patients with EF of 45% or less and OSA, there was an improvement in LV EF and a reduction in systolic BP.[52] In an RCT of continuous positive airway pressure (CPAP) therapy in 45 OSA patients with HFrEF there was increase in LV EF by 2.2% in patients treated with CPAP.[53] While the effects of CPAP have not been investigated in patients with HFpEF, they have been evaluated in patients with diastolic dysfunction. In a randomized placebo-controlled study, echocardiographic parameters of diastolic function improved after 12 weeks of CPAP therapy.[54] Further, in a study of 15 patients with severe OSA having received 6 months of nasal CPAP, there was regression of LV hypertrophy.[55] The role of CPAP was also investigated in patients with central sleep apnea. The Adaptive Servo-ventilation for Central Sleep Apnea in Systolic Heart Failure trial randomly assigned 1325 patients with central sleep apnea and an EF less than 45% to adapted servo-ventilation or usual care. This trial reported an increase in all-cause and cardiovascular mortality in the intervention arm. CPAP, as opposed to adapted servo-ventilation, was tested in a group of 258 patients with systolic HF and central sleep apnea in the largest trial to date of its kind. The use of CPAP not only improved overnight oxygenation but improved LV EF, peripheral adrenal stimulation, and the distance traveled in 6 minutes. It is, however, noteworthy that the quality of life, hospitalizations, and atrial natriuretic peptides did not differ with the control group.[56] While this study may suggest that CPAP is not effective in reducing major clinical end points in HFrEF patients, it has not been specifically evaluated in the HFpEF population and may be a focus of future research. Currently, the American College of Cardiology (ACC) recommends evaluation of OSA if there is a clinical suspicion and encourages its treatment (COR IIa, LOE B).[57] However, the use of adaptive servo-ventilation in patients with central sleep apnea is strongly discouraged and felt to cause harm (COR III, LOE B-R).

Renal Disease

Another comorbidity commonly associated with HFpEF is renal disease,[58] with a reported prevalence of 30% to 60% in HFpEF patients[59] In a meta-analysis of more than 1 million patients across 57 studies, there was a stronger association between renal failure and mortality in patients with HFpEF than with HFrEF.[60] In the I-PRESERVE trial, worsening renal function on presentation to hospital for the first episode of decompensated HFpEF was associated with an overall poor prognosis.[61] Renal disease appears to be independently associated with cardiac remodeling and impaired mechanics and can lead to perpetual activation of the RAAS with endothelial dysfunction.[62] The inability of the kidneys to maintain sodium and fluid balance also plays a major role in the development of symptomatic HF.[63,64] This bidirectional relationship between the heart and the kidneys is a putative pathophysiologic pathway in the cardiorenal syndrome (CRS). Although not currently recommended by the ACC, some advocate for early treatment of renal dysfunction and suggest favoring therapies that have shown benefit in the renal disease populations such as ACE inhibitors and ARBs when treating other comorbidities such as hypertension.[1,31] Clinicians often hold medications such as ACE inhibitors and ARBs in HFpEF patients who have acute or chronic renal dysfunction, and some advocate to slowly reintroduce diuretics first and to reintroduce ACE inhibitors and ARBs when clinical status and kidney function stabilize.[65] The Ultrafiltration in Decompensated Heart Failure with Cardiorenal Syndrome (CARRESS HF) trial, which randomized 188 patients hospitalized with acute heart failure (median EF 33%) and evidence of cardiorenal syndrome to either ultrafiltration or pharmacologic therapy, appeared to confirm that a stepwise introduction of medications was the strategy of choice to minimize adverse outcomes and worsening renal function when compared to ultrafiltration.[66]

Atrial Fibrillation

AFib is highly prevalent in elderly hypertensive patients and patients hospitalized for acutely decompensated HF.[67,68] Increased filling pressures result in LA structural remodeling that provides the necessary substrate for AFib.[31] A history of AFib was present in up to a third of patients in both the I-PRESERVE trial and the CHARM-Preserved trials.[69] In 41,446 patients from the Swedish Heart Failure registry, there was an AFib prevalence of 65% in patients with HFpEF, 60% in HF with midrange EF (HFmEF), and 53% in patients with HFrEF, despite similar age, sex, prior MI, and history of stroke among the three groups.[70] AFib is recognized as a poor prognostic indicator in HFpEF and is associated with increased hospitalizations independent of stroke risk and mortality.[70–72] Yet there is no specific therapy for AFib that has shown to be of clinical benefit in HFpEF patients.[73] Risk factor management, including BP control, treatment of ischemia, and management of diabetes and OSA, play a primary role.[74] AFib should be managed in accordance with the most recent iteration of the Heart Rhythm Society (HRS) guidelines.[75] An initial rate control strategy can optimize ventricular heart rate and decrease the paroxysms of rapid heart rate that are commonly associated with episodes of decompensated HF. In the Catheter Ablation for Atrial Fibrillation and Heart Failure (CASTLE AF) trial, 363 patients with AFib and HFrEF (EF ≤35%) were randomized to receive either medical therapy or catheter ablation for the management of AFib.[76] Ablation resulted in a 16.1% reduction in death and HF hospitalization as compared to the medical (rate or rhythm control) therapy arm. While there is a paucity of trials that investigated HFpEF and catheter-based procedures, some smaller studies were able to show improved diastolic function.[73,76,77] Thus catheter-based restoration of sinus rhythm in HFpEF patients with AFib may be a future therapy with promise.

Frailty

Frailty, a clinical syndrome characterized by unintentional weight loss, exhaustion, muscle weakness, abnormal gait speed, and overall low physical activity, is associated with functional decline, increased hospitalizations, and increased mortality.[78,79] After adjustment for cofounders, frailty has been shown to be more prevalent in HFpEF than HFrEF patients.[80] In a survey of 448 patients from three counties in Minnesota, frailty was an independent predictor of emergency department visits and hospitalizations in HFpEF and HFrEF patients.[80] In the TOPCAT registry, higher frailty index was associated with higher risk of adverse cardiovascular outcomes, including CV death and HF hospitalizations (HR 3.51, CI 2.6–4.61; $p = < 0.001$).[79] Treatment of frailty is multifactorial and commonly involves a comprehensive geriatric assessment and management plan. In a recent meta-analyses of 27 publications, supplemental vitamin D, nutrition, exercise training, and physiotherapy were the most useful interventions to treat frailty.[81] The European Society of Cardiology HF guidelines recommend that frailty be monitored and any reversible causes be addressed.[2] The ACC HF guidelines do not currently address treatment of frailty.[57]

SPECIFIC THERAPIES

Phase III RCTs in HFpEF patients are shown in Table 34.1.

Diuretics

Diuretics reduce intravascular volume and ventricular preload, lowering filling pressures in HFpEF patients. By lowering BP, diuretics can also reduce afterload, thus ameliorating ventricular output. Despite their being commonly used in HFpEF patients and recommended in current guidelines, there is paucity of RCT data demonstrating clinical efficacy in HFpEF patients. In the Hong Kong Diastolic Heart Failure study, 150 patients with HFpEF (LV EF >45%) were randomized to (a) diuretics alone, (b) diuretics plus irbesartan, or (c) diuretics plus ramipril.[82] The study demonstrated that diuretic therapy significantly improved symptoms and neither irbesartan nor ramipril had a significant additional effect. However, diuretics in combination with irbesartan or ramipril marginally improved LV systolic and longitudinal

TABLE 34.1 Phase III, Placebo-Controlled Trials of Medical Therapy in Patients With Heart Failure With Preserved or Mildly Reduced Left Ventricular Ejection Fraction

Trial Name/Year	Drug	Population	Mean Follow-Up	Primary End Point	Results
DIG trial[6] (2006)	Digoxin	988 patients with HF and LV EF > 45%	37 months	HF hospitalization or HF mortality	Primary end point in 102 patients (21%) in the digoxin group and 119 patients (24%) in the placebo group (HR 0.82; 95% CI 0.63–1.07; $p = 0.136$)
SENIORS[8] (2005)	Nebivolol	752 patients aged ≥70 years with a history of HF and EF > 35%	21 months	All-cause mortality or cardiovascular hospital admission	Primary outcome in 100 patients (17.6%) in nebivolol arm compared to 125 patients (21.9%) in the placebo arm (RRR 10%; $p < 0.05$)
PEP-CHF[7] (2006)	Perindopril	850 HF patients >70 years old, LV EF > 45%	26 months	Composite of all-cause mortality and unplanned HF hospitalization with a minimum follow-up of 1 year	Primary outcome in 107 patients (25.1%) assigned to placebo and 100 patients (23.6%) to perindopril (HR 0.92, 95% CI 0.70–1.21; $p = 0.545$) with annual incidence rates of 13.2% and 12.2%, respectively
CHARM-Preserved[5] (2003)	Candesartan	3023 HF patients NYHA Class II–IV, EF ≥ 40%	36.6 months	CV death or unplanned admission to hospital for HF	Primary outcome in 333 patients (22%) in the candesartan group and 366 patients (24%) in the placebo group (RRR 11%; $p = 0.118$), covariate adjusted HR 0.86 (CI 0.74–1.00; $p = 0.051$). HF hospitalization rates were 12.5% and 8.9% in the placebo and candesartan groups, respectively ($p = 0.018$). HR for recurrent HF hospitalization in treatment vs. placebo arms was 0.75 (95% CI 0.62–0.91; $p = 0.003$)
I-PRESERVE[9] (2008)	Irbesartan	4128 HF patients ≥60 years old, NYHA Class II–IV EF ≥ 45%	49.5 months	Composite of death from CV causes or CV hospitalization	Primary outcome occurred in 742 patients (36%) in the irbesartan group and 763 patients (37%) in the placebo group ($p = 0.35$). Rates of hospitalization for CV causes that contributed to the primary outcome were similar at 70.6 and 74.3 per 1000 patient-years, respectively (HR 0.95, 95% CI 0.85–1.08; $p = 0.44$)
TOPCAT[11] (2014)	Spironolactone	3445 HF patients, LV EF ≥ 45%	40 months	Composite of death from CV causes, aborted cardiac arrest, or hospitalization for HF	Primary outcome occurred in 320 of 1722 patients in the spironolactone group (18.6%) and 351 of 1723 patients in the placebo group (20.4%) (RRR 9%; $p = 0.14$). Greater reductions in primary end point for spironolactone at lower LV EF (<50%: HR 0.72, CI 0.5–1.0) and (<55%: HR 0.85, CI 0.61–1.18)

HF: heart failure; LV: left ventricle; EF: ejection fraction; CV: cardiovascular diastolic LV function, and lowered NT-proBNP over 1 year. A recently published phase II trial prospectively randomized 90 HFpEF patients hospitalized with acute HF within 24 hours of admission to one of four treatments: (1) intravenous bolus furosemide every 12 hours, (2) continuous infusion furosemide, (3) intermittent bolus furosemide with low-dose dopamine, and (4) continuous infusion furosemide with low-dose dopamine. The primary end point was change in creatinine from baseline to 72 hours. This trial showed that low-dose dopamine had no significant impact on renal function, and a continuous infusion diuretic strategy, compared to a bolus diuretic strategy, was associated with increased renal impairment.[83] The only other RCT in diuretic therapy was the Antihypertensive and Lipid-Lowering Treatment to Prevent Heart Attack Trial (ALL-HAT) trial, which evaluated treatment of hypertensive patients (stage A) and determined whether they developed clinical HF. In the ALL-HAT study, 42,418 high-risk hypertensive patients were randomized to chlorthalidone, amlodipine, lisinopril, or doxazosin to compare these treatments on the incidence of hospitalized HFpEF or HFrEF.[84] The trial showed that chlorthalidone significantly reduced the occurrence of new-onset hospitalized HF compared with amlodipine and doxazosin. Chlorthalidone also reduced the incidence of new-onset HFpEF compared with lisinopril. Because of these data, current guidelines recommend diuretics to decrease symptoms of volume congestion (COR 1, LOE C).

Digitalis

The main mechanism of action of digitalis is on the sodium-potassium adenosine triphosphatase of the myocyte, resulting in increased contractility and slowed conduction in the sinoatrial and atrioventricular nodes via a vagal mechanism.[85] The DIG trial randomized 988 patients with HF and LV EF greater than 45% to digoxin or placebo. At an average follow-up of 37 months there was no difference in morbidity or mortality end points between the two groups.[7] However, use of digoxin was associated with a trend toward a reduction in HF hospitalizations (HR = 0.79; 95% CI 0.59–1.04; $p = 0.094$). Thus in current guidelines digoxin is not recommended for use in HFpEF patients.

Beta Blockers

As in HFrEF patients in whom they are effective, there are several potential mechanisms by which beta blockers may improve clinical status in HFpEF patients: by treating concomitant CAD, reducing BP, lowering adrenergic tone, lowering heart rate to increase diastolic filling period, and augmenting LV relaxation. The SENIORS trial randomized 2128 HF patients age 70 years and older to nebivolol or placebo, with a prespecified analysis in patients with LV EF greater than 35%.[9] In the overall trial, the primary outcome of all-cause mortality or CV hospital admission was lower (HR = 0.86, 95% CI 0.74–0.99; $p = 0.039$) in the nebivolol compared placebo arms (absolute risk reduction [ARR] = 4.2%). In the 752 patients (36%) with LV EF greater than 35%, the reduction in the primary end point in the nebivolol compared to placebo groups was maintained (primary outcome in 100 patients [17.6%] in nebivolol arm compared to 125 patients [21.9%] in the placebo arm [relative risk reduction (RRR) = 10%, $p < 0.05$]). The J-DHF randomized 245 patients with HF and LV EF greater than 40% to carvedilol or placebo.[86] At a median 3.2-year follow-up, the primary end point (CV death and HF hospitalization) did not differ between the groups, occurring in 29 patients (24%) in the carvedilol group and in 34 patients (27%) in the control group (adjusted HR = 0.90, 95% CI 0.55–1.49; $p = 0.68$). A recent meta-analysis showed that all-cause mortality was reduced with beta blocker therapy compared with placebo (RR: 0.78, 95% CI 0.65–0.94, $p = 0.008$).[87] However, HFpEF was defined as LV EF greater than 40%, thus potential benefits in the HFmEF population may have influenced the findings. In addition, the only positive trial of the three in the meta-analysis was a small study randomizing 150 patients to propranolol or not to receive propranolol (i.e., not placebo), all of whom were post-MI and had clinical congestive HF with LV EF greater than 40%.[88] Thus current guidelines only recommend beta blockers to control BP in HFpEF patients (COR IIa, LOE C).

ACE Inhibitors

ACE inhibitor therapy has been the cornerstone of treatment of HFrEF patients for decades. In HFpEF patients, inhibition of the RAAS may also be expected to inhibit hypertrophy, vasoconstriction, and fibrosis. In the PEP-CHF study, 850 patients age 70 years and older with HF and LV EF of 45% and above were randomized to perindopril or placebo.[8] The trial showed no difference in mortality between the two groups, although HF hospitalization was marginally reduced in the perindopril arm at 1 year. A small RCT randomized 74 elderly patients (mean age 78 years) in the New York Heart Association (NYHA) Class II/III and normal or only mildly impaired LV systolic function (EF $\geq$40%) to quinapril or matched placebo for 6 months.[89] It found no significant differences in HF hospitalization rates or in several other surrogate outcomes. One arm of the Hong Kong Diastolic HF trial also included ramipril therapy (see Diuretics, earlier in chapter) but also found no difference in clinical outcomes. Based on these data, current guidelines only recommend ACE inhibitor therapy in HFpEF patients to control BP (COR IIa, LOE C).

Angiotensin Receptor Blockers

Like ACE inhibitors, ARBs also have been a cornerstone of treatment for HFrEF to reduce clinical end points. They also interrupt the RAAS and may be anticipated to reduce deleterious effects in HFpEF patients. In the CHARM-Preserved trial, which randomized 3023 HF patients with HF and LV EF of 40% and above to candesartan or placebo, there was no overall difference in the primary outcome of all-cause death between the two groups; however, HF hospitalizations were significantly lower in the candesartan compared to the placebo group.[6] More patients in the candesartan group developed hypotension, hyperkalemia, or renal insufficiency. A secondary analysis from CHARM showed that all-cause mortality and CV death declined with increasing EF until an LV EF of 45%, above which the risk of these outcomes remained relatively stable with increasing LV EF.[90] The I-PRESERVE trial randomized 4128 patients (predominantly elderly with hypertension) with HF with LV EF of 45% and above to irbesartan or placebo and found similar morbidity and mortality in the two groups at a 49.5-month follow-up.[10] As mentioned, the Hong Kong diastolic HF trial included an irbesartan (+ diuretic) arm, which showed no difference in clinical end points. Therefore current guidelines state that ARBs may be used to reduce HF hospitalizations in HFpEF patients (COR IIb, LOE B).

Mineralocorticoid Receptor Antagonists

MRAs act on the RAAS by blocking the aldosterone receptor, thereby counteracting the deleterious CV effects of circulating endogenous aldosterone.[91] By minimizing the sodium and fluid retention, vasoconstriction, and fibrotic effects of endogenous aldosterone, MRAs have been shown to be beneficial in patients with HFrEF. The TOPCAT study evaluated spironolactone versus placebo in patients with HFpEF ($\geq$45%) and did not show a significant difference in the composite primary end point in patients randomized to spironolactone or placebo, although HF hospitalizations were significantly reduced in the spironolactone arm.[12] There was also a suggestion of fewer events in patients with an EF less than 55%.[5] Post hoc analysis showed a reduction in the primary end point in patients recruited in the Americas (HR = 0.83) but not in Russia/Georgia (HR = 1.10); the latter, despite having been in the active treatment arm, had nondetectable levels of the metabolite spironolactone.[86] Based on these post hoc analyses, current guidelines suggest spironolactone may be used in HFpEF patients who satisfy the following criteria: symptomatic HFpEF (with ≥45%), elevated B-type natriuretic peptide level or HF admission within 1 year, estimated glomerular filtration rate greater than 30 mL/min, creatinine less than 2.5 mg/dL, and potassium less than 5.0 mEq/L (COR II, LOE IIB-R).

Long-Acting Nitrates

By decreasing preload, nitrates could potentially ameliorate symptoms and signs of HF in HFpEF patients. The INDIE-HFpEF trial randomized 105 patients in a crossover RCT design who inhaled inorganic nitrite, or placebo, for 4 weeks and evaluated peak oxygen consumption on exercise testing.[13] They found that nitrate therapy, compared with placebo, did not result in significant improvement in exercise capacity. In another RCT, 110 HFpEF patients were randomized to a 6-week dose-escalation regimen of isosorbide mononitrate (from 30 mg to 60 mg to 120 mg once daily) or placebo, with subsequent crossover to the other group for 6 weeks. They found patients who received isosorbide mononitrate were less active and did not have better quality of life or submaximal exercise capacity than did patients who received placebo.[92] Therefore, currently, long-acting nitrate therapy is not recommended for HFpEF patients to reduce clinical end points.

Phosphodiesterase Inhibitors

By resulting in vasodilation and lowering pulmonary artery pressure, phosphodiesterase inhibitors were thought to have a potential role in the treatment of HFpEF patients. In a prospective trial, 216 patients with HFpEF were randomized to silendifil or placebo. There was no difference in peak oxygen capacity, clinical status, or other surrogate end points at 24 weeks.[93] Therefore current guidelines do not recommend phosphodiesterase inhibitors in HFpEF patients.

KEY ONGOING PHASE III RCTS

Angiotensin Neprilysin Receptor Inhibitors

Endogenous natriuretic peptides, released from myocytes in response to pressure or volume overload, have beneficial effects, leading to natriuresis, diuresis, and vasodilation. The PARADIGM trial demonstrated that HFrEF patients randomized to sacubitril/valsartan (a commercially available ARNI) had reductions in CV mortality and HF hospitalization compared to patients treated with enalapril.[94] The PARAGON-HF trial prospectively randomized chronic HFpEF patients to sacubitril/valsartan who satisfy the following criteria: LV EF of 45% and above, NYHA Class II–IV, elevated natriuretic peptides, and evidence of structural heart disease.[4] The primary outcome was the composite of CV death and total (first and recurrent) HF hospitalizations. In this study, sacubitril–valsartan did not result in a significantly lower rate of total hospitalizations for heart failure and death from cardiovascular causes among patients with heart failure and an ejection fraction of 45% or higher.[95]

SGLT2 Inhibitors

An SGLT2 inhibitor, empagliflozin, by blocking absorption of glucose and sodium in the kidney, has been demonstrated in a large placebo-controlled RCT in diabetic patients to reduce the incidence of clinical HF. There is an ongoing large RCT of 4126 HFpEF patients who will randomize to empagliflozin or placebo, with the primary outcome being a combination of either CV mortality or HF hospitalization.[14] Follow-up will be 38 months, and the trial is expected to report sometime in 2020.

CASE STUDY CONCLUSION

While no specific underlying myopathy was diagnosed, this gentleman has poorly controlled BP, an elevated BMI, and a suboptimal volume status. Hydrochlorothiazide, bisoprolol, and spironolactone were prescribed. He was counseled on diet (including sodium restriction), exercise, and weight loss. At 3-month follow-up, his BP was better controlled (134/82 mmHg), jugular venous distention and peripheral edema had subsided, symptoms of dyspnea improved, and he did not suffer further HF hospitalizations or cardiac events.

FUTURE DIRECTIONS

HFpEF is an increasing patient population that suffers substantial morbidity and mortality; however, to date, RCTs have failed to demonstrate a specific therapy that reduces major CV events in this population. Thus current guidelines recommend treatment of volume status, hypertension, and comorbidities, with consideration of MRA or ARBs in specific patient subsets. Ongoing, large phase III trials with SGLT2 inhibitor may identify, at last, an effective, targeted therapy for this patient population.

KEY POINTS

- There are currently no RCTs demonstrating that any medical therapy significantly reduces major cardiac events in patients with HFpEF.
- General treatment guidelines recommend treatment of hypertension and diuresis with guideline-directed treatment of common comorbidities (e.g., CAD, diabetes, AFib, and sleep apnea).

REVIEW QUESTIONS

1. Atrial fibrillation is equally prevalent among HFrEF, HFmEF, and HFrEF patients.
   a. True
   b. False
2. The CHARM-Preserved trial showed that angiotensin receptor blockers, compared to placebo, decreased HF hospitalizations in patients with HF and EF greater than 40%.
   a. True
   b. False
3. In the TOPCAT study, spironolactone, compared to placebo, did not result in the reduction of any clinical outcome in HFpEF patients.
   a. True
   b. False

REFERENCES

1. Redfield M. Heart failure with preserved ejection fraction. *N Engl J Med.* 2016;375(19):1868–1877.
2. Ponikowski P, Voors AA, Anker SD, et al. 2016 ESC guidelines for the diagnosis and treatment of acute and chronic heart failure: the task force for the diagnosis and treatment of acute and chronic heart failure of the European Society of Cardiology (ESC). *Eur Heart J.* 2016;37(27):2129–2200.
3. Yancy CW, Jessup M, Bozkurt B, et al. 2017 ACC/AHA/HFSA focused update of the 2013 ACCF/AHA guideline for the management of heart failure: a report of the American College of Cardiology/American Heart Association task force on clinical practice guidelines and the Heart Failure Society of America. *Circulation.* 2017;136(6):e137–161.
4. Solomon SD, Rizkala AR, Gong J, et al. Angiotensin receptor neprilysin inhibition in heart failure with preserved ejection fraction: rationale and design of the PARAGON-HF trial. *JACC Heart Fail.* 2017;5(7):471–482.
5. Yusuf S, Pfeffer MA, Swedberg K, et al. Effects of candesartan in patients with chronic heart failure and preserved left-ventricular ejection fraction: the CHARM-Preserved trial. *Lancet (London, England).* 2003;362(9386): 777–781.
6. Ahmed A, Rich MW, Fleg JL, et al. Effects of digoxin on morbidity and mortality in diastolic heart failure: the ancillary digitalis investigation group trial. *Circulation.* 2006;114(5):397–403.
7. Cleland JGF, Tendera M, Adamus J, Freemantle N, Polonski L, Taylor J. The perindopril in elderly people with chronic heart failure (PEP-CHF) study. *Eur Heart J.* 2006;27(19):2338–2345.
8. Flather MD, Shibata MC, Coats AJS, et al. Randomized trial to determine the effect of nebivolol on mortality and cardiovascular hospital admission in elderly patients with heart failure (SENIORS). *Eur Heart J.* 2005;26(3):215–225.
9. Massie BM, Carson PE, McMurray JJ, et al. Irbesartan in patients with heart failure and preserved ejection fraction. *N Engl J Med.* 2008;359(23):2456–2467. https://doi.org/10.1056/NEJMoa0805450.
10. Yamamoto K, Origasa H, Hori M. Effects of carvedilol on heart failure with preserved ejection fraction: the Japanese Diastolic Heart Failure study (J-DHF). *Eur J Heart Fail.* 2013;15(1):110–118.
11. Pitt B, Pfeffer MA, Assmann SF, et al. Spironolactone for heart failure with preserved ejection fraction. *N Engl J Med.* 2014;370(15):1383–1392. https://doi.org/10.1056/NEJMoa1313731.
12. Borlaug BA, Anstrom KJ, Lewis GD, et al. Effect of inorganic nitrite vs placebo on exercise capacity among patients with heart failure with preserved ejection fraction: the INDIE-HFpEF randomized clinical trial. *JAMA.* 2018;320(17):1764–1773.
13. Zinman B, Wanner C, Lachin JM, et al. Empagliflozin, cardiovascular outcomes, and mortality in type 2 diabetes. *N Engl J Med.* 2015;373(22):2117–2128. https://doi.org/10.1056/NEJMoa1504720.
14. Kraigher-Krainer E, Shah AM, Gupta DK, et al. Impaired systolic function by strain imaging in heart failure with preserved ejection fraction. *J Am Coll Cardiol.* 2014;63(5):447–456.
15. Shah SJ, Katz DH, Selvaraj S, et al. Phenomapping for novel classification of heart failure with preserved ejection fraction. *Circulation.* 2015;131(3):269–279.
16. Lewis GA, Schelbert EB, Williams SG, et al. Biological phenotypes of heart failure with preserved ejection fraction. *J Am Coll Cardiol.* 2017;70(17):2186–2200.
17. Ezekowitz JA, O'Meara E, McDonald MA, et al. 2017 comprehensive update of the Canadian Cardiovascular Society guidelines for the management of heart failure. *Can J Cardiol.* 2017;33(11):1342–1433. https://doi.org/10.1016/j.cjca.2017.08.022.
18. Juillière Y, Venner C, Filippetti L, Popovic B, Huttin O, Christine S-S. Heart failure with preserved ejection fraction: a systemic disease linked to multiple comorbidities, targeting new therapeutic options. *Arch Cardiovasc Dis.* 2018;Dec;111(12):766–781.
19. Maurer MS, King DL, El-Khoury Rumbarger L, Packer M, Burkhoff D. Left heart failure with a normal ejection fraction: identification of different pathophysiologic mechanisms. *J Card Fail.* 2005;11(3):177–187.
20. Obokata M, Reddy YNV, Pislaru SV, Melenovsky V, Borlaug BA. Evidence supporting the existence of a distinct obese phenotype of heart failure with preserved ejection fraction. *Circulation.* 2017;136(1):6–19.
21. Adamson PB, Abraham WT, Bourge RC, et al. Wireless pulmonary artery pressure monitoring guides management to reduce decompensation in heart failure with preserved ejection fraction. *Circ Heart Fail.* 2014;7(6):935–944.
22. Heise T, Seewaldt-Becker E, Macha S, et al. Safety, tolerability, pharmacokinetics and pharmacodynamics following 4 weeks' treatment with empagliflozin once daily in patients with type 2 diabetes. *Diabetes Obes Metab.* 2013;15(7):613–621.
23. Borlaug BA. Heart failure with preserved and reduced ejection fraction: different risk profiles for different diseases. *Eur Heart J.* 2013;34(19):1393–1395. https://dx.doi.org/10.1093/eurheartj/eht117.
24. Norton GR, Woodiwiss AJ, Gaasch WH, et al. Heart failure in pressure overload hypertrophy. The relative roles of ventricular remodeling and myocardial dysfunction. *J Am Coll Cardiol.* 2002;39(4):664–671.
25. Little WC, Brucks S. Therapy for diastolic heart failure. *Prog Cardiovasc Dis.* 2005;47(6):380–388.
26. Schmieder RE, Martus P, Klingbeil A. Reversal of left ventricular hypertrophy in essential hypertension. A meta-analysis of randomized double-blind studies. *JAMA.* 1996;275(19):1507–1513.
27. Dahlof B, Devereux RB, Kjeldsen SE, et al. Cardiovascular morbidity and mortality in the Losartan Intervention For Endpoint reduction in hypertension study (LIFE): a randomised trial against atenolol. *Lancet (London, England).* 2002;359(9311):995–1003.
28. Wright JTJ, Williamson JD, Whelton PK, et al. A randomized trial of intensive versus standard blood-pressure control. *N Engl J Med.* 2015;373(22):2103–2116.
29. Beckett NS, Peters R, Fletcher AE, et al. Treatment of hypertension in patients 80 years of age or older. *N Engl J Med.* 2008;358(18):1887–1898.
30. James PA, Oparil S, Carter BL, et al. 2014 evidence-based guideline for the management of high blood pressure in adults: report from the panel members appointed to the Eighth Joint National Committee (JNC 8). *JAMA.* 2014;311(5):507–520.
31. Samson R, Jaiswal A, Ennezat P, Cassidy M, Jemtel T. Clinical phenotypes in heart failure with preserved ejection fraction. *J Am Hear Assoc.* 2016;Jan 25;5(1):e002477.
32. Owan TE, Hodge DO, Herges RM, Jacobsen SJ, Roger VL, Redfield MM. Trends in prevalence and outcome of heart failure with preserved ejection fraction. *N Engl J Med.* 2006;355(3):251–259.
33. Bhatia RS, Tu JV, Lee DS, et al. Outcome of heart failure with preserved ejection fraction in a population-based study. *N Engl J Med.* 2006;355(3):260–269.
34. Hwang S-J, Melenovsky V, Borlaug BA. Implications of coronary artery disease in heart failure with preserved ejection fraction. *J Am Coll Cardiol.* 2014;63(25 Pt A):2817–2827.
35. Lam CSP, Voors AA, de Boer RA, Solomon SD, van Veldhuisen DJ. Heart failure with preserved ejection fraction: from mechanisms to therapies. *Eur Heart J.* 2018;39(30):2780–2792.
36. Tavazzi L, Maggioni AP, Marchioli R, et al. Effect of rosuvastatin in patients with chronic heart failure (the GISSI-HF trial): a randomised, double-blind, placebo-controlled trial. *Lancet (London, England).* 2008;372(9645):1231–1239.
37. Fukuta H, Sane DC, Brucks S, Little WC. Statin therapy may be associated with lower mortality in patients with diastolic heart failure: a preliminary report. *Circulation.* 2005;112(3):357–363.
38. Ohte N, Little WC. Statins beneficial for heart failure with preserved ejection fraction but not heart failure with reduced ejection fraction? *Circ J.* 2015;79:508–509.
39. McHugh K, DeVore AD, Wu J, et al. Heart failure with preserved ejection fraction and diabetes. *J Am Coll Cardiol.* 2019;73(5):602–611. http://www.onlinejacc.org/content/73/5/602.
40. Aguilar D, Deswal A, Ramasubbu K, Mann DL, Bozkurt B. Comparison of patients with heart failure and preserved left ventricular ejection fraction among those with versus without diabetes mellitus. *Am J Cardiol.* 2010;105(3):373–377.
41. Kristensen SL, Mogensen UM, Jhund PS, et al. Clinical and echocardiographic characteristics and cardiovascular outcomes according to diabetes status in patients with heart failure and preserved ejection fraction: a report from the I-PRESERVE trial (irbesartan in heart failure with preserved ejection). *Circulation.* 2017;135(8):724–735.

42. Boulanger CM. Secondary endothelial dysfunction: hypertension and heart failure. *J Mol Cell Cardiol.* 1999;31(1):39–49.
43. Jia G, Whaley-Connell A, Sowers JR. Diabetic cardiomyopathy: a hyperglycaemia- and insulin-resistance-induced heart disease. *Diabetologia.* 2018;61(1):21–28.
44. Kenchaiah S, Evans JC, Levy D, et al. Obesity and the risk of heart failure. *N Engl J Med.* 2002;347(5):305–313.
45. Kishi S, Armstrong AC, Gidding SS, et al. Association of obesity in early adulthood and middle age with incipient left ventricular dysfunction and structural remodeling: the CARDIA study (coronary artery risk development in young adults). *JACC Heart Fail.* 2014;2(5):500–508.
46. Haass M, Kitzman DW, Anand IS, et al. Body mass index and adverse cardiovascular outcomes in heart failure patients with preserved ejection fraction: results from the Irbesartan in Heart Failure with Preserved Ejection Fraction (I-PRESERVE) trial. *Circ Heart Fail.* 2011;4(3):324–331.
47. Kitzman DW, Brubaker P, Morgan T, et al. Effect of caloric restriction or aerobic exercise training on peak oxygen consumption and quality of life in obese older patients with heart failure with preserved ejection fraction: a randomized clinical trial. *JAMA.* 2016;315(1):36–46.
48. Pandey A, Parashar A, Kumbhani D, et al. Exercise training in patients with heart failure and preserved ejection fraction: meta-analysis of randomized control trials. *Circ Heart Fail.* 2015;8(1):33–40.
49. Otto ME, Belohlavek M, Romero-Corral A, et al. Comparison of cardiac structural and functional changes in obese otherwise healthy adults with versus without obstructive sleep apnea. *Am J Cardiol.* 2007;99(9):1298–1302.
50. Bradley TD, Floras JS. Sleep apnea and heart failure: part I: obstructive sleep apnea. *Circulation.* 2003;107(12):1671–1678.
51. Khattak HK, Hayat F, Pamboukian SV, Hahn HS, Schwartz BP, Stein PK. Obstructive sleep apnea in heart failure: review of prevalence, treatment with continuous positive airway pressure, and prognosis. *Tex Hear I J.* 2018;45(3):151–161.
52. Kaneko Y, Floras JS, Usui K, et al. Cardiovascular effects of continuous positive airway pressure in patients with heart failure and obstructive sleep apnea. *N Engl J Med.* 2003;348(13):1233–1241.
53. Egea CJ, Aizpuru F, Pinto JA, et al. Cardiac function after CPAP therapy in patients with chronic heart failure and sleep apnea: a multicenter study. *Sleep Med.* 2008;9(6):660–666.
54. Arias MA, Garcia-Rio F, Alonso-Fernandez A, Mediano O, Martinez I, Villamor J. Obstructive sleep apnea syndrome affects left ventricular diastolic function: effects of nasal continuous positive airway pressure in men. *Circulation.* 2005;112(3):375–383.
55. Cloward TV, Walker JM, Farney RJ, Anderson JL. Left ventricular hypertrophy is a common echocardiographic abnormality in severe obstructive sleep apnea and reverses with nasal continuous positive airway pressure. *Chest.* 2003;124(2):594–601.
56. Bradley TD, Logan AG, Kimoff RJ, et al. Continuous positive airway pressure for central sleep apnea and heart failure. *N Engl J Med.* 2005;353(19):2025–2033.
57. Yancy CW, Jessup M, Bozkurt B, et al. 2013 ACCF/AHA guideline for the management of heart failure: a report of the American College of Cardiology Foundation/American Heart Association task force on practice guidelines. *Circulation.* 2013;128(16):e240–e327.
58. Khalid U, Ather S, Bavishi C, et al. Pre-morbid body mass index and mortality after incident heart failure: the ARIC Study. *J Am Coll Cardiol.* 2014;64(25):2743–2749.
59. Sharma K, Hill T, Grams M, et al. Outcomes and worsening renal function in patients hospitalized with heart failure with preserved ejection fraction. *Am J Cardiol.* 2015;116(10):1534–1540.
60. Damman K, Valente MAE, Voors AA, O'Connor CM, van Veldhuisen DJ, Hillege HL. Renal impairment, worsening renal function, and outcome in patients with heart failure: an updated meta-analysis. *Eur Heart J.* 2014;35(7):455–469.
61. Damman K, Perez AC, Anand IS, et al. Worsening renal function and outcome in heart failure patients with preserved ejection fraction and the impact of angiotensin receptor blocker treatment. *J Am Coll Cardiol.* 2014;64(11):1106–1113.
62. Bibbins-Domingo K, Pletcher MJ, Lin F, et al. Racial differences in incident heart failure among young adults. *N Engl J Med.* 2009;360(12):1179–1190.
63. Chrysant SG, Chrysant GS. New insights into the true nature of the obesity paradox and the lower cardiovascular risk. *J Am Soc Hypertens.* 2013;7(1):85–94.
64. Okin PM, Kjeldsen SE, Dahlof B, Devereux RB. Racial differences in incident heart failure during antihypertensive therapy. *Circ Cardiovasc Qual Outcomes.* 2011;4(2):157–164.
65. House AA. Management of heart failure in advancing CKD: core curriculum 2018. *Am J Kidney Dis.* 2018;72(2):284–295.
66. Bart BA, Goldsmith SR, Lee KL, et al. Cardiorenal rescue study in acute decompensated heart failure: rationale and design of CARRESS-HF, for the Heart Failure Clinical Research Network. *J Card Fail.* 2012;18(3): 176–182.
67. Maggioni AP, Dahlstrom U, Filippatos G, et al. EURObservational Research Programme: regional differences and 1-year follow-up results of the Heart Failure Pilot Survey (ESC-HF Pilot). *Eur J Heart Fail.* 2013;15(7):808–817.
68. Magnani JW, Rienstra M, Lin H, et al. Atrial fibrillation: current knowledge and future directions in epidemiology and genomics. *Circulation.* 2011;124(18):1982–1993.
69. Campbell RT, Jhund PS, Castagno D, Hawkins NM, Petrie MC, McMurray JJV. What have we learned about patients with heart failure and preserved ejection fraction from DIG-PEF, CHARM-Preserved, and I-PRESERVE? *J Am Coll Cardiol.* 2012;60(23):2349–2356.
70. Sartipy U, Dahlstrom U, Fu M, Lund LH. Atrial fibrillation in heart failure with preserved, mid-range, and reduced ejection fraction. *JACC Heart Fail.* 2017;5(8):565–574.
71. Zakeri R, Borlaug BA, McNulty SE, et al. Impact of atrial fibrillation on exercise capacity in heart failure with preserved ejection fraction: a RELAX trial ancillary study. *Circ Heart Fail.* 2014;7(1):123–130.
72. Mamas MA, Caldwell JC, Chacko S, Garratt CJ, Fath-Ordoubadi F, Neyses L. A meta-analysis of the prognostic significance of atrial fibrillation in chronic heart failure. *Eur J Heart Fail.* 2009;11(7):676–683.
73. Kotecha D, Lam C, Veldhuisen D, Gelder I, Voors A, Rienstra M. Heart failure with preserved ejection fraction and atrial fibrillation vicious twins. *J Am Coll Cardiol.* 2016;68(20):2217–2228.
74. Abed HS, Wittert GA, Leong DP, et al. Effect of weight reduction and cardiometabolic risk factor management on symptom burden and severity in patients with atrial fibrillation: a randomized clinical trial. *JAMA.* 2013;310(19):2050–2060.
75. January CT, Wann LS, Calkins H, et al. 2019 AHA/ACC/HRS focused update of the 2014 AHA/ACC/HRS guideline for the management of patients with atrial fibrillation: a report of the American College of Cardiology/American Heart Association task force on clinical practice guidelines and the heart. *J Am Coll Cardiol.* 2019; Jul 9;140(2):e125–e151.
76. Marrouche NF, Brachmann J, Andresen D, et al. Catheter ablation for atrial fibrillation with heart failure. *N Engl J Med.* 2018;378(5):417–427.
77. Machino-Ohtsuka T, Seo Y, Ishizu T, et al. Efficacy, safety, and outcomes of catheter ablation of atrial fibrillation in patients with heart failure with preserved ejection fraction. *J Am Coll Cardiol.* 2013;62(20):1857–1865.
78. Afilalo J, Alexander KP, Mack MJ, et al. Frailty assessment in the cardiovascular care of older adults. *J Am Coll Cardiol.* 2014;63(8):747–762.
79. Sanders NA, Supiano MA, Lewis EF, et al. The frailty syndrome and outcomes in the TOPCAT trial. *Eur J Heart Fail.* 2018;20(11):1570–1577. https://onlinelibrary.wiley.com/doi/abs/10.1002/ejhf.1308.
80. McNallan SM, Singh M, Chamberlain AM, et al. Frailty and healthcare utilization among patients with heart failure in the community. *JACC Heart Fail.* 2013;1(2):135–141.
81. Veninšek G, Gabrovec B. Management of frailty at individual level—clinical management: systematic literature review. *Zdr Varst.* 2018;57(2):106–115.
82. Yip GWK, Wang M, Wang T, et al. The Hong Kong diastolic heart failure study: a randomised controlled trial of diuretics, irbesartan and ramipril on quality of life, exercise capacity, left ventricular global and regional function in heart failure with a normal ejection fraction. *Heart.* 2008;94(5):573–580.
83. Sharma K, Vaishnav J, Kalathiya R, et al. Randomized evaluation of heart failure with preserved ejection fraction patients with acute heart failure and dopamine: the ROPA-DOP trial. *JACC Heart Fail.* 2018;6(10):859–870.

84. Davis BR, Kostis JB, Simpson LM, et al. Heart failure with preserved and reduced left ventricular ejection fraction in the antihypertensive and lipid-lowering treatment to prevent heart attack trial. *Circulation.* 2008;118(22):2259–2267.
85. Ehle M, Patel C, Giugliano RP. Digoxin: clinical highlights: a review of digoxin and its use in contemporary medicine. *Crit Pathw Cardiol.* 2011;10(2):93–98.
86. Pfeffer MA, Claggett B, Assmann SF, et al. Regional variation in patients and outcomes in the Treatment of Preserved Cardiac Function Heart Failure With an Aldosterone Antagonist (TOPCAT) trial. *Circulation.* 2015;131(1):34–42.
87. Zheng SL, Chan FT, Nabeebaccus AA, et al. Drug treatment effects on outcomes in heart failure with preserved ejection fraction: a systematic review and meta-analysis. *Heart.* 2018;104(5):407–415.
88. Aronow WS, Ahn C, Kronzon I. Effect of propranolol versus no propranolol on total mortality plus nonfatal myocardial infarction in older patients with prior myocardial infarction, congestive heart failure, and left ventricular ejection fraction > or = 40% treated with diuretics plus. *Am J Cardiol.* 1997;80(2):207–209.
89. Zi M, Carmichael N, Lye M. The effect of quinapril on functional status of elderly patients with diastolic heart failure. *Cardiovasc drugs Ther.* 2003;17(2):133–139.
90. Solomon SD, Anavekar N, Skali H, et al. Influence of ejection fraction on cardiovascular outcomes in a broad spectrum of heart failure patients. *Circulation.* 2005;112(24):3738–3744.
91. Mentz RJ, Bakris GL, Waeber B, et al. The past, present and future of renin-angiotensin aldosterone system inhibition. *Int J Cardiol.* 2013;167(5):1677–1687.
92. Redfield MM, Anstrom KJ, Levine JA, et al. Isosorbide mononitrate in heart failure with preserved ejection fraction. *N Engl J Med.* 2015;373(24):2314–2324.
93. Redfield MM, Chen HH, Borlaug BA, et al. Effect of phosphodiesterase-5 inhibition on exercise capacity and clinical status in heart failure with preserved ejection fraction: a randomized clinical trial. *JAMA.* 2013;309(12):1268–1277.
94. McMurray JJV, Packer M, Desai AS, et al. Angiotensin–neprilysin inhibition versus enalapril in heart failure. *N Engl J Med.* 2014;371(11): 993–1004. https://doi.org/10.1056/NEJMoa1409077.
95. Solomon SD, McMurray JJV, Anand IS, et al. Angiotensin-Neprilysin Inhibition in Heart Failure with Preserved Ejection Fraction. *N Engl J Med.* 2019;381(17):1609–1620. doi:10.1056/NEJMoa1908655.

35

Echo-Based Approach to the Management of Heart Failure With Preserved Ejection Fraction

Partho Sengupta and Christopher Michael Bianco

OUTLINE

Case Study

A 76-year-old female with a history of heart failure with preserved ejection fraction (HFpEF), type 2 diabetes mellitus, obesity, hypertension, and chronic back pain is referred to you from her primary care provider. She was diagnosed with HFpEF approximately 2 years ago and has been hospitalized once in the past year for a presumed HF exacerbation. She reports progressively worse dyspnea on exertion and intermittent lower extremity edema. She denies chest pain, palpitations, or syncope. On physical examination she is afebrile, her pulse is regular at 86 bpm, blood pressure (BP) 158/76 mmHg, respiration rate (RR) 16, and O_2 saturation 97%. Her cardiac examination is significant for jugular venous pressure (JVP) of 14 cm H_2O, regular rate and rhythm without murmur but with an S_4 gallop. Faint rales are heard at both lung bases. Her abdomen is nontender and obese. She has +2 lower extremity pulses and is normothermic; however, she has +1 lower extremity edema bilaterally. Laboratory tests: Na 134 mg/dL, K 3.7 mg/dL, Cl 103 mg/dL, HCO_3 24 mg/dL, BUN 19 mg/dL, SCR 0.8 mg/dL, BNP 199 pg/mL, HbA1c 8.4%. Her medications include amlodipine 5 mg once daily, hydrochlorothiazide 12.5 mg once daily, pravastatin 20 mg once daily, metformin 500 mg twice daily, sitagliptin 25 mg once daily, meloxicam 15 mg twice daily as needed, and potassium chloride 20 mEq twice daily. Select echocardiogram images are shown (Video 35.1; Figs. 35.1, 35.2, 35.3, 35.4). Left ventricular (LV) EF by modified biplane Simpson rule method was 58%, and no regional wall motion abnormalities or hemodynamically significant valvular disease were appreciated.

INTRODUCTION

Heart failure is a clinical syndrome resulting from structural and functional impairment of ventricular filling or ejection of blood. Patients with HF can be divided into those with reduced ejection fraction (HFrEF) or preserved ejection fraction (HFpEF), and recent literature has also defined an intermediate category of midrange ejection fraction (HFmrEF).[1] Diastolic dysfunction is a central derangement found within all HF patients, regardless of EF. Furthermore, although EF may be preserved, subtle systolic dysfunction is often present in HFpEF as evidenced by deformation imaging.[2] In addition to impairment in LV diastolic properties, those with HFpEF may suffer from a multitude of associated conditions, including right heart dysfunction, pulmonary hypertension (PH), ventricular-arterial uncoupling, left atrial (LA) dysfunction, chronotropic incompetence, atrial tachyarrhythmias, and maladaptive peripheral vascular and skeletal abnormalities. Complementary to the diastolic LV assessment, evaluation of several of these associated conditions makes echocardiography an essential tool in the management of HFpEF.

Heart failure is not a specific disease entity, instead it is a clinical syndrome that develops as a result of several potentially different forms of underlying cardiovascular (CV) disease. Risk factor acquisition and the subsequent response to risk mitigation strategies, combined with intrinsic individual factors, determine whether structural cardiac abnormalities will develop. Antecedent structural changes lead to the eventual development of symptoms and thus the clinical HF syndrome. With this in mind, the American College of Cardiology/American Heart Association (ACC/AHA) have developed a HF staging system (Table 35.1). Interventions are aimed at modifying risk factors (stage A), treating structural heart changes (stage B), and reducing morbidity and mortality (stages C and D). Although this conceptual framework has been largely adopted in the HFrEF realm, uptake of this concept into the management and study of HFpEF has been lacking despite widespread agreement that comorbid disease management is imperative in HFpEF treatment.

Contrary to common perception, mean survival for patients suffering from HFpEF is similar to those with HFrEF.[3] Mode of death in both HFpEF and HFrEF is most commonly related to CV causes, although non-CV causes of death likely represent a more sizable contributor in HFpEF than in HFrEF.[4] Comorbid disease states likely

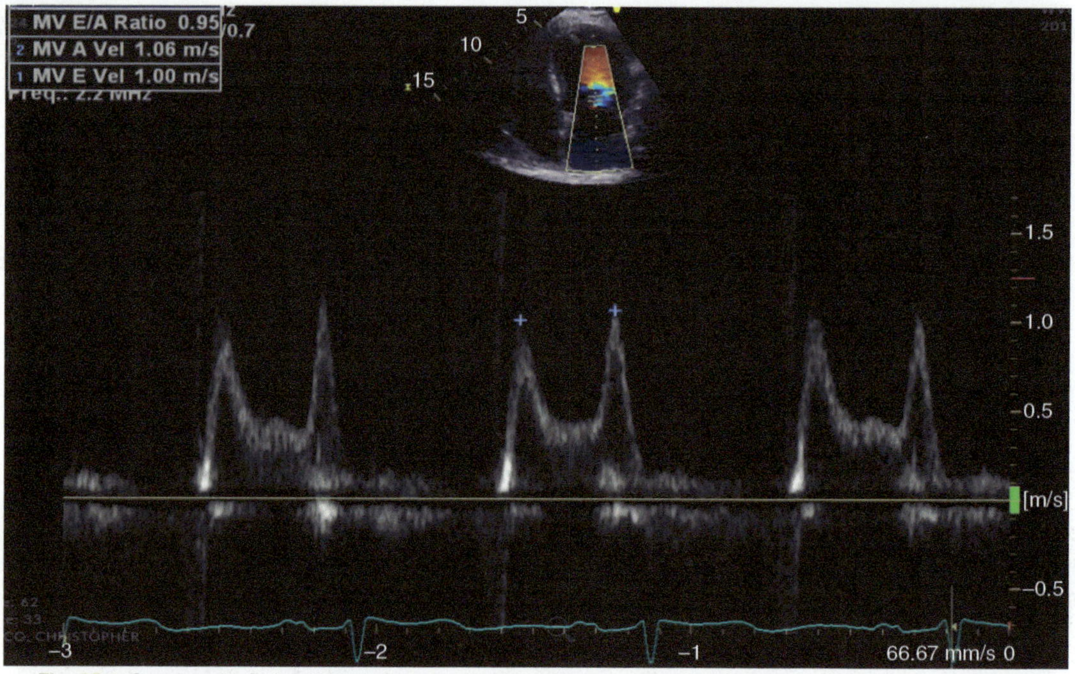

Fig. 35.1 **Case study: Pulsed-Wave Doppler LV Filling Pattern.** Falk RH, Alexander KM, Liao R, Dorbala S. Al (light-chain) cardiac amyloidosis: A review of diagnosis and therapy. J Am Coll Cardiol. 2016;68:1323-1341.

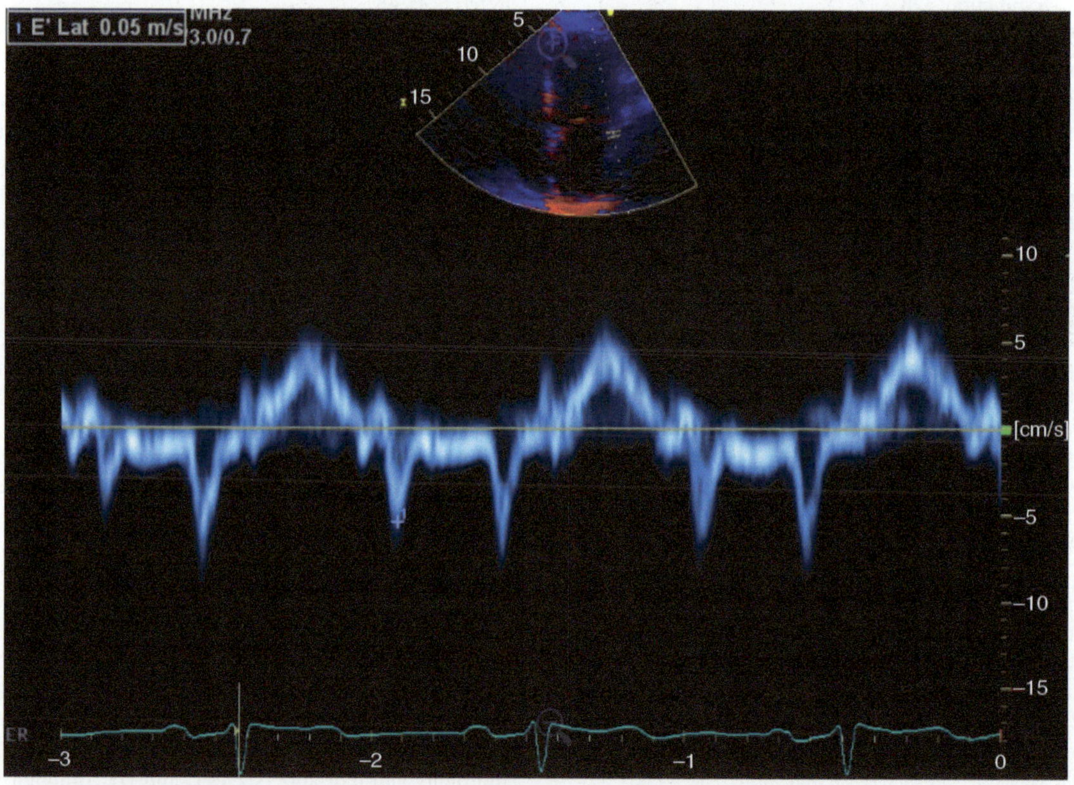

Fig. 35.2 **Case study: Lateral Mitral Annulus Tissue Doppler Imaging (TDI).** From DOI: 10.1161/CIR.0000000000000509, ACC/AHA 2017 updated heart failure guidelines.

contribute to both the development and progression of diastolic dysfunction, as well as predict recurrent hospitalizations and clinical deterioration.[5] Several echo-derived variables have been associated with increased risk of morbidity and mortality in HFpEF[6-9] (Box 35.1). Worsening of diastolic function on serial echocardiographic studies over time is an independent predictor of increased mortality.[10]

Optimal management strategies for HFpEF remain to be defined. Several large-scale phase III therapeutic clinical trials in HFpEF have been conducted, and all failed to meet their primary end point.[11-16] Lack of clear, beneficial evidence-based therapy of HFpEF represents one of the largest unmet needs in CV disease management. Several potential explanations for these neutral results exist, including

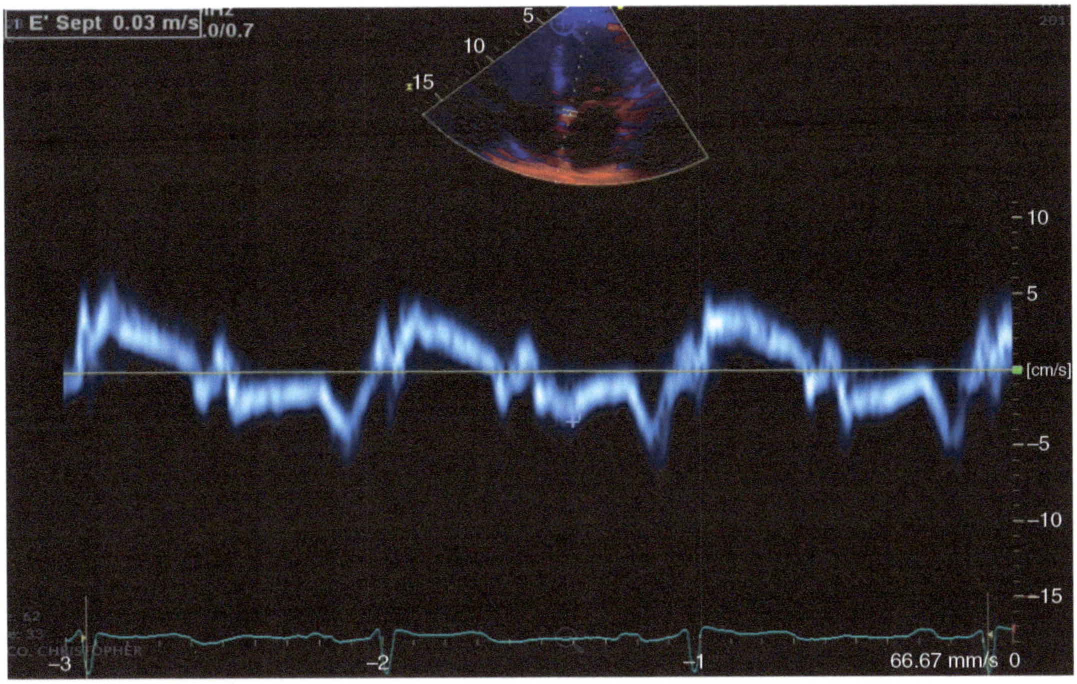

Fig. 35.3 Case study: Medial Mitral Annulus Tissue Doppler Imaging (TDI)

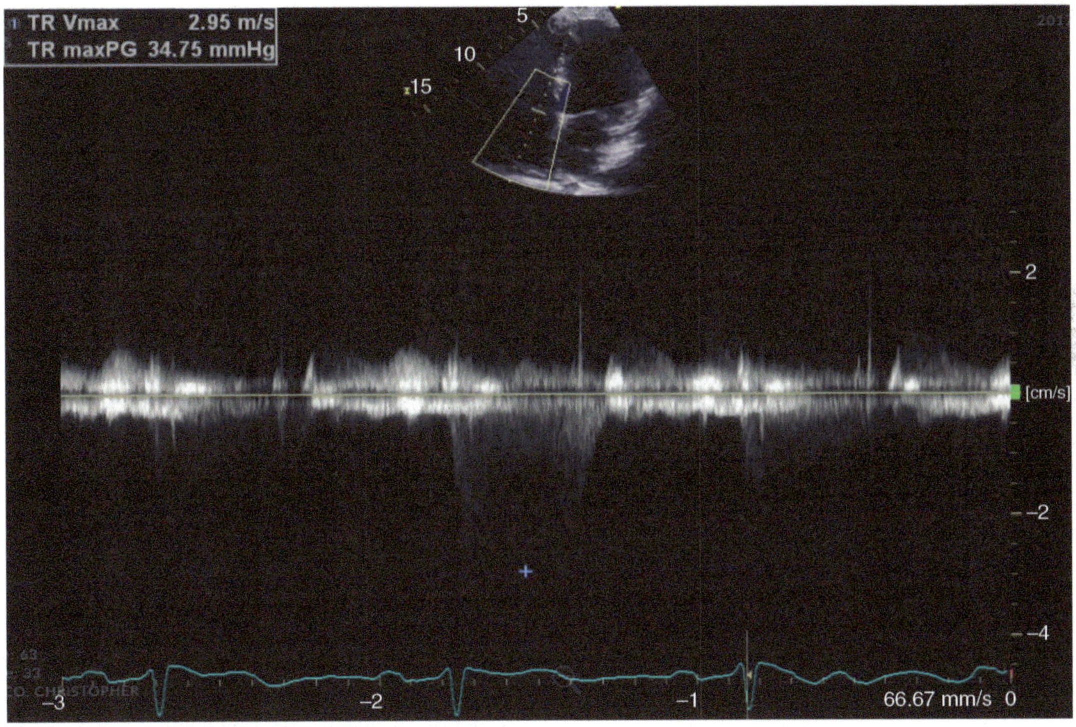

Fig. 35.4 Case study: Medial Mitral Annulus Tissue Doppler Imaging (TDI)

BOX 35.1 Prognostic Echocardiographic Features in HFpEF

- Reduced LV GLS
- Restrictive mitral inflow pattern
- Elevated E/e′
- LV hypertrophy
- LA enlargement
- Reduced LA strain
- Abnormal pulmonary vein S/D ratio
- Reduced TAPSE
- Reduced FAC
- Reduced RV free wall strain
- Reduced TAPSE/RVSP ratio
- Elevated TR peak velocity

Abbreviations: LV, left ventricle; GLS, global longitudinal strain; E/e′, early mitral inflow velocity to mitral annular early diastolic velocity ratio; LA, left atrium; S/D, systole to diastole ratio; TAPSE, Tricuspid annular plane systolic excursion; FAC, fractional area change; RV, right ventricle; RVSP, right ventricular systolic pressure; TR, tricuspid regurgitation.

TABLE 35.1 **Progression of HFpEF Through the ACC/AHA Stages**

Pathologic Description	Stage A Risk factors (e.g., HTN, DM, Obesity)	Stage B DD Without Clinical HF (Preclinical DD)	Stages C and D Clinical Syndrome of HFpEF
Diastolic dysfunction	n	↑	↑
Deposition (collagen, fibrosis)	↑	↑	↑↑
LV dimensions	n	n/↓	n/↓
LA dimensions	n	n/↑	↑
RH dysfunction	n	n/↑	n/↑
LV GLS	n/↓	n/↓	↓
LV GCS	n	n/↑	↑
LV GRS	n	n/↓	↓
LA GLS	n/↓	n/↓	↓
Primary treatment goal(s)	Risk factor modification	Comorbid disease management Treating structural heart disease	Reduce filling pressures Phenotype-specific therapy

n/↑/↓, relates to course/characteristic found in most patients; *AHA*, American Heart Association; *ACC*, American College of Cardiology; *DD*, diastolic dysfunction; *DM*, diabetes mellitus; *GLS*, global longitudinal strain; *GCS*, global circumferential strain; *GRS*, global radial strain; *HFpEF*, heart failure with preserved ejection fraction; *HTN*, hypertension; *LA*, left atrial; *LV*, left ventricular; *RH*, right heart.

inconsistent inclusion criteria with respect to the presence and severity of diastolic dysfunction by echocardiography, differing EF and circulating natriuretic peptide cutoff values, high representation of confounding comorbid conditions, and an overall heterogeneity of structural abnormalities within study populations.[17] The latter recognition of heterogeneity within HFpEF pathogenesis and characterization has led to the concept of phenotyping of distinct HFpEF subtypes.[18,19]

Although convincing clinical outcomes data are lacking, echocardiographic-derived diastolic function following specific treatment strategies may inform the provider of structural and functional response to therapy.[10,20,21] The echocardiographic-based approach to management of HFpEF can broadly be divided into the study of highly load-dependent variables related to real-time volume and pressure status versus relatively load-independent variables related to chronic structural remodeling. Furthermore, LA function, PH, right heart function, and ventricular-arterial coupling can readily be assessed with echocardiography; all are of great importance in HFpEF management.

PATHOPHYSIOLOGY

The field's understanding of HFpEF pathophysiology has exploded in recent years. Once viewed purely as a LV disease of impaired relaxation and increased elastic stiffness, we now know that a multitude of factors influence this condition. Broadly, the pathophysiology of HFpEF can be divided into central and peripheral mechanisms, several of which are readily assessed with echocardiography. Central mechanisms include impaired LV relaxation and progressive stiffness, subclinical LV systolic dysfunction, LA dysfunction, PH, right heart failure, atrial tachyarrhythmias, chronotropic incompetence, atrial dysfunction, coronary microvascular rarefaction, and endothelial dysfunction. Peripheral mechanisms include systemic hypertension, arterial endothelial dysfunction, renal insufficiency, and poor peripheral oxygen extraction by skeletal muscle. Emerging data support systemic inflammation as a principal driver of multiorgan dysfunction that leads to cardiac remodeling and arterial stiffening.

Cellular Dysfunction

LV cardiac myocytes from HFpEF patients are more calcium sensitive, the sarcomere protein titin undergoes hypophosphorylation and an isoform shift that leads to increased cell stiffness,[22] and maladaptive titin-actin[23] and actomycin[24] interactions develop. Although myocardial fibrosis was previously thought to be a major pathologic mechanism, both in vivo endomyocardial biopsy[22] and an autopsy study[25] have failed to show impressive fibrosis or collagen volume fraction. However, varying degrees of interstitial fibrosis may be seen, and more extensive hypertrophy and myofibrillar density are common.[22] Emerging echocardiographic techniques, including interactive backscatter analysis, can be used to estimate the degree of myocardial fibrosis but currently is largely restricted to the research arena.

Systolic LV Dysfunction

Ultrastructural changes also lead to concomitant systolic dysfunction in the presence of normal EF. Necessary restoring forces for normal diastolic function are created during systole and may be impaired with even subtle systolic dysfunction. Depressed global longitudinal strain (GLS) is an early marker of systolic dysfunction and is often present in HFpEF. Although GLS may be depressed, global circumferential strain (GCS) and LV twist remain unchanged or even increase, allowing a preserved LV EF.[26] Although LV twist remains preserved, the onset of LV untwist onset is delayed in those with diastolic dysfunction, which compromises the suction function in early diastole.[27] Furthermore, even normal resting LV untwist may become markedly compromised with exercise.[28] A reduced GLS in HFpEF is independently associated with reduced peak O_2 uptake and exercise capacity.[29] Therefore subclinical systolic dysfunction also plays a role in exertional symptoms in HFpEF.

LA Dysfunction

Abnormal diastolic suction function in HFpEF leads to impaired transmitral diastolic flow patterns apparent in traditional indices such as transmitral Doppler profile, as well as more sophisticated methods, including particle imaging velocimetry and vortex formation analysis.[30] Progressive LV diastolic dysfunction leads to impaired LA emptying resulting in LA dysfunction. Chronic LA dysfunction manifests with LA enlargement, thus LA size may be viewed as a potential biomarker of the severity and chronicity of diastolic dysfunction.[31] LA function has been divided into three phases: reservoir, conduit, and active contraction.[32] During reservoir phase the left atrium stores pulmonary venous return during LV contraction and isovolumetric relaxation. With mitral valve opening, the left atrium acts as a conduit transferring blood passively into the left ventricle. Finally, the left atrium actively contracts contributing to late LV filling. Three-dimensional (3-D) echocardiography allows quantification of LV filling volume resulting from each atrial

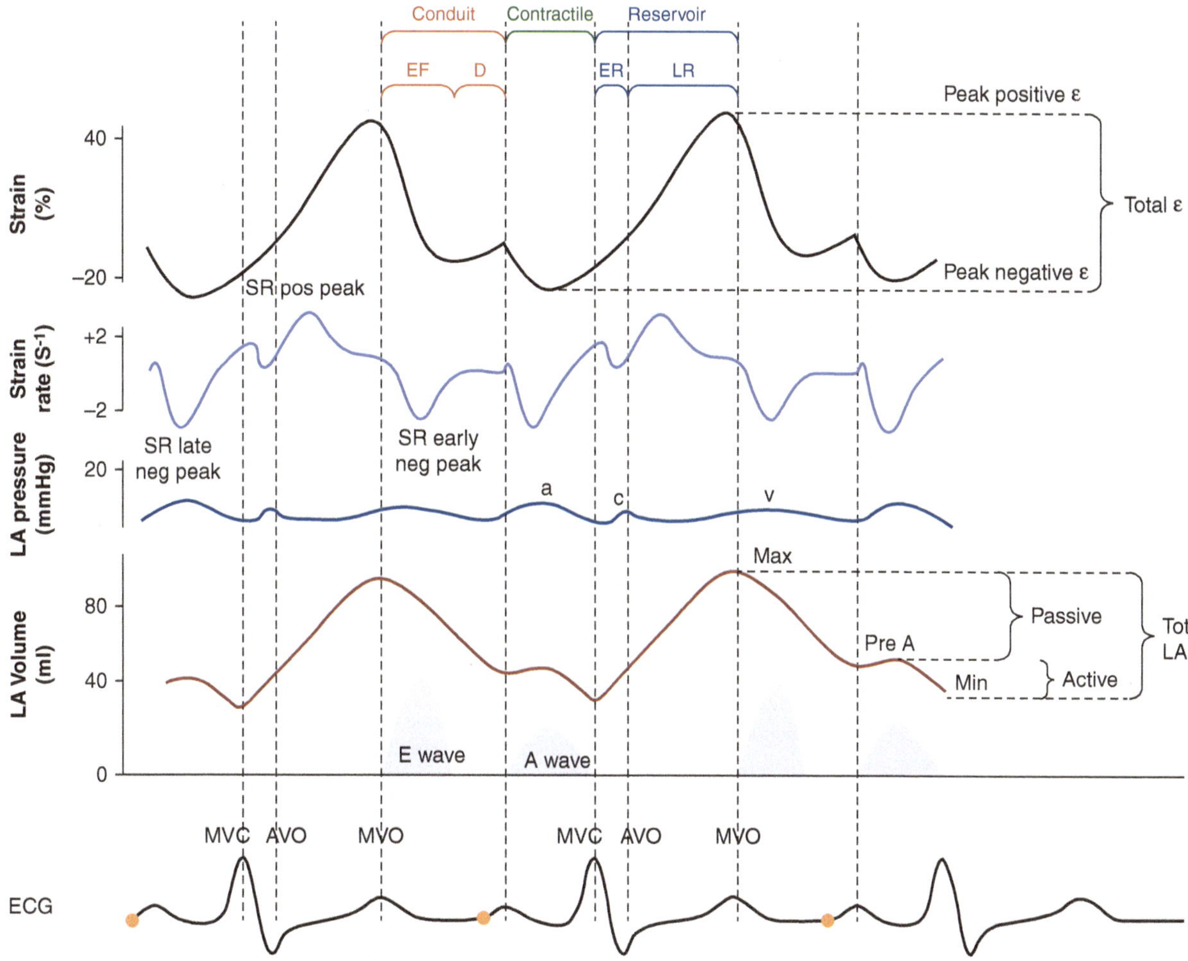

Fig. 35.5 Left Atrial Myocardial Mechanics. Figure Abbreviations: AVO, Aortic valve opening; D, diastasis, ECG, electrocardiogram; EF, early filling; ER, early reservoir; *ε*, strain; LASV, LA stroke volume; LR, late reservoir; Max, maximum; Min, minimum; MVC, mitral valve closure. MVO, mitral valve opening; SR, strain rate; SR ear neg peak, SR early negative peak; SR late neg peak, SR late negative peak; SR pos peak, SR positive peak.

phase, and deformation imaging allows further physiologic assessment of LA function (Fig. 35.5). The degree of decrement in peak LA strain measured during reservoir function has been associated with increasing degrees of diastolic dysfunction.[33] Depressed LA contractile function is associated with increased LV filling pressures,[34,35] and LA contraction contributes progressively less to LV filling volume with worsening grades of diastolic dysfunction.[36] Impaired LA strain response to exercise is associated with right ventricular (RV)–pulmonary artery (PA) uncoupling and exercise ventilation inefficiency.[37] Chronic LA hypertension and dysfunction lead to elevated pulmonary capillary wedge pressure (PCWP) and PH.

Pulmonary Hypertension and Right Heart Dysfunction

At least two-thirds of HFpEF patients will exhibit evidence of resting pulmonary hypertension (PH-HFpEF),[38,39] and pulmonary pressures may increase substantially with exercise, forming the basis of diastolic stress testing. A significant minority (12%) of PH-HFpEF patients will also develop a component of pulmonary vascular remodeling from long-standing pulmonary venous hypertension leading to combined precapillary and postcapillary PH.[40] PH-induced RV afterload, reflected by increased end-systolic elastance, eventually leads to RV dysfunction and RV-PA uncoupling. A reduced ratio (<0.36) of tricuspid annular plane systolic excursion/right ventricular systolic pressure (TAPSE/RVSP) reflects RV-PA uncoupling and is associated with worse prognosis.[41] Right heart dysfunction as measured by traditional echocardiographic indices (RV fractional area change [FAC], TAPSE, tricuspid annular systolic velocity [RV S′]) is present in at least one-fifth and potentially 30% to 50% of patients with HFpEF.[39,42] Furthermore, normal resting RV function may conditionally deteriorate with exercise and preload augmentation. Concomitant atrial fibrillation (AFib) may also contribute to right heart failure and is independently associated with RV dysfunction.[6] RV dilatation based on echo-derived basal RV linear diameter (>41 mm) is present in almost a third of cases.[39] RV hypertrophy may be present in up to 45% of patients with PH-HFpEF.[43] Pulmonary hypertension and right heart dysfunction may represent important treatment targets that are readily assessed with echocardiography.

Exercise Limitations

Chronotropic incompetence is common in HFpEF. During exercise, HFpEF patients display lower peak oxygen uptake (VO_2) coupled with blunted increases in heart rate, stroke volume, and EF, often coupled with a hypertensive exercise response.[44,45] A stronger relationship exists between exercise capacity and diastolic function than EF.[46,47] Abnormal global longitudinal LA and LV stain have both been associated with exercise intolerance.[29,37] Compounding central factors, skeletal muscle structural and biochemical changes ensue favoring decreased peripheral O_2 extraction, further limiting exercise tolerance.[48]

Endothelial Dysfunction

Increased arterial stiffness is common in HFpEF. Endothelial dysfunction related to a decrease in NO bioavailability is present in both the peripheral vasculature and the coronary microvasculature. Coronary microvasculature endothelial dysfunction and rarefaction lead to downstream effects, including myocyte hypertrophy and stiffening, as well as promoting inflammatory cell migration into the interstitial space.[49] Peripheral arterial endothelial dysfunction leads to decreased compliance and an abnormal vasodilator response to exercise.[45] Increased arterial stiffness leads to dramatic changes in BP with relatively small volume changes. Furthermore, reduced central aortic compliance contributes to LV-aortic uncoupling in HFpEF.[50] Carotid to femoral pulse wave velocity (PWV), a measure of aortic stiffness,[51] and pathologic wave reflection, a measure of late systolic wall stress,[52] are emerging Doppler echocardiography tools used to evaluate arterial stiffness in HFpEF.

Multisystem Dysfunction

Beyond direct central and peripheral CV system changes, an emerging model of HFpEF involves systemic inflammation as a principal disease driver. In this model, systemic inflammation leads to multiorgan dysfunction, including the lungs, kidneys, skeletal muscle, and hematologic system. Extramyocardial organ dysfunction drives cardiac remodeling and arterial stiffening, leading to diastolic dysfunction.

This appreciation of the complex pathogenesis combined with vast heterogeneity of remodeling patterns, stages of presentation, and comorbid conditions has led to the recognition of distinct HFpEF phenotypes originally identified by data-driven analytic strategies.[18] The phenogroup suffering from PH and right heart failure dysfunction is of particular interest as treatment response can be readily monitoring using serial echocardiographic indices of right heart function and RV-PA interactions. From a clinical perspective, phenotype-specific optimization of myocardial factors (CAD, atrial arrhythmias, chronotropic incompetence) and extramyocardial factors (renal insufficiency, pulmonary dysfunction, hypertension, metabolic disease, anemia, and skeletal muscle deterioration) are important treatment targets. Downstream treatment response can be monitored echocardiographically with assessment of preload-dependent indices reflecting real-time pressure-volume (P-V) relationships and with relatively load-independent variables reflecting longer standing remodeling responses, as well as indices reflecting LA dysfunction and right heart disease.

CLINICAL RELEVANCE

Stage A: At Risk

Our evolving knowledge of HFpEF implicates extracardiac comorbidities such as hypertension, renal insufficiency, obesity, and metabolic syndrome as central drivers of systemic inflammation and endothelial dysfunction, leading to LV remodeling and diastolic dysfunction. Therefore measures to prevent and adequately treat these implicated comorbidities may ultimately reduce the incidence of HFpEF.

LV hypertrophy secondary to hypertension is a known risk factor for the development of diastolic dysfunction and HF.[53] Antihypertensive therapy with angiotensin-converting enzyme (ACE) inhibitors more effectively prevents the development of LV hypertrophy than non-ACE inhibitor–based therapy in diabetic patients with hypertension.[54] Diuretic therapy may also play a protective role in prevention of symptomatic HF. In a secondary analysis of the Antihypertensive and Lipid-Lowering Treatment to Prevent Heart Attack Trial (ALL-HAT) study, diuretic therapy with chlorthalidone was associated with a decreased incidence of HF compared to lisinopril, amlodipine, or doxazosin.[55] Although these data suggest the potential merit of particular agents, overall BP control is likely the most important factor in preventing the development of LV hypertrophy and progression to structural remodeling.[56]

Renal insufficiency may contribute to worsening hypertension through volume expansion and promote diastolic dysfunction through several mechanisms, including accumulation of advanced glycation end products, uremic toxins, and systemic inflammation. Even mild chronic kidney disease (CKD), particularly when associated with albuminuria, is associated with endothelial dysfunction and changes in bone mineral handling that have been associated with the development of ventricular hypertrophy and fibrosis.[57] Although CKD, hypertension, and subsequent LV hypertrophy play important roles in the development of HF, diastolic dysfunction may actually precede the development of LV hypertrophy in some circumstances.[58] Extracellular matrix changes preceding gross hypertrophy and increased wall thickness may lead to increased ventricular stiffness.[59] Therefore risk factor modifications beyond hypertension therapy and prevention of LV hypertrophy play an important role in preventing diastolic dysfunction.

Metabolic disease, across the diabetic continuum of insulin resistance to frank diabetes mellitus, is strongly associated with the development of adverse remodeling and associated diastolic dysfunction. In most cases, changes in diastolic function are already present before the onset of diabetes and largely associated with the state of insulin resistance.[60] A strong association exists between obesity and the development of diastolic dysfunction.[61] Obesity leads to mitochondrial dysfunction, hyperinsulinemia with subsequent insulin resistance, and systemic inflammation in keeping with the extramyocardial hypothesis of inflammation driving HFpEF pathogenesis. Also obesity independently increases the risk for incident LV hypertrophy in hypertensive patients.[56] In those with established structural changes (stage B), weight loss leads to improved diastolic indices.[62] Although data for prevention of diastolic dysfunction are lacking, risk factor modification directed at comorbid conditions in known association with the development of diastolic dysfunction may prove efficacious.

Stage B: Preclinical Structural Disease

Approximately one-fourth of the adult US population have evidence of stage B, preclinical diastolic dysfunction.[63] Prevalence increases with older age and common cardiovascular comorbidities. Furthermore, even mild, asymptomatic diastolic dysfunction is associated with increased mortality.[64] Not surprising, persistent or worsening Doppler pattern of diastolic dysfunction on serial examinations in asymptomatic, stage B individuals increases the likelihood of progression to symptomatic, stage C disease.[65] Increasing age, along with the presence of comorbid hypertension, peripheral arterial disease, diabetes, or coronary disease also increases the likelihood of progression from preclinical diastolic dysfunction to symptomatic disease. Therefore treatment strategies addressing these highly prevalent comorbid conditions would seem prudent in preventing the development of clinical HF.

Hypertension is one of the strongest risk factors for progression from preclinical disease to clinical HF (stage C).[53] Regression of LV hypertrophy can be expected in hypertensive patients once adequate BP control is instituted. Although hypertension treatment with angiotensin receptor blockers (ARBs) has generally shown the highest rates of LV hypertrophy regression,[66,67] no particular antihypertensive agent has emerged superior for improvement of diastolic indices.[68,69]

Diastolic dysfunction worsens across the diabetic continuum, predominantly related to increasing degrees of insulin resistance.[60] E′ velocity tends to fall and E/e′ progressively rises as patients evolve from prediabetes to frank diabetes mellitus. In diabetic patients with preclinical diastolic dysfunction, elevated E/e′ ratio is associated with the subsequent development of HFpEF as well as increased mortality

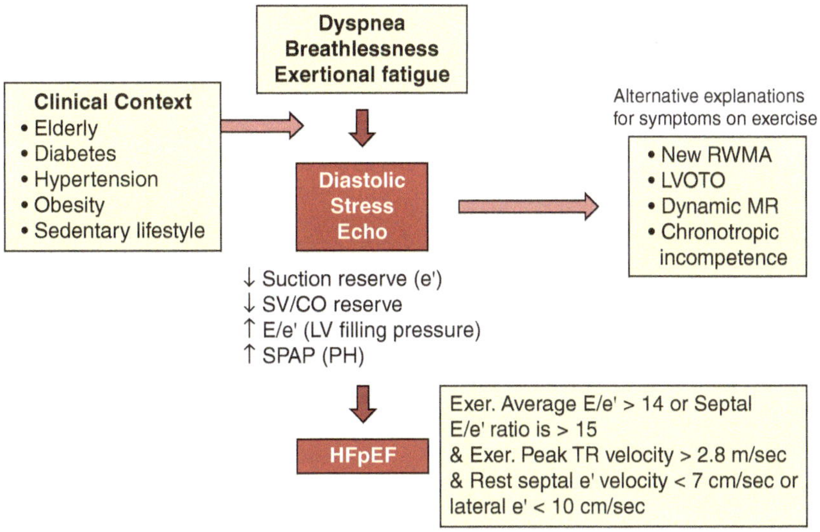

Indications

- When resting echocardiogram does not explain symptoms of heart failure or dyspnea, especially with exertion
- The most appropriate patients for diastolic exercise testing have grade 1 diastolic dysfunction with normal filling pressures or perhaps diastolic dysfunction with indeterminate filling pressures
- Generally not indicated for patients with completely normal resting diastolic parameter or those with clearly abnormal diastolic function and elevated filling pressures

Fig. 35.6 Diastolic stress testing. Abb: RWMA, regional wall motion abnormalities; LVOTO, left ventricular outflow tract obstruction; MR, mitral regurgitation; SV, stroke volume; CO, cardiac output; SPAP, systolic pulmonary arterial pressure; PH, pulmonary hypertension; TR, tricuspid regurgitation.

independent of hypertension, coronary disease, or other echocardiographic parameters.[70]

Coronary artery disease (CAD) is present in approximately half of patients with HFpEF.[71] Diastolic dysfunction, particularly associated with region wall motion abnormalities, should prompt consideration of underlying CAD. Revascularization of obstructive epicardial coronary disease is associated with improvements in diastolic indices.[72]

LA size has been described as a biomarker of CV disease and predicts CV risk.[31] Progression into symptomatic disease is largely mediated by either resting or effort-induced PH, which implies LA hypertension and dysfunction. Increased LA size is a late manifestation of long-standing LA dysfunction. Furthermore, LA size associated with diastolic dysfunction may be underestimated using standard two-dimensional (2-D) imaging, or LA compliance may be decreased despite a relatively normal LA size despite the presence of diastolic dysfunction. Modern echocardiographic techniques, including LA deformation imaging, provide further information regarding LA function. Impaired LA reservoir and conduit function are strongly associated with diastolic dysfunction in preclinical (stage B) disease.[73] Importantly, these parameters showed higher diagnostic accuracy in detecting early diastolic dysfunction compared with LA volume index and may serve as a more sensitive marker of diastolic dysfunction than frank LA enlargement.

Stages C and D: Heart Failure Syndrome

Diagnosis

The diagnosis of HFpEF may be challenging. At least one-fourth of the US adult population has echocardiographic evidence of diastolic dysfunction, and several etiologies for breathlessness and hypervolemia exist. The presence of nonspecific clinical signs and symptoms, as well as diastolic dysfunction, does not necessarily imply a diagnosis of HFpEF. Several diagnostic algorithms are available, the H2FPEF score incorporates both clinical (age >60, obesity, requiring two or more antihypertensive medications) and echocardiographic parameters (RVSP >35 mmHg, E/e′ >9), reflecting the need for an integrative approach to diagnosis.[74]

Conversely, some patients may have suggestive HF signs and symptoms, yet resting diastolic indices may seem out of proportion to symptoms. Diastolic stress testing may be of value in patients with borderline resting diastolic indices in which the diagnosis of HFpEF is being entertained (Fig. 35.6). Normal individuals are able to increase stroke volume without significantly increasing filling pressures due to concomitant augmentation of myocardial relaxation and diastolic suction. Increased diastolic suction and relaxation lead to a proportional increase in both the mitral early diastolic E velocity and annular velocity (e′) resulting in a preserved E/e′ relationship in those with a normal exercise response. Exercise-induced elevations in the E/e′ relationship associated with increased tricuspid regurgitation (TR) velocity suggest an abnormal diastolic response. The diastolic stress test (See Chapter 18) is considered definitely abnormal when the following three conditions are met: (1) average E/e′ greater than 14 or septal E/e′ ratio greater than 15 with exercise, (2) peak TR velocity greater than 2.8 m/sec with exercise and (3) septal e′ velocity less than 7 cm/sec if only lateral velocity is acquired, and lateral e′ less than 10 cm/sec at baseline.[75]

Differential Diagnosis

HFpEF is highly prevalent and associated with significant morbidity and mortality. That said, the clinical diagnosis is challenging, and several other conditions may mimic HFpEF. Echocardiography is a powerful tool in differentiating several states that may present clinically similar. A

Parameter	PAH	PVH
RV size	↑	n/↑
RV/LV size ratio	↑	n/↓
IVS position	Leftward	Midline/ Rightward
LVH	Uncommon	Common
RA size	↑	n/↑
LA size	n	n/↑
RA/LA size ratio	↑	n/↓
IAS position	Leftward	Midline/ Rightward
Lateral e'	n/↑	↓
E/e'	n/↓	↑
RVOT notching	Common	Rare

PAH = pulmonary arterial hypertension, PVH = pulmonary venous hypertension, RV = right ventricle, LV = left ventricle, IVS = interventricular septum, LVH = left ventricular hypertrophy, RA = right atrium, LA = left atrium, IAS = interatrial septum, e' = tissue Doppler derived early mitral annular velocity, E = pulsed-wave Doppler early mitral inflow velocity, RVOT = right ventricular outflow tract pulse wave Doppler, n = normal, ↑ = enlarged/increased, ↓ = smaller/reduced

Fig. 35.7 Pulmonary arterial hypertension (PAH) vs pulmonary venous hypertension (PVH).

diagnosis of pulmonary arterial hypertension (PAH) is certainly of concern, particularly when the overall degree of pulmonary hypertension and RV dysfunction appears out of proportion to the degree of left heart diastolic dysfunction. Helpful indices more suggestive of PAH include notching of the right ventricular outflow tract (RVOT) pulsed-wave Doppler profile, a peak TR velocity/RVOT velocity-time integral ratio greater than 0.18, an increased RA-to-LA size ratio, and interatrial or interventricular septal bowing toward the left-sided structures[76] (Fig. 35.7). Pericardial constriction should be considered in every patient before making a diagnosis of HFpEF (Fig. 35.8). Useful echocardiographic indices suggestive of constriction include respiration-related ventricular septal shift and variation in mitral and tricuspid inflow E velocity, increased medial mitral annular e′ velocity, annulus reversus, and hepatic vein expiratory diastolic reversal ratio.[77] Constriction is associated with constraint primarily of the subepicardial layer, leading to decreased circumferential motion evident by decreased circumferential strain, torsion, and untwisting velocity, while subendocardial longitudinal function is relatively preserved. On the other hand, HFpEF and restrictive cardiomyopathy are associated with reduced longitudinal function, while LV rotational motion is spared.[78] Potential hypertrophic cardiomyopathy or restrictive cardiomyopathy, including cardiac amyloidosis, should always be considered prior to making a diagnosis of HFpEF. The echocardiographic and clinical characteristics used in the recognition of these different forms of cardiomyopathy are outside the scope of this chapter; however, one must always consider these forms of cardiomyopathy when assessing for potential HFpEF. Furthermore, disorders such as advanced liver disease, kidney disease, and hypothyroidism may lead to fluid retention, increased filling pressures, and breathlessness and may be initially mistaken for HFpEF or may play a synergistic role in progression from preclinical disease to frank HF.

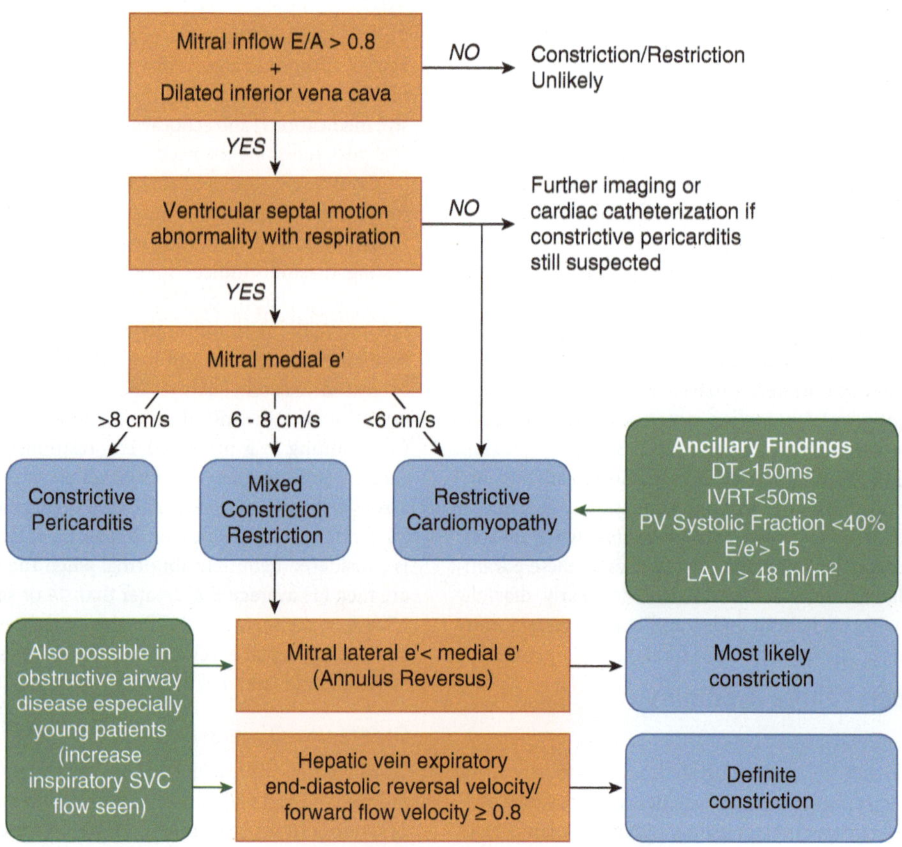

Fig. 35.8 Constrictive pericarditis (CP) vs restrictive cardiomyopathy (RCM). Diagnostic Algorithm (from reference 75)

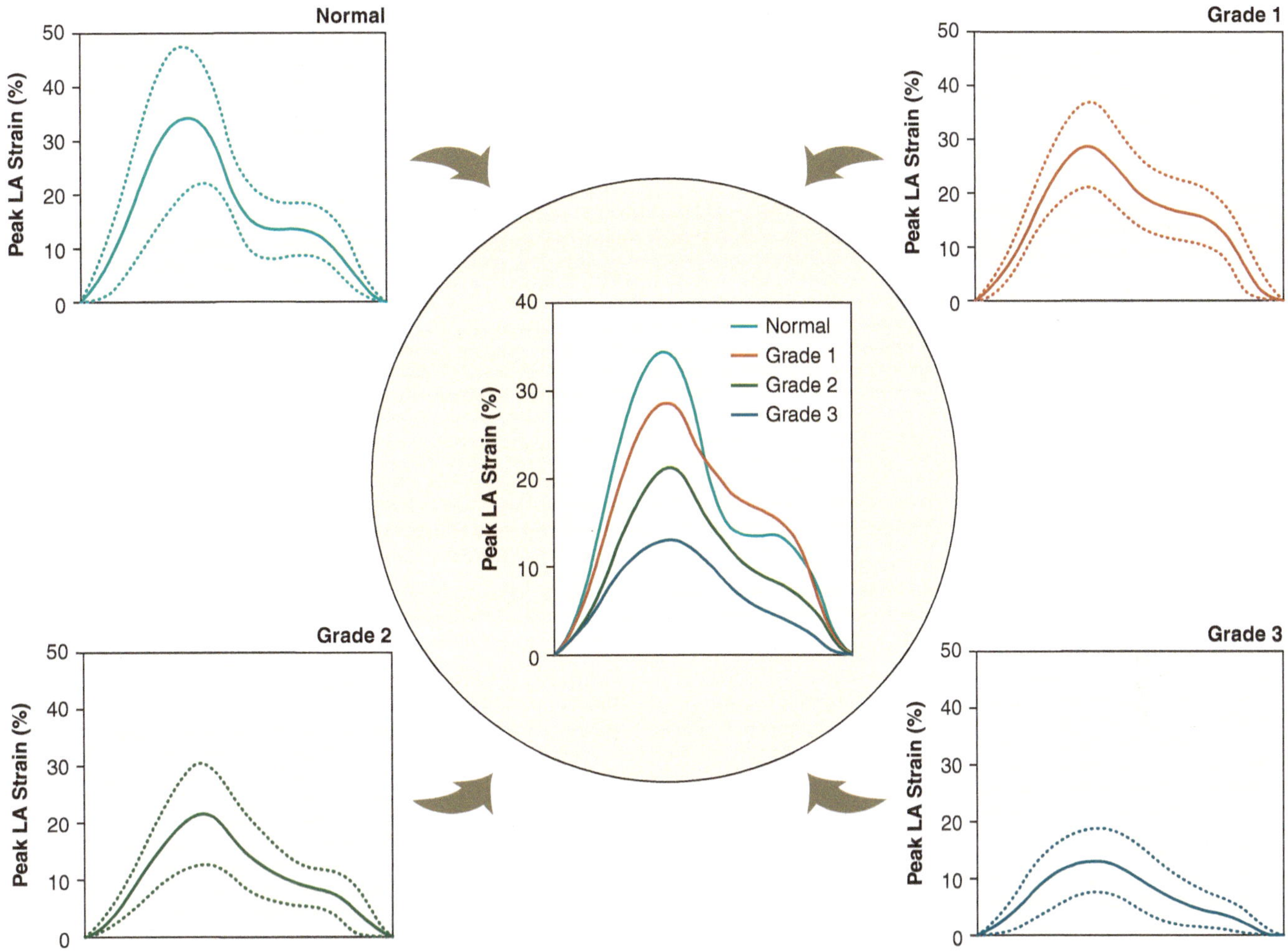

Fig. 35.9 LA strain by diastolic dysfunction (DD) grade. From: Singh et al (ref 33)

Emerging Diagnostic Parameters

The complex interrelated myocardial mechanics of systole and diastole in HFpEF can be further appreciated using deformation imaging. Subendocardial dysfunction leading to depressed GLS is often present. GCS and LV twist remain unchanged or may even increase in a compensatory nature allowing for a preserved LV EF.[26] However, LV untwist in early diastole is delayed, likely leading to impaired suction function for transmitral filling. With exercise both global longitudinal function and LV untwist may become markedly impaired, which likely further explains exercise intolerance and exercise-induced pulmonary congestion appreciated in the HFpEF population. In the TOPCAT trial, a reduction in GLS was the strongest echocardiographic predictor of CV death or HF.[9] Reduced GLS in HFpEF is independently associated with reduced peak O_2 uptake and reduced exercise capacity.[29]

The traditional assessment of diastolic dysfunction has been dominated by the examination of LV relaxation and stiffness properties. Although LA enlargement has long been recognized as a marker of cardiovascular risk and diastolic dysfunction, the assessment of LA function has undergone a renaissance in recent years with currently available imaging techniques. Speckle tracking of the LA walls allows for a physiologic assessment of LA reservoir, conduit, and contractile function. The degree of reduction in peak longitudinal LA strain has been associated with increasing degrees of diastolic dysfunction (Fig. 35.9).[33] Furthermore, depressed peak longitudinal strain, as well as LA contractile function, is associated with increased PCWP and may outperform E/e′ ratio in accuracy of estimating LV filling pressures.[34,35] The volumetric contribution of each atrial phase to LV filling can be assessed using 3-D echocardiography. The proportion of LV filling volume during the conduit phase becomes significantly higher with worsening diastolic dysfunction grade. As diastolic dysfunction progresses, conduit phase filling volume increases while filling volume secondary to LA contraction falls.[36] LA contraction volume more strongly correlates with E/e′ than other measures of LA volume.[79]

Echocardiographic-Based Treatment

Despite our evolving knowledge of the pathogenesis leading to and perpetuating the HFpEF syndrome, optimal treatment strategies remain to be defined (Table 35.2). Although convincing clinical outcomes data are lacking, echocardiographic-derived parameters (Box 35.2)

BOX 35.2 Potential Echocardiographic-Based Treatment Goals

- Improvement in mitral inflow pattern
- Reduction in TR velocity
- Reduction in E/e′ ratio
- Improvement in e′
- Reduction in LA size
- Reduction in RV dimensions
- Improvement in IVC size and collapsibility

Abbreviations: TR, tricuspid regurgitation; E/e′, ratio of early mitral inflow velocity to mitral annular early diastolic velocity; e′, mitral annular early diastolic velocity; LA, left atrium; RV, right ventricle; IVC, inferior vena cava.

TABLE 35.2 ACC/AHA Recommendations for the Pharmacologic Treatment of HFpEF

COR	LOE	Recommendation
I	B	Systolic and diastolic blood pressure should be controlled in patients with HFpEF in accordance with published clinical practice guidelines.
I	C	Diuretics should be used for relief of symptoms due to volume overload in patients with HFpEF.
IIa	C	The use of beta-blocking agents, ACE inhibitors, and ARBs is patients with HTN is reasonable to control blood pressure in patients with HFpEF.
IIb	B-R	In appropriately selected patients with HFpEF (with LV EF ≥45%, elevated BNP or HF admission within 1 year, estimated GFR >30 mL/min, creatinine <2.5 mg/dL, potassium <5.0 mEq/L), aldosterone receptor antagonists might be considered to reduce hospitalizations.
IIb	B	The use of ARBs might be considered to decrease hospitalizations for patients with HFpEF.
III: No benefit	B-R	Routine use of nitrates or phosphodiesterase-5 inhibitors to increase activity or QOL in patients with HFpEF is ineffective.
III: No benefit	C	Routine use of nutritional supplements is not recommended for patients with HFpEF.

Abbreviations: COR, Class of Recommendation; LOE, Level of Evidence; HFpEF, Heart Failure with Preserved Ejection Fraction; ACE, Angiotensin Converting Enzyme; ARB, Angiotensin II receptor blockers; HTN, hypertension; HF, Heart Failure; BNP, brain natriuretic peptide; GFR, Glomerular Filtration Rate; QOL, Quality of Life.

following specific treatment strategies may inform the provider of structural and functional responses to therapy.[10,20,21] Clinically useful echocardiographic parameters that predict disease manifestations extend past the LV diastolic assessment and include assessment of right heart function, pulmonary hypertension, ventricular-arterial coupling, and LA function.

Although diastolic dysfunction results from impaired active relaxation and increased passive stiffness, we are unable to independently quantify traditional indices of relaxation or stiffness separately. Furthermore, although the classic approach divided traditional indices into preload-independent variables and preload-dependent variables, we now know that this classification has significant limitations. Nonetheless, certain variables are highly load dependent and may change quickly related to real-time P-V relationships, while others are relatively load independent and likely signify chronic structural remodeling. Lastly, we have always divided the study of systolic function and diastolic function into separate assessments, yet we increasingly appreciate the interrelated nature of each phase of the cardiac cycle through modern imaging techniques. It is now uniformly accepted that all patients with depressed EF suffer from some degree of diastolic dysfunction. We now appreciate that many if not all patients with significant diastolic dysfunction also suffer from varying degrees of systolic dysfunction, despite a preserved EF.

Targeting filling pressures. One of the most important pieces of information that the echocardiographic examination can provide is an estimation of filling pressures (Fig. 35.10). Using the current American Society of Echocardiography/European Association of Cardiovascular Imaging (ASE/EACVI) recommendations in patients with establish diastolic dysfunction or myocardial dysfunction, those with an E/A ratio of 2 and above have elevated LA pressure, while those with an E velocity of 50 cm/sec or below and E/A of 0.8 or below have normal LA pressure. In the remaining patients, left-sided filling pressures can be determined using a multiparametric approach incorporating average E/e′ greater than 14, TR velocity greater than 2.8 m/sec, and LA volume index greater than 34 mL/m^2. If two or more of these parameters are met, the patient likely has elevated LA pressure. If two or more of these parameters are negative, the patient likely has normal LA pressure. In those in whom only two criteria are available, if one is positive and one negative, a determination of LA pressure cannot be made. In the absence of a clearly restrictive (E/A ≥2) or normal (E velocity ≤50 cm/sec and E/A ≤0.8) mitral inflow pattern, it is important that this multiparametric assessment take place because the accuracy of each component of the multiparametric assessment has limited independent predictive value for determining elevated filling pressures secondary to diastolic dysfunction. The use of E/e′ in predicting LV filling pressure in patients with preserved EF has been recently challenged and may correlate poorly with invasively obtained wedge pressure.[80] TR velocity may be increased secondary to a number of etiologies other than left-sided cardiac disease, or the Doppler signal may be reduced or absent in the presence of elevated left-sided filling pressures. LA enlargement may be absent in nearly half of HFpEF patients.[8] Despite the potentially poor accuracy of each parameter independently, if multiple parameters (TR velocity >2.8 m/sec, LA volume index >34 mL/m^2, E/e′ >14) are abnormal, the diagnostic accuracy of predicting elevated PCWP increases significantly.[81]

A restrictive patterns of mitral inflow (E/A ≥2) in patients with defined diastolic dysfunction is highly specific for elevated PCWP.[81] Likewise, an intermediate mitral inflow pattern associated with multiple abnormal indices of the multiparametric assessment is associated with elevated PCWP. Therapies directed at reduction in LV preload via diuresis or ultrafiltration can improve the mitral inflow pattern in the majority of individuals. Even with therapy, the mitral inflow pattern will never return to normal in most patients. Therefore continued fluid removal until the E/A is less than 1 with improvements in the E/e′ and TR jet velocity may serve as useful echocardiographic targets to define therapeutic success in decongestion.[82] In the CHAMPION trial, reduction in HFpEF hospitalizations may have been largely related to significant up-titration of diuretics in the PA pressure-guided treatment group compared to conventional management, highlighting the importance of diuretic therapy in the management of HFpEF.[83] An improvement in E/A ratio or TR jet velocity from baseline to follow-up was associated with a lower subsequent risk of first occurrence of HF hospitalization, aborted sudden death, or CV death in the TOPCAT study.[84] Abnormal peak atrial longitudinal strain and LA contractile function by LA strain both predict increased PCWP.[34,35] Composite indices incorporating both global LA strain and LV strain have also been shown to correlate with filling pressures.[85] The change in these variables with therapy has not been well studied but may serve as a future echocardiographic therapeutic target.

Right heart dysfunction is present in at least one-fifth of patients with HFpEF.[39,42] Assessment of the right-sided filling pressures can inform the clinician regarding right heart function and overall fluid status. Elevated central venous pressure transmits to the renal venous system causing worsening renal function via decreased renal blood flow and renal perfusion pressure, as well as increased tubular pressures and activation of the RAAS and the sympathetic nervous system.[86] Renal insufficiency leads to impaired natriuresis further potentiating a vicious cycle of renal dysfunction and volume overload. A distinct phenogroup of older HFpEF patients with right heart dysfunction and

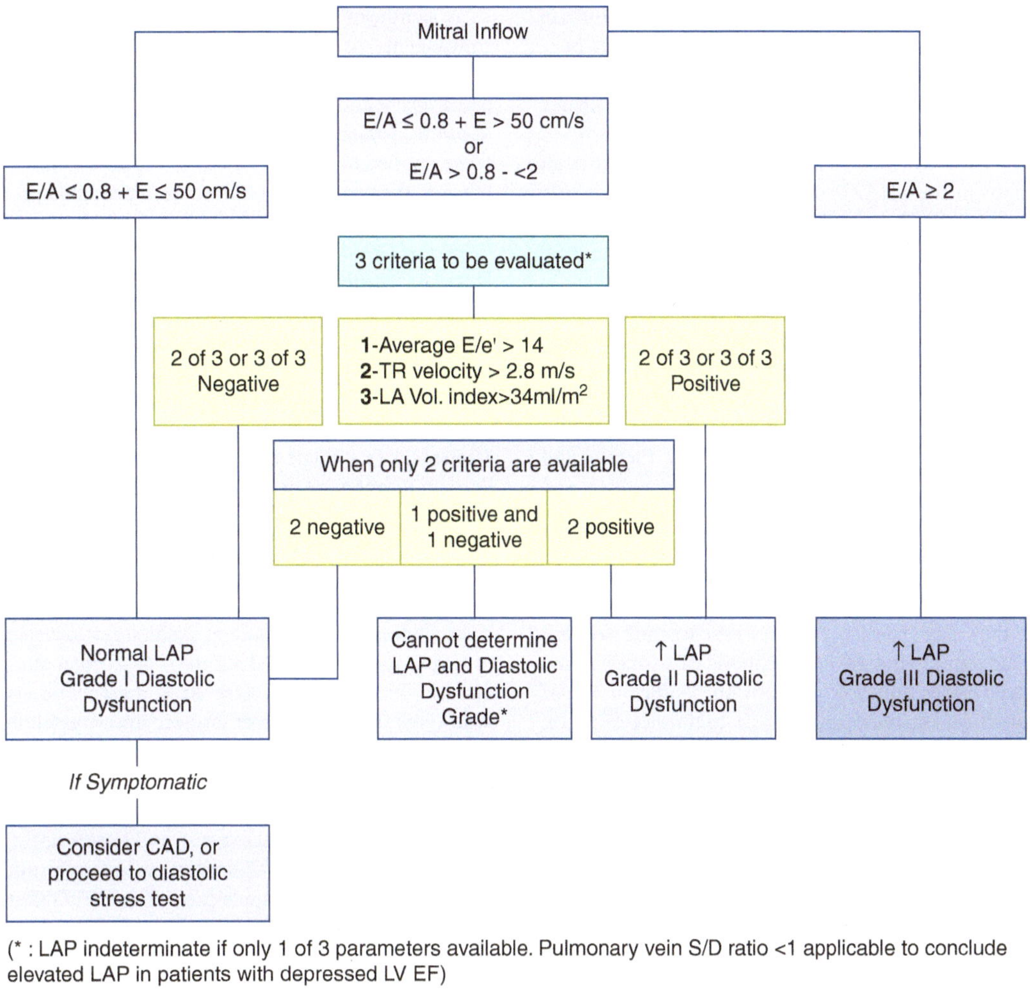

Fig. 35.10 ASE filling pressure and diastolic dysfunction (DD) grading. from ref 75

renal insufficiency has been identified.[87] Significant volume removal in the face of renal insufficiency may be an important treatment strategy in HFpEF, and serial echocardiographic assessments of the inferior vena cava (IVC) may help guide diuresis.

Targeting remodeling. LA enlargement is a well-established predictor of adverse outcomes and reflects the cumulative effect of diastolic dysfunction. A regression in LA volume at follow-up was associated with a lower risk of subsequent cardiac events in HFpEF-treated patients from the TOPCAT trial.[84] Notably the use of spironolactone in this trial was not associated with improvements in LA volume. Sacubitril-valsartan use in HFpEF was associated with a reduction in LA volume and natriuretic peptide levels in a phase II study[88] and is a promising agent being tested in randomized trials currently. Therapies directly addressing LA hypertension and dysfunction represent a potential paradigm shift in treatment, and serial assessment of LA size and function may play an important role in the evolving echocardiographic management of HFpEF.

Mitral annular early diastolic tissue velocity (e′) is generally referred to as a load-independent variable reflecting relaxation and restoring forces of the long axis of the left ventricle. However, it is affected by blood pressure, systolic function, and LV minimal pressure, and therefore is not truly load independent. Nonetheless, a reduction in e′ can be viewed as a marker of abnormal LV remodeling. In the absence of acute myocardial infarction or a rapidly progressive myocardial disorder such as myocarditis, e′ likely represents the cumulative effects of myocyte dysfunction and remodeling over time. Therefore long-term treatment strategies aimed to improve myocardial dysfunction may lead to improvements in diastolic tissue velocity. Improved treatment of hypertension, regardless of the medication used, has been shown to improve e′ in patients with hypertension and diastolic dysfunction.[69] Furthermore, the degree of BP reduction correlates with the degree of improvement in e′. However, it must be recognized that the improvement in e′ cannot be clearly attributed to improved diastolic function as afterload reduction is known to impact e′.

The impact of mineralocorticoid antagonists on cardiac remodeling and diastolic dysfunction has been inconsistent in the literature. ALDO-DHF, the largest study to investigate the echocardiographic impact of spironolactone on cardiac structure and function in HFpEF, demonstrated significant improvements in e′, E/e′ ratio, LV mass index, and LV size among patients treated with spironolactone.[20] Furthermore, the effects of spironolactone on E/e′ ratio remained statistically significant after adjustment for baseline and follow-up BP, suggesting that the reverse remodeling effects of spironolactone were independent of BP reduction. In TOPCAT, the use of spironolactone in HFpEF was associated with a nonsignificant 11% reduction in a combined primary clinical end point. Significant concerns regarding geographic differences in patients and study drug administration in this trial have been raised. On subgroup analysis restricted to the

Americas, spironolactone was associated with a significant reduction in the primary clinical outcome. TOPCAT failed to demonstrate beneficial effects of spironolactone on e′, E/e′, LV mass index, or LV size; however, less echocardiographic information was available in TOPCAT than ALDO-DHF.[84]

Therapy with the ARB candesartan was associated with reduction in HF hospitalizations in the CHARM-Preserved trial[12]; however, use of the irbesartan in the I-PRESERVE trial failed to improve mortality or hospitalization risks in HFpEF patients.[16] Although the trial evidence supporting ARB therapy in HFpEF is conflicting, there is notably no strong negative outcomes data to date associated with ACE inhibitor or ARB use. Treatment with ARBs and ACE inhibitors has generally shown the highest rates of LV hypertrophy regression in hypertension trials[66,67] and, along with other antihypertensive therapy, has been associated with improvements in mitral annular early diastolic tissue velocity (e′).[69] The combination of diuretic therapy and either ACE inhibitor or ARB therapy has been shown to improve e′ and natriuretic peptide levels to a greater extent than diuretic therapy alone.[89] Furthermore, registry data, which likely reflect more realistic, highly comorbid HFpEF patients, support ARB and ACE inhibitor use.[90] Caution must be taken when administering vasodilators to HFpEF patients, as they may experience greater BP reduction, less enhancement in cardiac output, and greater likelihood of stroke volume drop, reflecting a steep end-systolic P-V relationship.[91] Judicious use of diuretics, mineralocorticoid antagonists, and ACE inhibitors/ARBs are reasonable first choices to control BP in HFpEF based on the currently available data.

Extracellular matrix composition and homeostasis also impact diastolic function. Collagen synthesis, crosslinking, and degradation may play particularly important roles. Increased content of type I myocardial collagen and enhanced collagen crosslinking are associated with impaired e′ and E/e′, and collage overexpression correlates with reduced exercise capacity.[92] Furthermore, cardiomyocytes and myocardial extracellular matrix (ECM) are not completely independent compartments, and a close crosstalk exists such that abnormalities in one compartment may be accompanied by changes in the other.[93] Diuretic therapy with torsemide more favorably impacts ECM collagen crosslinking than furosemide, and limited clinical data suggest this translates into an improved LV chamber stiffness in patients with hypertensive heart disease.[94] Mineralocorticoid antagonist therapy in HFpEF has also been associated with significant improvement in markers of collagen homeostasis.[95] Several agents are currently being tested addressing ventricular remodeling and ECM homeostasis, in addition to improved cardiometabolic function on the myocyte level.

Targeting right heart function. Right heart dysfunction as measured by traditional echocardiographic indices (RV FAC, TAPSE, RV s′) is present in at least one-fifth and potentially 30% to 50% of patients with HFpEF.[39,42] Furthermore, normal resting RV function may deteriorate with exercise if pulmonary pressures rise significantly leading to RV-PA uncoupling. A reduced ratio (<0.36) of TAPSE/RVSP reflects RV-PA uncoupling and is associated with worse prognosis.[41]

The primary cause of right heart dysfunction in HFpEF is likely increased RV afterload secondary to postcapillary PH. At least two-thirds of HFpEF patients will exhibit evidence of resting PH,[38,39] and pulmonary pressures may increase substantially with exercise. Therefore therapies directed at left heart decongestion and improved ventriculoarterial coupling may prove advantageous in associated postcapillary PH and right heart dysfunction. A reduction in PA systolic pressure and right heart function as assessed by echocardiographic measures may serve as an echocardiographic treatment target in HFpEF therapy. An improvement in TR jet velocity from baseline to follow-up was associated with improved clinical outcomes in the TOPCAT study.[84]

A significant minority of PH-HFpEF patients will also develop a component of pulmonary vascular remodeling secondary to long-standing pulmonary venous hypertension leading to a combined precapillary and postcapillary PH phenotype.[40] The use of selective pulmonary vasodilator therapy has failed to show consistent benefit when applied to the overall HFpEF population.[96,97] However, targeted use of therapy in the combined precapillary and postcapillary PH-HFpEF phenotype has not been well studied. Observational data from the COMPERA registry showed improvements in New York Heart Association (NYHA) functional class, 6-minute walking distance, and plasma N-terminal pro-brain natriuretic peptide (NT-proBNP) after 3 and 12 months of therapy in patients with combined precapillary and postcapillary PH-HFpEF patients treated with selective pulmonary vasodilators.[98] Sildenafil therapy led to significant improvements in right heart function by echocardiographic and invasive assessment in a single center prospective study of patients with baseline significant right heart dysfunction and elevated pulmonary vascular resistance.[99] Ongoing research in this area will further inform the field on the use of selective pulmonary vasodilators in appropriate HFpEF phenotypes.

Targeting electromechanical function. Elevated heart rate is (in sinus rhythm) an independent predictor of adverse clinical outcomes in HFpEF patients.[100] Reduction of heart rate, in attempts to prolong diastole, has been advocated as a therapeutic strategy to mitigate symptoms. However, chronotropic incompetence is known to be highly prevalent in the HFpEF population and may contribute to exercise intolerance.[45] The use of selective heart rate slowing with ivabradine in HFpEF has been associated with worsening peak O_2 consumption at maximal exercise and significantly reduced submaximal exercise capacity.[101] Overall the evidence for therapeutic attempts at reductions in heart rate is poor. The SWEDIC study evaluated the use of carvedilol in HFpEF patients with predominantly grade 1 ($A > E$) mitral inflow patterns and noted a statistically significant improvement toward normalization of the E/A ratio without significant changes in other diastolic indices, including deceleration time, isovolumic relaxation time, and pulmonary vein S/D ratio. Notably no improvements in symptoms resulted from carvedilol use in this small study. Perhaps individualized use of rate control agents may be appropriate in select patients with an E/A ratio of less than 1. In this situation slowing the heart rate may allow for adequate time for LV filling and atrial contraction, which helps to lower the LA pressure and boost cardiac output. However, in patients with a high E/A ratio, the majority of LV filling occurs in early diastole; therefore slowing the heart rate may not help. In fact, slowing the heart rate may actually be harmful in patients with significant ventricular stiffness because stroke volume is often fixed in these patients, and tachycardia may be necessary to maintain cardiac output.[102]

AFib occurs in approximately two-thirds of HFpEF patients and portends a poorer prognosis.[103] Also, AFib independently leads to LA and LV remodeling, as well as greater exertional intolerance.[104] Furthermore, AFib is associated with RV dysfunction in HFpEF.[6] Management of AFib in HFpEF is outside the scope of this chapter but is an area of active interest. Limited data suggest that maintenance of sinus rhythm following ablation therapy is associated with improvements in LA volume index, LA emptying fraction, E/e′, LV GLS and strain rate, as well as ratios of early mitral inflow (E) and peak strain rate during isovolumetric relaxation period (SR_{IVR}) and early diastole (SR_E).[105] Given our increasing understanding of the role of LA dysfunction in HFpEF, therapies directed at improvements in LA function will continue to evolve and may include effort at maintenance of sinus rhythm. The study of AFib in HF is an exciting field that will continue to grow and inform the medical community on optimum future treatment strategies.

SUMMARY

HFpEF is responsible for approximately half of all HF hospitalizations. A lack of clearly beneficial evidence-based therapy represents one of the largest unmet needs in CV disease management. Echocardiography remains essential in the diagnosis of HFpEF. Furthermore, echocardiography serves as an ideal tool for the serial evaluations of diastolic parameters in the response to therapeutic interventions. With further study incorporating multiparametric characteristics, we may further refine the phenotypic identification and treatment of HFpEF.

FUTURE DIRECTIONS

The echocardiographic assessment of diastolic dysfunction and clinical diagnosis of HFpEF are both complex, multiparametric tasks. Although currently recommended diagnostic algorithms are available, they require a high level of expertise to be effectively used and might still misclassify a significant proportion of cases. Advanced analytic methods are now available that are well suited for dense, multidimensional data exploration. Machine learning approaches may allow for computer-driven interpretation of diastolic dysfunction and the diagnostic evaluation of HFpEF. Distinct clinical[87] and morphofunctional[85] phenotypes have already been described using data-driven analytic methods. Clinical phenomapping has identified mutually exclusive phenogroups of individuals with related comorbidities and pathophysiologies that have differential outcomes. The future of HFpEF management likely involves further refinement of HFpEF phenotypes with subsequent phenotype-directed management. Further refinement of phenotyping may include the incorporation of advanced imaging techniques such as deformation imaging and cardiac fluid dynamics, as well as an expanding pool of omics data, including genomics, proteomics, and metabolomics. The field of Big Data analytics utilizing artificial intelligence will allow for precision characterization and study of HFpEF.

KEY POINTS

- LA function, pulmonary hypertension, right heart function, and ventricular-arterial coupling can be readily assessed with echocardiography and are of great importance in HFpEF management.
- Depressed global longitudinal strain is an early marker of systolic dysfunction and is often present in HFpEF. Global circumferential strain and LV twist remain unchanged or even increase, allowing a preserved LV EF.
- Reduced GLS in HFpEF is independently associated with reduced peak O_2 uptake and exercise capacity and is a strong echocardiographic predictor of CV death or HF.
- A reduced ratio (<0.36) of TAPSE/RVSP reflects RV-PA uncoupling and is associated with worse prognosis in HF.
- In diabetic patients with preclinical diastolic dysfunction, elevated E/e′ ratio is associated with the subsequent development of HFpEF.
- An improvement in E/A ratio or TR jet velocity from baseline is associated with lower risk of HF hospitalization, aborted sudden death, or CV death.
- Regression of LA enlargement with medical therapy is associated with a lower risk of subsequent cardiac events in HFpEF.

REVIEW QUESTIONS

1. Reasonable changes to the medication regimen of the patient described in the case study would include
   a. discontinue her potassium supplementation and start spironolactone.
   b. discourage use of meloxicam and sitagliptin.
   c. consider the addition of candesartan.
   d. all of these.
2. Improvement in which echocardiographic parameter(s) following HFpEF treatment has been associated with improved clinical outcomes?
   a. Regression in LA volume
   b. Reduction in LV mass index
   c. Improvement in LV EF
   d. Both a and b
3. Echocardiographic evidence of RV dysfunction is present in approximately what percentage of HFpEF individuals?
   a. 10%
   b. 25%
   c. 60%
   d. 90%
4. Echocardiographic parameters associated with exercise intolerance in HFpEF patients include which of the following?
   a. Peak atrial longitudinal strain
   b. LV GLS
   c. LVH
   d. Both a and b
5. Treatment with which agent(s) has been associated with a reduction in HFpEF hospitalizations and carry a Class IIb recommendation in the 2017 ACC/AHA/Heart Failure Society of American (HFSA) heart failure guidelines focused update?
   a. Candesartan
   b. Isosorbide mononitrate
   c. Spironolactone
   d. Both a and c

REFERENCES

1. Ponikowski P, Voors AA, Anker SD, et al. 2016 ESC guidelines for the diagnosis and treatment of acute and chronic heart failure. *Eur Heart J.* 2016;37(27):2129–2200. http://eurheartj.oxfordjournals.org/content/37/27/2129.abstract.
2. Kraigher-Krainer E, Shah AM, Gupta DK, et al. Impaired systolic function by strain imaging in heart failure with preserved ejection fraction. *J Am Coll Cardiol.* 2014;63(5):447–456. doi: 10.1016/j.jacc.2013.09.052.
3. Shah KS, Xu H, Matsouaka RA, et al. Heart failure with preserved, borderline, and reduced ejection fraction: 5-year outcomes. *J Am Coll Cardiol.* 2017;70(20):2476–2486. doi: 10.1016/j.jacc.2017.08.074.
4. Vaduganathan M, Patel RB, Michel A, et al. Mode of death in heart failure with preserved ejection fraction. *J Am Coll Cardiol.* 2017;69(5):5560–5569. http://www.onlinejacc.org/content/69/5/556.abstract.
5. Arora S, Lahewala S, Hassan Virk HU, et al. Etiologies, trends, and predictors of 30-Day readmissions in patients with diastolic heart failure. *Am J Cardiol.* 2017;120(4):616–624. doi: 10.1016/j.amjcard.2017.05.028.

6. Mohammed SF, Hussain I, AbouEzzeddine OF, et al. Right ventricular function in heart failure with preserved ejection fraction. *Circulation.* 2014;130(25):2310–2320. http://circ.ahajournals.org/content/130/25/2310.abstract.
7. Zile MR, Gottdiener JS, Hetzel SJ, et al. Prevalence and significance of alterations in cardiac structure and function in patients with heart failure and a preserved ejection fraction. *Circulation.* 2011;124(23):2491–2501. http://circ.ahajournals.org/content/124/23/2491.abstract.
8. Shah AM, Claggett B, Sweitzer NK, et al. Cardiac structure and function and prognosis in heart failure with preserved ejection fraction. *Circ Heart Fail.* 2014;7(5):740–751. http://circheartfailure.ahajournals.org/content/7/5/740.abstract.
9. Shah AM, Claggett B, Sweitzer NK, et al. Prognostic importance of impaired systolic function in heart failure with preserved ejection fraction and the impact of spironolactone. *Circulation.* 2015;132(5):402–414. http://circ.ahajournals.org/content/132/5/402.abstract.
10. AlJaroudi W, Alraies MC, Halley C, et al. Impact of progression of diastolic dysfunction on mortality in patients with normal ejection fraction. *Circulation.* 2012;125(6):782–788. http://circ.ahajournals.org/content/125/6/782.abstract.
11. Pitt B, Pfeffer MA, Assmann SF, et al. Spironolactone for heart failure with preserved ejection fraction. *N Engl J Med.* 2014;370(15):1383–1392. doi: 10.1056/NEJMoa1313731.
12. Yusuf S, Pfeffer MA, Swedberg K, et al. Effects of candesartan in patients with chronic heart failure and preserved left-ventricular ejection fraction: the CHARM-Preserved trial. *Lancet (London, England).* 2003;362(9386):777–781. doi: 10.1016/S0140-6736(03)14285-7.
13. Yamamoto K, Origasa H, Hori M. Effects of carvedilol on heart failure with preserved ejection fraction: the Japanese Diastolic Heart Failure Study (J-DHF). *Eur J Heart Fail.* 2013;15(1):110–118. doi: 10.1093/eurjhf/hfs141.
14. Ahmed A, Rich MW, Fleg JL et al. Effects of digoxin on morbidity and mortality in diastolic heart failure: the ancillary digitalis investigation group trial. *Circulation.* 2006;114(5):397–403. doi: 10.1161/CIRCULATIONAHA.106.628347.
15. Cleland JGF, Tendera M, Adamus J, et al. The perindopril in elderly people with chronic heart failure (PEP-CHF) study. *Eur Heart J Case Rep.* 2006;27(19):2338–2345. doi: 10.1093/eurheartj/ehl250.
16. Massie BM, Carson PE, McMurray JJ, et al. Irbesartan in patients with heart failure and preserved ejection fraction. *N Engl J Med.* 2008;359(23):2456–2467. doi: 10.1056/NEJMoa0805450.
17. Kelly JP, Mentz RJ, Mebazaa A, et al. Patient selection in heart failure with preserved ejection fraction clinical trials. *J Am Coll Cardiol.* 2015;65(16):1668–1682. doi: 10.1016/j.jacc.2015.03.043.
18. Shah SJ, Kitzman DW, Borlaug BA, et al. Phenotype-specific treatment of heart failure with preserved ejection fraction: a multiorgan roadmap. *Circulation.* 2016;134(1):73–90. doi: 10.1161/CIRCULATIONAHA.116.021884.
19. Lewis GA, Schelbert EB, Williams SG, et al. Biological phenotypes of heart failure with preserved ejection fraction. *J Am Coll Cardiol.* 2017;70(17):2186–2200. http://www.onlinejacc.org/content/70/17/2186.abstract.
20. Edelmann F, Wachter R, Schmidt AG, et al. Effect of spironolactone on diastolic function and exercise capacity in patients with heart failure with preserved ejection fraction: the Aldo-DHF randomized controlled trial. *JAMA.* 2013;309(8):781–791. doi: 10.1001/jama.2013.905.
21. Deswal A, Richardson P, Bozkurt B, et al. Results of the randomized aldosterone antagonism in heart failure with preserved ejection fraction trial (RAAM-PEF). *J Cardiac Fail.* 2011;17(8):634–642. doi: 10.1016/j.cardfail.2011.04.007.
22. van Heerebeek L, Borbély A, Niessen HWM, et al. Myocardial structure and function differ in systolic and diastolic heart failure. *Circulation.* 2006;113(16):1966–1973. doi: 10.1161/CIRCULATIONAHA.105.587519.
23. Chung CS, Methawasin M, Nelson OL, et al. Titin based viscosity in ventricular physiology: an integrative investigation of PEVK-actin interactions. *J Mol Cell Cardiol.* 2011;51(3):428–434. doi: 10.1016/j.yjmcc.2011.06.006.
24. Sequeira V, Najafi A, McConnell M, et al. Synergistic role of ADP and Ca(2 +) in diastolic myocardial stiffness. *J Physiol.* 2015;593(17):3899–3916. doi: 10.1113/JP270354.
25. Mohammed SF, Hussain S, Mirzoyev SA, et al. Coronary microvascular rarefaction and myocardial fibrosis in heart failure with preserved ejection fraction. *Circulation.* 2015;131(6):550–559. doi: 10.1161/CIRCULATIONAHA.114.009625.
26. Claus P, Omar AMS, Pedrizzetti G, et al. Tissue tracking technology for assessing cardiac mechanics: principles, normal values, and clinical applications. *JACC Cardiovasc Imag.* 2015;8(12):1444–1460. doi: 10.1016/j.jcmg.2015.11.001.
27. Wang J, Khoury DS, Yue Y, et al. Left ventricular untwisting rate by speckle tracking echocardiography. *Circulation.* 2007;116(22):2580–2586. doi: 10.1161/CIRCULATIONAHA.107.706770.
28. Omar AMS, Vallabhajosyula S, Sengupta PP. Left ventricular twist and torsion: research observations and clinical applications. *Circ Cardiovasc Imag.* 2015;8(6):e003029. doi: 10.1161/CIRCIMAGING.115.003029. ii.
29. Hasselberg NE, Haugaa KH, Sarvari SI, et al. Left ventricular global longitudinal strain is associated with exercise capacity in failing hearts with preserved and reduced ejection fraction. *Eur Heart J Cardiovasc Imag.* 2015;16(2):217–224. doi: 10.1093/ehjci/jeu277.
30. Kheradvar A, Assadi R, Falahatpisheh A, et al. Assessment of transmitral vortex formation in patients with diastolic dysfunction. *J Am Soc Echocardiogr Off Pub Am Soc Echocardiogr.* 2012;25(2):220–227. doi: 10.1016/j.echo.2011.10.003.
31. Douglas PS. The left atrium: a biomarker of chronic diastolic dysfunction and cardiovascular disease risk. *J Am Coll Cardiol.* 2003;42(7):1206–1207.
32. Blume GG, Mcleod CJ, Barnes ME, et al. Left atrial function: physiology, assessment, and clinical implications. *Eur J Echocardiogr J Work Group Echocardiogr Eur Soc Cardiol.* 2001;12(6):421–430. doi: 10.1093/ejechocard/jeq175.
33. Singh A, Addetia K, Maffessanti F, et al. LA strain for categorization of LV diastolic dysfunction. *JACC Cardiovasc Imag.* 2017;10(7):735–743. doi: 10.1016/j.jcmg.2016.08.014.
34. Hewing B, Theres L, Spethmann S, et al. Left atrial strain predicts hemodynamic parameters in cardiovascular patients. *Echocardiography.* 2017;34(8):1170–1178. doi: 10.1111/echo.13595.
35. Cameli M, Sparla S, Losito M, et al. Correlation of left atrial strain and Doppler measurements with invasive measurement of left ventricular end-diastolic pressure in patients stratified for different values of ejection fraction. *Echocardiography.* 2016;33(3):398–405. doi: 10.1111/echo.13094.
36. Yamano M, Yamano T, Iwamura Y, et al. Impact of left ventricular diastolic property on left atrial function from simultaneous left atrial and ventricular three-dimensional echocardiographic volume measurement. *Am J Cardiol.* 2017;119(10):1687–1693. doi: 10.1016/j.amjcard.2017.02.002.
37. Sugimoto T, Bandera F, Generati G, et al. Left atrial function dynamics during exercise in heart failure. *JACC Cardiovasc Imag.* 2016;10:1253–1264. http://imaging.onlinejacc.org/content/early/2016/12/08/j.jcmg.2016.09.021.abstract.
38. Lam CSP, Roger VL, Rodeheffer RJ, et al. Pulmonary hypertension in heart failure with preserved ejection fraction: a community-based study. *J Am Coll Cardiol.* 2009;53(13):1119–1126. doi: 10.1016/j.jacc.2008.11.051.
39. Gorter TM, Hoendermis ES, van Veldhuisen DJ, et al. Right ventricular dysfunction in heart failure with preserved ejection fraction: a systematic review and meta-analysis. *Eur J Heart Fail.* 2016;18(12):1472–1487. doi: 10.1002/ejhf.630.
40. Gerges M, Gerges C, Pistritto AM, et al. Pulmonary hypertension in heart failure. Epidemiology, right ventricular function, and survival. *Am J Resp Crit Care Med.* 2015;192(10):1234–1246. doi: 10.1164/rccm.201503-0529OC.
41. Guazzi M, Bandera F, Pelissero G, et al. Tricuspid annular plane systolic excursion and pulmonary arterial systolic pressure relationship in heart failure: an index of right ventricular contractile function and prognosis. *Am J Physiol Heart Circ Physiol.* 2013;305(9):H1373–H1381. doi: 10.1152/ajpheart.00157.2013.
42. Gorter TM, van Veldhuisen DJ, Bauersachs J, et al. Right heart dysfunction and failure in heart failure with preserved ejection fraction: mechanisms and management. Position statement on behalf of the heart failure association of the European Society of Cardiology. *Eur J Heart Fail.* 2018;20(1):16–37. doi: 10.1002/ejhf.1029.

43. Thenappan T, Shah SJ, Gomberg-Maitland M, et al. Clinical characteristics of pulmonary hypertension in patients with heart failure and preserved ejection fraction. *Circ Heart Fail.* 2011;4(3):257–265. http://circheartfailure.ahajournals.org/content/4/3/257.abstract.
44. Abudiab MM, Redfield MM, Melenovsky V, et al. Cardiac output response to exercise in relation to metabolic demand in heart failure with preserved ejection fraction. *Eur J Heart Fail.* 2013;15(7):776–785. doi: 10.1093/eurjhf/hft026.
45. Borlaug BA, Melenovsky V, Russell SD, et al. Impaired chronotropic and vasodilator reserves limit exercise capacity in patients with heart failure and a preserved ejection fraction. *Circulation.* 2006;114(20):2138–2147. doi: 10.1161/CIRCULATIONAHA.106.632745.
46. Grewal J, McCully RB, Kanne GC, et al. Left ventricular function and exercise capacity. *JAMA.* 2009;301(3):286–294. doi: 10.1001/jama.2008.1022.
47. Davies SW, Fussell AL, Jordan SL, et al. Abnormal diastolic filling patterns in chronic heart failure—relationship to exercise capacity. *Eur Heart J.* 1992;13(6):749–757. doi: 10.1093/oxfordjournals.eurheartj.a060251.
48. Haykowsky MJ, Brubaker PH, John JM, et al. Determinants of exercise intolerance in elderly heart failure patients with preserved ejection fraction. *J Am Coll Cardiol.* 2011;58(3):265–274. doi: 10.1016/j.jacc.2011.02.055.
49. Paulus WJ, Tschope C. A novel paradigm for heart failure with preserved ejection fraction: comorbidities drive myocardial dysfunction and remodeling through coronary microvascular endothelial inflammation. *J Am Coll Cardiol.* 2013;62(4):263–271. doi: 10.1016/j.jacc.2013.02.092.
50. Borlaug BA, Kass DA. Ventricular-vascular interaction in heart failure. *Heart Fail Clin.* 2008;4(1):23–36. doi: 10.1016/j.hfc.2007.10.001.
51. Raso FM, Hofman A, Verwoert GC, et al. Determinants of pulse wave velocity in healthy people and in the presence of cardiovascular risk factors: "establishing normal and reference values". *Eur Heart J.* 2010;31(19):2338–2350. doi: 10.1093/eurheartj/ehq165.
52. Chirinos JA, Segers P, Rietzschel ER, et al. Early and late systolic wall stress differentially relate to myocardial contraction and relaxation in middle-aged adults: the Asklepios study. *Hypertension (Dallas, Texas).* 1979/2013;61(2):296–303. doi: 10.1161/HYPERTENSIONAHA.111.00530.
53. Correa de Sa DD, Hodge DO, Slusser JP, et al. Progression of preclinical diastolic dysfunction to the development of symptoms. *Heart.* 2010;96(7):528–532. http://heart.bmj.com/content/96/7/528.abstract.
54. Ruggenenti P, Iliev I, Costa GM, et al. Preventing left ventricular hypertrophy by ACE inhibition in hypertensive patients with type 2 diabetes: a prespecified analysis of the Bergamo Nephrologic Diabetes Complications Trial (BENEDICT). *Diabetes Care.* 2008;31(8):1629–1634. doi: 10.2337/dc08-0371.
55. Davis BR, Kostis JB, Simpson LM, et al. Heart failure with preserved and reduced left ventricular ejection fraction in the antihypertensive and lipid-lowering treatment to prevent heart attack trial. *Circulation.* 2008;118(22):2259–2267. doi: 10.1161/CIRCULATIONAHA.107.762229.
56. Izzo R, Losi MA, Stabile E, et al. Development of left ventricular hypertrophy in treated hypertensive outpatients. *Hypertension.* 2017;69(1):136–142. http://hyper.ahajournals.org/content/69/1/136.abstract.
57. Rostand SG, Drueke TB. Parathyroid hormone, vitamin D, and cardiovascular disease in chronic renal failure. *Kidney Int.* 1999;56(2):383–392. 10.1046/j.1523-1755.1999.00575.x.
58. Dupont S, Maizel J, Mentaverri R, et al. The onset of left ventricular diastolic dysfunction in SHR rats is not related to hypertrophy or hypertension. *Am J Physiol Heart Circ Physiol.* 2012;302(7):H1524–H1532. doi: 10.1152/ajpheart.00955.2010.
59. Hamdani N, Bishu KG, von Frieling-Salewsky M, et al. Deranged myofilament phosphorylation and function in experimental heart failure with preserved ejection fraction. *Cardiovasc Res.* 2013;97(3):464–471. doi: 10.1093/cvr/cvs353.
60. Fontes-Carvalho R, Ladeiras-Lopes R, Bettencourt P, et al. Diastolic dysfunction in the diabetic continuum: association with insulin resistance, metabolic syndrome and type 2 diabetes. *Cardiovasc Diabetol.* 2015;14:4. doi: 10.1186/s12933-014-0168-x.
61. Borlaug BA, Redfield MM, Melenovsky V, et al. Longitudinal changes in left ventricular stiffness: a community-based study. *Circ Heart Fail.* 2013;6(5):944–952. doi: 10.1161/CIRCHEARTFAILURE.113.000383.
62. Karimian S, Stein J, Bauer B, et al. Improvement of impaired diastolic left ventricular function after diet-induced weight reduction in severe obesity. *Diabetes Metab Syndr Obesity Targets Ther.* 2017;10:19–25. doi: 10.2147/DMSO.S124541.
63. Wan SH, Vogel MW, Chen HH. Pre-clinical diastolic dysfunction. *J Am Coll Cardiol.* 2014;63(5):407–416. doi: 10.1016/j.jacc.2013.10.063.
64. Redfield MM, Jacobsen SJ, Burnett JCJ, et al. Burden of systolic and diastolic ventricular dysfunction in the community: appreciating the scope of the heart failure epidemic. *JAMA.* 2003;289(2):194–202.
65. Kane GC, Karon BL, Mahoney DW, et al. Progression of left ventricular diastolic dysfunction and risk of heart failure. *JAMA.* 2011;306(8):856–863. doi: 10.1001/jama.2011.1201.
66. Klingbeil AU, Schneider M, Martus P, et al. A meta-analysis of the effects of treatment on left ventricular mass in essential hypertension. *Am J Med.* 2003;115(1):41–46.
67. Devereux RB, Dahlöf B, Gerdts E, et al. Regression of hypertensive left ventricular hypertrophy by losartan compared with atenolol: the Losartan Intervention for Endpoint Reduction in Hypertension (LIFE) trial. *Circulation.* 2004;110(11):1456–1462. doi: 10.1161/01.CIR.0000141573.44737.5A.
68. Devereux RB, Palmieri V, Sharpe N, et al. Effects of once-daily angiotensin-converting enzyme inhibition and calcium channel blockade-based antihypertensive treatment regimens on left ventricular hypertrophy and diastolic filling in hypertension: The Prospective Randomized Enalapril Study Evaluating Regression of Ventricular Enlargement (PRESERVE) Trial. *Circulation.* 2001;104(11):1248–1254. https://www.ahajournals.org/doi/full/10.1161/hc3601.095927.
69. Solomon SD, Janardhanan R, Verma A, et al. Effect of angiotensin receptor blockade and antihypertensive drugs on diastolic function in patients with hypertension and diastolic dysfunction: a randomised trial. *Lancet (London, England).* 2007;369(9579):2079–2087. doi: 10.1016/S0140-6736(07)60980-5.
70. From AM, Scott CG, Chen HH. The development of heart failure in patients with diabetes mellitus and pre-clinical diastolic dysfunction: a population-based study. *J Am Coll Cardiol.* 2010;55(4):300–305. doi: 10.1016/j.jacc.2009.12.003.
71. Steinberg BA, Zhao X, Heidenreich PA, et al. Trends in patients hospitalized with heart failure and preserved left ventricular ejection fraction: prevalence, therapies, and outcomes. *Circulation.* 2012;126(1):65–75. doi: 10.1161/CIRCULATIONAHA.111.080770.
72. Hedman A, Samad BA, Larsson T, et al. Improvement in diastolic left ventricular function after coronary artery bypass grafting as assessed by recordings of mitral annular velocity using Doppler tissue imaging. *Eur J Echocardiogr J Work Group Echocardiogr Eur Soc Cardiol.* 2005;6(3):202–209. doi: 10.1016/j.euje.2004.09.009.
73. Brecht A, Oertelt-Prigione S, Seeland U, et al. Left atrial function in preclinical diastolic dysfunction: two-dimensional speckle-tracking echocardiography-derived results from the BEFRI trial. *J Am Soc Echocardiogr Off Pub Am Soc Echocardiogr.* 2016;29(8):750–758. doi: 10.1016/j.echo.2016.03.013.
74. Reddy YNV, Carter RE, Obokata M, et al. A simple, evidence-based approach to help guide diagnosis of heart failure with preserved ejection fraction. *Circulation.* 2018;138:861–870. http://circ.ahajournals.org/content/early/2018/05/22/CIRCULATIONAHA.118.034646.abstract.
75. Nagueh SF, Smiseth OA, Appleton CP, et al. Recommendations for the evaluation of left ventricular diastolic function by echocardiography: an update from the American Society of Echocardiography and the European Association of Cardiovascular Imaging. *J Am Soc Echocardiogr Off Pub Am Soc Echocardiogr.* 2016;29(4):277–314. doi: 10.1016/j.echo.2016.01.011.
76. McLaughlin VV, Shah SJ, Souza R, et al. Management of pulmonary arterial hypertension. *J Am Coll Cardiol.* 2015;65(18):1976–1997. http://www.onlinejacc.org/content/65/18/1976.abstract.
77. Welch TD, Ling LH, Espinosa RE, et al. et al. Echocardiographic diagnosis of constrictive pericarditis: Mayo Clinic criteria. *Circ Cardiovasc Imag.* 2014;7(3):526–534. doi: 10.1161/CIRCIMAGING.113.001613.
78. Sengupta PP, Krishnamoorthy VK, Abhayaratna WP, et al. Disparate patterns of left ventricular mechanics differentiate constrictive pericarditis

from restrictive cardiomyopathy. *JACC Cardiovasc Imag.* 2008;1(1):29–38. doi: 10.1016/j.jcmg.2007.10.006.

79. Scherr J, Jung P, Schuster T, et al. Left ventricular diastolic function is strongly correlated with active emptying of the left atrium: a novel analysis using three-dimensional echocardiography. *Cardiovasc Ultrasound.* 2016;14(1):43. doi: 10.1186/s12947-016-0085-0.
80. Santos M, Rivero J, McCullough SD, et al. E/e' ratio in patients with unexplained dyspnea: lack of accuracy in estimating left ventricular filling pressure. *Circ Heart Fail.* 2015;8(4):749–756. doi: 10.1161/CIRCHEARTFAILURE.115.002161.
81. Andersen OS, Smiseth OA, Dokainish H, et al. Estimating left ventricular filling pressure by echocardiography. *J Am Coll Cardiol.* 2017;69(15):1937–1948. doi: 10.1016/j.jacc.2017.01.058.
82. Little WC, Oh JK. Echocardiographic evaluation of diastolic function can be used to guide clinical care. *Circulation.* 2009;120(9):802–809. doi: 10.1161/CIRCULATIONAHA.109.869602.
83. Adamson PB, Abraham WT, Bourge RC, et al. Wireless pulmonary artery pressure monitoring guides management to reduce decompensation in heart failure with preserved ejection fraction. *Circ Heart Fail.* 2014;7(6):935–944. doi: 10.1161/CIRCHEARTFAILURE.113.001229.
84. Shah AM, Claggett B, Sweitzer NK, et al. The prognostic importance of changes in cardiac structure and function in heart failure with preserved ejection fraction and the impact of spironolactone. *Circ Heart Fail.* 2015;8(6):1052–1058. doi: 10.1161/CIRCHEARTFAILURE.115.002249.
85. Omar AMS, Narula S, Abdel Rahman MA, et al. Precision phenotyping in heart failure and pattern clustering of ultrasound data for the assessment of diastolic dysfunction. *JACC Cardiovasc Imag.* 2017;10(11):1291–1303. doi: 10.1016/j.jcmg.2016.10.012.
86. Ter Maaten JM, Damman K, Verhaar MC, et al. Connecting heart failure with preserved ejection fraction and renal dysfunction: the role of endothelial dysfunction and inflammation. *Eur J Heart Fail.* 2016;18(6):588–598. doi: 10.1002/ejhf.497.
87. Shah SJ, Katz DH, Selvaraj S, et al. Phenomapping for novel classification of heart failure with preserved ejection fraction. *Circulation.* 2015;131(3):269–279. doi: 10.1161/CIRCULATIONAHA.114.010637.
88. Solomon SD, Zile M, Pieske B, et al. The angiotensin receptor neprilysin inhibitor LCZ696 in heart failure with preserved ejection fraction: a phase 2 double-blind randomised controlled trial. *Lancet (London, England).* 2012;380(9851):1387–1395. doi: 10.1016/S0140-6736(12)61227-6.
89. Yip GWK, Wang M, Wang T, et al. The Hong Kong diastolic heart failure study: a randomised controlled trial of diuretics, irbesartan and ramipril on quality of life, exercise capacity, left ventricular global and regional function in heart failure with a normal ejection fraction. *Heart.* 2008;94(5):573–580. doi: 10.1136/hrt.2007.117978.
90. Lund LH, Benson L, Dahlstrom U, et al. Association between use of renin-angiotensin system antagonists and mortality in patients with heart failure and preserved ejection fraction. *JAMA.* 2012;308(20):2108–2117. doi: 10.1001/jama.2012.14785.
91. Schwartzenberg S, Redfield MM, From AM, et al. Effects of vasodilation in heart failure with preserved or reduced ejection fraction implications of distinct pathophysiologies on response to therapy. *J Am Coll Cardiol.* 2012;59(5):442–451. doi: 10.1016/j.jacc.2011.09.062.
92. Kasner M, Westermann D, Lopez B, et al. Diastolic tissue Doppler indexes correlate with the degree of collagen expression and cross-linking in heart failure and normal ejection fraction. *J Am Coll Cardiol.* 2011;57(8):977–985. doi: 10.1016/j.jacc.2010.10.024.
93. Kakkar R, Lee RT. Intramyocardial fibroblast myocyte communication. *Circ Res.* 2010;106(1):47–57. doi: 10.1161/CIRCRESAHA.109.207456.
94. Lopez B, Querejeta R, Gonzalez A, et al. Impact of treatment on myocardial lysyl oxidase expression and collagen cross-linking in patients with heart failure. *Hypertension (Dallas, Texas).* 1979/2009;53(2):236–242. doi: 10.1161/HYPERTENSIONAHA.108.125278.
95. Pandey A, Garg S, Matulevicius SA, et al. Effect of mineralocorticoid receptor antagonists on cardiac structure and function in patients with diastolic dysfunction and heart failure with preserved ejection fraction: a meta-analysis and systematic review. *J Am Heart Assoc.* 2015;4(10):e002137. doi: 10.1161/JAHA.115.002137.
96. Redfield MM, Chen HH, Borlaug BA, et al. Effect of phosphodiesterase-5 inhibition on exercise capacity and clinical status in heart failure with preserved ejection fraction: a randomized clinical trial. *JAMA.* 2013;309(12):1268–1277. doi: 10.1001/jama.2013.2024.
97. Hoendermis ES, Liu LCY, Hummel YM, et al. Effects of sildenafil on invasive haemodynamics and exercise capacity in heart failure patients with preserved ejection fraction and pulmonary hypertension: a randomized controlled trial. *Eur Heart J.* 2015;36(38):2565–2573. doi: 10.1093/eurheartj/ehv336.
98. Opitz CF, Hoeper MM, Gibbs JSR, et al. Pre-capillary, combined, and post-capillary pulmonary hypertension: a pathophysiological continuum. *J Am Coll Cardiol.* 2016;68(4):368–378. doi: 10.1016/j.jacc.2016.05.047.
99. Guazzi M, Vicenzi M, Arena R, et al. Pulmonary hypertension in heart failure with preserved ejection fraction: a target of phosphodiesterase-5 inhibition in a 1-year study. *Circulation.* 2011;124(2):164–174. doi: 10.1161/CIRCULATIONAHA.110.983866.
100. Bohm M, Perez AC, Jhund PS, et al. Relationship between heart rate and mortality and morbidity in the irbesartan patients with heart failure and preserved systolic function trial (I-Preserve). *Eur J Heart Fail.* 2014;16(7):778–787. doi: 10.1002/ejhf.85.
101. Pal N, Sivaswamy N, Mahmod M, et al. Effect of selective heart rate slowing in heart failure with preserved ejection fraction. *Circulation.* 2015;132(18):1719–1725. doi: 10.1161/CIRCULATIONAHA.115.017119.
102. Mitter SS, Shah SJ, Thomas JD. A test in context: E/A and E/e' to assess diastolic dysfunction and LV filling pressure. *J Am Coll Cardiol.* 2017;69(11):1451–1464. doi: 10.1016/j.jacc.2016.12.037.
103. Zakeri R, Chamberlain AM, Roger VL, et al. Temporal relationship and prognostic significance of atrial fibrillation in heart failure patients with preserved ejection fraction: a community-based study. *Circulation.* 2013;128(10):1085–1093. 10.1161/CIRCULATIONAHA.113.001475.
104. Lam CSP, Rienstra M, Tay WT, et al. Atrial fibrillation in heart failure with preserved ejection fraction: association with exercise capacity, left ventricular filling pressures, natriuretic peptides, and left atrial volume. *JACC Heart Fail.* 2017;5(2):92–98. doi: 10.1016/j.jchf.2016.10.005.
105. Machino-Ohtsuka T, Seo Y, Ishizu T, et al. Efficacy, safety, and outcomes of catheter ablation of atrial fibrillation in patients with heart failure with preserved ejection fraction. *J Am Coll Cardiol.* 2013;62(20):1857–1865. doi: 10.1016/j.jacc.2013.07.020.

36

Future Therapies in HFpEF

Pavan Bhat and W.H. Wilson Tang

OUTLINE

INTRODUCTION

The treatment of diastolic heart failure (HF), also known as heart failure with preserved systolic function (HFpEF), has been challenging, partly because there is a lack of consensus regarding the definition of the disease entity as well as a paucity of large-scale clinical trials to demonstrate effective therapeutic strategies. Diastolic and systolic HF may have certain similar pathophysiologic processes in common, but there are also distinct differences in myocardial structure and function. Most treatment strategies for diastolic HF strive to alleviate signs and symptoms or prevent exacerbating factors rather than alter the underlying pathophysiologic abnormalities (such as improving active relaxation or reducing passive stiffness). Several lines of new investigations have identified regression of left ventricular (LV) hypertrophy as a potential target of therapy, while others hope to improve outcomes in patients with features of diastolic HF via novel targets. Some of these drugs have already been approved for other indications, and improvement in diastolic dysfunction is considered an ancillary property that may have potential for further clinical development. This chapter summarizes the ongoing efforts to develop future therapies targeting extrinsic or intrinsic factors in diastolic HF.

PATHOPHYSIOLOGY AND CLINICAL RELEVANCE

HFpEF patients have underlying diastolic stiffness, which can be attributed to excessive myocardial collagen deposition and cardiomyocyte stiffness. A new paradigm has been recently postulated that identifies a proinflammatory state in the endothelium induced by comorbidities as the origin of endothelial cell inflammation, which triggers the cardiac remodeling that is specific for HFpEF.

Targeting Intracellular Intrinsic Factors: Metabolic Modulation

NO-cGMP-PK Activators

The endothelium plays an important role in cardiovascular homeostasis by regulating cardiac function, vasomotor tone, and vascular permeability. The release of nitric oxide (NO) by the endothelium is crucial for normal function. The HFpEF-associated comorbidities lead to endothelial dysfunction through disruption of the intracellular nitrogen monoxide–cyclic guanosine monophosphate (cGMP)–protein kinase (NO-cGMP-PK) signal cascade.[1] A disorder in this signal cascade contributes to the development of remodeling, including increased cardiomyocyte stiffness that is characteristic of HFpEF. The disruption of the NO-cGMP-PK signal cascade has been showed to lead to disturbances in the regulation of titin and an increase in fibrosis. Specifically the decline of cGMP through a NO mediated signal cascade has been shown to be specific during HFpEF remodeling and differs from HFrEF.[2] Targeting the NO-cGMP-PK signal cascade offers new future therapeutic options to intervene in the remodeling that is characteristic of HFpEF. Possible future therapies that interfere with this signal cascade include endothelial NO-synthase (eNOS) activators, inorganic nitrates, neprilysin inhibition, phosphodiesterase-5 inhibition, or soluble guanylate cyclase stimulators, which will be discussed in the following sections.

Organic Nitrates and eNOS Activators

Direct NO donators such as isosorbide mononitrate are not seen as an effective treatment for HFpEF. A prior double-blinded crossover study with 110 patients with HFpEF showed that HFpEF patients on isosorbide mononitrate were less active and did not have a better quality of life compared to placebo.[3] However, eNOS activators such as the eNOS transcription amplifier AVE3085 have had favorable outcomes in animal models.[4] In this study HFpEF was induced in 60 salt-sensitive rats, with 30 treated with AVE3085 and 30 treated with placebo. Treatment with AVE3085 significantly increased eNOS messenger ribonucleic acid (mRNA) and protein levels in cardiac tissue in the test animals. Diastolic dysfunction as measured by invasive pressure-volume (P-V) loop measurements, were attenuated in the AVE3085 group. Additionally, cardiac hypertrophy as measured by LV mass measurements by echocardiography showed improvement compared to the untreated animals. Treatment with AVE3085 for improvement in cardiac hypertrophy appears promising, but since the majority of data have been in animal models up to this point, applicability to patients with HFpEF still remains to be proven.

Inorganic Nitrates, Nitrites, and Beetroot Juice

In addition to organic nitrates, inorganic nitrates also represent an important route to increase myocardial NO bioavailability in patients with HFpEF.[5] The prior evidence of benefit of inorganic nitrates is based in prior studies involving acute infusion of sodium nitrate. In this study 28 patients with HFpEF underwent invasive cardiac catheterization at rest and during exercise and were randomized to either receiving sodium nitrite or placebo. The infusion of sodium nitrite resulted in significant reduction in exercise pulmonary capillary wedge pressure (PCWP), improvement of cardiac output with exercise, and normalization in the increase of cardiac output relative to oxygen consumption.[6] Other studies showed similar effects by inhaled sodium nitrite.[7] Further studies have looked at inorganic nitrates, which are precursors to nitrite and converted within the body. A study looking at beetroot juice drink as a source of inorganic nitrates showed improved submaximal exercise endurance in patients with HFpEF who were given daily beetroot juice for 1 week.[8] Recently the trial INDIE-HFpEF looked at the effect of 4 weeks of administration of inhaled inorganic nitrates on exercise capacity in patients with HFpEF, showing no significant improvement in exercise capacity.[9] Overall the data have shown that inhaled inorganic nitrates show no definitive benefits in patients with HFpEF; however, other modes of inorganic delivery may show benefit in future studies. The currently ongoing Inorganic Nitrate and Exercise Performance in Heart Failure (iNIX-HF) study is looking at the effects of an orally delivered inorganic nitrate pill compared to a beet juice drink, which is a source of inorganic nitrates. If the results of this study are promising, this allows reliable oral delivery of inorganic nitrates, which could be crucial for future HFpEF therapy.

Angiotensin Receptor and Neprilysin Inhibition

Sacubitril/valsartan is an active drug of investigation for future HFpEF therapies. Prior studies suggest that sacubitril/valsartan can stimulate the NO-cGMP-PK signal cascades. Specifically, neprilysin prevents degradation of numerous vasoactive peptides, including brain natriuretic peptide (BNP), which are thought to stimulate the formation of cGMP, which is involved in the remodeling process within HFpEF. The phase II PARAMOUNT trial investigated the change in N-terminal proBNP (NT-proBNP) in patients with HFpEF and showed a significant reduction in NT-proBNP levels in patients with HFpEF treated with sacubitril/valsartan.[10] Clinical outcomes were not assessed in these patients in the PARAMOUNT trial. Recently completed, the PARAGON-HF trial examined the effect of sacubitril/valsartan on reduction of cardiovascular death and HF hospitalizations in patients with HFpEF.[11] The results of PARAMOUNT showed no benefit of sacubitril/valsartan in total hospitalization for heart failure and death from cardiovascular causes with ejection fraction > 45%. However, subgroup analysis showed possible benefit in HFpEF patients with low normal ejection fractions and women. Further studies are necessary to further study these subgroups. In this study, sacubitril–valsartan did not result in a significantly lower rate of total hospitalizations for heart failure and death from cardiovascular causes. Moreover, patients assigned to the sacubitril–valsartan group had a higher incidence of hypotension and angioedema.

Phosphodiesterease-5 (PDE5) Inhibitors

Many patients with primary pulmonary hypertension also have concomitant HFpEF. Prior studies with patients with HFpEF and pulmonary hypertension showed that treatment with the PDE5 inhibitor sildenafil led to decreased pulmonary arterial pressures and improved functional capacity and improved diastolic dysfunction.[12] However, the RELAX study looked at HFpEF patients without pulmonary hypertension and showed no improvement in exercise capacity or clinical status.[13] Similarly, the BADDHY study looked at patients with HFpEF and pulmonary hypertension and looked at bosentan versus placebo therapy and noted no beneficial effects in the bosentan group.[14] Further studies are ongoing looking at the combination of phosphodiesterase inhibitors with endothelin antagonists in patients with HFpEF and pulmonary hypertension; however, given the negative results of the BADDHY study and the lack of improvement in exercise capacity in the RELAX study, the future of PDE5 inhibitors in HFpEF remains in question.

Soluble Guanylate Cyclase Stimulators and Activators

Insufficient generation of cGMP by soluble guanylase cyclase (sGC) may contribute to the pathophysiology of HFpEF via NO-cGMP-PK signal cascade as described earlier in this chapter. Direct stimulators of sGC differ from the other agents discussed earlier targeting cGMP as they are NO independent in their capacity to increase sGC activity. Vericiguat is a sGC stimulator that was studied in the SOCRATES-PRESERVED study. In SOCRATES-PRESERVED, patients with HFpEF received vericiguat or placebo.[15] Vericiguat was well tolerated and associated with improvements in quality of life but did not change NT-proBNP. However, preliminary results from the recently completed VITALITY-HFpEF trial which randomized 789 patients in 1:1:1 fashion to either placebo, 10mg vericiguat, or 15mg vericiguat did not show any benefit compared to placebo. Specifically they noted no significant difference in symptoms as assessed by the Kansas City Cardiomyopathy Questionnaire Physical limitation score (KCCQ PLS) and no change in 6 minute walk.[16] Looking at other sGC stimulators, in the DILATE-1 study, patients with HFpEF and pulmonary hypertension were randomized to riociguat versus placebo. In that study, riociguat did not significantly effect mean pulmonary arterial pressures, but there was an increase in stroke volume and cardiac index and a decrease in systolic blood pressure (BP) and right ventricular end-diastolic area.[17] Further clinic studies are underway; however, all the data for vericiguat and riociguat so far have looked at improvement of indirect hemodynamic variables as opposed to exercise tolerance. At this point, further studies concentrating on HFpEF patients' exercise capacity are required to demonstrate the clinical utility of vericiguat and riociguat.

Endothelin Receptor Antagonism

Endothelin-1 (ET-1) antagonists are elevated and predict mortality in patients with HFrEF. ET-1 as well as both its receptors, ET-A and ET-B, are synthesized and secreted by cardiac myocytes. ET-1 is associated with abnormalities in endothelial function, vascular compliance, pulmonary hypertension, impaired diastolic relaxation, and myocardial fibrosis, which points toward ET-1 being involved in HFpEF pathophysiology. The ET-A antagonist sitaxsentan was examined in a phase II study involving 192 HFpEF patients.[18] Treatment with sitaxsentan was associated with increased exercise tolerance but no changes in LV mass or diastolic function in patients with HFpEF. Other studies looking at the dual ET-A/ET-B receptor antagonist macitentan in a murine model of HFpEF showed that macitentan decreased LV hypertrophy and significantly reduced wall thickness measured by echocardiogram.[19] In addition, the same study showed macitentan improved adverse cardiac remodeling but reduced the stiffer cardiac collagen-1 and titin N2B expression in the left ventricle. Further human studies are underway looking at the effects of dual ET-A/ET-B receptor antagonism in patients with HFpEF. Given the prior studies showing improvement in echocardiographic parameters, this remains a promising target for future therapies.

Inflammation and Cytokine Inhibition

The pathophysiology of HFpEF involves chronic myocardial inflammation. Prior studies that looked at endomyocardial biopsy samples of patients with HFpEF showed increased cardiac collagen and an increase in inflammatory cells in patients with HFpEF versus normal controls.[20] Other studies, using a cardiac fibroblast cell culture system, showed that mechanical stretch mimicking cardiac dilation in HF induces activation of fibroblasts. In addition to activation of fibroblasts, the cell cultures also upregulate chemokine production and trigger typical inflammatory pathways in vitro.[21] This points to one general mechanism where mechanical stretch of cardiac tissue leads to inflammation, which can cause permanent remodeling. Specifically, interleukin-1 (IL-1) has been a key proinflammatory cytokine that has been implicated in impaired myocardial relaxation. In the D-HART study, 12 patients with HFpEF were enrolled in a double-blind, randomized, placebo-controlled, crossover trial and assigned to receive anakinra (IL-1 antibody) or placebo. The results showed anakinra led to a statistically significant improvement in peak oxygen consumption and significant reduction in plasma C-reactive protein (CRP) levels. In conclusion, IL-1 blockade with anakinra significantly reduced systemic inflammatory response and improved the aerobic exercise capacity in patients with HFpEF.

Modulators of Intracellular Calcium Homeostasis

Chronic HFpEF is associated with increased sympathetic outflow, which through long-term neurohormonal activation induced significant damage to the heart. Specifically, it leads to multiple alterations in the β-adrenergic receptor (β-AR) signaling cascade. Activation of β-ARs increases cyclic adenosine monophosphate (cAMP) production and results in protein kinase A (PKA) phosphorylation of key regulators of contraction coupling such as L-type Ca^{2+} channels, phospholamban, troponin I, ryanodine receptors (RyR),[22] myosin-binding protein Cm, and protein phosphate inhibitor-1.[23] There is evidence that alterations in the sarcoplasmic reticulum (SR) Ca^{2+} cycling are a component of the impaired contractile performance of HFpEF patients. The abnormal intracellular calcium handling includes SR calcium leak through the RyR, decreased SR calcium uptake, and decreased SR content. RyR2 stabilizers such as JTV519 (K201), which stabilizes RYR2s and decreases SR Ca^{2+} leak, have been shown to improve diastolic function in vitro in murine experimental models.[24] Other studies have shown that SEA0400, an Na^{+}/Ca^{2+} exchanger (NCX) inhibitor, has improved diastolic relaxation in rat animal models with HFpEF. SEA0400 was also associated with improved cardiac remodeling when given chronically to rat models with HFpEF.[25] Overall both of these novel substances have only shown improvement in HFpEF in animal models and have not yet been tested in human subjects.

Targeting Extracellular Intrinsic Factors: Noncardiac Mechanisms

Glucose-Lowering Drugs

Sodium glucose cotransporter-2 (SGLT2) inhibitors. The EMPA-REG OUTCOME trial looked at empagliflozin, a SGLT2 inhibitor in patients with type 2 diabetes. The results showed a 38% relative risk reduction, 38% in death from cardiovascular causes, 35% relative risk reduction for hospitalization for HF, and a 32% relative risk reduction for death from any cause.[26] This study did not specifically look at patients with HFrEF or HFpEF, but rather patients with type 2 diabetes at increased cardiovascular risk. The mechanism of effect of the cardiovascular benefit of empagliflozin is that the drug induces a mild hyperketonemia. In this state ketones are taken up by the cardiac tissue and oxidized to fatty acids, which would improve the efficiency of oxygen consumption of cardiac mitochondria during work. This hypothesis is known as the "thrifty substrate hypothesis."[27] Given that the prior studies did not specifically look at patients with HFpEF, future studies targeting this population are required to determine the true benefit of this therapy.

Incretins. Incretins are a group of metabolic hormones that stimulate a decrease in blood glucose levels. Incretins are released after eating and augment the stimulation of insulin from the pancreatic beta islet cells. Glucagon-like peptide-1 (GLP-1) analogues and dipeptidylpeptidase 4 (DDP-4) inhibitors are two classes of medications that have been used to stimulate this metabolic pathway. GLP-1 is a hormone in the incretin family, and GLP receptors have been found in cardiac tissue.[28] Stimulation of cardiac GLP receptors leads to increased cardiac glucose intake, which activates myocyte glycolysis.[29] Specifically the GLP-1 analogue exenatide has been shown to improve cardiac diastolic function in patients with diabetes.[30,31] Similarly, DDP-4 inhibitors are currently being studied in regard to their effect on patients with HFpEF. The DDP-4 inhibitors linagliptin and sitagliptin have been shown to improve diastolic function in patients with diabetes, HFpEF, and chronic kidney disease.[32] Future studies are needed to further clarify the role that GLP-1 analogues and DDP-4 have in improving diastolic function in both diabetics and nondiabetics.

Szeto-Schiller (SS) Peptides

Therapies to treat HF focus on fixing the mismatch between adenosine triphosphate (ATP) supply and demand. There are multiple reasons why there might be a mismatch: ischemia producing increased workload, hypertension, diastolic dysfunction, and cellular malfunctions. The majority of current therapies on decreased ATP demand by decreasing workload. A different approach targeting mitochondrial function to improve ATP supply might provide new therapies for HFpEF. SS peptides are novel mitochondria-targeted antioxidant peptides that were developed to target the inner mitochondrial membrane with antioxidants. This reduces mitochondrial free radicals and prevents oxidant-induced cell death.[33] SS-31 is one such SS peptide, also named MTP-131 or elamipretide, which is currently being studied in phase II clinical trials for HFrEF and HFpEF.

Advanced Glycation End Product Crosslink Breakers

Inflammation can lead to oxidative stress, which leads to the formation of advanced glycation end products (AGEs). AGEs are where protein and carbohydrates form an interlinking crosslink with the extracellular matrix.[34] Alagebrium chloride is a compound described as a crosslink breaker. In a small study involving patients with HFpEF, 16 weeks of alagebrium chloride resulted in improved diastolic function.[35] Another therapeutic target in the AGE pathway is lysl oxidase-like 2 (LOXL2), which is an enzyme involved in the crosslinking of collagen and has been shown to be involved in the fibrosis of HF. Prior studies have shown that using a LOXL2-specific neutralizing monoclonal antibody to inhibit LOXL2 activity in mouse hearts decreases stress-induced fibrosis, ventricular dilation, and systolic and diastolic dysfunction.[36] Given the small number of patients recruited in the prior human studies, larger human studies need to be undertaken to determine the utility, but the data from these early studies appear promising.

Micro-RNA Regulation

Micro-RNAs (miRNAs) are small noncoding RNA (containing about 22 nucleotides) that function in RNA silencing and posttranscriptional regulation of gene expression. MiRNAs have been reported to regulate genes involved in many essential disease processes as well as HF.[37] Additionally, both HFrEF and HFpEF have been found to have different miRNA profiles.[38,39] In addition to their usefulness as a biomarker, miRNAs offer a potential therapeutic target for future drug therapy in HF. A prior study looking at the inhibition of miRNA-21 (miR-21) in rat cardiomyocytes in cell culture as a rat model of HFpEF showed that, after injection of a miR-21 antagonist, the cardiac atrophy and cardiac fibrosis typical of HFpEF was reduced.[40] Given the limited experience in miRNA therapy in humans overall, further testing showing the safety of miRNA therapies in humans needs to be undertaken before the clinical utility of inhibition miR-21 can be investigated.

Novel Device Therapies

Interatrial Septal Devices

One of the hemodynamic effects of treating HFpEF is reduction in the left atrial (LA) pressure.[41] The fundamental concept of interatrial septal devices (IASDs) depends on the Lutembacher syndrome, which is the observation that patients with untreated mitral stenosis and atrial defect with left to right shunt had better survival. A small pilot trial involving 11 patients with HFpEF was undertaken to assess the utility of IASDs. The inclusion criteria included an EF greater than 45%, PCWP greater than 15 mmHg (rest) or greater than 25 mmHg (exercise), and more than one hospitalization for HF within the last 12 months, or New York Heart Association (NYHA) Class III/IV symptoms. In these patients an IASD was implanted using percutaneous transseptal access via the femoral vein. At 30 days, LV pressures were significantly reduced by 5.5 mmHg, and NYHA class was improved by two classes in two patients, one class in five patients, and worsened by one class in one patient.[42] A larger study, the REDUCE LAP-HF, looked at 68 HFpEF patients who underwent IASD implantation. After 6 months 52% of patients had reduction in PCWP at rest, 58% had a lower PCWP during exertion, and 39% had both.[43] However, REDUCE LAP-HF had not looked if the lower PCWPs translate to improvements in symptoms, which is a concentration of further ongoing studies. The V-wave system is an interatrial shunt system that has been associated with improved clinical and functional status in patients with heart failure. A recent feasibly and safety study looked at 38 patients with HFpEF with NYHA class III symptoms after V-wave implantation. The overall result of the study showed no significant increase in device related adverse events, but a significant improvement in NYHA class, quality of life, and 6-minute walk distance.[44] Further larger randomized trials are currently underway to confirm these preliminary results with the V-wave system.

Cardiac Contractility Modulation

Cardiac contractility modulation (CCM) therapy is delivered by a pacemaker-like device that applies an electrical signal during the refractory period to the septum. Since the electrical signal is applied during the refractory period there is no cardiac muscle contraction; however, the electrical signals increase the influx of calcium ions in the cardiomyocytes potentially triggering molecular remodeling. This is thought to improve symptoms of HFrEF patients.[45] A case series looking at CCM therapy in patients with HFpEF found an improvement in NYHA classification, 6-minute walking distance, quality of life, improvement in diastolic filling parameters, and improvement in EF reserve.[46] A phase II trial investing the role of CCM in HFpEF patients is currently ongoing.

Renal Denervation and Baroreflex Activation Therapy

One of the underlying mechanisms of HFpEF is increased sympathetic tone. Reduction of sympathetic tone can be achieved by renal denervation. Prior studies looked at the effect of catheter-based renal denervation on LV hypertrophy and diastolic function in patients with resistant hypertension. In that study, 45 patients with resistant hypertension underwent bilateral renal denervation. Compared to controls, the intervention decreased LV mass and improved diastolic function in addition to improving BP.[47] The RDT-PEF study was a prospective trial that further investigated this effect.[48] In this trial 25 patients were randomized to renal denervation or medical therapy. There was no difference between intervention and control at 12 months for Minnesota Living with Heart Failure Questionnaire, peak VO_2 at exercise, BNP E/e′, or LV mass index. However, more patients in the intervention arm had improved peak VO_2, but this was not significant. Future larger studies may show that this is a significant difference and needs additional investigation.

Baroreflex activation therapy (BAT) works by stimulating the carotid sinus via an implanted electrode close to the carotid sinus region, which elicits a reflex through the sympathetic and vagal nervous system that reduces BP. Similar to renal denervation, this device has been primarily studied for resistant hypertension. This therapy has been studied in HFrEF in the Barostim HOPE4HF study.[49] In this study 146 patients with EF less than 35% and NYHA Class III symptoms were randomized to placebo and BAT in a 1:1 distribution. The results showed that BAT was safe and improved functional status, quality of life, and exercise capacity and reduced NT-proBNP in the intervention group. So far, all the research for BAT has concentrated on HFrEF patients, but dedicated studies concentrating on HFpEF are required to show if this can be a viable therapy in this patient population.

FUTURE DIRECTIONS

Drugs and devices developed to treat diastolic HF are thought to hold limited commercial promise because they are primarily add-on therapies in a study population in which treatment goals and treatment outcomes are not well defined. The therapeutic options discussed in this chapter are just some of the examples on which there are published data or that are currently in active clinical development. The fact that there are a limited number of pipeline drugs that specifically target diastolic HF brings home the point that we are in the infancy of understanding the underlying pathophysiology of diastolic HF. Furthermore, the association between improvements of echocardiographic indices of diastolic dysfunction may not relate directly to clinical efficacy. Although LV hypertrophy regression appears to be a good surrogate end point for diastolic HF, definitive proof for this is not yet available.

From what we understand now, drugs that affect calcium homeostasis will emerge as important players in this field, although existing neurohormonal antagonists will maintain their presence in the diastolic HF regimen. New targets will emerge, and new drug classes (e.g., AGE crosslink breakers) will be tested as we broaden our understanding of the diversity of diastolic HF. Metabolic modulation has also shown great promise as we begin to understand the close connections between myocardial and vascular metabolic derangements and diastolic dysfunction.

Device implantation for treating diastolic HF will need further development to reduce the procedural risks, invasiveness, and expense. Nevertheless, intracardiac hemodynamic monitoring devices will likely play an important role in guiding therapy in this population. The road to clinical development in diastolic HF is tortuous and demanding, but at the same time it is exciting and rewarding as it brings new ideas, new challenges, and new hopes.

KEY POINTS

- A proinflammatory state in the endothelium triggers cardiac remodeling, which is specific for HFpEF. Endomyocardial biopsy samples of patients with HFpEF show increased cardiac collagen and an increase in inflammatory cells.
- Inflammation can lead to oxidative stress, which leads to the formation of advanced glycation products.
- HFpEF-associated comorbidities lead to endothelial dysfunction through disruption of the intracellular NO-cGMP-PK signal cascade.

- In addition to organic nitrates, inorganic nitrates represent an important route to increase myocardial NO bioavailability in patients with HFpEF.
- Insufficient generation of cGMP by sGC may contribute to the pathophysiology of HFpEF.
- ET-1 antagonists are elevated and predict mortality in patients with HFrEF.
- IL-1 has been a key proinflammatory cytokine that has been implicated in impaired myocardial relaxation.
- Increased sympathetic outflow in HFpEF is associated with induced myocardial cell injury.
- SGLT2 inhibitors in patients with type 2 diabetes have shown a reduction in death and hospitalization for HF.
- Stimulation of cardiac GLP receptors lead to increased cardiac glucose intake, which has shown to improve cardiac diastolic function in patients with diabetes.
- Targeting mitochondrial function to improve ATP supply might provide new therapies for HFpEF.
- IASDs, to allow left to right shunt, have been shown to decrease LV filling pressures and improve NYHA class in HF patients.
- BAT may be helpful in hypertensive-induced HF by eliciting a reflex through the sympathetic and vagal nervous system that reduces BP.

REVIEW QUESTIONS

1. Endothelial dysfunction through disruption of the intracellular NO-cGMP-PK signal cascade results in
   a. increased myocardial relaxation.
   b. increased cardiomyocyte stiffness.
   c. reduced levels of titin.
   d. decreased generation of NT-proBNP.
2. Which of the following hemodynamic effects is expected during the infusion of sodium nitrite in HFpEP patients?
   a. Increased capillary wedge pressure
   b. Increased cardiac output
   c. Increased oxygen consumption relative to cardiac output
   d. Increased LV stiffness
3. Which of the following glucose-lowering drug classes has demonstrated reduction in cardiovascular death and HF hospitalization?
   a. Sodium glucose cotransporter-2 inhibitors
   b. Glucagon-like peptide analogues
   c. Biguanides
   d. Sulfonylureas

REFERENCES

1. Tschöpe C, Van Linthout S. New insights in (Inter)cellular mechanisms by heart failure with preserved ejection fraction. *Curr Heart Fail Rep.* 2014;11(4):436–444. doi:10.1007/s11897-014-0219-3.
2. Van Heerebeek L, Hamdani N, Falcão-Pires I, et al. Low myocardial protein kinase G activity in heart failure with preserved ejection fraction. *Circulation.* 2012;126(7):830–839. doi:10.1161/CIRCULATIONAHA.111.
3. Redfield MM, Anstrom KJ, Levine JA, et al. Isosorbide mononitrate in heart failure with preserved ejection fraction. *N Engl J Med.* 2015;373(24):2314–2324. doi:10.1056/NEJMoa1510774.
4. Westermann D, Riad A, Richter U, et al. Enhancement of the endothelial NO synthase attenuates experimental diastolic heart failure. *Basic Res Cardiol.* 2009;104(5):499–509. doi:10.1007/s00395-009-0014-6.
5. Shah AM, Claggett B, Loehr LR, et al. Heart failure stages among older adults in the community: the atherosclerosis risk in communities study. *Circulation.* 2017;135(3):224–240. doi:10.1161/CIRCULATIONAHA.116.023361.
6. Borlaug BA, Koepp KE, Melenovsky V. Sodium nitrite improves exercise hemodynamics and ventricular performance in heart failure with preserved ejection fraction. *J Am Coll Cardiol.* 2015;66(15):1672–1682. doi:10.1016/J.JACC.2015.07.067.
7. Simon MA, Vanderpool RR, Nouraie M, et al. Acute hemodynamic effects of inhaled sodium nitrite in pulmonary hypertension associated with heart failure with preserved ejection fraction. *JCI Insight.* 2016;1(18):e89620. doi:10.1172/JCI.INSIGHT. 89620.
8. Eggebeen J, Kim-Shapiro DB, Haykowsky M, et al. One week of daily dosing with beetroot juice improves submaximal endurance and blood pressure in older patients with heart failure and preserved ejection fraction. *JACC Heart Fail.* 2016;4(6):428–437. doi:10.1016/J.JCHF. 2015.12.013.
9. Borlaug BA, Anstrom KJ, Lewis GD, et al. Effect of inorganic nitrite vs placebo on exercise capacity among patients with heart failure with preserved ejection fraction. *JAMA.* 2018;320(17):1764. doi:10.1001/jama.2018.14852.
10. Solomon SD, Zile M, Pieske B, et al. The angiotensin receptor neprilysin inhibitor LCZ696 in heart failure with preserved ejection fraction: a phase 2 double-blind randomised controlled trial. *Lancet.* 2012;380(9851):1387–1395. doi:10.1016/S0140-6736(12)61227-6.
11. Solomon SD et al. PARAGON-HF Investigators and Committees. Angiotensin-neprilysin inhibition in heart failure with preserved ejection fraction. *N Engl J Med.* 2019;381:1609–1620. doi:10.1056/NEJMoa1908655.
12. Guazzi M, Vicenzi M, Arena R, Guazzi MD. PDE5 inhibition with sildenafil improves left ventricular diastolic function, cardiac geometry, and clinical status in patients with stable systolic heart failure results of a 1-year, prospective, randomized, placebo-controlled study. *Circ Heart Fail.* 2011;4(1):8–17. doi:10.1161/CIRCHEARTFAILURE.110.944694.
13. Redfield MM, Chen HH, Borlaug BA, et al. Effect of phosphodiesterase-5 inhibition on exercise capacity and clinical status in heart failure with preserved ejection fraction. *JAMA.* 2013;309(12):1268. doi:10.1001/jama.2013.2024.
14. Tschöpe C, Van Linthout S, Kherad B. Heart failure with preserved ejection fraction and future pharmacological strategies: a glance in the crystal ball. *Curr Cardiol Rep.* 2017;19(8):70. doi:10.1007/s11886-017-0874-6.
15. Pieske B, Maggioni AP, Lam CSP, et al. Vericiguat in patients with worsening chronic heart failure and preserved ejection fraction: results of the SOluble guanylate Cyclase stimulatoR in heArT failurE patientS with PRESERVED EF (SOCRATES-PRESERVED) study. *Eur Heart J.* 2017;38(15):1119–1127. doi:10.1093/eurheartj/ehw593.
16. Butler J, et al. Rationale and Design of the VITALITY-HFpEF Trial. *Circ Heart Fail.* 2019 May;12:e005998.doi:10.1161/CIRCHEARTFAILRE.119.005998.
17. Bonderman D, Pretsch I, Steringer-Mascherbauer R, et al. Acute hemodynamic effects of riociguat in patients with pulmonary hypertension associated with diastolic heart failure (DILATE-1): a randomized, double-blind, placebo-controlled, single-dose study. *Chest.* 2014;146(5):1274–1285. doi:10.1378/chest.14-0106.
18. Zile MR, Bourge RC, Redfield MM, Zhou D, Baicu CF, Little WC. Randomized, double-blind, placebo-controlled study of sitaxsentan to improve impaired exercise tolerance in patients with heart failure and a preserved ejection fraction. *JACC Heart Fail.* 2014;2:123–130. doi:10.1016/j.jchf.2013.12.002.
19. Valero-Munoz M, Li S, Wilson RM, Boldbaatar B, Iglarz M, Sam F. Dual endothelin-A/endothelin-B receptor blockade and cardiac remodeling in heart failure with preserved ejection fraction. *Circ Heart Fail.* 2016;9(11):e003381. doi:10.1161/CIRCHEARTFAILURE.116.003381.
20. Westermann D, Lindner D, Kasner M, et al. Cardiac inflammation contributes to changes in the extracellular matrix in patients with heart failure and normal ejection fraction. *Circ Heart Fail.* 2011;4(1):44–52. doi:10.1161/CIRCHEARTFAILURE.109.931451.
21. Lindner D, Zietsch C, Tank J, et al. Cardiac fibroblasts support cardiac inflammation in heart failure. *Basic Res Cardiol.* 2014;109(5):428. doi:10.1007/s00395-014-0428-7.

22. Currie S, Elliott EB, Smith GL, Loughrey CM. Two candidates at the heart of dysfunction: the ryanodine receptor and calcium/calmodulin protein kinase II as potential targets for therapeutic intervention—an in vivo perspective. *Pharm Ther.* 2011;131(2):204–220. doi:10.1016/J.PHARMTHERA. 2011.02.006.
23. Lompré AM, Hajjar RJ, Harding SE, Kranias EG, Lohse MJ, Marks AR. Ca^{2+} cycling and new therapeutic approaches for heart failure. *Circulation.* 2010;121(6):822–830. doi:10.1161/CIRCULATIONAHA.109.890954.
24. Sacherer M, Sedej S, Wakuła P, et al. JTV519 (K201) reduces sarcoplasmic reticulum Ca^{2+} leak and improves diastolic function in vitro in murine and human non-failing myocardium. *Br J Pharmacol.* 2012;167(3):493–504. doi:10.1111/j.1476-5381.2012.01995.x.
25. Primessnig U, Schönleitner P, Höll A, et al. Novel pathomechanisms of cardiomyocyte dysfunction in a model of heart failure with preserved ejection fraction. *Eur J Heart Fail.* 2016;18(8):987–997. doi:10.1002/ejhf.524.
26. Zinman B, Wanner C, Lachin JM, et al. Empagliflozin, cardiovascular outcomes, and mortality in type 2 diabetes. *N Engl J Med.* 2015;373(22):2117–2128. doi:10.1056/NEJMoa1504720.
27. Ferrannini E, Mark M, Mayoux E. CV protection in the EMPA-REG OUTCOME trial: a "thrifty substrate" hypothesis. *Diabetes Care.* 2016;39(7):1108–1114. doi:10.2337/dc16-0033.
27. Wei Y, Mojsov S. Tissue-specific expression of the human receptor for glucagon-like peptide-I: brain, heart and pancreatic forms have the same deduced amino acid sequences. *FEBS Letters.* 1995;358(3):219–224. doi:10.1016/0014-5793(94)01430-9.
29. Inzucchi SE, McGuire DK. New drugs for the treatment of diabetes: part II: incretin-based therapy and beyond. *Circulation.* 2008;117(4):574–584. doi:10.1161/CIRCULATIONAHA.107.735795.
30. Wang X, Han L, Yu YR, et al. Effects of GLP-1 agonist exenatide on cardiac diastolic function and vascular endothelial function in diabetic patients. *Sichuan Da Xue Xue Bao. Yi Xue Ban (J Sichuan Univ) Med Sci Ed.* 2015;46(4):586–590. http://www.ncbi.nlm.nih.gov/pubmed/26480664.
31. Scalzo RL, Moreau KL, Ozemek C, et al. Exenatide improves diastolic function and attenuates arterial stiffness but does not alter exercise capacity in individuals with type 2 diabetes. *J Diabetes Complicat.* 2017;31(2):449–455. doi:10.1016/J.JDIACOMP. 2016.10.003.
32. Connelly KA, Bowskill N, Advani S, et al. Dipeptidyl peptidase-4 inhibition improves le ventricular function in chronic kidney disease. *Clinical and Investigative Medicine. Medecine Clinique Et Experimentale.* 2014;37(3):e172–e185.
33. Nickel AG, von Hardenberg A, Hohl M, et al. Reversal of mitochondrial transhydrogenase causes oxidative stress in heart failure. *Cell Metab.* 2015;22(3):472–484. doi:10.1016/j.cmet.2015.07.008.
34. Hartog JWL, Voors AA, Bakker SJL, Smit AJ, van Veldhuisen DJ. Advanced glycation end-products (AGEs) and heart failure: pathophysiology and clinical implications. *Eur J Heart Fail.* 2007;9(12):1146–1155. doi:10.1016/j.ejheart.2007.09.009.
35. Little WC, Zile MR, Kitzman DW, Hundley WG, O'Brien TX, Degroof RC. The effect of alagebrium chloride (ALT-711), a novel glucose cross-link breaker, in the treatment of elderly patients with diastolic heart failure. *J Card Fail.* 2005;11(3):191–195. doi:10.1016/j.cardfail.2004.09.010.
36. Yang J, Savvatis K, Kang JS, Fan P, Zhong H, Schwartz K, et al. Targeting LOXL2 for cardiac interstitial fibrosis and heart failure treatment. *Nat Commun.* 2016;7:13710. doi:10.1038/ncomms13710.
37. Ohtani K, Dimmeler S. Control of cardiovascular differentiation by microRNAs. *Basic Res Cardiol.* 2011;106(1):5–11. doi:10.1007/s00395-010-0139-7.
38. Watson CJ, Gupta SK, O'Connell E, et al. MicroRNA signatures differentiate preserved from reduced ejection fraction heart failure. *Eur J Heart Fail.* 2015;17(4):405–415. doi:10.1002/ejhf.244.
39. Wong LL, Armugam A, Sepramaniam S, et al. Circulating microRNAs in heart failure with reduced and preserved left ventricular ejection fraction. *Eur J Heart Fail.* 2015;17:393–404. doi:10.1002/ejhf.223.
40. Dong S, Ma W, Hao B, et al. microRNA-21 promotes cardiac fibrosis and development of heart failure with preserved left ventricular ejection fraction by up-regulating Bcl-2. *Int J Clin Exp Pathol.* 2014;7(2):565–574. http://www.ncbi.nlm.nih.gov/pubmed/24551276. Accessed July 17, 2018.
41. Sinning D, Kasner M, Westermann D, Schulze K, Schultheiss HP, Tschöpe C. Increased left ventricular stiffness impairs exercise capacity in patients with heart failure symptoms despite normal left ventricular ejection fraction. *Card Res Pract.* 2011;2011:692862. doi:10.4061/2011/692862.
42. Søndergaard L, Reddy V, Kaye D, et al. Transcatheter treatment of heart failure with preserved or mildly reduced ejection fraction using a novel interatrial implant to lower left atrial pressure. *Eur J Heart Fail.* 2014;16(7):796–801. doi:10.1002/ejhf.111.
43. Hasenfuß G, Hayward C, Burkhoff D, et al. A transcatheter intracardiac shunt device for heart failure with preserved ejection fraction (REDUCE LAP-HF): a multicentre, open-label, single-arm, phase 1 trial. *Lancet.* 2016;387(10025):1298–1304. doi:10.1016/S0140-6736(16)00704-2.
44. Guimaraes L, et al. Interatrial shunt with the second-generation V-wave system for patients with advanced chronic heart failure. *EuroIntervention.* 2020;15:1426–1428. doi:10.4244/EIJ-D-19-00291.
45. Borggrefe M, Burkhoff D. Clinical effects of cardiac contractility modulation (CCM) as a treatment for chronic heart failure. *Eur J Heart Fail.* 2012;14(7):703–712. doi:10.1093/eurjhf/hfs078.
46. Tschöpe C, Van Linthout S, Spillmann F, et al. Cardiac contractility modulation signals improve exercise intolerance and maladaptive regulation of cardiac key proteins for systolic and diastolic function in HFpEF. *Int J Cardiol.* 2016;203:1061–1066. doi:10.1016/j.ijcard.2015.10.208.
47. Brandt MC, Mahfoud F, Reda S, et al. Renal sympathetic denervation reduces left ventricular hypertrophy and improves cardiac function in patients with resistant hypertension. *J Am Coll Cardiol.* 2012;59(10):901–909. doi:10.1016/J.JACC. 2011.11.034.
48. Patel HC, Rosen SD, Hayward C, et al. Renal denervation in heart failure with preserved ejection fraction (RDT-PEF): a randomized controlled trial. *Eur J Heart Fail.* 2016;18(6):703–712. doi:10.1002/ejhf.502.
49. Abraham WT, Zile MR, Weaver FA, et al. Baroreflex activation therapy for the treatment of heart failure with a reduced ejection fraction. *JACC Heart Fail.* 2015;3(6):487–496. doi:10.1016/j.jchf.2015.02.006.

REVIEW QUESTION ANSWERS

CHAPTER 1

1. a. Cardiac relaxation is regulated by NO. ROS can affect NO-related signaling at multiple sites. NO is generated by NO synthase (NOS), which requires tetrahydrobiopterin as a cofactor for the reaction. Hypertension and activation of the renin-angiotensin system lead to a depletion of tetrahydrobiopterin.
2. c. Transcriptional control of mRNA encoding procollagen I is one mechanism by which levels of secreted procollagen can increase. Procollagen maturation in the extracellular space requires cleavage of both the N and C terminal propeptides from the procollagen monomer. Other proteins secreted into the extracellular space influence the assembly of collagen into insoluble fibrils and include matricellular proteins such as SPARC and periostin as well as other collagen family members and proteoglycans.
3. d. Early infiltration of neutrophils is associated with detection of neutrophil extracellular traps (NETs) in the heart. The release of chromatin by neutrophils in the form of NETs is thought to be an antimicrobial defense mechanism.

CHAPTER 2

1. b. The patient has age-induced diastolic dysfunction without any evidence of HFpEF. Comorbidity management is the only needed management.
2. c. The patient has postoperative myocardial edema from the cardioplegia and pump run and has edema-induced increased LV diastolic stiffness in addition to AS-induced increased LV stiffness. To increase cardiac output and reduce inotrope dependency, she needs to recruit Starling forces by increasing LV diastolic wall stress (increased PCWP) as long as she can successfully oxygenate.
3. d. The PADP at insertion was significantly elevated, and the subsequent PADP rose further. Both the elevated baseline and change from baseline pressures predict increased morbidity (HF hosp) and mortality. Therapeutic interventions must be taken based on PADP independent of symptom status.

CHAPTER 3

1. c. The impairment of diastolic filling is continuous through the entire diastole in cardiac tamponade. The size of the effusion as well as its distribution may be variable in cardiac tamponade. Since the pericardium is relatively stiff, if a pericardial fluid collects quickly, such as in hemopericardium, the limit of pericardial stretch is reached soon with volumes of 200 to 300 mL. On the other hand, a slowly accumulating pericardial effusion allows the pericardium to stretch and become more distensible, allowing effusions to reach 1 to 2 L before the development of cardiac tamponade.
2. b. Constrictive pericarditis is a syndrome where the pericardium becomes relatively rigid and inelastic, may be thickened and calcified or not, and impairs mid- to late diastolic filling.
3. c. Ventricular interdependence leads to impairment of LV and RV filling in cardiac tamponade, constrictive pericarditis, and effusive constrictive syndromes. In tamponade, the rate of fluid accumulation determines pericardial distensibility, allowing larger volumes of fluid to accumulate before a significant increase in pericardial pressure if the rate is slow. Pericardial constriction is caused by increased pericardial rigidity, which is not necessarily related to increased thickness.

CHAPTER 4

1. a. Net mechanical work is the difference between the A and V loop areas. Options b and c are incorrect, as they require additional ventricular measurements. Option d is incorrect, as strain measures tissue deformation, not volume.
2. b. Option a is incorrect, as it is the definition of atrial compliance, not contractility. Option c is incorrect as several investigators have derived atrial P-V loops in human subjects. Option d is incorrect, as it is a measure of booster pump, not reservoir function.
3. d. This is the correct answer because it is one of the determinants of atrial reservoir function. Option a is incorrect, as it is the LV end-systolic, not diastolic volume that influences atrial reservoir function. Options b and c are incorrect, as they primarily modulate atrial booster pump function.
4. a. This is the correct answer, as it is the characteristic hemodynamic finding in the stiff LA syndrome. Option b is incorrect because, by definition, atrial compliance (the inverse of stiffness) is decreased. Option c is incorrect since the highest prevalence estimates of the stiff LA syndrome are in the range of 1% to 2%. Option d is incorrect because the diastolic transmitral velocity is increased, not decreased.
5. b. This is the correct answer since hemodynamic overload in animal and human atria results in a switch from the fast (a) to slow (b) myosin heavy chain isoform. This is associated with decreased myosin ATPase activity, increased LA stiffness, and increased mechanical work. Therefore options a, c, and d are incorrect.
6. c. This is the correct answer since the inotropic response to calcium infusion is markedly attenuated. Option a is incorrect because the relative reservoir/conduit function is decreased. Option b is incorrect since there is no hypertrophy in this model. Option d is incorrect because this model is associated with a marked increase in LA stiffness.

CHAPTER 5

1. b. Deceleration time is inversely proportional to chamber stiffness. Patch material has a much higher stiffness than a muscle—in other words, it lacks any stretchability. Because of that, deceleration time will decrease. The time constant of relaxation (τ) reflects active properties (i.e., only alive tissues that are capable of modulating the relaxation process affect it). Since patch material is not alive, it will not affect τ.
2. c. Time constant of relaxation (τ) will increase early LV diastolic pressure with almost no impact on LVEDP. Relaxation is an asymptotic process that almost completely dissipates after the time interval of ~3 τ. In other words, if τ is 60 msec, the relaxation process will have no effect on LV pressure after ~180 ms (i.e., 3 × τ) after closure of the aortic valve, or 120 msec after the opening of the mitral valve. Since filling time at rest is much longer that 120 msec, τ will not affect LV end-diastolic pressure.
3. a. E wave velocity is decreased if relaxation is impaired (slow), but is increased if the filling pressure and ventricular chamber stiffness are increased. Flow propagation velocity is decreased if relaxation is impaired, or if the left ventricle is dilated. Constrictive pericarditis patients have high E wave velocities, as relaxation is normal while filling pressures are normal or increased, and high flow propagation velocity as the left ventricle is small (tubular deformity of the left ventricle). Hypertrophic cardiomyopathy patients have low or normal E wave velocities, as relaxation is impaired while filling pressures are normal or elevated. Finally, in dilated cardiomyopathy, the left ventricle operates in the region of the diastolic pressure-volume relationship characterized by high chamber stiffness, and therefore has high E wave velocity. In contrast, when rapid initial inflow across the mitral valve meets a wide ventricle of dilated cardiomyopathy, flow propagation velocity slows down even if relaxation is normal. Think about what happens when a narrow Alpine creek meets a meandering river in the meadows.
4. a. The first event of relaxation is peak LV untwisting. The untwisting of the left ventricle in turn leads to the unmasking of restoring forces—namely, elastic forces within the left ventricle that aim to restore the left ventricle to its initial, unstressed size that is larger than the one observed in end systole (think about the force that returns your stress ball to spherical shape after you squeezed it). Restoring forces create an intraventricular pressure gradient (i.e., suction). Finally, suction opens the mitral valve and E wave occurs.

CHAPTER 6

1. b. End-systolic elastance represents the stiffness generated by the myocardium at end systole, the slope of which provides a load-independent measure of contractility but is in addition influenced by chamber geometry and remodeling. Therefore it represents a ventricular property. Effective arterial elastance provides a lumped measure of steady-state and pulsatile vascular load, total arterial compliance reflects pulsatile load, and systemic vascular resistance is a measure of steady-state load. The augmentation index quantitates the impact of reflected waves on increasing aortic systolic pressure and is an additional measure of vascular load.
2. b. Patients with HFpEF have a steep end-systolic elastance (Ees), and as a result, any change in effective arterial elastance with afterload reduction will lead to a large drop in systolic blood pressure, with a minimal improvement in stroke volume. This contrasts to patients with HFrEF, where for any degree of afterload reduction, there will be a minimal drop in blood pressure but a large improvement in stroke volume, reflecting the shallower Ees in these patients.
3. b. There is no randomized trial that has demonstrated a symptomatic benefit to afterload reduction in HFpEF patients, so blood pressure should be controlled primarily for cardiovascular risk reduction as advocated for by current guidelines. This in part likely reflects the greater drop in blood pressure with minimal improvement in forward flow that occurs with vasodilation in HFpEF due to their steep end-systolic elastance relationship. Patients with HFpEF frequently also demonstrate normal hemodynamics at rest (including afterload measures) that can markedly worsen during the stress of exercise, leading to exertional dyspnea in part from abnormal ventricular-vascular coupling during exercise.

CHAPTER 7

1. e. The risk of HFpEF increases sharply with age. Patients with HFrEF tend to be younger, with CAD, and predominantly men. While there are many attributable risk factors for the development of HFpEF, few have emerged as more likely to greatly augment the risk. Among these are hypertension, older age, and female sex. The 5-year mortality rate in patients with newly diagnosed heart failure is actually in the 50% range. Roughly 60% of these deaths are attributable to cardiovascular causes. While the mechanism of death is often times difficult to pinpoint in large registry data available, it remains clear that HFpEF is a highly morbid condition with a mortality similar to HFrEF. Natriuretic peptides have emerged as important biomarkers in both HFrEF and HFpEF. Levels are higher in women and in patients with renal failure.
2. d. In response to exercise, there will be an exaggerated elevation in systemic blood pressure and intracardiac filling pressure, making choices a and c incorrect. While a right heart catheterization may demonstrate normal hemodynamics, a right heart catheterization with exercise can often confirm a suspected diagnosis of HFpEF. For patients with normal hemodynamics at rest, a pulmonary artery systolic pressure with exercise of greater than 45 mmHg suggests a diagnosis of HFpEF with high

sensitivity. HFpEF is associated with a lack of chronotropic response, making choice e incorrect.

3. c. There have been several randomized controlled trials examining the effect of RAAS blockade in HFpEF. To the disappointment of the scientific community, all trials have been largely neutral. There has been much debate about the specifics of these trials, mostly about the lack of uniform diagnostic criteria for HFpEF. To date, however, there has been no trial definitively showing improved survival with neurohormonal therapy. Similarly, despite nearly 30% to 40% of all HFpEF deaths attributable to sudden cardiac death, there has been no trial showing ICD therapy is indicated in this cohort of patients. By far the most effective treatment strategy has been to target risk factors for the disease: hypertension, coronary disease, diabetes, and obesity. A promising target for HFpEF has been to condition the periphery and potentially reverse the maladaptive vascular remodeling through exercise. There have been several small, short-duration exercise trials conducted in HFpEF to date. Although results are difficult to interpret given the small numbers, the prevailing underpinning is that exercise is safe and does improve functional capacity and quality of life.

CHAPTER 8

1. d. Many patients with HFpEF display normal natriuretic peptide and echocardiogram, without apparent clinical congestion at rest. However, they develop abnormal increases in filling pressure during exercise. Noninvasive estimates of filling pressure, such as natriuretic peptides or echocardiography used in the current guidelines (average E/e′ >14 and LA volume index >34 mL/m^2), do not exclude the diagnosis of HFpEF due to poor sensitivity. Since this case has multiple typical comorbidities of HFpEF (obesity, hypertension, and atrial fibrillation), further testing should be considered. Invasive right heart catheterization during exercise has emerged as the gold standard to establish or exclude HFpEF and thus should be considered to bring out hemodynamic abnormalities that develop during exercise. Noninvasive diastolic stress echocardiography could be performed to rule out HFpEF. However, a positive exercise echocardiography does not establish HFpEF because of a high rate of false positive.
2. e. Incorrect wedge values can occur if the position of the catheter tip is incorrectly placed or if the balloon occlude is underinflated or overinflated. Intrathoracic pressure is transmitted to the pulmonary venous system. Values can oscillate dramatically and differ from atmospheric pressure in patients with severe dyspnea, air trapping, or receiving positive airway pressure ventilation. High-fidelity micromanometer-tipped catheters respond faster than fluid-filled catheters to rapid changes in pressure. These are not routinely used due to their much higher cost. Simultaneous recording of LV and capillary wedge pressure is required in some instances to establish the diagnosis of mitral stenosis or severe mitral regurgitation as the etiology of HF.
3. e. Even though by definition HFpEF patients have normal or near-normal EF, contractility is commonly impaired as demonstrated when using advanced quantitative imaging methods such as strain imaging. Pulmonary hypertension can occur not only secondary to increase LA pressure but as a result of chronic pulmonary vascular remodeling. This often leads to impaired RV function. Ventricular interdependence imposed by the pericardium can lead to elevation of LV filling pressures secondary to acute RV failure in conditions such as RV infarction, hypoventilation, and pulmonary embolism.

CHAPTER 9

1. b. The patient is young and has abnormal loading conditions with a very high cardiac output. The LVEDP is elevated as pulmonary venous A wave duration exceeds mitral A wave duration by 30 msec.
2. a. The evidence that LV filling is a normal pattern is the concordance of the E/A wave velocity ratio with the TDI MAM e′/a′ velocity ratio. Although the left atrium is enlarged because of the high cardiac output, there is no evidence of increased LA pressure by either LV IVRT or reduced pulmonary venous systolic flow.
3. a. A Valsalva maneuver that showed a decrease in both mitral E and A wave velocities with LA pressure reduction would have been confirmatory evidence of the normal LV relaxation present.
4. a. The patient is middle aged and has normal loading conditions at the time of his echo. There is no evidence of increased filling pressures.
5. b. Mitral filling pattern is abnormal with a long IVRT, reduced mitral E wave, and increased A wave, indicating impaired relaxation. His TDI MAM e′ and a′ also have a ratio consistent with decreased longitudinal function, which suggests LV hypertrophy from either HT or obesity.
6. b. As in the previous answer, this patient represents the large group of patients with early diastolic dysfunction due to impaired LV relaxation who have no increase in filling pressures. However, in long-term studies, they are at increased risk for progression of disease and future adverse CV events.
7. d. This elderly male has multiple risk factors for cardiac disease and systolic and diastolic dysfunction. He has moderate LV hypertrophy with stage III–IV chronic kidney disease and is significantly volume overloaded, as seen by his dilated IVC.
8. c. His increased LA volume, short LV IVRT, increased mitral E/A wave ratio, and short DT and A wave duration are all consistent with pseudonormal filling. His TDI e′ and a′ MAM also has a pattern (ratio <1) consistent with decreased longitudinal function, which suggests LV hypertrophy. The e′/a′ ratio less than 1 is discordant from the mitral filling pattern, which is also consistent with pseudonormal filling.

9. d. The elevated LA pressure masks the impaired LV relaxation, but is revealed by a Valsalva maneuver, which lowers the LA pressure. This shows that LV chamber compliance is likely reduced because of the volume overload more than myocardial stiffness. Therefore the patient's main diastolic abnormality is most likely impaired relaxation if loading conditions were normalized.
10.d. This elderly female fits the classic profile for HFpEF. She has long-standing HT with marked LV hypertrophy. Although her CVP is normal, she has HT with a very wide pulse pressure. As expected, her BNP is mildly elevated and left atrium enlarged.
11.c. This elderly female fits the classic profile for HFpEF. She has long-standing HT with marked LV hypertrophy. Although her CVP is normal she has HT with a very wide pulse pressure. As expected, her BNP is mildly elevated and left atrium enlarged.
12.d. As in the previous case, the elevated LA pressure masks the impaired LV relaxation. However, the rather modest changes in mitral inflow velocity with a Valsalva maneuver suggests the main problem here is increased myocardial stiffness, an advanced form of diastolic dysfunction. This is reflected in the blunted pulmonary venous systolic flow, which also indicates an elevated LA pressure even though preload is normal.
13.d. The reduced pulmonary venous systolic flow in a patient with pseudonormal filling is associated with a marked increase in CV mortality that is nearly similar to restrictive filling, as it indicates LA systolic function is failing. Therefore the patient's main diastolic abnormality is impaired relaxation if loading conditions could be normalized.

CHAPTER 10

1. d. Global longitudinal strain can be calculated from apical views (AP3, AP4, and AP2), while radial and circumferential strains are calculated from short axis views.
2. d. TDI-derived strain is less affected by segmental tethering and translational motion but is still limited by angle dependency, while 2-D speckle tracking–derived strain is angle-independent.
3. c. Global longitudinal strain represents the percentage change from end diastole to end systole in the length of the LV wall perimetry measured from one basal segment, around the apex, to the opposite basal segment averaged from the three apical views.

CHAPTER 11

1. d. Vp is a complex phenomenon that is determined by rate of LV relaxation, geometry, and intraventricular pressures and gradients. Abnormalities in those parameters will impair diastolic suction and slow down early ventricular flow propagation.
2. d. In normal conditions, it represents the motion of columnar flow from base to apex. Presence of vortices and convective forces influence Vp on a variety of clinical conditions.
3. a. In normal conditions Vp is relatively fast, above 45 cm/sec.
4. a. Severe LV hypertrophy typically has a small cavity with intracavitary flow acceleration depending more on the geometry of the cavity than the early diastolic properties. In cases of constrictive pericarditis, Vp can be particularly fast, as in the case shown at the beginning of this chapter. In restrictive cardiomyopathy and LV systolic dysfunction, velocity flow propagation is slow, particularly when there is also significant ventricular dilatation.

CHAPTER 12

1. c, d, e. The apical four-chamber image includes important information about cardiac structure and function in this case. The wall thickness is markedly increased in both left and right ventricles without cavitary dilatation. LV ejection fraction is visually preserved, and the inward motion is particularly preserved in the apical segment rather than the basal and midsegments (apical sparing). Furthermore, LA expansion is fairly limited during ventricular systole. The abnormal LA function could be evaluated by volumetric and strain analyses of the left atrium.
2. d. Transmitral inflow shows that E wave velocity is 94 cm/sec, A wave 21 cm/sec, and E/A 4.5, suggesting restrictive physiology. The decrease of A wave velocity might imply that LA systolic force is decreased.
3. b, d. Average peak systolic (s′), peak early diastolic (e′), and peak atrial systole (a′) mitral annular velocities are estimated as 4 cm/sec, 3 cm/sec, and 1 cm/sec, respectively. LV (longitudinal) systolic and diastolic functions are severely reduced. E/e′ is calculated as 31.3. In this patient, LV filling pressure is elevated, and LA booster function is impaired despite the sinus rhythm being maintained.
4. a, b, d, e. This patient was histologically diagnosed as cardiac amyloidosis. The P-P gating method is used for an estimation of LA strain, and the R-R gating method is used for LV strain. LA booster and reservoir strains are severely depressed probably due to amyloid deposition or fibrosis in the LA wall. LV apical sparing is one of the diagnostic findings of LV strain in patients with cardiac amyloidosis.

CHAPTER 13

1. b. The pre-A pressure reflects the diastolic pressure in the LV during the passive phase of filling and is within a few mmHg of the mean LAP or PCW pressure (as shown, Fig. 13.3).
2. d. In the presence of normal MV area, the transmitral E velocity relates directly with LV relaxation (i.e., suction effect) and early LA pressure (see Fig. 13.3). Because relaxation is impaired in the presence of any type of myocardial pathology, LA pressure becomes the primary force driving the E velocity. Consequently, in patients with elevated mean LAP, E is usually higher than 50 cm/sec.

3. a. Peak TR velocity provides an estimate of the instantaneous pressure gradient between the right ventricle and right atrium. In the absence of RV outflow obstruction, a peak velocity of 2.9 m/sec is converted with the $4V^2$ equation into a pressure gradient of 34 mmHg, which in the presence of a mean RAP of 4 mmHg or higher results in an estimated PA systolic pressure greater than 37 mmHg. When combined with an average E/e′ greater than 14 and/or a dilated left atrium, this finding is highly predictive of an elevated mean LAP. However, it is important to exclude intrinsic pulmonary vascular disease, which is usually accompanied by RV enlargement and dysfunction, septal flattening, and typical changes in RV outflow velocity (short acceleration with midsystolic notching).
4. c. The absence of atrial contraction and the varying R-R intervals makes the estimation of mean LAP difficult though not impossible. The combined findings of a shortened IVRT and DT with increased TR velocity and septal E/e′, although fairly specific for elevated LAP, are less sensitive in patients with normal EF. Consequently, the overall accuracy of these findings is higher when EF is less than 45%. In patients with normal EF, peak, TR greater than 2.8 has significant weight, given that with a normal EF and stroke volume, PASP exceeds 37 mmHg in most patients with elevated LAP.
5. b. The large regurgitant volume seen with moderate or severe MR caused by a primary valvular defect will increase E velocity and E/A, shorten IVRT, reduce the pulmonary vein S/D ratio, and preserve e′, particularly at the lateral annular corner. Consequently, ASE guidelines recommend abstaining from evaluating diastolic function in these patients. In contrast to primary MR, patients with functional or ischemic MR have myocardial disease, and as such, they have diastolic dysfunction. Although E velocity and E/A ratio may be increased by the regurgitant volume, studies have shown that the application of the ASE algorithm as a rule works well in the estimation of mean LAP.

CHAPTER 14

1. e. In RV systolic dysfunction, RV fractional area change is less than 35%, TAPSE less than 17 mm, RV free wall strain less than 25% (absolute value), and 3-D RV EF less than 45%.
2. d. Option a is consistent with normal mean RA pressure given an IVC maximum diameter of only 1.5 cm, with greater than 50% collapse with sniffing. A systolic to diastolic velocity ratio greater than 1 is consistent with normal RA pressure. Likewise, normal RA volume index is supportive of normal mean RA pressure. A tricuspid E/e′ ratio greater than 6 supports the conclusion of elevated RA pressure. Patients with increased systolic RV-RA pressure gradient can have normal RA pressure. Therefore the mere presence of pulmonary hypertension should not be equated to elevated RA pressure, and specific indices of RA mean pressure should be evaluated.
3. d. Peak PR velocity can be used to measure mean PA pressure, whereas end-diastolic velocity is of value in estimating PA diastolic pressure in conjunction with the estimation of mean RA pressure. PR pressure half time of 150 msec and less is consistent with RV involvement in patients with inferior wall myocardial infarction and predicts worse outcomes. An elevated end-diastolic PR velocity can occur in the presence of normal RA pressure. Therefore the mere presence of pulmonary hypertension should not be equated to elevated RA pressure, and specific indices of RA mean pressure should be evaluated.

CHAPTER 15

1. c. The electromagnetic forces of an MRI scanner can induce thermal and nonthermal effects that can be of significant clinical consequence in patients with ferromagnetic metallic devices. Mechanical heart valves and coronary stents are nonferromagnetic, and therefore it is safe to perform cardiac MRI for these patients. While pacemakers and defibrillators were previously absolute contraindications, MRI conditional devices are now frequently being implanted. It is therefore important to check a patient's device features before definitively ruling out cardiac MRI capability. Cochlear implants are an absolute contraindication due to the strong internal magnet within the device, which can be damaged by the external magnetic field of the scanner.
2. c. Transmitral flow (TMF) serves to directly quantify the filling gradient between the left atrium and the left ventricle. The normal filling pattern consists of two waves, E and A. The E wave correlates with the rapid LV filling in early diastole, while the A wave correlates with the late LV filling at end diastole after the atrial kick. The A wave amplitude and duration are related to LV stiffness and LA contractility. Numerous studies have shown sufficient correlation between cardiac MRI and TTE for measurement of flow velocities.[6–8] See Fig. 8.3. Pulmonary venous flow helps differentiate between normal TMF and pseudonormalization. In such cases, a normal TMF pattern where $E > A$ may actually be pseudonormalization. In patients with pseudonormal TMF, the duration of the pulmonary venous atrial reversal (AR) wave will be longer than that of the mitral A wave.[10–12] However, pulmonary venous flow by echocardiography can sometimes yield suboptimal results, as illustrated in this case. PVF by cardiac MRI can be measured in the majority of cardiac MRI cases, as opposed to only 68% of TTE cases due to improved image quality with cardiac MRI.[7]
3. b. The global diffuse hyperenhancement is most consistent with a diagnosis of cardiac amyloidosis. Patients with amyloidosis will typically demonstrate a diffuse pattern of LGE in a noncoronary distribution that can also extend into the right ventricle, interatrial septum, and atrial walls. Additionally, native T1 measurements and ECV measurements can identify cardiac amyloidosis at earlier stages and provide powerful prognostic risk stratification

in patients with both transthyretin amyloidosis and primary amyloidosis.

CHAPTER 16

1. d. The radionuclide assessment of the diastolic LV function is attained plotting the changes in radioactivity over time, which is proportional to changes in LV volume over time. This allows the calculation of ventricular filling rates, maximum filling timing, as well as time to peak filling rates. An adequate temporal sampling of the LV volume is crucial to capture the subtle alterations in diastolic filling requiring at least 16 to 32 frames per heart cycle. The presence of arrhythmias during the data acquisition reduces the quality and fidelity of the diastolic assessment. As any change in the R-R interval invariably introduces changes in the diastolic filling, beats with R-R interval that vary by more than ±10% from the mean R-R must be rejected, as well as the beat following the rejected beat. Finally, the evaluation of diastolic function using radionuclides techniques was initially conducted using the equilibrium and first-pass radionuclide angiocardiogram; however, myocardial perfusion studies are also able to adjunctively assess the diastolic function assuming an optimized data acquisition for this purpose as presented in this chapter.
2. b. The rate of volume change over time during early diastole provides the most important measurements of ventricular diastolic function. These measurements include the peak ventricular filling rate (PFR) and the time to peak filling rate (TPFR). Under normal conditions, the PFR is greater than 2.5 EDV/sec attained in less than 180 msec, otherwise an impaired diastolic dysfunction is suggested. Alterations in these parameters are highly sensitive but lack specificity, as they can be altered in the absence of pathology due to age, heart rate, systolic function, end-diastolic volume, adrenergic state, medications, and even changes in methods of acquisition and processing.
3. d. The high sensitivity of radionuclide techniques in the detection of diastolic dysfunction may allow the identification of certain clinical conditions such as hypertensive heart disease, chemotherapy-induced cardiotoxicity, or even microvascular dysfunction before the onset of symptoms. For instance, those patients with hypertensive heart disease present with diastolic impairments that appear to be dependent on myocardial mass rather than age or severity of hypertension. The presence of an impaired diastolic function despite a normal LV systolic function can suggest the presence of HFpEF in the right clinical context. Nevertheless, radionuclides techniques only detect diastolic dysfunction in less than 60% of patients with suspected HFpEF. This highlights the wide heterogeneity of pathology within these groups of patients. Finally, the adjunctive analysis of diastolic function during myocardial perfusion studies might be of help to ascertain the underlying pathology in patients presenting with cardiorespiratory symptoms with normal myocardial perfusion, as illustrated in the case study.

CHAPTER 17

1. d. This is a case example of cardiac amyloid. Classic features include marked LV and RV wall thickening, a small pericardial effusion, marked biatrial dilatation, and apical sparing on the GLS bull's eye plot. LV systolic function is normal with an LV EF of 60%. For LV diastolic function, in the setting of a normal LV EF, the assessment normally begins with algorithm A in Fig. 17.1. However, there is a significant increase in LV wall thickness, as well as abnormal GLS (−9.4%), indicating the presence of underlying myocardial disease. Therefore in this instance, analysis of LV diastolic grading begins with algorithm B. The transmitral inflow profile shows that the E/A ratio is greater than 2; this is consistent with grade III diastolic dysfunction and elevated LAP. To support this further, there is a marked reduction in both the septal and lateral e′ velocities (2.7 cm/sec and 4.1 cm/sec, respectively), an elevated average E/e′ ratio of 37, and a dilated left atrium (indexed LA volume 53 mL/m^2).
2. c. In this case, there is evidence of grade III diastolic dysfunction with an elevated LAP. When there is diastolic dysfunction, impaired relaxation is in most patients present across all grades. Both the IVRT and Vp are indices that reflect LV relaxation; hence it would be expected that both of these indices would be prolonged. However, while the Vp is relatively preload independent, the IVRT is preload dependent. This means that the IVRT is influenced by the LAP. Therefore in this case example, the Vp would be prolonged, but the IVRT would be shortened by the increased LAP. Remember that while LV relaxation is prolonged, because of the coexistent marked elevation in the LAP, the crossover between the LA and LV pressures occurs earlier and thus the mitral valve opens earlier than normal. This results in the shortening of the IVRT.
3. c. Grade III diastolic dysfunction is consistent with restrictive LV filling and a marked elevation in LAP. In these cases, the Valsalva maneuver may be performed to differentiate between reversible restrictive LV filling and irreversible restrictive LV filling. When there is reversible restrictive LV filling, following preload reduction, the profile is reversed to either a pseudonormal profile or even to an abnormal relaxation profile. When there is irreversible restrictive LV filling, following preload reduction, the profile remains unchanged, the E/A ratio remains high, and the DT remains short. An adequate Valsalva attempt is a 10% reduction in the peak transmitral E velocity from the baseline value. In the example shown, the peak transmitral E velocity decrease by just 3% (resting E velocity 1.26 m/sec and 1.22 m/sec with Valsalva); therefore this was a suboptimal Valsalva attempt.
4. a. This pulmonary venous trace was acquired at high PRF. This is identified by the appearance of a second sample volume along the Doppler beam (see figure). Therefore the displayed signal shows the pulmonary venous inflow signal from sample volume 1 (SV1) plus the transmitral inflow signal from sample volume 2 (SV2) superimposed

on the pulmonary venous trace; the pulmonary venous S velocity is seen below the zero baseline, while a combination of the transmitral E and the pulmonary venous D velocities are seen above and below the zero baseline. This occurs when the velocity scale is set too high and the high PRF mode is activated. Recall that in the low PRF mode, the transducer emits a pulse, and then waits for the returning signal before sending out the next pulse; this limits the maximum velocity that can be displayed. To increase the velocity scale further, the number of sample volumes can be increased by going into high PRF mode. In high PRF mode, the transducer does not wait for the first pulse to return to the transducer before sending out a second pulse, and this then increases the maximum displayed velocity. Decreasing the velocity scale will remove the second sample volume and eliminate contamination of the pulmonary venous signal by transmitral inflow.

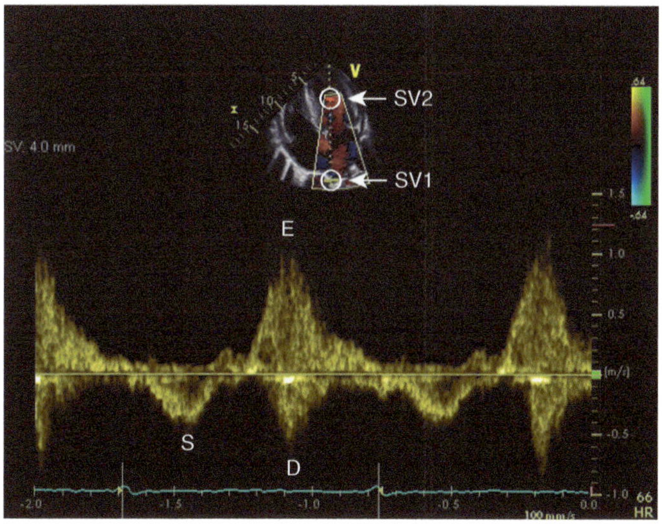

CHAPTER 18

1. c. Atrial pacing is a feasible and easy way of stressing the heart, especially in patients in whom physical exercise is not possible. However, it must be noted that the hemodynamic changes associated with atrial pacing are different from those associated with physical exercise. The main hemodynamic change with atrial pacing is a decrease in LV stroke volume due to a decrease in LV filling time that is not accompanied by an adequate compensatory increase in systemic venous return. Therefore to demonstrate an increase in LV filling pressure with stress, pacing is not a suitable technique. Dobutamine has been frequently used to pharmacologically stress the cardiovascular system. Similar to atrial pacing, dobutamine may not be a suitable technique to demonstrate an increase in LV filling pressure with stress. However, dobutamine administration may be helpful to evaluate myocardial longitudinal functional reserve in subjects with an inability to exercise. Physical exercise is the most physiologic means of gathering data regarding stress-induced elevation of LV filling pressure. These features may make exercise Doppler echocardiography during supine bicycle exercise the optimal approach to demonstrate the increase in LV filling pressures with exercise.
2. c. Diastolic stress echocardiography is indicated when resting echocardiography does not explain the symptoms of heart failure or exertional dyspnea. Patients with completely normal hearts and diastolic function at rest with preserved e′ velocity need not undergo stress testing, as it is highly unlikely that they will develop diastolic dysfunction and elevated filling pressures with exercise. Likewise, patients with abnormal findings at baseline consistent with elevated LV filling pressures should not be referred for stress testing, as the cardiac etiology for dyspnea has already been established and their filling pressures will almost certainly increase further with exercise. The most appropriate patient population for diastolic stress echocardiography is the group of patients with grade I diastolic dysfunction, which indicates delayed myocardial relaxation and normal LA mean pressure at rest.
3. d. Diastolic stress echocardiography is definitively normal if the septal E/e′ is less than 10 at rest and with exercise, and the peak tricuspid regurgitation (TR) velocity is less than 2.8 m/sec at rest and with stress. A study is definitively abnormal when the septal E/e′ ratio is above 15, peak TR velocity is greater than 2.8 m/sec with exercise, and the septal e′ velocity is less than 8 cm/sec at baseline.

CHAPTER 19

1. c. Algorithm 1 should be used from the ASE/EACVI 2016 guidelines. Of the four parameters used to evaluate LV diastolic function, three are positive: septal e′ less than 7 and lateral e′ less than 10, TR velocity greater than 2.8 m/sec, and LA volume greater than 34 mL/m^2. As more than 50% of the parameters are positive, there is reason to suspect diastolic dysfunction.
2. c. Algorithm 2 should be used since the patient has a cardiac history and myocardial disease. The first step in the evaluation of LV filling pressure is estimation of mitral flow velocities. This patient has a mitral E velocity of 65 cm/sec and an E/A ratio of 0.9, which places the patient in the intermediate group, where three additional parameters need to be evaluated. Two of these three additional parameters, TR velocity and E/e′, are below their respective cutoff values (2.8 m/sec and 14), whereas LA volume is above the cutoff value. Thus the majority of parameters are negative, the patient is considered to have grade I diastolic dysfunction, and LV filling pressure is assumed to be normal.
3. a, d. In patients with atrial fibrillation, there is normally dilatation of the left atrium, and thus elevated LA volume cannot be used to estimate LV filling pressure. As there is no atrial contraction, the E/A ratio cannot be estimated. E/e′ and TR velocity, on the other hand, correlate well with LV filling pressure also in patients with atrial

fibrillation, and these two parameters can thus be used in the evaluation of LV filling pressure.

4. b. In the guidelines from 2009, grade I diastolic dysfunction was defined as patients with echocardiographic evidence of diastolic function but normal LV filling pressure. In the updated version, four criteria are used to decide whether diastolic dysfunction is present or not in patients with normal systolic function. Only if three or four of these parameters are positive, the patient is said to have diastolic dysfunction. Three of these parameters are also used to decide whether LV filling pressure is elevated or not. Thus to be defined as having diastolic dysfunction, LV filling pressure is elevated. This is a more restrictive definition, defining fewer patients as having diastolic dysfunction than with the 2009 guidelines. Thus sensitivity (the ability of the test to be positive in patients with diastolic dysfunction) was reduced, whereas the specificity (the ability of the test to be negative in patients without the disease) was increased.

5. c. In the early stages of diastolic dysfunction, patients may have completely normal echocardiography at rest or evidence of delayed relaxation only. When heart rate increases with activity in healthy individuals, LV relaxation rate also increases. Patients with diastolic dysfunction may not be able to increase relaxation rate with exercise. This results in impairment of diastolic function with exercise. Thus in patients presenting mainly with symptoms of diastolic dysfunction with exercise but normal echocardiography at rest, a diastolic stress test is recommended.

CHAPTER 20

1. c. At the myocardial level, LV diastolic dysfunction is caused by incomplete and/or slowed relaxation and increased passive stiffness. Titin, along with extracellular matrix collagen, is responsible for the passive stiffness of the myocardium. In hypertensive patients with HFpEF, reduced phosphorylation of PKA/PKG sites on titin has been reported[14,15] and serves to increase titin's stiffness, and in turn reduce diastolic LV chamber compliance. Increased, not decreased, collagen has been reported in these patients and also contributes to diastolic dysfunction. Reduced $SERCA_2$ activity and reduced troponin I phosphorylation have not been reported.

2. c. The development of HFpEF has been attributed to multiple comorbidities, including, but not limited to, hypertension, obesity, diabetes, and chronic kidney disease.[4] Of all of these, hypertension is thought to be present in at least 90% of HFpEF patients,[5] and is thus the most common.

3. c. ACC/AHA guidelines recommend chlorthalidone as a first-line agent for blood pressure lowering in HFpEF patients.[17,19] This is based in part on the results of the ALL-HAT trial, which showed that chlorthalidone reduced the risk of cardiovascular events, including heart failure in hypertensive patients. The guidelines also support inhibition of the renin-angiotensin system (RAS) with ACE inhibitors or ARBs as first-line treatment for hypertension management, particularly in patients with T2DM. Beta blockers are not guideline-recommended first-line blood pressure–lowering agents in patients with HFpEF and may possibly contribute to diastolic dysfunction and adverse outcomes.[20,21] Hydralazine and nitrates are also not first-line treatments.

CHAPTER 21

1. e. The patient is clearly in heart failure (shortness of breath, pulmonary rales, peripheral edema, increased NT-proBNP). His LV EF is calculated at 45%, which is only mildly reduced, but his GLS is 9% (normal, 20%), which is severely reduced. GLS is a marker of both systolic and diastolic LV function. Since there are clear signs of diastolic dysfunction, this may explain some of the reduction in GLS, but GLS is also more sensitive to milder forms of systolic LV dysfunction than ejection fraction, in particular in patients with LV hypertrophy (as in this case). Degenerative mitral stenosis is mild with transmitral velocities not exceeding 1.4 m/sec; the mean gradient of 5 mmHg confirms mild stenosis. Such a stenosis can explain neither the considerable pulmonary hypertension nor the heart failure symptoms. Regarding the right ventricle, size and function are described as normal, although given the high right-sided pressures, there may still be silent RV dysfunction, which may manifest with physical exertion.

2. c. Several studies[6,7] have suggested in aortic stenosis patients that baseline LV diastolic function before valve intervention (surgical or transcatheter) affects postinterventional survival and quality of life, independently of LV systolic function. Of course, ejection fraction and, even more so, global longitudinal strain, as well as increased pulmonary pressures, are also strong predictors of prognosis.

3. b. Mitral regurgitation, due to the additional regurgitant volume passing through the mitral valve in diastole, increases E wave velocity. This in turn also leads to higher E/A and E/e′ ratios independently of myocardial diastolic function, although e′ may be commensurately elevated if the left ventricle contracts and relaxes more vigorously due to the extra volume load. RV pressures tend to increase due to backward propagation of high LA pressures caused by mitral regurgitation. Finally, systolic pulmonary venous flow is pushed back by the regurgitant blood entering the left atrium in systole, leading to a decreased S/D ratio. All of these parameters also change in the same direction in the presence of diastolic dysfunction (without mitral regurgitation). LV wall thickness, however, is not affected by mitral regurgitation.

CHAPTER 22

1. b. Based on the results of the CHAMPION trial in 2014 the FDA approved use of the CardioMEMS sensor in both patients with HFpEF and HFrEF, who had symptomatic

HF (NYHA Class III) and were on optimal medical therapy with a history of HF hospitalization within the last year.

2. c. The most recent ACC/AHA guidelines state that in select patients with HFpEF, the use of spironolactone may be considered to reduce hospitalizations (COR IIb, LOA B-R). No other pharmacologic interventions have been proven to improve mortality or readmissions in HFpEF.
3. d. The major concern with LVAD implantation in patients with HFpEF is obstruction of flow into the LV inflow cannula due to the smaller cavity size and thickness of the LV walls. Patients with HFpEF in the studies experience more frequent and difficult-to-manage suction events. The investigators suggested the need for technical modifications in the surgical procedure. An echocardiographic analysis of a cohort of HFpEF patients found that larger LVEDD is a marker of better outcome. LVEDD of 4.6 cm and below was associated with increased mortality post LVAD implantation.
4. b. The ACC/AHA guideline for the management of heart failure classifies disease progression into four stages: stage A includes patients with risk factors for HF but without structural heart disease, stage B includes those with structural heart disease without HF symptoms, stage C represents symptomatic HF associated with underlying structural heart disease, and stage D reflects refractory symptoms despite guideline-directed medical therapy (GDMT).
5. d. According to ACC/AHA guidelines, HFpEF is defined as the presence of the HF syndrome in an individual with a LV EF of 50% and above. Patients suffering from HFpEF where LV diastolic dysfunction predominates usually also exhibit LV systolic dysfunction as evident by abnormalities of longitudinal strain, LV end-systolic (Ees) stiffness (elastance), ventricular-arterial coupling (Ea/Ees ratio), and vasculoventricular coupling. In addition, chronotropic incompetence, abnormal vasorelaxation, right heart dysfunction, and abnormalities in the periphery are present in patients with HFpEF.
6. c. Compared to patients with HFrEF, those with HFpEF are older and more likely to be female. The incidence and prevalence of HFpEF increase sharply with age. The prevalence of HFpEF is increasing relative to HFrEF at a rate of 1% per year, suggesting that HFpEF may become the most common type of HF in the near future. The proportion of patients hospitalized with acute HF who had HFpEF increased from 33% in 2005 to 39% in 2010. At the same time, the proportion of HF hospitalizations due to HFrEF decreased from 52% to 47% in the United States.
7. c. COMPASS-HF, a randomized clinical trial testing the efficacy of Chronicle, enrolled 301 patients with NYHA Class III–IV symptoms regardless of LV EF but failed to show any significant effect on hospitalizations, as compared to the control group. LAPTOP-HF, a large randomized trial designed to test the safety and effectiveness of LA pressure-guided HF therapy, was terminated early by the study's data and safety monitoring board after randomization of only 486 patients because of a high number of implant-related complications. The CHAMPION trial found a 37% reduction in the primary end point of HF-related hospitalization compared to the control group.
8. c. Patients with HFpEF presenting with acute HF have higher systolic blood pressure values than those with HFrEF. Treatment with intravenous nitroprusside results in greater blood pressure reduction in HFpEF, less enhancement in cardiac output, and greater likelihood of stroke volume drop in HFpEF, as compared to HFrEF.
9. b. Based on the results of the CHAMPION trial in 2014, the FDA approved the use of the CardioMEMS sensor in both patients with HFpEF and HFrEF, who had symptomatic HF (NYHA Class III) and were on optimal medical therapy with a history of HF hospitalization within the last year.
10. c. The most recent ACC/AHA guidelines state that in select patients with HFpEF, the use of spironolactone may be considered to reduce hospitalizations (COR IIb, LOA B-R). No other pharmacologic interventions have been proven to improve mortality or readmissions in HFpEF.
11. d. The major concern with LVAD implantation in patients with HFpEF is obstruction of flow into the LV inflow cannula due to the smaller cavity size and thickness of the LV walls. Patients with HFpEF in the studies experienced more frequent and difficult-to-manage suction events. The investigators suggested the need for technical modifications in the surgical procedure. An echocardiographic analysis of a cohort of HFpEF patients found that larger LVEDD is a marker of better outcome. LVEDD less than or equal to 4.6 cm was associated with increased mortality postLVAD implantation.

CHAPTER 23

1. e. Recent studies suggest that ~1% of patients diagnosed with HCM actually have Fabry disease. Mimics of HCM are referred to as phenocopies and include many other infiltrative or storage diseases, such as Fabry disease, amyloidosis, and glycogen storage diseases. Fabry disease is an X-linked disease caused by a deficiency in the lysosomal enzyme α-galactosidase A, leading to accumulation of glycosphingolipids in various tissues, including the heart. Fabry disease should be suspected in patients diagnosed with HCM when there are systemic symptoms or signs, a family history of Fabry disease or cardiomyopathy with male predominance in severity, or suggestive echocardiographic or cardiac MRI findings. Systemic symptoms and signs include cornea verticillata, hypohidrosis, acroparasthesias, premature transient ischemic attack/stroke, kidney disease with proteinuria, and angiokeratoma. On echocardiography, patients are more often nonobstructers, with symmetric hypertrophy, and may have hypokinesis or thinning of the inferolateral basal wall. On cardiac MRI, the hallmark finding is low native T1 values.

2. d. The presence of extreme LV hypertrophy in a young male with the presence of ventricular preexcitation suggests alternative diagnoses other than HCM. The rare glycogen storage diseases (PRKAG2, Danon disease, and LAMP2 mutations) should be suspected with this clinical history. Danon disease is an X-linked dominant gene affecting primarily young males under the age of 20 years old. Noncardiac manifestations include skeletal myopathy, mental retardation or behavioral abnormalities, and ocular changes. Echocardiography may show massive hypertrophy, and electrocardiography may show preexcitation. Laboratory testing is notable for elevated CPK, LFTs, and troponin levels. Patients with Danon disease usually have a malignant clinical course, and if undetected are at risk of premature sudden death.
3. e. The clinical history, physical examination, laboratory testing, and echocardiogram are all consistent with idiopathic restrictive cardiomyopathy (IRCM). The clinical findings are consistent with biventricular diastolic heart failure. The echocardiogram is virtually diagnostic in this case. The ventricular wall thickness with IRCM is generally normal or at most mildly increased due to extensive fibrosis. There is severe diastolic dysfunction (grade III or restrictive filling pattern), with an elevated LA pressure (elevated E/e′ ratio, LA enlargement, and pulmonary hypertension). The slow color M mode propagation velocity, absence of respiratory variability, and prominence of atrial reversal in the hepatic veins with inspiration are consistent with a restrictive cardiomyopathy, not constrictive pericarditis. Cardiac catheterization hemodynamics, cardiac MRI, cardiac biopsy, and genetic testing may be helpful for confirming the diagnosis. The prognosis, particularly in the pediatric population, is poor and cardiac transplantation should be considered.

CHAPTER 24

1. b. The patient is presenting in the setting of a myocardial infarction with abnormal baseline echo, so likely has some degree of diastolic dysfunction. After using the recommended variables to evaluate LV diastolic function in the setting of preserved LV EF with structural disease, we next rely on E/A ratio and velocities. With septal E/e′ ratio less than 14, LA maximum volume index greater than 34 mL/m^2, and peak TR velocity less than 2.8 m/sec, she falls into the grade I diastolic dysfunction category with normal LV filling pressures.
2. c. Though pulmonary venous flow analysis was deemphasized in the 2016 ASE/ESE diastolic guideline document, valuable pathophysiologic insight is provided by these data. What is shown here is the absence of a pulmonary vein S wave and a remarkably D-dominant pattern. The differential diagnosis for this finding includes choices a through c; however, with the data furnished thus far, the most reasonable choice is c. The ECG described and the rhythm strip on the echo shows sinus rhythm. DT less than 140 msec is an independent predictor for in-hospital heart failure and cardiac death. E/e′ is another independent predictor of in-hospital events and follow-up LV EF. Option a is not correct because high LA pressure alone can blunt the S wave. Option b is an incorrect choice because the ECG tracing clearly shows a P wave. It is true, however, that the pulmonary vein S wave will be blunted in patients with atrial fibrillation because the first component of a pulmonary vein S wave depends on atrial relaxation. Option d is incorrect. While it is very likely that this patient has a high LVEDP, the A reversal duration on which this judgement depends is not clearly shown in this real-world example.

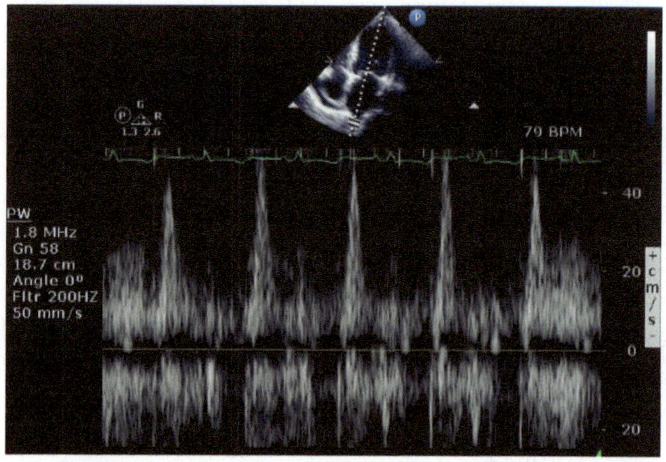

3. e. There is still evidence for elevated filling pressures by virtue of an elevated E/e′ ratio. According to the ASE guidelines, using the second grading algorithm (invoked here because of manifest LV dysfunction), this individual has grade II diastolic function. Even if one were to eschew the grade nomenclature, this patient has evidence of elevated filling pressures. Option a is an incorrect choice because the E/e′ ratio is elevated, denoting elevated mean LA pressure. Option b is incorrect because the presence of three of three abnormal criteria for the second algorithm denotes grade II or pseudonormal diastolic function. Options c and d are incorrect choices because of the marked reduction in E/A ratio, which is no longer greater than 2.

CHAPTER 25

1. c. Mutations related to HCM result in the production of abnormal myocardial sarcomeric proteins that have altered contraction and relaxation. Myosin heavy chain mutations in this region enhance contractility at the expense of impaired relaxation.
2. b. Coronary blood flow reserve is compromised in HCM through increased myocardial oxygen demand secondary to increased myocardial mass, myocyte disarray, the presence of interstitial fibrosis, and decreased oxygen supply due to abnormalities of the coronary microvasculature.
3. a. Peak myocardial systolic velocities, strain, and diastolic function parameters are preserved in an athlete's heart,

when compared to HCM. LV mass and LA volumes are often increased in both conditions. Concentric LV hypertrophy is more common in HCM.

CHAPTER 26

1. c. Prominent x and y descents are the classic venous wave morphology seen in patients with constrictive pericarditis (W sign). These are negative deflections (i.e., descents), in contrast to the large v wave seen in patients with severe tricuspid regurgitation. Cannon a waves are typically seen in patients with complete heart block or atrioventricular dissociation. The presence of markedly elevated venous pressure and blunted y descents is consistent with cardiac tamponade and reflects the impaired ventricular diastolic filling associated with increased intrapericardial pressures.
2. b. The Doppler signal shown illustrates the typical increased diastolic flow reversals during expiration seen in constrictive pericarditis. The proper timing in the respiratory cycle is identified by the simultaneous respirometer (upward deflections mark the beginning of inspiration, whereas the downward deflections mark the onset of expiratory) and the peak systolic forward flow velocities (highest at peak inspiration and lowest at peak expiration). Increased inspiratory flow reversals are seen in restrictive cardiomyopathy, whereas systolic flow reversals are typical for severe tricuspid regurgitation (note the preserved systolic forward flow in this patient; only trivial tricuspid regurgitation was present).
3. d. The presence of respirophasic septal shift is shown in the video; during inspiration, the ventricular septum moves toward the LV cavity with reciprocal changes occurring during expiration. This reflects the reciprocal changes in RV and LV preload due to the presence of pericardial restraint/constrictive pericardium. The inspiratory decrease in mitral E velocities reflects the presence of dissociation of intrathoracic-intracardiac pressures, where filling of the left heart decreases during inspiration. Signs of elevated filling pressures are demonstrated by the dilated inferior vena cava and the restrictive mitral inflow seen in constrictive pericarditis. Lastly, pulsus paradoxus is a consequence of the decreased inspiratory stroke volume of the left ventricle, due to a combination of both ventricular interdependence and dissociation of intrathoracic-intracardiac pressures.
4. b. His cardiac magnetic resonance demonstrates significant late gadolinium enhancement, consistent with ongoing pericardial inflammation. Although surgical pericardiectomy remains the definite therapy for patients with refractory or chronic constrictive pericarditis, anti inflammatory therapy should always be attempted initially in patients presenting with evidence of ongoing inflammation (elevated inflammatory markers or late gadolinium enhancement on cardiac MRI). Surgical pericardiectomy should be reserved for those presenting subacutely, who have failed medical therapy or in those where anti inflammatory therapy is felt to have low yield. Given the diagnostic bedside, echocardiographic, and cross-sectional findings, the diagnosis of constrictive pericarditis can be established, foregoing the need for cardiac catheterization.

CHAPTER 27

1. d. In aortic stenosis and other left obstructive lesions, development of endocardial fibroelastosis in fetal life contributes to a noncompliant left ventricle over and above myocardial fibrosis. A merged mitral inflow E and A wave is common in this scenario, when infants are tachycardic and complicate assessment of diastolic function using mitral inflow parameters. The left atrium may not be dilated due to unloading of the left atrium through the patent foramen ovale in fetal life and postnatally. LV systolic function may be significantly reduced in critical AS, but good systolic function does not preclude the presence of diastolic dysfunction.
2. c. The diastolic parameters are consistent with signs of delayed relaxation and decreased compliance (pseudonormal), with some parameters intermediate because of the opposed effects of impaired relaxation versus increased filling pressures. The presence of a mid-diastolic L wave is consistent with both delayed relaxation and increased filling pressures, especially the latter. While it is difficult to classify the diastolic function of this adolescent using adult criteria, he has abnormal diastolic function affecting both early and late diastole.
3. b. As the previous case demonstrates for the left ventricle, this case displays features of RV delayed relaxation and decreased compliance. While the clinical implications of antegrade end-diastolic flow in the main pulmonary artery are not totally clear, it is thought to reflect decreased RV compliance and not delayed relaxation. The E/e′ ratio does not accurately predict filling pressures in children, including those with congenital heart disease. Pulmonary regurgitation duration shortens with restrictive physiology.

CHAPTER 28

1. e. Diabetes mellitus dramatically increases HF. Data from the Framingham population demonstrated twofold to fivefold excess risk for developing new HF in individuals with diabetes mellitus.[5] If they are young, the excess risk is fourfold to eightfold.[5] The effect has a greater impact on women as compared to men,[5] which is also the case in patients with HFpEF.
2. b. Data are from Australian heart disease statistics, published by the National Heart Foundation of Australia.[6] A recent cohort study of 1.9 million persons found that heart failure and peripheral arterial disease are the initial cardiovascular presentations of diabetes[7] (see Introduction in Chapter 28).
3. d. See Table 28.1. From more than 8%, there is a significant increase in HF incidence. Of note, each 1% elevation in

HbA1c leads to an 8% to 15% increase in the frequency of HF independent of other risk factors.[9,10] Conversely, a 1% reduction of HbA1c levels is associated with a 16% reduced risk of developing HF and worsening outcome.[11]

4. b. See Imaging for Systolic Function section in Chapter 28. The myocardial strain imaging is a relatively new technique to determine the degree of myocardial deformation (strain and strain rate). In current practice, most are derived from two-dimensional speckle tracking echocardiography (2D STE) but can be derived from three-dimensional images (3D STE). Myocardial strain is defined as the change in the length of a segment divided by the original length of the segment, whereas the strain rate is the rate at which this deformation occurs during a cardiac cycle. GLS is calculated by averaging the strains of three apical views. Reduced GLS is a sensitive marker of systolic dysfunction, identifying diminished longitudinal deformation even while EF is preserved. A decrease in GLS was independently associated with all-cause death and hospitalization after adjusting for age, systolic BP, exercise capacity, and HbA1c (HR 1.12 [1.00–1.21]), as well as provided incremental prognostic value up to 10 years.[64]
5. a, e. See Management section in Chapter 28 and Table 28.2. Multiple studies have looked at the CV benefits of the antidiabetic medications. Metformin[120] and SGLT2i[14,130–132] being the only classes showing positive signals. Metformin and SGLT2i have protective effects, whereas thiazolidinediones increase HF. Insulin has similar HF incidence with placebo but more HF compared with other glucose-lowering drugs. Sulfonylureas are less favorable to metformin. Further trials are ongoing, which will shed more light on this area.

CHAPTER 29

1. b. In the normal heart, the complex process of LV myocardial deformation results from the oblique orientation of myocardial fibers, whereby endocardial ones are aligned more parallel to the long axis and relate primarily to longitudinal mechanics, versus epicardial fibers, responsible primarily for circumferential mechanics. Both layers contribute to LV rotation, and the sum of their deformation represents radial deformation. ASE guidelines do not strictly define normal ranges of GLS as the result of the wide heterogeneity of published data; however, values above −20% with a SD of ± 2% are suggested as normal reference. Both technical (clip selection, timing, vendor, image quality, etc.) and clinical (age, gender, volume status, hemodynamics, etc.) factors constitute potential sources of variability in the clinical application of speckle tracking strain. Limitations of tissue Doppler imaging in strain imaging include noise, angle dependency, and measurement of deformation between time points as opposed to deformation between original and measured length, factors not applicable to speckle tracking strain analysis.
2. c. Dyspnea is a rather complex complaint associated with a multiplicity of potential mechanisms and etiologies ranging from cardiac and musculoskeletal, to respiratory disorders. As such, a single parameter of LV performance cannot assess all these factors, particularly if measured in resting conditions. Remodeling processes in the ailing heart lead to impaired myocardial relaxation and contractility causing either systolic or diastolic dysfunction regardless of the LV EF or the underlying disease mechanism. Hypertrophic cardiomyopathy encroaches the LV cavity during diastolic filling, thereby reducing end-diastolic volume and increasing the EF; changes in stroke volume and contractility in this setting do not necessarily impact EF. Since EF is influenced by preload and afterload (markers of pressure/volume interactions), it cannot be used as a reliable reproducible marker of contractility.
3. a. Despite absent or subtle LV mechanics abnormalities at rest, many patients with HFpEF exercise testing may unmask abnormal LV untwisting and longitudinal strain indices (in addition to reduced mitral annular motion) that are invariably correlated with peak VO_2 max and elevated filling pressures.
4. d. Patients with HFpEF have a normal EF despite reduced longitudinal strain. Increased LV volume, reflecting remodeling, is the main difference between HFpEF and HFrEF; in the former, there is LV stiffness that largely depends on volume, which explains why the pressure-volume loop is shifted up and to the left. The reason patients with HFpEF have a normal EF despite reduced longitudinal strain is the presence of preserved circumferential strain and twist that compensates for the reduced shortening of subendocardial fibers.

CHAPTER 30

1. d. This patient's HR of 64 is indicative of chronotropic incompetence in the setting of cardiogenic shock. ECMO cannulation, while indicated for refractory cardiogenic shock, is not the correct answer for this patient given his partial response to pharmacologic therapies and several less invasive/morbid additive therapies still available. Option b is a reasonable answer if the patient remains in cardiogenic shock after his chronotropic incompetence is corrected and if his peripheral artery disease permits insertion. Option c is incorrect because while an echocardiogram should be performed urgently, the patient should be stabilized first. Additionally, there are no signs on the physical exam of aortic valve incompetence.
2. c. Doppler echo-guided AV optimization studies are designed to optimize the diastolic filling period of the cardiac cycle. Typically this is done by programming an inappropriately short AV delay, and then progressively

prolonging the AV delay until the A wave fully emerges in the diastolic interval. The A wave should terminate just after the onset of the QRS (within 40 msec) most closely approximating normal electrical-mechanical delay. These characteristics allow the atria to contribute to ventricular filling, thereby maximizing cardiac output. Abbreviation of the E wave by the A wave is representative of the passive filling stage of diastole being cut short by a premature atrial contraction.

3. a. Available series show up to 6.7% of HBP leads will require revision after implant due to loss of capture or increasing thresholds. This failure rate is improving with improved equipment but still prevents the widespread adoption of this technology. The HBP does not lead to increased rates of TV disruption, and in most cases can be affixed to the atrial side of the TV. The initial success rates for HBP implant are over 90% in modern series and will likely continue to improve as delivery sheaths and the leads themselves are improved. There are many series demonstrating the restoration of AV/VV synchrony and downstream improvements in EF and LVESV/LVEDV in patients utilizing HBP compared to those with a traditional RVA pacing system.

CHAPTER 31

1. c. The patient has TTE findings indicative of diastolic dysfunction but no objective evidence of volume overload or lung congestion by exam. The clinical definition of HFpEF requires additional confirmatory findings such as lung congestion on chest x-ray and/or elevated BNP.
2. b. The TTE findings at rest are consistent with grade I diastolic dysfunction. One may, however, consider an exercise study to determine if the symptoms of dyspnea are related to worsened hemodynamics during exercise.
3. b. The cardiopulmonary exercise can determine the degree of exercise intolerance as well as to differentiate cardiac versus ventilatory failure as the etiology of symptoms.
4. d. ASE diastolic function set cutoffs for e′ velocities of 10 cm/sec for lateral annulus and 8 cm/sec for septal annulus. In Amil Shah's 2016 analysis of ARIC, 82% of subjects ages 67 to 90 years had an abnormal septal e′ and 91% had an abnormal lateral e′. As expected, subjects below this cutoff did not have an increased risk of heart hospitalization or death.
5. b. Aging in itself appears to prolong LV relaxation. Markers of relaxation in lifelong exercisers, such as e′ velocities or isovolumetric relaxation time, are more similar to their sedentary peers than young controls. On the other hand, compliance curves in lifelong exercisers are superimposable with the young controls, and sedentary seniors are shifted to the left. While compliance declines with sedentary aging, this appears to be primarily related to fitness and lifestyle and is preventable. Systolic function does not decline with age, though more data on systolic mechanics are needed.
6. c. Aging results in an expected sarcopenia that can result in deconditioning and fatigue on exertion. Other changes that occur include a decrease in oxygen carrying capacity (VO_2max), decrease in lung function, and alterations of diastolic function. Ejection fraction and elevated resting cardiac filling pressures are not expected to change with healthy age.
7. c. HFpEF is highly prevalent in the elderly population and often presents later in life. In 2008, Tribouilloy et al. demonstrated that the incidence of HFpEF overtakes HFrEF in the seventh decade of life.
8. b. With aging, the heart undergoes alterations that may compromise longitudinal function, such as myocardial remodeling and becoming more spheroid. A recent study using speckle tracking echocardiography found reduced longitudinal strain in sedentary seniors compared to sedentary young participants, but this difference was ameliorated in seniors with a committed level of lifelong exercise.

CHAPTER 32

1. c. Tricuspid regurgitation does not significantly affect the assessment of LV filling pressures. With mitral annular calcification, the restriction of the mitral annulus by calcification renders tissue Doppler imaging of the mitral annulus inaccurate in reflecting LV filling dynamics. Additionally, transmitral flow (E/A ratio, Vp) is more reflective of valvular pathology than the intrinsic relaxation of the left ventricle. Similarly, increased LA pressures in patients with severe primary mitral regurgitation will result in an increase in the transmitral E wave velocity and blunting or reversal of the S wave during assessment of pulmonary vein flow. Similarly, the E/e′ ratio has not been shown to reliably predict LV filling pressures in patients with primary mitral regurgitation. Finally, studies of diastolic assessment in patients with hypertrophic cardiomyopathy have not been shown to reliably predict LV filling pressures.
2. b. Diastolic dysfunction has been demonstrated to be most strongly predictive of death and atrial fibrillation following coronary artery bypass grafting. This patient with grade III diastolic dysfunction would have an approximately 28-fold increase in his risk for postoperative atrial fibrillation. The proposed mechanism of this increased risk is a decrease in LV compliance, resulting in increased LA pressure, which promotes stretch, fibrosis, and the development of atrial arrhythmias.
3. a. Ventricular pacing has a variable effect on indices of diastolic function, depending on the specific site of pacing. In general, studies assessing the effect of ventricular pacing on diastolic function show a mostly deleterious effect. Patients receiving DDD, DOO, and VVI pacing will all typically receive ventricular pacing. In contrast, patients paced in AAI mode will only receive atrial pacing, which has not been shown to dramatically alter indices of diastolic function.

CHAPTER 33

1. d. Echocardiography demonstrates findings consistent with HFpEF physiology. The parasternal long and short axis views demonstrate a normal LV EF. There is Doppler and 2-D evidence of pulmonary hypertension. The estimated RA pressure is in excess of 15 mmHg, given the markedly dilated inferior vena cava without collapse on inspiration. The peak tricuspid regurgitant velocity of 3.7 m/sec suggests the pulmonary artery systolic pressure is in excess of 70 mmHg. Despite the significant elevation in the RA pressure, there appears to be relative equivalence of atrial pressures as the intraatrial septum swings to the left and to the right throughout the cardiac cycle. This elevation in LA pressure is supported by the mitral inflow pattern that has a short deceleration time and a high lateral E/e′ ratio.
2. d. The hemodynamics are consistent with postcapillary PH with a markedly elevated pulmonary capillary wedge pressure; however, there are also features of a precapillary component with an elevated pulmonary vascular resistance at 5 WU.
3. a. In the setting of marked volume overload in a patient not responding to loop diuretics, the addition of metolazone would be the next logical step. Metoprolol is not indicated in the absence of myocardial ischemia or systemic hypertension. Sildenafil is not recommended in the management of any patients with HFpEF, including those with PH. Ultrafiltration will only be indicated for volume management if the patient is unresponsive to diuretics.

CHAPTER 34

b. False. AF appears to be more prevalent in patients with HFpEF than in the other HF phenotypes. In 41,446 patients from the Swedish Heart Failure Registry, there was an AF prevalence of 65% in patients with HFpEF, 60% in HF with midrange EF (HFmrEF), and 53% in patients with HFrEF, despite similar age, sex, prior myocardial infarction, and history of stroke among the three groups.[70]

a. True. In the CHARM-Preserved trial, which randomized 3023 HF patients with HF and LV EF greater than 40% to candesartan or placebo, there was no overall difference in the primary outcome of all-cause death between the two groups; however, HF hospitalizations were significantly lower in the candesartan compared to the placebo group. More patients in the candesartan group developed hypotension, hyperkalemia, or renal insufficiency.[6]

b. False. The TOPCAT study evaluated spironolactone versus placebo in patients with HF with preserved EF (>45%). While it did not show a significant difference in the primary end point (a composite of death from cardiovascular causes, aborted cardiac arrest, or hospitalization for the management of HF) in patients randomized to spironolactone or placebo, hospitalizations for the management of HF were significantly reduced in the spironolactone arm.[12]

CHAPTER 35

1. d. Current guidelines recommend control of hypertension in patients with HFpEF in accordance with published clinical practice guidelines. Both spironolactone and candesartan are associated with antihypertensive effects. Furthermore, each has also been associated with a reduction in HFpEF hospitalizations and both carry a IIb recommendation in the updated 2017 ACC/AHA/HFSA guidelines. The use of NSAIDs and DDP-4 inhibitors in heart failure patients should be discouraged and are associated with fluid retention and increased heart failure hospitalizations.
2. a. In the TOPCAT trial, a reduction in LA volume at follow-up was associated with a lower risk of subsequent occurrence of the primary composite outcome (CV death, HF hospitalization, or aborted cardiac arrest).[84]
3. b. A large systematic review and meta-analysis, including 38 studies of HFpEF, published in the *European Heart Journal* in 2016 reported the prevalence of echocardiographic RV dysfunction by TAPSE was 28%, by FAC was 18%, and by RV S′ was 21%.[39]
4. d. In HFpEF, an impaired LA strain response is a key hemodynamic trigger for RV-to-PC uncoupling and exercise ventilation inefficiency.[37] LV GLS correlates independently to peak VO_2 in patients with preserved EF and was found to be superior to other echocardiographic parameters in identifying patients with reduced exercise capacity.[29] LVH has not been found to correlate with exercise intolerance in HFpEF patients.
5. d. In 2017, a focused update of the 2013 ACC/AHA/HFSA guidelines was released. Based on the CHARM-Preserved Trial, the use of ARBs continued to receive a IIb LOE B recommendation to decrease hospitalization for patients with HFpEF. Based on a post hoc analysis of the TOPCAT trial, the use of aldosterone receptor antagonists received a IIb LOE B-R recommendation for appropriately selected individuals with HFpEF to decrease hospitalizations. It was found that in patients studied in the Americas, rates of the primary end point were fourfold higher than those in Russia/Georgia; in the Americas population, treatment with spironolactone was efficacious in reducing the trial's primary end point. The routine use of nitrates or phosphodiesterase-5 inhibitors to increase activity or quality of life received a Class III (no benefit) recommendation based on the results of the NEAT-HFpEF trial and RELAX, respectively.

CHAPTER 36

1. b. The endothelium plays an important role in cardiovascular homeostasis by regulating cardiac function, vasomotor tone, and vascular permeability. The HFpEF-associated comorbidities lead to endothelial dysfunction through disruption of the intracellular NO-cGMP-PK signal cascade. A disorder in this signal cascade contributes to the development of remodeling, including increased cardiomyocyte stiffness that is characteristic of HFpEF. The disruption of the NO-cGMP-PK signal cascade has been

shown to lead to disturbances in the regulation of titin and an increase in fibrosis.

2. b. In a study of patients with HFpEF undergoing invasive cardiac catheterization at rest and during exercise, the infusion of sodium nitrite resulted in significant reduction in exercise pulmonary capillary wedge pressure, improvement of cardiac output with exercise, and normalization in the increase of cardiac output relative to oxygen consumption.

3. a. The EMPA-REG OUTCOME Trial looked at empagliflozin, a SGLT2 inhibitor in patients with type 2 diabetes. The results showed a 38% relative risk reduction, 38% in death from cardiovascular causes, 35% relative risk reduction for hospitalization for heart failure, and a 32% relative risk reduction for death from any cause. More recently, other SGLT2 inhibitors have demonstrated similar results.

INDEX

Page numbers followed by *b* denote boxes, those followed by *f* denote figures, and those followed by *t* denote tables.

E

M

N

O

P

Q

R

S

W

X